PEDIATRIC ANESTHESIA

PEDIATRIC ANESTHESIA

A PROBLEM-BASED LEARNING APPROACH

EDITED BY

Kirk Lalwani, MD, FRCA, MCR
PROFESSOR OF ANESTHESIOLOGY AND PEDIATRICS
OREGON HEALTH AND SCIENCE UNIVERSITY
VICE-CHAIR FOR FACULTY DEVELOPMENT
DIRECTOR, PEDIATRIC ANESTHESIOLOGY FELLOWSHIP PROGRAM
DOERNBECHER CHILDREN'S HOSPITAL

Ira Todd Cohen, MD, MEd
PROFESSOR OF ANESTHESIOLOGY AND PEDIATRICS
GEORGE WASHINGTON UNIVERSITY
DIRECTOR OF EDUCATION
DEPARTMENT OF ANESTHESIOLOGY AND PAIN MEDICINE
CHILDREN'S NATIONAL MEDICAL CENTER

Ellen Y. Choi, MD
ASSISTANT PROFESSOR
CLINICAL DIRECTOR, PEDIATRIC ANESTHESIOLOGY
DEPARTMENT OF ANESTHESIA AND CRITICAL CARE
UNIVERSITY OF CHICAGO

Vidya T. Raman, MD
ASSOCIATE PROFESSOR
DIRECTOR OF PREOPERATIVE ASSESSMENT TESTING
DEPARTMENT OF ANESTHESIA AND PAIN MEDICINE
THE OHIO STATE UNIVERSITY
NATIONWIDE CHILDREN'S HOSPITAL

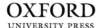

OXFORD
UNIVERSITY PRESS

OXFORD
UNIVERSITY PRESS

Oxford University Press is a department of the University of Oxford. It furthers
the University's objective of excellence in research, scholarship, and education
by publishing worldwide. Oxford is a registered trade mark of Oxford University
Press in the UK and certain other countries.

Published in the United States of America by Oxford University Press
198 Madison Avenue, New York, NY 10016, United States of America.

© Oxford University Press 2018

CIP data is on file at the Library of Congress
ISBN 978–0–19–068515–7

This material is not intended to be, and should not be considered, a substitute for medical or other professional advice. Treatment for the
conditions described in this material is highly dependent on the individual circumstances. And, while this material is designed to offer accurate
information with respect to the subject matter covered and to be current as of the time it was written, research and knowledge about medical
and health issues is constantly evolving and dose schedules for medications are being revised continually, with new side effects recognized and
accounted for regularly. Readers must therefore always check the product information and clinical procedures with the most up-to-date published
product information and data sheets provided by the manufacturers and the most recent codes of conduct and safety regulation. The publisher
and the authors make no representations or warranties to readers, express or implied, as to the accuracy or completeness of this material. Without
limiting the foregoing, the publisher and the authors make no representations or warranties as to the accuracy or efficacy of the drug dosages
mentioned in the material. The authors and the publisher do not accept, and expressly disclaim, any responsibility for any liability, loss or risk that
may be claimed or incurred as a consequence of the use and/ or application of any of the contents of this material.

1 3 5 7 9 8 6 4 2

Printed by Sheridan Books, Inc., United States of America

DIGITAL MEDIA ACCOMPANYING THE BOOK

Individual purchasers of this book are entitled to free personal access to accompanying digital media in the online edition. Please refer to the access token card for instructions on token redemption and access.

These online ancillary materials, where available, are noted with iconography throughout the book.

 Test

The corresponding media can be found on *Oxford Medicine Online* at: http://oxfordmedicine.com/pediatricanesthesiaPBL
If you are interested in access to the complete online edition, please consult with your librarian.

CONTENTS

PREFACE

"We do not learn from experience . . . we learn from reflecting on experience." —John Dewey

In 1902, the renowned American philosopher, psychologist, and educational reformer John Dewey argued that "in order for education to be most effective, content must be presented in a way that allows the student to relate the information to prior experiences, thus deepening the connection with this new knowledge." Today, we know that linking existing knowledge to new knowledge that is presented in the form of a case or a problem results in better retention of the knowledge and improves the ability of the learner to apply that knowledge to solve real problems. This problem-based learning (PBL) method was introduced into medical education at McMaster University in Ontario, Canada, in 1969. Since then it has been widely incorporated into secondary, undergraduate, and graduate education in a variety of disciplines worldwide.

The hallmarks of PBL include active, self-directed learning in small groups, building on prior knowledge with critical thinking, problem-solving, and reflection on what has been learned. A moderator guides the discussion using open-ended questions that stimulate discourse and encourage higher levels of application, analysis, and evaluation of knowledge, thereby creating new knowledge.

We are excited to present this review of pediatric anesthesia that utilizes the PBL approach. Trainees and educators in anesthesia and pediatric anesthesia will be the core users of this book. Each chapter deals with commonly encountered conditions and problems in pediatric anesthesia practice presented as a case stem with questions to encourage critical thinking, followed by an evidence-based discussion and multiple-choice questions for self-assessment.

We encourage learners and educators to utilize this book to review an upcoming clinical case or as a PBL tool. The "Stem Case and Key Questions" section could be provided to groups of learners for independent study in advance of a PBL session and the "Discussion" section withheld until after the PBL session. The case could form the basis of an interactive learning experience for a study group. Alternatively, the book covers a wide range of important topics in pediatric anesthesia for the solitary learner attempting a broad yet in-depth clinical review of the subspecialty. Finally, the self-assessment questions can be answered before and after the session as a measure of knowledge acquisition or simply as a question bank to prepare for examinations. The self-assessment questions are provided without the adjacent answers via the online resource that accompanies this book.

It is unrealistic to expect that this or any other publication will cover every condition or complication that a pediatric anesthesia practitioner will encounter in practice. Alas, the complexity of the human body and the conditions that afflict it are simply too numerous and too complex to be held within the mundane confines of two paper covers. With that in mind, we have selected and presented a broad systems-based tour of commonly encountered clinical cases in pediatric anesthesia based on our collective experience. The authors hail from a variety of pediatric institutions of repute across the breadth of the country, and many of them are experts in their field.

We hope this book provides you with much food for thought; to quote Dewey once again, "We only think when confronted with a problem." The clinical problems outlined in this book are presented in a format designed to stimulate critical thinking and discussion, and we hope you will analyze, discuss, and reflect, and encourage your learners to do so as well.

We would like to dedicate this book to all those who toiled before us in the pursuit of knowledge, the advancement of science, and the education of the next generation. We have all been benefactors of these great clinicians, scientists, and educators. As a small token of gratitude for their contributions, we are honored to be able to contribute all editorial royalties from this book to the Patient Safety, Education and Research Fund of the Society for Pediatric Anesthesia, which awards the annual Young Investigator Research Grants in pediatric anesthesia. Last but not least, we dedicate this book to our young patients, whose courage and strength in the face of daunting odds never ceases to amaze and humble us every single day.

Kirk Lalwani
Ellen Y. Choi
Ira Todd Cohen
Vidya T. Raman

CONTRIBUTORS

I. Aliason, MD
Pediatric Anesthesiologist
Valley Children's Healthcare
Madera, CA

Staci N. Allen, MD
Pediatric Anesthesiology Fellow
Children's Hospital Colorado
University of Colorado
Boulder, CO

Jennifer L. Anderson, MD
Visiting Associate Professor of Clinical Anesthesiology
University of Illinois Medical Center
Department of Anesthesiology
Chicago, IL

Lydia Andras, MD
Attending Physician
Assistant Professor of Clinical Anesthesiology
Keck School of Medicine of USC
Children's Hospital of Los Angeles
Los Angeles, CA

Caitlin Aveyard, MD
Clinical Associate
Department of Anesthesia and Critical Care
University of Chicago
Chicago, IL

Graciela Argote-Romero, MD
Clinical Assistant Professor
Department of Anesthesiology and Pain Medicine
Nationwide Children's Hospital
The Ohio State University, Wexner Medical Center
Columbus, OH

Ihab Ayad, MD
Clinical Professor
Department of Anesthesiology and Perioperative Medicine
University of California Los Angeles
Los Angeles, CA

Heather Ballard, MD
Instructor in Anesthesiology
Northwestern University's Feinberg School of Medicine
Department of Pediatric Anesthesiology
Ann and Robert H. Lurie Children's Hospital of Chicago
Chicago, IL

Ralph J. Beltran, MD
Clinical Assistant Professor
Department of Anesthesiology and Pain Medicine
Nationwide Children's Hospital
The Ohio State University, Wexner Medical Center
Columbus, OH

Paul Bhalla, MBChB, FRCA, FFPMRCA
Acting Assistant Professor
Department of Anesthesiology and Pain Medicine
Harborview Medical Center
Seattle, WA

Sanjay Bhananker MD, FRCA
Professor
Department of Anesthesiology and Pain Medicine
Harborview Medical Center and Seattle Children's Hospital
Seattle, WA

Eric Boudreau, MD
Anesthesiologist
Capitol Anesthesiology Association
Austin, TX

Christina Brown, MD
Fellow, Pediatric Anesthesiology
Department of Anesthesiology and Perioperative Medicine
Oregon Health & Science University
Portland, OR

Jason Bryant, MD
Clinical Assistant Professor
Department of Anesthesiology and Pain Medicine
Nationwide Children's Hospital
The Ohio State University, Wexner Medical Center
Columbus, OH

Nelson Burbano-Vera, MD
Associate in Cardiac Anesthesia
Boston Children's Hospital
Instructor in Anaesthesia
Harvard Medical School
Boston, MA

Alyssa M. Burgart, MD, MA
Clinical Assistant Professor
Division of Pediatric Anesthesia
Department of Anesthesia
Stanford University Hospital
Stanford, CA

Candice Burrier, MD
Attending Anesthesiologist
Clinical Assistant Professor
Department of Anesthesiology and Pain Medicine
Nationwide Children's Hospital
The Ohio State University
Columbus, OH

Patrick M. Callahan, MD
Assistant Professor
Department of Anesthesiology and Perioperative Medicine
University of Pittsburgh Medical Center
Pittsburgh, PA

Yonmee Chang, MD
Anesthesiologist
Children's National Health System
Washington, DC

Debnath Chatterjee, MD, FAAP
Associate Professor of Anesthesiology
Children's Hospital Colorado/University of Colorado
School of Medicine
Director of Fetal Anesthesia, Colorado Fetal Care Center
Aurora, CO

Kristin Chenault, MD
Pediatric Anesthesiologist
Clinical Assistant Professor
Department of Anesthesiology and Pain Medicine
Nationwide Children's Hospital
Wexner Medical Center
Columbus, OH

Ellen Y. Choi, MD
Assistant Professor
Department of Anesthesia and Critical Care
University of Chicago
Chicago, IL

Franklyn P. Cladis, MD
Associate Professor
Director, Pediatric Anesthesiology Fellowship Program
Department of Anesthesiology and Perioperative Medicine
University of Pittsburgh Medical Center
Pittsburgh, PA

Andrew J. Costandi, MD
Assistant Professor of Clinical Anesthesiology
Keck School of Medicine of USC
Los Angeles, CA

Ajay D'Mello, MD
Department of Anesthesiology and Pain Medicine
Nationwide Children's Hospital
The Ohio State University
Columbus, OH

Pikulkaew Dachsangvorn, MD
Assistant Professor
Oregon Health and Science University
Portland, OR

Priti G. Dalal, MD, FRCA
Professor
Division of Pediatric Anesthesia
Penn State Health Children's Hospital
Hershey, PA

Samuel David Yanofsky
Children's Hospital of Los Angeles
USC Keck School of Medicine
Los Angeles, CA

Sarah Deverman, MD
Assistant Professor of Anesthesiology and Perioperative
Medicine
Oregon Health & Sciences University Hospital
Portland, OR

Nina Deutsch, MD
Associate Professor of Anesthesiology and Pediatrics
Division of Anesthesiology, Pain, and Perioperative Medicine
Children's National Medical Center
Washington, DC

Christina D. Diaz, MD, FASA, FAAP
Associate Professor
Medical College of Wisconsin
Children's Hospital of Wisconsin
Milwaukee, WI

Laura A. Downey, MD
Assistant Professor of Anesthesiology and Pediatrics
Emory University School of Medicine
Children's Healthcare of Atlanta
Atlanta, GA

Elizabeth C. Eastburn, DO
Assistant in Peroperative Anesthesia
Boston Children's Hospital
Instructor in Anaesthesia
Harvard Medical School
Boston, MA

Brian Egan, MD
Associate Professor of Anesthesiology
Columbia University Medical Center
New York, NY

Jamey E. Eklund, MD
Associate Professor of Clinical Anesthesiology
University of Illinois Medical Center
Department of Anesthesiology
Chicago, IL

Nicole M. Elsey, MD
Pediatric Anesthesiologist
Clinical Assistant Professor
Department of Anesthesiology and Pain Medicine,
Nationwide Children's Hospital
The Ohio State University
Wexner Medical Center
Columbus, OH

Thomas O. Erb, MD, MHS, DEAA
Head, Department of Anesthesiology
University Children's Hospital Beider Basel
University of Basel
Basel, Switzerland

Lynne R. Ferrari, MD
Chief, Perioperative Anesthesia
Medical Director, Operating Rooms and Perioperative
Program

John E. Fiadjoe, MD
Associate Professor of Anesthesiology and Critical Care
Hospital of the University of Pennsylvania and the Children's
Hospital of Philadelphia
Department of Anesthesiology and Critical Care Medicine
Philadelphia, PA

Louise K. Furukawa, MD
Clinical Associate Professor
Department of Anesthesiology, Perioperative and Pain
Medicine
Stanford University School of Medicine
Stanford, CA

Annery Garcia-Marcinkiewicz, MD
Clinical Associate of Anesthesiology and Critical Care
Attending Anesthesiologist, The Children's Hospital of
Philadelphia
Department of Anesthesiology and Critical Care Medicine
Philadelphia, PA

Shannon M. Grap, MD
Assistant Professor
Division of Pediatric Anesthesiology
Penn State Health Children's Hospital
Hershey, PA

Nina A. Guzzetta, MD, FAAP
Professor of Anesthesiology and Pediatrics
Emory University School of Medicine
Children's Healthcare of Atlanta
Atlanta, GA

Denise Hall-Burton MD, FAAP
Assistant Professor of Anesthesiology
Children's Hospital
University of Pittsburgh Medical Center
Pittsburgh, PA

Michelle Keese Harvey, MD
Assistant Clinical Professor
Department of Anesthesiology and Perioperative Medicine
University of California Los Angeles
Los Angeles, CA

Michael R. Hernandez, MD
Instructor in Anaesthesia
Department of Anesthesiology
Perioperative and Pain Medicine
Boston Children's Hospital
Harvard Medical School
Boston, MA

Jimmy Hoang
Children's Hospital of Los Angeles
USC Keck School of Medicine
Los Angeles, CA

Anita Honkanen, MD, MS
Clinical Professor of Anesthesia
Department of Anesthesiology
Perioperative and Pain Medicine
Stanford University School of Medicine
Stanford, CA

Jared Hylton, MD
Assistant Professor of Anesthesiology
University of Wisconsin School of Medicine
Pediatric Anesthesiologist
American Family Children's Hospital
Madison, WI

Rebecca S. Isserman, MD
Department of Anesthesiology and Critical Care Medicine,
The Children's Hospital of Philadelphia
Assistant Professor of Anesthesiology
Perelman School of Medicine
University of Pennsylvania
Department of Anesthesiology and Critical Care
Philadelphia, PA

Andrea Johnson, DO
Assistant Professor of Anesthesiology and Perioperative Medicine
Oregon Health & Sciences University Hospital
Portland, OR

Zeev N. Kain, MD
Chancellor's Professor
Executive Director, Center on Stress and Health
Department of Anesthesiology and Perioperative Care
University of California Irvine
Irvine, CA

Komal Kamra, MBBS, MMI
Clinical Associate Professor
Pediatric Cardiac Anesthesia
Department of Anesthesiology
Perioperative and Pain Medicine
Stanford University School of Medicine
Stanford, CA

Joelle Karlik, MD
Assistant Professor
Oregon Health Sciences
Department of Anesthesiology and Perioperative Medicine
Oregon Health & Science University
Portland, OR

Meredith Kato, MD
Assistant Professor, Pediatric Anesthesiology
Department of Anesthesiology and Perioperative Medicine
Oregon Health & Science University
Portland, OR

Sabina A. Khan, MD
Assistant Professor
Department of Anesthesiology
McGovern Medical School
The University of Texas Health Science Center
Houston, TX

Adele King, MBChB, FRCA
Department of Anesthesiology & Pain Medicine
Nationwide Children's Hospital
Columbus, OH

J. Koh, MD, MBA
Professor of Anesthesiology and Perioperative Medicine
Oregon Health & Science University
Portland, OR

Mary Landrigan-Ossar, MD, PhD
Senior Associate in Perioperative Anesthesia
Boston Children's Hospital
Assistant Professor of Anaesthesia
Harvard Medical School
Boston, MA

Alina Lazar, MD
Assistant Professor
Department of Anesthesia and Critical Care
University of Chicago
Chicago, IL

Jennifer K. Lee, MD
Johns Hopkins University
Department of Anesthesiology and Critical Care Medicine
Division of Pediatric Anesthesiology
Baltimore, MD

Lisa Lee, MD
Clinical Instructor
Department of Anesthesiology and Perioperative Medicine
University of California Los Angeles
Los Angeles, CA

Matthew Lilien, MD
Pediatric Cardiac Anesthesia Fellow
Emory University
Atlanta, GA

Justin L. Lockman, MD, MSEd
Director, Pediatric Anesthesiology Fellowship Program
Associate Director of Education
Department of Anesthesiology and Critical Care Medicine,
The Children's Hospital of Philadelphia
Associate Professor of Anesthesiology and Critical Care
Perelman School of Medicine, University of Pennsylvania
Philadelphia, PA

Aaron Low, MD
Fellow in Pediatric Anesthesiology
Seattle Children's Hospital
Seattle, WA

Marcus Malek, MD, FAAP
Assistant Professor of Surgery
Children's Hospital
University of Pittsburgh School of Medicine
Pittsburgh, PA

Thomas J. Mancuso, MD, FAAP
Senior Associate in Anesthesia, Critical Care
and Pain Medicine
Boston Children's Hospital
Associate Professor of Anaesthesia
Harvard Medical School
Boston, MA

Darlene Mashman, MD
Assistant Professor of Anesthesiology
Emory University School of Medicine
Atlanta, GA

Andrew J. Matisoff, MD
Cardiac Anesthesiology
Department of Anesthesiology, Pain and Perioperative
Medicine
Children's National Health System
Washington, DC

Carmen Mays, MD
Assistant Professor of Anesthesiology
Emory University School of Medicine
Attending Anesthesiologist
Children's Healthcare of Atlanta
Atlanta, GA

Christopher McKee, MD
Clinical Associate Professor
Director Education
Department of Anesthesiology and Pain Medicine
Nationwide Children's Hospital
The Ohio State University, Wexner Medical Center
Columbus, OH

Petra M. Meier, MD, DEAA
Senior Associate in Perioperative Anesthesia
Department of Anesthesiology, Perioperative and Pain
Medicine
Boston Children's Hospital
Harvard Medical School
Boston, MA

Pilar Mercado, MD
Associate Professor of Clinical Anesthesiology
University of Illinois Medical Center
Department of Anesthesiology
Chicago, IL

M. Navaratnam, MD
Assistant Clinical Professor
Department of Anesthesiology and Perioperative Medicine
David Geffen School of Medicine at UCLA
Los Angeles, CA

Jonathon Nelson, MD
Anesthesiologist
Children's National Health System
Washington, DC

Khoa N. Nguyen, MD
Assistant Professor
Department of Anesthesiology and Perioperative Medicine
University of Pittsburgh Medical Center
Pittsburgh, PA

Sarah Nizamuddin, MD
Assistant Professor
Department of Anesthesia and Critical Care
University of Chicago
Chicago, IL

Alyssa Padover, MD
Johns Hopkins University
Department of Anesthesiology and Critical Care Medicine
Division of Pediatric Anesthesiology
Baltimore, MD

Arati Patil, MD
Clinical Assistant Professor
Division of Pediatric Anesthesia
Department of Anesthesiology, Perioperative Care, and Pain Medicine
NYU Langone Medical Center
New York University School of Medicine
New York, NY

Sophie Pestieau, MD
Anesthesiologist, Children's Research Institute
Children's National Health System
Assistant Professor of Anesthesiology
School of Medicine and Health Sciences
George Washington University
Washington, DC

Andrew Pittaway, MD
Associate Professor,
Seattle Children's Hospital
Seattle, WA

C. Ramamoorthy, MD
Assistant Clinical Professor
UCLA Department of Anesthesiology and Perioperative Medicine
David Geffen School of Medicine at UCLA
Los Angeles, CA

Vidya T. Raman, MD, FAAP, FASA
Clinical Associate Professor
Director, Preoperative Assessment Testing
Department of Anesthesiology & Pain Management
Nationwide Children's Hospital
The Ohio State University, Wexner Medical Center
Columbus, OH

Justin D. Ramos, MD
Pediatric Anesthesiology Fellow
Department of Anesthesiology and Perioperative Medicine
Oregon Health & Science University
Portland, OR

Srijaya K. Reddy, MD, MBA
Anesthesiologist
Children's National Health System
Washington, DC

Bobbie Riley, MD, FAAP
Associate in Anesthesiology
Perioperative and Pain Medicine
Boston Children's Hospital
Instructor in Anaesthesia,
Harvard Medical School
Boston, MA

Jamie E. Rubin, MD
Assistant Professor
Oregon Health and Science University
Portland, OR

Haleh Saadat, MD, FAAP
Integrated Anesthesia Associates
Clinical Associate Professor of Anesthesiology
Frank H. Netter MD School of Medicine
Quinnipiac University
Hamden, CT

Annette Y. Schure, MD, FAAP, DEAA
Senior Associate in Cardiac Anesthesia
Boston Children's Hospital
Instructor in Anaesthesia
Harvard Medical School
Boston, MA

Evan R. Serfass, MD, PhD
Assistant Professor
Department of Anesthesiology and Perioperative Medicine
Oregon Health & Science University
Portland, OR

Navil Sethna, MD, FAAP
Associate in Pain Medicine
Senior Associate in Perioperative Anesthesia
Boston Children's Hospital
Associate Professor of Anesthesiology
Harvard Medical School
Boston, MA

Monica Shah, MD
Assistant Professor
Department of Anesthesiology
Pain and Perioperative Medicine
George Washington University
Children's National Health System
Washington, DC

Ravi Shah, MD
Associate Professor in Anesthesiology
Northwestern University's Feinberg School of Medicine
Department of Pediatric Anesthesiology
Ann and Robert H. Lurie Children's Hospital of Chicago
Chicago, IL

Anshuman Sharma, MD, MBA
Professor of Anesthesiology
Washington University in St. Louis
St. Louis, MO

Erica Sivak MD
Assistant Professor
Department of Anesthesiology
Children's Hospital of Pittsburgh
University of Pittsburgh Medical Center
Pittsburgh, PA

Ashley Smith, MD
Attending Anesthesiologist,
Department of Anesthesiology and Pain Medicine,
Nationwide Children's Hospital
Clinical Assistant Professor,
Department of Anesthesiology,
The Ohio State University,
Columbus, OH

Jamey J. Snell, MD
Director of Sedation Services, Children's Hospital of
Michigan/Detroit Medical Center
Clinical Assistant Professor, Wayne State University
School of Medicine
Clinical Assistant Professor, Michigan State University
College of Osteopathic Medicine
Detroit, MI

Amy Soletta, MD
Assistant Professor of Pediatric Anesthesiology
Oregon Health & Science University Hospital
Portland, OR

Elizabeth Q. Starker, MD
Pediatric Anesthesiology Fellow
Children's Hospital Colorado/University of Colorado
Denver, CO

Joel Stockman, MD
Associate Clinical Professor
Department of Anesthesiology and Perioperative Medicine
University of California Los Angeles
Los Angeles, CA

Santhanam Suresh, MD
Professor in Anesthesiology
Northwestern University's Feinberg School of Medicine
Department of Pediatric Anesthesiology
Ann and Robert H. Lurie Children's Hospital of Chicago
Chicago, IL

Tori N. Sutherland, MD
Assistant Professor
Department of Anesthesiology and Critical Care
Children's Hospital of Philadelphia (CHOP)
Philadelphia, PA

Mehdi Trifa, MD
Department of Anesthesiology and Pain Medicine
Nationwide Children's Hospital
The Ohio State University
Columbus, OH

Joshua C. Uffman, MD, MBA
Clinical Associate Professor
Vice Chairman, Quality Improvement
Department of Anesthesiology and Pain Medicine
Nationwide Children's Hospital
The Ohio State University, Wexner Medical Center
Columbus, OH

Caroll N. Vazquez-Colon, MD
Anesthesiologist
Anesthesiology, Pain, and Perioperative Medicine
Department
Children's National Health System
Washington, DC

Bistra G. Vlassakova, MD
Associate in Perioperative Anesthesia
Boston Children's Hospital
Instructor in Anaesthesia
Harvard Medical School
Boston, MA

Andrew T. Waberski, MD
Assistant Professor of Anesthesiology and Pediatrics
Division of Anesthesiology, Pain, and Perioperative
Medicine
Children's National Medical Center
Washington, DC

Nitin Wadhwa, MD
Assistant Professor
Department of Anesthesiology
McGovern Medical School
The University of Texas Health Science Center
Houston, TX

David Waisel, MD
Professor, Harvard Medical School
Department of Anesthesiology, Perioperative and Pain
Medicine
Boston Children's Hospital
Boston, MA

Tammy Wang, MD
Clinical Assistant Professor of Anesthesia
Department of Anesthesiology, Perioperative and Pain
Medicine
Stanford University School of Medicine
Stanford, CA

Steven J. Weisman, MD, FAAP
Professor
Medical College of Wisconsin
Medical Director, Pain Management
Children's Hospital of Wisconsin
Milwaukee, WI

Meghan Whitley, DO
Assistant Professor
Division of Pediatric Anesthesia
Penn State Health Children's Hospital
Hershey, PA

Glyn D. Williams, FFA(SA)
Professor, Pediatric Cardiac Anesthesia
Department of Anesthesiology, Perioperative and Pain
Medicine
Stanford University School of Medicine
Stanford, CA

Jocelyn Wong, MD
Resident in Anesthesia
Department of Anesthesiology, Perioperative and Pain
Medicine
Stanford University School of Medicine
Stanford, CA

David A. Young, MD, MEd, MBA
Professor of Anesthesiology
Baylor College of Medicine
Texas Children's Hospital
Houston, TX

SECTION 1

PREMATURITY AND NEONATAL SURGERY

1.

NECROTIZING ENTEROCOLITIS

Jared Hylton and Sarah Deverman

STEM CASE AND KEY QUESTIONS

You are called to the neonatal intensive care unit (NICU) to evaluate a 10-day old infant. The baby was born at 29 weeks to a G2P1001 mother with pregnancy complicated by severe preeclampsia and chorioamnionitis. The infant was initially intubated at birth due to poor tone and low APGARs (appearance, pulse, grimace, activity, and respiration) but was successfully extubated. The infant is on high flow nasal cannula 0.21% in the NICU and weighs 1.4 kg. The neonatologist notes that over the past day the baby has developed increased work of breathing and feeding intolerance with increased amount of gastric regurgitation. In addition, the physical exam is concerning for a distended abdomen.

WHAT IS IN THE DIFFERENTIAL DIAGNOSIS? WHAT IS NECROTIZING ENTEROCOLITIS (NEC)? WHAT ARE THE MEDICAL MANAGEMENT OPTIONS FOR NEC?

Enteral feeds are stopped, and a nasogastric tube is placed and left on low-pressure continuous suction. The infant is started on intravenous fluid and broad spectrum antibiotics after sending off blood and urine cultures. General surgery is consulted. An abdominal X-ray is ordered, which shows abdominal distention. The infant continues to deteriorate despite the current care regimen and is subsequently intubated by the neonatologist due to worsening respiratory status with a 3.0 cuffed endotracheal tube. A repeat abdominal film is ordered, which shows free air in the intestinal wall as well as free air within the abdomen.

WHAT ARE THE INDICATIONS FOR SURGICAL INTERVENTION? WHAT ARE THE SURGICAL MANAGEMENT OPTIONS FOR NEC?

The surgeons want to proceed to the operating room (OR) immediately. Prior to transporting to the OR, you note that the infant has an umbilical arterial and venous catheter line and one 24 g peripheral intravenous (IV) drip. The infant is intubated on pressure control with rate of 40, peak inspiratory pressure (PIP) 15, positive end-expiratory pressure (PEEP) 5, and fraction of inspired oxygen (FiO$_2$) 50%. A nasogastric tube is in place and the infant is receiving D10 ½ normal saline (NS) at maintenance. The monitors are transferred to the OR. You induce with fentanyl 2 mcg/kg and rocuronium 0.6 mg/kg and continue the preoperative ventilator settings. The surgeon tells you that the umbilical arterial and venous catheter line will need to be removed as it is in the operating field. After induction, you place an additional 24 g peripheral IV in the left saphenous vein and a 24 g arterial line in the right radial artery.

WHAT ARE YOUR ANESTHETIC CONSIDERATIONS FOR MANAGING THIS NEONATE? WHAT INTRAOPERATIVE MONITORS WILL YOU UTILIZE FOR THIS PATIENT? WHAT IS THE IDEAL ANESTHETIC FOR A NEONATE WITH NEC?

As the case proceeds, the surgeon notifies you that there are multiple areas of bowel ischemia that will likely need resection. You have given a total of 5 mcg/kg of fentanyl in addition to the rocuronium. The infant is currently on minimal sevoflurane with minimum alveolar concentration of 0.3 and has already received 40 mL/kg of crystalloid in addition to a maintenance infusion of D10 ½ NS at 4 mL/kg/hr. You have difficulty maintaining the patient's blood pressure within an acceptable range. To maintain stable hemodynamics, you start the patient on dopamine at 5 mcg/kg/min. You also note that your ventilation settings have increased with PIP of 18 and PEEP 8. At the conclusion of the case, you transport the patient directly back to the NICU while intubated and sedated on fentanyl and versed.

WHAT ARE YOUR CONCERNS FOR THE POSTOPERATIVE PERIOD?

Throughout the first postoperative day the patient's arterial blood gases show ongoing difficulties with ventilation and oxygenation despite adjustments to ventilator parameters. A chest X-ray shows air space opacification and pleural effusions. In addition, the patient shows diffuse anasarca.

HOW WILL THIS NEONATE BE MANAGED POSTOPERATIVELY?

Ventilation and oxygenation improve over the next few days and the patient is extubated to HFNC. The infant remains on bowel rest and total parental nutrition (TPN) until a contrast enema is obtained to confirm absence of stricture formation. Antibiotics are continued for a total of ten to fourteen days.

DISCUSSION

OVERVIEW

NEC is a life-threatening condition mainly found in preterm neonates. The incidence is 5% to 15% in infants less than 1,500 g with the mortality rate ranging from 10% to as high as 50% if surgery is required.[1] The pathophysiology remains poorly understood but thought to be multifactorial. While medical management allows some infants to recover without sequelae, infants requiring surgical intervention are at higher risk for morbidity and mortality. The anesthetic management remains a challenge to the pediatric anesthesiologist.

PATHOGENESIS

The pathogenesis of NEC is multifactorial and incompletely understood. An initial insult results in an exaggerated inflammatory response. Current theories suggest that the disease may be initiated by perinatal insults such as formula feeding, abnormal bacterial colonization of the immature gut, lack of appropriate gut colonization with commensal organisms, hypoxia, and hypoperfusion. In response to an epithelial injury, inflammatory mediators are released causing intestinal inflammation.[2]

Intestinal immaturity plays a key role in the pathogenesis of this disease. Intestinal motility develops during the third trimester of pregnancy when the migrating motor complexes first appear around week 34 of gestation. Decreased motility increases exposure to noxious substances as well as decreased digestion and absorption. In addition, intestinal epithelium normally acts as a barrier to potential pathogens. Yet, in preterm infants, tight junctions are incompletely developed leading to increased intestinal permeability.[2] Excessive intestinal inflammation in response to intestinal stimulation may also play a role in this disease process. The serum levels of several cytokines and chemokines that recruit inflammatory cells have been reported to be higher in patients in NEC. One of these cytokines, interleukin-8, is produced by epithelial cells and mediates the migration of neutrophils to the site of inflammation and can cause necrosis and increased production of acute-phase proteins in the gut.[3] An additional hypothesis is that premature infants may have inappropriate microbial colonization leading to NEC. Premature infants are at risk for abnormal bacterial colonization due to their time spent in the NICU and exposure to nosocomial flora. The balance between pathogenic and beneficial bacteria in the intestines may tip to favor the pathogens thus exposing the infant to intestinal injury.[2]

RISK FACTORS

In a recent systematic review of prognostic studies, the following were found to be associated with an increased risk of NEC: small for gestational age, low gestational age, assisted ventilation, sepsis, hypotension, premature rupture of membranes, and black ethnicity.[4] Low birth weight is the most commonly reported significant factor for NEC among neonates in the current literature. In the National Institute of Child Health and Human Development Neonatal Research Network cohort, rates of NEC were inversely proportional to birth weight, with NEC affecting 11.5% of infants weighing 401 to 750 g, 9% of infants weighing 751 to 1,000 g, 6% of infants weighing 1,001 to 1,250 g, and 4% of infants weighing 1,251 to 1,500 g.[2]

Morbidity associated with NEC includes short-gut syndrome, sepsis, and adhesions associated with bowel obstructions.[1] Mortality rates remain high, ranging from 10% to 50%, with the majority of mortality occurring in cases managed surgically. The highest rates of mortality occur in very low birth weight (VLBW) infants who are black and male.[2]

CLINICAL PRESENTATION AND DIAGNOSIS

Early signs of NEC include feeding intolerance, increased work of breathing, lethargy, and temperature instability. Later signs may include hypotension, abdominal distention, apnea, thrombocytopenia, coagulopathy, and multisystem organ failure. In addition, infants may have metabolic and hematologic abnormalities including hyperglycemia, thrombocytopenia, coagulopathy, and anemia.[1]

PREVENTATIVE APPROACHES

While surgical techniques to manage NEC have not changed in recent years, preventative strategies have become the new focus to improve outcome for infants with NEC. Feeding strategies, the role of oral antibiotics, and use of probiotics are all potential preventative measures under investigation. Prolonged withholding of enteral feeds may be dangerous due to the reliance of parenteral nutrition and subsequent intestinal atrophy, increased inflammation, and late-onset sepsis. An alternative approach is to provide small boluses of breast milk plus fortified milk, which may result in a lower incidence of NEC.[3] The use of probiotics remains controversial. In a recent prospective, randomized study in *Pediatrics*, it was suggested that the use of probiotics for six weeks in VLBW infants (*Lactobacillus* and *Bifidobacterium*) decreased the incidence of NEC. However, there seemed to be a higher incidence of sepsis in infants receiving probiotics if birth weight was less than 750 g.[5] Additional research remains to be seen on preventative strategies for NEC.

MEDICAL MANAGEMENT

When NEC is first suspected in the NICU, it is important for the neonatologist to implement immediate medical management. The first steps include bowel rest and decompression by placing an orogastric or nasogastric tube on low intermittent suction. Fluid resuscitation should be started as well as broad spectrum intravenous antibiotics after cultures have been taken.[2] A key component of medical management is close observation and serial abdominal examinations.

SURGICAL MANAGEMENT

Relative indications for surgery are fairly nonspecific and may be controversial. They include oliguria, hypotension, metabolic acidosis, thrombocytopenia, ventilatory failure, deterioration of clinical status, portal venous gas, fixed abdominal masses, persistently dilated loops of bowel, and abdominal wall erythema. The only universally accepted absolute indication for surgery for NEC is evidence of intestinal perforation.[2]

Surgical management consists of either peritoneal drainage or a laparotomy with resection of necrotic bowel. Primary peritoneal drainage requires a small surgical incision and can be done at bedside so it is typically reserved for VLBW infants or infants deemed "too sick" for laparotomy. In a randomized, multicenter trial (NECSTEPS), infants with perforated NEC with birth weight <1,500 g were randomized to either primary peritoneal drainage or laparotomy. There was no difference in mortality at 90 days between the two groups.[2]

PREOPERATIVE ANESTHETIC ASSESSMENT

In approaching the preoperative assessment of a neonate with NEC, the pediatric anesthesiologist is confronted with a multitude of considerations including but not limited to prematurity, sepsis, hemodynamic instability, acid-base and electrolyte abnormalities, coagulopathy and platelet dysfunction, temperature instability, and hypovolemia. NEC is rare in full-term infants.[6] The "classic" neonate with NEC will be a preterm baby weighing less than 1,500 g and often less than 1,000 g. The signs and symptoms of NEC in more than 90% of cases appear between the first and tenth days of life.[7] It is paramount for the pediatric anesthesiologist to determine the severity of critical illness, appropriately prepare for the case, mobilize necessary resources, and determine whether any preoperative patient clinical optimization is necessary prior to surgery.

The first step in preoperative preparation should involve chart review and assessment to identify all pertinent laboratory and imaging data that elucidate the patient's current clinical status. A specific focus on trends in acid-base status, electrolytes, blood gases, glucose, hematocrit, platelet count, and coagulation status will help to identify specific areas of concern that may need optimization prior to surgery. Abdominal plain film imaging may reveal dilated loops of bowel and in advanced NEC, pneumatosis and/or gas in the portal venous system can indicate more severe disease (Figure 1.1). During the initial review, it is also important to note any comorbid conditions often associated with prematurity that may affect anesthetic management such as congenital cardiac disease, craniofacial abnormalities, or intraventricular hemorrhage.

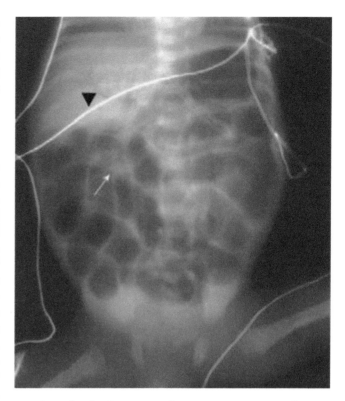

Fig. 1.1 Reproduced with permission from Cote CJ, Lerman J, Anderson BJ. *Cote and Lermans A Practice of Anesthesia for Infants and Children*. Philadelphia, PA: Elsevier/Saunders; 2013: 762.

In addition to laboratory and imaging data, it is also important to review the medical management of the patient prior to the decision to go to surgery. Without frank evidence or suspicion for intestinal necrosis or perforation, the initial treatment for NEC is nonoperative. The patient will most often be managed with gastrointestinal decompression with an orogastric tube, no enteral feeding, administration of fluids, glucose, and electrolytes, which can include parenteral nutrition, administration of broad spectrum IV antibiotics, and correction of any coagulation abnormalities. As the condition worsens, these neonates will often need hemodynamic support with inotropic agents and steroids as well as ventilatory support. Given this progression of medical management, it is important for the pediatric anesthesiologist to note what medications the patient is currently receiving, current ventilator settings, urine output, and specific information regarding volume and type of blood products that have been administered. Ventilatory status is of special importance. Depending on the neonate's clinical status, the decision to bring the NICU ventilator for transport and use during the surgery may be necessary, or the anesthesiologist may deem the baby stable enough to be ventilated with the anesthesia workstation ventilator.

After collecting and synthesizing all pertinent information with regards to the neonate's clinical status two main decisions need be considered: where to operate and when to operate. If the patient is deemed too unstable to transport from the NICU to the OR, then the possibility of a bedside procedure in the NICU needs to be considered. The decision of when to operate will also depend upon the consideration of the baby's overall clinical status and need for medical optimization prior to surgery. These decisions need to be made during open and ongoing discussions between the surgeons, NICU team, and pediatric anesthesiologist.

Lastly, prior to proceeding to surgery, it is important to ensure that blood products including packed red blood cells (PRBC), platelets, and fresh frozen plasma are all available and in the OR prior to incision.

INTRAOPERATIVE ANESTHETIC MANAGEMENT

The choice of surgical technique (exploratory laparotomy vs percutaneous intraabdominal drain placement) will influence many decisions regarding intraoperative anesthetic management. This discussion will focus on the anesthetic management for an exploratory laparotomy with possible bowel resection.

Intraoperative monitors should include standard American Society of Anesthesiologists monitors. Central venous and arterial access lines should be placed to closely monitor hemodynamics and fluid status and facilitate close monitoring of arterial blood gases and glucose management. In addition, if not already present a central venous line is often desired by the NICU team for postoperative parenteral nutrition and hemodynamic support with inotropic medications, if needed. While abdominal near-infrared spectrometry (NIRS) has been examined in the NICU setting to monitor and identify neonates at risk for NEC, to our knowledge the use of cerebral, abdominal, or flank NIRS has unclear utility within the intraoperative setting for exploratory laparotomy for NEC.[8]

Anesthetic considerations of the NEC patient should follow the same considerations for any surgery involving neonatal patients including very low or extremely low birth weight infants.[9] Meticulous attention to temperature management is critical to prevent complications associated with either hypo- or hyperthermia. It is well known that volatile anesthetics are potent inhibitors of brown adipose tissue thermogenesis and that general anesthesia utilizing volatile anesthetics places low birth weight infants at higher risk for hypothermia.[10] The patient should be warmed during transport to and from the OR. The OR should be warmed and other warming devices such as an underbody forced air warming blanket and heating lamps should be utilized when necessary. Ideally, both core (rectal) and skin temperatures should be monitored. The literature demonstrates that retinopathy of prematurity (ROP) occurs only in premature infants and the severity of ROP is inversely proportional to birth weight and gestational age.[11] Given this consideration, ideally the FiO_2 should be kept below 40% with goal oxygen saturations between 85% and 94%. The reported incidence of patent ductus arteriosus (PDA) is approximately 45% in neonates weighing less than 1,750 g at birth and 80% in infants weighing less than 1,200 g at birth.[12] Left to right shunting through the PDA can cause excessive pulmonary blood flow and decreased systemic circulation leading to decreased coronary and systemic perfusion as well as increased risk for pulmonary hemorrhage. The pediatric anesthesiologist should be mindful of the potential presence of a PDA and manage the neonate accordingly to prevent circulatory overload of the pulmonary vasculature. A final critical

consideration regarding neonatal anesthesia is regarding glucose management. Hypoglycemia is defined as a plasma glucose concentration of less than 25 mg/dL in the low birth weight neonate and less than 35 mg/dL in the term infant up to 72 hours of age. After 72 hours of age, plasma glucose concentration should be greater than 45 mg/dL.[13] A continuous source of intravenous glucose should be provided to the neonate throughout the perioperative course, and plasma glucose levels should be checked on a regular basis. Term neonates require 5–8 mg/kg/min of glucose whereas premature, small for gestational age neonates, and neonates of diabetic mothers may need 8 to 15 mg/kg/min of glucose.[14] An infusion of D10W at standard maintenance rates will deliver approximately 7 mg/kg/min of glucose and, in most cases, is adequate to prevent hypoglycemia. Of note, the high glucose content of PRBC may remove the need for an additional exogenous source of glucose.

The choice of anesthetic technique will focus on maintaining cardiovascular stability and optimum operating conditions for the surgeon. No well-designed randomized trial has established a superior anesthetic technique in this scenario. Traditionally, the most common technique has utilized high dose fentanyl (20–50 mcg/kg total for case) or other opiates, titrated as tolerated hemodynamically, along with non-depolarizing neuromuscular blockade. Depending on the baby's clinical status, volatile inhalational agents can be poorly tolerated and are often utilized only at low concentrations to help supplement a mainly opiate technique. It is advisable to avoid nitrous oxide, especially in the presence of free air in the GI tract (pneumatosis intestinalis) or portal venous system. Given that these neonates present to the OR only after failure of medical management, these patients are often on the verge of hemodynamic collapse. Vasoactive medications, such as dopamine and epinephrine, should be readily available for continuous hemodynamic support.

Fluid, electrolyte, and blood product management bears special mention as exploratory laparotomy for NEC subjects the neonate to significant insensible fluid losses due to the open belly and bowel manipulation, blood loss often necessitating transfusion, and coagulopathy with the possibility of disseminated intravascular coagulation. For this surgery, the patient may require as much as 10 mL/kg/hr in fluid replacement to correct ongoing third space and insensible losses. Further fluid replacement to replace blood loss can be done at a 1:1 ratio with colloid (5% albumin or whole blood) or 3:1 ratio with isotonic crystalloid. It is important to maintain ongoing communication with the surgeon, frequently inspect the surgical field to assess for clinically relevant coagulopathy, and check hematocrit and coagulation labs at appropriate intervals or if clinical concern arises. As a general rule of thumb, 10 mL/kg of PRBC will raise the hematocrit by 10%, 10 to 15 mL/kg of fresh frozen plasma will increase plasma clotting factors by 15% and fibrinogen by 40 mg/dL, and 5 to 10 mL/kg of platelets will raise the platelet count by 50,000.[14] A use of 0.17 U/kg of cryoprecipitate will raise the fibrinogen by 100 mg/dL but the use of cryoprecipitate significantly increases the risk of delivery of blood-borne pathogens and should be utilized only for specific indications. For a surgery such as NEC where ongoing coagulopathy and intravascular hypovolemia can simultaneously pose problems, the utilization of fresh frozen plasma is likely a better choice initially to treat both hypovolemia and coagulopathy. Lastly, it is well known that neonatal cardiac myocytes are immature in their ability to efficiently sequester and utilize calcium and these myocytes are more dependent upon adequate plasma calcium levels for contraction and inotropy.[15,16] Given this consideration, it is reasonable to prepare for ongoing calcium replacement to assist in support of hemodynamics, especially in the setting of administration of citrate-containing blood products. Institution of a calcium chloride infusion (10–20 mg/kg/hr) or intermittent bolus dosing of IV calcium chloride or calcium gluconate are both reasonable approaches, provided that the plasma ionized calcium levels are checked at appropriate intervals.

At the conclusion of surgery, these neonates should be transported with a warming device, continuous monitors, and intubated and sedated directly back to NICU. Depending upon ventilatory status in the OR, it may be advisable to call a respiratory therapist to help transport the baby on a NICU vent. Many pediatric anesthesiologists would also recommend redosing neuromuscular blockade just prior to transport to the NICU to help prevent any patient movement that may risk dislodgement of the endotracheal tube, arterial line, or venous lines during transport.

POSTOPERATIVE MANAGEMENT

After transport to the NICU, primary responsibility and postoperative care is resumed by the neonatologist after a thorough handoff. The patient may still require hemodynamic support and ongoing intestinal decompression until evidence of intestinal function is confirmed.

CONCLUSION

NEC remains a challenging disease of neonates that may require both medical and surgical management. While management and surgical outcomes have not changed much over recent years, the focus is now on prevention to hopefully minimize the number of neonates that require surgery. As NEC is a disease of premature neonates, the pediatric anesthesiologist must be prepared to manage prematurity, sepsis, hemodynamic instability, acid-base and electrolyte abnormalities, coagulopathy and platelet dysfunction, temperature instability, and hypovolemia, among other things. Anesthetic management should focus on fluid management, ventilatory strategies, temperature regulation, and optimization prior to surgery.

REVIEW QUESTIONS

1. Which of the following birth weights most closely describes an "extremely low birth weight" infant?

    A. <750 g
    B. <1,000 g
    C. <1,500 g
    D. <2,500 g

Answer: B
Low birth weight is defined as <2,500 g and very low birth weight is <1,500 g.[9]

2. Of the following conditions, which is **STRONGEST** indication for surgery for a neonate with suspected NEC?

    A. abdominal wall erythema
    B. metabolic acidosis
    C. pneumoperitoneum
    D. portal venous gas

Answer: C
Various authors have described absolute and relative indications for surgery in neonates with suspected NEC.[7,17] Certain markers of disease severity, such as degree of thrombocytopenia, remain controversial as proposed indications for surgery.[7] While there is some controversy and slight variations between what different authors consider absolute and relative indications, certain clinical scenarios are, in general, universally accepted absolute indications (Table 1.1). The relative indications for surgery in NEC are far broader but worth noting.

3. An ex-30-week gestational age, 10-day-old neonate in the NICU develops apnea, bradycardia, and temperature instability. He previously had high gastric residuals and mild abdominal distention but now has developed grossly bloody stools and worsening abdominal distention but without abdominal wall edema or palpable loops of bowel. A plain film of his abdomen demonstrates an ileus gas pattern with several dilated loops of bowel and focal pneumatosis. NEC is suspected. What is the **MOST** appropriate designation for this presentation on the Modified Bell's Staging for NEC?

    A. Stage I
    B. Stage IIA
    C. Stage IIB
    D. Stage IIIB

Table 1.1 **INDICATIONS FOR SURGERY IN NECROTIZING ENTEROCOLITIS**

ABSOLUTE INDICATIONS	RELATIVE INDICATIONS
Pneumoperitoneum	Clinical deterioration prior to maximal medical management • Metabolic acidosis • Ventilatory failure • Oliguria • Thrombocytopenia • Leukocytosis • Hypotension
Intestinal gangrene (positive paracentesis)	Portal venous gas
Clinical deterioration despite maximal medical treatment	Erythema of abdominal wall
Abdominal mass with persistent intestinal obstruction or sepsis	Persistently dilated bowel loop
	Abdominal mass without persistent obstruction or sepsis

Answer: B

Given the clinical scenario as presented, this neonate has a presumptive diagnosis of NEC with a Modified Bell's Stage IIA. In 1978, Bell and colleagues first described a simple staging scheme for NEC, which subsequently became central to the reporting and capture of NEC cases utilized for clinical studies and prospective databases.[18] The field of neonatology and pediatric surgery have used this staging scheme with only minor subsequent modifications (Table 1.2).

4. What finding is the **MOST** "classic" for NEC on radiographic imaging?

    A. double bubble sign
    B. distended bowel
    C. normal X-ray
    D. pneumatosis intestinalis

Answer: D

Pneumatosis intestinalis, or gas in the intestinal wall, is a key finding in infants with NEC. While they may also have distended bowel, that could also be found in other abdominal pathology.[1] Double bubble sign (dilatation of the proximal duodenum and stomach) is a finding on X-ray for duodenal atresia or volvulus.

5. Which of the following is **MOST** recognized risk factor for NEC?

    A. Caucasian ethnicity
    B. hypertension
    C. large for gestational age
    D. low birth weight

Answer: D

Low birth weight is the most commonly reported significant prognostic factor for NEC. The incidence is 5% to 10% of infants born with VLBW, which is defined as less than 1,500 g. Other risk factors include low gestational age, black ethnicity, hypotension, sepsis, and premature rupture of membranes.[4]

6. An ex-37-week gestation, 5-week-old male infant presents to the emergency room with reports of feeding intolerance, lethargy, and repeated bilious vomiting. His laboratory results show that the infant is hypochloremic, alkalotic, and hypokalemic. Abdominal physical examination is remarkable for an olive-shaped mass between the midline and right upper quadrant. What is the **MOST** likely diagnosis?

    A. duodenal atresia
    B. hypertrophic pyloric stenosis
    C. NEC
    D. pancreatitis

Answer: B

Pyloric stenosis usually manifests between weeks 2 and 6 of life and occurs most frequently in first-born males. The classic clinical presentation is repeated, protracted bilious vomiting with feeding intolerance, dehydration, and lethargy. The classic "olive-shaped" mass, indicative of a hypertrophied pylorus, can be difficult to palpate on an awake infant. The diagnosis is most often confirmed with ultrasound or, rarely, a barium swallow study.

7. A 9-day-old ex-31-week gestational age female infant is in the NICU with abdominal distention and feeding intolerance. Which of the following is the **LEAST** likely next step in her management?

    A. intravenous fluid resuscitation
    B. nil per os for bowel rest
    C. orogastric tube for decompression
    D. peritoneal drain placement

Answer: D

Peritoneal drainage is a surgical intervention for NEC. Medical management consists of bowel rest and decompression with nasogastric or orogastric tube to low-intermittent suction. Intravenous fluids for resuscitation should be started, and broad spectrum antibiotics are also indicated after blood, sputum, and urine cultures are obtained.[2]

Table 1.2 **MODIFIED BELL'S STAGING FOR NECROTIZING ENTEROCOLITIS**

BELL'S STAGES	GENERAL CLINICAL FINDINGS	ABDOMINAL RADIOGRAPHIC RESULTS	GASTROINTESTINAL SIGNS
I	Temperature instability, apnea, bradycardia	Normal gas pattern or mild ileus	Stool with occult blood, mild abdominal distention, gastric residuals
IIA	Temperature instability, apnea, bradycardia	One or more dilated loops, ileus gas pattern, focal pneumatosis	Moderate to severe abdominal distention, absent bowel sounds, stool with gross blood
IIB	Mild metabolic acidosis, thrombocytopenia	Generalized pneumatosis, ascites, portal venous gas	Palpable bowel loops, generalized tenderness, abdominal wall edema
IIIA	Mixed acidosis, hypotension, oliguria, coagulopathy	No free air, moderate to severe ascites, prominent bowel loops	Severe wall edema, induration, erythema
IIIB	Marked derangements in laboratory values, frank shock	Pneumoperitoneum	Perforated bowel

Source. Adapted from RM Kliegman, MC Walsh. Neonatal necrotizing enterocolitis: pathogenesis, classification, and spectrum of disease. *Curr Probl Pediatr.* 1987;17(4):243–288.

QUESTIONS AND ANSWERS

This chapter has accompanying questions and answers which are available to subscribers as part of the Oxford eLearning platform. To access the questions, go to ✅ http:// oxfordmedicine. com/pediatricanesthesiaPBL

REFERENCES

1. Cote CJ, Lerman J, Anderson BJ. *Cote and Lermans: a practice of anesthesia for infants and children*. Philadelphia, PA: Elsevier/ Saunders; 2013.
2. Henry MCW, Moss RL. Necrotizing enterocolitis. *Annu Rev Med*. 2009;60:111–124. doi:10.1146/annurev.med.60.050207.092824
3. Neu J, Walker WA. Necrotizing enterocolitis. *N Engl J Med*. 2011;364:255–264.
4. Samuels N, van de Graaf RA, de Jonge CJ, Reiss IKM, Vermeulen MJ. Risk factors for necrotizing enterocolitis in neonates: a systematic review of prognostic studies. *BMC Pediatrics*. 2017;17:105. doi:10.1186/s12887-017-0847-3
5. Lin HC, Hsu CH, Chen HL, et al. Oral probiotics prevent necrotizing enterocolitis in very low birth weight preterm infants: a multicenter, randomized, controlled trial. *Pediatrics*. 2008;122:693–700.
6. Hsueh W, Caplan MS, Qu XW, et al. Neonatal necrotizing enterocolitis: clinical considerations and pathogenetic concepts. *Pediatr Dev Pathol*. 2003 Jan–Feb;6(1):6–23.
7. Davis PJ, Cladis FP, Motoyama EK. *Smith's anesthesia for infants and children*, 8th ed. St. Louis, MO: Mosby; 2011.
8. Patel AK, Lazar DA, Burrin DG, et al. Abdominal near-infrared spectroscopy measurements are lower in preterm infants at risk for necrotizing enterocolitis. *Pediatr Crit Care Med*. 2014 Oct;15(8):735–741.
9. Kinouchi K. Anaesthetic considerations for the management of very low and extremely low birth weight infants. *Best Pract Res Clin Anaesthesiol*. 2004;18:273–290.
10. Ohlson KBE, Mohell N, Cannon B, et al. Thermogenesis in brown adipocytes is inhibited by volatile anesthetic agents: a factor contributing to hypothermia in infants? *Anesthesiology*. 1994;81:176–183.
11. Whitfill CR, Drack AV. Avoidance and treatment of retinopathy of prematurity. *Semin Pediatr Surg*. 2000;9:103–105.
12. Moore P, Brook MM, Heymann MA. In: Allen HD, Gutgesell HP, Clark EB, et al. (eds.), Ch 30. *Patent ductus arteriosus*, 6th ed. Moss and Adam's Heart Disease in Infants, Children, and Adolescents Including the Fetus and Young Adults, Vol. 1. Philadelphia: Lippincott Williams & Wilkins; 2001:652–669.
13. Cornblath M, Reisner SH. Blood glucose in the neonate and its clinical significance. *N Engl J Med*. 1965;273:378.
14. Brusseau R, McCann ME. Anaesthesia for urgent and emergency surgery. *Early Hum Dev*. 2010 Nov;86(11):703–714.
15. Jarmakani JM, Nakanishi T, George GL, et al. Effect of extracellular calcium on myocardial mechanical function in the neonatal rabbit. *Dev Pharmacol Ther*. 1982;5(1–2):1–13.
16. Nayler WG, Fassold E. Calcium accumulating and ATPase activity of cardiac sarcoplasmic reticulum before and after birth. *Cardiovasc Res*. 1977 May;11(3):231–237.
17. Pierro A. The surgical management of necrotising enterocolitis. *Early Hum Dev*. 2005 Jan;81(1):79–85.
18. Bell MJ, Ternberg JL, Feigin RD, et al. Neonatal necrotizing enterocolitis: therapeutic decisions based upon clinical staging. *Ann Surg*. 1978;187:1–7.

2.

NEONATAL STRIDOR

Aaron Low and Andrew Pittaway

STEM CASE AND KEY QUESTIONS

A 1-month-old infant is admitted from an outside hospital with a history of increasingly noisy and labored breathing. Following a premature birth at 30 weeks gestation, she quickly developed signs of respiratory distress associated with persistent pulmonary hypertension (PPHTN) that necessitated intubation. High-frequency oscillatory ventilation with added nitric oxide was instituted for 2 days and then converted to "conventional" ventilation for a further 5 days. At that time, she was successfully extubated and subsequently transferred to a facility closer to the parental home for ongoing care.

At the time of readmission, she had been extubated for 1 week, had received 1 dose of intravenous (IV) steroids and is breathing oxygen 2 L/minute via nasal cannulae. She has received nebulized epinephrine for a "croupy" sounding cough. Repeat echocardiograms performed in the emergency room reveals resolution of her PPHTN. Her hematocrit is 30.

Examination reveals a pink neonate in obvious respiratory distress. Pertinent clinical findings include a respiratory rate of 60 breaths per minute with significant sternal and subcostal recessions. In addition, she makes a loud inspiratory noise and has coarse rhonchi scattered throughout both lung fields. She last ate formula 6 hours previously and has a nasogastric tube in situ. She has a 24-gauge IV cannula in her foot through which she is receiving a dextrose/saline infusion.

DEFINE THE TERM STRIDOR AND LIST THE DIFFERENT TYPES OF STRIDOR THAT MAY OCCUR. DESCRIBE THE UNDERLYING PHYSICS THAT EXPLAIN STRIDOR. HOW DO STRIDOR AND WHEEZE DIFFER? WHAT IS THE DIFFERENTIAL DIAGNOSIS FOR STRIDOR IN A NEONATE?

The otolaryngology surgeon wishes to perform urgent direct laryngoscopy and bronchoscopy, possibly with lasering for a presumed subglottic stenosis.

WHAT ARE THE POSSIBLE ANESTHETIC APPROACHES TO THIS CASE, THEIR ADVANTAGES AND DISADVANTAGES?

With standard ASA (American Society of Anesthesiologists) monitoring in place, the infant is transported to the operating room (OR) and anesthesia is induced.

IN ADDITION TO ROUTINE ANESTHESIA SETUP, WHAT ADDITIONAL EQUIPMENT AND MEDICATIONS WOULD YOU HAVE PREPARED IN ADVANCE? HOW MIGHT YOU INDUCE THIS INFANT? DESCRIBE THE ADVANTAGES AND DISADVANTAGES OF THE INDUCTION TECHNIQUES CONSIDERED.

Following an uneventful induction, a surgical timeout is completed, and the OR bed is rotated 90 degrees. The otolaryngology surgeon takes over mask ventilation of the infant.

DESCRIBE YOUR PLAN FOR MAINTENANCE OF ANESTHESIA.

A suspension laryngoscope is positioned, and a rigid bronchoscope is then advanced through the laryngoscope. The vocal cords are easily visualized and normal in appearance. The laryngoscope is then advanced through the vocal cords to visualize the trachea. An area of subglottic stenosis is observed.

During this examination, the infant demonstrates increasing evidence of respiratory difficulty with obvious intercostal and sternal notch retractions. An asynchronous (seesaw) breathing pattern of the chest and abdomen is noted. This is followed by rapid oxygen desaturation and bradycardia <60 bpm so you ask the circulating nurse to call a code as you take over the airway from the surgeon.

DESCRIBE YOUR RESUSCITATION ALGORITHM.

Help arrives, and circulation and ventilation are restored. You decide to intubate the infant. A styletted 3.0 endotracheal tube (ETT) will not advance beyond the tracheal stricture. A 2.5 uncuffed ETT is placed with no leak audible at a pressure of 40 cm H_2O. After discussion, a decision is made to perform a tracheostomy prior to transfer from OR to the intensive care unit.

HOW WILL YOU MANAGE
AN ANESTHETIC FOR TRACHEOSTOMY
SURGERY? DESCRIBE THE TYPE
OF TRACHEOSTOMY TUBES
USED IN PEDIATRICS. WHAT ARE
THE POTENTIAL COMPLICATIONS
OF TRACHEOSTOMY?

Tracheostomy is completed without further complication, and the infant is transported to the intensive care unit in stable condition.

WHAT FURTHER MEDICAL OR
SURGICAL INTERVENTIONS MAY BE
CONSIDERED FOR TREATMENT OF THE
TRACHEAL STENOSIS?

DISCUSSION

INTRODUCTION

This is a complex and common clinical scenario in pediatric anesthesia. In addition to all the usual concerns relevant to neonatal anesthesia, the practitioner must also surrender exclusive right to the airway—a stressful prospect for even the most experienced provider. Fortunately, reports in the literature are gradually defining what might be the optimal technique for such cases.[1] Before considering these, it is important to properly evaluate the significant features of this case.

UPPER AIRWAY OBSTRUCTION

The history of prolonged intubation is suggestive of an iatrogenic cause for the observed inspiratory stridor. Certainly, acquired subglottic stenosis (Figure 2.1) caused by ischemic injury to the cricoid mucosa is high on the list of differential diagnoses; congenital subglottic stenosis (e.g., Down syndrome) causes similar symptoms: stridor (often biphasic), recurrent croup/lower respiratory tract infection, and exertional dyspnea.

Acquired subglottic stenosis in infants is most commonly caused by use of too large an endotracheal tube and is associated with prolonged intubation.[2] Laryngomalacia (Figure 2.2) is another possibility causing some 50% stridor in (nonintubated) infants.[3,4] Stridor caused by laryngomalacia is similar in many ways to that due to other causes. It is often present from birth, worsened by crying and improved by prone positioning. This worsening with agitation can be explained by

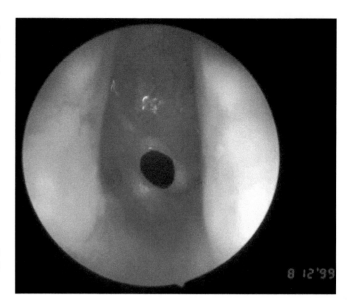

Fig. 2.1 Acquired subglottic stenosis.

a combination of the Bernoulli and Venturi effects. Bernoulli's principle states that an increase in velocity leads to decrease in pressure, while the Venturi effect explains the reduction of pressure when flow is directed through a constricted orifice. This is why stridor may not be present in the comfortable, nonagitated patient but may become severe in the agitated, tachypneic patient. The majority of neurologically normal children with laryngomalacia do not demonstrate the feeding difficulties encountered in neurologically impaired children with the same condition—unless unusually severe.[5] Laryngomalacia usually improves with age but may persist up to the age of 5 years. Tracheobronchomalacia is usually a far more serious condition requiring early tracheostomy and prolonged ventilation.

Although stridor is relatively common in infancy, significant airway pathology is likely if it is severe, persistent, or

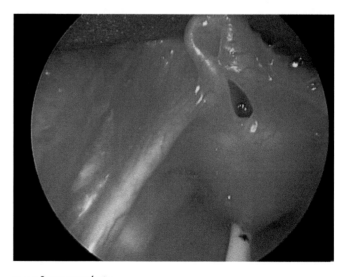

Fig. 2.2 Laryngomalacia.

associated with apnea, failure to thrive, an abnormal cry, and prior intubation. Three types of stridor are recognized:

- Inspiratory
- Expiratory
- Biphasic (or mixed)

All are a result of partial airway obstruction that results in turbulent air flow across the narrowing and hence production of a high-pitched noise; however, differences in timing related to the breathing cycle give important clues to the precise anatomic location of the airway narrowing.

In this case, the stridor occurs during the inspiratory phase of breathing; this usually correlates with obstruction of the extrathoracic airway—that is, above the thoracic inlet (encircled by first thoracic vertebra, first ribs and costal cartilages, and manubrium). During inspiration, the intraluminal pressure of the extrathoracic airway becomes more negative because of chest expansion. Transluminal pressure from surrounding soft tissues thus increases causing increased narrowing of the already partially occluded airway and worsens the stridor. During expiration, intraluminal pressure increases, briefly relieving the obstruction and improving stridor.

Expiratory stridor implies obstruction of the *intrathoracic* airway. During inspiration, intraluminal pressure exceeds the surrounding intrathoracic pressure, dilating the airway and improving stridor. During expiration, the reverse happens, and stridor worsens.

Biphasic stridor implies midtracheal obstruction (at the thoracic inlet), as occurs with tracheomalacia or stenosis. A combination of the described pathophysiological processes results in noises throughout the breathing cycle.

Patent ductus arteriosus (PDA) is relevant in this case for several reasons—the circulation of PPHTN is PDA-dependent, and although the repeat echocardiogram suggests its near-resolution, it may become significant once again in the context of sudden increases in pulmonary vascular resistance (PVR). Consideration of some of those factors known to raise PVR—hypoxia, hypercapnea, and hypothermia—makes it imperative that any anesthetic technique chosen be meticulous in minimizing these derangements. Unfortunately, this case is at risk for all of these by virtue of the limitations imposed by the planned surgery. Also of significance in this case, increased PVR can be abruptly precipitated by airway manipulation under an inadequate depth of anesthesia—a real possibility.

TREATMENT OPTIONS

Subglottic tracheal stenosis is quite common in this patient population, especially following prolonged intubation, or intubation with an ETT that is too large. Grade 1 or 2 subglottic stenosis may not require treatment and may only become symptomatic in the setting of an upper respiratory infection or patient exertion. Grade 3 and 4 subglottic stenosis should be surgically managed. If mild to moderate with symptoms limited to feeding difficulties, upright positioning, anti-reflux medications and a thickened-liquid diet may suffice. Surgically, management may include rigid bronchoscopy with subsequent dilation. Incision with a carbon dioxide laser with subsequent dilation is gaining popularity. In severe cases, tracheal reconstruction with cartilaginous grafting (often from a rib), anterior cricoid split, or cricotracheal reconstruction may be necessary.

ANESTHETIC PRACTICALITIES

A careful history should enquire about symptoms of obstruction; their onset, timing, and severity; and recognized aggravating and alleviating factors. Physical examination should be tailored to elicit signs of respiratory distress. One must plan for a lost airway, difficult mask ventilation, or a code situation when preparing for airway surgery.

The anesthesiologist and should have a firm grasp of Neonatal Resuscitation Program (NRP) algorithms as set forth by the American Academy of Pediatrics. To this end, code and subcode doses of epinephrine (10 mcg/kg and 1 mcg/kg) and atropine (20 mcg/kg) should be drawn up and available. Since most neonatal cardiac arrests are due to hypoxemia, a plan in conjunction with the surgeon should be made to as how to address a lost airway. It is vital to remember that the neonate's oxygen requirements are higher (7 mL/kg/min) and that closing capacity approaches functional residual capacity. This is reflected in the NRP guidelines that emphasize control of oxygenation and ventilation. A complete discussion of the algorithm is beyond the scope of this discussion, but key components are addressed here. This includes positive pressure ventilation as a first step to addressing bradycardia (heart rate <100 bpm), troubleshooting a poor mask ventilation scenario (MRSOPA: adjust the mask, reposition to a "sniffing" position, suctioning of the mouth and nose, opening the mouth and moving the jaw forward to relieve an obstructing tongue, increasing pressure to achieve chest rise, and considering an airway alternative) and early intubation, especially if bradycardia does not improve. Airway adjuncts (nasal pharyngeal airways, oral pharyngeal airways, and supraglottic airway devices) should be readily available to address difficult mask ventilation, and high continuous positive airway pressure may be required to ventilate the patient with tracheal stenosis.

Because of the neonate's limited cardiac reserve—low intrinsic intracellular calcium stores and poor lusitropy (which renders their cardiac output heart rate dependent), chest compressions should be initiated and epinephrine administered for a heart rate <60 bpm.

This patient arrived in the operating theatre with an IV catheter but if one is not present, epinephrine may be administered via an endotracheal tube at 10 times the IV dose (100 mcg/kg); however, a more dilute solution should be used (1:10,000 is recommended). For airway surgery in the tenuous neonate, emergency airway equipment (including that required for a surgical airway) must be immediately available, as should the surgeon. With tracheal stenosis, a feared scenario

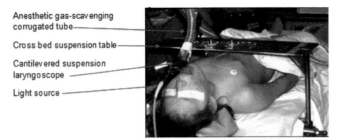

Anesthetic gas-scavenging
corrugated tube
Cross bed suspension table
Cantilevered suspension
laryngoscope
Light source

Fig. 2.3 Suspension laryngoscopy.

is not inability to obtain a Cormack-Lehane laryngoscopic view as much as inability to pass an ETT due to the obstruction. Thus, small endotracheal tubes, including uncuffed 2.5 and 2.0 tubes should be available. Sometimes, continuous positive airway pressure and high positive pressure will improve mask ventilation and temporize the situation. Assisting spontaneous ventilation with positive pressure may be more successful than attempting to ventilate a completely apneic infant. Rigid bronchoscopy by the surgeon may allow passage of a small ETT. If all else fails, an emergency surgical airway may need to be performed distal to the obstruction to re-establish oxygenation.

The surgeon will frequently wish to perform *suspension laryngoscopy*, during which the glottis is observed during spontaneous breathing for evidence of abnormal movement or collapse (Figures 2.3, 2.4 and 2.5). Note the arrangement (in a much larger patient) of the cross-bed "Mustard" low table upon which the suspension laryngoscope is cantilevered (Figure 2.3). Figure 2.4 is a close-up of the proximal end of the suspension laryngoscope.

This arrangement also provides optimal unimpeded conditions for subsequent use of the CO_2 laser (although its use is beyond the remit of this discussion). Sudden airway loss under anesthesia in such cases is much safer if spontaneous breathing is preserved and is mandatory in cases where a potentially difficult airway is being examined. The only option to maintain oxygenation in cases where apnea is either deliberately induced or accidentally supervenes is intermittent ventilation through either a face mask, jet ventilator, or endotracheal tube placed by the surgeon. On occasions where a rigid bronchoscope is employed instead, continuous ventilation is possible using either a ventilating (usually Storz™) or Venturi™ scope.[6]

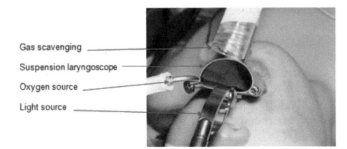

Gas scavenging
Suspension laryngoscope
Oxygen source
Light source

Fig. 2.4 Suspension laryngoscopy.

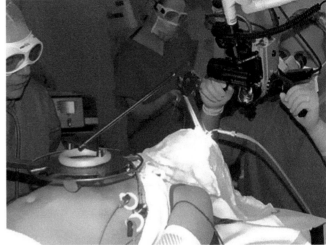

Fig. 2.5 Suspension laryngoscopy with CO_2 laser in place.

The Sanders jet-ventilating device utilized with the latter instrument is *not* recommended for children weighing <40 kg because of the potential for pulmonary barotrauma.

Possible anesthesia techniques include

- Spontaneous/controlled ventilation with volatile agent delivered via the sidearm of the scope/ventilating rigid bronchoscope.

- Total IV anesthesia.

- Apnea with intermittent intubation and controlled ventilation—risks hypoventilation, repeated interruptions to surgery, and glottic edema from numerous intubations.

- Jet ventilation with a Sanders injector/Venturi bronchoscope combination—some authors recommend its use in larger children only, and it requires experience and vigilant skill to keep the jet aimed at the glottic opening.

Sedative premedication is best avoided because it risks turning partial into complete upper airway obstruction. Glycopyrrolate 10 to 20 mcg/kg is given IV to dry secretions, enhance topicalization, and counteract any bradycardia. Dexamethasone 0.5 mg/kg (maximum 12 mg) may be given IV if airway edema is anticipated.

One popular technique employs a mask induction with sevoflurane in oxygen, followed by IV maintenance with a propofol infusion (100–300 mcg/kg/hr) supplemented by judicious bolus doses of alfentanil (5–10 mcg/kg/dose).[7] Remifentanil is sometimes used for this purpose elsewhere[8] (0.05–0.1 mcg/kg/min). Anesthesia can be supplemented with further volatile agent if deemed necessary via the breathing circuit/bronchoscope sidearm connection. The rate is carefully adjusted to sustain a depth of anesthesia sufficient to permit both surgery and spontaneous breathing. Crucial to the success of this technique is prelaryngoscopy topicalization of the glottis and vocal cords under direct vision with lidocaine. This can be achieved either with 2% lidocaine delivered via a "Cass" (an 18-gauge angle-tip side-hole) needle (2–3 mg/kg in neonates; up to 4 mg/kg in older children) or by the ingenious "atomizer" technique described by Fahy.[9] In the latter, a 3-way tap is connected simultaneously to an oxygen supply set at 10 L/minute, the syringe containing lidocaine and to the plastic catheter of a 20-gauge IV cannula. When the lidocaine is injected, it is effectively "atomized" into a fine mist that coats the glottis, providing good topical anesthesia and reducing both maintenance agent requirements and coughing or unwanted movements. Children should remain nil per os for 2 hours after such treatment. Disadvantages of this approach include risk of aspiration, hypoventilation/hypoxemia, and coughing/movement.

Although the quoted incidence of complications following pediatric rigid bronchoscopy varies, overall it appears to be low[10] (7.6%) and is usually associated with attempts to retrieve inhaled foreign bodies. The incidence of pneumothorax (the most common severe complication) can be reduced by avoiding the right middle and (left) lingular lobes of the lung[11] with the bronchoscope.

Although not relevant to our case, it is worth considering how these techniques might be modified in the case of an even smaller neonate requiring the same procedure. Premature infants of between 1 and 2 kg require a size 2.5 Storz™ bronchoscope—which confusingly has internal and external diameters of 3.2 mm and 4.0 mm, respectively. Attempts at ventilation can, however, generate dangerously high airway pressures and risk barotrauma. An *apneic* technique involving periods of hyperventilation with 100% oxygen through the side arm of the bronchoscope followed by bouts of apnea/instrumentation is preferred. The optical telescope may then be carefully introduced through the bronchoscope ensuring continuous escape of the 1 L/min oxygen continuously delivered via the side arm (*apneic oxygenation*) through the proximal end of the instrument. In even smaller infants, the airway will admit the telescope only (outer diameter 2.7 mm). A similar apneic technique can be used as described, or a spontaneously ventilating alternative in which sevoflurane in 100% oxygen is delivered via a nasopharyngeal airway connected to the anesthesia circuit.

Extubation should only be performed at the conclusion of surgery (following discussion with the surgeon) once it is established that airway swelling is *not* anticipated to cause significant airway compromise. Remember that Poiseuille's law states that airflow resistance is inversely related to fourth power of the airway radius; that is, small changes in airway radius have disproportionately large effects on resistance. The child should be awake before extubation and should be closely monitored in a proximate, high-acuity environment afterwards. The child should remain nil by mouth for 2 hours afterwards if the glottis was topicalized with lidocaine.

Tracheostomy in a neonate is sometime needed when stenosis is so severe that only a very small ETT can be passed or if the neonate will not successfully wean from mechanical ventilation due to the stenosis. As with any airway surgery, anesthetic management of this procedure requires close communication with the surgeon and presents challenges unique to this patient age group. If tracheostomy is to be undertaken, it is preferably undertaken in a controlled, preplanned scenario as opposed to an emergency or rescue scenario. As such, preoperative evaluation to ensure that the patient is medically optimized from a cardiorespiratory standpoint is important. Furthermore, imaging to ensure that tracheostomy will bypass the obstruction and the location of any aberrant vasculature structures (e.g., high riding innominate vein) that may make the surgical technique difficult is important. Generally, when placing a tracheostomy, parameters of the tracheostomy tube that need to considered include length, diameter, curvature, size, and whether a cuff is needed. Ideally, the length of the tube should extend at least 2 cm beyond the stoma, and the tip should be no closer than 1–2 cm from the carina (the authors are aware of a patient who, for anatomic reasons, had only 0.5 cm of tracheostomy tube in her trachea and decannulated and arrested with alarming frequency). A cuffed tracheostomy tube should be considered if one thinks that high airway pressures are going to be required for ventilation or oxygenation or if there is high risk of aspiration. Fenestrated tracheostomy tubes are designed to facilitate translaryngeal airflow and phonation; however, they are not usually used in the pediatric population. Finally, some tracheostomy tubes have adjustable lengths that may be considered in lieu of, or prior to, insertion of a customized tracheostomy.

The anesthetic management of surgery for tracheostomy placement depends on the reason for placement. If the patient cannot be intubated via an oral or nasotracheal route, then maintenance of spontaneous ventilation is of paramount importance. This is analogous to the "awake trach" in older patients that historically is managed via local anesthetic infiltration by the surgeon and gentle titration of sedative medications with maintenance of spontaneous ventilation by the anesthesia team. Oxygen is insufflated via a small ETT or nasal pharyngeal airway inserted into the side of the mouth or through a nares. Dexmedetomidine may be used as a sedative as spontaneous ventilation is typically maintained with little change in tidal volumes. It is important to keep in mind that even with dexmedetomidine, relaxation of upper airway musculature resulting in obstruction may occur. In the neonate who cannot be intubated from above (e.g., craniofacial abnormalities), maintenance of spontaneous ventilation is also important—whether this is achieved via total intravenous anesthesia or insufflation of a volatile anesthetic through a suspension laryngoscope side port. A rigid bronchoscope permits delivery of intermittent breaths throughout the procedure. Insufflation of 100% oxygen through either a suspension laryngoscopy side port, nasally placed ETT, or nasal airway should be employed. If intubation is possible, then ventilation can be controlled until the airway is entered surgically. Just prior to surgical entry into the trachea, the cuff on the ETT, if present, is deflated so as not to violate the cuff. Once the surgeon has visualized the ETT, it is very slowly withdrawn under direct visualization by the surgeon until it is just no longer visible but still within the trachea. This not only allows room for the surgeon to place the tracheostomy tube but also allows the anesthesia team to advance the ETT past the stoma and ventilate the patient if complications arise. Once the tracheostomy tube is in place, it is connected to the anesthesia circuit and breath sounds, adequate tidal volumes, and end-tidal carbon dioxide are all confirmed. Only then is the ETT removed from the patient's trachea.

Plans should be made beforehand to manage complication that may arise during tracheostomy surgery. If electrocautery is used, fraction of inspired oxygen (FiO_2) should be decreased as much as possible prior to tracheal entry to minimize risk of an airway fire. Prior to starting, management of an airway fire should be discussed—including simultaneously flooding the operative field with saline, extubating the trachea, and turning off fresh gas flows. Once the fire is extinguished, the trachea should be reintubated as quickly as possible.

Another potential complication is creation of a false passage through which ventilation can cause subcutaneous emphysema, worsen pre-existing obstruction, and make ventilation more difficult. If the tracheostomy tube is not parallel to the trachea and is directed posteriorly or anteriorly, it can abut a tracheal wall causing erosion into the esophagus or innominate artery causing life-threatening hemorrhage or a suction event precluding ventilation. Pneumothorax and pneumomediastinum occur with higher frequency in children as their pleural apices are higher than in adults. Finally, if a tracheostomy is absolutely necessary and the patient is requiring very high ventilator settings (positive end-expiratory pressure, FiO_2, peak inspiratory pressure) and has a difficult airway, one might consider having veno-venous extracorporeal membranous oxygenation on standby.

Postoperative complications include granuloma formation (most common), infection, obstruction of the cannula, and accidental decannulation. Granuloma formation is most common if the tracheostomy tube abuts either the anterior or the posterior tracheal wall. As previously stated, erosion into the esophagus or a major vascular structure is also possible. Long-term tracheostomy is associated with *Pseudomonas aeruginosa* and *Staphyloccocus aureus* colonization.

REVIEW QUESTIONS

1. Of the following conditions, which is **LEAST** likely to result in stridor?

    A. brachial cleft cyst
    B. laryngomalacia
    C. laryngeal cleft
    D. vascular ring

Answer: A

2. Which principle of physics **BEST** explains the causes of stridor?

    A. Bernoulli's Law
    B. Venturi Effect
    C. Boyle's Law
    D. Both A and B

Answer: D

3. Of the following physiological states, which will **LEAST** likely cause right to left shunting through a patent ductus arteriosus?

    A. hypercapnia
    B. hyperthermia
    C. hypoxemia
    D. hypothermia

Answer: B

4. What physiological measurement, which is increase in neonates as compared with adults, is **MOST** responsible for their rapid desaturation?

    A. body surface area
    B. cardiac output
    C. hemoglobin level
    D. metabolism rate

Answer: D

5. In neonatal resuscitation, after "warm, dry, and stimulate," if the heart rate is less than 100 bpm, what is the **BEST** next course of action?

    A. bag-mask ventilation
    B. chest compressions
    C. endotracheal intubation
    D. epinephrine administration

Answer: A

6. Which intervention is the **LEAST** appropriate in managing an airway fire?

    A. endotracheal extubation.
    B. fresh gas flows termination.
    C. nitrous oxide insufflation.
    D. surgical field saline saturation.

Answer: C

7. Which of the following occurs **MORE** commonly during tracheostomy in children, as compared to adults?

    A. airway fire
    B. cardiac arrest
    C. hemorrhage
    D. pneumomediastinum

Answer: D

QUESTIONS AND ANSWERS

This chapter has accompanying questions and answers which are available to subscribers as part of the Oxford eLearning platform. To access the questions, go to ✓ http:// oxfordmedicine. com/pediatricanesthesiaPBL

REFERENCES

1. Brett CM, Zwass MS. Eyes, ears, nose, throat and dental surgery. In: Gregoray GA, ed. *Principles of Pediatric Anesthesia*. 4th ed. New York: Churchill Livingstone; 2002:687–688.

2. Austin J, Ali T. Tracheomalacia and bronchomalacia in children: pathophysiology, assessment, treatment and anaesthetic management. *Pediatr Anesth.* 2003;13(1):3–11.

3. Holzki J, Laschat M, Stratmann C. Stridor in the neonate and infant. implications for the pediatric anaesthetist. Prospective description of 155 patients with congenital & acquired stridor in early infancy. *Pediatr Anesth.* 1998;8(3):221–227.

4. Roberts S, Thornington R. Paediatric bronchoscopy. *Contin Educ Anaesthes Crit Care Pain.* 2005;5(2):41–44.

5. Marc T, Susan G. Laryngomalacia: review and summary of current clinical practice in 2015. *Paediatr Respir Rev.* 2016;17:3–8.

6. Gregory D, Eller RL, Thomas RF. Diagnosing aerodynamic supraglottic collapse with rest and exercise flexible laryngoscopy. *J Voice.* 2012;26(6):779–784.

7. Holinger L. Etiology of stridor in the neonate, infant and child. *Ann Otol Rhinol Laryngol.* 1980;89:397–400.

8. Orr R. Anesthesia for microlaryngoscopy. *Pediatr Anesth.* 2005;15(1):81.

9. de Trey L, Lambercy K, Monnier P, Sandu K. Management of severe congenital laryngeal webs—a 12 year review. *Int J Pediatr Otorhinolayrngol.* 2016 Jul;86:82–86.

10. Weiner G, Zaichkin J. *Textbook of Neonatal Resuscitation.* 7th ed. Itasca, IL: American Academy of Pediatrics; 2016.

11. Davis PJ, Cladis FP, Motoyama EK, eds. *Smith's Anesthesia for Infants and Children.* 8th ed. St. Louis, MO: Mosby; 2010.

12. Reynolds P, Weatherly R. Laser therapy for laryngeal papillomas. In: Stoddart P, Lauder G, eds. *Problems in Paediatric Anaesthesia.* 1st ed. London: Dunitz; 2004:93–97.

13. Fahy C. Topical airway anaesthesia for paediatric bronchoscopy. *Pediatr Anesth.* 2003;13(9):844.

14. Tomaske M, Gerber AC, Weiss M. Anesthesia and peri-interventional morbidity of rigid bronchoscopy for tracheobronchial foreign body diagnosis and removal. *Pediatr Anesth.* 2006;16(2):123–129.

15. Brownlee K, Crabbe D. Paediatric bronchoscopy. *Arch Dis Child.* 1997;77(3):272–275.

16. Campisi P, Forte V. Pediatric tracheostomy. *Semin Pediatr Surg.* 2016;25:191–195.

17. Dal'Astra A, Quirino, AV, de Sousa Caixêta, JA, Gomes Avelino MA. Tracheostomy in childhood: review of the literature on complications and mortality over the last three decades. *Brazil J Otorhinolaryngol.* 2017;83(2):207–214.

3.

CHARGE SYNDROME

Pilar Mercado, Jamey E. Eklund, and Jennifer L. Anderson

STEM CASE AND KEY QUESTIONS

At 38-weeks gestation, a 3.2 kg neonate is born to a G1P1 mother. She had poor prenatal care and did not receive an ultrasound. Delivery is unremarkable with an initial APGAR (appearance, pulse, grimace, activity, and respiration) score of 7. The baby is pink, and the pulse is 130 bpm. She has reflexes with strong stimulation, has some flexion, and has a weak irregular cry. The neonate is brought to the infant bed, stops crying, and becomes cyanotic. After about 15 seconds, she begins to cry again, and her color improves. A team member comments that the baby's ears look abnormally wide, low set, and cup-shaped.

HOW IS CHOANAL ATRESIA DIAGNOSED AND TREATED?

The care team stimulates the baby and actively suctions the mouth and nose. A murmur is heard on chest auscultation, but the result of a lung exam is normal. As the baby calms down, her breathing becomes obstructed, and she becomes cyanotic again; sternal retractions are also noted. Again, after stimulation, she begins crying, and her color improves. A soft suction catheter is inserted into each nare, and resistance is met after 1 to 1.5 cm. Bilateral choanal atresia is suspected. An oral airway is placed to temporarily keep the oral passage open for respiration.

The patient is brought to the neonatal intensive care unit (NICU) for stabilization and further management. Oxygen saturation gradually increases as expected in the neonatal period, but she intermittently desaturates as low as 80%. These episodes resolve spontaneously. The oral airway is exchanged for a McGovern nipple, and the end is cut off. It is tied around the infant's head and secured at the occiput. Given the concern for choanal atresia and her ear anomalies, a computed tomography (CT) scan of the head is ordered with attention to the temporal bones. CT scan reveals bilateral choanal atresia and ossicular malformations.

WHAT STUDIES ARE INDICATED TO AID IN THE DIAGNOSIS OF CHARGE SYNDROME IN THE NEONATAL PERIOD AND TO RULE OUT SERIOUS ANOMALIES?

Although choanal atresia is usually an isolated anomaly, CHARGE syndrome must be ruled out. An electrocardiogram,

echocardiogram, and cranial and renal ultrasound are scheduled. Genetic testing for a mutation in CHD7 is sent. The parents are counseled that further testing as their child matures may be necessary.

The transthoracic echocardiogram reveals moderate pulmonary valve stenosis and an atrial septal defect with normal function. The ultrasound of the abdomen, ordered for renal anomalies, is normal. The multidisciplinary team is assembled to decide how to manage the patient's choanal atresia in light of the pulmonary stenosis. After considering the risks and benefits of various options, the team agrees that the patient should undergo a balloon valvuloplasty prior to repair of the choanal atresia.

WHAT SPECIALISTS SHOULD BE CONSULTED TO CARE FOR THIS PATIENT?

Otolaryngology is immediately consulted regarding treatment options for the choanal atresia. Given that choanal atresia and ear anomalies can be associated with CHARGE syndrome or other genetic syndromes, a geneticist is also consulted. Cardiology has already been consulted. Opthomology and neurology and other specialists may need to be consulted as the child's symptoms manifest.

WHAT LAB TESTS ARE USEFUL TO HAVE PRIOR TO ANESTHESIA?

Blood urea nitrogen, creatinine, and electrolytes are sent to evaluate and monitor renal function and to exclude hypocalcemia. Complete blood count with differential is a starting point for assessing immune function.

WHAT IS AN APPROPRIATE ANESTHETIC PLAN FOR THE VALVULOPLASTY? WHAT EQUIPMENT SHOULD BE IMMEDIATELY AVAILABLE?

The anesthesiologist is aware that difficulty with ventilation and intubation is of concern in this patient. She has different size oral airways and endotracheal tubes at hand. A video-assisted laryngoscope and various supraglottic airways are in the room. She has specifically asked the otolaryngologist to be present on induction in case her expertise is needed.

The infant is brought to the cardiac catheterization lab. On induction, bag-mask ventilation becomes difficult but improves after placement of an oral airway. The child is intubated, and analgesia is provided with minimal opioid dosing. The neonate remains hemodynamically stable throughout the procedure. Pulmonary artery pressures after the procedure measure close to normal.

WHAT ISSUES SHOULD BE CONSIDERED AT THE END OF THE CASE IN TERMS OF AIRWAY MANAGEMENT?

The anesthesiologist decides to keep the patient intubated at the end of the procedure. The child can fully emerge from the anesthetic in the NICU and regain adequate respiratory function. Also, if the child remains stable, choanal atresia repair may occur within the next several days. Although, keeping the child intubated does carry some risk, it would help prevent aspiration and provide a secure airway for this infant.

The patient remains stable after valvuloplasty, and the team decides to repair the choanal atresia 3 days later. The child is brought to the operating room (OR) intubated. The procedure is uneventful. At the end of the surgery, nasal stents are placed. The baby emerges from anesthesia and is extubated fully awake. The child recovers for 2 days in the NICU with close monitoring. She is then transferred to a floor bed for several days. Although feeding is difficult at times, she successfully recovers and goes home 1 week later.

Testing reveals she meets the criteria for CHARGE syndrome. She has an associated CHD7 mutation. She has no renal involvement but has ocular coloboma causing visual impairment, ear anomalies, hearing impairment, and abnormal genitalia, for which assessment of the pituitary gonadal axis is performed.

Over the next several months she develops clinical symptoms of reflux and two episodes of aspiration pneumonia requiring hospitalization. At 13 months of age, a swallow study is performed and reveals uncoordinated swallowing and aspiration.

As a result, she is scheduled for a gastrostomy tube placement. During the preoperative assessment, the anesthesiologist discovers that the patient is scheduled for bilateral myringotomies and tube placement in the next month and that cardiologists plan for a transthoracic echocardiogram within the next 3 months to assess the status of her pulmonary valve, atrial septal defect, and cardiac function. The anesthesiologist takes steps to coordinate the completion of these procedures under one anesthetic.

IS IT ADVANTAGEOUS TO DO MULTIPLE SURGERIES UNDER ONE ANESTHETIC FOR THESE CHILDREN?

Although it is uncommon for otolaryngology, general surgery, and cardiology to schedule OR time on the same day, it is necessary to accommodate extenuating circumstances. The coordinating anesthesiologist holds a preoperative multidisciplinary meeting to review perioperative management of patients with CHARGE. The care team agrees that the risk of postoperative complications are decreased if the patient undergoes only one anesthetic. A block of OR time is scheduled in advance for the bilateral myringotomies and tube placement, gastrostomy tube placement, and transthoracic echocardiogram.

IS IT APPROPRIATE FOR PATIENTS WITH CHARGE SYNDROME TO UNDERGO PROCEDURES IN AN OUTPATIENT SETTING?

During the planning meeting, one of the surgeons requests these short procedures occur at an outpatient center. The head anesthesiologist at the surgery center denies this request. He explains that, due to the concern for postoperative respiratory complications in this patient, even small procedures should be done in a hospital setting.

The now 14-month-old child arrives in the preoperative area at the children's hospital to undergo these procedures 1 month later.

While interviewing the parents, the anesthesiologist scheduled to care for her that day is reminded by the family that the child is both hearing and visually impaired. She is also developmentally delayed. In addition, although the child is currently healthy, she has had several episodes of aspiration pneumonia in the past.

SHOULD THE PATIENT BE GIVEN ANY PREMEDICATION PRIOR TO ENTERING THE OR?

The patient is fussy in the preoperative area. The nurse requests an order for oral midazolam for the patient. Given the history of aspiration pneumonia and copious secretions, the anesthesiologist decides against premedication.

SHOULD PARENTAL PRESENCE FOR INDUCTION BE CONSIDERED?

Because no premedication is given, the anesthesiologist asks if a parent is willing to be present in the OR for induction. Typically, at this hospital, parental presence for induction is denied due to insufficient staffing. The child life specialist offers a tablet computer for distraction instead. Unfortunately, a tablet is of limited utility for a visually and hearing-impaired child with developmental delay. The pediatric anesthesiologist discusses the situation with the OR staff and explains why an exception needs to be made. Having someone familiar to the child be present for induction may be the best way to help keep the child calm. Furthermore, the mother might be one of the only people capable of communicating with the child. Nonetheless, the mother should be briefed about the mask induction process including nuances observed during stage 2, such as disconjugate gaze, involuntary movements, and agitation. After learning about these issues, the OR staff agree and coordinate to allow the mother to be present for induction.

The child undergoes an uneventful anesthetic for the three procedures. She is extubated at the end of the case.

WHERE SHOULD THE CHILD BE RECOVERED FROM ANESTHESIA?

The child is brought to the PICU for recovery given her high risk for aspiration. The anesthesiologist was judicious in the use of pain medication during the operation so as to not produce excessive sedation postoperatively. The child appears alert and is brought to the PICU lying on her side. Over the next hour, her respiratory status becomes tenuous. She has copious secretions and periodically coughs and desaturates to 70% to 80%. Continuous suction is instituted overnight, and these episodes gradually decrease.

HOW DO YOU ASSESS PAIN IN A CHILD WITH CHARGE SYNDROME?

While in the PICU, in addition to ongoing respiratory issues, the patient becomes tachycardic and is making repetitive motions with her arms on postoperative day (POD) 2. The nurse asks if pain medications can be given. One of the team members comments that it is difficult to determine whether a developmentally delayed child is in pain. The nurse notes that in the past she has referred to the Non-Communicating Children's Pain Checklist (NCCPC), a pain scale for nonverbal children. After reviewing the scale, the team and parents agree it may be a useful tool. They find the scale helps them tease out her level of pain, and they use it to help provide treatment for her discomfort.

She gradually improves overall and is back to baseline by POD 3. The child remains in the PICU until POD 4 to monitor her respiratory status. She remains stable with oxygen saturation (SpO$_2$) >93% on room air and is transferred to a regular floor bed. The remainder of her hospital stay is uneventful.

The child recovers, and her overall health improves with the initiation of tube feeding. She goes on to require several other anesthetics. The multidisciplinary team remains engaged in her care.

DISCUSSION

CHARGE syndrome comprises a pattern of congenital anomalies affecting multiple organ systems that can pose significant challenges to the anesthesia provider (Figures 3.1 and 3.2). The condition benefits from a long-term multidisciplinary approach to patient care. Mortality has historically been described as highest in the first year of life.[1,2] This is especially significant since, not only will the majority of children with CHARGE syndrome require major surgery in their first year, but surviving children will also likely undergo multiple operations and diagnostic procedures in their lifetimes.[1] Given the complexity and rarity of this syndrome, an overview of its workup is presented along with implications for the anesthesia provider.

ETIOLOGY AND PATHOGENESIS

CHARGE syndrome is a rare disorder, with an incidence of approximately one in 8,500–10,000 live births and results, in most cases, from a sporadic autosomal dominant loss-of-function mutation of the CHD7 gene on chromosome 8.[3,4] These mutations are genetically heterogeneous, and no clear genotype/phenotype relationship has been found.[5] A clue to CHARGE syndrome's high degree of phenotypic variability lies in the CHD7 nuclear protein, which belongs to the family of chromodomain helicase DNA-binding proteins that affect transcription by altering chromatin structure. Its precise function is mostly unknown. Mutations are sporadic; although, rare evidence of parent-to-child transmission has been observed[6] as well as an empiric recurrence rate of 1% to 2% and an association with increasing paternal age.[7] Data on frequency of the presence of a mutation when diagnostic criteria are met varies in the literature. Anywhere from 5% to 40% of individuals with the diagnosis have no observable genetic mutation.[8,9]

DIAGNOSIS AND MANAGEMENT

Since its first description in 1979[10,11] and later coinage by Pagon et al.[12] of the acronym CHARGE, the clinical criteria for diagnosis have undergone significant modifications based on a better understanding of the pathogenesis of the disorder. Blake et al.[13] proposed changes to the clinical criteria in 1998 and have since updated them further. Verloes[14] elegantly describes the specific embryological events that occur early in the first trimester that form the basis for his proposed criteria and provides definitions of atypical and partial CHARGE. These three sets of criteria form the backbone of the CHARGE diagnosis and are outlined in Table 3.1. Both Blake et al.'s and Verloes's criteria are primarily used today.

With the considerable and varied disorders that can accompany this diagnosis, the importance of a multidisciplinary approach to medical and surgical management cannot be overemphasized to limit the number of anesthetics each child will undergo. Table 3.2 highlights the myriad problems that children with CHARGE syndrome face. Complex cardiac defects, brain anomalies, bilateral choanal atresia, esophageal atresia, and severe T-cell deficiency can be life-threatening in the neonatal period.[2]

Presentation of the syndrome can occur very early or later in life. Some patients with bilateral choanal atresia present with respiratory distress at birth. In these cases, management options include placing an intraoral airway or intubation. A McGovern nipple with the end removed can be placed orally and tied in place at the occiput to temporarily relieve obstruction until definitive repair, or tracheostomy can be performed.[15] Suspicion of CHARGE syndrome involves ruling out associated abnormalities and establishing a baseline for subsequent follow-up, especially as new or persistent symptoms become apparent. Once clinical diagnosis is made or suspected, genetic evaluation of CHD7 mutations by direct sequencing is performed. Exclusion of other multiple congenital anomaly syndromes, such as 22q11.2 deletion syndrome,

Table 3.1 CLINICAL CRITERIA

	MAJOR CRITERIA	MINOR CRITERIA	INCLUSION RULE
Pagon et al.[12]	1. Choanal atresia 2. Ocular coloboma	1. Heart defects of any type 2. Retardation (of growth and/or of development) 3. Genital anomalies 4. Ear anomalies (abnormal pinnae or hearing loss)	4 criteria out of 6 and at least 1 major
Blake et al.[13]	1. Coloboma—of iris, retina, choroid, disc; microphthalmia 2. Choanal atresia—unilateral/bilateral, membranous/bony, stenosis/atreasia 3. Characteristic ear abnormalities—external ear (lop- or cup-shaped), middle ear (ossicular malformations, chronic serous otitis), mixed deafness, cochlear defects 4. Cranial nerve dysfunction—facial palsy (unilateral or bilateral), sensorineural deafness and/or swallowing problems	1. Genital hypoplasia—males: micropenis, cryptorchidism; females: hypoplastic labia; both males and females: delayed, incomplete pubertal development 2. Developmental delay—delayed motor milestones, language delay, mental retardation 3. Cardiovascular malformations—all types, especially conotruncal defects (e.g., Tetralogy of Fallot), atrioventricular canal defects, and aortic arch anomalies 4. Growth deficiencies—short stature, growth hormone deficiency 5. Orofacial cleft—cleft lip and/or palate 6. Tracheoesophageal fistula/defects of all types 7. Characteristic face—sloping forehead, flattened tip of nose	4 majors or 3 majors + 3 minors
Verloes	1. Ocular coloboma 2. Choanal atresia 3. Hypoplasia of semicircular canals	1. Rhombencephalic dysfunction (brainstem and cranial nerve III–XII anomalies, including sensorineural deafness) 2. Hypothalamo-hypophyseal dysfunction (including growth hormone and gonadotropin defects) 3. Malformation of the ear (internal or external) 4. Malformation of mediastinal organs (heart, esophagus) 5. Mental retardation	Typical CHARGE: 3 majors or 2 majors + 2 minors Partial CHARGE: 2 majors + 1 minor Atypical CHARGE: 2 majors but no minors or 1 major + 2 minors

Source. Reprinted with permission from Sanlaville D, Verloes A. CHARGE syndrome: an update. *Eur J Hum Genet.* 2007;15:389–399.

Kabuki syndrome, and VACTERL, is essential given significant clinical overlap.[16]

The team approach to the care of these complex patients involves consultation with genetics, otolaryngology, ophthalmology, neurology, endocrinology, and cardiology services, depending on the symptomatology. Workup includes echocardiogram, renal ultrasound, magnetic resonance imaging (MRI) and/or CT scan of the head, auditory testing, cranial nerve testing, chemistry labs, and endocrine and immunologic testing.[17]

ANESTHETIC IMPLICATIONS

Morbidity and early mortality is significant in the CHARGE syndrome population and is related not only to the severity of congenital abnormalities and their sequelae but also to underlying laryngeal and pharyngeal incoordination leading to aspiration.[1,2,6] This is of particular significance because both feeding difficulties and gastroesophageal reflux disease (GERD) are seen in the majority of CHARGE patients. As important causes of post-neonatal death are respiratory, circulatory, and perioperative in nature, and since most surviving patients will undergo multiple procedures, the anesthesia provider is uniquely situated to serve as a patient advocate.

Given their comorbidities, patients with CHARGE are likely to undergo multiple surgeries, often beginning early in life. In a review of 9 patients, Blake et al.[18] found that the first surgery occurred within 1 and 52 days of life and that these patients underwent between 6 and 40 operations. A thorough medical history with particular attention to history of GERD, airway anomalies, tracheostomy, feeding or swallowing difficulties, and other evidence of brainstem dysfunction is

Table 3.2 PHENOTYPE AND ATTENDANT CHALLENGES

	DYSFUNCTION OR DEFECT	COMMON PROCEDURES	ANESTHETIC CONCERNS
Central nervous system	Brainstem dysfunction manifested as cranial nerve palsies, sucking or swallowing problems, difficulty handling secretions, pharyngoesophageal dysmotility, respiratory problems, vagal overactivity; arhinencephaly or hypoplasia of olfactory bulbs	Extensive multidisciplinary assessment of cranial nerve function; feeding/swallowing studies	Difficult airway Respiratory aspiration Thermal dysregulation Osteoporosis in older patients Risks unique to particular surgery Postoperative airway events O_2 desaturation Excess secretions Airway obstruction Crackles, wheezing Stridor Erratic breathing Failed extubation
Cardiac	Congenital heart defects; rarely dysrhythmia	Palliative shunts; total repair of cyanotic heart defects (Tetralogy of Fallot is most common); patent ductus arteriosus ligation	•
Respiratory tract	Choanal atresia; laryngo-tracheomalacia; laryngeal cleft; subglottic stenosis; tracheoesophageal fistula (TEF); micrognathia; cleft lip/palate	Repair of choanal atresia, cleft lip/palate; tracheostomy; bronchoscopy/laryngoscopy/naso-pharyngoscopy; cochlear implants; TEF repair; myringotomies	
Gastrointestinal tract	Esophageal atresia; gastroesophageal reflux	Feeding tube; esophagoscopy; Nissen fundoplication; esophageal repair	
Eyes	Coloboma; strabismus; retinal detachment	Examinations and repair	
Genitourinary	Cryptorchidism; hypospadias; vesicoureteral reflux	Examinations and repair	
Endocrine	Growth deficiencies; delayed/absent puberty	Orthopedic correction	
Immune system	Primarily T-cell dysfunction		
Psychosocial	Variable intellectual ability (mental retardation >70%); delayed motor milestones; potentially low adaptive behavior skills		
Musculoskeletal	Limb and vertebral anomalies; scoliosis; hypotonia		

paramount to anticipate potential perioperative problems and to ensure adequate postoperative observation.

Challenging airway management should be anticipated, especially in emergency situations. In addition to choanal atresia or cleft lip/palate, up to 56% of patients have other upper airway abnormalities.[19,20] These can include midface hypoplasia, micrognathia, laryngomalacia, small mouth, subglottic stenosis, laryngeal cleft, recurrent laryngeal nerve palsy, tracheomalacia, and tracheo-oesophageal fistula.[17] Up to 50% of CHARGE patients will need a tracheotomy due to abnormal airway, inability to manage saliva, swallowing disorders, and high risk of chronic aspiration.[21]

Because of neurologic issues and the potential for chronic aspiration, preoperative assessment of recent respiratory illness in these children is important. In addition to glossopharyngeal (CN IX) and vagal nerve (CN X) palsy, truncal or axial hypotonia is present in up to 93% of cases.[6] These deficits can lead to a high risk of aspiration and influence respiratory mechanics postoperatively. Therefore, lower respiratory issues should be optimized preoperatively. Preoperative treatment with anticholinergics and Botox injections into salivary glands may be useful to help control secretions.[18–20,22] Prolonged intubation may be required in patients with laryngomalacia, frequent aspiration, or truncal hypotonia. In a review by Blake et al.[18] of anesthetics performed in a single tertiary care center, up to 35% resulted in postoperative airway events, including oxygen desaturation requiring intervention and reintubation for airway obstruction by excessive secretions. The highest risk of airway events has been shown to occur after procedures involving the heart, gastrointestinal tract, and diagnostic scopes in the airway (laryngoscopy, bronchoscopy, and nasopharyngoscopy). Extra caution regarding respiratory support after these procedures may be indicated, and postoperative ventilatory support may be needed.

All patients suspected with CHARGE syndrome should have a cardiology consult and echocardiogram. Conotruncal abnormalities including septal defects and Tetralogy of Fallot as well as other anomalies are found in these patients. Arrhythmias have also been described. It should be noted that mortality is more often due to aspiration than from cardiac causes.[20] Other common mediastinal abnormalities include esophageal atresia with or without tracheal fistula.

Genitourinary, renal, ocular, otolaryngologic, endocrine, and immunologic issues in patients with CHARGE syndrome are listed in Table 3.2. Anesthetics for examinations and procedures related to these defects may be needed, thus increasing exposure to the perioperative risks as described.

In addition to these physical abnormalities, patients with CHARGE have a wide spectrum of developmental delay. When coupled with deafness and blindness, communication with these patients can be extremely difficult. Sedatives, if not contraindicated, may help calm patients prior to proceeding to the OR. Parental presence for induction is advocated in this population because tactile sensation by someone familiar may be the primary means of providing comfort for these children.

Developmental delay, blindness, and deafness can also lead to difficulty in assessing the patient's level of pain in the postoperative period. Gaining input from parents or guardians may be useful. In addition, pain scales for nonverbal patients may be useful for this population. Both the Pediatric Pain Profile (PPP) and the NCCPC are validated scales that may be useful.[23–26] In fact, Stratton and Hartshorne developed the CHARGE Non-Vocal Pain Assessment Scale in 2012, based on the PPP and NCCPC. This scale takes into consideration changes in eating habits and other behaviors, the presence of obsessive compulsive-type behaviors, the frequency of rubbing or touching of body parts, and whether the patient is turning the mouth down or puckering his or her lips.[27]

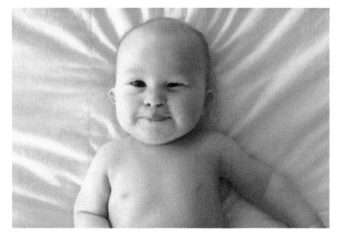

Fig. 3.1 Infant with CHARGE syndrome. Photo supplied with permission by The CHARGE Syndrome Clinical Database Project, Meg Hefner, MS (PI), Saint Louis University IRB #22507.

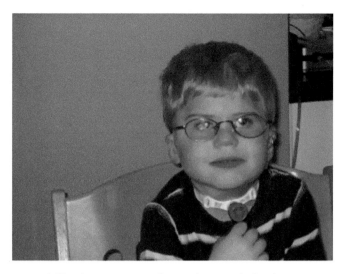

Fig. 3.2 Child with CHARGE syndrome. Photo supplied with permission by The CHARGE Syndrome Clinical Database Project, Meg Hefner, MS (PI), Saint Louis University IRB #22507.

Given the number of surgical procedures CHARGE patients are likely to require and the risk of postoperative respiratory issues, it is appropriate, if not imperative, to argue for a consolidation of multiple procedures under one anesthetic.

REVIEW QUESTIONS

1. A 3.2-kg baby is born to a mother who received limited prenatal care. The baby is born via caesarean section. The baby does well initially but then becomes cyanotic. Rescue breaths are attempted with an Ambu® bag, and the nose and mouth are suctioned. Attempts to pass a catheter through both nares are unsuccessful. Before bag-mask ventilation to improve oxygenation (if needed), what is the **BEST** next step in managing this neonate?

    A. Insert an endotracheal tube.
    B. Insert a McGovern airway.
    C. Insert an oral airway.
    D. Insert a supraglottic airway.

Answer: C
The inability to pass a suction catheter through both nares indicates this patient may have choanal atresia. As an obligate nasal breather, the infant attempts to breathe through the nose, but is unable because of obstruction. Cyanosis ensues, and the child begins to cry, opening up an oral passage for air movement. The cyanosis improves, and the cycle repeats itself. If not stabilized, this can be a life threatening emergency. The best initial treatment is to place an oral airway to break the seal formed by the tongue against the palate. Bag mask ventilation can then be employed as indicated. If the child is stabilized with this method, a McGovern nipple (with the end cut-off) can be placed in the mouth and secured with ties around the occiput. If the child remains unstable with an oral airway, intubation may be necessary. Close monitoring in an intensive care

unit setting is indicated until definitive repair or tracheostomy can be completed.[15]

2. You are scheduled to take care of a 4-year-old girl for a surgical procedure. Her chart indicates she has CHARGE syndrome. Of the following abnormalities, which one is **NOT** associated with this CHARGE syndrome?

    A. immunologic issues
    B. heart defects
    C. liver dysfunction
    D. swallowing difficulties

Answer: C

CHARGE is an acronym for **C**oloboma, **H**eart disease, **A**tresia choanae, **R**etarded growth and development, **G**enital hypoplasia, and **E**ar anomalies/deafness. This acronym leaves out the important common characteristic of cranial nerve palsies and immunologic problems that are often found in these patients.[7] Patients with CHARGE syndrome may have hepatic disease, but it is not associated with the syndrome. Criteria for CHARGE syndrome according to Blake et al.[13] are the following:

Major Criteria	Minor Criteria
Ocular coloboma	Heart defects
Choanal atresia/stenosis	Genital hypoplasia
Cranial nerve anomalies	Cleft lip/palate
Characteristic ear anomalies	Tracheoesophageal fistula
	Distinctive CHARGE facies
	Growth deficiency
	Developmental delay

According to criteria proposed by Blake, patients with all four major criteria or three major and three minor criteria are highly likely to have CHARGE syndrome.[7] Alternate criteria proposed by Verloes[14] may be used to make the diagnosis. Both systems are used as diagnostic tools today (Table 3.1).

3. You are caring for a 2-week-old infant scheduled for an inguinal hernia repair. He has low set ears, cleft palate, and echocardiogram revealed an atrial septal defect. A syndrome is suspected, but the diagnosis is not confirmed. Which of the following studies will be the **LEAST** helpful in a possible diagnosis of CHARGE syndrome?

    A. chest radiography
    B. genetic testing
    C. nasal endoscopy
    D. temporal bone imaging

Answer: A

When cardiac, ear, and facial anomalies are present, the clinician should be suspicious of CHARGE syndrome. Further clinical tests aid in diagnosis and management of the individual patient. Abdominal ultrasound and voiding cystourethrogram should be performed to rule out renal anomalies. Cranial CT

scan with temporal bone imagining investigates the presence and extent of otologic involvement. Bilateral choanal atresia is likely to present clinically at birth, but if unilateral or incomplete, nasal endoscopy may help define the presence of stenosis. Genetic testing for CHD7 mutation and to rule out other syndromes is indicated.[17] A chest X-ray is not useful in the diagnosis of CHARGE syndrome.

4. A 10-day-old male infant is scheduled for an MRI of the brain. The ordering physician suspects a syndrome and requests that an anesthesiologist manage the airway. The infant has a cleft palate and ear anomalies. No diagnosis has been confirmed. Which of the following studies or physical findings **BEST** differentiates 22q11.2 deletion syndrome from CHARGE syndrome?

    A. abdominal ultrasound
    B. calcium level
    C. echocardiogram
    D. genital hypoplasia

Answer: C

Clinical features of CHARGE syndrome are present in other disorders and proper testing can help delineate which syndrome is present. 22q11.2 deletion syndrome (DiGeorge syndrome) has many features of CHARGE including cardiac anomalies, hearing abnormalities, ear abnormalities, renal abnormalities, developmental delay, cleft palate, and immunologic abnormalities. Given the other overlapping features as listed, abdominal ultrasound and presence of a patent ductus arteriosus will not aid in distinguishing these syndromes. Older resources indicate that hypocalcemia, commonly associated with 22q11.2 deletion syndrome, could distinguish between CHARGE syndrome and 22q11.2 deletion syndrome. However, a study by Jyonouchi et al.[28] revealed that hypocalcemia is commonly present in both sets of patients. In the retrospective review, hypocalcemia was present in 72% of 25 children with CHARGE syndrome and in only 26% of 357 children with 22q11.2 deletion syndrome. It was noted that the presence of hypocalcemia led some of the multidisciplinary teams to diagnose patients with CHARGE as having 22q11.2 deletion initially. Therefore, calcium levels cannot be used to distinguish these syndromes. Information in this study supports obtaining calcium levels perioperatively in children with CHARGE syndrome, such that proper replacement can be initiated. Although hypocalcemia did not distinguish the two syndromes, Jyonouchi found a much higher percentage of genital hypoplasia in male patients with CHARGE syndrome (78%) than those with 22q11.2 deletion syndrome (2%).[28]

5. You are performing a preoperative evaluation of a 4-year-old male patient with failure to thrive, developmental delay, hearing deficits, and persistent nasal drainage. The mother notes that he had a small ventricular septal defect that closed on its own as an infant. He is scheduled to undergo a nasal endoscopy/laryngoscopy. You suspect CHARGE syndrome. You explain to the mother that you would like to get a genetics consult. She asks why you are getting this consult. What is the **BEST** statement regarding genetic testing for CHARGE?

A. Her son is displaying all of the typical signs of CHARGE syndrome, and, therefore, he should have genetic testing to verify its presence.
B. Approximately 50% to 80% of cases of CHARGE syndrome are caused by autosomal recessive mutations in the KMT2D gene.
C. Genetic testing for mutations in the CHD7 gene, although not definitive, can aid in the diagnosis of CHARGE syndrome.
D. Genetic testing is definitive because all patients with CHD7 mutation have CHARGE syndrome.

Answer: C
CHARGE syndrome results in most cases from a sporadic autosomal dominant mutation of the CHD7 gene on chromosome 8. It is a rare disorder, with an incidence of approximately 1 in 8,500–10,000 live births. No clear genotype/phenotype relationship has been found.[5] Not all patients with CHARGE have this genetic mutation. Research varies, but studies indicate that 5% to 40% of patients with the diagnosis have no observable genetic mutation.[8,9] Kabuki syndrome is caused by an autosomal recessive mutation in the KMT2D gene.

6. An anesthesiologist is working at a busy, free-standing ambulatory surgery center. The next patient is a 3-year-old with CHARGE syndrome, scheduled for laryngoscopy and tonsillectomy. The patient has no known cardiac disease, but she does have a gastrostomy tube. The **MOST** appropriate management step is to:

A. Do the case after suction the gastrostomy tube and glycopyrrolate.
B. Do the case with 4-hour observation in the postanesthesia care unit.
C. Do the case with no special precautions.
D. Reschedule the case for when a pediatric anesthesiologist is available.

Answer: D
Patients with CHARGE syndrome are at increased risk for postoperative airway and respiratory complications. Reflux and aspiration due to cranial nerve defects along with upper airway abnormalities make these patients high risk for respiratory issues postoperatively. Up to 56% of these patients have upper airway abnormalities. Blake et al.[18] found up to 35% of these patients have some type of respiratory issue postoperatively. Due to these concerns, surgery at an outpatient center should not be considered. Moreover, Blake et al. found that patients undergoing laryngoscopy, gastrointestinal procedures, or cardiac procedures have the highest risk of these events. Although prolonged monitoring in the postanesthesia care unit and use of glycopyrrolate may be useful, due to the potential for respiratory sequelae, all procedures should be done in a setting where reintubation and overnight monitoring in an intensive care units are immediately available. Only option c provides for this level of care.[17] Patients with CHARGE should have surgical procedures at major hospital centers equipped with multidisciplinary teams knowledgeable about CHARGE syndrome, including pediatric otolaryngologists, pediatric anesthesiologists, and pediatricians. These patients are not candidates for surgery at free-standing ambulatory surgery centers.

7. A 3-year-old patient with CHARGE syndrome presents to the preoperative area. He is scheduled to undergo a gastrostomy tube revision and cystoscopy for recurrent urinary tract infections. The mother mentions to you that the patient is scheduled to undergo a cochlear implant in 3 weeks. He is a known difficult airway. What is the **MOST** appropriate way to proceed?

A. Coordinate with surgeons to do procedures all under one anesthetic.
B. Proceed with gastrostomy tube revision and reschedule the cystoscopy.
C. Proceed with today's cases and keep cochlear implant as scheduled.
D. Proceed with today's case and reschedule cochlear implant for next month.

Answer: A
CHARGE syndrome patients have an increased risk postoperative airway and respiratory events. They also have an increased risk of difficult airway, difficult mask ventilation, and difficult intubation. By combining multiple procedures into one anesthetic, the risk of airway complications per anesthetic declines. Blake et al.[18] presented a study of 147 anesthetics in CHARGE patients. About one third of the cases resulted in postanesthetic airway complications. However, combining multiple procedures into one anesthetic did not increase the risk of airway complications. Therefore, by combining procedures, the incidence of respiratory issues will be reduced.

8. A 4-year-old patient with CHARGE syndrome presents for a dental procedure, eye exam, and cystoscopy. The patient has copious oral secretions, repaired choanal atresia, extensive hearing loss, developmental delay, and partial blindness. He has signs and symptoms of severe obstructive sleep apnea. The child appears very anxious and agitated. What is the **LEAST** appropriate way to provide anxiolysis for induction in the OR?

A. parental presence
B. child life specialist present
C. oral midazolam via gastrostomy tube
D. intramuscular ketamine

Answer: D
There is no "safest" premedicine for CHARGE patients. Anxiolysis should be tailored to each patient, taking into consideration the child's constellation of symptoms. Midazolam may be useful in some patients. However, because it can contribute to increased risk of obstructive symptoms postoperatively in patients with obstructive sleep apnea, it should be dosed accordingly. Having a child life specialist present for induction may be helpful, given hearing impairment, developmental delay, and visual impairment. Having parents or primary caregivers present may be very useful in calming these patients who have limited ability to communicate

during induction. Ketamine may produce sedation, but it can increase salivation and increase risk of aspiration in these patients who have poor swallowing ability.

9. A 6-year-old patient with CHARGE syndrome, who is blind, hearing impaired, and developmentally delayed, was in a motor vehicle accident and suffered a femur fracture. She underwent a complex open repair of the femur. It is now POD 1, and you are the pain specialist rounding on this patient. What is the **LEAST** appropriate method to assess the level of this patient's pain?

    A. Consult with regular nurses regarding the patient's behavior.

    B. Ask the parent whether the child's actions or moods are indicative of discomfort.

    C. Use a pain scale that has been developed for nonverbal children.

    D. Use your own best judgement; you're pain specialist.

Answer: D

Assessing the level of pain in nonverbal patients with CHARGE syndrome can be challenging. Typical indicators of pain may not be present in this patient population. Multiple criteria should be considered when evaluating and treating pain in this population. Gaining input from the parent or guardians may be useful. Regular care providers such as nurses or parents may have insight into what behaviors seem to indicate discomfort in these patients. In addition, using pain scales such as the PPP, NCCPC, or the CHARGE Non-Vocal Pain Assessment scale may be useful in developmental delayed CHARGE patients.[25–27]

QUESTIONS AND ANSWERS

This chapter has accompanying questions and answers which are available to subscribers as part of the Oxford eLearning platform. To access the questions, go to ✓ http://oxfordmedicine. com/pediatricanesthesiaPBL

REFERENCES

xx Blake KD, Hartshorne TS, Lawand C, Dailor AN, Thelin JW. Cranial nerve manifestations in CHARGE syndrome. *Am J Med Genetics Part A*. 2008;146(5):585–592.

1. Blake KD, Blake KD, Russell-Eggitt IM, Morgan DW, Ratcliffe JM, Wyse RK. Who's in CHARGE? Multidisciplinary management of patients with CHARGE association. *Arch Dis Child*. 1990;65(2):217–223.

2. Bergman JE, Blake KD, Bakker MK, du Marchie Sarvaas GJ, Free RH, Ravenswaaij-Arts V. Death in CHARGE syndrome after the neonatal period. *Clin Genet*. 2010;77(3):232–240.

3. Vissers LE, van Ravenswaaij CM, Admiraal R, et al. Mutations in a new member of the chromodomain gene family cause CHARGE syndrome. *Nat Genet*. 2004;36(9):955–957.

4. Bergman JE, Janssen N, Hoefsloot LH, Jongmans MC, Hofstra RM, van Ravenswaaij-Arts CM. CHD7 mutations and CHARGE syndrome: the clinical implications of an expanding phenotype. *J Med Genet*. 2011;48(5):334–342.

5. Jongmans MC, Admiraal RJ, Van Der Donk KP, et al. CHARGE syndrome: the phenotypic spectrum of mutations in the CHD7 gene. *J Med Genet*. 2006;43(4):306–314.

6. Tellier AL, Cormier-Daire V, Abadie V, et al. CHARGE syndrome: report of 47 cases and review. *Am J Med Genet Part A*. 1998;76(5):402–409.

7. Blake KD, Prasad C. CHARGE syndrome. *Orphanet J Rare Dis*. 2006;1(1):34.

8. Sanlaville D, Verloes A. CHARGE syndrome: an update. *Eur J Hum Genet*. 2007;15(4):389–399.

9. Hsu P, Ma A, Wilson M, Williams G, Curotta J, Munns CF, Mehr S. CHARGE syndrome: a review. *J Paediatr Child Health*. 2014;50(7):504–511.

10. Hall BD. Choanal atresia and associated multiple anomalies. *J Pediatr*. 1979;95(3):395–398.

11. Hittner HM, Hirsch NJ, Kreh GM, Rudolph AJ. Colobomatous microphthalmia, heart disease, hearing loss, and mental retardation-a syndrome. *J Pediatr Ophthalmol Strabismus*. 1979;16(2):122–128.

12. Pagon RA, Graham JM, Zonana J, Yong SL. Coloboma, congenital heart disease, and choanal atresia with multiple anomalies: CHARGE association. *J Pediatr*. 1981;99(2):223–237.

13 Blake KD, Davenport SL, Hall BD, Hefner MA, Pagon RA, Williams MS, Lin AE, Graham Jr JM. CHARGE association: an update and review for the primary pediatrician. *Clin Pediatr*. 1998;37(3):159–173.

14. Verloes A. Updated diagnostic criteria for CHARGE syndrome: a proposal. *Am J Med Genet Part A*. 2005;133(3):306–308.

15. Kwong KM. Current updates on choanal atresia. *Front Pediatr*. 2015;3:52.

16. Wong MT, Schölvinck EH, Lambeck AJ, van Ravenswaaij-Arts CM. CHARGE syndrome: a review of the immunological aspects. *Eur J Hum Genet*. 2015 Oct 1;23(11):1451–1459.

17. Anesthesia recommendations for patients suffering from CHARGE syndrome. http://www.orphananesthesia.eu/en/component/docman/doc_download/92-charge-syndrome.html. Accessed November 2, 2017.

18. Blake K, MacCuspie J, Hartshorne TS, Roy M, Davenport SL, Corsten G. Postoperative airway events of individuals with CHARGE syndrome. *Int J Pediatr Otorhinolaryngol*. 2009;73(2):219–226.

19. Stack CG, Wyse RK. Incidence and management of airway problems in the CHARGE Association. *Anaesthesia*. 1991;46(7):582–585.

20. Wyse RK, Al-Mahdawi S, Burn J, Blake K. Congenital heart disease in CHARGE association. *Pediatr Cardiol*. 1993;14(2):75–81.

21. Naito Y, Higuchi M, Koinuma G, Aramaki M, Takahashi T, Kosaki K. Upper airway obstruction in neonates and infants with CHARGE syndrome. *Am J Med Genet Part A*. 2007;143(16):1815–1820.

22 Blake KD, MacCuspie J, Corsten G. Botulinum toxin injections into salivary glands to decrease oral secretions in CHARGE syndrome: prospective case study. *Am J Med Genet Part A*. 2012;158(4):828–831.

23. Hunt A, Goldman A, Seers K, Crichton N, Mastroyannopoulou K, Moffat V, Oulton K, Brady M. Clinical validation of the paediatric pain profile. *Dev Med Child Neurol*. 2004;46(1):9–18.

24. Breau L, McGrath P, Finley A, Camfield C. Non-communicating Children's Pain Checklist-Revised (NCCPC-R). https://barnepalliasjon.no/wp-content/uploads/2016/02/NCCPC-P-og-PV.pdf. Accessed November 2, 2017.

25. Validation of the non-communicating children's pain checklist–postoperative version. *J Am Soc Anesthesiolog*. 2002;96(3):528–535.

26. Hunt A. *Paediatric Pain Profile*. London: University College London/Institute of Child Health and Royal College of Nursing Institute; 2003.

27. Stratton and Hartshorne. CHARGE Non-Vocal Pain Assessment (CNVPA). https://www.chargesyndrome.org/wp-content/uploads/2016/03/non-vocal-pain-assessment.pdf. Accessed October 30, 2017.

28. Jyonouchi S, McDonald-McGinn DM, Bale S, Zackai EH, Sullivan KE. CHARGE (coloboma, heart defect, atresia choanae, retarded growth and development, genital hypoplasia, ear anomalies/deafness) syndrome and chromosome 22q11. 2 deletion syndrome: a comparison of immunologic and nonimmunologic phenotypic features. *Pediatrics*. 2009 May 1;123(5):e871–e877.

4.

OMPHALOCELE AND BECKWITH-WIEDEMANN SYNDROME

Pikulkaew Dachsangvorn

STEM CASE AND KEY QUESTIONS

You are consulted to the bedside of a male infant who was just born to a 30-year-old G1P1 female, at 36-weeks gestational age via cesarean section. The infant has prenatal ultrasound findings of polyhydramnios and a large abdominal wall defect. You are told the baby is hypotonic and has an abnormally large tongue but is breathing spontaneously. APGAR (appearance, pulse, grimace, activity, and respiration) scores at 1 and 5 minutes of life were 7 and 8, respectively.

WHAT IS HYPOTONIA? WHAT ARE THE DIFFERENTIAL DIAGNOSES FOR HYPOTONIA IN A NEWBORN?

The neonatal intensive care unit (NICU) team did not attempt to access umbilical vessels and instead tried several times to obtain peripheral intravenous (IV) access. After access is obtained, blood is sent for complete blood count, blood gas, and electrolytes. A nasogastric tube is placed. As the neonatologist wraps the protruding abdominal content in a plastic wrap, you notice that the defect is midline with intact peritoneal covering, consistent with omphalocele.

HOW DOES OMPHALOCELE DIFFER FROM GASTROSCHISIS?

The surgeon insists that the baby be taken to the operating suite emergently due to the large defect. She is concerned about hypothermia, fluid loss, and sepsis. The neonatologist is no longer available for input. The nurse asks that you wait for the blood work results and other work-up.

SHOULD YOU WAIT? WHAT IF THE PERITONEUM HAS RUPTURED? HOW SHOULD ONE EVALUATE A BABY WITH OMPHALOCELE?

You decide to examine the baby before making a decision. The baby is quite large for his age (3.5 kg or 97th percentile). He is lethargic and floppy but displayed no evidence of respiratory distress or cyanosis. His facial features are notable for midface hypoplasia, infraorbital creases, ear pits, and macroglossia. A bedside glucose level measures 25 mg/dL. A preliminary diagnosis of Beckwith-Wiedemann syndrome (BWS) is made. The neonatologist, surgeon, and you agree that the baby should be stabilized and receive a full workup before proceeding to the operating suite.

DESCRIBE OTHER ORGAN SYSTEMS THAT MAY BE AFFECTED BY THIS SYNDROME.

The baby is now day of life 2 with stable cardiopulmonary function, vital signs, and urine output. He is nil per os and receiving peripheral parenteral nutrition with a stable blood glucose level. His workup reveals normal head ultrasound and anatomically normal echocardiogram. His abdominal ultrasound is significant for hepatomegaly, splenomegaly, and enlarged kidneys. His blood work is significant for slight polycythemia with no evidence of hypothyroidism. Alpha-fetoprotein assay is still pending.

WHAT ARE THE RISKS OF ANESTHESIA IN PATIENTS WITH BWS? WHAT SURGICAL OPTIONS ARE AVAILABLE FOR CLOSURE OF OMPHALOCELE?

The surgeon re-examines the defect and measures the diameter to be 4 cm with only small intestine in the sac. The omphalocele-to-head ratio from prenatal ultrasound was 0.20. With this information, she plans to do a primary closure.

HOW WOULD ONE MANAGE ANESTHESIA FOR OMPHALOCELE CLOSURE INTRA AND POSTOPERATIVELY? WHAT INTRAOPERATIVE FINDING MIGHT PREVENT THE SURGEON FROM CLOSING THE FASCIA PRIMARILY? WHAT RISKS WOULD YOU DISCUSS WITH THE PARENTS?

You discuss the risks of anesthesia, including respiratory complications from difficult airway and post-operative mechanical ventilation with the parents. The surgeon is able to close the defect with minimal changes in ventilation pressures. The baby returns to the NICU uneventfully.

DISCUSSION

HYPOTONIA

Hypotonia is the inability to achieve postural control and sustain movement against gravity. This is different from weakness, which is the reduction in strength (reduced maximum power). Hypotonia may be due to central or peripheral causes. Central causes account for up to 80% of cases and include a variety of intracranial, chromosomal/genetic, metabolic, and multisystem disorders. Infants with central etiologies do not track visually, lack facial expression, and can appear lethargic. They may also have other central symptoms such as seizure or irregular breathing. Peripheral causes may involve abnormality in the motor unit, peripheral nerve, neuromuscular junction, or the muscles. A hypotonic infant who is alert and has appropriate facial responses is more likely to have a peripheral etiology.[1]

Evaluation of hypotonic infants should include family history and prenatal, perinatal, and neonatal assessments. The course of the disease (static, progressive, or fluctuating) should also be elicited. The etiology of hypotonia is important as many of the causes can involve other organs, including cardiovascular and respiratory systems. Other causes such as hypoglycemia may require prompt treatment to prevent further complications.

OMPHALOCELE

Omphalocele and gastroschisis are the two most common congenital abdominal wall defects that present in the neonatal period. The main differences between the two entities are outlined in Table 4.1. Both of these defects are usually detected via routine prenatal maternal serum screening and fetal ultrasound. Distinguishing between the two entities is important as omphalocele carries a much higher rate of morbidity and mortality due to associated congenital anomalies.

Omphalocele occurs in the midline with the umbilical cord rising from the middle of the defect. It is a protrusion of intra-abdominal organs through the base of the umbilical cord and is covered by the peritoneal sac without skin. Omphalocele can be categorized into small (does not contain liver), giant (defect larger than 5 cm and/or contain liver), and ruptured.[2] Surgical repair of omphalocele should occur only after the neonate has been adequately resuscitated and evaluated for comorbidities.

EMBRYOLOGY AND PATHOPHYSIOLOGY

Normal gastrointestinal formation involves the following stages[3]:

- At 4 weeks gestation, the primordial gut is formed from the yolk sac and is divided into the foregut, the midgut, and the hindgut. The midgut gives rise to the distal part of the duodenum, ileum, cecum, appendix, ascending colon, and the right portion of the transverse colon.

- At 6 weeks gestation, the midgut undergoes a period of rapid growth and herniates into the umbilical cord. While there, it rotates counterclockwise 90 degrees.

- At 10 and 11 weeks gestation, the midgut loop rotates another 90 degrees as it returns to the abdominal cavity. It finally rotates a final 90 degrees, for a total 270 degrees rotation.

Failure of the somatic folds to complete the formation of anterior abdominal wall or failure of the intestinal loop to migrate back into abdominal cavity results in omphalocele. Omphalocele has a high rate of associated anomalies because it occurs as a result of abnormal embryologic development.

PRENATAL CORRELATIONS

There are higher rates of omphalocele in male infants born to mother older than 35 years or younger than 20 years of age. Multiple gestations are twice as likely as singletons to have omphalocele.[4]

ASSOCIATED ANOMALIES AND OUTCOMES

Omphalocele is found in 1 in 1,100 pregnancies, but the incidence reduces to 1 in 4,000 to 6,000 live births.[5] There is a high rate of associated anomalies that affects 75% to 78% of fetuses with omphalocele.[4,6] Many fetuses with serious anomalies do not survive beyond the prenatal period. Some of these anomalies can be attributed to a single gene disorder, chromosomal abnormalities, or genetic syndrome.

Table 4.1 **OMPHALOCELE VERSUS GASTROSCHISIS**

	OMPHALOCELE	GASTROSCHISIS
Incidence[3,9,16,17]	1:3,000 to 1:4,000 live births	1:10,000
Location	Central defect in the umbilical ring	Lateral (right) to the umbilical cord
Peritoneal sac	Present	Absent
Herniated organs	Bowel and sometimes liver	Bowel only
Embryology	Failure of intestinal loop to return to the abdominal cavity or failure of somatic folds to complete abdominal wall formation	Controversial but suspected to be due to vascular abnormality
Associated anomalies	Frequent (higher than 50%)	Rare
Prognostic factors	Associated anomalies	Condition of bowel
Prognosis	70%–90% survival	90%–95% survival

Note. See Brett and Peter.[17]

Congenital anomalies can involve any organ system, but the most common systems are cardiac, cranial, and urogenital. Table 4.2 lists common anomalies found in newborns with omphalocele. Preterm neonates account for 33% of neonates with omphalocele.[7]

Outcomes of neonates with omphalocele are poor but are more favorable in isolated cases. However, clinicians should not be falsely reassured when prenatal ultrasound indicates an isolated omphalocele. Up to 39% of the isolated anomalies can have postnatally diagnosed anomalies, with BWS being one of the most frequently missed diagnoses.[8]

Isolated omphalocele has a 1-year survival rate of 90%. In comparison, infants with co-occurring chromosomal defect, central nervous system defect, and congenital heart defect have 1-year survival rates of 30%, 55%, and 75%, respectively. Seventy-five percent of all deaths occurred in the first 28 days of life.

Omphalocele diagnosed prenatally can carry a higher mortality rate. This is largely because larger omphaloceles and fetus with multiple anomalies are easier to detect via ultrasound imaging.[9] Of note, neonates born with very low birth weight have the lowest 1-month survival rate (33.9%) compared to low birth weight (68.9%) and normal weight neonates (91.2%).[4] Additionally, pulmonary hypoplasia with associated pulmonary hypertension and respiratory insufficiency have been suggested to be independent risk factors of mortality in infants with omphalocele.[10] Since severe pulmonary hypoplasia is present in 54% of infants with giant omphalocele, they are at a much higher risk of mortality.[11] Neonates with omphalocele who require extracorporeal membrane oxygenation (ECMO) for pulmonary hypertension have a much higher mortality rate than those who are on ECMO for other medical conditions.[12] A study reviewing the Extracorporeal Life Support Organization for 1992–2015 found that overall mortality rate for infants with omphalocele who required ECMO was 82%.[12]

PRENATAL WORKUP AND PERIPARTUM MANAGEMENT FOR FETUS WITH OMPHALOCELE

Prenatally, abdominal wall defects are associated with elevated maternal alpha-fetoprotein levels. Omphalocele is commonly diagnosed on routine second trimester ultrasound.[3,13] Omphalocele to head ratio greater than 0.21 or omphalocele to abdominal circumference greater than 0.26 may be used to predict the need for staged closure and respiratory insufficiency.[14,15] Once diagnosed, a comprehensive fetal ultrasound and fetal echocardiogram, should be performed.[3,13,16] Karyotype is recommended to screen for chromosomal abnormality. Serial ultrasounds are performed due to the increased risk of polyhydramnios and fetal growth restriction. The presence of pulmonary hypoplasia from Pentalogy of Cantrell, trisomy 13 or 18, or triploidy carries a very poor prognosis.

There is no consensus on the preferred mode of delivery, but delivery should occur at a tertiary care center. Fetus with giant omphalocele have been recommended to be delivered via cesarean section to decrease the risk of sac rupture and trauma to the viscera.[2]

MANAGEMENT AND ASSESSMENT OF NEWBORN WITH OMPHALOCELE

Initial management of neonates with omphalocele should focus on cardiopulmonary status since some infants can have pulmonary hypoplasia or pulmonary insufficiency that requires immediate intubation and ventilation. Peripheral IV access and IV fluid therapy should be initiated. Due to high fluid loss, these neonates may need as much as 3 to 4 times the usual maintenance rate.[17] A gastric tube is inserted and placed on suction to decompress the stomach and reduce the risk of aspiration. Umbilical vessels can be used if needed during resuscitation but can be difficult to cannulate, plus other peripheral access will be needed during the perioperative period.[18] The herniated sac should be handled with care and in a sterile fashion to avoid distorting the vascular supply to the bowel and causing reflux of stomach contents and pulmonary aspiration. The sac should be stabilized and wrapped to minimize heat and fluid loss. Newborns with ruptured omphalocele are at a particularly high risk for fluid loss, temperature instability, bowel injury, and sepsis as ruptured omphaloceles are often large.[5] These neonates require immediate fluid resuscitation and protection of the bowel by placing it into a bowel bag. Left lateral decubitus position may be useful for hypotension, tachycardia, or evidence of bowel vascular compromise.

Table 4.2 ASSOCIATED ANOMALIES

ORGAN SYSTEM	PERCENTAGE IN NEWBORN	COMMON ANOMALIES
Craniofacial	20	Cleft palate[3]
Central nervous system	4–8	Spina bifida and anencephaly[4,34]
Cardiac	18–30	Ventricular septal defect and atrial septal defect, but can include high risk cardiac lesions[16]
Pulmonary	3–9	Pulmonary hypoplasia and pulmonary hypertension[34]
Gastrointestinal	3–20	Malrotation, Meckel's diverticulum[5,24]
Genitourinary	6–20	Hydronephrosis, bladder extrophy[3,24,34]
Musculoskeletal	7	Limb deformities[4]
Chromosomal	49 in fetus[9] 17 in neonate[4]	Trisomy 18, 13, 21 (in the order of frequency)[4,9]
Syndromes		Beckwith-Wiedemann syndrome (8%–10%),[8,16] Pentalogy of Cantrell, Prune belly syndrome, OEIS (omphalocele, exstrophy of the cloaca, imperforate anus, and spine abnormalities)[35]

Physical exam should include evaluation for evidence of craniofacial defects or syndromic features, careful cardiac examination, and thorough pulmonary assessment. The size of the omphalocele should be assessed as a neonate with a giant omphalocele carries a higher risk of pulmonary hypoplasia and pulmonary hypertension.[19] Testing should include complete blood count, electrolytes, glucose level, blood gas, and type and crossmatch. Echocardiogram and abdominal ultrasound are performed to look for associated cardiac and renal anomalies.

Once stable, primary concerns for infants with omphalocele are fluid resuscitation, minimizing heat loss, treating sepsis, and avoiding trauma to the herniated organs.[17] Fluid replacement and IV antibiotics are required. Ongoing assessment of fluid status and temperature as well as corrections of any hemodynamic derangements are paramount.

SURGICAL TECHNIQUES

Depending on the size of the omphalocele, gestational age, and associated comorbidities, surgical repair is divided into 3 categories: primary, staged, and delayed closure.[20,21]

Primary closure is generally plausible in small to moderate sized defects (2–4 cm) and reported to have good surgical outcomes. Survival of these patients is dependent on associated defects. Some giant omphaloceles can undergo primary closure successfully. Advantages to primary closure are a low rate of infection and possibility of early enteral feeding. However, there is a higher risk of abdominal compartment syndrome (ACS).[22]

Staged closure is classified into two methods. One uses serial inversion of the amnion sac; the other method involves excising the amnion sac and replacing with mesh. The defect is then closed over time. Different techniques are employed to facilitate fascial closure. They include silo bag, external compression, tissue expander, synthetic and biological mesh, acellular dermal matrices, component separation technique, and vacuum-assisted closure device.[20] The most commonly used method is the silo bag, which allows gradual reduction of the sac in the NICU without the need for anesthesia.

Delayed closure ("paint and wait") is used in cases where the omphalocele is too large or the neonate has significant cardiac or pulmonary issues that would preclude successful closure. This method also allows early feeding, but it can involve longer hospital stays and a longer period where patient is at risk for infection. Additionally, the patient is left with a ventral hernia that can be difficult to repair in the future. In this approach, the sac is painted with a nontoxic agent that promotes an eschar formation over the intact amnion sac. The most common agents are silver sulfadiazine, povidone-iodine solution, silver impregnated dressings, neomycin, and polymixin/bacitracin ointments. The sac epithelializes over 4 to 10 weeks to form a ventral hernia. Most patients eventually undergo closure of the ventral hernia between 1 and 5 years of age. The technique can be primary fascial closure, component separation, stage repair with tissue expander, or mesh repair.[20]

Repair of a large ruptured omphalocele is challenging and not a commonly encountered clinical situation. Therefore, there is no consensus on the approach to these patients.

ANESTHETIC MANAGEMENT OF NEONATES WITH OMPHALOCELE

Surgical repair in the operating suite can be considered once the neonate is medically stable and thorough evaluation for associated anomalies has been completed.[17] Regardless of associated anomalies, all neonates with omphalocele are at risk for temperature instability, hypovolemia, bowel injury and ischemia, and sepsis. Preoperative assessment of volume status and sepsis should include assessment of temperature, heart rate, blood pressure, central venous pressure (if available), urine output, blood gas, serum electrolytes, and respiratory status. Arterial and central venous catheters can be helpful in assessing fluid and acid-base status and should be considered in neonates with large omphalocele and those with cardiopulmonary comorbidities.

During transport, neonates can lose a significant amount of heat. Cold stress can lead to increased oxygen consumption, metabolic acidosis, and increased pulmonary vascular resistance and should be avoided. Rapid sequence induction and full muscle relaxation should be used for induction. The endotracheal tube should have an air leak between 18 to 30 cm H_2O as a lower cuff leak may not provide sufficient ventilation after fascial closure.[23] During and after fascial closure, ACS can develop, and it is critical to maintain communication with the surgeon to avoid this serious complication. ACS can impair ventilation, decrease cardiac preload, decrease renal perfusion, and decrease perfusion to the lower extremities. The most commonly employed method to prevent ACS is using peak inspiratory pressure (PIP) as a guideline during fascial approximation. Fascial closure is not recommended if PIP is greater than 25 to 30 cm H_2O.[24] Others recommend that a change in central venous pressure less than 4 mmHg and intragastric pressure less than 20 mmHg are reliable measure to avoid ACS.[25] Even in the absence of ACS, cardiovascular collapse can result from distortion of the hepatic vein or hemorrhage from liver injury during dissection of the sac.[5] After primary closure, neonates usually remain intubated for 24 to 48 hours.[17]

Preoperative: Minimize heat and fluid loss. Avoid bowel injury during patient transfer.

Monitors: Standard American Society of Anesthesiologists monitors with arterial catheter if needed. Central venous pressure monitoring for high-risk patients.

Lines: Large bore peripheral IV access in the upper extremity.

Induction: Rapid sequence induction.

Maintenance: Volume resuscitation with isotonic fluid (may require 50–100 mL/kg for the case).[24]

Administer 20 mL/kg fluid bolus at the beginning of the procedure. Continue to administer dextrose-containing IV fluid to avoid hypoglycemia. Maintain maximal muscle relaxation. Watch for ACS and hypovolemia due to fluid loss, fluid shift, and blood loss.

Postoperative: Minimize heat loss during transport. Watch for ACS.

BECKWITH-WIEDEMANN SYNDROME

Beckwith-Wiedemann syndrome is the most common congenital overgrowth syndrome with an estimated incidence between 1:13,700 to 1:66,000 live births.[26,27] It is a clinical spectrum in which affected individuals have abnormally accelerated growth and can present at birth or later in life. Characteristic findings during pregnancy are polyhydramnios, placental hyperplasia, and umbilical cord elongation.[26] When presented in the neonatal period, it is characterized by neonatal hypoglycemia, macrosomia, macroglossia, and omphalocele. Other anomalies include hemihyperplasia, embryonal tumors, visceromegaly, adrenocortical cytomegaly, renal abnormalities, and ear creases/pits. Birth weight is around 75th to 95th percentile. Nearly 50% of BWS are associated with polyhydramnios and fetal macrosomia.[28]

GENETIC INHERITANCE AND PATHOGENESIS

Most cases are sporadic. However, familial autosomal dominant inheritance accounts for 15%.[27] Familial type involves chromosome 11p15 and has variable expressivity, incomplete penetrance, and preferential maternal transmission. The 11p15 chromosome region contains genes that involve growth promotion and tumor suppression. Genetic anomaly in this region causes increased expression of the insulin-like growth factor-2 gene.[26]

CLINICAL MANIFESTATION OF BWS

Other than the characteristic features previously mentioned, 30% to 50% of newborns with BWS have severe hypoglycemia, most commonly in the first 72 hours of life.[29,30] This is due to hyperinsulinemia from pancreatic hyperplasia. Historically, BWS has a mortality rate of 20%. However, the mortality rate is better due to earlier detection and treatment of hypoglycemia. When not treated, the hypoglycemia can lead to seizure, permanent brain injury, and long-term neurologic sequelae. Neurogenic signs and symptoms of hypoglycemia present earlier (at higher blood glucose level) and result from activation of the adrenergic nervous system in response to hypoglycemia. These symptoms include sweating, pallor, temperature instability, irritability, hunger, tremulousness, tachycardia, and vomiting. Neuroglycopenia results from the lack of glucose in the central nervous system and is an ominous development that presents later. Features include apnea, hypotonia, seizure, and coma that may progress to death.[31]

Other less common findings include hearing loss, hypothyroidism, hyperlipidemia, brain anomaly, and polycythemia. These children generally have normal development unless there is a chromosomal or brain anomaly or a perinatal insult. They have increased risk of mortality associated with neoplasia, which usually presents around 7 to 8 years of age.

DIAGNOSTIC CRITERIA

There are no consensus diagnostic criteria for BWS. However, suggestive findings are listed in Table 4.3. Because BWS is a clinical spectrum, some individuals may only have one or two suggestive features. Diagnosis is made if an individual has three major criteria or has two major plus one minor criteria.[32] Prenatal diagnosis is possible in the third trimester. Alternatively, molecular genetic testing is also diagnostic.[33]

MANAGEMENT OF PATIENTS WITH BWS

Initial management during neonatal period should focus on treating hypoglycemia to reduce the risk of insult to the central nervous system. Neonate with compromised airway

Table 4.3 **SUGGESTIVE FINDINGS IN BECKWITH-WIEDEMANN SYNDROME**

MAJOR FINDINGS	MINOR FINDINGS
• Macrosomia (weight and length/height >97th percentile) • Macroglossia • Hemihyperplasia (asymmetric overgrowth of one or more regions of the body) • Omphalocele or umbilical hernia • Embryonal tumor (Wilms tumor, hepatoblastoma, neuroblastoma, rhabdomyosarcoma) in childhood • Visceromegaly involving one or more intra-abdominal organs including liver, spleen, kidneys, adrenal glands, and/or pancreas • Cytomegaly of the fetal adrenal cortex (pathognomonic) • Renal abnormalities including structural abnormalities, nephromegaly, nephrocalcinosis, and/or later development of medullary sponge kidney • Anterior linear ear lobe creases and/or posterior helical ear pits • Cleft palate (rare in Beckwith-Wiedemann syndrome) • Positive family history of Beckwith-Wiedemann syndrome	• Pregnancy-related findings including polyhydramnios and prematurity • Neonatal hypoglycemia • Vascular lesions including nevus simplex (typically appearing on the forehead, glabella, and/or back of the neck • Characteristic facies including midface retrusion and infraorbital creases • Structural cardiac anomalies or cardiomegaly • Diastasis recti • Advanced bone age (common in overgrowth/endocrine disorders)

Note. See Shuman et al.[32] and Weksberg et al.[36]

due to macroglossia may require endotracheal intubation. All equipment for a difficult airway should be prepared, including a fiberoptic bronchoscope. These patients may need surgical interventions such as repair of omphalocele or umbilical hernia and reduction glossectomy for macroglossia. Later, these children may need orthopedic procedures for leg length discrepancy or craniofacial surgery due to hemihyperplasia.

ANESTHETIC MANAGEMENT OF NEONATE WITH BWS

Caution: Difficult to ventilate, difficult to intubate, hypoglycemia, prematurity.

Preoperative: Assessment of airway and blood glucose. Abdominal ultrasound.

Induction: Prepare for difficult airway. For omphalocele surgery, balance the risk of aspiration in a potentially difficult to ventilate/intubate patient.

Maintenance: As appropriate for the procedure. Continue to monitor and treat hypoglycemia.

Postoperative: Increased risk of upper airway obstruction if extubated. May remain intubated postoperatively particularly after omphalocele or tongue reduction surgery.

CONCLUSIONS

- Omphalocele is one of the most common surgical abdominal wall defects that present in infancy. Unlike its counterpart (gastroschisis), omphalocele has a high rate of association with other anomalies. A thorough workup, including an echocardiogram, must be performed prior to surgical intervention.

- Management of patients with omphalocele center around ongoing vigilance to maintain euthermia, euvolemia and to avoid sepsis and bowel injury. Neonates with associated comorbidities have increased risk of mortality, which requires individualized surgical and anesthetic plan.

- Neonates with giant omphalocele, pulmonany hypoplasia, chromosomal anomaly, central nervous system and cardiac anomalies, low birth weight, and those on extracorporeal membrane oxygenation have much higher mortality rates than those with isolated omphalocele.

- Neonates with BWS have the additional risk of airway complication due to macroglossia and other complications from hypoglycemia. The risk of aspiration must be weighed against a difficult airway in this population.

REVIEW QUESTIONS

1. A 3.2-kg boy is born with a midline abdominal wall defect with intact peritoneum covering. Which of the following is the **LEAST** likely to be required prior to surgical repair of the defect?

    A. antibiotic
    B. bladder pressure
    C. echocardiogram
    D. electrolytes

Answer: B
Omphalocele is a midline herniation of abdominal organ with peritoneum covering. It is commonly associated with cranial, cardiac, and genitourinary defects. These patients are also at risk for sepsis, heat loss, and fluid loss. Preoperative assessment should include thorough assessment for associated anomalies. Testing should include complete blood count, electrolytes, and glucose level. IV fluid and antibiotic should be started as soon as possible as there is no skin covering and the bowel is exposed to nonsterile environment during and after birth. Echocardiogram is required to rule out any associated congenital heart defect. Bladder pressure is used to help diagnose ACS, which generally does not occur in patients with unrepaired omphalocele and therefore not required preoperatively. See the discussion of the management and assessment of newborn with omphalocele and anesthetic management.

2. Which of the follow is the **MOST** consistent with a gastroschisis diagnosis?

    A. associated with anomalies
    B. Defect is midline.
    C. Peritoneal sac is absent.
    D. Prognosis is poor.

Answer: C
Gastroschisis is a common abdominal wall defect that occurs lateral to the umbilical cord and does not contain peritoneal covering. Herniated organ includes bowel only. Associated anomalies are rare. Prognosis is favorable and is largely dependent on the condition of herniated bowel. In contrast, omphalocele is a central defect that herniates through umbilical ring. It can contain bowel and liver and is frequently associated with congenital anomalies. Prognosis is poor and is dependent on associated anomalies. See Table 4.1.

3. A 4-kg, 2-day-old boy with macroglossia is scheduled for repair of omphalocele. Immediately after transferring the patient to the operating room table, he displayed tonic-clonic seizure. Which of the following is the **MOST** appropriate next step?

    A. blood glucose check
    B. hyperventilation
    C. pentobarbital injection
    D. midazolam infusion

Answer: A
The infant in this question stem displayed three classic characteristics of neonate with BWS: macrosomia, macroglossia, and

omphalocele.[26] Hypoglycemia occurs in up to 50% of neonates with BWS. Therefore, all neonates with suspected BWS and should be monitored for hypoglycemia and treated promptly to avoid secondary complications.[30] Midazolam infusion and pentobarbital are not treatment of choice for neonate seizure caused by suspected hypoglycemia. Hyperventilation strategy is employed in certain situations with increased intracranial pressure, not for hypoglycemia. See discussion of the clinical manifestations of BWS.

4. During primary fascial closure of an omphalocele, which measurement is the **MOST** predictive of surgical failure?

    A. central venous pressure up by 10 mmHg
    B. diastolic blood pressure up by 10 mmHg
    C. heart rate increased by 10 beats/min
    D. systolic blood pressure up by 10 mmHg

Answer: A
ACS is a feared complication of large abdominal defect closure, including omphalocele closure. ACS can impair ventilation, decrease cardiac preload, decrease renal perfusion, and decrease perfusion to the lower extremities. PIP >25 cm H_2O, central venous pressure increase greater than 4 mmHg, or intragastric pressure >20 mmHg puts patient at increased risk for ACS. PIP of 10 cm H_2O is appropriate for neonates. Heart rate and blood pressure increases can have multiple causes but is not indicative of unfavorable facial closure. See discussion of anesthetic management of neonates with omphalocele.

5. Which of the following is **LEAST** likely to be present during an anesthetic for omphalocele repair in a neonate with BWS?

    A. aspiration
    B. difficult airway
    C. hypothermia
    D. micrognathia

Answer: D
Neonates with BWS have a difficult airway due to macroglossia, not micrognathia. Infants with omphalocele are at risk for aspiration due to herniated bowel and at risk for hypothermia due to the lack of skin, which covers the abdominal wall defect. See the discussion of anesthetic management of neonate with BWS and anesthetic management of neonates with omphalocele.

6. During primary repair of gastroschisis, in an otherwise healthy 3.5-kg newborn, the ventilator alarms "tidal volume not achieved." Which of the following is the **MOST** appropriate next step?

    A. Change alarm settings.
    B. Decrease the tidal volume.
    C. Notify the general surgeon.
    D. Switch to pressure support.

Answer: C
Repair of large abdominal wall defect such as gastroschisis and omphalocele carries a risk of acute ACS. ACS is a clinical situation in which the intra-abdominal pressure is so high that it interferes with venous return to the heart,

perfusion to the kidneys and lower extremities, and ventilatory mechanics. The inability to achieve tidal volume during the repair should alert the clinician of the possibility of ACS. The surgeon should be informed, and the anesthesiologist should look for possible causes for the ventilation change. Ignoring the alarm or decreasing the tidal volumes is not appropriate (answers A and D, respectively). Pressure support ventilation (answer B) is not appropriate in gastroschisis repair as the patient should be paralyzed and, thus, would not be able to maintain spontaneous breathing. See the discussion of anesthetic management of neonates with omphalocele.

QUESTIONS AND ANSWERS

This chapter has accompanying questions and answers which are available to subscribers as part of the Oxford eLearning platform. To access the questions, go to ✔ http://oxfordmedicine. com/pediatricanesthesiaPBL

REFERENCES

1. Peredo DEH, Mark C. The floppy infant. *Pediatr Rev.* 2009;30(9):e66–e76.
2. Mann S, Blinman Ta Fau–Douglas Wilson R, Douglas Wilson R. Prenatal and postnatal management of omphalocele. *Prenat Diagn.* 2008;28(7):626–632.
3. Martin CR, Fishman SJ. Omphalocele. In: Hansen AR, Puder M, eds. *Manual of Neonatal Surgical Intensive Care.* 2nd ed. Shelton, CT: Peoples Medical Publishing House; 2002:238–244.
4. Marshall J, Salemi JL, Tanner JP, et al. Prevalence, correlates, and outcomes of omphalocele in the United States, 1995–2005. *Obstet Gynecol.* 2015;126(2):284–293.
5. Desai AA, Iqbal CW. Omphalocele. In: Mattei P, Nichol PF, Rollins IIMD, Muratore CS, eds. *Fundamentals of Pediatric Surgery.* 2nd ed. Cham: Springer International; 2017:575–580.
6. Perretta J. Abdominal defects. In: Perretta J, ed. *Neonatal and Pediatric Respiratory Care.* Philadelphia: F. A. Davis; 2014:213–305.
7. Diu MW, Mancuso TJ. Pediatric diseases. In: Hines RL, Marschall KE, eds. *Stoelting's Anesthesia and Co-existing Disease.* 6th ed. Elsevier; 2012:596–598.
8. Cohen-Overbeek TE, Tong WH, Hatzmann TR, et al. Omphalocele: comparison of outcome following prenatal or postnatal diagnosis. *Ultrasound Obstet Gynecol.* 2010;36(6):687–692.
9. Brantberg A, Blaas HGK, Haugen SE, Eik-Nes SH. Characteristics and outcome of 90 cases of fetal omphalocele. *Ultrasound Obstet Gynecol.* 2005;26(5):527–537.
10. Baerg JE, Thorpe DL, Sharp NE, et al. Pulmonary hypertension predicts mortality in infants with omphalocele. *J Neonatal Perinatal Med.* 2015;8(4):333–338.
11. Charlesworth P, Ervine E Fau–McCullagh M, McCullagh M. Exomphalos major: the Northern Ireland experience. *Pediatr Surg Int.* 2009;2577–81,
12. Baerg JE, Thirumoorthi A, Hopper AO, Tagge EP. The use of ECMO for gastroschisis and omphalocele: two decades of experience. *J Pediatr Surg.* 2017;52:984–988.
13. Christison-Lagay ER, Kelleher CM, Langer JC. Neonatal abdominal wall defects. *Semin Fetal Neonatal Med.* 2011;16(3):164–172.
14. Montero FJ, Simpson LL, Brady PC, Miller RS. Fetal omphalocele ratios predict outcomes in prenatally diagnosed omphalocele. *Am J Obstet Gynecol.* 2011;205(3):281–287.

15. Fawley JA, Peterson EL, Christensen MA, Rein L, Wagner AJ. Can omphalocele ratio predict postnatal outcomes? *J Pediatr Surg.* 2016;51(1):62–66.

16. Baird PA, MacDonald EC. An epidemiologic study of congenital malformations of the anterior abdominal wall in more than half a million consecutive live births. *Am J Hum Genet.* 1981;33(3):470–478.

17. Brett CD, Peter J. Anesthesia for general surgery in the neonate. In: Davis PJC, Franklyn P, Motoyama, Etsuro K, eds. *Smith's Anesthesia for Infants and Children.* 8th ed. Philadelphia: Elsevier; 2011:562–567.

18. Ledbetter DJ. Congenital abdominal wall defects and reconstruction in pediatric surgery. *Surg Clin North Am.* 2012;92(3):713–727.

19. Partridge EA, Hanna BD, Panitch HB, et al. Pulmonary hypertension in giant omphalocele infants. *J Pediatr Surg.* 2014;49(12):1767–1770.

20. Islam S. Advances in surgery for abdominal wall defects. *Clin Perinatol.* 2012;39(2):375–386.

21. Pacilli M, Spitz L Fau–Kiely EM, Kiely Em Fau–Curry J, Curry J Fau–Pierro A, Pierro A. Staged repair of giant omphalocele in the neonatal period. *J Pediatr Surg.* 2005;40:785–788.

22. Mack AJ, Rogdo B. Giant omphalocele: current perspectives. *Res Rep Neonatol.* 2016;2016(6):33–39.

23. Dutta S, Smith BM, Albanese C, Claure RE, Golianu B, Hammer GB. Pediatric general surgery. In: Jaffe RA, Samuels SI, eds. *Anesthesiologist's Manual of Surgical Procedures.* 4th ed. Philadelphia: Wolters Kluwer; 2009:1296–1300.

24. Chin WA. Gastroschisis/omphalocele (Chapter 172). In: Atchabahian A, Gupta R, eds. *The Anesthesia Guide.* New York: McGraw-Hill; 2013. http://accessanesthesiology.mhmedical.com.liboff.ohsu.edu/content.aspx?bookid=572&sectionid=42543763. Accessed June 27, 2018.

25. Yaster M, Rossberg MI. Anesthesia for newborn surgical emergencies (Chapter 63). In: Longnecker DE, Brown DL, Newman MF, Zapol WM, eds. *Anesthesiology.* 2nd ed. New York: McGraw-Hill; 2012.

26. Bissonnette B, Luginbuehl I, Marciniak B, Dalens BJ. Beckwith-Wiedemann syndrome. In: Bissonnette B, Luginbuehl I, Marciniak B, Dalens BJ. eds. *Syndromes: Rapid Recognition and Perioperative Implications.* New York: McGraw-Hill; 2006. http://accessanesthesiology.mhmedical.com.liboff.ohsu.edu/content.aspx?bookid=852&sectionid=49517273. Accessed June 27, 2018.

27. Beckwith–Wiedemann syndrome. In: Chen H, ed. *Atlas of Genetic Diagnosis and Counseling.* New York: Springer; 2012:203–212.

28. Elliott M, Maher ER. Beckwith-Wiedemann syndrome. *J Med Genet.* 1994;31(7):560–564.

29. Tobias JD, Lowe S, Holcomb GW. Anesthetic considerations of an infant with Beckwith-Wiedemann syndrome. *J Clin Anesth.* 1992;4(6):484–486.

30. Mussa A, Di Candia S, Russo S, et al. Recommendations of the Scientific Committee of the Italian Beckwith–Wiedemann Syndrome Association on the diagnosis, management and follow-up of the syndrome. *Eur J Med Genet.* 2016;59(1):52–64.

31. Thompson-Branch AH, Thomas. Neonatal hypoglycemia. *Pediatr Rev.* 2017;38(4):147–157.

32. Shuman C, Beckwith JB, Weksberg R. Beckwith-Wiedemann syndrome. In: Pagon RA, Adam MP, Ardinger HH, et al., eds. *GeneReviews(R).* Seattle; 2011.

33. Kominiarek MA, Zork N Fau–Pierce SM, Pierce Sm Fau–Zollinger T, Zollinger T. Perinatal outcome in the live-born infant with prenatally diagnosed omphalocele. *Am J Perinatol.* 2011;28(8):627–634.

34. Corey KM, Hornik CP, Laughon MM, McHutchison K, Clark RH, Smith PB. Frequency of anomalies and hospital outcomes in infants with gastroschisis and omphalocele. *Early Hum Dev.* 2014 Aug; 90(8):421–424.

35. Hwang P-J, Kousseff BG. Omphalocele and gastroschisis: an 18-year review study. *Genet Med.* 2004;6(4):232–236.

36. Weksberg R, Shuman C, Beckwith JB. Beckwith–Wiedemann syndrome. *Eur J Hum Genet.* 2010;18(1):8–14.

5.

EX UTERO INTRAPARTUM TREATMENT PROCEDURE FOR GIANT FETAL CERVICAL TERATOMA

Debnath Chatterjee

STEM CASE AND KEY QUESTIONS

A 28-year-old G2P1 female with a singleton pregnancy at 34 weeks gestational age is referred to your institution for evaluation of a giant fetal neck mass. She has received no prenatal care and presents to her obstetrician with polyhydramnios. An ultrasound examination reveals a singleton fetus in the breech position with a large asymmetric left-sided fetal neck mass that is predominantly solid with some cystic areas. The fetal neck mass has well defined borders and is causing significant distortion of airway anatomy. Other findings include hyperextension of the fetal neck, absence of stomach bubble, and maternal polyhydramnios. A presumptive diagnosis of fetal cervical teratoma is made.

WHAT ARE THE CAUSES OF FETAL AIRWAY OBSTRUCTION? WHAT IS THE DIFFERENTIAL DIAGNOSIS FOR FETAL NECK MASSES? WHAT IS THE CAUSE OF MATERNAL POLYHYDRAMNIOS? WHAT OTHER DIAGNOSTIC STUDIES SHOULD BE PERFORMED?

The maternal fetal care center at your institution holds a multidisciplinary team meeting to discuss the care of this patient and a decision is made to perform an ex utero intrapartum treatment (EXIT) procedure at 36 weeks gestational age to secure the fetal airway on placental support.

WHAT IS AN EXIT PROCEDURE? WHAT ARE THE COMMON INDICATIONS FOR AN EXIT PROCEDURE? WHAT ARE THE GUIDING PRINCIPLES OF AN EXIT PROCEDURE? HOW IS AN EXIT PROCEDURE DIFFERENT THAN A CESAREAN SECTION?

After the multidisciplinary team meeting, it is now your turn as the anesthesiologist to perform a preoperative assessment. The patient tells you that she is otherwise healthy, other than gastroesophageal reflux disease symptoms. She also complains of progressively worsening shortness of breath and swelling of her lower extremities. She is nervous about the EXIT procedure and is concerned about future pregnancies.

WHAT ARE THE ESSENTIAL COMPONENTS OF THE PREOPERATIVE EVALUATION? WHAT LABORATORY TESTS SHOULD BE ORDERED BEFORE THE EXIT PROCEDURE? WHAT ANESTHETIC TECHNIQUE WOULD YOU RECOMMEND FOR THE EXIT PROCEDURE? WHAT ADDITIONAL OPERATING ROOM SET UP IS NECESSARY FOR AN EXIT PROCEDURE?

On the morning of surgery, the patient is admitted to the fetal care center and an 18-gauge peripheral intravenous (IV) catheter is inserted. After administering aspiration prophylaxis medications, the patient is taken to the operating room.

HOW WOULD YOU INDUCE GENERAL ANESTHESIA IN THIS PATIENT? WHAT PRECAUTIONS MUST BE TAKEN WHILE POSITIONING THIS PATIENT? DOES SHE NEED ANY ADDITIONAL MONITORS DURING THE EXIT PROCEDURE? HOW WOULD YOU MAINTAIN GENERAL ANESTHESIA? WHAT ARE THE HEMODYNAMIC GOALS DURING AN EXIT PROCEDURE? HOW WOULD YOU MONITOR THE FETUS DURING AN EXIT PROCEDURE?

A transverse abdominal incision is made and the uterus is exposed. The surgeon requests adequate uterine relaxation.

HOW WOULD YOU ACHIEVE ADEQUATE UTERINE RELAXATION?

The surgeons proceed to map the placental borders with ultrasound guidance and then perform a hysterotomy. As soon as the hysterotomy is performed, they notice uterine contractions.

HOW WOULD YOU STOP THE UTERINE CONTRACTIONS? WHY IS IT IMPORTANT TO PREVENT UTERINE CONTRACTIONS DURING AN EXIT PROCEDURE?

The fetus is then partially delivered through the hysterotomy. The pediatric cardiologist monitoring the fetus announces that the fetal heart rate is 80 bmp.

WHAT IS THE SIGNIFICANCE OF FETAL BRADYCARDIA? WHAT IS THE MOST LIKELY CAUSE OF FETAL BRADYCARDIA, AND HOW WOULD YOU TREAT IT?

After treating the bradycardia, the surgeons are ready to secure the fetal airway.

HOW SHOULD THE FETAL AIRWAY BE SECURED? WHAT IS THE BACK-UP PLAN, SHOULD DIRECT LARYNGOSCOPY BE UNSUCCESSFUL?

Despite rigid bronchoscopy, the surgeon is not able to secure the fetal airway.

WHAT ADDITIONAL MANEUVERS MAY BE PERFORMED TO FACILITATE ENDOTRACHEAL INTUBATION?

After securing the fetal airway, the surgeons clamp the umbilical cord and deliver the newborn. While the neonatology team is caring for the newborn, the surgeons notice a large amount of hemorrhage from a boggy uterus.

HOW WOULD YOU MANAGE THIS MASSIVE HEMORRHAGE? IN ADDITION TO OXYTOCIN, WHAT OTHER UTEROTONIC DRUGS SHOULD BE ADMINISTERED? WHAT BLOOD PRODUCTS SHOULD BE USED FOR TRANSFUSION? IS THERE A ROLE FOR ANTIFIBRINOLYTIC AGENTS?

The surgeon is done with skin closure, and the patient has been extubated.

WHAT ARE YOUR PLANS FOR POSTOPERATIVE ANALGESIA?

DISCUSSION

FETAL AIRWAY OBSTRUCTION

Advances in the field of prenatal diagnostic imaging, including 3-dimensional ultrasonography and fetal magnetic resonance

Table 5.1 FETAL LESIONS CAUSING EXTRINSIC AND INTRINSIC AIRWAY OBSTRUCTION

EXTRINSIC AIRWAY OBSTRUCTION	INTRINSIC AIRWAY OBSTRUCTION
Oral	Congenital High Airway Obstruction Syndrome (CHAOS)
Epignathus (oropharyngeal teratoma)	
Epulis (gingival granular cell tumor)	
Severe micrognathia	Laryngeal web or cyst
Cervical	Laryngeal atresia or stenosis
Teratoma	Tracheal atresia or stenosis
Lymphatic malformation	
Vascular malformation	
Congenital goiter	
Thoracic	
Congenital pulmonary airway malformation	
Bronchogenic cyst	
Mediastinal teratoma	

Source. Adapted from G Ryan, S Somme, TM Crombleholme. Airway compromise in the fetus and neonate: prenatal assessment and perinatal management. *Semin Fetal Neonatal Med.* 2016;21:230–239.

imaging (MRI) have allowed the accurate diagnosis of several fetal anomalies. Lesions that cause fetal airway obstruction can be identified on prenatal imaging and can be broadly categorized into extrinsic and intrinsic causes[1-5] (Table 5.1). Extrinsic causes of fetal airway obstruction include cervical teratoma, epignathus (oropharyngeal teratoma), epulis (gingival granular cell tumor), severe micrognathia, lymphatic malformation, hemangioma, goiter, and intrathoracic masses such as congenital pulmonary airway malformation and bronchogenic cyst.[1-3] These lesions can cause significant distortion of airway anatomy, putting the newborn at risk for hypoxia and life-threatening airway compromise after birth. In addition, by compressing the fetal esophagus and impeding fetal swallowing, they can cause maternal polyhydramnios, predisposing to preterm delivery.

Cervical teratomas are large, bulky tumors in the anterior neck with representation of all three germ layers.[1-3] They are typically irregular masses with both solid and cystic components. Calcification is seen in 50% of cervical teratomas. They have well-defined borders and can cause hyperextension of the fetal neck secondary to mass effect. Other fetal neck masses include lymphatic or vascular malformations and congenital goiter. Lymphatic malformations are usually multiloculated cystic structures with poorly defined borders that infiltrate the normal structures of the neck. Vascular malformations may be both solid and cystic but do not have calcifications. Doppler imaging often reveals the extensive vascularity of these lesions.

Prenatal imaging should include a comprehensive fetal ultrasound examination looking for other anatomical defects.[1-3] An ultrafast fetal MRI should also be performed for a more detailed evaluation of the level and degree of airway obstruction (Figure 5.1). These imaging studies can be used to predict which fetuses are at an increased risk for airway compromise after birth. Other diagnostic studies should include amniocentesis for karyotype and microarray to rule out chromosomal abnormalities and fetal echocardiography to rule out congenital heart disease.

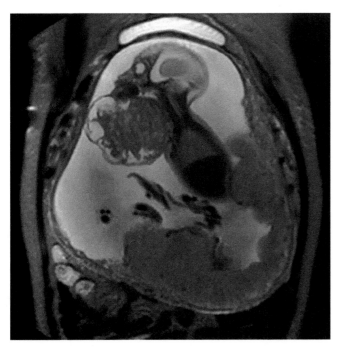

Fig. 5.1 Fetal MRI showing large oropharyngeal teratoma. (Photo courtesy of David M Mirsky, MD, Children's Hospital Colorado).

If significant fetal airway obstruction is suspected, the mother should be referred to a fetal treatment center with experience in the diagnosis and delivery management of fetuses with airway obstruction.[1-5] A multidisciplinary team of specialists including maternal-fetal medicine, fetal/pediatric surgery, otolaryngology surgery, anesthesiology, neonatology, radiology, nursing, and social work should be actively involved in the counseling of the mother and her family. All management options including expectant management, palliative care, and pregnancy termination should be discussed. Risks and benefits of each option should be discussed, and the parents should be given realistic expectations for their baby's prognosis and postnatal course.

EXIT PROCEDURE

The EXIT procedure has allowed securing the fetal airway and performing other life-saving fetal interventions in a controlled fashion, while still on uteroplacental circulation.[2-5] The EXIT procedure was initially described to secure the airway in fetuses with severe congenital diaphragmatic hernia that had undergone in utero fetal tracheal clipping to promote lung growth. Over the years, the indications for an EXIT procedure have evolved.[2-5] While EXIT-to-airway in fetuses with life-threatening airway obstruction remains the most common indication, EXIT procedures are also being performed for the resection of fetal lung and mediastinal masses causing intrathoracic airway obstruction and extra corporeal membrane oxygenation cannulation while still on placental support (Table 5.2). This chapter will focus on EXIT-to-airway for a giant fetal cervical teratoma.

Table 5.2 INDICATIONS FOR AN EXIT PROCEDURE

TYPE	SOURCE OF OBSTRUCTION	EXAMPLES
EXIT-to-airway	Extrinsic obstruction	Cervical teratoma Epignathus Hemangioma Congenital goiter Giant ranula
	Intrinsic obstruction	Congenital high airway obstruction syndrome
	Iatrogenic	Following fetal tracheal occlusion for CDH
	Miscellaneous	Severe micrognathia
EXIT-to-resection		Congenital pulmonary airway malformation Bronchopulmonary sequestration Bronchogenic cyst Mediastinal teratoma Fetal lobar interstitial tumor
EXIT-to-ECMO		Severe CDH with poor prognostic indicators
EXIT-to-separation		Conjoined twins

Note. EXIT = ex utero intrapartum treatment; ECMO = extra corporeal membrane oxygenation; CDH = congenital diaphragmatic hernia.

Source. Adapted from Walz PC, Schroeder JW. Prenatal diagnosis of obstructive head and neck masses and perinatal airway management: the ex utero intrapartum treatment procedure. *Otolaryngol Clin North Am.* 2015;48:191–207.

The guiding principles of an EXIT procedure are as follows[2]:

1. Maintaining adequate uteroplacental blood flow and stable maternal hemodynamics.

2. Achieving adequate uterine relaxation prior to hysterotomy and during fetal intervention.

3. Reversing uterine relaxation prior to clamping of the umbilical cord and delivery of newborn.

4. Preserving uterine volume during fetal intervention by partially delivering the fetus and amnioinfusion.

5. Minimizing fetal cardiac dysfunction and monitoring fetal cardiac function.

Unlike a cesarean section, one of the central tenets of an EXIT procedure is achieving adequate uterine relaxation and preventing uterine contractions prior to hysterotomy and during the fetal intervention.[2] Traditionally, high doses of volatile anesthetic agents are used to maintain uterine relaxation. In addition to the transplacental passage of volatile anesthetic agents administered to the mother, fetal analgesia and immobilization is ensured by the direct fetal intramuscular administration of a narcotic and muscle relaxant, once the fetus has been partially delivered.

PREOPERATIVE EVALUATION

A detailed history and a targeted physical examination must be performed to rule out maternal comorbidities that increase anesthetic risk.[2,3] Any issues with prior pregnancies or deliveries must be investigated. Preoperative laboratory testing should include a complete blood cell count and a type and crossmatch. In addition, leukocyte reduced, irradiated O negative blood, crossmatched to the mother should be readily available for the fetus. Fetal evaluation should include a detailed evaluation of all prenatal diagnostic studies including ultrasonography, fetal MRI, fetal echocardiography, and karyotype analysis. The anesthesiologist should pay attention to the fetal airway anatomy, estimated fetal weight (for drug dosing), baseline fetal heart rate and cardiac function, placental location, and presence of fetal hydrops.

ANESTHESIA FOR EXIT PROCEDURES

EXIT procedures are typically performed under maternal general anesthesia.[2-6] Preoperatively, aspiration prophylaxis medications are administered, and a lumbar epidural catheter is inserted for postoperative analgesia. In the operating room, the patient is positioned supine and a wedge is used to maintain uterine displacement. After adequate preoxygenation, a rapid sequence induction is performed to facilitate endotracheal intubation. In addition to standard American Society of Anesthesiologists monitors, a second large bore IV access is obtained, and a radial arterial catheter is inserted for close hemodynamic monitoring. General anesthesia is maintained with either volatile anesthetic agents or IV anesthetic agents such as propofol and remifentanil infusions. Maternal hemodynamics are closely monitored and supported with phenylephrine or ephedrine, if necessary.

After maternal laparotomy, the uterus is exposed, and the placental borders are mapped with a sterile ultrasound probe. At this point, achieving adequate uterine relaxation is critical. Traditionally, high doses (2–3 minimal anesthetic concentration) of volatile anesthetic agents have been used for achieving uterine hypotonia. However, this can result in significant fetal cardiac dysfunction. Alternatively, supplementing volatile anesthetic agents with IV anesthetic agents (propofol and remifentanil infusions) has allowed lowering the dose of volatile anesthetic agents, thereby minimizing fetal cardiac dysfunction.[7,8] A hemostatic hysterotomy is then performed using a specialized absorbable uterine stapler. To maintain uterine volume, a catheter is inserted through the hysterotomy into the uterine cavity to continuously infuse warm lactated Ringers solution. The fetus is then partially delivered through the hysterotomy to expose the fetal head, upper extremities, and torso. To ensure adequate fetal analgesia and immobilization, an intramuscular fetal cocktail of fentanyl, muscle relaxant, and atropine is administered into the fetal shoulder.

FETAL MONITORING

Fetal echocardiography every 3 to 5 minutes is an essential part of an EXIT procedure.[2] A pediatric cardiologist uses a sterile ultrasound probe to monitor fetal heart rate, ventricular function, and ductal patency. In addition, a sterile pulse oximeter is placed on a fetal hand after partially delivering the fetus to monitor fetal oxygen saturation. The normal range for fetal oxygen saturation is 30% to 70%. Accuracy of the fetal pulse oximeter probe is limited by light interference and vasoconstriction.

MANAGEMENT OF FETAL BRADYCARDIA

Fetal bradycardia (fetal heart rate <100 bpm) is a sign of fetal distress that warrants immediate attention. The most common cause of fetal bradycardia is mechanical compression or kinking of the umbilical cord. The surgeons must be immediately notified; the fetus must be repositioned, and uterine volume, increased. Other causes of fetal bradycardia include uterine contractions, placental separation, fetal hypovolemia, and maternal hypotension. Uterine contractions decrease uteroplacental blood flow and should be immediately treated by increasing the concentration of the volatile anesthetic agent and administering a bolus of nitroglycerin. Maternal hypotension should be aggressively treated with fluids and vasopressors. The placental unit must be examined with ultrasound to rule out placental separation. If these initial measures are not successful, fetal intramuscular administration of epinephrine and atropine must be considered. If necessary, the surgeon might have to perform chest compressions on the fetus. If hemodynamic instability persists, the next step is emergent fetal delivery and neonatal resuscitation.

FETAL AIRWAY MANAGEMENT

Regardless of the indication for the EXIT procedure, the fetal airway must be secured first should the EXIT procedure be terminated early.[2,3] Additional equipment for alternative airway management techniques should be readily available. In fetuses with large neck masses, direct laryngoscopy and endotracheal intubation is usually the first option for securing the fetal airway (Figure 5.2). If direct laryngoscopy is unsuccessful, a rigid bronchoscopy is then attempted. Additional maneuvers such as elevating the mass off the airway, release of neck strap muscles, and partial resection of the neck mass may be necessary to increase the chances of successful endotracheal intubation.[2,3] If these maneuvers fail, a tracheotomy with retrograde wire intubation may be necessary.

After the fetal airway is secured, the position of the endotracheal tube or tracheostomy tube is confirmed using flexible bronchoscopy and surfactant is administered, if clinically indicated. To prevent accident dislodgement, the endotracheal tube is usually sutured to the maxillary ridge. It is important to note that ventilation of the lungs is not initiated at this stage, as that would initiate the process of transitional

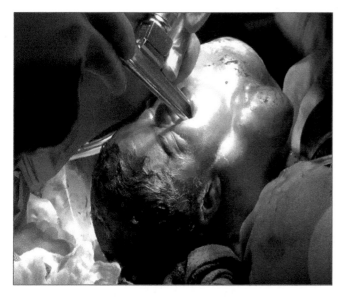

Fig. 5.2 Direct laryngoscopy during an EXIT-to-airway for a giant fetal cervical teratoma. Reproduced with permission from Chatterjee D, Galinkin JL. Fetal medicine and anesthesia for fetal surgery. In: Holzman RS, Mancuso TJ, Polaner DM, eds. *A practical Approach to Pediatric Anesthesia*. 2nd ed. Philadelphia, PA: Wolters Kluwer; 2016: 703–725. (Photo courtesy of Timothy M Crombleholme, MD, Children's Hospital Colorado).

circulation and placental separation. Subsequently, other planned fetal interventions such as extra corporeal membrane oxygenation cannulation or thoracotomy and resection of intrathroacic masses are performed, while still on placental support.

TERMINATION OF EXIT PROCEDURE

Upon completion of the planned fetal intervention, the volatile anesthetic agent is discontinued to allow return of uterine tone. Close communication between the surgeons and anesthesiologists is critical at this stage. Immediately after cutting the umbilical cord and delivering

the newborn, an oxytocin infusion is started, and uterine massage is performed by the surgeon. Additional uterotonic drugs should be readily available for excessive maternal hemorrhage.

NEONATAL RESUSCITATION AND BACK-UP TEAM

The initial resuscitation of the newborn is usually performed by the neonatology team. Umbilical arterial and venous catheters are obtained, as clinically indicated. The newborn is then transferred to the neonatal intensive care unit for further monitoring and management. A separate surgical team that includes a pediatric surgeon, anesthesiologist, and scrub nurse should be readily available in an adjoining operating room for completion of surgery on the newborn, should the EXIT procedure be terminated early.

UTERINE ATONY

Failure to allow sufficient time for return of uterine tone before clamping the umbilical cord and delivering the newborn may result in massive maternal hemorrhage from uterine atony. The first line of therapy for uterine atony is administration of an oxytocin infusion and manual uterine massage by the surgeon. The second line of therapy includes other uterotonic drugs such as methylergonovine, carboprost, and misoprostol (Table 5.3). Early mobilization of resources and aggressive hemostatic resuscitation by activating the massive transfusion protocol is recommended.[9] Hemostatic resuscitation involves limiting the administration of crystalloids and transfusing packed red blood cells in a 1:1:1 ratio with fresh frozen plasma and platelets. In a recently published randomized, double-blind placebo-controlled World Maternal Antifibrinolytic (WOMAN) trial, early IV administration of 1 g of tranexamic acid within 3 hours of giving birth significantly reduced maternal mortality due to bleeding from postpartum hemorrhage without any side effects.[10] Other surgical options include insertion of a

Table 5.3 UTEROTONIC DRUGS FOR THE MANAGEMENT OF UTERINE ATONY

MEDICATION	DOSAGE	EFFECTS	CAUTION
Oxytocin (Pitocin)	20-40 U/L as IV infusion	Vasodilation, hypotension, hyponatremia	IV infusion preferred to boluses
Methylergonovine (Methergine)	0.2 mg IM	Vasoconstriction, hypertension, increased PA pressures, coronary vasopasm	Avoid in patients with pre-eclampsia, pulmonary hypertension and coronary artery disease
Carboprost- Prostaglandin $F_{2\alpha}$ analog (Hemabate)	0.25 mg IM	Bronchospasm, V/Q mismatch, increased PA pressures, nausea, vomiting	Avoid in patients with severe asthma and pulmonary hypertension
Misoprostol Prostaglandin E1 analog (Cytotec)	200-800 mcg buccal, vaginal or rectal	Fever, abdominal pain, diarrhea	None

Note. PA = pulmonary artery; V/Q = ventilation/perfusion.

Bakri balloon for uterine tamponade, uterine compression sutures, arterial embolization in interventional radiology, and hysterectomy.

EMERGENCE FROM ANESTHESIA

Upon completion of the EXIT procedure and delivery of the newborn, the epidural catheter is bolused with local anesthetic. After reversing paralysis and administering prophylactic anti-emetics, the mother is extubated when fully awake. Postoperative analgesia is achieved using an epidural infusion of local anesthetic and narcotic. Additional pain medications are administered as needed.

COMPLICATIONS OF AN EXIT PROCEDURE

Common pitfalls and potential complications during an EXIT procedure are listed in Table 5.4.

REVIEW QUESTIONS

1. Which of the following is the **MOST** common cause for fetal bradycardia during an EXIT procedure?

   A. maternal aortocaval compression
   B. maternal hypotension
   C. placental abruption
   D. umbilical cord compression

Table 5.4 COMMON PITFALLS AND POTENTIAL COMPLICATIONS DURING AN EXIT PROCEDURE

PITFALLS	COMPLICATIONS
Failure to position with uterine displacement	Compromised uteroplacental blood flow
Failure to maintain maternal blood pressure	Compromised uteroplacental blood flow
Failure to achieve uterine relaxation	Uterine contractions resulting in compromised uteroplacental blood flow
Failure to maintain uterine volume	Placental abruption
Failure to recognize cord compression	Unrecognized fetal bradycardia and distress
Failure to monitor fetal hemodynamics	Unrecognized fetal bradycardia and distress
Failure to have back up plan for airway management	Loss of fetal airway resulting in hypoxia and fetal demise
Failure to allow sufficient time for return of uterine tone	Uterine atony and maternal hemorrhage

Source. Adapted from Marwan A, Crombleholme TM. The EXIT procedure: principles, pitfalls and progress. *Semin Pediatr Surg.* 2006;15:107–115.

Answer: D
Fetal bradycardia is a sign of fetal distress and must be treated immediately. The most common cause of fetal bradycardia during an EXIT procedure is mechanical compression or kinking of the umbilical cord. When fetal bradycardia is identified, the surgeon must be informed immediately, and the fetus must be repositioned. Other less common causes of fetal bradycardia include placental abruption or compromised uteroplacental blood flow secondary to maternal hypotension, uterine contractions, or aortocaval compression.

2. Which of the following anesthetic considerations for the management of an EXIT procedure is different from a cesarean section performed under general anesthesia?

   A. avoidance of maternal hypotension
   B. avoidance of aortocaval compression during positioning
   C. uterine relaxation prior to hysterotomy
   D. maximizing uterine tone after delivery

Answer: C
The EXIT procedure is not a glorified cesarean section. One of the central tenets of an EXIT procedure is achieving adequate uterine relaxation prior to hysterotomy and during the fetal intervention. EXIT procedures are typically performed under general anesthesia and, like a cesarean section, aortocaval compression should be avoided during positioning. Maintaining adequate uteroplacental blood flow and maximizing uterine tone after delivery of the newborn are like a cesarean section.

3. Which of the following uterotonic drugs is **MOST** important to avoid in patients with pre-eclampsia?

   A. oxytocin
   B. methylergonovine
   C. misoprostol
   D. carboprost

Answer: B
Methylergonovine is a semisynthetic ergot derivate that is used as a second-line uterotonic agent for refractory uterine atony. The most common side effect of methylergonovine is hypertension due to vasoconstriction. Therefore, it should be avoided in patients with pre-eclampsia. The use of methylergonovine in patients with coronary artery disease may result in acute coronary syndrome or infarction. The other uterotonic drugs do not cause hypertension.

4. Which of the following uterotonic drugs is **MOST** important to avoid in patients with severe asthma?

   A. carboprost
   B. methylergonovine
   C. misoprostol
   D. oxytocin

Answer: A
Carboprost is an analog of prostaglandin $F_{2\alpha}$ that may be used as a second-line uterotonic agent for refractory uterine atony. Frequent side effects include nausea, vomiting, and diarrhea. Carboprost may precipitate bronchospasm, increase

intrapulmonary shunt fraction, and cause V/Q mismatch. Asthmatic patients can experience life-threatening broncho-spasm after administration of carboprost.

QUESTIONS AND ANSWERS

This chapter has accompanying questions and answers which are available to subscribers as part of the Oxford eLearning platform. To access the questions, go to ✓ http:// oxfordmedicine. com/pediatricanesthesiaPBL

REFERENCES

1. Ryan G, Somme S, Crombleholme TM. Airway compromise in the fetus and neonate: prenatal assessment and perinatal management. *Semin Fetal Neonatal Med.* 2016;21:230–239.
2. Marwan A, Crombleholme TM. The EXIT procedure: principles, pitfalls and progress. *Semin Pediatr Surg.* 2006;15:107–115.
3. Walz PC, Schroeder JW. Prenatal diagnosis of obstructive head and neck masses and perinatal airway management: the ex utero intrapartum treatment procedure. *Otolaryngol Clin North Am.* 2015;48:191–207.
4. Bouchard S, Johnson MP, Flake AW, et al. The EXIT procedure: experience and outcome in 31 cases. *J Pediatr Surg.* 2002;37:418–426.
5. Liechty KW. Ex-utero intrapartum therapy. *Semin Fetal Neonatal Med.* 2010;15:34–39.
6. Lin EE, Moldenhauer JS, Tran KM, Cohen DE, Adzick NS. Anesthetic management of 65 cases of Ex Utero Intrapartum Therapy: a 13-year single-center experience. *Anesth Analg.* 2016;123:411–417.
7. Boat A, Mahmoud M, Michelfelder EC, et al. Supplementing desflurance with intravenous anesthesia reduces fetal cardiac dysfunction during open fetal surgery. *Paediatr Anaesth.* 2010;20:748–756.
8. Ngamprasertwong P, Vinks AA, Boat A. Update in fetal anesthesia for the EXIT procedure. *Int Anesthesiol Clin.* 2012;50:26–40.
9. Pacheco LD, Saade GR, Costantine MM, et al. An update on the use of massive transfusion protocols in obstetrics. *Am J Obstet Gynecol.* 2016;214:340–344.
10. Shakur H, Roberts I, Fawole B, et al. Effect of early tranexamic acid administration on mortality, hystrectomy, and other morbidities in women with post-partum haemorrhage (WOMAN): an international, randomised, double-blind, placebo-controlled trial. *Lancet.* 2017;389:2105–2116.

SECTION 2

CARDIOVASCULAR SYSTEM

6.

PATENT DUCTUS ARTERIOSUS

Priti G. Dalal and Shannon M. Grap

STEM CASE AND KEY QUESTIONS

A 6-month-old male is scheduled for closure of patent ductus arteriosus (PDA) using the transcatheter approach. He was born premature at 34-weeks gestation and was in the neonatal intensive care unit (NICU) for 6 weeks for feeding difficulties and initially needed continuous positive airway pressure (CPAP). He was discharged to home on an apnea and bradycardia monitor, but it has never alarmed. His weight is 4 kg, and he has failure to thrive.

DESCRIBE THE ROLE OF THE PDA IN FETAL CIRCULATION. WHAT IS THE NATURAL HISTORY OF NORMAL ANATOMIC AND PHYSIOLOGIC CLOSURE OF THE PDA? HOW MIGHT A PDA CONTRIBUTE TO FAILURE TO THRIVE IN INFANTS?

Although he initially required CPAP in NICU, he no longer requires respiratory assistance or supplemental oxygen since his discharge home.

WHAT ARE THE INDICATIONS TO ATTEMPT MEDICAL CLOSURE OF A PDA DURING THE NEONATAL PERIOD? WHAT TYPES OF PHARMACOLOGIC INTERVENTION MAY BE USED?

The patient does have a persistent continuous murmur on exam since birth. He remains below fifth percentile for weight despite adequate nutritive intake, falling from 20th percentile at birth. Parents report that he occasionally "turns blue" with severe crying episodes.

WHAT ARE THE CLINICAL MANIFESTATIONS AND PHYSICAL EXAM FINDINGS SIGNIFICANT OF A PERSISTENT PDA? WHAT FURTHER DIAGNOSTIC TESTING SHOULD BE OBTAINED, IF ANY?

An echocardiogram reveals a large PDA with a peak gradient of 15 mmHg PDA and an estimated mean pulmonary pressure of 25 mmHg at rest with mostly left to right flow. The heart is otherwise structurally normal with a normal shortening fraction. There is intermittent diastolic flow reversal of the abdominal aorta.

DESCRIBE EISENMENGER'S SYNDROME AND THE CLINICAL IMPLICATIONS. WHAT ARE THE ANESTHETIC CONCERNS FOR THIS PATIENT WITH THE ECHO RESULTS AS DESCRIBED AND CLINICAL CYANOSIS?

While in the preoperative area prior to the planned catheterization procedure, the patient is agitated and fussy. A colleague suggests oral midazolam as a premedication.

DISCUSS THE RISKS AND BENEFITS OF AN ORAL PREMEDICATION IN A PATIENT WITH PULMONARY HYPERTENSION. WOULD YOU CHOOSE PARENTAL PRESENCE FOR INDUCTION OF THIS CHILD? WHY OR WHY NOT?

You plan for a spontaneous inhalational induction via face mask with oxygen and sevoflurane, with a peripheral intravenous catheter to be placed following induction.

WHAT ADDITIONAL MEDICATIONS, IF ANY, WILL YOU PROVIDE ON INDUCTION? WOULD YOU ADVISE AGAINST THE USE OF NITROUS OXIDE?

Following induction and intravenous catheter placement, intravenous rocuronium 1 mg/kg and fentanyl 1 mcg/kg are administered to facilitate tracheal intubation. The airway is secured without any incidence of hypoxia or hypercarbia with stable hemodynamics.

WHAT MONITORS WILL YOU USE? DO YOU NEED INVASIVE ARTERIAL MONITORING? WILL YOU CHOOSE TO PLACE AN ARTERIAL LINE IN ADDITION TO THE FEMORAL ARTERIAL CATHETER ACCESS USED FOR THE PROCEDURE IN THIS PATIENT? WHY OR WHY NOT?

The interventional cardiologist places the femoral catheter successfully and requests normocarbia and room air for pre-procedural intracardiac pressure measurements. The mean pulmonary pressure is 28 mmHg and the PDA is visualized on radiopaque injection.

WHAT HEMODYNAMIC CHANGES MIGHT YOU EXPECT TO OCCUR DURING DEVICE OCCLUSION? HOW WILL YOU PREPARE FOR DEVICE OCCLUSION DEPLOYMENT?

Following successful device occlusion of the PDA, the femoral catheter is removed. Pressure is applied on the femoral arterial access site to achieve adequate hemostasis.

WHAT ARE YOUR PLANS FOR EMERGENCE? DO YOU PLAN FOR AN AWAKE OR DEEP EXTUBATION? WHAT ARE THE RISKS OF EACH IN THIS PATIENT?

The patient arrives following an uneventful extubation to the post anesthesia care unit. After approximately 20 minutes, the patient awakens with severe agitation. The cardiologist recommends that the patient must lay flat for 4 hours postcatheterization. A colleague suggests the use of intravenous dexmedetomidine for treatment of emergence delirium.

WHAT ARE THE RISKS AND BENEFITS OF USING DEXMEDETOMIDINE IN THIS PATIENT FOR EMERGENCE DELIRIUM? WOULD MIDAZOLAM BE A BETTER OPTION? WHY OR WHY NOT? WHAT STRATEGIES COULD YOU USE PRIOR TO EMERGENCE TO PLAN FOR A PROLONGED RECOVERY IN THE SUPINE POSITION FOR THIS PATIENT?

After a further uneventful post-anesthesia care unit stay, the patient is discharged the following morning in stable condition.

WHY MIGHT A TRANSCATHETER APPROACH BE UTILIZED RATHER THAN AN OPEN SURGICAL APPROACH TO CLOSE A PDA? FOR A PATIENT RECEIVING A THORACOTOMY FOR AN OPEN SURGICAL APPROACH, WHAT ARE THE ANESTHETIC CONCERNS? DISCUSS THE SIGNIFICANCE OF PRELIGATION CLAMPING DURING THE SURGICAL APPROACH.

A transthoracic echocardiogram after 1 month follow-up shows resolution of the pulmonary hypertension and no further PDA flow.

DISCUSSION

The ductus arteriosus (DA) is a vascular connection between the pulmonary artery and the descending aorta. During the fetal state, it facilitates blood flow from the right ventricle and pulmonary artery to the aorta, thus bypassing the nonfunctional lungs. Its common site of origin is at the aorta, just distal to the left subclavian artery, and it communicates with the pulmonary artery. Normally following birth, the DA functionally closes at 10 to 15 hours, but anatomical closure may take 2 to 3 weeks. Failure of the ductus to close will lead to the condition referred to as PDA, which results in shunting of blood from aorta to pulmonary artery. PDA is defined as a persistent patent DA in term infants older than 3 months or in preterm infants >1 year of age.[1,2]

ETIOLOGY AND PATHOGENESIS

The incidence of isolated persistent PDA is 1:2,500 live births. In the case of preterm infants, the incidence is much higher. However, spontaneous delayed closure occurs in 79% of premature infants with very low birth weight. It is twice as common in females and accounts for 10% of all congenital heart defects. Prenatal exposure to rubella in the first trimester may be associated with this condition. The DA is a remnant of the sixth branchial arch. It is structurally different from the aorta and pulmonary artery in that the inner media layer is composed of longitudinal and circumferential fibers, which constrict on exposure to higher PaO_2. Permanent closure of the DA occurs by several mechanisms.[1,3] The initial functional closure is due to vasoconstriction. Subsequent anatomical closure is due to proliferation of the intima and fibrosis. In the fetal state, the DA diverts blood from the right ventricle to the descending aorta, thus bypassing the lungs, which are nonfunctional in the fetal state. After birth, the baby starts breathing, the lungs are functional, and there is decreasing hypoxemia. The clamping of the umbilical cord leads to a decrease in the circulating prostaglandins in the neonate that were secreted by the placenta in the fetal state. Shortly after birth, decreased prostaglandin E2 levels and a rise in arterial oxygen partial pressure induce an increase in endothelin-1 in ductal smooth muscles, thereby causing constriction of the DA.[1,4] After birth, due to decreased pulmonary vascular resistance and increase in left sided pressures, there is left to right shunting. Hemodynamically, the degree of left to right shunt is determined by the capacity of the ductus to impede flow from the aorta to pulmonary artery.

FAILURE TO THRIVE AND PDA

Failure to thrive is a state of undernutrition due to inadequate caloric intake or absorption, or increased caloric expenditure.[5] Although malnutrition is often a common cause of failure to thrive in infants, congenital heart disease, including PDA should also be suspected.[5,6] The workup for failure to thrive should include a physical exam and suspicion for congenital heart disease, including auscultation for murmurs and oxygen saturation determination. Congenital heart defects may lead to failure to thrive through low energy intakes and high energy requirement.[6] This may be due to increased oxygen demand. Feeding problems may be due to fatigue related to hypoxia and breathlessness. Malabsorption may be due to venous congestion and edema. There may be persistent acidosis leading to underutilization of nutrients and an increased basal metabolic rate, thereby further increasing oxygen requirements.[6] Hypoxia may lead to fatigue and feeding problems.

CLINICAL MANIFESTATIONS OF PDA

Shunting of blood from left to right causes an increase in pulmonary blood flow with left atrial and left ventricular overload. This may progress to pulmonary hypertension, and if left untreated, eventual reversal of blood flow across the shunt. Diastolic run-off into the pulmonary artery may result in systemic hypoperfusion. Premature infants are at risk for respiratory distress, necrotizing enterocolitis, renal impairment, and intracranial hemorrhage. The signs and symptoms include tachypnea, decreased exercise tolerance, failure to thrive, recurrent respiratory infection, and congestive heart failure. On physical exam, a continuous murmur is heard at the first and second intercostal space of the left sternal border, which gets louder throughout systole and softer throughout diastole. There is a wide pulse pressure and a bounding pulse. Investigations include electrocardiogram (left ventricular or right ventricular hypertrophy depending on severity) and chest radiography (increased pulmonary vascular markings, prominent aortic knob, and left heart enlargement). The mainstay of diagnosis is echocardiography. It helps in confirming presence of the ductus and identifying the aortic end, flow, and characteristics of the ductus. Based on the clinical findings, hemodynamic and angiographic size, the PDA may be classified as shown in Table 6.1.[2] Although there is no universal echocardiographic definition for a hemodynamically significant ductus, a left atrium to aortic root diameter ratio ≥1.4, a DA diameter ≥1.4 mm/kg body weight, left ventricular enlargement, and holodiastolic flow reversal in the descending aorta indicate a hemodynamically significant ductus.[7] Angiography is useful for a detailed diagnosis, further grading and therapy.[8,9]

Indications for closure of PDA include:

1. Patients with left ventricular overload

2. Pulmonary hypertension

3. Patients with a small PDA and continuous murmur to avoid risks of open PDA complications (pulmonary hypertension and subacute bacterial endocarditis or infective endarteritis).

Clinically, a silent PDA refers to a small PDA detected with echocardiography, but without a murmur on auscultation. Although the PDA closure in the case of silent PDA is avoided, this may be weighed against the risk of infective endarteritis and the risk of transcatheter closure.[9] The complications of untreated PDA may include prolonged ventilation, pulmonary hemorrhage, bronchopulmonary dysplasia, necrotizing enterocolitis, intraventricular hemorrhage, failure to thrive, ventricular overload, pulmonary hypertension, renal impairment, and subacute bacteria endocarditis. Older infants and children may suffer from recurrent respiratory tract infections, and if left untreated, severe pulmonary hypertension and reversal of shunt (Eisenmengerization). The overall management is shown in Table 6.2.

PHARMACOLOGICAL MANAGEMENT

Administration of nonselective cyclo-oxygenase inhibitors, such as indomethacin or ibuprofen, is the mainstay of pharmacological treatment of neonates with PDA.[10] Administration of these drugs results in successful closure of the ductus in 75% to 93% of the cases. However, these are not without side effects. Recently, successful use of intravenous acetaminophen has been described in the literature.[10,11] Approximately half of extremely premature infants need indomethacin for closure of the ductus and about 12% will need surgical closure following failure of indomethacin therapy.[12]

Table 6.1 **CLASSIFICATION OF PATENT DUCTUS ARTERIOSUS BASED ON SEVERITY**

PDA TYPE	CLINICAL	HEMODYNAMIC QP:QS MINIMAL PULMONARY HYPERTENSION	ANGIOGRAPHIC PDA SIZE IN MM
Silent	No murmur	Minimal Shunt detected on routine e chocardiography	<1
Small	Continuous murmur No signs of volume overload	<1.5:1 Mild PAH	>1–1.5
Moderate	Continuous murmur Signs of volume overload	>1.5–2.2:1 Moderate PAH	>1.5–3
Severe	Continuous murmur Signs of severe volume overload Mitral diastolic flow murmur	>2.2:1 Severe PAH Reversal of shunt to right to left may occur— Eisenmegerization of PDA	>3–5

Note. PDA = patent ductus arteriosus. PAH = pulmonary arterial hypertension.

Table 6.2 OVERALL MANAGEMENT OPTIONS OF PATIENT WITH PATENT DUCTUS ARTERIOSUS

TYPE OF MANAGEMENT	AGE GROUP	TECHNIQUE	COMMENTS
Medical	Used in neonates	Indomethacin or Ibuprofen Acetaminophen use has been described	Inhibition of prostaglandin forming cyclooxygenase enzymes
Transcatheter technique	Infants and children Use in younger infants has also been described	Large PDAs closed with the Amplatzer device Small PDAs occluded with coils	Weight limitation due to the size of femoral sheath Recent studies with use in neonates have been reported
Surgical management—bedside	Neonates	Bedside PDA ligation in intensive care unit, left lateral thoracotomy	Use in critically neonates not stable for transport
Surgical management—operating room	Neonates, infants and children	Left lateral thoracotomy or video-assisted thoracoscopy	Neonates, infants, and children stable to be transported to the operating room

Note. PDA = patent ductus arteriosus.

NONSURGICAL MANAGEMENT

Transcatheter PDA occlusion is currently the treatment of choice for most PDA in term infants, children, and even adults. In the asymptomatic patient, the technique is usually delayed until a few years of age due to risks of femoral artery injury. However, safe use of this technique was recently reported in 24 patients with ages ranging from 5 to 80 days and weight ranging from 755 gm to 2380 g with a success rate of 88%.[13] Various devices and transcatheter techniques for closure of the PDA have been described. These include the coiling device and the duct occluder. The choice of the device depends on the morphology and size of the ductus. Coil occlusion entails use of Gianturco coils to obliterate the ductus. It is generally used in cases of a small ductus with minimal ductal

diameter of <2 mm at its narrowest point via a transvenous or retrograde arterial approach (Figure 6.1). Following an angiogram, the coil is advanced into the ampulla of the DA and across the narrowest proximal aspect typically within the distal main pulmonary artery. A selective angiogram is done to check for residual leaks, in which case additional coils may be deployed. Device occlusion entails use of an occluder. The Amplatzer duct occluder is most commonly used. This device is used for a large PDA with a sufficient aortic ampulla, also using a transvenous approach (Figure 6.2). A wire, followed by a delivery sheath, are passed from the main pulmonary artery through the ductus and into the descending aorta. The device occluder is partially deployed into the descending aorta and then pulled back into the aortic ampulla. Delayed closure may

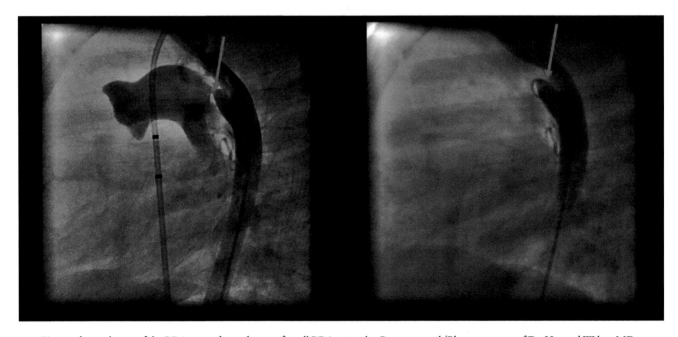

Fig. 6.1 Transcatheter closure of the PDA pre and postclosure of small PDA using the Gianturco coil (Photo courtesy of Dr. Howard Weber, MD, Division of Pediatric Cardiology, Penn State Health Children's Hospital, Hershey, PA).

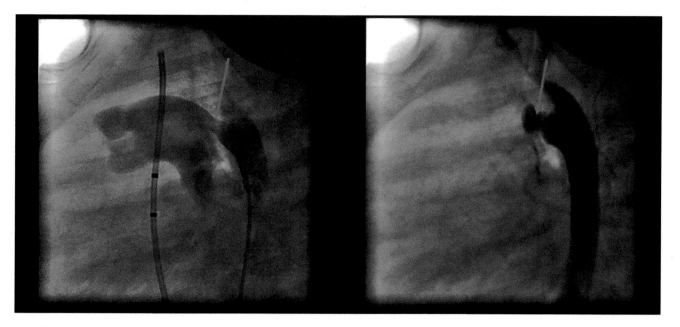

Fig. 6.2 Transcatheter closure of the PDA pre- and postclosure of large PDA using the Amplatzer duct occluder. (Photo courtesy of Dr. Howard Weber, MD, Division of Pediatric Cardiology, Penn State Health Children's Hospital).

be expected with the occluder device; however, with the coil device, it is very important to ensure absence of any residual leak before actually leaving the catheterization laboratory. Complications of the transcatheter techniques, albeit rare, include residual shunting and the need for repeated procedures, hemolysis, device embolization, and device-induced left pulmonary artery stenosis or aortic arch obstruction. In one study,[14] complete shunt occlusion was documented in 89% of patients on day 1 postcatheterization and 99.7% at 1 year with the occluder device.

ANESTHETIC MANAGEMENT FOR TRANSCATHETER TECHNIQUE

With the advent of newer techniques, the management of patients with PDA has transitioned from primarily surgical to interventional transcatheter techniques. Administration of anesthesia in catheterization laboratories is challenging because these are usually at remote locations. However, the same standards of care apply as in the operating room. The expert consensus statement by a multisociety panel made recommendations for monitoring in the pediatric cardiac catheterization laboratory.[15] The problems that the anesthesiologists may encounter include:

1. Restricted space for the anesthesia machine, monitors and equipment.

2. Limited access to the patient due to the radiology equipment, moving procedure table, use of heavy lead gowns and lead screens, thus increasing the risk of dislodging anesthesia circuits and accidental extubation— adequately securing and taping of the endotracheal tube, and use of long or expandable anesthetic circuits is important.

3. Visibility is affected due to darkened room for the cardiologist to view clear images.

4. Risk of hypothermia to the patient as the laboratory is set at a lower ambient temperature to prevent overheating of the electronic equipment; also, cold saline flushes used by the cardiologist as a part of the procedure.

The anesthetic management must take into consideration the patient's pathophysiological status. A balanced anesthetic technique should be used. Premedication may be needed in older infants and children. The anesthetic management considerations are similar to those mentioned for the surgical technique in the following discussion. The general anesthesia technique with endo tracheal intubation is preferred, as it ensures a secure airway and controlled ventilation. It is important that the child is absolutely still during key portions of the procedure; hence, neuromuscular blockade may be useful in this situation. An initial diagnostic angiogram is done to assess the severity of the PDA. Diagnostic angiogram and hemodynamic studies involve measuring intracardiac pressures, intravascular pressures, and systemic and pulmonary blood flow ratios (Qp:Qs). Hemodynamic calculations are performed with patient breathing room air. Arterial blood gases and activated clotting time (if heparin is used) measurements are made throughout the case. Postprocedure, the patient may be extubated if stable. The cardiologist may request smooth emergence, which may be facilitated by the deep extubation technique or administration of opioid to minimize coughing and struggling at extubation. Smooth emergence ensures that there is no dislodgement of the femoral clot; else, there is risk of development of hematoma at the site of the femoral puncture. Use of intravenous dexmedetomidine has been described for smooth extubation in pediatric patients although this may still be a matter of controversy.[16,17]

SURGICAL TECHNIQUES

Surgical closure remains the treatment of choice in neonates or children where prostaglandin inhibitors have failed (usually two failed cycles of pharmacotherapy with cyclo-oxygenase inhibitors) or are contraindicated and patient is unstable for transport,[18] as well as in infants and children with a large or aneurysmal ductus that is too large for device closure. While the timing and outcome of surgical ligation of PDA is still controversial, a recent report revealed lower mortality in those neonates who underwent surgical ligation versus medical treatment of the PDA.[19] Complications of surgery include vocal cord palsy, diaphragmatic paralysis, pneumothorax, and chylothorax.[18,20] Recently, postligation syndrome has also been described where patients experience hemodynamic instability, left ventricular dysfunction, and pulmonary edema following PDA ligation due to inability of the neonatal myocardium to tolerate acute increase in afterload.[7,13] In the past, concerns have been raised regarding association of surgical ligation with worse neurodevelopmental outcomes, increased retinopathy of prematurity, and bronchopulmonary dysplasia.[19,20] A recent multicenter outcomes study[19] demonstrated that compared with medical management, surgical ligation of a hemodynamically significant PDA is associated with lower mortality, without increased risk of chronic lung disease, retinopathy of prematurity, and neurodevelopmental impairment. Further, a systematic review and meta-analysis[21] comparing clinical outcomes of surgical ligation versus catheter occlusion demonstrated both treatment modalities to be comparable although re-intervention was more common with the transcatheter technique.

Surgical approaches described include ligation of the ductus through a thoracotomy, video-assisted thoracoscopic surgery and robotically assisted closure. A systematic review suggested no difference in the early clinical outcomes between the video-assisted thoracoscopic surgery and conventional thoracotomy group.[22] Surgical closure allows complete closure in 94% to 100% cases with mortality rate of 0% to 2%.[9]

The surgical technique for closure of PDA entails a left thoracotomy performed in the third and fourth intercostal space. Incision is made in the anterior axillary line and extends posteriorly. After the ductus is identified, either a clip is placed (Figure 6.3), or the ductus is ligated and divided. It is important to monitor the pulse oximetry and blood pressure in the upper and lower extremity as there is a risk of inadvertently ligating or clamping the aorta.

ANESTHETIC MANAGEMENT FOR SURGICAL CLOSURE

Patients who are greater than 6 months of age may need premedication with midazolam 0.5 mg/kg orally. General endotracheal anesthesia is the anesthetic of choice, although use of high spinal and epidural in neonates has been described in literature.

Spontaneous inhalational induction with sevoflurane may be considered in stable patients without intravenous access. In severely ill patients, intravenous induction with etomidate fentanyl and muscle relaxant may be considered. Temperature monitoring and avoidance of hypothermia is very important. Maintenance with inhalational agents is appropriate for patients who are stable. However, in patients with congestive heart failure or moribund patients an opioid based (typically fentanyl) anesthetic maintenance with low-dose inhalational agents and muscle relaxant may be considered. Choice of anesthetic depends on multiple factors such as patient condition, prematurity, birth weight, co-existing disease, and the surgical procedure. Besides standard American Society of Anesthesiologists monitoring, pre- and postductal oxygen saturations should be measured. Preductal oxygen saturation is measured in the right upper extremity, and postductal saturations are measured in the left upper extremity or either lower extremity. Either invasive or noninvasive monitoring may be used in both preductal and postductal extremities. Invasive arterial monitoring may be considered in patients

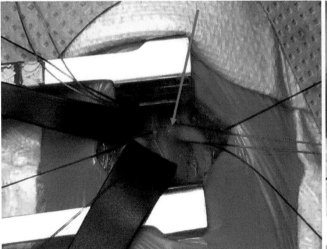 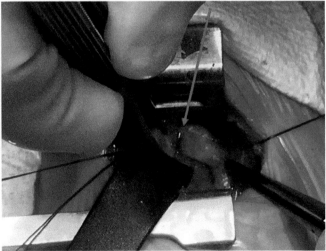

Fig. 6.3 Pre- and postsurgical ligation of the PDA using a clip. (Photo courtesy of Dr. Joseph B. Clark, MD, Division of Pediatric Cardiothoracic Surgery, Dr. Carolyn Barbieri, MD, Division of Pediatric Anesthesiology, Penn State Health Children's Hospital, Hershey, PA).

with congestive heart failure or other co-morbidities. In patients with other co-existing conditions and congestive heart failure, central venous monitoring may be considered.

Inadvertent ligation of the aorta or pulmonary artery may manifest as a decrease in the postductal saturation signal as seen on pulse oximetry. Hence, it is very important to monitor the postductal saturations.

After the ligation of the ductus, there should be an increase in diastolic pressure as there is absence of run-off to the lungs. If there is a decrease or absence of postductal blood pressure, the descending aorta may have been ligated. A pre- and postductal gradient may indicate a pre-existing coarctation of the aorta or may have been caused following the surgical procedure. If the child is already intubated, one may consider leaving the child intubated postoperatively with transport back to the intensive care unit. If the child is stable and otherwise without any co-morbidities extubation may be considered at the end of the procedure. Factors that may guide the decision to extubate include age, birth weight, prematurity, and other co-morbidities.

The procedure may be safely done in the NICU by the bedside in certain situations where the baby is unstable for transport to the operating room.[23] In this situation, the challenges are similar to anesthesia at remote locations needing special consideration for associated co-morbidities. Usually a fentanyl-based anesthesia with neuromuscular paralysis is the technique of choice.[12]

INFECTIVE ENDOCARDITIS PROPHYLAXIS

Recommendations for antimicrobial prophylaxis against infective endocarditis (subacute bacterial endocarditis) were last revised in 2007 with updated guidelines from the American Heart Association (AHA).[24] This update was in response to the recognition that acute endocarditis is dependent upon bacterial exposure and adherence to cardiac structures causing bacterial vegetation. Antibiotic administration to prevent infective endocarditis is no longer recommended for all patients receiving dental, genitourinary, or gastrointestinal procedures and is limited to only those at highest risk with dental procedures. Prophylaxis may be administered to high-risk patients for respiratory tract procedures in which an open incision is performed or biopsy and is not recommended for bronchoscopy alone.[24] Recognizing that certain types of congenital heart disease and associated repairs may increase the risk of infective endocarditis with dental and incisional airway procedures, including tonsillectomy and adenoidectomy, antimicrobial prophylaxis is recommended for the lesions listed in the 2007 AHA guidelines.

Cardiac conditions requiring antimicrobial prophylaxis for infective endocarditis prophylaxis per the 2007 AHA guidelines are:

1. Prosthetic cardiac valve or prosthetic material in valvular repair

2. Previous infective endocarditis

3. Congenital heart disease, including the following:

    a. Unrepaired cyanotic lesion, including palliative shunts and conduits
    b. Within the first 6 months of completely repaired defect with prosthetic material or device, including surgical repair or catheter intervention
    c. Repaired lesion with residual defects at or adjacent to site of prosthetic patch or device

4. Cardiac transplant recipients with valvulopathy

For the prevention of subacute bacterial endocarditis, oral amoxicillin 50 mg/kg up to 2 g is the recommended antimicrobial agent. For patients unable to take orally, intravenous ampicillin 50 mg/kg up to 2 g or cefazolin 50 mg/kg up to 1 g may be administered. Ceftriaxone 50 mg/kg up to 1 g may be administered as an intramuscular injection. For patients allergic to penicillin, intravenous clindamycin 20 mg/kg up to 600 mg may be used.[24]

CONCLUSIONS

- DA is an important physiological and anatomical connection between the pulmonary artery and aorta in the fetal life. Failure of the ductus to close leads to the condition persistent PDA.

- PDA may become hemodynamically significant causing a left to right shunt with subsequent pulmonary overcirculation and systemic hypoperfusion. If untreated it may lead to immediate and long-term complications including failure thrive and infective endocarditis.

- The choice of treatment depends on multiple factors including gestation age, timing, and associated co-morbidities.

- Anesthesia for surgical ligation may be challenging. Surgery may be performed in the NICU by bedside in case of unstable patients or in the operating room if stable. It is important to measure pre- and postductal saturations via pulse oximetry and blood pressures.

- Transcatheter technique for PDA closure is increasing in popularity with the advent of devices that can be used in infants as well. Anesthesia in the catheterization lab can be challenging and entails careful positioning of the anesthesia equipment and circuits with smooth extubation techniques where appropriate.

REVIEW QUESTIONS

1. A 32-week gestational age, 2.5-kg preterm neonate at 2 days of age has a persistent PDA. If the ductus becomes hemodynamically significant, the **MOST** appropriate management of the neonate is:

    A. extreme fluid restriction with close observation

B. immediate ligation of the ductus in the operating room
C. immediate ligation of the ductus by bed side in NICU
D. indomethacin for pharmacotherapy

Answer: D

Approximately one third of very low birth weight infants are actually diagnosed with a persistent PDA in the neonatal intensive care unit. Of these, 70% of the infants less than 28 weeks gestational age may be affected with persistent PDA.[3] The indication and timing of treatment in the premature age group is still controversial. The strategies that can be used in the treatment of a hemodynamically significant PDA include either prophylactic treatment (within 24 hours of birth with indomethacin) or symptomatic treatment (early with indomethacin or ibuprofen <72 hours after birth or late symptomatic with ibuprofen >72 hours after birth).[3] Surgical ligation should be limited to PDA with clinical signs persisting after 2 courses of failed pharmacotherapy in a hemodynamically significant ductus[11]; therefore, answers B and C are incorrect. Answer A is incorrect, as extreme fluid restriction may be detrimental to the systemic flow.[3,11]

2. Prostaglandin E1 infusion is **MOST** appropriate for which of the following lesions:

    A. atrial septal defect
    B. incomplete vascular ring
    C. transposition of the great arteries
    D. ventricular septal defect

Answer: C

Prostaglandin E1 is indicated when maintaining the patency of the DA is beneficial to the neonate.[25] If ductal closure causes significant decrease in systemic circulation the condition is termed *ductus dependent systemic flow*. Systemic flow dependent lesions include coarctation of aorta, interrupted aortic arch, and hypoplastic left heart. Similarly, if ductal closure causes decrease in pulmonary circulation, the condition is termed *ductus dependent pulmonary flow*. Pulmonary blood flow dependent lesions include pulmonary atresia, severe pulmonary stenosis, and Fallot's tetralogy with severe pulmonary stenosis. Answers A, B, and D are incorrect, as vascular ring, atrial septal defect, and isolated ventricular septal defect, respectively, are not a ductus dependent lesions.

3. A 2-day old premature neonate is diagnosed with a hemodynamically significant PDA. Which of the following complication is **MOST** likely associated with untreated hemodynamically significant DA in this scenario?

    A. necrotizing enterocolitis
    B. periventricular leukomalacia
    C. postrenal failure
    D. subdural hematoma

Answer: A

A large PDA shunting left to right is associated with several adverse outcomes.[7] The increase in pulmonary blood flow can result in pulmonary edema and its sequelae. Additionally, the "ductal steal" phenomenon will reduce the systemic perfusion. This will lead to hypoperfusion of vital organs such as the intestines and kidney increasing risk of necrotizing enterocolitis (answer A) and prerenal failure (not postrenal failure; answer C). Systemic hypotension, altered intracerebral blood flow, and intraventricular hemorrhage have all been associated with a persistent PDA.[7] The effect of PDA on periventricular leukomalacia is not known (answer B).[7] Answer A is incorrect, as prophylactic surgical ligation has not been shown to significantly decrease the risk of intraventricular hemorrhage. Perhaps, prophylactic indomethacin may reduce the risk of intraventricular hemorrhage.[7,26]

4. A neonate born at 28-weeks gestation is diagnosed with a persistent PDA. Which of the following is **MOST** accurate regarding a PDA?

    A. Anatomical closure occurs at 18–21 days.
    B. Functional closure occurs in the first hour of life.
    C. Incidence in 28-week preterm infants is almost 100%.
    D. Incidence is directly proportional to gestational age.

Answer: A

Premature infants have a higher incidence of persistent PDA (up to 60% if born before 28 weeks gestation and up to 20% if born after 32 weeks of gestation)[27,28]; therefore, answers C and D are incorrect. Functional closure of the ductus occurs at 12–18 hours after birth and anatomical closure at 2 to 3 weeks[2]; thus, answer B is incorrect, and answer A is correct.

5. Complications of surgical ligation of PDA is **MOST** likely to result in injury to which of the following structures?

    A. external laryngeal nerve
    B. left recurrent laryngeal nerve
    C. right recurrent laryngeal nerve
    D. superior laryngeal nerve

Answer: B

Surgical complications of PDA ligation include vocal cord paralysis due to recurrent laryngeal nerve injury, diaphragmatic paralysis, pneumothorax, and chylothorax.[18,20] The recurrent laryngeal nerve passes inferior and posterior to the DA; therefore, answer B is correct. The right recurrent laryngeal nerve, phrenic nerve, external laryngeal nerve, and superior laryngeal nerve do not pass near the DA, and, thus, answers A, C, and D are incorrect. Other complications that have been implicated are neurodevelopmental outcomes and retinopathy of prematurity, but results from a meta-analysis suggest no difference in these outcomes compared to medical management of PDA.[19] Early surgical closure in premature infants has been associated with shortened delay to full feeding and improved growth compared to delayed surgical closure.[29]

6. A 3-month old is scheduled for ligation of the PDA because of a hemodynamically significant ductus. Which of the following statements regarding surgical ligation of the PDA is **MOST** likely to be true?

    A. Arterial line is absolutely necessary for monitoring.
    B. Aorta may need to clamped during surgical dissection.
    C. Blood pressure monitoring in right upper limb is sufficient.
    D. Sternotomy and cardiopulmonary bypass are needed.

Answer: B

For ligation of isolated PDA, the incision is a left muscle-sparing posterolateral thoracotomy,[30] and answer D is incorrect as sternotomy and cardiopulmonary bypass are not necessary. Blood pressure as well as pulse oximetry should be measured in both upper and lower extremities during surgical ligation; therefore, answer C is incorrect. A successful ductal ligation results in elevation of the diastolic blood pressure due to elimination of the diastolic run-off. Answer A is incorrect, as an arterial line is not necessary unless the patient's other co-morbidities warrants its use. If control of aortic end of the ductus is lost, the surgeon may have to place a clamp on the aorta[30] (answer B).

7. A 2-year-old patient presents for a procedure under general anesthesia. He had a successful transcatheter PDA closure 3 months ago with coil occlusion device. Which of the following procedures is **MOST** at risk for causing endocarditis prophylaxis in this patient?

    A. bronchoscopic biopsy
    B. dental radiography
    C. umbilical herniorraphy
    D. ureter reimplantation

Answer: A

The 2007 AHA guidelines for infective endocarditis prophylaxis list cardiac conditions that are associated with highest risk for infective endocarditis.[24] Completely repaired congenital heart defects with prosthetic material or device placed by surgery or transcatheter technique during the first 6 months are at highest risk. Antibiotic prophylaxis is not indicated for bronchoscopy unless it involves incision of the respiratory tract mucosa[24] (answer D). Answer B is incorrect: Taking dental radiographs does not require subacute bacterial endocarditis prophylaxis. Additionally, answers C and D are incorrect as antibiotic prophylaxis is no longer recommended for genitourinary or gastrointestinal procedures. In patients with native PDA, infective endocarditis is seen in second or third decade of life.[28]

8. A 2-week-old premature neonate born at 26 weeks has a hemodynamically significant PDA. Which of the following is **MOST** likely to be true regarding surgical ligation, as compared to pharmacotherapy, as treatment options?

    A. less expensive
    B. less protective
    C. more benign
    D. more successful

Answer: D

Both pharmacotherapy with COX inhibitors and surgical ligation are associated with risks and complications[20]; therefore, answer C is incorrect. Controversies still remain around the optimal timing of therapy and what constitutes a hemodynamically significant ductus.[7] Surgery is indicated in case of a hemodynamically significant ductus when either pharmacotherapy has failed (answer D) or there are contraindications to use of NSAIDS (e.g., necrotizing enterocolitis, renal impairment, platelet dysfunction). Pharmacotherapy is typically less

expensive than surgical therapy; therefore, answer A is incorrect. Answer B is incorrect in light of a recent retrospective cohort study, which reported lower mortality with PDA ligation without increased risk of chronic lung disease, retinopathy of prematurity, and neurodevelopmental impairment.[19]

QUESTIONS AND ANSWERS

This chapter has accompanying questions and answers which are available to subscribers as part of the Oxford eLearning platform. To access the questions, go to ✔ http:// oxfordmedicine. com/pediatricanesthesiaPBL

REFERENCES

1. Forsey JT, Elmasry OA, Martin RP. Patent arterial duct. *Orphanet J Rare Dis.* 2009;4:17.
2. Anilkumar M. Patent ductus arteriosus. *Cardiol Clin.* 2013;31(3):417–430.
3. Sallmon H, Koehne P, Hansmann G. Recent advances in the treatment of preterm newborn infants with patent ductus arteriosus. *Clin Perinatol.* 2016;43(1):113–129.
4. Coceani F. Control of the ductus arteriosus—a new function for cytochrome P450, endothelin and nitric oxide. *Biochem Pharmacol.* 1994;48(7):1315–1318.
5. Cole SZ, Lanham JS. Failure to thrive: an update. *Am Fam Physician.* 2011;83(7):829–834.
6. Menon G, Poskitt EM. Why does congenital heart disease cause failure to thrive? *Arch Dis Child.* 1985;60(12):1134–1139.
7. Hamrick SE, Hansmann G. Patent ductus arteriosus of the preterm infant. *Pediatrics.* 2010;125(5):1020–1030.
8. Krichenko A, Benson LN, Burrows P, Moes CA, McLaughlin P, Freedom RM. Angiographic classification of the isolated, persistently patent ductus arteriosus and implications for percutaneous catheter occlusion. *Am J Cardiol.* 1989;63(12):877–880.
9. Baruteau AE, Hascoet S, Baruteau J, et al. Transcatheter closure of patent ductus arteriosus: past, present and future. *Arch Cardiovasc Dis.* 2014;107(2):122–132.
10. Sivanandan S, Agarwal R. Pharmacological closure of patent ductus arteriosus: selecting the agent and route of administration. *Paediatr Drugs.* 2016;18(2):123–138.
11. Mitra S, Ronnestad A, Holmstrom H. Management of patent ductus arteriosus in preterm infants—where do we stand? *Congenit Heart Dis.* 2013;8(6):500–512.
12. Janvier A, Martinez JL, Barrington K, Lavoie J. Anesthetic technique and postoperative outcome in preterm infants undergoing PDA closure. *J Perinatol.* 2010;30(10):677–682.
13. Zahn EM, Peck D, Phillips A, et al. Transcatheter closure of patent ductus arteriosus in extremely premature newborns: early results and midterm follow-up. *JACC Cardiovasc Interv.* 2016;9(23):2429–2437.
14. Pass RH, Hijazi Z, Hsu DT, Lewis V, Hellenbrand WE. Multicenter USA Amplatzer patent ductus arteriosus occlusion device trial: initial and one-year results. *J Am Coll Cardiol.* 2004;44(3):513–519.
15. Odegard KC, Vincent R, Baijal R, et al. SCAI/CCAS/SPA expert consensus statement for anesthesia and sedation practice: recommendations for patients undergoing diagnostic and therapeutic procedures in the pediatric and congenital cardiac catheterization laboratory. *Catheter Cardiovasc Interv.* 2016;88(6):912–922.
16. Chen JY, Jia JE, Liu TJ, Qin MJ, Li WX. Comparison of the effects of dexmedetomidine, ketamine, and placebo on emergence agitation after strabismus surgery in children. *Can J Anaesth.* 2013;60(4):385–392.
17. Riveros R, Makarova N, Riveros-Perez E, et al. Utility and clinical profile of dexmedetomidine in pediatric cardiac catheterization

procedures: a matched controlled analysis. *Semin Cardiothorac Vasc Anesth*. 2017:1089253217708035.

18. Vida VL, Lago P, Salvatori S, et al. Is there an optimal timing for surgical ligation of patent ductus arteriosus in preterm infants? *Ann Thorac Surg*. 2009;87(5):1509–1515; discussion 1515–1516.

19. Weisz DE, Mirea L, Rosenberg E, et al. Association of patent ductus arteriosus ligation with death or neurodevelopmental impairment among extremely preterm infants. *JAMA Pediatr*. 2017;171(5):443–449.

20. Weinberg JG, Evans FJ, Burns KM, Pearson GD, Kaltman JR. Surgical ligation of patent ductus arteriosus in premature infants: trends and practice variation. *Cardiol Young*. 2016;26(6):1107–1114.

21. Lam JY, Lopushinsky SR, Ma IW, Dicke F, Brindle ME. Treatment options for pediatric patent ductus arteriosus: systematic review and meta-analysis. *Chest*. 2015;148(3):784–793.

22. Stankowski T, Aboul-Hassan SS, Marczak J, Cichon R. Is thoracoscopic patent ductus arteriosus closure superior to conventional surgery? *Interact Cardiovasc Thorac Surg*. 2015;21(4):532–538.

23. Avsar MK, Demir T, Celiksular C, Zeybek C. Bedside PDA ligation in premature infants less than 28 weeks and 1000 grams. *J Cardiothorac Surg*. 2016;11(1):146.

24. Wilson W, Taubert KA, Gewitz M, et al. Prevention of infective endocarditis: guidelines from the American Heart Association: a guideline from the American Heart Association Rheumatic Fever, Endocarditis, and Kawasaki Disease Committee, Council on Cardiovascular Disease in the Young, and the Council on Clinical Cardiology, Council on Cardiovascular Surgery and Anesthesia, and the Quality of Care and Outcomes Research Interdisciplinary Working Group. *Circulation*. 2007;116(15):1736–1754.

25. Danford DA, Gutgesell HP, McNamara DG. Application of information theory to decision analysis in potentially prostaglandin-responsive neonates. *J Am Coll Cardiol*. 1986;8(5):1125–1130.

26. Kabra NS, Schmidt B, Roberts RS, et al. Neurosensory impairment after surgical closure of patent ductus arteriosus in extremely low birth weight infants: results from the Trial of Indomethacin Prophylaxis in Preterms. *J Pediatr*. 2007;150(3):229–234, 34 e1.

27. Siassi B, Blanco C, Cabal LA, Coran AG. Incidence and clinical features of patent ductus arteriosus in low-birthweight infants: a prospective analysis of 150 consecutively born infants. *Pediatrics*. 1976;57(3):347–351.

28. Chugh R, Salem MM. Echocardiography for patent ductus arteriosus including closure in adults. *Echocardiography*. 2015;32(Suppl 2): S125–S139.

29. Jaillard S, Larrue B, Rakza T, Magnenant E, Warembourg H, Storme L. Consequences of delayed surgical closure of patent ductus arteriosus in very premature infants. *Ann Thorac Surg*. 2006;81(1):231–234.

30. Mavroudis C, Backer CL, Gevitz M. Forty-six years of patient ductus arteriosus division at Children's Memorial Hospital of Chicago. Standards for comparison. *Ann Surg*. 1994;220(3):402–409; discussion 409–410.

7.

VENTRICULAR SEPTAL DEFECT

Evan R. Serfass and Justin D. Ramos

STEM CASE AND KEY QUESTIONS

A 3-month-old boy who was born at term presents to the hospital with diaphoresis, tachypnea, and decreased oral intake with less frequent wet diapers. His vitals are notable for respiratory rate of 60 breaths per minute, heart rate 155 bpm, blood pressure 80/45 mmHg, and oxygen saturation 94%. On exam, rales are audible in bilateral lung fields. There is lateral displacement of the cardiac apex, but there is no audible murmur upon auscultation. He was born at normal weight (60th percentile) but has begun to fall off of his growth curve (now 10th percentile). Echocardiography reveals a large nonrestrictive perimembranous ventricular septal defect (VSD) with wide open left-to-right flow across the defect. The left atrium is enlarged, and the left ventricle (LV) is moderately dilated. The right ventricle (RV) demonstrates mild hypertrophy and mild dilation. The valvular structures and the aorta are normal. No atrial septal defect is visualized.

WHAT EXAM FINDINGS ARE EXPECTED IN A PATIENT WITH AN ISOLATED VSD? WHY IS THERE NO AUDIBLE MURMUR IN THIS CHILD?

Exam findings may include evidence of a large LV leading to lateral displacement of the cardiac apex. The intensity of a pansystolic murmur depends on the velocity of flow across the defect, with smaller defects being associated with murmurs with higher intensity due to higher velocities. Some large defects may not be associated with audible murmurs due to low-velocity, nonturbulent flow across a large defect as in this infant.[1]

HOW SHOULD THIS PATIENT BE MEDICALLY MANAGED AT THIS TIME?

Diuretics, digoxin, and potentially an afterload reducing agent (e.g., angiotensin converting enzyme inhibitor) should be initiated as treatment for congestive heart failure. The patient's blood pressure and kidney function must be monitored during medical treatment.[1,2] Any concurrent respiratory infection should be treated as indicated. Due to the infant's failure to thrive, nutrition should be supplemented enterally via nasogastric tube or parenterally as indicated to optimize growth.

The infant is admitted to the pediatric intensive care unit (ICU). Diuretics and digoxin therapy are initiated. A nasogastric feeding tube is placed, and a course of antibiotic therapy is completed for a lower respiratory infection. The child begins to gain some weight over several weeks.

WHAT ARE INDICATIONS FOR SURGICAL CORRECTION OF A VSD? WHEN SHOULD SURGERY BE SCHEDULED?

Infants with large lesions may present with symptoms of heart failure in the first weeks to months of life. Infants with intractable heart failure symptoms and failure to thrive despite medical management may be indicated for early surgical treatment.[2,3] Medical management of heart failure and failure to thrive might allow more time for the infant to grow and gain weight. For infants younger than six months of age, lower weight is associated with increased risk of morbidity following surgery; however, lower weight was not associated with poorer outcomes in children older than 6 months of age.[4]

The child is now 5 months old and is readmitted for tachypnea and respiratory distress. Despite initially good weight gain, he currently weighs 5.9 kg (below second percentile). A repeat echocardiogram demonstrates increased RV dilation, though ventricular function appears normal. A multidisciplinary team convenes to discuss, and the decision is made to proceed with surgical repair given the child's failure to thrive despite medical management for heart failure.

THE PATIENT IS ADMITTED FOR SURGERY. HOW SHOULD WE INDUCE ANESTHESIA FOR THIS PATIENT? HOW WILL YOU MANAGE THE PATIENT'S OXYGENATION AND VENTILATION?

Given our patient's preserved ventricular function, an inhalational induction should be well tolerated. The safest approach in cases of severe pulmonary hypertension or impaired ventricular function may be an intravenous induction. During intubation, fraction of inspired oxygen (FIO_2) can be increased temporarily, but after securing the airway, it is prudent to lower minute ventilation and restrict FIO_2. To minimize pulmonary overcirculation, it is important to maintain pulmonary vascular tone by avoiding hypocarbia and excessive oxygenation. Maintenance of normo- to mild hypercapnia while weaning FIO_2 as low as possible, keeping SpO_2 in the mid-90s or above, is a reasonable approach.

AFTER INDUCTION AND PLACEMENT OF INVASIVE LINES, THE BABY BECOMES HYPOTENSIVE. HOW WILL YOU ASSESS AND TREAT THE PATIENT'S HYPOTENSION?

In addition to typical considerations such as volume status and depth of anesthesia, low systemic blood pressure in the setting of left-to-right shunt merits careful consideration of the ratio between pulmonary and systemic circulation (Qp:Qs ratio). High oxygen saturation or low end-tidal carbon dioxide may indicate that pulmonary vascular tone is too low. Low pulmonary vascular resistance (PVR) can lead to pulmonary overcirculation at the expense of systemic blood flow, which may manifest as systemic hypotension and metabolic acidosis. Vasoactive agents that selectively increase systemic vascular resistance should generally be avoided because they will increase afterload on the left heart and worsen left-to-right shunt at the expense of systemic perfusion. During this period prior to repair, pulmonary vascular tone should be maintained by managing ventilation to avoid hyperventilation and hyperoxygenation. If necessary, a drug with inotropic properties such as dopamine or epinephrine may be considered if needed to raise cardiac output, understanding that systemic vascular resistance is also likely to increase.

HOW SHOULD WE MAINTAIN ANESTHESIA DURING SURGERY? HOW SHOULD WE TREAT PAIN? SHOULD WE PLAN TO EXTUBATE THIS PATIENT IN THE OPERATING ROOM, SOON AFTER ARRIVAL IN THE PEDIATRIC ICU OR MUCH LATER?

We decide to maintain anesthesia with volatile anesthetic, a moderate to high dose of fentanyl (between 15–25 mcg/kg for the case), and muscle relaxation with a non-depolarizing neuromuscular relaxant. Opioids, benzodiazepines, dexmedetomidine, and volatile anesthetics are all reasonable agents for the maintenance of anesthesia during pediatric cardiac surgeries. Pain control after a low-dose fentanyl-only technique may be inferior to a high-dose fentanyl technique if other analgesic adjuncts are not utilized. High-dose opioid techniques may be associated with decreased stress response and decreased detectable inflammatory markers.[5] However, adjuncts such as dexmedetomidine (0.5 mcg/kg/hr) or neuraxial techniques with caudal morphine[6–8] may help facilitate tracheal extubation with adequate pain control and a reasonable total fentanyl dose soon after completion of surgery.

Older children with isolated VSDs are good candidates for tracheal extubation soon after the end of surgery.[1,2,9] However, given our infant's young age, low weight and significant risk of pulmonary hypertension, the decision is made to delay tracheal extubation for later after arrival in the ICU.

WHAT CONCERNS AND CONTINGENCIES SHOULD WE PREPARE FOR AS WE SEPARATE FROM CARDIOPULMONARY BYPASS?

Prevention and treatment of pulmonary hypertension is important as we prepare for separation from cardiopulmonary bypass. Given our patient's preoperative RV dilation and risk for pulmonary hypertension, agents such as inhaled nitric oxide, inhaled iloprost, or milrinone may be necessary for pulmonary vasodilation.[2] The patient should be ventilated initially with 100% oxygen, and further weaning of inspired oxygen fraction (FIO_2) should be undertaken slowly and carefully. Right heart failure could develop if pulmonary hypertension is uncontrolled, and epinephrine, dobutamine, or isoproterenol may be required. With significant right ventricular dilation from preoperative shunt, the RV is also less able to tolerate hypovolemia after closure. Volume status should be monitored closely, and significant volume loading may be necessary to maintain adequate preload to the dilated RV.

ON TRANSESOPHAGEAL ECHOCARDIOGRAPHY, A RESIDUAL VSD IS VISUALIZED. WHAT ARE OPTIONS FOR NEXT STEPS?

Smaller VSDs are sometimes not evident on preoperative echocardiography because the effects of larger lesions can obscure their presence.[3] Residual VSDs that are small and less hemodynamically significant have the potential to close naturally over time and may not warrant additional repair. Percutaneous device closure at a later time could also be considered in patients who are appropriately sized for percutaneous devices or immediately in the operating room following bypass where this hybrid interventional capability exists.[10] The benefit of fixing a potentially hemodynamically significant residual VSD must be weighed against the risk of additional time on cardiopulmonary bypass, which may contribute to increased coagulopathy, ventricular dysfunction, and inflammatory response.

The surgeons decide to go back on bypass and attempt to repair the residual defect because it appears hemodynamically significant.

THE SURGEONS DISCUSS DELAYING STERNAL WOUND CLOSURE. WHY WOULD THEY CONSIDER THIS? WHAT, PRECISELY, DOES IT MEAN TO "LEAVE THE CHEST OPEN"? HOW DOES AN OPEN CHEST AFFECT RESPIRATORY PHYSIOLOGY?

The sternum is sometimes left open after complex neonatal surgery, procedures with long cardiopulmonary bypass times, and in cases with significant bleeding, edema, or tenuous hemodynamic status that may necessitate postoperative extracorporeal membrane oxygenation (ECMO) such as severe pulmonary hypertension or ventricular outflow tract obstruction.[11,12] Closing the skin incision (or patching with synthetic material) and dressing the wound without closing the sternum allows for significantly increased pulmonary system compliance, which may aid in sustaining hemodynamic and respiratory stability. This strategy may be employed electively after complex procedures or on an as needed basis for ongoing or anticipated hemodynamic instability, bleeding, cardiac edema, or pulmonary edema. Delayed sternal closure facilitates rapid wound re-exploration or institution of ECMO if necessary and avoidance of cardiac tamponade in the setting of bleeding. The infant must undergo sternal wound closure after several days. Delayed closure increases the risk of infectious complications (i.e., sepsis, pneumonia, mediastinitis, wound infection, wound dehiscence), and the risk of infection must be weighed against the benefit of improved hemodynamic stability. A review of the Society of Thoracic Surgery Congenital Heart Surgery database published by Nelson-McMillan et al.[12] in 2016 revealed increasing infection risk with increased duration of time with the sternum left open, but no association between location of sternal wound closure and infection outcome (operating room vs ICU). The majority of patients (67%) had their sternal wounds closed in the ICU after several days.

WHAT RHYTHM ABNORMALITIES IS THIS PATIENT AT RISK FOR? HOW OFTEN DO THESE ABNORMALITIES OCCUR, AND WHY?

Temporary or permanent atrioventricular (AV) block is a risk associated with surgical VSD repair. Though historically the incidence of AV block requiring permanent pacemaker placement was as high as 3% to 8%, more recent case series indicate an incidence of heart block and pacemaker placement between 0.5% and 1.9% of patients.[3,4,13–15] Patient size less than 4 kg was correlated with a higher incidence of surgical AV block requiring pacemaker placement.[13] The anatomic location of the VSD also affects the risk of heart block, as inlet VSDs are associated with higher incidence of AV block due to their proximity to the AV conduction axis.[3,13] The need for ventriculotomy to approach certain anterior or muscular VSDs is also thought to increase the risk of conduction disturbances.[2] Though the majority of patients do not require permanent pacing, temporary pacing wires are typically left in place for all patients due to the significant risk of conduction abnormalities.[3,4,13] The incidence of at least transient AV block ranges approximately 5.6% to 7.7% of all patients in case series.[4,13,16] Patients are also at risk for junctional ectopic tachycardia, which occurred in up to 7.5% of VSD repair patients in a retrospective analysis of cases between 2001 and 2009, which was consistent with previously published series.[13]

AFTER CORRECTION, IS ENDOCARDITIS PROPHYLAXIS INDICATED?

Antibiotic prophylaxis is recommended for 6 months after complete surgical closure of VSD and prior to dental procedures and other procedures involving the respiratory tract or infected soft tissues. If there is a residual defect related to patch material, then antibiotic prophylaxis may be indicated indefinitely. Antibiotic prophylaxis solely to prevent infective endocarditis is not recommended for most gastrointestinal or genitourinary tract procedures. The American Heart Association guidelines stress the importance of good dental hygiene, as the risk of infectious endocarditis from activities of daily living is higher than infective endocarditis associated with discrete dental or surgical procedures.[17]

HOW WOULD YOU MANAGE THIS PATIENT IF HE HAD DOWN'S SYNDROME AND PRESENTED AT 2 MONTHS OF AGE FOR GASTROSTOMY TUBE PLACEMENT PRIOR TO REPAIR OF HIS LARGE PERIMEMBRANOUS VSD?

Patients with Down's syndrome (trisomy 21) are at increased risk for early development of pulmonary hypertension, and these patients may not exhibit the normal physiologic decline in pulmonary vascular tone during the first 3 months of life that is thought to precipitate heart failure symptoms in other neonates due to worsening left-to-right shunt. In the presence of a large VSD, this maintained or increased pulmonary vascular tone may limit shunt and prevent heart failure symptoms; however, if left uncorrected, permanent changes to the pulmonary vasculature may lead to vascular occlusive disease, shunt reversal, and cyanosis constituting Eisenmenger's syndrome.[1,2]

During an anesthetic for this patient, pulmonary vascular tone should be maintained by avoiding hyperventilation and hyperoxygenation to limit pulmonary overcirculation at the expense of systemic circulation. However, oxygenation, ventilation, temperature, acid-base status, and pain must also be managed to avoid excessive pulmonary vascular tone, which could result in shunt reversal (right to left or dynamic) and cyanosis if pulmonary pressures approach or exceed systemic pressures. Injection of air bubbles into the venous circulation should be carefully avoided due to the risk of paradoxical air embolism with dynamic shunt. Given the patient's uncorrected cardiac lesion, it would be prudent to arrange for recovery in the ICU.

HOW SHOULD WE MANAGE A 5-YEAR-OLD CHILD WITH AN UNTREATED, UNCORRECTED, WIDE OPEN VSD WHO WAS JUST ADOPTED FROM A FOREIGN COUNTRY? AN ECHOCARDIOGRAM REVEALS SEVERE PULMONARY HYPERTENSION WITH NEAR-SYSTEMIC PRESSURES AND DYNAMIC SHUNT ACROSS THE DEFECT. THE PATIENT DOES NOT TAKE ANY PULMONARY VASODILATORS.

This patient has developed Eisenmenger's syndrome due to uncorrected left-to-right shunt leading to pulmonary vascular occlusive disease and perhaps permanent remodeling of the pulmonary vascular bed. In the past, treatment was solely supportive as surgical repair did not address the morbidity from permanent vascular remodeling and pulmonary hypertension. More recent pharmacologic advances have revealed that pulmonary vasodilators targeted at the pulmonary endothelium may have clinical benefits in both symptom management and survival for these patients. Pharmacologic treatments include bosentan, a dual-endothelin receptor antagonist, and sildenafil, a phosphodiesterase inhibitor that increases cGMP levels. In some cases, good pharmacologic response may restore operability in patients previously deemed inoperable. As such, this patient should have close follow-up and be maintained on pulmonary vasodilators.[1,2]

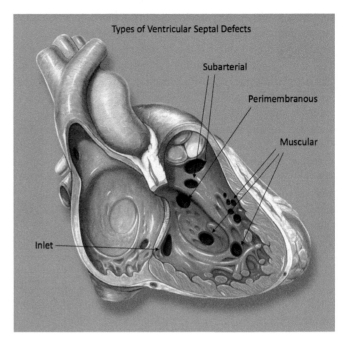

Fig. 7.1 Types of ventricular septal defects. An anatomic view of the right ventricle and right atrium with example VSDs. Patrick J. Lynch, medical illustrator (https://commons.wikimedia.org/wiki/File:Heart_right_vsd.jpg), Heart right VSD. Labels added to image by Justin D. Ramos, https://creativecommons.org/licenses/by/2.5/legalcode.

HOW WOULD YOU MANAGE A 3-YEAR-OLD CHILD WITH AN UNTREATED, UNCORRECTED VSD WHO IS PRESENTING FOR ELECTIVE NONCARDIAC SURGERY? HER DEFECT IS SMALL, RESTRICTIVE, AND SHE APPEARS ASYMPTOMATIC.

Small, restrictive VSDs are often managed conservatively with routine cardiology follow-up and monitoring. Most small VSDs require no intervention if patients do not exhibit heart failure symptoms, pulmonary hypertension, or secondary effects of the VSD such as valvular insufficiency.[1,2,18] Teenagers and adults with small, restrictive, unrepaired VSDs have near-normal survival although a small minority of patients eventually develop pulmonary hypertension or ventricular enlargement requiring late repair.[19] Most patients with small, restrictive VSDs have normal exercise tolerance and tend to tolerate standard anesthetic management for noncardiac surgeries.[1] Restrictive VSDs tend to have high velocity left-to-right flow, reducing the risk of paradoxical emboli from the right-sided circulation.

DISCUSSION

BACKGROUND

VSD is the most common congenital cardiac lesion, and VSDs are present in up to 40–50% of all children with congenital cardiac malformations. Ventricular septal defects are isolated lesions in up to 20% of children with congenital heart disease.[1,2,18] Underlying etiologies are varied and likely multifactorial. VSDs are associated with congenital syndromes such as CHARGE (coloboma, heart anomaly, choanal atresia, retardation, and genital and ear anomalies), VACTERL (vertebral, anal, cardiac, tracheoesophageal fistula, renal, and limb anomalies) and chromosomal abnormalities such as DiGeorge (22q11 deletion), Turner's syndrome (45x), and trisomies 13, 18, and 21. Many VSDs close within the first year of life, though the rate of spontaneous closure varies with size and anatomic location.[2,18]

ANATOMIC CLASSIFICATIONS

Ventricular septal defects are classified by their location, though there is not one universal consensus for classification and naming[1,2,18] (see Figure 7.1).

- Subarterial VSDs (also called infundibular, subpulmonary, supracristal, or conal) are found within the outlet septum above the crista supraventricularis. These comprise roughly 5% of all VSDs. Due to their proximity to the valvular leaflets, a Venturi effect from flow through the defect may cause prolapse of one of the aortic cusps resulting in aortic insufficiency.[1,2]

- Perimembranous VSDs are located in the area near the membranous septum of the heart and the fibrous connections between the aortic, mitral, and tricuspid valves. These are the most common subtype, comprising 80% of all lesions.[1,2] Perimembranous VSDs are less likely to close spontaneously, closing roughly 12% of the time.[20]

- Inlet VSDs make up about 10% of all ventricular septal defects. They are located beneath the septal leaflet of the tricuspid valve near the posterior part of the septum.[20]

- Muscular VSDs are located within the muscular interventricular septum. There can be multiple muscular defects present, and these comprise about 2% to 7% of all VSDs.[1,2] Muscular VSDs are the most likely to close, closing at a rate of up to 40%.[20]

PATHOPHYSIOLOGY

Isolated VSDs create a left-to-right shunt across the interventricular septum during systole. The degree of shunting or interventricular flow is the primary determinant of the physiologic effect of the VSD. Larger defects are considered nonrestrictive, as they do not significantly limit flow and are typically associated with a high degree of left-to-right shunt. In nonrestrictive defects, the degree of shunting between the pulmonary and systemic circulations (Qp:Qs ratio) is predominantly determined by the relative resistances of the pulmonary and systemic vascular beds (PVR:SVR ratio). In smaller, restrictive defects the size of the defect provides intrinsic resistance to flow through the defect. In utero, the pressures in the left and right ventricles are normally essentially equal. In the neonatal period, high PVR may limit left-to-right shunting, but symptoms may worsen as PVR decreases over the first three months of life resulting in worsening left-to-right shunt and heart failure symptoms due to pulmonary overcirculation. Over time, increased volume loading of both ventricles may lead to eccentric hypertrophy or dilation of both ventricles. These changes are more likely in patients with larger, nonrestrictive defects. In some patients, especially those with trisomy 21, pulmonary vascular tone may be maintained beyond the neonatal period or pulmonary hypertension may develop. If the defect remains uncorrected, permanent changes in the pulmonary endothelium may develop, resulting in the constellation of vascular occlusive disease, reversal of shunt and cyanosis, which is termed Eisenmenger's syndrome.[1,2,18]

Ventricular septal defects may also be associated with secondary structural anomalies. Aortic valve prolapse with regurgitation may be associated with VSDs near the aortic valve due to Venturi forces associated with high velocity VSD jets affecting the aortic leaflets. Significant right ventricular hypertrophy may cause mid-cavity obstruction of the RV, resulting in a "double-chambered RV" with a proximal high-pressure chamber and a distal low-pressure chamber within the ventricle.[2]

DIAGNOSIS

Patients with VSD have a wide range of age at presentation and variation in symptoms depending on the anatomy, size, and hemodynamic effects of the defect. Patients may be asymptomatic for many years, or they may present in infancy with signs and symptoms of congestive heart failure of varying degrees. In symptomatic patients, recurrent respiratory infections, tachypnea, diaphoresis, or failure to thrive may develop.[1–3,18,21] Physical exam findings associated with VSD include lateral displacement of the cardiac apex from volume loading of the LV, a pansystolic murmur from flow across the VSD or diastolic rumble at the apex from increased mitral inflow. The murmur is of varying intensity depending on the velocity of flow through the defect. Large defects may have lower velocity, less turbulent flow, and less audible murmur or no detectable murmur. Smaller defects are typically associated with higher velocity flow and higher intensity murmurs, perhaps with an associated thrill.[1] Though nonspecific, chest radiographs may demonstrate prominent pulmonary vascularity or cardiomegaly. The left atrium may be enlarged on radiograph with a normal sized aorta.[3,9] Electrocardiogram may reveal LV or RV hypertrophy. Patients who have developed Eisenmenger's syndrome may present with clubbing, cyanosis, an RV heave, and typically with no murmur.[1]

Echocardiography is the mainstay of diagnosis and evaluation of VSD, as it allows for assessment of the location, size, and flow across the defect[1,2] (see Figure 7.2). Prenatal diagnosis is also possible with prenatal echocardiography, though as many as one third of prenatally diagnosed VSDs close spontaneously by birth or early postgestational ultrasound.[22] Cardiac MRI is also a useful modality for the assessment of complex lesions, such as a double-chambered RV.[1,2] Velocity encoded phase-contrast images above the semilunar valves can also be used to calculate pulmonary flow (Qp) and systemic flow (Qs) and the Qp:Qs ratio.[9]

TREATMENT

Most infants with large, nonrestrictive VSDs will develop symptoms of congestive heart failure by 3 months of age,[2] and uncontrolled congestive heart failure with associated failure to thrive is the most common indication for surgical repair in the first year of life.[4] For children younger than 6 months of age, lower patient weight was associated with increased risk of complications; however, infants older than 6 months of age did not demonstrate the same association between weight and complication rate.[4] As such, medical management of heart failure symptoms in young infants with diuretics, digoxin, or afterload reducing therapy with careful monitoring of blood pressure and renal function are appropriate strategies to bridge patients with congestive heart failure symptoms to surgery.[1]

Surgical repair via patch closure using cardiopulmonary bypass and median sternotomy is the gold standard for repair.[2,3] With modern surgical, anesthetic, and cardiopulmonary bypass technique, surgical repair of VSD has very low morbidity and mortality. Mortality is typically lower than 1%, and the rate of serious complications such as reoperation, need for ECMO, residual VSD, or complete heart block requiring permanent pacemaker placement is around 5%.[2,4,14,21] The typical approach is via a right atriotomy, with the VSD visible through the open tricuspid valve, though a right ventriculotomy may be necessary to approach certain muscular VSDs.[1,3] Pulmonary banding may still be employed

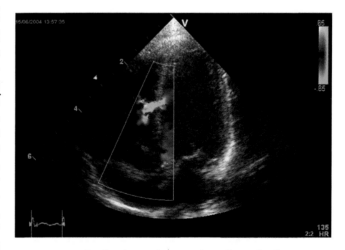

Fig. 7.2 VSD visualized with transthoracic echocardiography. (https://commons.wikimedia.org/wiki/File:Ventricular_Septal_Defect.jpg)

in the case of multiple muscular VSDs to decrease left-to-right shunting and allow the patient to grow until surgical or transcatheter repair can be attempted when the patient is older or larger.[2,3] Percutaneous techniques are also now being employed in certain centers, with success rates that are comparable to surgical repair. Concerns over an increased risk of heart block after transcatheter closure initially limited the implementation of early percutaneous devices,[14,23] though larger and older patients seem to have safe outcomes after percutaneous closure with new devices and an incidence of complete AV block in the range of 1.7%. Hospital length of stay, rate of blood transfusion, and other complication rates are also low with percutaneous closure in appropriately selected patients.[10]

ANESTHETIC CONSIDERATIONS

A thorough understanding of the patient's cardiac anatomy, degree of shunting, ventricular function, secondary lesions, and degree of pulmonary hypertension must inform the anesthetic management of a patient undergoing surgical VSD repair. Oxygenation and ventilation must be optimized with regard to the ratio of pulmonary to systemic flow (Qp:Qs). Hyperventilation and hyperoxygenation may lead to increased pulmonary flow (Qp) at the expense of systemic circulation(Qs), which may manifest as systemic hypotension and metabolic acidosis.[2]

Patients who had signs of pulmonary hypertension preoperatively may be at increased risk of pulmonary hypertension after repair and during separation from cardiopulmonary bypass. These patients may respond to pulmonary vasodilators like inhaled nitric oxide or iloprost.[1,2] They should be ventilated with 100% oxygen during separation from cardiopulmonary bypass. Hypercarbia and metabolic acidosis should be avoided to keep pulmonary vascular tone low. Weaning of inspired oxygen fraction (FIO_2) should be undertaken slowly and carefully. Right heart failure could develop if pulmonary hypertension is uncontrolled, and milrinone, epinephrine, dobutamine or isoproterenol may be required.[2] Volume status should be monitored closely after repair, and significant volume loading may be necessary to maintain adequate preload to the dilated RV.

Maintenance of anesthesia and management of pain should be tailored to accomplish early extubation in appropriate cases. A majority (up to 80% or more) of patients having uncomplicated VSD repairs can be extubated soon after the end of surgery.[4] Techniques utilizing some volatile anesthetic with high opioid (25 mcg/kg total) or low opioid (10 mcg/kg total) and adjuncts such as dexmedetomidine infusion and neuraxial opioids (i.e., caudal morphine) have been described and can all lead to successful early extubation in the operating room[6] or soon after arrival in the ICU.[4,6,7]

Due to the significant risk of conduction abnormalities after VSD repair, temporary pacing wires are typically left in place. Patients are also at significant risk of arrhythmias such as junctional ectopic tachycardia, which occurred in up to 7.5% of patients postoperatively in some series.[14]

CONCLUSIONS

Ventricular septal defect is the most common congenital cardiac lesion, and the natural history and pathophysiology of VSD varies by patient age, patient size, anatomic location, and size of the defect. Though many small lesions close spontaneously, patients who have large defects and significant left-to-right shunt resulting in heart failure symptoms or failure to thrive may be indicated for early surgical repair. Patients with significant unrepaired shunt may develop pulmonary hypertension that may progress to Eisenmenger's syndrome, which consists of permanent pulmonary vascular remodeling, progressive pulmonary hypertension, and subsequent shunt reversal and cyanosis. Anesthetic management should consider that the relative resistances of the pulmonary and systemic vascular beds (PVR:SVR ratio) determines the degree of shunting across larger defects. Intraoperatively, pulmonary vascular tone should be maintained by avoiding hyperventilation and excessive oxygenation to prevent pulmonary overcirculation and systemic undercirculation. The risk of pulmonary hypertension should be considered during separation from cardiopulmonary bypass. Early extubation can be accomplished in the majority of patients. Despite risk of arrhythmia and conduction abnormalities, surgical repair of VSD is accomplished routinely with low morbidity and very low mortality.

REVIEW QUESTIONS

1. Which type of VSD is **MOST** likely to close on its own?

    A. inlet
    B. muscular
    C. perimembranous
    D. supracristal

Answer: B
Muscular, with up to 40% of defects closing spontaneously. Perimembranous, supracristal, and inlet defects are less likely to close spontaneously.[1,2,20]

2. Which statement regarding VSDs and valves is **MOST** accurate?

    A. accessory tricuspid valve tissue often occludes perimembranous VSDs
    B. muscular VSDs are associated with mitral regurgitation
    C. subarterial VSDs are associated with aortic stenosis
    D. subarterial VSDs are associated with pulmonic insufficiency

Answer: A
Accessory tricuspid valve tissue often partially covers or may even completely occlude perimembranous VSDs.[18,20] Subarterial VSDs are associated with aortic insufficiency (not pulmonic insufficiency or aortic stenosis) due to prolapse of the right coronary leaflet of the aortic valve through the VSD into the RV.[2,20] Muscular VSDs are not associated with any particular valvular lesions.

2. The absence of a murmur in a patient with a VSD, **MOST** likely indicates which of the following flow dynamics across the defect?

A. hemodynamically insignificant
B. limit by a small defect
C. low in velocity
D. reversed by Eisenmenger syndrome

Answer: C
Murmurs are caused by high-velocity flow; therefore, the absence of a murmur indicates that flow across the VSD is low velocity.[1] This often occurs with large VSDs in neonates, as in the case described, but can also occur later as pulmonary hypertension develops, RV pressures increase, and flow velocity across the VSD decreases. Answer A is incorrect because VSDs without murmurs are likely to be large, and large defects are unlikely to be hemodynamically insignificant. Answer B is incorrect because patients with small VSDs usually have large LV–RV pressure gradients and thus high flow velocity across the VSD. Answer D is one possible explanation for the lack of a murmur, but other explanations are possible; therefore, lack of a murmur does not mean Eisenmenger's syndrome has developed.

4. An infant with trisomy 21 is found to have a nonrestrictive VSD. Clinically, he appears well, with normal vital signs, and his growth charts have been tracking around the 50th percentile. Which of the following statements **BEST** describes his cardiac status?

A. Cardiac function is worsening.
B. Left ventricular dilation is increasing.
C. Pulmonary hypertension is developing.
D. Shunting is from right to left.

Answer: C
His normal growth and lack of heart failure symptoms suggest his pulmonary and systemic flow ratio (Qp:Qs) is relatively balanced; given the nonrestrictive nature of his VSD, this implies high pulmonary artery pressures. In addition, children with trisomy 21 and heart defects are known to be at higher risk of developing pulmonary hypertension.[18] Answer A is incorrect because his normal growth and well appearance are not consistent with a diagnosis of heart failure. Answer D is incorrect because his vital signs are normal—with right-to-left shunting his SpO_2 would be decreased. Answer B is incorrect because LV dilation occurs with a high Qp:Qs ratio, which is not supported by his growth and well appearance.[2]

5. Which statement about postoperative arrhythmia following VSD repair is **MOST** accurate?

A. Atrioventricular blocks are most likely permanent.
B. Muscular VSDs have the highest risk for arrhythmia.
C. Junctional ectopic tachycardia is common in older children.
D. Permanent pacemakers are rarely needed.

Answer: D
Atrioventricular block is the most common arrhythmia following VSD repair; however, most cases resolve within 10 days, and need for permanent pacing is low, at roughly 1% of patients undergoing VSD repair.[13,15] Junctional ectopic tachycardia is possible following repair of a simple VSD; however, it is more likely to occur in children whose repair is performed at less than one year of age.[2] Muscular VSDs are typically remote from the conduction system, and thus injury to it is unlikely during repair of these lesions.

6. For which of the following VSD patients would antibiotic prophylaxis against subacute bacterial endocarditis be the **LEAST** indicated for dental cleaning?

A. 14-month old with patch closure 8 months ago of a perimembranous VSD
B. 3-year old with an unrepaired VSD, clubbing, and perioral cyanosis
C. 5-year old with primary closure 4 years ago, complicated by bacterial endocarditis
D. 9-year old with closure at 8 years ago, with a tiny leak at her patch's the superior border

Answer: A
Dental cleaning, which involves manipulation of the gingiva, is considered a high-risk procedure for seeding the bloodstream with bacteria, and thus patients at risk for subacute bacterial endocarditis should receive antibiotic prophylaxis. Currently, criteria include presence of a prosthetic heart valve; history of bacterial endocarditis, as in answer C; cyanotic congenital heart disease, as in answer B; completely repaired congenital heart defect (whether by surgery or catheter-based device) within the first 6 months after repair; repaired congenital heart defect with a defect at or adjacent to the site of the repair, as in answer D; and in recipients of cardiac transplants who have valvular disease.[17]

7. A 3-month-old boy with a large VSD is scheduled for gastrostomy tube placement due to failure to thrive. Following mask induction using sevoflurane and 100% oxygen, peripheral intravenous line placement, and intubation, the vital signs are heart rate 170 bpm, SpO_2 100%, blood pressure 52/28 mmHg, and respitory rate 30 breaths per minute with $ETCO_2$ of 43 mmHg and end-tidal sevoflurane of 2% on pressure control ventilation. Which of following interventions is the **MOST** appropriate first step?

A. FiO_2 reduction
B. lactated ringers bolus
C. phenylephrine injection
D. respiratory rate increase

Answer: A
In the presence of a nonrestrictive VSD, high FiO_2 results in low PVR and an increase in the Qp:Qs ratio, which decreases cardiac output to the systemic circulation. In this situation the initial measure to take would be to lower the FIO_2 significantly—ideally to 21% if tolerated—to decrease the Qp:Qs ratio.[2] Administration of phenylephrine might increase measured noninvasive blood pressure but would likely decrease systemic cardiac output (and thus oxygen delivery) further by increasing Qp:Qs and is thus a poor choice. Increasing the respiratory rate would reduce PVR and thus

also increase the Qp:Qs ratio. Administration of intravenous fluid and reduction in inhaled agent may be appropriate steps to take if reduction in FIO$_2$ is ineffective at significantly increasing the blood pressure.

8. In patients, who have just undergone cardiac surgery, delayed sternal closure is **LEAST** likely for which of the following indications?

    A. cardiovascular stability
    B. infectious avoidance
    C. respiratory function
    D. extracorporeal membrane oxygenator support

Answer: B

A review of the Society of Thoracic Surgery Congenital Heart Surgery database published by Nelson-McMillan et al.[12] in 2016 revealed increasing infection risk with increased duration of time with the sternum left open but no association between location of sternal wound closure and infection outcome (operating room vs ICU). Each day of delayed closure was associated with a slightly higher risk of infectious complication, though the risk seemed to increase more dramatically after the sixth day. Sternal closure can result in inadequate space in the chest cavity to accommodate effective respiration, unobstructed systemic venous return, postsurgical bleeding, and postsurgical edema. For these reasons, following neonatal surgeries or especially prolonged or complex surgeries in older children, delayed sternal closure is often chosen. Typically, tissue swelling has resolved enough and hemodynamic status stabilized to the point where sternal closure can be performed, often in the ICU, 2 to 4 days after the initial surgery. In patients whose hemodynamics are tenuous following repair or who are at risk of pulmonary hypertensive crisis and in whom ECMO support may be required, delayed sternal closure may be chosen to reduce the time to ECMO initiation during an emergency.

9. Which of the following is the **BEST** indication for echocardiography for a patient with a VSD?

    A. preoperative postcatheterization check
    B. Qp:Qs measurements and calculations
    C. spontaneous VSD closure serial assessments
    D. unseen VSD identification after large VSD closure

Answer: D

Closure of a moderate to large VSD may result in flow across smaller VSDs that were not previously seen due to left-to-right shunting occurring exclusively via the low-resistance, larger VSD.[3] Answer A is incorrect as most patients with VSD can be adequately characterized preoperatively with echocardiography alone.[1,3] Answer B is incorrect as echocardiography cannot accurately measure flow quantity, just flow velocity; if accurate information about Qp:Qs is needed, MRI or cardiac catheterization would need to be performed.[1] Answer C is incorrect as serial echocardiograms are also very important for evaluating effects of the VSD on valvular and ventricular size and function, and pathologic changes may spur repair even if the VSD is shrinking in size.[1]

10. Which statement about VSD closure, in regard to pulmonary hypertension, is the **LEAST** accurate?

    A. Delayed sternal closure can be advantageous for patient with pulmonary hypertension.
    B. Eisenmenger's syndrome patients will experience decreased pulmonary pressures.
    C. Residual atrial septal defect/patent foramen ovale may be advantageous for patients at risk for pulmonary hypertension.
    D. Trisomy 21 patients are at increased risk for pulmonary hypertension with VSD closure.

Answer: B

Once Eisenmenger's syndrome has developed the pulmonary vascular changes that cause pulmonary hypertension are not completely reversible, although current treatments with pulmonary vasodilators may lead to some improvement.[1] Management of pulmonary hypertension postcardiopulmonary bypass focuses on lowering PVR, with the initial measures being 100% oxygen, modest hyperventilation, and possibly inhaled nitric oxide.[2] In patients at high risk for postoperative pulmonary hypertension, an atrial septal defect, or patent foramen ovale may be left to allow for right-to-left shunting at the atrial level and maintenance of adequate cardiac output (at the expense of reduced systemic oxygen saturation) during pulmonary hypertensive crisis. Delaying sternal closure following VSD repair can be used in patients at risk of pulmonary hypertensive crisis to decrease the time to institution of extracorporeal membrane oxygenation.[11,12] Patients with trisomy 21 are at increased risk of pulmonary hypertension.[18]

QUESTIONS AND ANSWERS

This chapter has accompanying questions and answers which are available to subscribers as part of the Oxford eLearning platform. To access the questions, go to ✓ http://oxfordmedicine. com/pediatricanesthesiaPBL

REFERENCES

1. Penny DJ, Vick GW. Ventricular septal defect. *Lancet.* 2011;377(9771):1103–1112.
2. Walker S. Anesthesia for left-to-right shunt lesions. In: Andropoulos DB, Stayer SA, Mossad EB, et al. (eds.), *Anesthesia for congenital heart disease*, 3rd ed. New York: John Wiley; 2015:461–496.
3. Van Doorn C, De Leval MR. Ventricular septal defects. In: Stark JF, Leval MR, Tsang VT, eds. *Surgery for Congenital Heart Defects*. 3rd ed. New York: John Wiley; 2006:355–371.
4. Anderson BR, Stevens KN, Nicolson SC, et al. Contemporary outcomes of surgical ventricular septal defect closure. *J Thorac Cardiovasc Surg.* 2013;145(3):641–647.
5. Naguib AN, Tobias JD, Hall MW, et al. The role of different anesthetic techniques in altering the stress response during cardiac surgery in children: a prospective, double-blinded, and randomized study. *Pediatr Crit Care Med.* 2013;14(5):481–490.

6. Garg R, Rao S, John C, et al. Extubation in the operating room after cardiac surgery in children: a prospective observational study with multidisciplinary coordinated approach. *J Cardiothorac Vasc Anesth.* 2014;28(3):479–487.

7. Leyvi G, Taylor DG, Reith E, Stock A, Crooke G, Wasnick JD. Caudal anesthesia in pediatric cardiac surgery: does it affect outcome?. *J Cardiothorac Vasc Anesth.* 2005;19(6):734–738.

8. Stuth EA, Berens RJ, Staudt SR, et al. The effect of caudal vs intravenous morphine on early extubation and postoperative analgesic requirements for stage 2 and 3 single-ventricle palliation: a double blind randomized trial. *Paediatr Anaesth.* 2011;21(4):441–453.

9. Rojas CA, Jaimes C, Abbara S. Ventricular septal defects: embryology and imaging findings. *J Thorac Imaging.* 2013;28(2):W28–W34.

10. Butera G, Piazza L, Saracino A, Chessa M, Carminati M. Transcatheter closure of membranous ventricular septal defects—old problems and new solutions. *Interv Cardiol Clin.* 2013;2(1):85–91.

11. Bojan M, Pouard P. Hemodynamic management. In: Andropoulos DB, Stayer SA, Mossad EB, et al., eds. *Anesthesia for Congenital Heart Disease.* 3rd ed. New York: John Wiley; 2015:375–403.

12. Nelson-McMillan K, Hornik CP, He X, et al. Delayed sternal closure in infant heart surgery—the importance of where and when: an analysis of the STS Congenital Heart Surgery Database. *Ann Thorac Surg.* 2016;102(5):1565–1572.

13. Siehr SL, Hanley FL, Reddy VM, Miyake CY, Dubin AM. Incidence and risk factors of complete atrioventricular block after operative ventricular septal defect repair. *Congenit Heart Dis.* 2014;9(3):211–215.

14. Scully BB, Morales DL, Zafar F, Mckenzie ED, Fraser CD, Heinle JS. Current expectations for surgical repair of isolated ventricular septal defects. *Ann Thorac Surg.* 2010;89(2):544–549.

15. Liberman L, Silver ES, Chai PJ, Anderson BR. Incidence and characteristics of heart block after heart surgery in pediatric patients: a multicenter study. *J Thorac Cardiovasc Surg.* 2016;152(1):197–202.

16. Anderson HO, de Leval MR, Tsang VT, et al. Is complete heart block after surgical closure of ventricular septum defects still an issue? *Ann Thorac Surg.* 2006;82:948–956

17. Wilson W, Taubert KA, Gewitz M, et al. Prevention of infective endocarditis: guidelines from the American Heart Association: a guideline from the American Heart Association Rheumatic Fever, Endocarditis, and Kawasaki Disease Committee, Council on Cardiovascular Disease in the Young, and the Council on Clinical Cardiology, Council on Cardiovascular Surgery and Anesthesia, and the Quality of Care and Outcomes Research Interdisciplinary Working Group. *Circulation.* 2007;116(15):1736–1754.

18. Minette MS, Sahn DJ. Ventricular septal defects. *Circulation.* 2006;114(20):2190–2197.

19. Soufflet V, Van de bruaene A, Troost E, et al. Behavior of unrepaired perimembranous ventricular septal defect in young adults. *Am J Cardiol.* 2010;105(3):404–407.

20. Eroglu AG, Atik SU, Sengenc E, Cig G, Saltik IL, Oztunc F. Evaluation of ventricular septal defect with special reference to the spontaneous closure rate, subaortic ridge, and aortic valve prolapse II. *Pediatr Cardiol.* 2017;38(5):915–921.

21. Danford DA, Martin AB, Danford CJ, Kaul S, Marshall AM, Kutty S. Clinical implications of a multivariate stratification model for the estimation of prognosis in ventricular septal defect. *J Pediatr.* 2015;167(1):103–107.

22. Mosimann B, Zidere V, Simpson JM, Allan LD. Outcome and requirement for surgical repair following prenatal diagnosis of ventricular septal defect. *Ultrasound Obstet Gynecol.* 2014;44(1):76–81.

23. Yang J, Yang L, Yu S, et al. Transcatheter versus surgical closure of perimembranous ventricular septal defects in children: a randomized controlled trial. *J Am Coll Cardiol.* 2014;63(12):1159–1168.

8.

TETRALOGY OF FALLOT

Matthew Lilien and Anshuman Sharma

STEM CASE AND KEY QUESTIONS

Tetralogy of Fallot (TOF) is the most common form of cyanotic heart disease and accounts for approximately 10% of all congenital heart defects. The word *tetralogy* refers to a combination of four abnormalities observed in the morphology of the heart, namely, (i) an unrestrictive ventricular septal defect (VSD), (ii) right ventricular outflow tract (RVOT) obstruction, (iii) aorta overriding the ventricular defect, and (iv) right ventricular hypertrophy. This combination of defects produces an obstruction to the flow of pulmonary blood and results in shunting of deoxygenated blood from the right (pulmonary) circulation to the left (systemic) circulation, thereby producing desaturation of the blood in the systemic circulation. The degree of right to left shunting and hence its clinical presentation depends entirely on the degree of obstruction to the flow of pulmonary blood. Many additional cardiac and extracardiac defects are often seen in children born with TOF. While primary definitive surgical care is the treatment of choice, in some children anatomical constraints will enforce a palliative procedure before definitive surgery can be carried out. Many long-term physiological abnormalities such as free pulmonary insufficiency, progressive right ventricular dilatation, and conduction defects are frequently seen consequences of the surgical repair and continue to affect the lives of survivors. These children often undergo multiple surgical procedures related to their cardiac and extracardiac defects. A thorough preoperative assessment, deep understanding of patient's anatomy and physiology, and careful anesthetic planning is essential even for minor surgical procedures.

A 2-month-old male child presented to the emergency room with incarceration of a hernia on the left side. The hernia was manually reduced in the emergency room, and the patient was admitted for a complete repair of the defect. The surgical plan was to repair the hernia on the left side and perform laparoscopic assessment of the right inguinal area.

Patient's history was significant as he was diagnosed prenatally with TOF. With his dysmorphic features, a genetic workup was conducted and diagnosis of 22-q11 microdeletion syndrome was confirmed. He was monitored at home with pulse oximeter, and, according to his parents, his oxygen saturation generally stayed around 93%. However, they also mentioned noticing bluish discoloration around his lips especially during feeding and crying. He was feeding well but his weight remained at the 30th percentile. He was scheduled to undergo definitive repair of his heart defect at the age of 3 months.

WHAT WERE THE FINDINGS ON THE PHYSICAL EXAM?

Patient was small for his age, weighing only 4.1 kg. Child had some dysmorphic features with a relatively small chin. A detailed airway examination identified a cleft in the hard palate. His preoperative saturations were recorded at 91% on room air. On auscultation, a harsh crescendo-decrescendo murmur was auscultated on the left sternal border. Lungs were clear bilaterally.

WHAT WERE THE SIGNIFICANT FINDINGS REPORTED IN THE LAST ECHOCARDIOGRAM?

A transthoracic echocardiogram was performed soon after birth. A large, unrestrictive, malaligned VSD and a small pulmonary valve with dysplastic leaflets were seen. Branch pulmonary arteries were small but confluent. A few muscle bundles were seen obstructing the right ventricular tract outflow, producing a peak flow velocity of 4 m/sec. A generalized right ventricular hypertrophy was also present. A small foramen ovale, with flow of blood from the left atrium to the right atrium was also seen.

WHAT ARE THE COMMON ANOMALIES ASSOCIATED WITH THE TOF? SHOULD THE ANESTHESIA TEAM HAVE ANTICIPATED A DIFFICULT AIRWAY?

With his dysmorphic features, cleft palate, and hypocalcemia his pediatrician considered the diagnosis of DiGeorge syndrome. The diagnosis of 22q micro-deletion was then confirmed, first by fluorescence in situ hybridization test and subsequently by chromosomal microarray testing. Patient was put on oral calcium and vitamin D supplementation. Complete blood workup and blood chemistry tests were obtained a night prior to surgery and serum calcium levels were within normal limits. Targeted assessment of the airway suggested a mild retrognathia. A complete cleft palate was also present.

HOW WILL YOU INDUCE THE GENERAL ANESTHETIC FOR THIS CHILD?

Patient was anesthetized with inhalational induction using Sevoflurane, and intravenous access was obtained. Direct laryngoscopy was performed using Miller 1.5 blade but providers were unable to clearly visualize the laryngeal inlet. Intubation was finally accomplished using a video-laryngoscope. A caudal block was also performed with 4 cc of 0.2% Ropivacaine. During induction, oxygen saturations and blood pressure remained stable.

WHAT POTENTIAL COMPLICATIONS CAN BE EXPECTED DURING SURGERY? WHAT IS A TET SPELL?

Within 15 minutes after surgical incision, patient's oxygen saturation decreased from 94% to 74%. Patient's hemodynamics remained stable at noninvasive blood pressure of 75/45 and heart rate of 123 beats per minutes. After increasing the inspired oxygen fraction to 100%, the anesthesia care team decided to administer a bolus of 40 mL of 5% albumin. In the face of persistent desaturations to mid-70s, after ruling out common causes of hypoxemia, the anesthesia team correctly made the diagnosis of a Tet spell and decided to increase the systemic vascular resistance, and phenylephrine (1 mcg/kg) was administered through the peripheral intravenous line. These measures resulted in significant improvement in the systemic oxygen saturation levels. Surgery was then successfully completed and the patient was extubated at the end of the procedure. The patient was admitted postoperatively to the cardiac intensive care unit for continuous monitoring. During the postoperative period, the child developed 2 more episodes of persistent desaturations, requiring treatment with fluid boluses, morphine, and boluses of phenylephrine. A repeat transthoracic echocardiogram demonstrated a significant increase in muscle bundles obstructing the RVOT, producing peak velocity of more than 5 m/sec across the pulmonary valve. As frequent episodes of desaturations continued throughout the night, a decision was made to proceed with a definitive repair of the TOF the next day. Patient was finally discharged to home after 2 weeks without any major complications.

DISCUSSION

Tetralogy of Fallot is the most common cyanotic congenital heart defect accounting for 3% to 9% of all children born with congenital heart defects.[1,2] The classic lesion, as described initially by Neal Stenson in 1673 and then by Etienne-Louis Arthur Fallot in 1888,[2] is a combination of four discrete abnormalities: (i) a nonrestrictive VSD, (ii) an aortic valve that overrides the interventricular septum, (iii) RVOT obstruction of varying degrees, and (iv) right ventricular hypertrophy that results from obstruction to the pulmonary blood flow.

Although most cases are sporadic in nature, about one third of children with TOF have chromosomal abnormalities such as 22q11 micro-deletion, trisomy of chromosomes 11, 13, and 18.[3,4] While additional cardiac and extracardiac abnormalities can influence the nature and timing of the surgical interventions and anesthetic management, the degree of obstruction to the pulmonary blood flow remains the key determinant of the clinical presentation and the approach to surgical treatment. Cyanosis is generally the main feature but the onset and severity of cyanosis varies widely. Some children, appropriately called "pink Tets," have relatively mild obstruction to the RVOT and display only mild cyanosis. At the other end of the spectrum are defects where the pulmonary valve is completely atretic. In these children, pulmonary blood flow becomes critically dependent on the patency of ductus arteriosus or existence of direct aortopulmonary collaterals.

In most children, a definitive and complete repair of the defect during early infancy is preferred. The ideal age for definitive surgery is not agreed upon, but most surgeons prefer to conduct surgical repair during 1 to 6 months of age. In children with severe obstruction to pulmonary outflow, prostaglandin E_2 is often needed to keep the ductus patent until the time an alternative source of blood flow to the lungs can be surgically established. In these children, a systemic-pulmonary shunt such as Blalock-Taussig shunt becomes necessary to (i) establish adequate pulmonary blood flow and (ii) facilitate growth of pulmonary arteries until a comprehensive repair can be performed.

ANATOMY AND MORPHOLOGY

The essential phenotype of the tetralogy consists of four cardiac anatomical defects previously outlined. All four defects however, result from an anterior and cephalad deviation of the infundibular part of the interventricular septum. As a result, the aorta appears to be straddling over the two limbs of the septomarginal band, creating a large and unrestrictive VSD (Figure 8.1). This anterior migration of the septum also creates an obstruction to the flow of blood through the right ventricular outflow. During the first few months of life, hypertrophy of the septoparietal trabeculations, which are normally present in the anterior wall of the RVOT, further increases RVOT obstruction. In children with TOF, reduced blood flow through the pulmonary circulation throughout the fetal life compromises the growth of branch pulmonary arteries and the rest of the pulmonary vasculature.

The VSD in TOF is always unrestrictive and lies between the two limbs of the septomarginal band. The aortic valve is typically seen encroaching over the right ventricle but in patients with TOF, continuity between aortic and mitral valve is maintained.

ANATOMICAL VARIANTS OF TOF

In extreme cases of right ventricular tract obstruction, the pulmonary valve and the main pulmonary artery are completely atretic, and branch pulmonary arteries are rudimentary and nonconfluent (Figure 8.2). In these patients, pulmonary blood flow is supplied by a number of collaterals directly coming from the aorta (Figure 8.3). One commonly seen variant of TOF lacks pulmonary valve leaflets. This variant of TOF has significant impact on the anesthetic management. The lack of leaflets

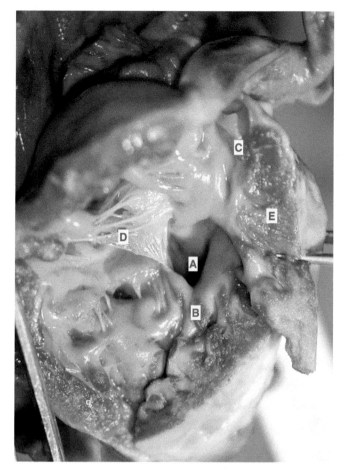

Fig. 8.1 Specimen of the heart with TOF. Right ventricular free wall has been cut open to demonstrate a large ventricular septum defect (A) situated between the two limbs of septomarginal band (B). Pulmonary annulus is small and valve appears to be thickened (C). Septal leaflet (D) of the tricuspid valve has been lifted to show the full extent of the VSD. Right ventricle wall is hypertrophied (E).

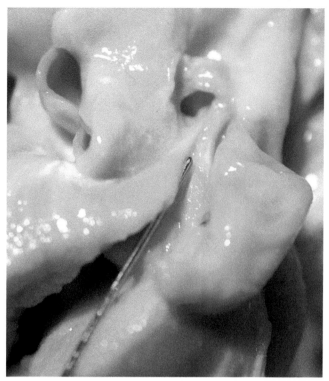

Fig. 8.2 Specimen of the heart of TOF with atretic pulmonary valve and rudimentary main pulmonary artery.

in pulmonary valves produces severe pulmonary insufficiency. The constant to and fro movement of the blood results in markedly dilated pulmonary arteries, which, in turn, cause significant compression of the major airways. Most patients with this variant develop significant tracheabronchomalacia that can persist for months and years even after definitive repair has been completed. Another variant is seen in children with trisomy 21. In this type of cardiac morphology, atrioventricular canal defects are seen in combination with components of TOF. The surgical repair of this variant is relatively complex and is generally performed beyond the first 6 months of life.

ASSOCIATED ANOMALIES

A number of cardiac and extra cardiac anomalies can be associated with the diagnosis of TOF. These defects can significantly impact the anesthetic management of a child with TOF. Most significantly, facial dysmorphism and structural airway abnormalities such as small jaw, laryngo-tracheomalacia, complete tracheal rings, and cleft palate make for a challenging day in the operating room. Hypocalcemia

due to hypoparathyroidism is considered a cardinal feature of DiGeorge syndrome and can be particularly severe during the neonatal period. A long list of additional extracardiac malformations affecting the abdominal wall, central nervous system, and renal system are sporadically seen in patients with TOF.

Tetralogy of Fallot is also the most common congenital heart defect found in patients of CHARGE syndrome. CHARGE syndrome is a nonrandom association of defects that include coloboma, heart defect, atresia of choanae, retarded growth, genital hypoplasia, and ear anomalies.

Another complex syndrome associated with TOF is VACTERL syndrome. Similar to CHARGE syndrome, a number of organs are affected nonrandomly. A variety of combinations of any three of the following major defects can be present: scoliosis due to vertebral defects, esophageal atresia with trachea-esophageal fistula, anal atresia, absence of radius, and renal abnormalities can be present along with cardiac defects of the tetralogy. These children require frequent anesthetics for a variety of noncardiac and cardiac problems. The dysmorphic features, difficult venous access, and complex physiology can pose anesthetic challenges even for experienced anesthesia care providers.

A number of additional cardiac abnormalities can have implications for the surgical repair the TOF. As a result from the abnormal rotation of the aortic root, up to 10% of patients may have an anomalous origin of coronary arteries.[5] An abnormal origin of left anterior descending or left main coronary from the right coronary artery that crosses the RVOT may limit the extent of the incision to relieve right ventricular

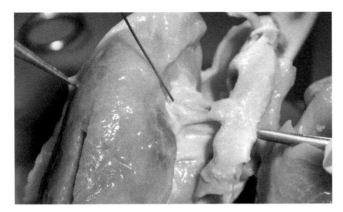

Fig. 8.3 Specimen of the heart and the left lung in a patient with TOF. A large aorto-pulmonary collateral can be seen directly originating from the descending aorta to supply pulmonary blood flow to the left lung.

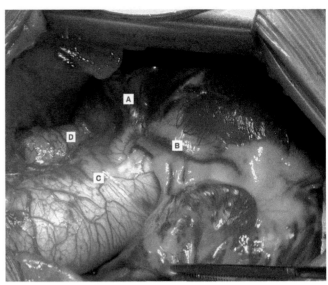

Fig. 8.4 Abnormal origin of left coronary artery (A) from the right coronary artery (B) can be seen across the right ventricular outflow tract. Also seen is relatively large aortic root (C) compared to visibly smaller main pulmonary artery (D).

obstruction (Figure 8.3). In these patients, a definitive repair may require right ventricular to pulmonary artery conduit.[6] Other common cardiac defects such as right aortic arch, persistent left-sided superior vena cava, or muscular VSDs may also affect surgical decision-making.

PHYSIOLOGY AND HEMODYNAMIC CONSEQUENCES OF THE LESION

The presence of a large VSD and obstruction to the blood flow out of the right ventricle results in shunting of deoxygenated blood to the systemic side, thus producing systemic desaturation. The amount of right to left shunting is a function of the cumulative resistance at subvalvar, valvar, or postvalvar level relative to the systemic vascular resistance. Any decrease in systemic vascular resistance, as caused by anesthetic agents, will facilitate right to left shunting and thereby worsen systemic oxygen desaturation. Conversely, increasing systemic vascular resistance with the help of α-agonists will reduce right to left shunting and thereby increase systemic oxygen saturation. While rarely encountered in developed nations, if TOF remains unrepaired, consequences of long-term hypoxemia such as severe polycythemia, clubbing of the fingers and toes (Figure 8.4), and stunted growth are clearly seen.[7]

HYPERCYANOTIC OR TET SPELLS

Some children born with the classic form of TOF develop acute, often unprovoked, episodes of severe cyanosis associated with hyperpnoea and loss of conscious. These "tet spells," also known as hypercyanotic spells, result from intense spasm of hypertrophic muscle bundles in the RVOT and commonly happen during high catecholaminergic situations such as extreme anxiety, pain, or crying. These spells begin early during infancy and often result in temporary loss of consciousness and even stroke. New onset of "tet spells" is a strong indication for earlier surgical intervention. During the intraoperative period, high catecholaminergic surge resulting from pain or the stress of endotracheal intubation, combined with vasodilatory effects of anesthetic agent can precipitate "tet spells."

A number of measures such as ensuring adequate hydration, maintenance of adequate depth of anesthetic, and avoiding drugs that induce significant vasodilatation can help prevent these episodes. Aggressive measures should be taken to treat even brief episodes of desaturation. These include hyperventilation with 100% oxygen, deepening the plane of anesthetics with drugs like morphine or ketamine, and the use of an α-agonist such as phenylephrine. Short acting beta blockers such as esmolol are sometimes required to treat desaturation episodes that prove resistant to other measures.[8] In few cases with refractory hypoxemia, palliative surgery may be urgently needed.

TREATMENT

Most patients born with the diagnosis of TOF will require surgical treatment. The single definitive repair requires the use of cardiopulmonary bypass and remains the preferred approach. In most children, complete repair is electively performed between the ages of 1 to 5 months.[9-11] Staged repair with initial palliative intervention to ensure adequate pulmonary blood flow is sometimes needed in those children with (i) duct dependent pulmonary blood flow such as tetralogy with complete pulmonary atresia, (ii) extremely underdeveloped pulmonary arteries, (iii) small birth weight, or (iv) specific anatomical defects that make definitive surgical repair a challenge in an infant such as aberrant left anterior descending coronary artery crossing the RVOT.

PALLIATIVE SURGERY

Shunt palliation involves creation of a systemic to pulmonary artery connection to ensure or augment pulmonary blood flow. A modified Blalock-Taussig shunt is the most common approach and typically involves placing a tube graft for connecting a systemic vessel (generally the innominate artery on the side opposite to the aortic arch) to the pulmonary artery. Other type of shunts, which are placed more centrally by connecting descending aorta to the left pulmonary artery (Pott's shunt) or ascending aorta to right pulmonary artery (Waterston shunt), are sometimes needed in children with severely underdeveloped pulmonary arteries. There are a number of potential disadvantages of the staged approach. These include complications resulting from (i) continued high right ventricle pressure with associate ventricular hypertrophy, (ii) persistent hypoxemia, (iii) myocardial dysfunction, and (iv) surgical palliation such as excessive pulmonary blood flow, partial or complete occlusion of the shunt, or narrowing of the branch pulmonary artery.

DEFINITIVE REPAIR

The definitive repair of the TOF involves closure of the VSD(s) and ensuring pulmonary blood flow by relieving obstruction at subvalvar, valvar, or postvalvar regions. Specifically, the VSD is closed through an atrial approach and muscle bundles in the outflow tract are resected through an incision in pulmonary artery. The decision to place a transannular patch to augment the pulmonary valve is taken after careful deliberations. Incision through the pulmonary valve will inevitably result in free pulmonary insufficiency. While relatively well tolerated in the immediate postoperative period, severe pulmonary insufficiency has significant long-term consequences. The volume overload created by an incompetent pulmonary valve results in progressive right ventricular dilatation and eventually leads to right ventricular failure. For these very reasons, the current surgical approach aims to preserve the function of the pulmonary valve and accepts higher right ventricular pressures. In patients with small branch pulmonary arteries, patch augmentation of these structures is also carried out as far as possible into the hilum of the lungs. Whenever high right ventricular pressures are anticipated, surgeon often leaves a communication at the atrial level or a fenestration in the VSD patch is created to work as a "pop off" for the right ventricle.

LONG-TERM OUTCOMES

Following a complete repair, most children will catch up with their peers and achieve normal height and weight within the first 5 years. More than 90% of patients will survive more than 30 years if operated on prior to the age of 5 years.[12] A number of sequelae persist into the adulthood and impact the quality of life as well as life expectancy.[13] Historically, surgical efforts were directed at minimizing residual obstruction to the pulmonary blood flow and any residual pulmonary insufficiency was considered inconsequential. However, long-term follow-up of the survivors has made it evident that free pulmonary insufficiency created by incising the pulmonary valve produces chronic volume overload for the right ventricle and results in the irreversible dilatation and failure of the right ventricle.[14]

ANESTHETIC MANAGEMENT FOR A NONCARDIAC SURGERY IN CHILDREN WITH TOF

Intraoperative management of a child with an unrepaired or palliated TOF can be challenging even for minor surgical procedures. Whenever possible, noncardiac surgeries should be deferred until a definitive repair has been successfully completed. Ideally, these patients should be cared for at a tertiary care hospital by an anesthesia care team that has significant expertise in managing children with complex congenital cardiac defects.

A thorough preoperative examination should include the review of a recent transthoracic echocardiogram to assess cardiac morphology, especially any changes in the RVOT obstruction. Muscle bundles in the right outflow tract can hypertrophy rapidly during the first few months of life, worsening the RVOT obstruction. Cardiac catheterization is usually reserved for those cases where a balloon valvuloplasty of the pulmonary valve could potentially be sufficient to augment pulmonary blood flow. Any change in patient symptoms or oxygenation should merit a repeat echocardiogram. A thorough assessment of the airway to anticipate difficult airways must be conducted, especially in patients with chromosomal anomalies.

In children with unrepaired TOF, anesthetic management is directed toward minimizing pulmonary resistance while maintaining high systemic vasculature. One of the biggest concerns for the anesthesiologist is the development of a "tet spell" during intra- or postoperative period. A number of events can potentially trigger episodes of severe hypoxemia during the course of the anesthetic. Anesthetic drugs that decrease systemic vascular resistance (inhaled anesthetic agents, propofol, etc) will facilitate right to left shunting and therefore worsen hypoxemia. Similarly, high catecholamine levels, resulting from intubation or surgical stimulation can also trigger spasm of the muscle bundles in the RVOT, thereby causing an increase in right to left shunting of blood. The resulting hypoxemia further worsens the situation by increasing pulmonary vascular resistance. Therefore, any desaturation should be promptly detected and aggressively treated. Usual steps will include (i) increasing inspired oxygen concentration, (ii) hyperventilation, (iii) fluid boluses to optimize right heart filling pressures, (iv) deepening the anesthetic with opioids and anesthetics like ketamine, and (v) use of α-agonists to increase systemic vascular resistance. If hypoxemia persists, a short-acting beta blocker such as esmolol (50–100 mcg/kg) may be used to treat infundibular spasm; however, in few cases, persistent, severe hypoxemia necessitates an urgent aortopulmonary shunt.

Tetralogy of Fallot patients, who have been palliated with aortopulmonary shunts, are at high risk of a major morbidity during routine noncardiac surgical procedures. Shunt thrombosis is a major concern and, if not promptly diagnosed, can quickly result in unresponsive and extreme desaturations, leading to cardiac arrest and often death. A loss of holosystolic shunt murmur in the clinical setting of unexplained hypoxemia should raise suspicion of shunt occlusion and should be quickly confirmed by a transthoracic echocardiogram. Once diagnosed, an emergent cardiac catheterization is needed to restore patency of the obstructed shunt.

Most children and adult survivors remain in New York Heart Association functional class I or II, and can undergo noncardiac surgical procedures without major complications. The anesthesia team, however, must be cognizant of the common long-term sequelae of the surgical repair. Residual pulmonary insufficiency is usually well tolerated for years, but volume overload on the right ventricle from the regurgitant jet eventually results in a progressive dilatation of the right ventricle, producing ventricular dysfunction and reduced exercise tolerance. Right ventricular dilatation and progressive widening of the QRS complex in the electrocardiogram is a risk factor for ventricular tachycardia and sudden cardiac arrests. A QRS width more than 180 millisecond, or rate of increase in QRS duration of more than 3.5 millisecond per year, are strong indicators for the treatment of pulmonary insufficiency.[15] Recently, cardiac magnetic resonance imaging has become the gold standard for assessing regurgitant volume, right ventricular function, and size. With recent improvements in the transcatheter pulmonary valves techniques, more patients with pulmonary insufficiency are being treated in the cardiac catheterization lab. A specially designed heart valve, made from a bovine jugular vein attached to an expandable wireframe, is guided through a major vein and is placed across the pulmonary annulus (Figure 8.5). These techniques have shown good mid-term outcomes and can be performed with minimal morbidity and mortality.[16]

CONCLUSIONS

Tetralogy of Fallot is the most common cyanotic heart defect. The right-to-left shunting of the blood produced by the obstruction to the pulmonary blood flow is the hallmark of the defect. Anesthesiologists can be asked to provide care to children who have unrepaired, palliated, or repaired cardiac defect. Anesthesiologists must be aware of the physiological alterations caused by the defect and its surgical repair.

REVIEW QUESTIONS

1. Which of the following statement is the **MOST** accurate regarding tetralogy of Fallot?

    A. Right ventricular pressure is less than left ventricular pressure.
    B. Septal anterocephalad deviation causes outflow tract obstruction.
    C. Septomarginal trabeculations worsen outflow tract obstruction.
    D. VSD is restrictive to the flow of blood.

Answer: B

The primary defect in the cardiac morphogenesis is the anterior and cephalad migration of the outlet septum and as a result aortic outlet appears to straddle over the two limbs of septo-marginal trabeculation. Further hypertrophy of muscle bundles in the RVOT can occur and worsen the degree of RVOT obstruction. As the VSD is always large nonrestrictive, right ventricular pressures are equal to the left ventricular pressure. Patient's saturations in the unrepaired TOF will depend of the degree of RVOT obstruction.

2. A 3-month child with unrepaired tetralogy of Fallot develops intraoperative persistent desaturation. Which one of the following interventions is **MOST** important to avoid?

    A. afterload reduction with milrinone
    B. preload optimization with lactated ringers
    C. RVOT infundibular spasm relief with esmolol
    D. systemic vascular resistance hike with phenylephrine.

Answer: A

The goal of the treatment is to reduce right to left shunting of the blood and is achieved by increasing the systemic vascular resistance and reducing the pulmonary vascular resistance. Use of drugs such as milrinone and sodium nitroprusside will facilitate right-to-left shunting and thereby worsen the desaturation. Increasing inspired oxygen concentration and optimizing preload by fluid therapy will improve oxygen carrying capacity. Beta blockers such as esmolol and propranolol are helpful in treating the spasm of the infundibular muscles in the RVOT.

3. Which of the following is the **MOST** accurate statement about tetralogy of Fallot?

    A. Trachea-esophageal fistula are commonly seen.
    B. Chromosome 22 q11 deletion is the underlying cause.
    C. Hypercalcemia often appears in older children.
    D. Turner syndrome is a known association.

Answer: A

While TOF has been strongly associated with the microdeletion of q11 section of 22nd chromosome, TOF is not caused by the defect in this chromosome. Most cases of TOF are sporadic in nature but TOF has been associated

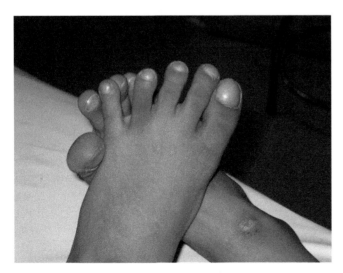

Fig. 8.5 Extreme clubbing of toes in an older child with unrepaired TOF.

with DiGeorge syndrome. Many other syndromes such as CHARGE and VACTRL syndromes can be seen with TOF but Turner syndrome is not one of them. Patients with DiGeorge syndrome develop hypocalcemia at an early age and require oral supplements of calcium and vitamin D.

4. Which of the following statements is **MOST** accurate regarding Blalock-Taussig shunts?

A. Blalock-Taussig shunt is the treatment of choice.
B. Diastolic pressures is elevated.
C. Oxygen saturation is normal.
D. Shunt occlusion is an emergency.

Answer: D

Blalock-Taussig or other systemic-pulmonary shunts are used only for palliation in children, when definitive, single-stage repair cannot be accomplished. Blood flows through the shunt during the entire cardiac cycle, thereby lowering the diastolic pressure. Any occlusion can be potentially life threatening and should be addressed urgently.

5. A child with unrepaired TOF is scheduled to undergo elective surgery. His room air is 93% oxygen. Which of the following situation is **MOST** important to avoid?

A. fraction of inspired oxygen 1.0
B. hyperventilate
C. acidosis
D. alkalosis

Answer: C

High concentration of inspired oxygen, hyperventilation, and respiratory alkalosis will reduce pulmonary vascular resistance and thereby reduce right to left shunting of the deoxygenated blood.

6. A 16-year-old male is scheduled to undergo posterior spinal fusion surgery for the correction of idiopathic scoliosis. He had undergone definitive repair of TOF defect at the age of 6 months. A transannular patch was placed at the time of surgery to relieve RVOT obstruction. Which of the following abnormalities is **MOST** likely to be seen in this child?

A. free pulmonary insufficiency
B. left ventricular dilatation
C. severe mitral regurgitation
D. prolonged PR interval

Answer: A

A definitive repair that involves an incision through the pulmonary valve placement of transannular patch invariably results in severe insufficiency of the pulmonary valve and over the course of time will lead to the dilatation of the right ventricle. Prolongation of the QRS interval can be predictive of ventricular arrhythmias and sudden death.

QUESTIONS AND ANSWERS

This chapter has accompanying questions and answers which are available to subscribers as part of the Oxford eLearning platform. To access the questions, go to ✓ http://oxfordmedicine. com/pediatricanesthesiaPBL

REFERENCES

1. Apitx, C, Anderson RA, and Redington AN. Tetralogy of Fallot with pulmonary stenosis. In: Anderson RH, Baker, EJ, Penny, DJ, Redington AN, Rignby ML, Wernovsky G eds. *Paediatric Cardiology.* London: Churchill Livingstone; 2010:753–774.
2. Apitz C, Webb GD, Redington AN. Tetralogy of Fallot. *Lancet.* 2009;374(9699):1462–1471.
3. Goldmuntz E. DiGeorge syndrome: new insights. *Clin Perinatol.* 2005;32(4):963–978.
4. Michielon G, Marino B, Formigari R, et al. Genetic syndromes and outcome after surgical correction of tetralogy of Fallot. *Ann Thorac Surg.* 2006;81(3):968–975.
5. Kapur S, Aeron G, Vojta CN. Pictorial review of coronary anomalies in tetralogy of Fallot. *J Cardiovasc Comput Tomogr.* 2015;9(6):593–596.
6. Sharkey AM, Sharma A. Tetralogy of Fallot: anatomic variants and their impact on surgical management. *Semin Cardiothorac Vasc Anesth.* 2012;16(2):88–96.
7. Loh TF, Ang YH, Wong YK, Tan HY. Fallot's tetralogy—natural history. *Singapore Med J.* 1973;14(3):169–171.
8. Kothari SS. Mechanism of cyanotic spells in tetralogy of Fallot—the missing link? *Int J Cardiol.* 1992;37(1):1–5.
9. Dodge-Khatami A, TulevskiII, Hitchcock JF, de Mol BA, Bennink GB. Neonatal complete correction of tetralogy of Fallot versus shunting and deferred repair: is the future of the right ventriculo-arterial junction at stake, and what of it? *Cardiol Young.* 2001;11(5):484–490.
10. Alassal M, Ibrahim BM, Elrakhawy HM, Hassenien M, Sayed S, Elshazly M, Elsadeck N. Total correction of tetralogy of Fallot at early age: a study of 183 cases. *Heart Lung Circ.* 2018;27:248–253.
11. Starr JP. Tetralogy of fallot: yesterday and today. *World J Surg.* 2010;34(4):658–668.
12. Hickey EJ, Veldtman G, Bradley TJ, et al. Late risk of outcomes for adults with repaired tetralogy of Fallot from an inception cohort spanning four decades. *Eur J Cardiothorac Surg.* 2009;35(1):156–164; discussion 164.
13. Dennis M, Moore B, Kotchetkova I, Pressley L, Cordina R, Celermajer DS. Adults with repaired tetralogy: low mortality but high morbidity up to middle age. *Open Heart.* 2017;4(1):e000564.
14. Davlouros PA, Karatza AA, Gatzoulis MA, Shore DF. Timing and type of surgery for severe pulmonary regurgitation after repair of tetralogy of Fallot. *Int J Cardiol.* 2004;97(Suppl 1):91–101.
15. Gatzoulis MA, Balaji S, Webber SA, et al. Risk factors for arrhythmia and sudden cardiac death late after repair of tetralogy of Fallot: a multicentre study. *Lancet.* 2000;356(9234):975–981.
16. Cheatham JP, Hellenbrand WE, Zahn EM, et al. Clinical and hemodynamic outcomes up to 7 years after transcatheter pulmonary valve replacement in the US Melody Valve Investigational Device Exemption Trial. *Circulation.* 2015;131(22):1960–1970.

9.

HYPOPLASTIC LEFT HEART SYNDROME

M. Navaratnam and C. Ramamoorthy

STEM CASE AND KEY QUESTIONS

A 3 kg neonate (36-weeks gestation) with a prenatal diagnosis of hypoplastic left heart syndrome (HLHS) was delivered by cesarean section 6 hours ago for premature labor and is currently being medically managed in the neonatal intensive care unit. Prostaglandin E1 (PGE1) infusion was started at 0.01 mcg/kg/min soon after birth. When the baby was delivered the preductal O_2 sat was 70% on room air. Over the last hour the baby has become increasingly tachypneic and more desaturated with respiratory rate of 60 to 70 breaths per minute and mild intercostal and subcostal retractions. The preductal peripheral capillary oxygen saturation (SpO_2) is now 60% despite being on high flow nasal cannula at 6l per minute. The baby has an umbilical artery catheter (UAC) line and a double lumen umbilical vein catheter (UVC) line. Blood pressure measured from the UAC is 50/28 with a mean arterial pressure of 35 mmHg and heart rate is 174 bpm. Cerebral near infrared spectroscopy is 40%. She has cool peripheries. The baby's core temperature is 35.8 degrees Celsius; arterial blood gas: pH 7.25, PCO_2 32, PO_2 28, B-8, HCO_3 18.6, lactate 5.4; hematocrit 43.3, hemoglobin 14.6, white blood cell count 9.1; blood urea nitrogen: urea 9, creatinine 0.8.

Transthoracic echo shows anatomy consistent with mitral atresia and aortic atresia and a severely hypoplastic left ventricle (LV). There is a restrictive atrial septum and enlarged left atrium (LA). There is mild to moderately reduced right ventricle (RV) function but no significant atrioventricular valve regurgitation. There is a patent ductus arteriosus (PDA) with bidirectional flow.

Chest X-ray shows increased interstitial markings suggestive of pulmonary congestion.

WHAT IS HLHS? DESCRIBE HOW OXYGENATED BLOOD FROM THE LUNGS GETS TO THE SYSTEMIC CIRCULATION IN NEONATES BORN WITH HLHS? HOW IS THE NEONATE WITH HLHS MEDICALLY MANAGED PRIOR TO THE NORWOOD PROCEDURE? WHAT ARE THE CAUSES OF METABOLIC ACIDOSIS IN A NEONATE BORN WITH HLHS? HOW WILL PH AFFECT PULMONARY-TO-SYSTEMIC FLOW RATIO (QP:QS)? WHAT ARE THE SURGICAL OPTIONS FOR A BABY BORN WITH HLHS? WHAT PREOPERATIVE FACTORS ARE ASSOCIATED WITH DECREASED SURVIVAL AFTER STAGE I PALLIATION? BRIEFLY DESCRIBE STAGE II AND III PALLIATION FOR HLHS.

You have been asked to take this baby to the cardiac catheterization lab for an urgent atrial septostomy to improve intracardiac mixing and arterial oxygenation.

DESCRIBE HOW CARDIAC PHYSIOLOGY IN HLHS IS ALTERED BY THE SIZE OF THE ATRIAL SEPTAL DEFECT (ASD). WHAT ARE THE OPTIONS FOR ENLARGING THE ASD? WHAT ARE YOUR CONCERNS FOR TRANSPORTING THIS BABY?

You decide to start the baby on milrinone at 0.5 mcg/kg/min and dopamine at 5 mcg/kg/min to augment cardiac output and oxygen delivery and actively warm the baby with a heating pad. You transport the baby on high flow nasal cannula with the intention of intubating him in the catheterization lab. After transferring him onto the cardiac catheterization table you establish routine American Society of Anesthesiologists monitoring and transduce the UAC and UVC line.

You successfully intubate the baby with 3.5 uncuffed endotracheal tube (ETT) after administering ketamine and rocuronium. After securing the ETT and checking depth with fluoroscopy you start positioning the baby for the cardiac procedure. The catheterization lab nurse shows you that the prostaglandin E (PGE) infusion has become disconnected from the patient. You are not sure when exactly this happened.

HOW DOES PGE1 WORK? WHAT ARE THE POTENTIAL SIDE EFFECTS? WHAT ARE YOUR CONCERNS REGARDING THE PROSTAGLANDIN INTERRUPTION?

You change the tubing of the PGE infusion, clean the intraveneous (IV) port with alcohol and restart the PGE at a higher rate of 0.05 mcg/kg/min to compensate for the disconnection. You ask the cardiologist to perform a quick transthoracic echocardiogram (TTE) to assess ductal patency. The TTE shows bidirectional flow through the PDA confirming ductal patency. The baby's groin is then sterilized and draped and the interventional cardiologist obtains access to the right femoral vein with a 5F sheath. The atrial septum is punctured with a Brockenbrough needle and a 6Fr transeptal sheath is advanced over the needle. After deployment of a stent across the septum the baby becomes bradycardic and hypotensive with a heart rate of 80 bpm and blood pressure of 35/20 and loss of waveform on pulse oximetry.

You give 10 mcg/kg epinephrine IV and start cardiopulmonary resuscitation (CPR) according to pediatric advanced life support algorithm and call a code blue.

WHAT IS THE DIFFERENTIAL DIAGNOSIS?

The cardiologist performs an angiogram and says that the wire appears to be sticking out of the back of the LA. TTE shows a pericardial effusion. The cardiologist is concerned that they have perforated the LA. An extracorporeal membrane oxygenation (ECMO) code is called and you continue with CPR. The surgeon, perfusionist, and ECMO team arrive. The surgeon performs a median sternotomy, relieves the pericardial tamponade, and cannulates the right atrium and main pulmonary artery and initiates veno-arterial (VA) ECMO. The tear in the LA is repaired and an atrial septectomy is performed. Bilateral pulmonary artery (PA) bands are placed to control pulmonary blood flow. The baby is stabilized with blood transfusion, calcium, and bicarbonate bolus and an epinephrine infusion, and you prepare to transport the baby back to the cardiovascular intensive care unit (CVICU) on ECMO.

WHAT IS THE DIFFERENCE BETWEEN VENO-ARTERIAL (VA) AND VENO-VENOUS (VV) ECMO VENO-VENOUS (VV) ECMO? WHAT ARE YOUR VENTILATION GOALS DURING ECMO? WHAT ARE YOUR CONCERNS AND PRIORITIES WHEN TRANSPORTING THE BABY BACK TO CVCIU ON ECMO?

The patient was successfully weaned off ECMO after 5 days. One week later the baby underwent a Norwood procedure with a RV–PA conduit.

DISCUSSION

WHAT IS HLHS?

Hypoplastic left heart syndrome has a reported incidence of 2 per 10,000 live births[1] and accounts for 2% to 3% of all congenital heart defects.[2] This condition occurs due to the failure of development of left-sided heart structures in utero resulting in a hypoplastic left-sided ventricle and hypoplasia of the aortic arch. The aortic and mitral valves may be severely stenotic or atretic (no antegrade blood flow). The inadequately developed left heart structures are unable to support the systemic circulation. There are 4 recognized anatomical subtypes of HLHS with varying degrees of underdevelopment of the left heart structures:

1. Mitral stenosis/aortic stenosis (MS/AS)

2. Mitral stenosis /aortic atresia (MS/AA)

3. Mitral atresia/aortic atresia (MA/AA)

4. Mitral atresia/aortic stenosis (MA/AS)

Of the four anatomic subtypes, there are emerging data that MS/AA may be associated with a worse outcome.[3] This may be due to the higher incidence for ventricular-coronary communications (coronary sinusoids and fistulae) in addition to a generalized thickening of the LA and pulmonary veins.[4]

SYSTEMIC CIRCULATION OF OXYGENATED BLOOD

When a neonate with HLHS is born, preoperative survival depends on an ASD and a PDA. Oxygen-rich blood returning from the lungs to the LA must pass through the ASD to the right atrium where it mixes with deoxygenated blood returning from the systemic venous circulation. The "mixed" blood then passes to the right ventricle and is ejected via the pulmonary artery. A proportion of blood from the pulmonary artery flows to the lungs and a proportion via the PDA to the descending aorta to supply the lower body. Depending on the anatomic subtype of HLHS (e.g., aortic atresia), the upper extremities, brain, and coronary arteries are perfused by retrograde blood flow through the PDA into the aortic arch (Figure 9.1).

In the HLHS circulation, the RV is burdened with the extra workload of pumping blood to both the lungs and the systemic circulation via the PDA. The balance of pulmonary vascular resistance (PVR) and systemic vascular resistance (SVR) determines whether blood pumped from the RV travels preferentially to the pulmonary (Qp) or systemic circulation (Qs). This ratio of blood flow is referred to as Qp:Qs and reflects the amount of pulmonary blood flow compared to systemic blood flow. In a physiologically normal neonate, this ratio is 1:1. In a neonate with HLHS, this ratio can be as high as 2:1, 3:1, or more, if there is little right-to-left flow through the PDA. All factors that decrease PVR will increase pulmonary blood flow at the expense of systemic blood flow resulting in significant metabolic acidosis (Figure 9.2).

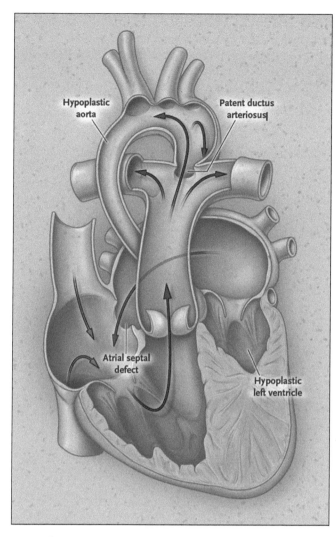

Fig. 9.1 Reproduced from Ohye RG, Sleeper LA, Mahony L, et al. Pediatric Heart Network Investigators. Comparison of shunt types in the Norwood procedure for single-ventricle lesions. *N Engl J Med.* 2010;362:1980–1992.

MEDICALLY MANAGING HLHS PRIOR TO THE NORWOOD PROCEDURE

A neonate born with HLHS must be medically optimized prior to undergoing the Norwood procedure. Preoperative

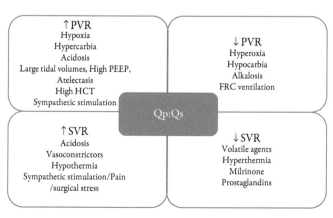

Fig. 9.2 Factors affecting PVR and SVR.

stabilization is associated with improved outcomes.[5] After initial assessment, immediate treatment in the delivery room for known HLHS babies involves:

1. Institution of PGE1: Closure of the PDA is incompatible with life and, therefore, must be kept patent with a prostaglandin infusion.

2. Placement of UA and UVC catheter.

3. Ideally, the baby should be spontaneously ventilating in room air so that she can self-regulate her Qp:Qs. Peripheral oxygen SpO_2 should be as close as possible to 80% with inspired oxygen concentration close to room air.

4. Transfer to neonatal intensive care unit or CVICU.

5. Postnatal TTE to confirm diagnosis and assess other anatomy such as atrioventricular valve regurgitation, restrictive atrial septum, size of the LV, presence of anomalous pulmonary venous return, presence of coronary artery fistulae, or sinusoids to the LV.

6. 15% to 30% of HLHS neonates have extracardiac anomalies or genetic syndromes such as CHARGE, Turner, and Noonan, and a thorough evaluation for these problems should also be performed since they are associated with a worse 5-year survival.[6]

The distribution of cardiac output in these neonates depends on the relative resistances in the pulmonary and systemic circuits. After birth, the PVR slowly decreases over hours or days and the Qp:Qs may increase to 2:1, 3:1, or more. If the PDA is large, there may be excessive pulmonary blood flow whereas a more restrictive PDA may limit pulmonary overcirculation. Excessive pulmonary blood flow may cause a decrease in systemic cardiac output and oxygen delivery resulting in anaerobic metabolism, lactic acidosis, and end-organ dysfunction such as coronary ischemia, acute tubular necrosis, gastrointestinal ischemia,[7] cerebral ischemia, and liver failure. Insufficient pulmonary blood flow will result in a lower arterial oxygen content and decreased oxygen delivery to the vital organs with a potential for hypoxic insult.

Overall, the goal is adequate oxygen delivery to tissues, which can be assessed with pulse oximetry and cerebral and/or renal near infrared spectroscopy and arterial blood gases.

Adequate oxygen delivery to the tissues depends on both adequate cardiac output and arterial oxygen content (CaO_2), which depends on normal HgB conc and arterial oxygen saturation (SaO_2).

Recall the equation:

$$CaO_2 = (SaO_2 \times Hb \times 1.34) + 0.003(PaO_2)$$

Extrapolating from the Fick equation and ignoring the amount of dissolved oxygen that contributes to oxygen content, we can simplify and calculate Qp:Qs as

$$Qp / Qs = (SaO_2 - SmvO_2) / (SpvO_2 - SaO_2)$$

Assuming a mixed venous oxygen saturation ($SmvO_2$) of 60% and pulmonary vein oxygen saturation (pvO_2) of 100%, an arterial saturation (SaO_2) of 80% suggests a balanced Qp:Qs of 1:1.

Arterial oxygen saturation >85% suggests excessive pulmonary blood flow and this may be at the expense of systemic flow.[8] It is important to correlate SpO_2 with blood pressure and markers of end-organ perfusion.

If there is excessive pulmonary blood flow, the Qp:Qs balance can be altered by

- Agents that increase PVR such as hypoxic or hypercapnic gas mixtures. Published data suggest that hypoxic gas mixtures may not provide as adequate cerebral and tissue oxygenation as hypercapnic gas mixtures for the ventilated patient.[8–12]

- Decrease SVR by avoiding hypothermia and using agents such as Milrinone.[13–15]

- Nasal continuous airway pressure (CPAP) on room air may help to relieve respiratory distress and elevate the PVR whilst maintaining spontaneous ventilation.

- Severe respiratory distress from pulmonary overcirculation may necessitate intubation, sedation, and ventilation to allow for a slight respiratory acidosis to increase PVR.

- Diuretics to treat pulmonary edema.

- Total cardiac output should be maintained with adequate preload and heart rate. If right heart function is compromised, this can be supported with inotropes.

- Early surgery in the first few days of life.

In neonates with decompensated HLHS, physical signs include listlessness, poor peripheral pulses, cool extremities, systemic hypotension, tachypnea, hepatomegaly, and lab abnormalities include acidosis, hyperkalemia, and hypoglycemia.

CAUSES OF METABOLIC ACIDOSIS

Metabolic acidosis suggests a maldistribution of cardiac output and insufficient oxygen delivery to tissues leading to anaerobic metabolism and lactic acidosis.[9] Clinical values that can be used to assess metabolic acidosis include pH, acid-base status, and lactate. Early studies indicated that preoperative metabolic acidosis was a risk factor for increased postoperative mortality.[16]

Metabolic acidosis may either be due to inadequate cardiac output or inadequate arterial oxygen content.

EFFECT OF PH ON QP:QS

Inadequate cardiac output leading to metabolic acidosis may result if there is excessive pulmonary blood flow at the expense of systemic blood flow(Qp:Qs >2:1) with a concomitant high arterial oxygen saturation (>85%).

Inadequate arterial oxygen content leading to metabolic acidosis may result from decreased pulmonary blood flow or inadequate mixing of oxygenated and deoxygenated blood such as occurs with a severely restrictive ASD. Hypoxemia may be further exacerbated by pulmonary congestion. Acidosis will also increase the PVR and, therefore, reduce pulmonary blood flow and worsen the hypoxemia.

Figure 9.2 illustrates how pH can affect Qp: Qs.

SURGICAL OPTIONS

Over the past 20 years, due to significant advancements in surgical techniques, cardiopulmonary bypass, medical therapy, anesthesia care, and interstage care, there is an expectation that 70% of these patients should survive into adulthood.[17]

The 3 main surgical options available are

1. Neonatal Norwood procedure.

2. Neonatal Hybrid procedure.

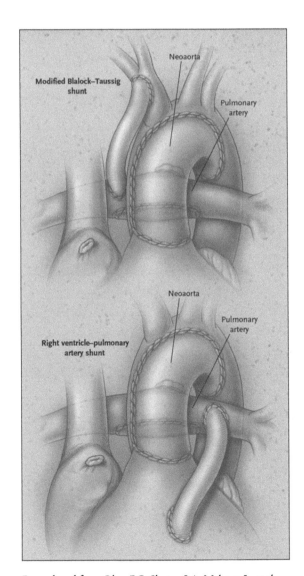

Fig. 9.3 Reproduced from Ohye RG, Sleeper LA, Mahony L, et al. Pediatric Heart Network Investigators. Comparison of shunt types in the Norwood procedure for single-ventricle lesions. *N Engl J Med.* 2010;362:1980–1992.

3. Neonatal heart transplant.

The Neonatal Norwood Stage I procedure involves three main components (Figure 9.3):

1. Reconstruction of the ascending aorta +/− arch and creation of a neoaorta by constructing an outflow from the systemic RV through the pulmonary valve. This neoaorta also provides blood flow to the native aortic root and coronary arteries.

2. Transection and oversewing of the main pulmonary artery. A reliable source of pulmonary blood flow is achieved with a polytetrofluroethylene shunt either via the systemic to pulmonary route (right innominate or subclavian artery to right PA—modified Blalock-Taussig shunt) or via a RV to PA conduit, popularly referred to as the Sano shunt.

3. Ensuring a nonrestrictive ASD.

The initial postoperative period appears to be more stable with a RV–PA conduit than with a Blalock-Taussig shunt.[18] In the RV–PA conduit, the lack of diastolic run-off from the systemic circulation to the pulmonary circulation leads to a higher diastolic blood pressure, increased coronary blood flow, and enhanced postoperative stability. Theoretical disadvantages of the RV–PA conduit include less favorable pulmonary artery growth and right ventricle dysfunction from the surgical ventriculotomy. The single ventricle reconstruction trial showed no difference in 3-year survival between the RV–PA conduit and the Blalock-Taussig shunt.[19]

PREOPERATIVE FACTORS FOR DECREASED SURVIVAL AFTER STAGE I PALLIATION

Reported risk factors for increased morbidity and mortality during and after Norwood stage I palliation include

1. Patient-specific factors: gestational age <34weeks,[6] birth weight <2.5 kg,[20,21] and associated genetic or noncardiac abnormalities.[6]

2. Anatomic factors: restrictive atrial septum, significant tricuspid regurgitation,[9,11] ascending aorta size <2 mm,[22] and MS/AA.[3]

3. Preoperative factors: shock,[21] poor ventricular function, and ECMO.[6,23]

The hybrid procedure was developed as an alternative first-stage palliation to treat these high-risk neonates and involves a PDA stent, surgical placement of bilateral PA bands via median sternotomy, and stenting of the atrial septum if restrictive. The potential advantage of the hybrid procedure is that it avoids the adverse effects of cardiopulmonary bypass during the neonatal period. However, this is at the expense of a more complex stage II palliation at 4 to 6 months, which consists of stent removal, aortic arch reconstruction, pulmonary artery reconstruction, and bidirectional cavopulmonary anastomosis (bidirectional Glenn). Centers committed to the hybrid stage I approach achieve similar results to the Norwood stage 1 approach.[24]

STAGES II AND III PALLIATION FOR HLHS

Due to the widespread shortage of neonatal heart donors, most pediatric cardiac centers opt for a three-stage palliation starting with either the neonatal Norwood or hybrid procedure.

Second-stage palliation

Creating the superior vena cava to right pulmonary artery anastomoses around 3 to 6 months of age resulting in a bi-directional cavopulmonary shunt (Glenn shunt). The goal of the second stage is to start volume unloading the RV as early as possible and reduce the duration of pulmonary bed exposure to systemic pressures. The patient continues to remain desaturated since deoxygenated blood from the lower extremity still returns to the heart via the inferior vena cava and mixes with oxygenated blood.

Third-stage palliation

Creating the inferior vena cava to right pulmonary artery anastomosis (Fontan circulation), using an external conduit, between 2 and 4 years of age. The end goal of palliation is to restore an "in series" circulation, complete the RV volume unloading and normalize oxygen saturation. Deoxygenated blood returns to the lungs by passive flow via a total cavopulmonary connection, is oxygenated, and returns to the heart via pulmonary veins and the RV pumps this oxygenated blood to the body.

There is now improved understanding of the Fontan circulation as an altered physiological state with a high rate of late complications. Current consensus guidelines recommend lifelong care with an adult congenital heart disease specialist and a proactive approach to surveillance and treatment of anticipated problems.[25] Although some patients may survive into early adult years without significant medical intervention, many patients develop right ventricular dysfunction over time and may require orthotopic heart transplantation.

SIZE OF ASD AND CARDIAC PHYSIOLOGY

In patients with mitral atresia or severe mitral stenosis, oxygenated blood from the pulmonary veins has to get from the LA to the right side of the heart to get to the systemic circulation. This mandates an interatrial shunt.

Unrestrictive ASD

As PVR falls in the first few days of life, a large ASD in combination with a large PDA will lead to pulmonary overcirculation, which may lead to decreased systemic perfusion. An additional risk from the increased total cardiac output (from a high Qp:Qs) may be an increased volume work on the RV and a high output cardiac failure.

Highly restrictive ASD

A highly restrictive ASD will lead to LA hypertension and, consequently, excessive limitation of pulmonary blood flow. A chest X-ray may show increased pulmonary congestion (a sign of pulmonary venous hypertension). Instead of the typical partial pressure arterial oxygen (PaO_2) of 40 mmHg seen in HLHS, in the setting of restrictive ASD and LA hypertension, PO_2 may be 20 mmHg or lower. Hypoxemia and acidemia can eventually lead to depressed myocardial function and heart failure.

Approximately 10% to 20% of fetuses diagnosed with HLHS have a restrictive ASD.[26] Intact or restrictive ASD has been well described as a risk factor for increased early and late morbidity and mortality.[20,21,27] This may be due to pulmonary vein hypertension cause by the obstruction to blood flow coming back from the lungs.[27] Several studies have shown that pulmonary vein hypertension causes rapid histological and vascular changes that may trigger irreversible pulmonary hypertension[28,29] and increased PVR. PVR is an important parameter for determining whether HLHS patients reach and survive the Fontan palliation.

Options for enlarging the ASD

There is no uniform consensus on the optimal management of HLHS with an intact or severely restrictive interatrial communication. Techniques include bedside balloon septostomies, surgical septostomies in the operating room, and cardiac catheter lab based approaches such as percutaneous blade septostomy, Brockenbrough transseptal needle septoplasties, and radiofrequency perforation with or without atrial stent placement.

SIDE EFFECTS OF PGE1

PGE1 (also known as alprostadil) is a prostaglandin that was first noted to be a potent relaxant of the ductus arteriosus in 1973[30] and was approved for clinical use by the Food and Drug Administration in 1981. Its use has revolutionized preoperative survival for babies born with ductal-dependent congenital heart disease such as HLHS. The onset of action is 15 minutes to 3 hours, and it is rapidly metabolized by the lungs. The metabolites are excreted by the kidney and its half-life is 5 to 10 minutes.

Frequently reported short-term side effects include apnea, hypoventilation, hypotension, rhythm disturbances, vasodilation, flushing, diarrhea, seizures, and hyperpyrexia.[31–33] Frequent apneas may necessitate intubation of the neonate. The short-term effects of PGE1 are easily reversed when the infusion is switched off.

Reported long-term effects include gastric outlet obstruction, metabolic derangements, platelet dysfunction, and cortical hyperostosis.

The traditional starting dose ranges from 0.05 mcg/kg/mn up to 0.4 mcg/kg/mn, decreasing to 0.01 mcg/kg/mn once the desired effect is achieved. Many centers are now starting with lower doses of 0.001 to 0.02 mcg/kg/mn. Because the incidence of side effects appears to be dose dependent.

Since PGE1 has a very short half-life, interruption of the infusion may lead to constriction of the ductus arteriosus. Once the PDA starts to constrict an increasing amount of blood is driven into the pulmonary circulation at the expense of hypotension and circulatory shock.

VA VERSUS VV ECMO

Since its successful adoption in the 1970s to support neonates with severe respiratory distress, ECMO has become an important modality of cardiorespiratory support for pediatric and neonatal patients with cardiac and/or respiratory disease. In 2015, 446 neonates, 319 infants (age: >30 days to <1 year), and 281 children (age: 1 to <16 years) with cardiac disease requiring ECMO support were reported to the Extracorporeal Life Support Organization registry with survival to discharge of 45%, 55%, and 61%, respectively.[34] There is a reported 5% to 20% incidence of ECMO support following stage I palliation.[18,35] As the complexity of congenital heart surgery increases across the United States, the use of ECMO in neonates and children for cardiac indications is expected to grow.[34]

During ECMO support blood is drained from the venous system into a mechanical pump with an oxygenator where the blood becomes fully saturated with oxygen and CO_2 is removed. Oxygenation is determined by flow rate, and CO_2 elimination can be controlled by adjusting the rate of countercurrent gas flow through the oxygenator.[36] Blood is then reinfused into the body via a vein (VV ECMO) or into the arterial side (VA ECMO; Figure 9.4.

In neonates and pediatric patients <25 kg, ECMO can be established via peripheral cannulation in the neck (right internal jugular to right atrium and right common carotid into aortic arch) using Seldinger or cut-down techniques. Transthoracic cannulation via a sternotomy is also a technique used especially for small babies or those with complex anatomy. Transthoracic cannulation usually involves placement of a venous cannula in the right atrial appendage and an arterial cannula in the aortic arch.

Patients over 25 kg with favorable anatomy can be cannulated peripherally via the groin vessels.

Table 9.1 summarizes the differences between VV and VA ECMO. The main difference is that VA ECMO provides both respiratory and hemodynamic support whereas VV ECMO only provides respiratory support.

VENTILATION DURING ECMO

The goal of ventilation for patients supported with VA or VV ECMO is to allow the lungs to rest and facilitate lung protection and recovery. The goal of ventilation is to prevent atelectasis and avoid barotrauma to the lungs. The mode of ventilation chosen (e.g., pressure regulated volume mode)

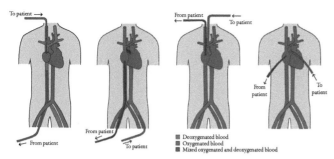

Fig. 9.4 Cannulation sites for V-V and V-A ECMO (Gaffney AM, Wildhirt SM, Griffin MJ, Annich GM, Radomski MW. Extracorporeal life support. BMJ. 2010;341:c5317. doi: 10.1136/bmj.c5317).

should avoid barotrauma and volutrauma. Tidal volumes of 1–4 mL/kg with plateau pressures not exceeding 20–24 mmHg and a positive end-expiratory pressure of 10 to 15 can be used to aid lung recruitment. Ventilation rate can be set low varying from 10 to 20 breaths per minute depending on the age of the patient. Fraction of inspired oxygen (FiO_2) should be <50% to avoid oxygen free radical-induced lung injury and absorption atelectasis.

TRANSPORTING TO CVICU ON ECMO

Neonates and children supported with ECMO may require intrahospital transport (IHT) as an important part of their successful management, for example, transporting to the catheterization lab for balloon atrial septostomy to relieve left atrial hypertension and pulmonary edema. Studies have shown that IHT to the catheterization lab for diagnostic or therapeutic intervention resulted in a change in management in 83% of patients.[37,38] However, there are significant risks inherent to transporting critically ill patients supported on ECMO. Potential problems during transport include

1. Cannulae migration/displacement from major blood vessels

2. Multiple infusion pumps that require long tubing

3. Significant bleeding from sternotomy and cannulae site

4. ECMO pump failure

5. Hypotension

6. Comprehensive coordination of multiple personnel and chaos minimization

A recent publication described focusing on 3 phases to facilitate successful ECMO transport: preparatory phase, transport phase, and posttransport stabilization.[38]. The authors described the use of a checklist and an ECMO coordinator to ensure safety during transport. Checklist items included review of sedation, muscle relaxation, monitors, back-up battery, gas supply, blood products, and an emergency resuscitation cart. Their reported time for preparation before IHT was approximately 30 minutes.

Table 9.1 DIFFERENCES BETWEEN VENO-ARTERIAL AND VENO-VENOUS EXTRACORPOREAL MEMBRANE OXYGENATION

	VA ECMO	VV ECMO
Cannulation	Venous + Arterial	Venous (single or double)
Cardiac support	Provides cardiac support (both LV and RV)	No cardiac support
Pulmonary blood flow	Bypasses pulmonary circulation	Maintains pulmonary blood flow
RV support	Supports RV failure	Does not support RV failure
End organ perfusion	Depends on ECMO flow and native cardiac output	Depends on native cardiac output
ECMO flow	Lower perfusion rate (e.g., 80–100 mL/kg/mn)	Higher perfusion rate (e.g.,100–120 mL/kg/mn)
PA pressures	Decreased	Elevated
Arterial SpO_2	Controlled by ECMO flow; higher PaO_2 achieved	80%–95%; lower PaO_2 achieved
Configuration	ECMO circuit in parallel to heart and lungs	ECMO circuit in series to heart and lungs

Note. ECMO = extracorporeal membrane oxygenation; LV = left ventricle; RV = right ventricle; PA = pulmonary artery.

Successful transport is a labor-intensive process involving multidisciplinary teamwork and communication. However, despite the risks and logistics involved published reports have shown that IHT can be carried out safely and without major complications.[37,38]

CONCLUSIONS

Neonates born with HLHS can be successfully managed both pre- and postoperatively provided careful attention is paid to balancing the Qp:Qs, avoiding metabolic acidosis, and ensuring adequate end-organ perfusion. An understanding of ECMO management and transport is also required because ECMO remains an important rescue modality following stage I palliation.

REVIEW QUESTIONS

1. Of the following conditions, which is the **LEAST** likely to decrease PVR?

A. alkalosis
B. FiO_2 1.0

C. hypocapnia
D. polycythemia

Answer: D

2. Of the following preoperative factors, which is the **LEAST** associated with decreased survival after stage I palliation for HLHS?

    A. birth weight less than 2.5 kg
    B. metabolic acidosis
    C. restrictive ASD
    D. trivial tricuspid valve regurgitation

Answer: D

3. Which one of the following will **MOST** likely decrease Qp:Qs?

    A. alkalosis
    B. hypothermia
    C. milrinone
    D. oxygen

Answer: C

4. Which one of the following statements **BEST** describes VA ECMO?

    A. bypasses pulmonary circulation
    B. elevates pulmonary artery pressures
    C. does not support end organ perfusion
    D. effective only in supporting left heart failure

Answer: A

5. In a neonate born with HLHS, if the peripheral oxygen saturation is 90%, the Qp:Qs is **MOST** likely

    A. 0.8:1.
    B. 1:1.
    C. <2:1.
    D. 3:1.

Answer: D

QUESTIONS AND ANSWERS

This chapter has accompanying questions and answers which are available to subscribers as part of the Oxford eLearning platform. To access the questions, go to ✔ http:// oxfordmedicine. com/pediatricanesthesiaPBL

REFERENCES

1. Botto LD, Correa A, Erickson JD. Racial and temporal variations in the prevalence of heart defects. *Pediatrics.* 2001;107:E32.
2. Morris CD, Outcalt J, Menashe VD. Hypoplastic left heart syndrome: natural history in a geographically defined population. *Pediatrics.* 1990;85:977–983.
3. Vida VL, Bach EA, LArrazabal A, Gauvreau K. Surgical outcome for patients with the mitral stenosis-aortic atresia variant of hypoplastic left heart syndrome. *J Thorac Cardiovasc Surg.* 2008 Feb;135(2):339–346.
4. Shillingford M, Ceithaml E, Bleiweis M. Surgical considerations in the management of hypoplastic left heart syndrome. *Semin Cardiothorac Vasc Anesth.* 2013 Jun;17(2):128–136.
5. Mahle WT, Clancy RR, Moss EM, et al. Neurodevelopmental outcome and lifestyle assessment in school-aged and adolescent children with hypoplastic left heart syndrome. *Pediatrics.* 2000;105:1082–1089.
6. Jacobs JP, Obrien SM, Chai PJ, Morell VO, Lindberg HL, Quintessenza JA. Management of 239 patients with hypoplastic left heart syndrome and related malformations from 1993 to 2007. *AnnThorac Surg.* 2008;85:1691–1697.
7. McElhinney DB, Hedrick HL, Bush DM, et al. Necrotizing enterocolitis in neonates with congenital heart disease: risk factors and outcomes. *Pediatrics.* 2000;106:1080–1087.
8. Mora GA, Pizarro C, Jacobs ML, Norwood WI: Experimental model of single ventricle: influence of carbon dioxide on pulmonary vascular dynamics. *Circulation.* 1994; 90:43–46.
9. Stieh J, Fischer G, Scheewe J, et al. Impact of preoperative treatment strategies on the early perioperative outcome in neonates with hypoplastic left heart syndrome. *J Thorac Cardiovasc Surg.* 2006;131:1122–1129.
10. Tabbutt S, Ramamoorthy C, Montenegro LM, et al. Impact of inspired gas mixtures on preoperative infants with hypoplastic left heart syndrome during controlled ventilation. *Circulation.* 2001;104:159–164.
11. Johnson BA, Mussatto K, Uhing MR, Zimmerman H, Tweddell J, Ghanayem N. Variability in the preoperative management of infants with hypoplastic left heart syndrome. *Pediatr Cardiol.* 2008;29:515–520.
12. Ramamoorthy C, Tabbutt S, Kurth CD, et al. Effects of inspired hypoxic and hypercapnic gas mixtures on cerebral oxygen saturation in neonates with univentricular heart defects. *Anesthesiology.* 2002;96:283–288.
13. Krushansky E, Burbano N, Morell V, Moguillansky D, Kim Y, Orr R, Chrysostomou C, Munoz R. Preoperative management in patients with single-ventricle physiology. *Congenit Heart Dis.* 2012 Mar-Apr;7(2):96–102.
14. Shime N, Hashimoto S, Hiramatsu N, Oka T, Kageyama K, Tanaka Y. Hypoxic gas therapy using nitrogen in the preoperative management of neonates with hypoplastic left heart syndrome. *Pediatr Crit Care Med.* 2000;1:38–41.
15. Graham EM, Bradley SM, Atz AM. Preoperative management of hypoplastic left heart syndrome. *Expert Opin Pharmacother.* 2005;6:687–693.
16. Bando K, Turrentine MW, Sun K, et al. Surgical management of hypoplastic left heart syndrome. *Ann Thorac Surg.* 1996;62:70–76.
17. Feinstein JA, Benson DW, Dubin AM, et al. Hypoplastic left heart syndrome: current considerations and expectations. *J Am Coll Cardiol.* 2012;59(1 Suppl):S1–S42.
18. Ohye RG, Sleeper LA, Mahony L, et al. Pediatric Heart Network Investigators. Comparison of shunt types in the Norwood procedure for single-ventricle lesions. *N Engl J Med.* 2010;362:1980–1992.
19. Newburger JW, Sleeper LA, Frommelt PC, et al. Transplantation-free survival and interventions at 3 years in the single ventricle reconstruction trial. *Circulation.* 2014;129:2013–2020.
20. Gaynor JW, Mahle WT, Cohen MI, et al. Risk factors for mortality after the Norwood procedure. *Eur J Cardiothorac Surg.* 2002;22:82–89.
21. Tabbutt S, Dominguez TE, Ravishankar C, et al. Outcomes after the stage I reconstruction comparing the right ventricular to pulmonary artery conduit with the modified Blalock Taussig shunt. *Ann Thorac Surg.* 2005;80:1582–1591.
22. Ashburn DA, McCrindle BW, Tchervenkov CI, et al. Outcomes after the Norwood operation in neonates with critical aortic stenosis or aortic valve atresia. *J Thorac Cardiovasc Surg.* 2003;125:1070–1082.
23. Tabbutt S, Ghanayem N, Ravishankar C, et al. Pediatric Heart Network Investigators. Risk factors for hospital morbidity and mortality after the Norwood procedure: a report from the Pediatric Heart Network Single Ventricle Reconstruction Trial. *J Thorac Cardiovasc Surg.* 2012;144:882–895.
24. Baba K, Kotani Y, Chetan D, et al. Hybrid versus Norwood strategies for single-ventricle palliation. *Circulation.* 2012;126(suppl 1):S123–S131.

25. Warnes CA, Williams RG, Bashore TM, et al. ACC/AHA 2008 guidelines for the management of adults with congenital heart disease: executive summary: a report of the American College of Cardiology/American Heart Association Task Force on Practice Guidelines (writing committee to develop guidelines for the management of adults with congenital heart disease). *Circulation.* 2008;118(23):2395–2451.

26. Twite MD, Ing RJ. Anesthetic considerations in infants with hypoplastic left heart syndrome. *Semin Cardiothorac Vasc Anesth.* 2013 Jun;17(2):137–145.

27. Lowenthal A, Kipps AK, Brook MM, Meadows J, Azakie A, Moon-Grady AJ. Prenatal diagnosis of atrial restriction in hypoplastic left heart syndrome is associated with decreased 2-year survival. *Prenat Diagn.* 2012;32:485–490.

28. Grant CA, Robertson B. Microangiography of the pulmonary arterial system in "hypoplastic left heart syndrome." *Circulation.* 1972;45(2):382–388.

29. Rychik J, Rome JJ, Collins MH, DeCampli WM, Spray TL. The hypoplastic left heart syndrome with intact atrial septum: atrial morphology, pulmonary vascular histopathology and outcome. *J Am Coll Cardiol.* 1999;34(2):554–560.

30. Coceani F, Olley PM. The response of the ductus arteriosus to prostaglandins. *Can J Physiol Pharmacol.* 1973;51:220e5.

31. Freed MD, Heymann MA, Lewis AB, Roehl SL, Kensey RC. Prostaglandin E1 infants with ductus arteriosus-dependent congenital heart disease. *Circulation.* 1981;64:899–905.

32. Hallidie-Smith KA. Prostaglandin E1 in suspected ductus dependent cardiac malformation. *Arch Dis Child.* 1984;59:1020–1026.

33. Lewis AB, Freed MD, Heyman MA Roehl SL, Kensey RC. Side effect of therapy with prostaglandin in infants with critical congenital heart defects. *Circulation.* 1981;64:893–898.

34. Thiagarajan RR, Barbaro RP, Rycus PT, Mcmullan DM, Conrad SA, Fortenberry JD, Paden ML. Extracorporeal Life Support Organization Registry international report 2016. *ASAIO J.* 2017 Jan/Feb;63(1):6067.

35. Fernandez RP, Joy BF, Allen R, Stewart J, Miller-Tate H, Miao Y, Nicholson L, Cua CL. Interstage survival for patients with hypoplastic left heart syndrome after ECMO. *Pediatr Cardiol.* 2017 Jan;38(1):50–55.

36. Schmidt M, Tachon G, Devilliers C, et al. Blood oxygenation and decarboxylation determinants during venovenous ECMO for respiratory failure in adults. *Intensive Care Med.* 2013;39:838–846.

37. Booth KL, Roth SJ, Perry SB, et al: Cardiac catheterization of patients supported by extracorporeal membrane oxygenation. *J Am Coll Cardiol.* 2002;6(40):1681–1686

38. Prodhan P, Fiser RT, Cenac S, et al. Intrahospital transport of children on extracorporeal membrane oxygenation: indications, process, interventions, and effectiveness. *Pediatr Crit Care Med.* 2010 Mar;11(2):227–233.

10.

TRANSPOSITION OF THE GREAT ARTERIES

Andrew T. Waberski and Nina Deutsch

STEM CASE AND KEY QUESTIONS

Five hours after birth, a 38-week-old baby boy develops prominent cyanosis. He was born by caesarean section for breech position to a G1P0 mother with limited prenatal care. Initial APGARs (appearance, pulse, grimace, activity, and respiration) were 6 and 8 with stimulation. Mother reports two family members with a history of congenital cardiac disease.

At birth, the patient's oxygen saturation was 90%. During the course of the newborn stay, the child has developed lower oxygen saturations to both pre- and postductal pulse oximeters. Current vital signs are weight 3.1 kg, heart rate 145 bpm, right arm blood pressure 65/32 mmHg, left leg blood pressure 62/34 mmHg, respiratory rate 45 breaths per minutes, preductal oxygen saturation 60%, and postductal oxygen saturation 62%. Physical examination shows prominent perioral and periorbital cyanosis, diminished second heart sound and a 2/6 systolic ejection murmur. The patient has normal facial and skeletal features and no hepatosplenomegaly.

WHAT TESTS SHOULD YOU ORDER? WHAT IS THE FIRST LINE OF TREATMENT FOR A PERSISTENTLY HYPOXIC NEWBORN WITHOUT IMPROVEMENT FROM OXYGEN SUPPLEMENTATION?

After institution of prostaglandin E1 (PGE1) the patient's oxygen saturation elevates to 73%. Chest radiography shows a narrow mediastinum and ovoid shape of the heart, no cardiomegaly, and increased pulmonary vasculature. Electrocardiogram shows right axis deviation and normal sinus rhythm.

Urgent 2-dimensional echocardiography shows transposition of the great arteries (TGA), situs solitus, d-loop ventricles, and d-loop great arteries, small atrial secundum defect, small patent foramen ovale, bidirectional patent ductus

arteriosus (PDA), normal biventricular function, and intact ventricular septum.

WHAT IS THE ANATOMICAL CLASSIFICATION OF TGA? WHAT IS THE TYPICAL PRESENTATION AND CLINICAL FEATURES OF TGA? HOW COMMON IS TGA AS A CONGENITAL CARDIAC DISEASE? WHAT ARE THE FEATURES OF DEXTRO-TGA (D-TGA)? WHAT ARE THE LESIONS ASSOCIATED WITH TGA? WHAT IS THE NORMAL POSITION OF THE CORONARY ANATOMY? HOW DOES THE CORONARY ANATOMY IN TGA DIFFER FROM NORMAL CORONARY ANATOMY? WHAT IS CONGENITALLY CORRECTED TGA, AND HOW DOES IT DIFFER FROM UNCORRECTED D-TGA? DESCRIBE THE PATHOPHYSIOLOGIC CIRCULATION ASSOCIATED WITH THIS CARDIAC LESION. WHY DOES THE PATIENT'S SATURATION IMPROVE WITH PGE1?

The patient is intubated and mechanically ventilated without resolution of cyanosis despite the initiation of intravenous PGE1.

IN THIS PATIENT, WHAT METHODS ARE TYPICALLY INSTITUTED TO OXYGENATE AND STABILIZE THE PATIENT WITH RESTRICTIVE ATRIAL COMMUNICATION AND D-TGA IF PGE1 IS NOT EFFECTIVE?

Interventional cardiologists perform an emergency balloon atrial septostomy (BAS) in the intensive care unit without event. Oxygen saturation improves to 88% on upper and lower extremities. The patient's sedation and mechanical ventilator are weaned, and the patient is extubated the next day.

WHAT IS THE PURPOSE OF A BAS PROCEDURE, AND WHY DOES THE SATURATION IMPROVE? HOW DOES PULMONARY VASCULAR DISEASE DEVELOP IN UNTREATED PATIENTS WITH TRANSPOSITION? WOULD THE PROGRESSION IN DISEASE ALTER WITH THE PRESENCE OF A VENTRICULAR SEPTAL DEFECT (VSD)?

The patient is taken to the operating room at day 4 of life for repair of transposition of the great arteries. During the course of the intensive care stay, the patient has been orally fed without episodes of cyanosis, maintaining a saturation of 88% to 95%, systolic blood pressures from 55 to 65 mmHg, and capillary refill time of less than 2 seconds. An infusion of PGE1 at 0.01 mcg/kg/min has been continued.

WHAT ARE THE CURRENT AND HISTORICAL SURGICAL REPAIRS FOR TGA? WHY IS TIMING OF THE SURGICAL REPAIR FOR D-TGA WITHIN THE FIRST WEEKS OF LIFE? WHAT IS AN APPROPRIATE INDUCTION TECHNIQUE FOR THIS PATIENT? IS THIS THE ONLY OPTION FOR INDUCTION? WHAT VENTILATOR SETTING SHOULD BE SET FOR THE PATIENT, INCLUDING FRACTION OF INSPIRED OXYGEN (FIO$_2$)? WHY IS THIS IMPORTANT? WHAT MONITORS ARE NECESSARY? WHAT ARE THE RISKS OF PLACING A CENTRAL VENOUS CATHETER IN A NEWBORN?

Induction with fentanyl, sevoflurane, and rocuronium is uneventful, and the patient is intubated without difficulty. Ventilation is instituted at 6 mL/kg tidal volumes with FiO$_2$ of 30%. A radial artery catheter and additional peripheral intraveneous lines are placed. Transition to bypass is uneventful with single atrial cannulation, and the patient is cooled to deep hypothermia of 16 degrees Celsius. Circulatory arrest is instituted for closure of the atrial septal defect.

WHY IS SINGLE VENOUS CANNULATION ON BYPASS PREFERRED OVER BICAVAL CANNULATION? WHICH BYPASS STRATEGY IS TYPICALLY INSTITUTED IN THE NEWBORN POPULATION WITH RESPECT TO BLOOD GAS MANAGEMENT? WHAT ARE THE BENEFITS TO PH STAT MANAGEMENT?

A left atrial pressure line is placed prior to transition from cardiopulmonary bypass, and an infusion of dopamine is started at 5 mcg/kg/min. Shortly after transition from bypass with mechanical ventilation at 100% FiO$_2$, the SpO$_2$ is 100%, radial artery blood pressure is 65/33 mmHg, and left atrial pressure is 10 mmHg. However, during echocardiographic evaluation, the cardiologist notes new mitral regurgitation directed posteriorly. At this time the left atrial pressure rises to 18 mmHg and the blood pressure is 45/22 mmHg.

WHAT IS THE ETIOLOGY OF NEW ONSET MITRAL VALVE REGURGITATION? WHAT IS THE PATHOPHYSIOLOGIC CONSEQUENCE OF THE POSITIVE FEEDBACK LOOP? WHAT IS THE MANAGEMENT FOR ELEVATED ATRIAL PRESSURES AND DECREASING BLOOD PRESSURE IN THIS SETTING?

Cardiopulmonary bypass is reinstituted to further repair the coronary anastomosis. Following repair, discontinuation of bypass is again attempted on dopamine and low-dose epinephrine with improved vital signs and no mitral regurgitation. The total bypass time now totals over 250 minutes.

WHAT ARE THE IMPLICATIONS OF PROLONGED CARDIOPULMONARY BYPASS IN A NEONATE? WHAT MANAGEMENT STRATEGIES NEED TO BE IN PLACE TO TREAT THESE?

Following treatment with multiple blood products, there is improvement in bleeding, and the patient remains stable on dopamine and low-dose epinephrine. The patient is returned to the intensive care unit for further management.

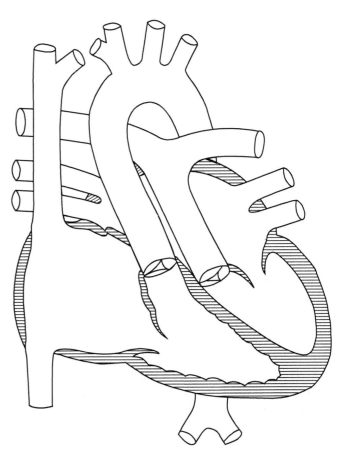

Fig. 10.1 Schematic drawing of dextro-transposition of the great arteries.

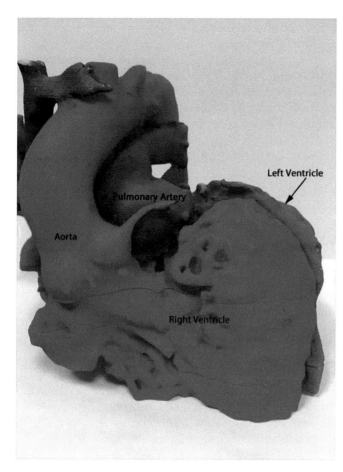

Fig. 10.2 Three-dimensional reconstruction model of uncorrected dextro-transposition of the great arteries.

WHAT ARE POSSIBLE COMPLICATIONS THAT COULD ARISE IN THE FIRST 24 HOURS FOLLOWING SURGERY?

Approximately 12 hours after arrival in the intensive care unit, the patient has a slight decrease in blood pressure, requiring an escalation of the epinephrine dose. Echocardiogram demonstrates a mild decrease in heart function. This improves over the following 24 hours.

DISCUSSION

EMBRYOLOGY AND ANATOMY

Transposition of the great arteries stems from the inability of the septum between the great arteries to properly spiral. This is considered a conotruncal anomaly with tetralogy and double outlet right ventricle being the opposite end of the scale. The consequence is concordance between the mitral valve and pulmonary valve. Anatomically, this results in 2 circulatory systems in parallel, separating the pulmonary circulation, which is fed by the left ventricle, from the systemic circulation, which is pumped from the right ventricle. Mixing between the 2 systems must occur to support life. Optimal mixing occurs as an unrestricted atrial or ductal shunt.[1]

Transposition of the great arteries most frequently presents as d-TGA or dextro-TGA (Figures 10.1 and 10.2), which is the normal embryologic cardiac tube looping of the ventricles. L-TGA, or levo-TGA, is also referred to as congenitally-corrected transposition, where the morphologic left ventricle is positioned on the right and supplies the pulmonary artery.[1]

The arterial switch operation occurs in the neonatal period, with outcomes reliant on unobstructed coronary blood flow. Normal anatomy positions both the right and left main coronary arteries in the right and left coronary cusps, respectively, facing the pulmonary artery anteriorly. In TGA, however, the coronaries are positioned posteriorly and have a more tortuous path, which may make them more difficult to reimplant. In addition to aortocoronary position, aberrant coronaries may be stenotic, atretic, intramural, or singular. These variations have severe implications on coronary reimplantation. The anesthesiologist should be mindful of the long, tortuous, and restrictive pathways in which the coronaries are positioned, as this can have direct implications on the required coronary perfusion pressure after repair. Following repair, the poorly perfused coronary will be evident by two-dimensional echocardiography with regional wall motion abnormality or atrioventricular valve regurgitation directed toward the affected coronary. The Leiden classification is most commonly used to represent coronary artery positioning.

In addition to coronary anomalies and atrial septal defects, TGA occurs with VSD 20% to 40% of the time. Left ventricular outflow tract obstruction has an incidence of 5%, with aortic coarctation and Taussig-Bing malformations occurring even less frequently. With a significant VSD, the added pulmonary blood flow may result in elevated pulmonary artery pressures and potentially pulmonary vascular disease. Where there is left ventricular outflow obstruction, cyanosis will be present due to a decrease in pulmonary blood flow.[1,2]

PATHOPHYSIOLOGY

In the normal heart, blood flow occurs in series from systemic circulation to the right side of the heart then to the pulmonary circulation followed by the left side of the heart and systemic circulation. The consequence of TGA is a parallel system that circulates deoxygenated blood systemically and oxygenated blood through the pulmonary circulation. Without adequate mixing, this circulation is fatal. Suitable mixing occurs through the PDA, atrial septal defect (ASD), or VSD. Importantly, the degree of mixing is dependent on both anatomic and physiologic components. The size and location of these shunts as well as the relative resistances met across the shunts determine the level of mixing. Unrestrictive shunts or communication at one or multiple sites allows for adequate mixing of blood between these two systems.

Mixing at the atrial level appears to be beneficial due to the relative differences in atrial pressures between the two sides of the heart. Because of this pressure gradient, oxygenated blood is shunted systemically, from the high pressure left atrium to the right atrium, through the right ventricle, and out the aorta. However, with ventricular or ductus arteriosus mixing, both of which are under higher pressure overall, bidirectional flow may occur throughout different stages of the cardiac cycle and thereby limit the relative blood flow.

Early repair prevents pulmonary overcirculation and associated heart failure. Furthermore, it allows for adequate priming of the left ventricle by not allowing the wall to thin considerably from exposure to low afterload. In this manner, it is better able to handle the expected systemic load after the arterial switch procedure.[1] If pulmonary over-circulation is left unchecked, the patient will progressively develop pulmonary vascular disease, most likely due to prolonged hypoxemia, persistently elevated pulmonary blood flow, higher pulmonary artery pressures, and polycythemia.[3]

CLINICAL PRESENTATION

The most common presentation of a previously undiagnosed patient with d-TGA is cyanosis and acidosis shortly after birth due to inadequate mixing of the two parallel systems. This is especially true in the patient with intact ventricular septum and minimal mixing at the level of the atrium or the ductus arteriosus. Conversely, if mixing is widely unrestricted, then the patient is at higher risk of developing congestive heart failure and higher pulmonary blood flow. If a coarctation is present, differential cyanosis will present with higher oxygen saturation in the lower extremity and lower saturation on limbs proximal to the ductus.

Restricted mixing, pulmonary hypertension, and prematurity are all risk factors for mortality prior to surgical repair.

Chest x-ray will demonstrate a reduction in the width of the superior mediastinum due to the anteriorly displaced aorta, typical known as an "egg-on-a-string" appearance.[1] Two-dimensional echocardiography is diagnostic in d-TGA. It is imperative for the cardiologist to sufficiently qualify coronary anatomy and associated anomalies. If this is not possible, then other imaging modalities such as cardiac magnetic resonance imaging are warranted.

PREOPERATIVE MANAGEMENT

In this cardiac lesion, mixing can occur at the PDA, ASD, or VSD. If inadequate mixing is causing hypoxemia, the patient may require mechanical ventilation and/or institution of a prostaglandin infusion. PGE1 is a vasodilatory agent that acts on vascular smooth muscle and effectively maintains patency of the PDA, thereby providing mixing of parallel systems. The bidirectional shunting of the PDA should provide adequate mixing and antegrade systemic flow. If, however, the ductus is not bidirectional, the decreasing pulmonary resistance and increased pulmonary blood flow may result in hypoperfusion of the abdominal organs and an increase in left atrial pressure. Furthermore, prostaglandins may have limited efficacy on those patient with TGA and an intact ventricular septum due to elevated pulmonary vascular resistance that will limit pulmonary blood flow. At this point, measures to decrease pulmonary vascular resistance, including sedation and mechanical ventilation strategies aimed at mild respiratory alkalosis, will potentially help improve PaO_2.

If these measures still do not improve oxygenation, decompression with balloon atrial septostomy is performed. As stated before, the atrial level of communication and mixing allows for oxygenated blood to pass from a high-pressure left atrium to a low-pressure right atrium throughout the cardiac cycle. Septostomy is typically performed in the intensive care unit or catheterization lab.[3]

INTRAOPERATIVE MANAGEMENT

Anesthetic induction and maintenance

Due to the need to infuse continuous PGE1, all patients coming to the operating room for repair will have an intravenous line in place. Prior to induction, noninvasive monitors should be in place, including electrocardiogram, noninvasive blood pressure cuff and pre- and postductal pulse oximeters. Intravenous induction with a combination of an opiate, muscle relaxant, and a small amount of an inhalation agent is typically the induction method of choice. Once the patient is asleep, the airway is secured with endotracheal intubation. In many centers, the tube is placed nasally to allow for better stability and patient comfort as well as to decrease the potential for oral dislodgement with manipulation of the transesophageal echo.

Ventilator settings should be set to mimic the preoperative state. Typically, a tidal volume of 6 mL/kg with an FiO_2 of 21% to 30% is appropriate. Too much oxygen has the potential to decrease pulmonary vascular resistance (PVR) and lead to pulmonary overflow at the expense of systemic perfusion. However, if there is a consistent drop in saturations below 75%, then the typical causes of poor oxygenation, including decreased ventilation or cardiac output, should be addressed. While increasing FiO_2 may briefly improve saturations, this will lead to worsening cardiac output over a prolonged period of time. Therefore, it is important to move quickly to the initiation of bypass before this can occur.

Maintenance of anesthesia usually consists of a higher dose opioid in combination with a low-dose inhalation agent. While significantly higher doses of opioid have been used in the past, fentanyl dosing of 25 mcg/kg has been shown to adequately blunt the stress response as well as induce less coagulopathy and need for transfusion.[4,5] If possible, two large bore peripheral intravenous catheters should be placed as well for transfusion and medication administration.

Intraoperative monitoring

Following induction, invasive monitors need to be placed. When no other associated anomalies are present, the arterial line can be placed in either the upper extremities or in the femoral artery. Placement of a central line is often institution dependent. While many institutions opt to place a right internal jugular central line, this is not without risk. Due to the small size of the vessel, there is a high rate of thrombosis as well as the potential for interference with bicaval cannulation. Furthermore, with a primary sternotomy, there is less likelihood of difficulty entering the chest and the need for central venous access for inotropic infusions or transfusion prior to bypass. With this in mind, many institutions place transthoracic lines in both the right and left atrium prior to separation from bypass rather than percutaneous central lines. This not only allow for access for inotropic infusions, it further allows for the ability to measure left atrial pressures for signs of ventricular dysfunction following repair.

BYPASS STRATEGIES

Bypass strategy is institution dependent. Typically, arterial cannulation is carried out in the normal fashion unless there is an aortic interruption or obstruction that needs to be addressed. In centers in which deep-hypothermic circulatory arrest is employed to close the ASD or VSD, a single venous cannula is placed. This allows for less discrepancy in drainage from the superior vena cava cannula and decreases the potential for upper body edema. However, other institutions repair septal defects on bypass, requiring 2 venous cannulas to be placed. Then, both the ASD and VSD (if present) are closed through a right atrial incision.[6]

While institutions will vary in their bypass management strategies, all share a common goal of maintaining adequate systemic perfusion. Once on bypass, an age-appropriate mean arterial pressure must be maintained. By using cerebral oximetry, one can also detect inadequate cerebral perfusion or drainage with a significant decrease in cerebral saturation values, which should prompt adjustment of the venous cannulas to improve flow. Protocolized techniques for management of hematocrit and FiO_2 are also followed to improve outcomes.

Acid-base management strategies also vary. However, most institutions employ pH-stat management when temperatures are in the hypothermic range. By using this temperature-corrected strategy, the PCO_2 is unchanged from 37 degrees Celsius or 40 mmHg with the addition of CO_2 to the circuit.[7] This then allows for cerebral vasodilation and improved cerebral cooling/protection.

SEPARATION FROM CARDIOPULMONARY BYPASS

In preparation for separation from bypass, an inotropic agent will be initiated. The agents of choice vary between centers, but typically consist of dopamine 3 to 10 mcg/kg/min and epinephrine 0.03 to 0.05 mcg/kg/min, either alone or in combination. Milrinone can also be added to improve afterload reduction. Some institutions will start a low-dose nitroglycerine infusion with the idea that this can help to maximally dilate the coronary arteries and reduce preload.[8]

Once the patient is off bypass, evaluation of the patient includes interpretation of arterial blood pressure and left atrial pressures in the setting of transesophageal echo findings. In light of the surgery performed, the main concern following the arterial switch procedure is compromise of coronary perfusion and left ventricular dysfunction. This can manifest in several ways (Table 10.1).

If coronary compromise is suspected, then a return to bypass for correction of the issue is warranted. This should be done sooner rather than later to limit damage to the heart from ongoing ischemia. Once any coronary issues are corrected, then another attempt at separation from bypass should occur, often with improved hemodynamics and less inotropic support needed.

POST-BYPASS MANAGEMENT

The post-bypass period can be challenging to manage for several reasons. First, these patients are at significant risk of coagulopathy and bleeding. This is due to the dilutional coagulopathy produced by the bypass priming volume relative to the circulating volume of the neonate, prolonged bypass times, and the use of deep hypothermia. Second, patients can have significant hemodynamic compromise secondary to the inflammatory response produced by bypass and the fluid shifts that occur with bleeding and product replacement. Finally, the newly repaired heart is extremely sensitive to extreme changes in both preload and afterload due to the deconditioning of the left ventricle that occurs after birth.

With this in mind, the hemodynamic goals for the patient should be to achieve an adequate cardiac output with the lowest left atrial pressure possible.[8] The need to rapidly replace blood and coagulation factors must be balanced with the need to not stretch the myofibrils of the heart and result in overdistention of the left ventricle. When this occurs, reimplanted coronary arteries can be stretched and lead to a cycle of ischemia that then produces worsening cardiac distention.[6] Therefore, a more controlled replacement of blood products must be undertaken in which left atrial pressures do not rise above 10 mmHg.

Due to the numerous suture lines and the reasons for coagulopathy previously stated, large amounts of blood products and coagulation factors are often needed following the arterial switch operation. This can further add to edema of the myocardium and lungs. Therefore, the surgeon will often opt to leave the chest open until this edema has improved, and there is less chance of hemodynamic compromise. Even if the chest is closed, early extubation is often not appropriate since the potential for hemodynamic instability is high in these patients postoperatively.

POSTOPERATIVE MANAGEMENT

With significant myocardial and pulmonary edema, the potential for ongoing bleeding, coagulopathy, and hemodynamic instability, the first 24 hours following surgery are critical. Studies have shown that this edema and a prolonged cross clamp time contribute to the development of a decrease in global myocardial function within 6 to 12 hours after surgery.[9] Therefore, one should avoid aggressive weaning off of inotropic support in anticipation of this phenomenon. In fact, inotropic requirements may increase during this period. There should also be continued vigilance looking for signs of coronary compromise, such as new onset arrhythmias, ST segment abnormalities, or mitral regurgitation. If this occurs, then

Table 10.1 MAJOR CONCERNS FOLLOWING THE ARTERIAL SWITCH PROCEDURE

DIAGNOSTIC TOOL	FINDING
Transesophageal echo	Global myocardial dysfunction
	Regional wall motion abnormalities (rare)
	New onset mitral valve insufficiency
Electrocardiogram	ST and T wave changes consistent with ischemia
	New onset arrhythmias
Left atrial pressure	Increased (typically greater than 15 mmHg
Arterial pressure	Hypotension

an echocardiogram should be done looking at wall motion abnormalities and global function.[6]

REVIEW QUESTIONS

1. A 6-hour old neonate in the newborn nursery is noted to have an oxygen saturation of 75%. Despite intubation and 100% oxygen, there is no significant improvement in saturations. Heart rate is 160 bpm and blood pressure is 64/32. Which of the following medications is **MOST** appropriate at this time?

    A. epinephrine bolus
    B. dopamine infusion
    C. inhaled nitric oxide
    D. prostaglandin infusion

Answer: D

In neonates with significant hypoxia, despite adequate oxygenation and ventilation, there is the potential for congenital heart disease. In cyanotic heart disease, adequate pulmonary blood flow must be established. Therefore, PGE1 is typically started in cyanotic neonates until an echocardiogram is performed to assess the definitive anatomy (latham). Epinephrine and dopamine are not appropriate in this setting in light of the patient's normal heart rate and blood pressure. While inhaled nitric oxide will lower pulmonary vascular resistance, it will not allow for opening of a narrow ductus arteriosus and improved pulmonary blood flow, which is needed in this scenario.

2. Following BAS for cyanosis, a neonate with d-TGA on PGE1 at 0.01 mcg/kg/min has an oxygen saturation of 98% and a blood pressure of 48/27. The ventilator is set as follows: pressure control with peak inspiratory pressure 20, positive end-expiratory pressure 5, and FiO_2 50%. What is the **MOST** appropriate next step in management of the patient?

    A. Decrease FiO_2.
    B. Discontinue prostaglandin.
    C. Increase positive end-expiratory pressure.
    D. Initiate epinephrine.

Answer: A

Following BAS, neonates with d-TGA will have appropriate intracirculatory mixing. Therefore, with lower PVR relative to systemic vascular resistance (SVR), there will be an increase in pulmonary blood flow at the expense of systemic blood flow. This can result in hypotension, tachypnea, and metabolic lactic acidosis. To improve the relative systemic blood flow, maneuvers that will increase PVR and shunt blood away from the lungs will result in an improvement in blood pressure, with a goal SpO_2 of 75% to 85%. Prostaglandin should be maintained in the patient until surgical correction. While epinephrine will increase blood pressure due to its vasoconstrictor effects, it will potentially increase SVR as well and result in increased pulmonary blood flow. Increasing positive end-expiratory pressure will cause a slight increase in PVR, but it will typically improve oxygenation and have less effect on improving shunting than a decrease in FiO_2 will.

3. A neonate arrives in the operating room for repair of d-TGA. Which of the following induction agents is **MOST** appropriate for this patient?

    A. ketamine 2 mg/kg
    B. nitrous oxide 70%
    C. propofol 3 mg/kg
    D. sevoflurane 8%

Answer: A

While there is not 1 induction technique that is appropriate for all patients with d-TGA, typically a balanced technique of a low-dose inhalation agent in combination with an opioid and muscle relaxant is employed in light of their fragile hemodynamics. High-dose sevoflurane and propofol have the potential to significantly decrease SVR and acutely worsen blood pressure. Nitrous oxide, while limiting FiO_2, is often avoided in these patients. Ketamine allows for adequate induction while maintaining heart rate and without significantly decreasing SVR.

4. Following initiation of cardiopulmonary bypass, the cerebral oximeter shows a near-infrared spectroscopy value of 98 on the right and 52 on the left. What is the **MOST** appropriate next step?

    A. Adjust the superior vena cava cannula.
    B. Discontinue bypass immediately.
    C. Increase FiO_2 delivered on bypass.
    D. Nothing; this is expected.

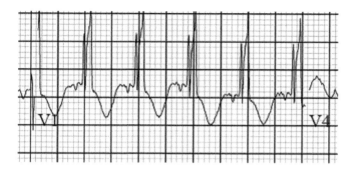

Fig. 10.3 Electrocardiogram post-bypass.

Answer: A

Inconsistent near-infrared spectroscopy values between the 2 sides of the head are indicative of inappropriate cannula placement until proven otherwise. Surgeon notification is imperative so that adjustments can be made. However, this can be done without the need to discontinue bypass. Increasing FiO_2 will not address the differential oxygenation between the 2 sides.

5. A neonate undergoing an arterial switch operation is at the end of the bypass period. He is currently on dopamine 8 mcg/kg/min and epinephrine 0.03 mcg/kg/min. Following discontinuation of bypass, the patient's vital signs are blood pressure 65/42, heart rate 150 bpm, leukocyte alkaline phosphatase (LAP) 7 mmHg, and electrocardiogram normal sinus rhythm. What is the **MOST** appropriate next step?

    A. Add milrinone 0.25 mcg/kg/min.
    B. Bolus albumen 10 mL/kg.
    C. Continue to observe.
    D. Increase epinephrine to 0.05 mcg/kg/min.

Answer: C

The vital signs in the patient are normal at this time, and no intervention is required. However, the hemodynamics will definitely vary with changes in fluid volume due to bleeding and the need to administer blood and coagulation factors. Therefore, continuous observation and the need to intervene with future changes are imperative.

6. Figure 10.3 shows the rhythm seen on electrocardiogram after discontinuation from bypass. What is the most likely associated finding?

    A. arterial BP of 70/42
    B. hyperdynamic LV
    C. LAP of 18 mmHg
    D. tricuspid regurgitation

Answer: C

New onset ST segment changes and arrhythmia are indications of coronary compromise following the arterial switch operation until proven otherwise. This is associated with elevated LAP, mitral regurgitation, decreased myocardial function, and hypotension. The treatment of choice in this setting is to return to bypass and address the cause of coronary compromise.

7. Following bypass for an arterial switch operation, a neonate is on dopamine 8 mcg/kg/min and epinephrine 0.05 mcg/kg/min. The arterial blood pressure is 48/30 and the LAP is 2 mmHg. Which of the following is the **MOST** appropriate next step?

    a. Administer 10 mL/kg fluid bolus.
    b. Administer calcium gluconate 30 mg/kg.
    c. Increase the epinephrine to 0.07 mcg/kg/min.
    d. Initiate milrinone 0.25 mcg/kg/min.

Answer: A

In the presence of both hypotension and a low LAP, the patient is most likely in need of a fluid bolus due to underresuscitation. In the presence of significant ongoing bleeding, this could be in the form of packed red blood cells or other blood products such as platelets or cryoprecipitate. However, all fluid administration should be done carefully to avoid overexpansion of the heart and coronary compromise. If there were signs of decreased cardiac function associated with hypotension, increasing epinephrine or administering calcium would be appropriate. The addition of milrinone may result in acute hypotension due to afterload reduction.

8. Approximately 10 hours after the arterial switch operation, a neonate is on dopamine 5 mcg/kg/min. Over the course of 1 hour, the blood pressure has drifted down to 48/32, and the LAP has increased from 6 to 12 mmHg. What is the **MOST** appropriate intervention at this time?

    a. Administer a fluid bolus.
    b. Bolus milrinone.
    c. Increase dopamine.
    d. Obtain an echocardiogram to rule out ischemia.

Answer: C

Commonly, following a prolonged bypass time, patients will develop a decrease in myocardial function. This typically occurs 6 to 12 hours following bypass and is thought to be due to post-bypass myocardial edema and a prolonged cross-clamp time.[9] In this scenario, one would expect to see a decrease in blood pressure associated with an increased LAP. Increasing inotropic support with an agent such as dopamine or epinephrine is the treatment of choice. Milrinone will potentially cause a worsening of hypotension if bloused at this time. Fluid administration will potentially increase the LAP and stretch the heart, potentially leading to an ischemia cycle. If, with increasing the inotropic agent, there is still no improvement in vital signs, an echocardiogram to assess function is indicated.

QUESTIONS AND ANSWERS

This chapter has accompanying questions and answers which are available to subscribers as part of the Oxford eLearning platform. To access the questions, go to ✅ http://oxfordmedicine. com/pediatricanesthesiaPBL

REFERENCES

1. Jonas RA. *Comprehensive Surgical Management of Congenital Heart Disease.* 2nd ed. New York: Oxford University Press; 2014.

2. Warnes CA. Transposition of the great arteries. *Circulation.* 2006;114:3699–3709.

3. Soongswang J, Adatia I, Newman C, et al. Mortality in potential arterial switch candidates with transposition of the great arteries. *J Am Coll Cardiol.* 1998;32:753–757.

4. Naguib AN, Tobias JD, Hall MW, et al. The role of different anesthetic techniques in altering the stress response during cardiac surgery in children: a prospective, double-blinded, and randomized study. *Pediatr Crit Care Med.* 2013;14:481–490.

5. Anand KJ, Hickey PR. Halothane-morphine compared with high-dose sufentanil for anesthesia and postoperative analgesia in neonatal cardiac surgery. *N Engl J Med.* 1992;326:1–9.

6. Latham GJ, Joffe DC, Eisses MJ, et al. Anesthetic considerations and management of transposition of the great arteries. *Semin Cardiothorac Vasc Anesth.* 2015;19:233–242.

7. Gertler R, Andropoulos D. Cardiopulmonary bypass. In: Andropoulos D, ed. *Anesthesia for Congenital Heart Disease.* 2nd ed. Oxford: Wiley Blackwell; 2010:93–120.

8. Rouine-Rapp K. Anesthesia for transposition of the great vessels. In: Andropoulos D, ed. *Anesthesia for Congenital Heart Disease.* 2nd ed. Oxford: Wiley Blackwell; 2010:443–455.

9. Wernovsky G, Wypij D, Jonas RA, et al. Postoperative course and hemodynamic profile after the arterial switch operation in neonates and infants: a comparison of low-flow cardiopulmonary bypass and circulatory arrest. *Circulation.* 1995;92:2226–2235.

11.

WILLIAMS-BEUREN SYNDROME

Yonmee Chang and Andrew J. Matisoff

STEM CASE AND KEY QUESTIONS

A 2-year old 10-kg boy presents for a cardiac magnetic resonance imaging (MRI) to evaluate for patency of coronary arteries, cardiac function, and renal vasculature prior to surgery. His history is significant for Williams-Beuren syndrome (WS) and hypertension managed with oral propranolol twice a day. General appearance is significant for a broad forehead, wide-set eyes with epicanthal folds, depressed nasal bridge with an upturned nose, long philtrum, and a hypoplastic mandible in an alert and friendly boy. Physical examination is otherwise unremarkable other than a grade 3/6 systolic ejection murmur at right upper sternal border. Electrocardiogram (EKG) shows regular rate and rhythm with left ventricular hypertrophy and correct QT interval (QTc) of 420 ms. Two-dimensional echocardiogram shows moderate supravalvar aortic stenosis (SVAS) with a gradient of 40 mmHg, mild branch pulmonary artery stenosis, mild left ventricular hypertrophy (LVH), poor visualization of coronary arteries, and normal biventricular function. Vital signs in are blood pressure (BP) 120/76, heart rate (HR) 107 bpm, peripheral capillary oxygen saturation (SpO$_2$) 100% on room air, and respiratory rate 20 breaths per minute.

WHAT ARE THE ANESTHETIC CONCERNS FOR PATIENTS WITH WS? WHAT ARE THE CARDIOVASCULAR EFFECTS OF COMMON ANESTHETIC DRUGS?

The patient has an intravenous (IV) catheter placement prior to sedation. An infusion of half normal saline at 20 mL/hr is started in preparation for his scheduled cardiac MRI. For sedation he receives, midazolam 1 mg (0.1 mg/kg) IV, followed by intravenous infusion of propofol at 200 mcg/kg/min, and Ketamine at 1 mg/kg/hr. Spontaneous ventilation is maintained while supplemental oxygen is delivered at 2 L/min via nasal cannula. The patient's vital signs as well as SpO$_2$, end-tidal carbon dioxide (EtCO$_2$), and EKG are monitored from the control room using an Invivo™ MRI-compatible monitor.

DISCUSS THE UNIQUE RISKS AND ANESTHETIC APPROACH FOR CARDIAC MRI.

With the level of sedation confirmed and the patient in stable condition, the study commences. Immediately after giving IV contrast via a power injection, the patient becomes progressively tachycardic to a HR of 160 bpm and starts to move. The anesthesiologist attempts to give small bolus dose of propofol for immediate sedation but recognizes that it is very hard to push through the IV line. The patient continues to move, and HR is increased to the 180s bpm with precipitously decreasing SpO2. There is also irregular breathing pattern on capnography. The anesthesiologist requests that the patient be taken out of the MRI scanner when IV extravasation is noticed in the right forearm. Vital signs are BP 76/38, HR 192 bpm, and SpO$_2$ 84% on 2L/m via nasal cannula. The patient is agitated and is moving his chest and abdomen in a paradoxical breathing pattern. No EtCO$_2$ is present on the monitor and the patient's lips appear cyanotic.

WHAT IS YOUR DIAGNOSIS AND RESPONSE? WHAT MAY HAVE CAUSED THIS? IS INHALATION WITH INHALED ANESTHESIA GAS AN OPTION TO DEEPEN THE PLANE OF ANESTHESIA AND MANAGE THIS SITUATION?

The anesthesiologist, in rapid succession, performs a jaw thrust maneuver, tilts the head, places an oropharyngeal airway and initiates positive pressure bag/mask ventilation with 100% oxygen. Diagnosing laryngospasm, the anesthesiologist requests additional help and intramuscularly injects succinylcholine 40 mg (4 mg/kg) and atropine 0.2 mg (20 mcg/kg), while the nurse tries to establish peripheral IV access. The patient becomes more tachycardic with ST depression noted on the EKG. While waiting for help, the anesthesiologist is now able to support ventilation. Finally, help arrives and after a few attempts, a peripheral IV access is obtained in the left saphenous vein. At this point, a wide complex rhythm with a heart rate of 90 bpm is noted on the EKG, and there is no palpable pulse.

Table 11.1 CLASSIFICATION OF RISKS OF WILLIAMS-BEUREN SYNDROME

LOW RISK	MODERATE RISK	HIGH RISK
Normal EKG	Mild stenosis of a branch of the pulmonary artery	Severe SVAS (>40 mmHg)
Normal Echocardiogram	Hypertension	Symptoms or EKG signs consistent with ischemia
Minimal extracardiac anomalies	Mild to moderate SVAS (<40 mmHg)	Coronary disease demonstrated in imaging
	Other mild cardiac anomalies (e.g., ventricular septal defect)	Severe left ventricular hypertrophy
	Repaired SVAS or SVPS without residual gradients	Biventicular outflow tract disease
	Mild left ventricular hypertrophy	Prolonged QTc on EKG
	Mild to moderate SVPS in isolation	
	Significant extracardiac disease such as difficult airway or severe gastroesophageal reflux	

Note. EKG= electrocardiogram. SVAS = supravalvar aortic stenosis. SVPS = supravalvar pulmonary stenosis.

Source. Reprinted with permission from Matisoff AJ, Olivieri L, Schwartz JM, et al. Risk assessment and anesthetic management of patients with Williams syndrome: a comprehensive review. *Pediatr Anesth.* 2015;25:1207–1215.

DISCUSS MANAGEMENT OF PULSELESS VENTRICULAR TACHYCARDIA (VT). WOULD YOU PERFORM THIS IN THE MRI SCANNER ROOM?

Patient is quickly evacuated from the MRI scanner with continued airway support and continuous monitoring to the designated resuscitation area. A code blue is called, and full resuscitative measures following Pediatric Advanced Life Support protocol is initiated by the code team. Endotracheal intubation is carried out by the anesthesiologist. VT progresses to pulseless electrical activity despite repeated rounds of defibrillation, epinephrine, and amiodarone. Patient is noted to be refractory to resuscitative efforts.

Table 11. 2 CARDIOVASCULAR EFFECTS OF COMMON ANESTHETIC DRUGS

DRUG	SVR	MYOCARDIAL DEPRESSION	TACHYCARDIA AND INCREASED MYOCARDIAL OXYGEN CONSUMPTION	DYSRHYTHMIAS	RESPIRATORY DEPRESSION WITH POSSIBLE REDUCED OXYGEN DELIVERY
Propofol	↓↓	↓	—	—	↓↓
Inhalational anesthetics (sevoflurane, isoflurane, desflurane)	↓↓	↓	—	—	↓↓
Barbiturates (thiopental, pentobarbital)	↓↓	↓	—	—	↓↓
Ketamine	—	—	↑↑	↑↑	—
Chloral hydrate	—	—	↑	↑↑	↓
Benzodiazepines (midazolam, lorazepam)	↓	↓	—	—	↓↓
Etomidate	—	—	—	—	↓

Note. SVR = systemic vascular resistance.

Source. Reprinted with permission from Matisoff AJ, Olivieri L, Schwartz JM, et al. Risk assessment and anesthetic management of patients with Williams syndrome: a comprehensive review. *Pediatr Anesth.* 2015;25:1207–1215.

Table 11.3 ANESTHETIC MANAGEMENT OF HIGH-RISK WILLIAMS-BEUREN SYNDROME PATIENTS

PREANESTHESIA PLANNING	INDUCTION AND MAINTENANCE OF ANESTHESIA	ANESTHESIA EMERGENCE AND DISPOSITION
1. Cardiac anesthesia team involved in care 2. Continue beta-blockers on day of anesthesia 3. Induction of anesthesia in an area suitable for resuscitation (operating room, catheterization lab, intensive care unit) 4. ECMO team aware and clear-primed ECMO circuit nearby 5. Resuscitation drugs including vasopressors immediately available	1. IV placed for prehydration 2. May need oral premedication prior to IV placement with small doses of midazolam, ketamine, or pentobarbital 3. Full ASA monitors including 5-lead EKG 4. IV induction with Etomidate, Fentanyl, or Ketamine 5. Balanced anesthetic with drugs which reduce myocardial oxygen consumption and minimize reductions in SVR 6. Consider direct monitoring of myocardial contractility with TEE in more complicated or prolonged cases 7. Treat ST changes with vasopressors 8. Monitor status of resuscitation with echocardiogram to evaluate contractility 9. Early ECMO deployment if standard resuscitation measures unsuccessful	1. Monitor for emergence tachycardia and EKG changes 2. Manage post-op pain and shivering aggressively to reduce oxygen consumption 3. Recover in high acuity setting with capability for resuscitation and ECMO deployment 4. Monitor after anesthesia for at least 6 hours and preferably overnight prior to discharge

Note. ECMO = extracorporeal membrane oxygenation. ASA = American Association of Anesthesiologists. EKG = electrocardiogram. SVR = systemic vascular resistance. TEE = transesophageal echocardiography.

Source. Reprinted with permission from Matisoff AJ, Olivieri L, Schwartz JM, et al. Risk assessment and anesthetic management of patients with Williams syndrome: a comprehensive review. *Pediatr Anesth.* 2015;25:1207–1215.

WHAT ELSE CAN BE DONE? DISCUSS THE ANESTHESIOLOGIST'S ROLE IN EXTRACORPOREAL CARDIOPULMONARY RESUSCITATION (E-CPR).

With chest compressions ongoing, the patient is positioned with his neck extended and rotated to the left. After sterile preparation and draping, the patient is given 1,500 units (150 units/kg) of heparin. The patient is cannulated onto extracorporeal membrane oxygenation (ECMO) via the right internal jugular vein and carotid artery, and ECMO flows are slowly increased to 100 mL/kg/min to achieve adequate flow. Chest compressions are discontinued, and the patient is transported to the cardiac intensive care unit in critical condition.

DISCUSSION

ETIOLOGY AND PATHOGENESIS

Williams-Beuren syndrome, commonly known as Williams syndrome, results from a deletion on the long arm of chromosome 7q11.23, which codes for elastin gene. Elastin gene encodes tropoelastin, which is involved in vascular wall fiber assembly.[1] Loss of elastin results in loss of aortic distensibility and secondary thickening of large arteries, leading to obstructive hyperplastic intimal lesions.[1] Deletions or point mutations limited to the elastin gene result in nonsyndromic EA (i.e., sporadic or familial), whereas deletions spanning approximately 42 genes including the elastin gene, results in WS.[2]

Approximately 80% of patients with WS have cardiovascular disease, and 40% of those cases require an intervention or surgery.[1]

DIAGNOSIS

The gold standard for WS laboratory diagnosis is the fluorescence in situ hybridization, which can be very expensive. There are other options such as multiplex ligation-dependent probe amplification, which allows the detection of deletions in specific target sequences or microarray-based comparative genomic hybridization, which can detect chromosomal alterations (deletions and duplications) not visible under a light microscope.[3] WS diagnosis is mostly clinical given the cost of these tests.[3]

MANIFESTATIONS OF WS

- Cardiac
  - SVAS: occurs in 45%–75%, aortic narrowing at sinotubular junction due to reduced elasticity causing left ventricular outflow tract obstruction[1]
  - Diffuse narrowing of ascending aorta
  - Supravalvular pulmonic stenosis (SVPS): present in 83%[1], improves with time[4]
  - Obstructive coronary disease (Figure 11.1)[5]
  - Diffuse aortic stenosis
  - Increased risk of myocardial infarction (MI) from reduced coronary artery blood flow[4]
  - LVH: from left ventricular outflow tract obstruction[1]

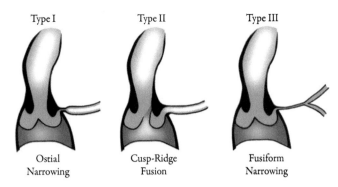

Type I   Type II   Type III

Ostial Narrowing   Cusp-Ridge Fusion   Fusiform Narrowing

Fig. 11.1 Classification of LMCA obstruction in SVAS. Reprinted with permission from: *The Journal of Thoracic and Cardiovascular Surgery.* Dec 2000;120(6):1040–1046.

- Prolonged QTc caused by MI from microvascular perfusion defects[1]

- Extracardiac vascular anomalies
  - Renal artery stenosis[1]
  - Systemic hypertension
  - Thoracic aortic stenosis or middle aortic syndrome: risk factor for coronary ostial stenosis[1]

- Facial appearance and airway
  - Elfin-like facies
  - Broad forehead, wide set eyes, short palpebral fissures, epicanthal folds, depressed nasal bridge, upturned nose, long philtrum, periorbital fullness/pouting lips[3]
  - Mandibular hypoplasia
  - Dental anomalies[4]
  - Hoarse voice (bilateral vocal cord dysfunction secondary to elastin abnormality)

- Cognitive and developmental traits
  - Developmental delay: average IQ 41–80[1]
  - Hypersociability: loquacious, outgoing, strong interest in others[3]
  - Anxiety

- Gastrointestinal
  - Feeding difficulties/failure to thrive
  - Gastroesophageal reflux disease

- Endocrine disease
  - Hypercalcemia: presenting as irritability, hypercalciuria, nephrocalcinosis, and EKG abnormalities. Presents usually in infancy, resolves by age 4, cause unknown.[6]
  - Hypothyroidism

- Neuromuscular disease
  - Hypotonia and joint laxity
  - Poor coordination

PREOPERATIVE WORKUP OF WS

- Cardiac assessment

- EKG: assess for LVH, ST-T wave abnormalities, prolonged QTc
- Echo: assess the severity of LVH, SVAS or pulmonary stenosis, wall motion abnormality, cardiac function
- Cardiac catheterization with aortic and coronary angiography or cardiac MRI/computer tomography: helpful in delineating obstruction to coronary blood flow
- Volume status: pre-induction hydration
- Highest risk: biventricular outflow tract obstruction (see Table 11.1), <3 years of age

- Airway assessment: mandibular hypoplasia and dental anomalies

- Lab: hypercalcemia, hypothyroidism

ANESTHETIC IMPLICATIONS OF WS

- Possibility of undiagnosed coronary disease may exist in all patients with WS (Figure 11.1).[5]

- Any medications that further impair coronary blood flow, provoke outflow tract obstruction, or lead to increased oxygen consumption will increase the risk of cardiac arrest (Table 11.2).

- Elective procedures requiring anesthesia should be planned only after consideration by all participants of the potential extreme hazards of anesthetizing patients with WS (Table 11.3).

- Preservation of sinus rhythm: dysrhythmias may interfere with diastolic perfusion time.

- Cardioversion (regardless of systemic BP) may be preferable to pharmacologic interventions (i.e., esmolol or adenosine), which may cause hypotension in this situation.

- Maintenance of age appropriate heart rate, preload, contractility, diastolic blood pressure, coronary perfusion pressure, and systemic vascular resistance/pulmonary vascular resistance.

- Phenylephrine and vasopressin are first-line vasopressor agents to treat hypotension.

Although there are insufficient data to recommend a specific anesthetic technique in these patients, the best approach would involve using a combination of drugs in incremental doses and titrating to effect over time.[7]

CARDIAC ARREST IN WS

- High risk of sudden death with severe biventricular outflow tract obstruction and coronary artery obstructions (refer to Table 11.1)

- ECMO/intensive care unit (ICU) capability, immediate use of echo to guide resuscitation efforts (refer to Table 11.3)

- Typical presenting symptoms at the time of arrest are hypotension and bradycardia[7]

- Mechanisms for sudden death include MI, decreased CO, and ventricular arrhythmias

- Cardiac arrest can occur on the day after anesthesia

- Unfortunately, many patients are refractory to resuscitation protocols when cardiac arrest occurs

EXTRACORPOREAL CARDIOPULMONARY RESUSCITATION

- The use of e-CPR, also known as ECMO, allows clinicians to potentially rescue patients unresponsive to traditional cardiopulmonary resuscitation (CPR).[8]

- ECMO involves partially removing blood from a patient, adding oxygen and removing carbon dioxide through an extracorporeal membrane and returning this blood back to the patient.

- Consideration for e-CPR is given to individuals with witnessed cardiac arrest who receive traditional high-quality CPR within 5 minutes of arrest and fail to achieve return of spontaneous circulation within 15–30 minutes and who can get ECMO cannulation within 30–60 minutes.[8]

- Extracorporeal circuits pre-primed with crystalloid solution only (no albumin or blood products) may be prepared ahead of time and on stand-by for e-CPR.[8]

- Venous-venous (VV) ECMO is used to support patients with respiratory failure whereas veno-arterial (VA) ECMO is used to support patients with cardiac failure or both cardiac and respiratory failure.

- Cannulation can be central (via median sternotomy, usually reserved for postcardiotomy or for those with peripheral vascular disease) or peripheral (via percutaneous or surgical).
  - Central: aorta-right atrium, aorta-bicaval
  - Peripheral: femoral vein–femoral artery, femoral vein–axillary artery, internal jugular vein–carotid artery, internal jugular vein–axillary artery

- Therapeutic anticoagulation required

- Bleeding is the most common complication with the most common site being cannulation sites.

CONCLUSIONS

Decreased elastin function is known to be the underlying etiology for the cardiovascular lesions found in WS. Sudden cardiac death during minor procedures even in the absence of gross cardiovascular pathology is the most dreaded complication in these patients. In many ways, the goals for induction in a patient with severe WS are similar to those with severe aortic stenosis. However, in contrast to aortic stenosis, the presence of an obstructive lesion above the coronary ostia creates a gradient between the ascending aorta and the coronary ostia further worsening the adverse effect of hypotension on coronary blood flow. In short, anesthesia should be individually tailored to the patient, and no one technique is guaranteed. Early intervention and decisive postoperative planning are crucial in life-saving care for patients with WS.

REVIEW QUESTIONS

1. Which of the following statements, in regard to caring for patients undergoing magnetic resonance imaging, is **MOST** accurate?

    A. Anesthesia machines are designed to be compatible for use in the MRI environment.
    B. Conventional laryngoscopes can be used in emergency airway situations in most MRIs.
    C. Evacuation and resuscitation plans should be in place and rehearsed in all MRI environments.
    D. Standard anesthesia monitors are acceptable for short periods of time in the MRI environment.
    E. Superconducting currents can be modified for certain patients with metallic devices.

Answer: C
There may be significant challenges to anesthetic administration and monitoring capabilities in the MRI environment due to very strong static magnetic field, high-frequency electromagnetic (radiofrequency) waves, and a time-varied (pulsed) magnetic field. Regular anesthesia machines and equipment such as conventional laryngoscopes are not compatible in MRI suite because the energy of the magnetic field can pull the steel devices into the magnet. Similarly, certain equipment necessary for code blue situations are not compatible in the MRI environment. Hence, a designated plan for evacuation and resuscitation of patients undergoing MRI scans should be in place and rehearsed in facilities that perform MRI scan with anesthesia.[9]

2. Which of the following conditions represents the **BEST** physiologic state in the management of aortic stenosis?

    A. elevated heart rate and afterload
    B. elevated heart rate and reduced SVR
    C. normal sinus rhythm and reduced afterload
    D. normal sinus rhythm and stable SVR
    E. reduced preload and afterload

Answer: D
Hemodynamic goal for aortic stenosis should be full, slow, and tight. To paraphrase, the physiologic goals in patients with aortic stenosis include preserving an adequate preload, maintenance of normal sinus rhythm with avoidance of tachycardia, and preservation of afterload (SVR). In aortic

stenosis, slow heart rate limits cardiac output as they have fixed stroke volume through a stenotic valve whereas fast heart rate decreases diastolic filling time for myocardial perfusion. Systemic hypotension can lead to myocardial ischemia by reducing coronary perfusion pressure. Maintaining adequate intravascular volume is also important as it ensures higher left ventricular end diastolic volume/left ventricular end diastolic pressure in the setting of aortic stenosis.

3. Which of the following anesthetic agents is the **MOST** appropriate to use in patients with severely reduced myocardial function?

    A. etomidate
    B. ketamine
    C. midazolam
    D. propofol
    E. sevoflurane

Answer: A

Etomidate is the drug of choice in patients with myocardial dysfunction. Caution should be taken in patients at risk for the development of adrenal insufficiency due to its suppression of the adrenal cortical axis. Midazolam, propofol, and all currently available inhaled halogenated volatile anesthetics cause myocardial depression and a decrease in SVR to some degree.[1] Ketamine can cause increases in systemic and pulmonary blood pressures, heart rate, cardiac output, cardiac work, and myocardial oxygen requirements from dose dependent direct stimulation of the central nervous system but does have a direct negative cardiac inotropic effect so it would not be an ideal drug to use in a patient with severely reduced myocardial function (Table 11.2).

4. Which finding on 2-dimensional echocardiogram signifies the **GREATEST** risk for perioperative mortality for patients with WS?

    A. biventricular outflow tract obstruction
    B. mild LVH with pulmonary artery stenosis
    C. moderate supravalvar aortic stenosis
    D. moderate supravalvar pulmonary stenosis
    E. ventricular septal defect

Answer: A

Patients with severe SVAS, symptoms or EKG consistent with ischemia, biventricular outflow tract disease, severe LVH, or documented coronary anomalies should be treated as high risk. Those patients with WS and QTc prolongation should also be considered at high risk for ischemia and ventricular dysrhythmias. The presence of biventricular outflow tract obstruction in combination with coronary artery abnormalities carries the highest risk of sudden cardiac death (Table 11.1).[10]

5. After induction with etomidate, a 5-year-old boy with WS has hypotension, tachycardia, and EKG changes consistent with myocardial ischemia. What is the next **BEST** step in his management?

    A. nitroglycerin
    B. phenylephrine

    C. epinephrine
    D. ECMO
    E. ephedrine

Answer: B

Nitroglycerin will worsen the hypotension, further reducing coronary perfusion pressure so it would not be the best choice. Epinephrine and ephedrine will improve the hypotension but will also increase the heart rate and worsen the myocardial ischemia by increasing myocardial oxygen consumption so it is not the best management. ECMO can be considered for refractory resuscitation efforts after temporizing measures to optimize hemodynamics have been attempted. Phenylephrine would be the best option in this scenario as it will treat hypotension and slow the heart rate thereby reducing myocardial oxygen consumption.

6. A 3-year-old boy with WS presents for an outpatient repair of an inguinal hernia. No cardiac data are available, but his mother states that he is healthy. Which of the following approaches is the **MOST** appropriate in this situation?

    A. Perform case with spinal anesthesia to avoid the physiologic risks associated with general anesthesia.
    B. Proceed with case if no cardiac murmur is heard on auscultation.
    C. Proceed with case if vital signs are within normal range.
    D. Proceed with case if recent EKG and echocardiogram are within normal range.
    E. Cancel case because all WS require ICU admission and ECMO standby.

Answer: D

In view of the reports of sudden cardiac deaths during minor diagnostic procedures in WS patients, all patients should have thorough cardiac workup including at a minimum a recent EKG and echocardiogram, along with a thorough history and physical exam. WS patients with moderate to severe cardiac disease can be refractory to standard resuscitation protocols when cardiac arrest occurs. Hence, elective procedures on moderate and high risk patients should be performed in institutions capable of providing ICU care and ideally have the capability of ECMO in the event that traditional resuscitation protocols fail.[7] Spinal anesthesia would be a poor choice in a WS patient as it would increase the risk of cardiac arrest by decreasing preload and worsening myocardial oxygen supply and demand.

7. An echocardiogram (Figure 11.2) from 3 months ago shows mild SVAS with a gradient of 20 mmHg and is otherwise unremarkable. EKG is normal. You decide to proceed with the anesthetic in a hospital setting. Of the following treatment plans, which is the **MOST** appropriate for this patient?

    A. ephedrine to maintain elevated heart rate and high afterload
    B. furosemide to reduce preload by venodilation and diuresis
    C. milrinone to maintain cardiac contractility while reducing afterload

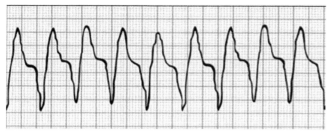

Fig. 11.2

D. nitroglycerin to decrease cardiac filling pressures and maintain vascular dilation

E. vasopressin to maintain in SVR while assuring adequate anesthesia

Answer: E

Again, physiologic goals in patients with aortic stenosis should be full, slow, and tight so preservation of adequate preload, maintenance of normal sinus rhythm with avoidance of tachycardia, and preservation of afterload (SVR) are important considerations in minimizing anesthetic risks. Afterload reduction from milrinone, elevated heart rate from ephedrine, vascular dilation with nitroglycerin, or preload reduction with furosemide would not produce favorable outcomes in a patient with SVAS. Use of vasopressors such as vasopressin or phenylephrine in this scenario fulfills the physiologic goals for a patient with SVAS.

8. During your anesthetic of the 3-year-old male described in question 7, the child develops the rhythm shown in the following figure. The patient's pulse is not palpable. After initiating chest compression, which is the **MOST** appropriate next step in this patient's management?

A. Epinephrine IV 0.12 mg (0.01 mg/kg) bolus

B. Chest compressions followed by immediate defibrillation at 2–4 Joules/kg

C. Amiodarone IV 60 mg (5 mg/kg) bolus followed by chest compressions

D. Esmolol 6 mg (500 mcg/kg) IV followed by an infusion of 50 mcg/kg/min to reduce myocardial demand and slow heart rate

E. Adenosine 1.2 mg (0.1 mg/kg) rapid IV push

Answer: B

Following the VF/VT Pediatric Cardiac Arrest Algorithm, one should start with high quality CPR followed by immediate defibrillation for shockable rhythm. The time to initial defibrillation in a shockable rhythm is inversely related to survival so defibrillation must not be delayed for administration of drug therapy such as Epinephrine or Amiodarone. If defibrillation does not terminate the refractory VF/ pulseless VT, this should be followed by high quality CPR and then drug therapy such as Epinephrine 0.01 mg/kg or Amiodarone 5 mg/kg bolus. Adenosine may be indicated for SVT but not for pulseless VT.

9. Of the following conditions, which is the **MOST** appropriate use for VA ECMO?

A. acute respiratory distress syndrome with progressive multiorgan failure

B. cardiac arrest from an ongoing intracranial hemorrhage

C. hypothermic cardiac arrest from cold water drowning

D. non-recoverable cardiac failure not eligible for a ventricular assist device

E. Severe aortic regurgitation with pulmonary edema

Answer: C

E-CPR is now the treatment of choice for deep hypothermic (<20 °C) cardiac arrest refractory to conventional resuscitation efforts.[8] It has been shown to provide good survival and neurological outcomes far superior in comparison with conventional methods of rewarming, particularly in adults. ECMO should only be considered if there is reasonable hope for a transplant, recovery, or long-term cardiac-assist device.[11] Because systemic anticoagulation is required for ECMO, any contraindication to anticoagulation or uncontrolled bleeding is contraindicated.[8] VA ECMO is contraindicated in those with more than moderate aortic regurgitation because of the potential for left ventricular distension.[11]

QUESTIONS AND ANSWERS

This chapter has accompanying questions and answers which are available to subscribers as part of the Oxford eLearning platform. To access the questions, go to ✓ http:// oxfordmedicine. com/pediatricanesthesiaPBL

REFERENCES

1. Matisoff AJ, Olivieri L, Schwartz JM, et al. Risk assessment and anesthetic management of patients with Williams syndrome: a comprehensive review. *Pediatr Anesth.* 2015;25:1207–1215.
2. Latham GJ, Ross FJ, Eisses MJ, et al. Perioperative morbidity in children with elastin arteriopathy. *Pediatr Anesth.* 2016;26:926–935.
3. Leme DE, Souza DH, Mercado G, et al. Assessment of clinical scoring systems for the diagnosis of Williams-Beuren syndrome. *Genet Mol Res.* 2013;12(3):3407–3411.
4. Pober BR, Johnson M, Urban Z. Mechanisms and treatment of cardiovascular disease in Williams-Beuren syndrome. *J Clin Invest.* 2008;118(5):1606–1615.
5. Thistlethwaite PA, Madani MM, Kriett JM, et al. Surgical management of congenital obstruction of the left main coronary artery with supravalvular aortic stenosis. *J Thorac Cardiovasc Surg.* 2000;120(6):1040–1046.
6. Deka S, Das J, Khanna S, et al. A child of Williams-Beuren syndrome for inguinal hernia repair: perioperative management concerns. *Indian Anaesthetists Forum.* 2016;17(2):62–64.
7. Burch T, McGowan F, Kussman B, et al. Congenital supravalvular aortic stenosis and sudden death associated with anesthesia: what's the mystery? *Anesth Analg.* 2008;107:1848–1854.
8. Conrad SA, Rycus PT. Extracorporeal membrane oxygenation for refractory cardiac arrest. *Ann Card Anaesth.* 2017;20:S4–S10.
9. Practice Advisory on Anesthetic Care for Magnetic Resonance Imaging. *Anesthesiology.* 2015;122:495–520.
10. Kussman B. Williams syndrome, supravalvar aortic stenosis and cardiac arrest during anesthesia. *SPA Newsl.* 2004;17(3).
11. Schmidt M, Brechot N, Combes A. Ten situations in which ECMO is unlikely to be successful. *Intensive Care Med.* 2016;42:750–752.

12.

CARDIOMYOPATHY AND HEART FAILURE

Komal Kamra and Glyn D. Williams

STEM CASE AND KEY QUESTIONS

An 11-month-old male (10 kg), who had no significant past medical history, presented to the emergency room with fussiness, decreased appetite, and vomiting. Recently, he had a runny nose and cough, followed by fever for 4 days. The parents treated him with acetaminophen without any significant improvement. In the emergency room, he was found to be pale, diaphoretic, tachypneic, and tachycardic. His physical exam also revealed cool limbs, prolonged capillary refill time, eyelid edema, and hepatomegaly. Electrocardiogram elicited low voltage QRS complexes. Chest X-ray demonstrated cardiomegaly and enhanced pulmonary venous markings. Echocardiogram showed an increased left atrium and left ventricle (LV) size, severe mitral regurgitation, increased LV filling pressures, severely decreased LV ejection fraction of 20%, and low LV diastolic function. Origins and proximal course of coronary arteries were normal. Lab tests revealed hyponatremia, lactic and respiratory acidosis, increased transaminases, troponin and N-terminal probrain natriuretic peptide (NT-proBNP) level. Results of viral titers to rule out viral myocarditis are pending. Patient was admitted to intensive care unit for close monitoring and treatment of congestive heart failure. He was placed on diuretics, an angiotensin-converting enzyme inhibitor (ACEI) and an intravenous milrinone infusion. As the patient's clinical status did not improve after 48 hours, he was scheduled to undergo endomyocardial biopsy (EMB) and placement of peripherally inserted central catheter (PICC) line for diagnosis and management.

HOW DO YOU DEFINE AND CLASSIFY CARDIOMYOPATHIES?

The American Heart Association has defined cardiomyopathy as "heterogeneous group of diseases of the myocardium associated with mechanical and/or electrical dysfunction that usually (but not invariably) exhibit inappropriate ventricular hypertrophy or dilation and are due to a variety of causes that frequently are genetic."[1] The American Heart Association classifies cardiomyopathies into 2 categories based on the predominant involvement of an organ. Primary cardiomyopathies affect myocardium dominantly whereas secondary cardiomyopathies impact myocardium and other organs. Primary cardiomyopathies are further subgrouped by etiology into genetic, mixed (genetic and nongenetic), and acquired. The main subgroups of cardiomyopathies are depicted in Figure 12.1 and Table 12.1.[1]

WHAT IS THE USUAL CLINICAL PRESENTATION OF HEART FAILURE IN A CHILD?

The clinical presentation in this patient is consistent with acute heart failure. Functional status of the child should be carefully assessed based on the clinical presentation and diagnostic studies to formulate a safe anesthetic plan. Acute heart failure in children can be grouped into 4 different subclasses by pulmonary congestion and perfusion as highlighted in Table 12.2.[2]

Common presenting symptoms and signs of presentation of acute heart failure are shown in Figure 12.2.[3]

HOW WOULD YOU ASSESS THE SEVERITY OF HEART FAILURE IN THIS CHILD?

Ross classification as depicted in Table 12.3 can be used to classify the severity of heart failure in infants and young children based on prevailing symptoms. This system has been modified for different age groups of children. The criteria used to score the severity of heart failure are feeding, weight gain, breathing rate and pattern, heart rate and perfusion, presence and extent of hepatomegaly, NT-proBNP levels, ejection fraction, and atrioventricular valvar insufficiency. Based on this classification, this patient shows characteristics of severe heart failure.[4]

Ross classification does not take into account the progression of disease overtime and effect of treatment on the course of the disease. So, a staging system was developed for heart failure to complement Ross classification. As highlighted in Table 12.4, this staging system proposes that the patient's heart failure will progress from 1 stage to the next unless interrupted or slowed by treatment.[5]

THE CARDIOLOGIST WANTS THE PATIENT TO UNDERGO EMB TO ARRIVE AT A DIAGNOSIS AND FOR FURTHER MANAGEMENT. WHICH PATIENTS WITH HEART FAILURE SHOULD BE CONSIDERED FOR EMB?

EMB is considered in any pediatric patient with unexplained cardiomyopathy where the diagnosis of type of

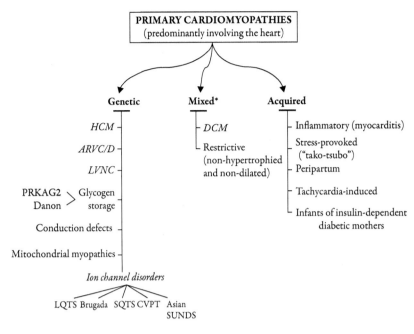

Fig. 12.1 Primary cardiomyopathies.[1]

cardiomyopathy cannot be confirmed by routine diagnostic tests (e.g., echocardiography, electrocardiography, chest X-ray and coronary angiography). An algorithm (Figure 12.3) for diagnostic workup and treatment of suspected myocarditis in children was suggested by Das et al.[6] EMB can guide the appropriate treatment in case of acute myocarditis that will eventually result in functional recovery. However, the risks of the procedure and anesthesia have to be taken into consideration.

YOU ARE ASKED TO PROVIDE ANESTHESIA FOR THE EMB. WHAT ARE YOUR CONCERNS, AND WHAT WILL BE YOUR ANESTHETIC PLAN?

It is recommended that the multidisciplinary team caring for the patient discuss the relative risks and benefits of EMB under anesthesia because periprocedural complications are more likely in patients with severe congestive heart failure. Rescue options, postoperative destination, and future procedures could be considered when planning coordination of care. Parents and patient should be appropriately informed of anesthetic concerns and plan. Anesthetic plan may vary depending on the type of cardiomyopathy and its pathophysiology. Different pathophysiological changes occur in cardiomyopathy. These changes for main types of cardiomyopathies and hemodynamic goals for intraoperative management of major cardiomyopathies are highlighted in Tables 12.5 and 12.6, respectively.[7]

The goal of the anesthesia in a patient with congestive heart failure is to prevent further myocardial depression, maintain normal to increase heart rate and preload but low afterload, and increase contractility. Diastolic pressure should be preserved within normal range to facilitate coronary perfusion. Arrhythmias should be treated promptly. Fluid overload can precipitate or worsen pulmonary edema while fluid restriction can impede cardiac output.

The goal of utilizing mechanical ventilation in a patient with heart failure is to decrease the work of breathing. Mechanical ventilation at a higher tidal volume results in a decline in venous return, hence jeopardizing cardiac output. Application of positive-end expiratory pressure can either increase or decrease the cardiac output depending on high versus low pulmonary capillary wedge pressure. Positive pressure during mechanical ventilation decreases right ventricular preload and left ventricular afterload. Change to right ventricular afterload with positive pressure ventilation is dependent on end expiratory lung volume to functional residual capacity relationship and recruitment of pulmonary vasculature and alveoli. Any modification to left ventricular preload with positive pressure ventilation is determined by right ventricular cardiac output and ventricular interdependence. Mechanical ventilation with adequate titration of positive end-expiratory pressure can also help diminish the extravascular lung water, improve recruitment, and prevent atelectasis.

General anesthetics can lead to systemic hypotension due to their effects on myocardial contractility, pulmonary and systemic vascular resistance, and heart rate and rhythm. Usually these patients are admitted in the hospital for the management of congestive heart failure and therefore may have intravenous access in situ. Slow, controlled, and monitored induction with etomidate, ketamine, benzodiazepines, and/or narcotics along with low-dose volatile agents and dexmedetomidine can be used to maintain anesthesia and hemodynamic stability. Due to its lack of effect on systemic vascular resistance, myocardial contractility, and heart rate, etomidate tends to keep the patients hemodynamically stable. Ketamine augments the heart rate, blood pressure, and cardiac output. Dexmedetomidine increases the blood pressure and decreases the heart rate if given as a bolus dose. Dexmedetomidine infusion decreases heart rate, systemic vascular resistance, and

Table 12.1 SECONDARY CARDIOMYOPATHIES

Infiltrative[b]	Amyloidosis (primary, familial autosomal dominant,[a] senile, secondary forms)
	Gaucher disease[a]
	Hurler's disease[a]
	Hunter's disease[a]
Storage[c]	Hemochromatosis
	Fabry's disease[a]
	Glycogen storage disease[a] (type II, Pompe)
	Niemann-Pick disease[a]
Toxicity	Drugs, heavy metals, chemical agents
Endomyocardial	Endomyocardial fibrosis
	Hypereosinophilic syndrome (Löeffler's endocarditis)
Inflammatory (granulomatous)	Sarcoidosis
Endocrine	Diabetes mellitus[a]
	Hyperthyroidism
	Hypothyroidism
	Hyperparathyroidism
	Pheochromocytoma
	Acromegaly
Cardiofacial	Noonan syndrome[a]
	Lentiginosis[a]
Neuromuscular/neurological	Friedreich's ataxia[a]
	Duchenne-Becker muscular dystrophy[a]
	Emery-Dreifuss muscular dystrophy[a]
	Myotonic dystrophy[a]
	Neurofibromatosis[a]
	Tuberous sclerosis[a]
Nutritional deficiencies	Beriberi (thiamine), pellagra, scurvy, selenium, carnitine, kwashiorkor
Autoimmune/collagen	Systemic lupus erythematosis
	Dermatomyositis
	Rheumatoid arthritis
	Scleroderma
	Polyarteritis nodosa
Electrolyte imbalance	
Consequence of cancer therapy	Anthracyclines: doxorubicin (adriamycin), daunorubicin
	Cyclophosphamide
	Radiation

[a]Genetic (familial) origin.

[b]Accumulation of abnormal substances between myocytes (i.e., extracellular).

[c]Accumulation of abnormal substances within the myocytes (i.e., intracellular).

Source. Maron BJ, Towbin JA, Thiene G, et al. Contemporary definitions and classification of the cardiomyopathies: an American Heart Association Scientific Statement from the Council on Clinical Cardiology, Heart Failure and Transplantation Committee; Quality of Care and Outcomes Research and Functional Genomics and Translational Biology Interdisciplinary Working Groups; and Council on Epidemiology and Prevention. *Circulation.* 2006;113(14):1807–1816. Copyright 2006 Wolters Kluwer Health, Inc. Adapted with permission

blood pressure. Propofol reduces systemic vascular resistance, mean arterial pressure, and myocardial contractility; it should be used cautiously in patients with heart failure. Large doses of benzodiazepine can also reduce blood pressure by decreasing the systemic vascular resistance. Opioids such as fentanyl can cause peripheral vasodilation and bradycardia by affecting the brainstem vasomotor centers. Although intravenous induction and preinduction arterial pressure monitoring may be the most prudent way to induce patient with moderate to severe heart failure, inhalational agents can also be used judiciously for induction in a patient with mild to moderate heart failure but no intravenous (IV) access. Most halogenated inhalational agents lower cardiac output and mean arterial blood pressure mainly by reducing the systemic vascular resistance. They also tend to increase heart rate; exceptions are sevoflurane, halothane, and xenon. Isoflurane, halothane, and desflurane cause coronary dilation.[8,9]

WHAT PREOPERATIVE DIAGNOSTIC TESTS ARE GENERALLY PERFORMED ON A PATIENT WITH HEART FAILURE AND WHAT INFORMATION DO THESE TESTS PROVIDE?

The diagnostic tests help ascertain the cause of heart failure, assess any associated pathologies, establish prognosis or severity of the disease, and assist with heart failure management by observing the impact of medications and additional treatment. The common diagnostic tests performed in a pediatric patient with heart failure include

- Laboratory tests such as complete blood count; rental, liver, and thyroid function tests; serum electrolytes; mixed venous oxygen saturation and blood lactate level; and B-type natriuretic peptide (BNP) and prohormone NT-proBNP levels. BNP and prohormone NT-proBNP are used to diagnose heart failure and predict severity and assess responsiveness to treatment.

- A 12-lead electrocardiogram identifies baseline rhythm and establishes the presence of any arrhythmia and myocardial ischemia.

- Chest radiography displays heart size, reveals presence of pulmonary edema, and depicts any associated respiratory anomalies or compression due to increased chamber size.

- Echocardiography delineates the cause and severity of heart failure, identifies structural abnormalities, evaluates ventricular cavity size and function, assesses left atrial volume and diastolic function, estimates pulmonary artery pressures, identifies concomitant pathophysiology, observes impact of medications and other treatment, and helps with prognosis.

- Cardiac magnetic resonance imaging MRI delineates anatomy, estimates ventricular function and regional wall motion abnormality, and measures ventricular volume,

Table 12.2 **PROFILE OF RESTING HEMODYNAMICS**

	No congestion	Congestion
Adequate perfusion	"Warm and dry"	"Wet and dry"
	A	B
	Optimal profile: focus on prevention of disease progression and decompensation	Diuresis with continuation of standard therapy
Critical hypoperfusion	"Cold and dry"	"Wet and cold"
	L	C
	Limited further options for therapy	Diuresis and redesign of regimen with other standard therapies

Note. The letter L represents the group with low output without congestion. Patients frequently progress from profile A to profile B. When that occurs, profile C commonly occurs after profile B. For the less common profile of low output without congestion, the letter L was chosen rather than the letter D to avoid the implication that this profile necessarily follows profile C or is a less desirable profile than C. In fact, the prognosis of profile C may be worse than that of profile L.

Source. Adapted from Grady KL, Dracup K, Kennedy G, et al. Team management of patients with heart failure: a statement for healthcare professionals from the Cardiovascular Nursing Council of the American Heart Association. Circulation. 2000;102(19):2443–2456. Copyright 2000 Wolters Kluwer Health, Inc. Adapted with permission.

mass, and strain. Gadolinium enhancement can define the cause and prognosis in cardiomyopathy by identifying cardiac inflammation and fibrosis.

- Cardiac computed tomography assesses anatomy of great vessels, pulmonary veins, and coronary arteries; evaluates pulmonary parenchyma and extrinsic compression of airways due to cardiomegaly; identifies bleeding,

thromboembolism and infection; and assists with neurologic evaluation.[10]

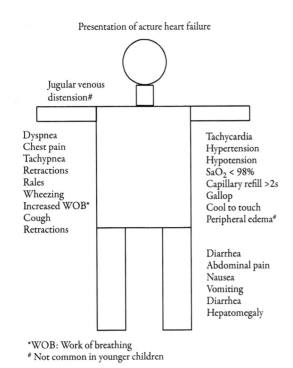

Presentation of acture heart failure

Jugular venous distension#

Dyspnea
Chest pain
Tachypnea
Retractions
Rales
Wheezing
Increased WOB*
Cough
Retractions

Tachycardia
Hypertension
Hypotension
SaO$_2$ < 98%
Capillary refill >2s
Gallop
Cool to touch
Peripheral edema#

Diarrhea
Abdominal pain
Nausea
Vomiting
Diarrhea
Hepatomegaly

*WOB: Work of breathing
Not common in younger children

Fig. 12.2 Common presentation of acute heart failure.

WHAT ARE THE COMMON MEDICATIONS THAT A HEART FAILURE PATIENT IS ON? WHAT IS THEIR ROLE IN PATIENT MANAGEMENT?

Medications used to manage heart failure in children fall under 3 major categories: diuretics, afterload reducing agents, and inotropes. These medications are intended to alleviate and minimize deterioration of symptoms related to heart failure, promote better exercise capacity, and improve survival. Diuretics decrease systemic and pulmonary fluid retention with the goal of making the patient euvolemic. Hyponatremia and hypokalemia can result from diuretics. Inotropes improve end-organ perfusion and provide symptomatic relief. Dopamine, dobutamine, and epinephrine increase cardiac output and heart rate. The increased heart rate results in enhanced myocardial oxygen consumption. Milrinone and levosimendan are inotropes that increase cardiac output and heart rate but do not affect myocardial oxygen consumption. Levosimendan, a calcium sensitizing agent, has the potential to reduce afterload. After short-term use of inotropes, a determination should be made whether to wean the inotropic support, convert to mechanical support, or consider cardiac transplant. Angiotensin-converting enzyme inhibitor and angiotensin II receptor blockers affect ventricular remodeling and reduce afterload. Aldosterone receptor antagonists optimize LV remodeling and LV diastolic filling. Hence, they are used in patients with systolic dysfunction of systemic ventricle. Beta-blockers can also be used in patients with left ventricular dysfunction. They act by

Table 12.3 ROSS CLASSIFICATION

CLASS	INTERPRETATION
I	Asymptomatic
II	Mild tachypnea or diaphoresis with feeding in infants. Dyspnea on exertion in older children
III	Marked tachypnea or diaphoresis with feeding in infants. Prolonged feeding times with growth failure due to heart failure. In older children, marked dyspnea on exertion.
IV	Symptoms such as tachypnea, retractions, grunting, or diaphoresis at rest.

Note. Ross classification is used for grading heart failure in infants and younger children.

Source. Adapted from Rosenthal D, Chrisant MR, Edens E, et al. International Society for Heart and Lung Transplantation: practice guidelines for management of heart failure in children. *J Heart Lung Transplant.* 2004;23(12):1313–1333. Copyright © 2004 International Society for Heart and Lung Transplantation. Published by Elsevier Inc.

Table 12.4 DISEASE STAGING FOR INFANTS AND CHILDREN WITH HEART FAILURE

STAGE	DESCRIPTION
Stage A	Patients with increased risk of developing HF, but who have normal cardiac function and no evidence of cardiac chamber volume overload. Examples: previous exposure to cardiotoxic agents, family history of heritable cardiomyopathy, univentricular heart, congenitally corrected transposition of the great arteries
Stage B	Patients with abnormal cardiac morphology or cardiac function, with no symptoms of HF, past or present. Examples: aortic insufficiency with LV enlargement, history of anthracycline with decreased LV systolic function.
Stage C	Patients with underlying structural or functional heart disease, and past or current symptoms of HF.
Stage D	Patients with end-stage HF requiring continuous infusion of inotropic agents, mechanical circulatory support, cardiac transplantation or hospice care.

Note. HF = heart failure. LV = left ventricular.

Source. Adapted from Rosenthal D, Chrisant MR, Edens E, et al. International Society for Heart and Lung Transplantation: practice guidelines for management of heart failure in children. *J Heart Lung Transplant.* 2004;23(12):1313–1333. Copyright © 2004 International Society for Heart and Lung Transplantation. Published by Elsevier Inc.

counteracting the chronic sympathetic load and ventricular modeling.[11]

THE PATIENT IS SCHEDULED TO UNDERGO EMB AND PICC LINE PLACEMENT. WHAT IS THE ROLE OF CARDIAC CATHETERIZATION IN THESE PATIENTS?

Primary objective of cardiac catheterization in patients with dilated cardiomyopathy is to perform EMB and to determine ventricular filling pressures, cardiac output (using thermodilution or Fick methods), and pulmonary vascular resistance (PVR). Elevated PVR can result from left atrial hypertension due to ventricular failure. In the early stages, PVR is reversible but eventually pulmonary vascular remodeling occurs that culminates into irreversible increase in PVR.[10]

PATIENT WAS MAINTAINED ON PROPOFOL AND KETAMINE INTRAVENOUS ANESTHETIC. DURING THE BIOPSY, THERE WAS A SLOW DECLINE IN BLOOD PRESSURE. WHAT COULD BE THE CAUSE AND HOW WOULD YOU MANAGE IT?

There can be several causes of hypotension associated with an anesthetic including anesthetic drugs, preoperative medications, blood products, and physiological changes due to procedure, ventilation strategies, arrhythmia, and so on. Hypotension was initially treated with fluid bolus. Despite giving the patient repeated doses of vasopressors such as ephedrine and phenylephrine, the blood pressure did not approach normal values. A preoperative, medication was suspected as the cause of hypotension.

Preoperative medication of the patient included ACEIs. Refractory hypotension may be a consequence of angiotensin-axis blockade, which is common in patients on ACEIs or angiotensin-receptor blockers. Angiotensin-axis blockade can result in both a sympatholytic condition in a patient and a dominant parasympathetic system. Concurrently, the arterial baroreceptors are set to lower level thus manifesting a diminished response to hypotension and exogenous catecholamines. Moreover, depleted levels of circulating and tissue levels of Angiotensin II, aldosterone, and arginine vasopressin are found in patients on ACEIs. Of note, patients on angiotensin-receptor blockers demonstrated a diminished amount of aldosterone and arginine vasopressin. Additionally, general anesthesia accentuates sympatholysis culminating in refractory hypotension. Glycopyrrolate can be used to treat hypotension in this case due to its effect on heart rate and vagal tone attributable to its parasympatholytic properties. Preload should be optimized by fluid bolus. Phenylephrine is the drug of choice if the cardiac output is adequate. If not, ephedrine is the first line of treatment. Repeated doses of vasopressors may be necessary. If hypotension is unresponsive to repeated doses of ephedrine and phenylephrine, then vasoconstrictors such as norepinephrine, epinephrine and methylene blue can be considered. Other treatment options like arginine vasopressin and terlipressin have been used in adult population.[12]

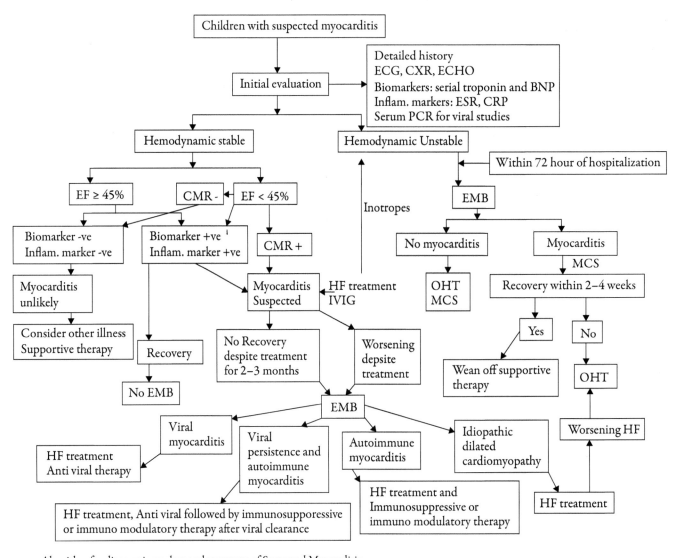

Fig. 12.3 Algorithm for diagnostic workup and treatment of Suspected Myocarditis
Source: Adapted from Das BB. Role of endomyocardial biopsy for children presenting with acute systolic heart failure. *Pediatr Cardiol.* 2014;35(2):191–196.

DURING THE EMB, ADVANCEMENT OF THE GUIDEWIRE PRECIPITATED INTRACTABLE VENTRICULAR ARRHYTHMIA. WHAT IS THE ROLE OF MECHANICAL CIRCULATORY SUPPORT IN PEDIATRIC PATIENTS WITH HEART FAILURE? WHAT ARE THE CRITERIA FOR SELECTING MECHANICAL CIRCULATORY SUPPORT DEVICES IN THIS PATIENT POPULATION?

In this patient with cardiogenic shock due to intractable arrhythmia, extracorporeal life support can enable hemodynamic stability and recuperation of end-organs. Extracorporeal life support optimizes oxygen delivery to the myocardium, minimizes myocardial workload, decreases the requirement of vasopressor and inotropic support, lessens intrathoracic pressure and pulmonary barotrauma, maximizes perfusion and oxygen delivery to the end-organs, and alleviate acidosis.[13]

Mechanical circulatory support in pediatric patients with end-stage heart failure reduces mortality while awaiting heart transplant. Device selection is determined by 3 main criteria: (a) type of support required—cardiopulmonary versus cardiac, (b) duration of support required, and (c) body surface area. Extracorporeal membranous oxygenation provides biventricular cardiopulmonary support and serves well if emergent cardiac support is necessary after cardiac arrest or failure of medical resuscitation. It is generally a temporary support as after 2 weeks there is an elevated risk of bleeding, thrombosis, and other complications.

Outcome of extracorporeal membranous oxygenation can be threefold: (a) pulmonary recovery leading to insertion of long-term cardiac support, (b) cardiopulmonary recovery leading to decannulation, and (c) no recovery leading to withdrawal of support. Patients with pulmonary recovery can be bridged with short-term or long-term ventricular assist devices. Ventricular assist devices can serve as a bridge-to-recovery, destination therapy, bridge-to-bridge, and bridge-to-transplant.[14–16]

Table 12.5 PATHOPHYSIOLOGICAL CHANGES IN KEY CARDIOMYOPATHIES

PATHOPHYSIOLOGICAL CHANGES	DILATED CARDIOMYOPATHY	HYPERTROPHIC CARDIOMYOPATHY	RESTRICTIVE CARDIOMYOPATHY	ARRHYTHMOGENIC RIGHT VENTRICULAR CARDIOMYOPATHY
Myocytes	Injured	Hypertrophy	Stiff myocardium	Fibrous and fatty tissue replaces right ventricular myocardium
Contractility	Decreased	Increased	Normal or decreased	Decreased right ventricular contractility
Stroke volume	Decreased	Decreased	Fixed	Decreased right ventricular stroke volume
Diastolic relaxation	May be impaired	Impaired	Impaired	
Ventricular filling pressures	Increased		Increased	
Left ventricular end diastolic pressure		Increased	Increased	
Chambers	Dilated left ventricle	Left ventricular hypertrophy May obliterate left ventricular outflow tract	Dilation of atria and pulmonary veins	Right ventricular enlargement, akinesia, dyskinesia, or right ventricular aneurysm.
Valves	Mitral regurgitation	Mitral regurgitation		
Cardiac output	Decreased	Decreased and cannot increase cardiac output with exertion	Decreased and heart rate dependent	
Mixed venous Oxygen consumption		Increased		
Arrhythmias		Ventricular		Ventricular
Systolic pressure		Increased		

DISCUSSION

INDICATIONS FOR TRANSPLANT IN PEDIATRIC HEART FAILURE PATIENTS

Heart transplant is advised in patients with end-stage heart failure who are unresponsive to surgical and medical management. Heart failure due cardiomyopathy and congenital heart disease is a predominant indication for transplant in pediatric population.[17]

EVALUATION OF TRANSPLANT RECIPIENTS

The pretransplant screening of pediatric heart transplant patient encompasses appraisal of risks associated with transplant surgery, surgical or nonsurgical ameliorative interventions, patient's prevailing state of health, and impact on patient's survival without transplant. A collaborative multidisciplinary team-based management strategy is effective in addressing the healthcare challenges of this critically ailing population. Several issues need to be addressed before

Table 12.6 HEMODYNAMIC GOALS FOR INTRAOPERATIVE MANAGEMENT OF MAJOR CARDIOMYOPATHIES

PARAMETER	DILATED	HYPERTROPHIC	RESTRICTED	ARVD
Heart rate	Normal/increase	Decrease	Increase	Normal/decrease
Preload	Normal/increase	Normal/increase	Increase	Normal
Afterload	Decrease	Increase	Normal/increase	Normal
Contractility	Increase	Decrease	Normal/increase	Normal/increase
Rhythm	Sinus	Sinus	Sinus	Sinus

listing a patient for heart transplant. First, an extensive assessment of patient's heart disease and all available medical and surgical management alternatives must be performed. Second, any associated comorbidities that will have ramification on survival and quality of life posttransplant should be accounted for. Third, psychological status of the patient and the family should be evaluated for adequate knowledge, commitment and provision of support structure. Lastly, any contraindications to the heart transplant should be investigated.[18–20] Patient evaluation should include the following.

ANATOMICAL EVALUATION

History and physical examination should include assessment of vascular access for monitoring, administration of medications, and resuscitation during and after transplant. Multiple previous catheterizations and prolonged hospital stay can obstruct the vessels and make vascular access challenging. Imaging studies such as chest radiography, echocardiography, cardiac catheterization, and computed tomography can ascertain comprehensive anatomy and physiological parameters of the heart and great vessels.

ASSESSMENT OF PULMONARY VASCULAR RESISTANCE

A fixed Pulmonary Vascular Resistance Index of upwards of 9 IU is considered as high risk for acute donor right heart failure and early death and is recognized as a contraindication for isolated heart transplantation. Preoperatively, inotropes, and vasodilator therapy can be used for evaluation of treatment and responsiveness of PVR as well as risk stratification of the patients.[21]

LABORATORY INVESTIGATIONS

Evaluation for heart transplant involves blood typing for ABO compatibility and human lymphocyte antigen testing. However, infants and young children who have insignificant anti-A and anti-B isohemagglutinins titers can receive ABO-incompatible donor heart. Human lymphocyte antigen testing is significant in patients that have previously received blood products and/or an organ transplant. Blood transfusion, previous homograft implantation, and organ transplantation can induce allosensitization in recipients. Allosensitization can result in cardiac allograft dysfunction, acute cellular and antibody-regulated rejection, and vasculopathy of transplanted heart. Panel reactive antibody screen is utilized to screen for antibodies to human lymphocyte antigen. Patients with high panel reactive antibody undergo plasmapheresis, receive intravenous immunoglobin and rituximab to lower the panel reactive antibody levels, and improve graft survival and decrease mortality.[22]

Generally, serologic testing for infectious disease encompasses screening for cytomegalovirus (CMV), Epstein-Barr virus, herpes simplex virus, varicella, toxoplasma gondii, HIV, measles, and hepatitis viruses A, B, C, and D. The screening discerns presence of any chronic viral infective agents such as hepatitis B or C and/ or HIV, and other acute viral, bacterial, and fungal infections that deter heart transplantation. Immunosuppression can reactivate hepatitis C infection. Serologic testing of CMV may direct prophylactic and diagnostic evaluation of posttransplant fever and occurrence and course of postoperative CMV infection. Immunosuppression to prevent graft rejection also puts the recipient at risk for posttransplant lymphoproliferative disease, frequently resulting from Epstein-Barr virus and CMV. Seronegativity to both Epstein-Barr virus and CMV are risk factors for development of posttransplant lymphoproliferative disease. A thorough evaluation of immunization history is also essential prior to transplant to update any pending immunization and minimize use of live viral vaccines posttransplant.[23]

PREOPERATIVE ANESTHETIC EVALUATION

Preoperatively, the clinical summary of the recipient from transplant coordinator provides information about medical and surgical history, demographics, vitals, status of venous access, immunosuppression and CMV status, medical and device management, and last cardiac catheterization data of the patient. A preoperative "huddle" facilitates knowledgeable, safe, and effective clinical care to these critical patients and usually involves anesthesiologists, intensivists, surgeons, and transplantation cardiologists. At the "huddle" specifics of immunosuppression, allosensitization, plasmapheresis, vascular access, coagulation management, infection prophylaxis, renal protection, and other crucial elements of the procedure are discussed. Perioperative challenges are identified and plans made on how to mitigate them. If the patient is on mechanical circulatory support, a transport plan should be devised with appropriate personnel. Pacemaker or implantable cardioverter-defibrillators should be evaluated and reprogrammed as necessary for the procedure. The perfusionist must be fully prepared for urgent transition to cardiopulmonary bypass if the patient decompensates after anesthesia induction. Overall, careful preoperative planning and preparation is vital for a successful outcome of the transplant surgery.[24,25]

REVIEW QUESTIONS

1. Primary cardiomyopathies predominantly involve the heart muscle, whereas secondary cardiomyopathies affect other organs besides the myocardium. Which one of the following **LEAST** fits into this group of cardiomyopathy?

    A. dilated cardiomyopathy
    B. hypertrophic cardiomyopathy
    C. noonan
    D. takotsubo

Correct Answer: C
Noonan syndrome is a form of secondary cardiomyopathy with dysmorphic facial features and involvement of cardiovascular, gastrointestinal, genitourinary, hematological, skeletal,

neurologic, and lymphatic systems. Hypertrophic and dilated cardiomyopathies are forms of primary cardiomyopathies. Takotsubo is a rare form of primary cardiomyopathy, which is more prevalent in adult population. The cardiomyopathy is characterized by LV dysfunction and apical ballooning and is provoked by physical or emotional stress.

2. A 10-month-old, 11-kg female with no significant past medical history presented to her primary physician with a recent complaint of decreased appetite. Her physical examination demonstrated dyspnea, rales, and peripheral edema. She seemed cold upon touching, and her capillary refill time was more than 2 seconds. Based on her physical examination, which of the following terminology **BEST** describes this patient's heart failure?

    A. cold and dry
    B. wet and cold
    C. warm and dry
    D. wet and warm

Correct Answer: B
Based on the physical exam, she falls into the "wet and cold" category of acute heart failure. She may have progressively worsened from "warm and dry" to her current state. She will benefit from inotropic and vasoactive support, which would improve her perfusion and optimize her circulation.

3. A 6-year old, 25-kg male presents with abdominal pain, vomiting, tachycardia, dyspnea on exertion, marked tachypnea, and increased work of breathing. He had a history of viral illness about a week prior to this presentation. He also had a family history of a sibling's death due to heart failure. Which classification **BEST** fits the severity of heart failure in this child?

    A. class I
    B. class II
    C. class III
    D. class IV

Correct Answer: B
This patient presented with marked tachypnea and dyspnea on exertion. Based on these symptoms, this patient falls under class III of Ross classification.

4. Which of the following is/are **LEAST** indicated in the evaluation of myocarditis?

    A. brain natriuretic peptide level
    B. echocardiogram
    C. electrocardiogram
    D. pulmonary function tests

Correct Answer: D
Pulmonary function tests are not used in the evaluation of myocarditis. BNP and prohormone NT-proBNP are used to diagnose heart failure and predict severity and assess responsiveness to treatment. Echocardiography delineates the cause and severity of heart failure; identifies structural abnormalities; evaluates ventricular cavity size and function; assesses left atrial volume and diastolic function; estimates pulmonary artery pressures; identifies concomitant pathophysiology; observes

impact of medications and other treatment; and helps with prognosis. A 12-lead electrocardiogram identifies baseline rhythm and establishes the presence of any arrhythmia and myocardial ischemia.

5. Of the main intraoperative hemodynamic goals for the management of dilated cardiomyopathy, which of following would be **LEAST** advantageous?

    A. afterload: increase
    B. contractility: increase
    C. heart rate: normal/increase
    D. preload: normal/increase

Correct Answer: A
Afterload reduction in dilated cardiomyopathy helps improve stroke volume and ejection fraction of the failing ventricle.

6. Which of the following drugs is **LEAST** like an ACEI?

    A. captopril
    B. enalaprilat
    c. levosimendan
    D. lotensin

Correct Answer: C
Levosimendan is a calcium-sensitizing drug with inotropic and vasodilating properties. It increases cardiac contractility and cardiac output without increasing the oxygen demand of the myocardial cells. Levosimendan decreases preload and afterload and improves tissue perfusion.

7. During a cardiac catheterization, what is the **BEST** location to get a mixed venous gas sample in a patient with dilated cardiomyopathy and absence of cardiac shunt?

    A. inferior vena cava
    B. pulmonary Artery
    C. right atrium
    D. superior vena cava

Correct Answer: B
In the absence of a shunt, there is complete mixing of the superior vena cava, inferior vena cava, and coronary sinus blood in the right-sided chambers before it reaches the pulmonary artery. As the blood reaches the pulmonary capillaries after traversing the pulmonary artery, it will get mixed with oxygenated pulmonary capillary blood. So, pulmonary artery serves as the best location for drawing a mixed-venous oxygen saturation sample.

QUESTIONS AND ANSWERS

This chapter has accompanying questions and answers which are available to subscribers as part of the Oxford eLearning platform. To access the questions, go to ✔ http://oxfordmedicine. com/pediatricanesthesiaPBL

REFERENCES

1. Maron BJ, Towbin JA, Thiene G, et al. Contemporary definitions and classification of the cardiomyopathies: an American Heart

Association Scientific Statement from the Council on Clinical Cardiology, Heart Failure and Transplantation Committee; Quality of Care and Outcomes Research and Functional Genomics and Translational Biology Interdisciplinary Working Groups; and Council on Epidemiology and Prevention. *Circulation*. 2006;113(14):1807–1816.

2. Grady KL, Dracup K, Kennedy G, et al. Team management of patients with heart failure: a statement for healthcare professionals from the Cardiovascular Nursing Council of the American Heart Association. *Circulation*. 2000;102(19):2443–2456.

3. Macicek SM, Macias CG, Jefferies JL, Kim JJ, Price JF. Acute heart failure syndromes in the pediatric emergency department. *Pediatrics*. 2009;124(5):e898–e904.

4. Ross RD. The Ross classification for heart failure in children after 25 years: a review and an age-stratified revision. *Pediatr Cardiol*. 2012;33(8):1295–1300.

5. Rosenthal D, Chrisant MR, Edens E, et al. International Society for Heart and Lung Transplantation: practice guidelines for management of heart failure in children. *J Heart Lung Transplant*. 2004;23(12):1313–1333.

6. Das BB. Role of endomyocardial biopsy for children presenting with acute systolic heart failure. *Pediatr Cardiol*. 2014;35(2):191–196.

7. Johnson PC, Dec GW, Lilly LS. The cardiomyopathies. In: Lilly LS, ed. *Pathophysiology of Heart Disease: A Collaborative Project of Medical Students and Faculty*. 6th ed. Philadelphia: Lippincott Williams & Wilkins; 2016:249–267.

8. Johnson JS, Loushin MK. The effects of anesthetic agents on cardiac function. In: Iaizzo PA, ed. *Handbook of Cardiac Anatomy, Physiology, and Devices*. Cham: Springer International; 2015:295–306.

9. Page RL 2nd, O'Bryant CL, Cheng D, et al. Drugs that may cause or exacerbate heart failure: a scientific statement from the American Heart Association. *Circulation*. 2016;134(6):e32–e69.

10. Kirk MA. Cardiac catheterization and endomyocardial biopsy. In: *ISHLT Guidelines for the Management of Pediatric Heart Failure* (ISHLT Monograph Series Book 8). Addison, TX: International Society for Heart & Lung Transplantation; 2014.

11. Hussey AD, Weintraub RG. Drug treatment of heart failure in children: focus on recent recommendations from the ISHLT guidelines for the management of pediatric heart failure. *Paediatr Drugs*. 2016;18(2):89–99.

12. Mets B. Management of hypotension associated with angiotensin-axis blockade and general anesthesia administration. *J Cardiothorac Vasc Anesth*. 2013;27(1):156–167.

13. Di Nardo M, MacLaren G, Marano M, Cecchetti C, Bernaschi P, Amodeo A. ECLS in pediatric cardiac patients. *Front Pediatr*. 2016;4:109.

14. Gournay V, Hauet Q. Mechanical circulatory support for infants and small children. *Arch Cardiovasc Dis*. 2014;107(6–7):398–405.

15. Byrnes J, Villa C, Lorts A. Ventricular assist devices in pediatric cardiac intensive care. *Pediatr Crit Care Med*. 2016;17(8 Suppl 1):S160–S170.

16. Mascio CE. The use of ventricular assist device support in children: the state of the art. *Artif Organs*. 2015;39(1):14–20.

17. Thrush PT, Hoffman TM. Pediatric heart transplantation—indications and outcomes in the current era. *J Thorac Dis*. 2014;6(8):1080–1096.

18. Smith AL, Sims DB. Patient selection and indications for heart transplantation. In: Kirk AD, ed. *Textbook of Organ Transplantation*. West Sussex, UK: John Wiley; 2014:30.

19. Mehra MR, Kobashigawa J, Starling R, et al. Listing criteria for heart transplantation: International Society for Heart and Lung Transplantation guidelines for the care of cardiac transplant candidates—2006. *J Heart Lung Transplant*. 2006;25(9):1024–1042.

20. Mehra MR, Canter CE, Hannan MM, et al. The 2016 International Society for Heart Lung Transplantation listing criteria for heart transplantation: a 10-year update. *J Heart Lung Transplant*. 2016;35(1):1–23.

21. Chiu P, Russo MJ, Davies RR, Addonizio LJ, Richmond ME, Chen JM. What is high risk? Redefining elevated pulmonary vascular resistance index in pediatric heart transplantation. *J Heart Lung Transplant*. 2012;31(1):61–66.

22. Asante-Korang A, Jacobs JP, Ringewald J, et al. Management of children undergoing cardiac transplantation with high panel reactive antibodies. *Cardiol Young*. 2011;21(Suppl 2):124–132.

23. Patel UD, Thomas SE. Evaluation of the candidate. In: Fine RN, Webber SA, Olthoff, KM, Kelly DA, Harmon WE, eds. *Pediatric Solid Organ Transplantation*. 2nd ed. Oxford: Blackwell; 2007:265–270.

24. Williams GD, Hammer GB. Cardiomyopathy in childhood. *Curr Opin Anaesthesiol*. 2011;24(3):289–300.

25. Williams GD, Ramamoorthy C, Sharma, A. Anesthesia for cardiac and pulmonary transplantation. In: Andropoulos DB, Stayer, Mossad EB, Miller-Hance WC, eds. *Anesthesia for Congenital Heart Disease*. 3rd ed. Hoboken, NJ: John Wiley; 2015:636–660.

13.

PEDIATRIC HEART TRANSPLANTATION

Nelson Burbano-Vera and Annette Y. Schure

STEM CASE AND KEY QUESTIONS

A 4-year-old boy with a history of neonatal critical aortic stenosis and multiple previous cardiac surgeries/interventions (fetal and postnatal aortic valve dilations, Ross procedure, mitral and pulmonary valve repair and replacements) presents for orthotopic heart transplantation. He is listed as United Network for Organ Sharing (UNOS) status 1A for stage D heart failure and had been doing well at home on a continuous milrinone infusion.

WHAT ARE THE MOST COMMON INDICATIONS FOR HEART TRANSPLANTATION IN CHILDREN? HOW LONG IS THE AVERAGE TIME ON THE WAIT LIST? WHAT ARE TYPICAL BRIDGING THERAPIES? WHAT DOES UNOS STATUS 1A MEAN? WHAT ARE IMPORTANT QUESTIONS FOR THE PREOPERATIVE EVALUATION?

Six months ago, during his pretransplant workup, cardiac catheterization showed a low normal cardiac index, significant tricuspid regurgitation, mild mitral stenosis, and right ventricular and pulmonary hypertension (HTN) with mean pulmonary arterial pressure of 39 mmHg, a transpulmonary gradient of 21 mmHg, a pulmonary vascular resistance (PVR) of 6.4 WU, a wedge pressure of 23 mmHg and significant diastolic dysfunction (left ventricular end diastolic pressure 18 mmHg). Vasodilator testing revealed an adequate response to oxygen and nitric oxide. His laboratory test results are remarkable for a panel reactive antibody (PRA) of 24%.

WHAT ARE THE MAIN ANESTHETIC CONCERNS FOR THIS PATIENT? HOW WOULD YOU MONITOR THIS PATIENT? WHAT MEDICATIONS WOULD YOU USE TO INDUCE GENERAL ANESTHESIA?

The patient receives supplemental oxygen and a carefully titrated intravenous (IV) premedication while being continuously monitored during transport to the operating room. After an uneventful IV induction with fentanyl, ketamine, and rocuronium, the patient is orally intubated without any problems. A radial arterial line and additional peripheral IV catheters are inserted. During positioning for the central venous line, blood pressure and end-tidal CO_2 suddenly decrease, and within seconds the heart rate drops to the mid-50s.

WHAT IS THE DIFFERENTIAL DIAGNOSIS FOR HYPOTENSION AND BRADYCARDIA IN THIS SITUATION? WHAT ARE TYPICAL CHALLENGES IN THE PRE-BYPASS PERIOD?

The patient responds to hyperventilation, increased fraction of inspired oxygen and inotropic support. A 5 French double-lumen central line is placed in the right jugular vein without further complications. Bilateral near infrared spectroscopy sensors and a transesophageal echo (TEE) probe are added for monitoring. The incision is well tolerated by the patient, but 15 minutes into the surgery, during the median sternotomy, the blood pressure suddenly decreases to the mid-60s; the heart rate is 110 bpm.

WHAT ARE TYPICAL EVENTS DURING THE SURGICAL DISSECTION PHASE? HOW DO YOU PREPARE FOR THESE COMPLICATIONS?

After volume replacement, blood transfusion and surgical repair of a perforation in the left innominate vein, the surgical dissection of the dense mediastinal adhesions continues. The donor heart arrives in the operating room 30 minutes later.

WILL THIS PATIENT REQUIRE ANYTHING SPECIAL BEFORE CARDIOPULMONARY BYPASS IS INITIATED? HOW IS THE DONOR HEART PREPARED? DO YOU HAVE ANY CONCERNS REGARDING THE TIMING?

Once the dissection is finished, the aorta and both caval veins are cannulated. Given the elevated PRA, cardiopulmonary bypass is started with an exchange transfusion to decrease the antibody load. A bicaval technique is used to transplant the prepared donor heart into the recipient. After release of the aortic cross clamp the transplanted heart is re-perfused. The patient is ventilated, and low-dose inotropic support with epinephrine started. Despite adequate reperfusion time, the initial TEE shows a dilated right ventricle (RV) with severe dysfunction and tricuspid regurgitation. The left ventricle (LV) function is moderately depressed.

WHAT ARE THE MAIN CONCERNS FOLLOWING CARDIOPULMONARY BYPASS AFTER HEART TRANSPLANTATION? HOW WOULD YOU MANAGE THE VENTRICULAR DYSFUNCTION IN THIS PATIENT?

The inotropic support is increased, the ventilation is optimized, and inhaled nitric oxide started. The RV function is slowly improving. Protamine is given slowly, followed by transfusions of platelets and cryoprecipitate. The activated clotting time is normal, but there is diffuse bleeding in the field. With ongoing volume resuscitation, the blood pressure is 65/45 mmHg and the central venous pressure 22 mmHg.

HOW DO YOU ASSESS AND TREAT COAGULOPATHY AFTER CARDIOPULMONARY BYPASS? WHAT ARE TYPICAL SURGICAL COMPLICATIONS AFTER THIS PROCEDURE?

Thromboelastography demonstrates a decreased maximal amplitude, and the coagulopathy is corrected with additional platelets. The bleeding eventually slows, and the surgeon can close the chest without major hemodynamic problems. The patient is transferred to the intensive care unit and successfully extubated on the third postoperative day.

POSTTRANSPLANT PERIOD

One year after transplant the patient presents for follow-up endomyocardial biopsy and first surveillance coronary angiography. He has been doing well at home on standard immunosuppressive medications. The last endomyocardial biopsy was consistent with grade 0 cellular rejection. The most recent transthoracic echocardiogram showed good biventricular function, trivial tricuspid regurgitation, mild mitral regurgitation, and mildly elevated right ventricular pressure.

WHAT ARE THE MAIN ANESTHETIC CONCERNS FOR PATIENTS WITH TRANSPLANTED HEARTS? WHAT INFORMATION IS IMPORTANT FOR THE PREOPERATIVE EVALUATION? WHAT IS THE BEST ANESTHESIA TECHNIQUE FOR ENDOMYOCARDIAL BIOPSIES AND CORONARY ANGIOGRAPHY IN SMALL CHILDREN?

After a thorough review of his medications and laboratory results, the patient receives an oral premedication with midazolam and is taken to the catheterization suite for an inhalational induction and placement of a peripheral IV line. Venous access is very difficult and multiple attempts are necessary.

ARE THERE ANY ALTERNATIVE OPTIONS? WHAT KIND OF ACCESS IS NECESSARY FOR ENDOMYOCARDIAL BIOPSIES WITH CORONARY ANGIOGRAPHY? WHAT ARE THE POTENTIAL COMPLICATIONS OF THESE PROCEDURES?

Peripheral access is established, and after a small bolus of propofol, rocuronium, and fentanyl, the patient is orally intubated with a 4.5 ID-cuffed endotracheal tube. Five minutes later the blood pressure is 65/40 mmHg.

WHAT IS THE DIFFERENTIAL DIAGNOSIS? WHAT IS THE BEST WAY TO TREAT HYPOTENSION IN PATIENTS WITH TRANSPLANTED HEARTS? ARE THERE ANY PREFERRED MEDICATIONS?

Once the cardiology team successfully accessed the right femoral vein and artery, the right heart catheterization is started. During passage of the balloon catheter, the heart rate suddenly jumps from 100 bpm to 200 bpm, and the blood pressure drops form 90/50 mmHg to 75/45 mmHg. The electrocardiogram tracing shows a narrow complex tachycardia.

WHAT ARE THE TREATMENT OPTIONS FOR SUPRAVENTRICULAR TACHYCARDIA? ARE THERE ANY SPECIAL CONCERNS FOR PATIENTS WITH TRANSPLANTED HEARTS?

After the right-heart catheterization and endomyocardial biopsies, the cardiologists proceed with the coronary angiography. Immediately after the contrast injection, the ST segments are elevated, there are short runs of ventricular tachycardia, and the patient is hypotensive.

WHAT COULD HAVE HAPPENED? WHAT IS THE BEST MANAGEMENT FOR ACUTE ST ELEVATION DURING THE CORONARY ANGIOGRAM?

The rest of the procedure is uneventful, and after removal of the sheaths and adequate hemostasis, the patient is ready for extubation. The train-of-4 is 3 out of 4.

WOULD YOU REVERSE THE NEUROMUSCULAR BLOCKADE?

DISCUSSION

The International Society for Heart and Lung Transplantation (ISHLT) is an important source for trends and developments in the transplant field. ISHLT collects worldwide data in a special registry and publishes annual reports with the latest analyses.

Every year about 500–600 pediatric heart transplantations are reported to the ISHLT. This number has been relatively stable over the last 5–10 years.[1]

INDICATIONS FOR HEART TRANSPLANTATION IN CHILDREN

As shown in Figure 13.1, the typical indications for pediatric heart transplantations vary by age: congenital heart disease is the most common indication during infancy whereas in older children dilated cardiomyopathy is the predominant diagnosis.[1,2]

According to the American Heart Association, pediatric heart failure can be classified in 4 stages (A, B, C, and D).[2] Please refer to Table 13.1 for further details.

Class I indications for pediatric heart transplantation are defined as[2]

- Stage D heart failure associated with systemic ventricular dysfunction in patients with cardiomyopathies or congenital heart disease.

- Stage C heart failure in pediatric heart disease with severe limitation of exercise and activity (maximal oxygen uptake <50% predicted), near sudden death and/or life-threatening arrhythmias untreatable with medications or an implantable defibrillator, and restrictive cardiomyopathy disease associated with reactive pulmonary HTN.

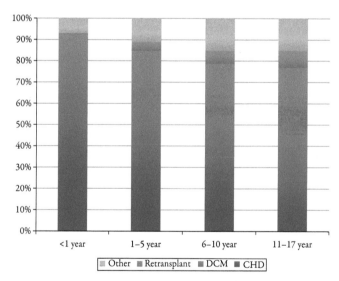

Fig 13.1 Recipient diagnosis by age group. CHD: congenital heart disease (hypoplastic left heart syndrome, valvular heart disease, etc.). DCM: dilated cardiomyopathy (idiopathic or caused by Adriamycin, alcohol, myocarditis, etc.). Retransplant: acute or chronic rejection, graft vasculopathy. Other: arrhythmogenic RV dysplasia, cancer, coronary artery disease, myopathy, hypertrophic or restrictive cardiomyopathy. Modified from Rossano JW, Dipchand AI, Edwards LB, et al. The Registry of the International Society for Heart and Lung Transplantation: Nineteenth Pediatric Heart Transplantation Report 2016; Focus theme: primary diagnostic indications for transplant. *J Heart Lung Transplant*. 2016;35(10): 1185–1195.

- Stage C heart failure associated with systemic ventricular dysfunction in patients with cardiomyopathies or congenital heart disease and significant growth failure attributable to the heart disease.

- After heart transplant with abnormal ventricular function and at least moderate graft vasculopathy.

Based on Organ Procurement and Transplantation Network data as of September 1, 2017, the overall median waiting time in the United States for children <18 years old is about 130 days. The time on the wait list is highly dependent on factors such as blood type (shortest for AB; longest for O), age (shortest for 11–17 years; longest for 1–5 years), UNOS status, and ethnicity. The Organ Procurement and Transplantation Network website offers a wealth of information about transplantation (http://optn.transplant.hrsa.gov).

While on the waiting list, the patients are usually managed with maximized heart failure therapy: diuretics, angiotensin-converting enzyme inhibitors, pulmonary vasodilators, and often additional continuous inotropic support (milrinone). Some children require electrophysiological interventions (implantable cardioverter-defibrillator or biventricular pacemaker for resynchronization therapy). Other bridging therapies include mechanical support with extracorporeal membrane oxygenation (short-term support), ventricular assist device (VAD), or special pediatric intra-aortic balloon pumps (for infants >4 kg).[1,3–8]

The UNOS is a private, nonprofit organization, contracted by the federal government to manage the organ transplant system in the United States. As presented in Table 13.2, UNOS has 3 different status assignments for pediatric patients on the waiting list: status 1A reflects the highest medical urgency for transplant (https://www.transplantpro.org).

PREOPERATIVE EVALUATION

Most patients presenting for heart transplantation had a thorough workup before being listed. This usually includes various imaging studies (echo, cardiac catheterization, etc.), liver biopsy, and a system-by-system assessment to search for dysfunction of other organs that could impact the posttransplant outcome. Box 13.1 lists common extracardiac comorbidities encountered in pediatric patients presenting for heart transplantation.[9,10]

A full report or at least a detailed summary, including history, baseline physical exam, social evaluation, laboratory, and important cardiopulmonary data should be available for review. The preoperative evaluation should otherwise focus on the interval history, recent changes in functional status or medications, anticoagulation, possible infections, vascular access, and nil per os status. Close communication with the surgical team regarding timing for induction and line placement is extremely important, especially for patients with multiple previous surgeries and potentially prolonged dissection. The plan for vascular access and emergency cannulation sites should also be discussed in

Table 13.1 HEART FAILURE STAGING IN PEDIATRIC PATIENTS

A	At risk for developing heart failure (i.e., presence of congenital heart defect)
B	Abnormal cardiac structure and/or function with no symptoms of heart failure (i.e., univentricular heart)
C	Abnormal cardiac structure and/or function with past or present symptoms of heart failure (i.e., repaired congenital heart defect)
D	Abnormal cardiac structure and/or function, continuous infusion of intravenous inotropes or prostaglandin E1 to maintain patency of a ductus arteriosus, mechanical ventilator and/or mechanical circulatory support

Modified from Canter CE, Shaddy RE, Bernstein D, et al. Indications for heart transplantation in pediatric heart disease: a scientific statement from the American Heart Association Council on Cardiovascular Disease in the Young; the Councils on Clinical Cardiology, Cardiovascular Nursing, and Cardiovascular Surgery and Anesthesia; and the Quality of Care and Outcomes Research Interdisciplinary Working Group. *Circulation.* 2007;115(5):658–676.

advance and an appropriate number of blood products ordered from the blood bank.

Unfortunately, the anesthesiologist has often little information about the donor heart during the preoperative evaluation. Box 13.2 highlights some valuable information.[11,12]

INTRAOPERATIVE MANAGEMENT

As illustrated in Table 13.3, patients presenting for heart transplantation have a wide variety of potential anesthetic concerns.[13,14] The use of premedication will depend on the age of the patient and the hemodynamic state. The combination of hypoxemia, hypercarbia, increased PVR, systemic vasodilation, and hypotension related to oversedation may be catastrophic, especially in patients with pulmonary HTN and significant right ventricular dysfunction. On the other hand, after multiple surgeries or weeks or months in the hospital, many transplant patients not only have significant levels of anxiety or even posttraumatic stress disorder but also high tolerance for sedatives and opioids. If premedication is necessary, it should be carefully titrated together with the administration of supplemental oxygen.

Standard noninvasive monitors should be placed before induction of general anesthesia. Invasive blood pressure monitoring, central venous access, and TEE are added after induction and endotracheal intubation. Some experts avoid using the right internal jugular vein for central venous line placement due to the future need of this vessel as the route for endomyocardial biopsies. Cerebral oximetry with near infrared spectroscopy, thromboelastography, and monitoring of pulmonary artery pressure are optional.

Rapid sequence induction is not ideal due to the tenuous hemodynamic state of these patients but should be considered when clinically indicated. There is no single "magic recipe" for anesthesia induction and maintenance, and, like in any other case, the anesthetic strategy should be customized for each patient. The general rule is "keep the patient where she or he lives" (preoperative vital signs when the patient is clinically well compensated). In general, hemodynamic goals for induction of anesthesia are:

- Preload: It is important to avoid acute changes in preload. Although the patient with end-stage heart failure is normally preload dependent, the preload state during induction will depend on the efficacy of the anticongestive/diuretic therapy. Patients may present to the operating room in a hypervolemic state (due to inadequate diuretic therapy or diuretic resistance despite complete tubular blockade) or intravascular depleted from overaggressive anticongestive therapy. In congestive patients, additional increases in preload only further increase left atrial pressure and pulmonary congestion without increasing cardiac output (abnormal preload recruitable stroke work relationship). In depleted patients,

Table 13.2 UNITED NETWORK FOR ORGAN SHARING PEDIATRIC HEART STATUS ASSIGNMENTS

CATEGORY	DESCRIPTION
Status 1A	Less than 18 years old with at least 1 of the following: • Requires continuous mechanical ventilation • Requires assistance of an intra-aortic balloon pump • Has ductal dependent pulmonary or systemic circulation, with ductal patency maintained by stent or prostaglandin infusion • Has a hemodynamically significant congenital heart disease diagnosis, requires infusion of multiple intravenous inotropes or a high dose of a single intravenous inotrope • Requires assistance of a mechanical circulatory support device
Status 1B	Less than 18 years old with at least 1 of the following: • Requires infusion of one or more inotropic agents but does not qualify for pediatric status 1A • Is less than 1 year old and has diagnosis of hypertrophic or restrictive cardiomyopathy
Status 2	Less than 18 years old and does not meet the criteria for pediatric status 1A or 1B but is suitable for transplant.

Source. Modified from (https://www.transplantpro.org)

- Central nervous system: seizure and stroke

- Endocrine: hypothyroidism (related to chronic amiodarone use)

- Pulmonary: pulmonary HTN (related to end-stage heart failure or congenital heart disease), intrinsic lung disease (frequently seen in cyanotic heart defects after multiple open heart procedures)

- Gastrointestinal: liver dysfunction (related to Fontan physiology or chronic heart failure) and malnutrition (related to end stage heart failure or protein loosing enteropathy in Fontan physiology)

- Genitourinary: chronic kidney disease (related to end stage heart failure or nephrotoxic immunosuppressants in patients presenting for re-transplant)

- Hematologic: deep venous thrombosis, intracardiac thrombosis, anemia of chronic disease, acquired antithrombin III (AT III) deficiency and chronic antiplatelet or other anticoagulation therapy, platelet dysfunction with chronic milrinone therapy.

- Immunologic: sensitization and concurrent infections.

  - Sensitization, allosensitization or humoral sensitization: panel reactive antibodies >10% to donor human leucocyte antigens. The PRA measures the presence of preformed circulating antibodies to HLA in the recipient. Sensitization is a risk factor for acute rejection, late rejection and mortality. It is caused by previous transfusions (surgery, extracorporeal membrane oxygenation, VAD) and exposure to homograft material (congenital heart surgery).
  - Infections: active infections (relative contraindication to transplant), CMV, and Epstein-Barr virus. CMV negative (−) recipients who receive a heart from a CMV positive (+) donor are at risk of clinical CMV disease.

preload augmentation may place the myocardium in a more favorable position of the Frank-Starling curve and increase the cardiac output.

- Cardiac contractility: The goal is to preserve contractility if necessary with early use of inotropic support and by avoiding myocardial depressants (high concentration of volatile anesthetics, high dose propofol, or ketamine with its direct cardiac depressant effects, potentially "demasked" in the setting of low catecholamine reserve).

- Heart rate: It is often beneficial to maintain normal/high heart rate and avoid bradycardia. Due to the intrinsic myocardial limitation to increase cardiac output at expense of stroke volume, the blood pressure becomes more dependent than normal on an adequate heart rate.

Box 13.2 KEY POINTS FOR DONOR HEART

- Chest trauma, cardiopulmonary resuscitation, low dose inotropic support or donations after cardiac death are not contraindications for donation.

- ABO compatibility should be confirmed before accepting and procuring the donor heart.

- Size matching of the organ is based on weight. Although the ideal donor/recipient ratio is 0.8–2.0, a wide range of donor/recipient ratios is acceptable (children with cardiomyopathy can accept larger hearts).

- Total ischemic time should be less than 3.5 hours.

- Infectious screening of the donor is vital.

- Cardiovascular assessment should include:

  - Electrocardiogram: frequently observed non-specific T wave and ST segment changes (neurogenic, electrolytes, catecholamines) do not increase mortality after heart transplantation
    - Chest radiograph.
    - Echocardiogram: cardiac dysfunction (LV ejection fraction <50% on inotropic support), significant valve regurgitation or pericardial effusion are red flags.
    - Cardiac enzymes: mild elevations in cardiac enzymes do not increase mortality.
  - Coronary angiography (i.e., adult donor with high risk of coronary artery disease for adolescent recipient).

Pre-bypass	Difficult vascular access
	Decreased cardiopulmonary reserve
	Hemodynamic instability
	Pulmonary hypertension
	Right ventricle dysfunction
	Aspiration
	Increased risk of infection with invasive monitoring
	Massive bleeding during repeat sternotomy
	Arrhythmias during dissection phase
Post-bypass	Elevated pulmonary vascular resistance
	Right ventricle dysfunction
	Left ventricle dysfunction
	Sinus node dysfunction
	Denervated heart
	Vasoplegia
	Renal dysfunction
	Acute lung injury
	Coagulopathy
	Hyperacute rejection

- Cardiac rhythm: The preservation of sinus rhythm and the "atrial kick" can be extremely important. Depending on the degree of diastolic dysfunction, the loss of sinus rhythm can lead to significant hemodynamic instability.

- Afterload: Normal or slightly lower afterload will promote anterograde flow and systemic perfusion, but hypotension must be avoided. The failing ventricle is very sensitive to decreases in coronary perfusion; low blood pressure can be detrimental. When myocardial depression is avoided, general anesthesia typically increases the cardiac output mainly due to its effect on decreasing afterload for the failing ventricle.

- PVR: PVR reflects the afterload for the RV and must be minimized. The importance of avoiding excessive increases in PVR during the transition from negative to positive pressure ventilation in the setting of a failing RV cannot be stressed enough. Factors that increase PVR include hypoxemia, hypercarbia, acidosis, low lung volume (due to high resistance to flow in extra-alveolar vessels, mainly larger arteries and veins), high lung volume (due to high resistance to flow in alveolar vessels, mainly pulmonary capillaries), positive intrathoracic pressure

(mean airway pressure can be used as a surrogate of intrathoracic pressure), and sympathetic activation.

AIRWAY MANAGEMENT

Selection of the mechanical ventilation mode and settings should be tailored toward minimizing PVR and afterload to the RV (typically the LV benefits from switching from negative pressure to positive pressure ventilation). In general, pressure control ventilation or hybrid modes that guarantee tidal volumes of 6–8 mL/kg, low respiratory rate, prolonged expiratory time (inspiratory:expiratory ratio 1:3), and minimal or no extrinsic positive end expiratory pressure are preferred by the authors to achieve ideal functional residual capacity and minimize PVR (PVR is the lowest when lung volume is close to functional residual capacity) while keeping intrathoracic pressure low. A useful way to monitor the effect of positive pressure ventilation on the intrathoracic pressure is by looking at the mean airway pressure which should be kept below 10 cm H_2O at all times and ideally below 5–6 cm H_2O in cases of significant RV dysfunction. Anesthesia maintenance is generally achieved with a balanced technique of low dose volatile agents, opioids, and muscle relaxants.

BLEEDING

Bleeding during the surgical dissection phase is a common problem, especially in anticoagulated patients with multiple previous surgeries or significant collaterals. Adequate vascular access, availability of cell saver, rapid infusion equipment, and close communications with the surgeons and the blood bank are essential.

TIMEOUT

See Figure 13.2 for the necessary timeout upon arrival of the donor heart.

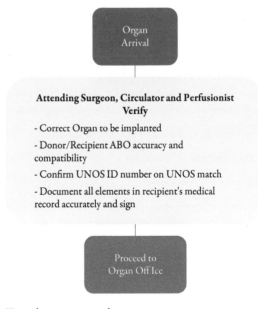

Fig. 13.2 Transplant organ arrival timeout.

CARDIOPULMONARY BYPASS MAINTENANCE

Cardiopulmonary bypass maintenance is not different from other pediatric open-heart procedures. Fresh-frozen plasma may be added to the bypass prime for patients with a ventricular assist device on anticoagulation. Bicaval-aortic cannulation is required. Most cases are done under mild hypothermia (>30°C) and alpha-stat blood gas management. If moderate hypothermia (25–30°C) is to be used, pH-stat blood gas management is indicated. Cardioplegia is not normally needed for the recipient or donor heart (the donor heart receives cardioplegia immediately before harvesting). It may be decided to administer cardioplegia before reperfusion of the donor heart if the ischemic time has been prolonged (>4 hours). High doses of methylprednisolone are typically used at the beginning of the bypass and before reperfusion of the graft. Intraoperative exchange transfusion or plasmapheresis may be performed for allosensitized patients to remove circulating human leukocyte antigen antibodies. At the author's institution, exchange transfusion is used more frequently than plasmapheresis, reserving the latter for larger patients. Exchange transfusion involves previous notification and request of an exchange volume to the blood bank (typically 2 times the estimated patient blood volume in red blood cells and plasma), modification of the perfusion circuit (Y in the venous line and an additional cardiotomy reservoir to drain and collect the blood volume of the patient), clear communication with the surgeon regarding the plan for the blood volume of the patient after it has been removed (it can be discharged or cell salvaged), and timing for use of pump suckers (use of wall sucker until after the exchange transfusion is complete). Patients with persistent aortopulmonary collaterals present an additional challenge due to the risk of systemic hypoperfusion and inadequate cerebral blood flow. Lower temperature, pH-stat blood gas management, higher pump flow, and hematocrit levels may be required during the bypass.

SEPARATION FROM CARDIOPULMONARY BYPASS

Separation from cardiopulmonary bypass is a critical part of the intraoperative anesthetic management. Right ventricular dysfunction is perhaps the most common hemodynamic problem in the post-bypass period. The best treatment strategy is prevention, early recognition, and intervention. Adequate preoperative donor evaluation, myocardial protection, and shortening of ischemic time are powerful tools to prevent ventricular dysfunction. The 3 pillars of right ventricular dysfunction treatment are (a) inotropic support, (b) low PVR, and (c) maintenance of coronary perfusion pressure. Epinephrine, dopamine, and milrinone are frequently used to provide inotropic support to the failing ventricle in the operating room. Although milrinone has the additional advantage of decreasing PVR, its use is frequently accompanied with systemic hypotension. Loading doses should be avoided after the patient is separated form cardiopulmonary bypass because hypotension may be severe. Continuous infusions without a loading dose should be started early enough during

the case if its pharmacologic effect is desired in the operating room. The combination of milrinone with norepinephrine is frequently used in some centers to contrast the hypotensive effect of milrinone. The goal of the mechanical ventilation strategy is to achieve a normal functional residual capacity while maintaining a low intrathoracic pressure and mean airway pressure. This can be obtained with the use of a normal-high tidal volume, low respiratory rate, and prolonged expiratory time strategy. Inhaled as opposed to systemic pulmonary vasodilators are preferred at the authors' institution to avoid the systemic hypotensive effect of these agents. Pharmacologic options include nitric oxide and prostaglandin I2 (Flolan, Veletri). The failing RV is very sensitive to ischemia, and the combination of high PVR and low coronary perfusion pressure may initiate a positive feedback loop characterized by rapid hemodynamic deterioration →hypotension + high PVR → RV dysfunction + RV dilation + tricuspid regurgitation → left shifting of ventricular septum → decreased filling of LV → low seminal vesicle stroke volume, CO, and blood pressure → further decrease in coronary perfusion pressure → further RV dysfunction.

Ongoing bleeding after separation from bypass and heparin reversal with protamine is often a major problem. Dysfunctional platelets after long bypass runs or chronic milrinone therapy, hemolysis, extensive suture lines, and collaterals can require multiple rounds of blood products. The constant volume resuscitation is a challenge for the struggling RV and leads to further dilation and decreased cardiac output. Thrombelastography can help to identify the coagulopathy and guide the therapy. Occasionally prothrombin complex factor concentrates are used to minimize the volume load for the dilated RV.

Typical surgical complications after heart transplantation include stenotic anastomoses of the pulmonary arteries, pulmonary veins or the caval veins. Significant increases in the central venous pressures measured via an internal jugular venous catheter despite an empty right atrium or adequate RV function should trigger direct measurements and surgical explorations. Minor SVC stenosis can be later treated in the cardiac catheterization laboratory.

POSTTRANSPLANT PERIOD

Over the last decades survival rates for pediatric heart transplant recipients have significantly improved. According to the most recent report from the ISHLT, the median survival for patients who were transplanted as an infant is currently 20.7 years, for children age 1–5 years, it is 18.2 years.[1] This progress is based on sophisticated new immunosuppression with different induction and maintenance therapies, strict surveillance protocols, intense antirejection therapy, and aggressive treatment of long-term morbidity.

Pediatric anesthesiologists will be increasingly involved in the care of patients with transplanted hearts for various diagnostic and surgical procedures. A thorough preoperative evaluation and basic understanding of the altered physiology, the pharmacologic implications, and procedure are important for safe anesthetic management.

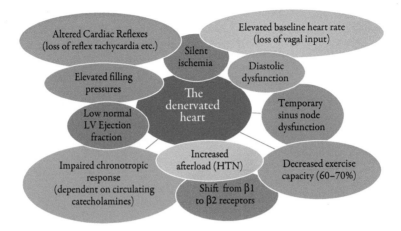

Fig. 13.3 Physiology of the denervated heart. Modified from Cotts WG, Oren RM. Function of the transplanted heart: unique physiology and therapeutic implications. *Am J Med Sci.* 1997;314:164–172.

PHYSIOLOGY OF THE TRANSPLANTED HEART

Acute denervation, physiologic adjustments and potential reinnervation

After loss of sympathetic and parasympathetic innervation, the transplanted heart is dependent on an intact Frank Starling mechanism and circulating endogenous catecholamines to increase cardiac output. The afferent denervation results in a lack of chest pain with ischemia. Reflex mechanisms involving cardiac baro- and mechano-receptors are altered (loss of reflex tachycardia during hypovolemia, increased blood volume due to decreased natriuresis, loss of nocturnal blood pressure changes, etc.). Baseline heart rate and filling pressures are elevated, and the exercise capacity is decreased (60%–70%). Additional characteristic changes are illustrated in Figure 13.3.[15,16]

Months to years after the transplant, partial and regionally heterogenous reinnervation is possible, but only occurs in 40%–70% of recipients. Reinnervation can improve basal heart rate, blood flow regulation, ventricular function, and exercise performance.[16]

Altered response to medications

As shown in Table 13.4, the denervation also changes the response to certain medications: Indirect-acting sympathomimetics like dopamine and ephedrine are less effective; parasympatholytics like atropine and glycopyrrolate or digoxin have no effect on heart rate. In contrast, direct-acting sympathomimetics like epinephrine or norepinephrine can have an exaggerated response due to the lack of presynaptic uptake and need to be carefully titrated. The denervated heart is also "supersensitive" to Ca-channel-, β-blockers and especially to adenosine. A regular dose given for the treatment of supraventricular tachycardia can lead to prolonged asystole. For transplant patients, it is recommended to reduce the initial dose by at least 50%.[15,17,18] Due to the lack of reflex tachycardia, direct vasodilators such as nitroprusside, nitroglycerine, or hydralazine can cause profound hypotension.

IMMUNOSUPPRESSION

The consequences of lifelong immunosuppression can have significant anesthetic implications.

Induction therapy

Currently, 70% of patients will receive an induction therapy to delay the use of nephrotoxic maintenance agents or reduce the need for high dose steroids. Thymoglobin or basiliximab, an interleukin-2 receptor antagonist, are often used for induction therapy. They deplete lymphocytes or prevent T-cell proliferation. See Table 13.5 for further details. Opportunistic infections can be a major problem.

Maintenance therapy

After the induction therapy, the immunosuppression can be maintained with various combinations of steroids, calcineurin

Table 13.4 **ALTERED RESPONSE TO MEDICATIONS**

DECREASED RESPONSE	EXACERBATED RESPONSE (SUPERSENSITIVITY)
Indirect acting sympathomimetics Dopamine, ephedrine - depleted NA storage in cardiac nerve endings	Direct acting sympathomimetics Epinephrine, norepinephrine - Lack of presynaptic uptake
Atropine and glycopyrrolate - No heart rate response	Ca-channel or β-blocker, Adenosine - Profound bradycardia/ asystole
Digitalis	Direct vasodilators Nitroprusside, nitroglycerine, hydralazine - Lack of reflex tachycardia

Source. Modified from Cotts WG, Oren RM. Function of the transplanted heart: unique physiology and therapeutic implications. *Am J Med Sci.* 1997;314:164–172.

Table 13.5 INDUCTION THERAPY

MEDICATION	MECHANISM	SIDE EFFECTS

Antilymphocyte antibodies
 - Polyclonal antithymocyte globulin
 - Monoclonal antibodies:
  - Muromonab-CD3,
  - alemtuzumab-CD52
	Lymphocyte depletion
	Multiple cell surface antigens
	Single T-cell surface antigen
		Opportunistic infections, malignancies?
		"serum sickness," leukopenia, thrombocytopenia
		"cytokine release syndrome,"
		fever, anaphylaxis, aseptic meningitis

Anticytokine receptor antibodies - Basiliximab, daclizumab	IL-2 receptor antagonists prevent T cell proliferation	Opportunistic infections

Source. Modified from Singh RK, Humlicek T, Jeewa A, Fester K. Pediatric Cardiac Intensive Care Society 2014 consensus statement: pharmacotherapies in cardiac critical care immune therapy. *Pediatr Crit Care Med.* 2016;17:S69–S76.

inhibitors like tacrolimus or the newer mechanistic target of rapamycin (mTOR) inhibitors sirolimus and an antiproliferative agent like mycophenolate mofetil. They all have multiple side effects, which are described in Table 13.6.

Rejection therapy

During episodes of acute rejections, therapy is often intensified and high-dose steroids added. Depending on the type of rejection, humoral or cellular, occasionally plasmapheresis, IV immunoglobulin, or monoclonal antibodies are necessary. As shown in Table 13.7, infections and infusion-related symptoms like fever or bronchospasm can complicate treatment.[19]

LONG-TERM MORBIDITY

Graft failure, cardiac allograft vasculopathy (CAV), renal dysfunction, HTN, and malignancies are common long-term problems associated with pediatric cardiac transplantation.[1,13,20,21]

1. Graft failure: Progressive heart failure can be caused by ischemia secondary to coronary artery disease or by acute or chronic rejections.

2. CAV: CAV is present in about 30%–40% of recipients 10 years posttransplant. It usually involves the distal coronary arteries and is mainly diagnosed during the annual angiography. Statins and mTOR inhibitors like sirolimus are used for prophylaxis. Treatment options include balloon dilations, stents, and antiplatelet therapy, but eventually it will require another transplant.

3. Renal dysfunction: Depending on the age at transplant (infants and small children less than adolescents), 5%–15% of patients have severe renal dysfunction (creatinine >2.5 mg/dL or renal replacement therapy) 10 years posttransplant.

4. HTN: HTN is a common finding; it can be a side effect of medications or caused by renal dysfunction and fluid retention.

5. Posttransplant lymphoproliferative disorder occurs in up to 10% of late survivors. It is characterized by an abnormal proliferation of B-cells in various degrees, 87% of cases are Ebstein-Barr virus positive. The primary location is often the gastrointestinal tract or the lungs. Treatment usually involves reduced immunosuppression monoclonal antibodies like rituximab and occasionally chemotherapy.

Table 13.6 MAINTENANCE THERAPY

MEDICATION	MECHANISM	SIDE EFFECTS
Corticosteroids	Inhibition of IL-1,2,3,6, TNF	Emotional instability, adrenocortical suppression, DM, HTN, fluid retention, weight gain, growth suppression, osteoporosis, glaucoma, infections, abdominal discomfort etc.
Cyclosporin Tacrolimus	Calcineurin Inhibitors Prevention of T cell proliferation	Nephrotoxicity, HTN, hyperlipidemia, DM, neurotoxicity, hypertrichosis, gingival hyperplasia Better with tacrolimus: no hypertrichosis or gingival hyperplasia
Sirolimus Everolimus	mTOR Inhibitors Rapamycin - Proliferation Signal - Serine/Threonine Protein Kinase Inhibition of smooth muscle cell and endothelial cell proliferation	Hyperlipidemia, hypertriglyceridemia, anemia, cytopenia, poor wound healing
Azathioprine Mycophenolate mofetil	Antiproliferative agents	Bone marrow suppression, nausea and vomiting, hepatotoxicity, pancreatitis

Source. Modified from Singh RK, Humlicek T, Jeewa A, Fester K. Pediatric Cardiac Intensive Care Society 2014 consensus statement: pharmacotherapies in cardiac critical care immune therapy. *Pediatr Crit Care Med.* 2016;17:S69–S76.

Table 13.7 **REJECTION THERAPYW**

A) Intensification or changes of current immunosuppression
B) High-dose intravenous steroids (3–5 days), followed by oral pulsed steroids
C) Plasmapheresis and intravenous immunoglobulin for antibody- mediated rejection
D) Antirejection Medications

MEDICATION	MECHANISM	SIDE EFFECTS
Rituximab	Monoclonal antibody—inhibits B cell proliferation and causes cellular apoptosis	FDA black box warning: HBV reactivation, PML Infusion-related reactions: bronchospasm, hypotension, neutropenia, thrombocytopenia
Eculizumab	Monoclonal antibody Inhibits complement C5	FDA black box warning: meningococcal infection risk. Infusion related reactions
Bortezomib	Proteasome inhibitor Cell cycle arrest and apoptosis	Peripheral neuropathy, infectious complications

Note. FDA = Food and Drug Administration. HBV = Hepatitis B virus. PML = progressive multifocal leukoencephalopathy.

Source. Modified from Singh RK, Humlicek T, Jeewa A, Fester K. Pediatric Cardiac Intensive Care Society 2014 consensus statement: pharmacotherapies in cardiac critical care immune therapy. *Pediatr Crit Care Med.* 2016;17:S69–S76.

SURVEILLANCE

Early detection of rejection and immediate treatment are important factors for improved survival after pediatric heart transplantations. The gold standard is currently serial endomyocardial biopsies and annual coronary angiography for early detection of CAV. The frequency of biopsies is highly dependent on the individual institution and can vary between 2–9 per year (first year posttransplant) to annually or "on cause" basis (after third year).[22] The choice of vascular access is influenced by age, size, anatomy, and indication: the femoral vessels are usually used for infants and toddlers or when coronary studies are planned. In older children and adolescents, the right internal jugular vein is preferred to minimize the recovery time (no bedrest).

Depending on patient age, comorbidities, and functional status, various anesthetic techniques have been used for endomyocardial biopsies, ranging from simple sedations, total IV anesthesia with propofol and natural airways, and laryngeal mask airways to general anesthesia with endotracheal intubation.

Severe adverse events occur in about 1% of procedures and are mainly caused by atrial or ventricular arrhythmias, vessel trauma, hemato- or pneumothorax, hypotension, hypoxia, and/ or airway issues. Atrial arrhythmias are often self-limited or can be terminated with catheter manipulations, adenosine (in reduced dose), or synchronized cardioversions. Sustained ventricular arrhythmias may require chest compressions and defibrillation or temporary pacing for complete heart block. The addition of coronary angiography increases the risk for complications significantly. Air bubbles during the contrast dye injection, vasospasm, or coronary dissections are potential complications and can lead to sudden ST changes. Treatment options include intra-arterial nitroglycerin, stents, and occasionally bypass surgery.[23]

ANESTHETIC CONSIDERATIONS

Pediatric heart transplant patients may present with unique challenges.

Difficult IV access

After multiple surgeries and hospitalizations, these patients often have poor venous access. The use of new technologies (infrared or ultrasound guidance), search in atypical locations (upper arm, leg), and close cooperation with the cardiologist (sharing access) are sometimes necessary.

Neurocognitive deficits and behavioral problems

Children with congenital heart disease frequently have neurocognitive deficits and developmental delays, and there is growing evidence that pediatric heart transplant recipients can experience significant adjustment and behavioral problems, resulting in poor compliance and lack of cooperation.[24–26] Even minor procedures can require heavy premedication, deep sedation, or general anesthesia.

Episodes of rejection

Signs of acute rejection can range from subtle variations in exercise tolerance to sudden onset of life-threatening arrhythmia and acute heart failure. Prior to any endomyocardial biopsy, elective or urgent, a careful history and physical examination should specifically address any recent changes in functional status, syncopal episodes, or adjustments of medications.

Previous biopsy results, current medications, and long-term morbidity

A thorough review of previous biopsy results, current immunosuppression or heart failure therapy, recent pulse steroids, evidence of liver, bone marrow or renal dysfunction, and long-term morbidity (CAV; posttransplant lymphoproliferative disease) is an important part of every preoperative evaluation.

Increased risk for infection and fractures

Chronic immunosuppression and repeated high-dose steroid pulses predisposes these patients to infections and bone fractures. Aseptic techniques and careful positioning are essential.

Choice of medications

The unique physiology of the denervated heart and the altered response to certain medications can influence the anesthetic course and the choice of rescue drugs.

- Physiology of denervated heart
  - Loss of cardiac reflexes, dependent on preload and circulating catecholamines
- Altered response to medications
  - No heart rate response to atropine, glycopyrrolate, and digitalis
  - Exaggerated response to Ca-channel blockers, β-blockers, and adenosine
  - Exaggerated response to direct acting sympathetic agents
  - Decreased response to indirect acting agents like dopamine and ephedrine

Hypotension is best treated with a careful fluid bolus and titration of a direct-acting sympathomimetic. For postoperative pain management, nonsteroidal anti-inflammatory drugs are usually avoided due to concerns about renal dysfunction. There are several case reports of cardiac arrests in association with reversal of neuromuscular blockade, but no common underlying cause could be established.[27] A recent investigation at a large tertiary center did not find any significant heart rate changes with neostigmine and glycopyrrolate.[28] Careful preoperative evaluation and assessment for potential rejection and CAV seem to be more important factors.

REVIEW QUESTIONS

1. A 3-year-old boy with a LVAD due to dilated cardiomyopathy is in the operating room to receive an orthotropic heart transplant. Immediately after IV induction with midazolam, fentanyl, ketamine and rocuronium, the LVAD starts alarming and the perfusionist correctly states that it is due to a "suction event." What is the BEST initial treatment?

A. Decrease the revolutions per minute of the LVAD.
B. Do nothing, as it is a self-limiting event.
C. Increase the revolutions per minute of the LVAD.
D. Increase Trendelenburg position.
E. Reverse Trendelenburg position.

Answer: A
"Suction events" are common in the operating room in patients with VADs. They typically occur when there is a rapid decrease in the preload of the ventricle (venodilation from anesthesia induction, bleeding, decreased venous return during pneumoperitoneum in abdominal laparoscopic surgery, etc.) while the pump flow (RPMs) remains constant. This is followed by a decrease in the LV diastolic volume and diameter and mechanical obstruction of the inflow cannula of the VAD by the ventricular wall or papillary muscles. The best initial approach is to decrease the flow of the VAD to relieve the obstruction and normalize the ventricular diameter, flow of the VAD (there is transient interruption of flow during the suction event) and systemic perfusion. It should be followed by IV volume administration. The diagnosis can be readily confirmed with transthoracic or transesophageal echocardiography, which will show collapse of the left ventricular cavity, left septal deviation, and turbulent flow at the level of the inflow cannula (typically placed at the apex of the LV). Position changes are ineffective methods to change the preload of small children.

2. Which of the following is LEAST likely to be seen as a contraindication to single heart transplantation?

A. active malignant neoplasmic diseases
B. allosensitization to human leucocyte antigens (HLA)
C. severe, irreversible end-organ or systemic disease
D. irreversible PVR (>6)
E. uncontrolled gram negative diplococci infection

Answer: B
Allosensitization or sensitization is defined as a PRA >10% to donor HLA. The PRA measures the presence of circulating preformed antibodies to HLA in the recipient. Although this humoral sensitization is a risk factor for early graft failure, coronary artery vasculopathy and even mortality, it is not considered a contraindication to heart transplantation. Although the presence of end-stage organ disease is still considered a contraindication to single heart transplant, combined kidney–heart or liver–heart transplants have been performed successfully in some institutions. PVR >6 Wood units/m² and transpulmonary gradient >15 mmHg that does not response to high fraction of inspired oxygen or pulmonary vasodilators, uncontrolled infection, and active neoplasm are also considered contraindications to heart transplantation.

3. Death, 1-year posttransplant, is MOST likely due to which of the following causes?

A. acute cellular rejection
B. antibody-mediated rejection
C. coronary allograph vasculopathy
D. lymphoproliferative disease
E. nosocomial infection
F. severe renal dysfunction

Answer: A
The leading causes of death during the first year after pediatric heart transplantation are acute cellular rejection and infection. Rejection peaks at 1–2 months posttransplant and approximately 40% of all the pediatric transplanted patients have had an episode of rejection during the first year after the transplant. Severe renal dysfunction is seen in about 10% of pediatric heart transplant recipients within 10 years

posttransplant and typically is not a common cause or early death. Posttransplant lymphoproliferative disorder includes benign and malignant disorders, is more common in children than in adults after transplant, and typically occurs during the first year posttransplant. CAV is the leading cause of late death and graft loss in pediatric patients after heart transplantation.

4. Regarding pulmonary HTN in the pediatric patient candidate for heart transplantation, which of the following is **MOST** accurate statement?

    A. For biventricular physiology it is defined as PVR >6 Wood units/m^2 and mean pulmonary artery pressure (PAP) >25 mmHg

    B. left-sided heart disease is typically the cause of pulmonary HTN

    C. positive vasodilator response is defined as a fall in mean PAP and PVR by 10%

    D. For univentricular physiology it is defined as PVR >3 Wood units/m2, even if mean PAP <25 mmHg

Answer: D
In 2011 The Pulmonary Vascular Research Institute Pediatric Taskforce defined the criteria for pediatric pulmonary hypertensive vascular disease following a cavopulmonary anastomosis (answer D). In the setting of nonpulsatile pulmonary blood flow, significant pulmonary hypertensive vascular disease may still be present even though the mean PAP is less than 25 mmHg. Pulmonary HTN is typically due to left heart disease in cases of cardiomyopathy but not in cases of congenital heart disease where it is caused by a combination of multiple factors (increased pulmonary blood flow due to left to right shunting, pulmonary vein obstruction, lung disease, chronic hypoxia, etc.). The correct definition of pulmonary HTN for a biventricular physiology (children and adults) includes mean PAP >25 mmHg and PVR >3 Wood units/m^2. PVR of 6 Wood units/m^2 when irreversible typically corresponds to the cut-off value when heart transplantation is deemed contraindicated. A positive vasodilator response typically is considered as a fall in mean PAP and PVR >20% of the baseline value. The absence of pulmonary HTN before the institution of cardiopulmonary bypass does not rule out its presence during the postbypass period.

5. A 10-year-old girl who weighs 30 kg is presenting for her regular surveillance endomyocardial biopsy. She underwent an uneventful heart transplantation for a dilated cardiomyopathy 9 months ago. Her previous biopsies were all negative, and she had no significant episode of rejection. She is currently treated with tacrolimus and mycophenolate mofetil. Clinically she is doing very well. She has been nil per os for 12 hours and "insists" on a mask induction. Her heart rate is 90 beats per minute, and her baseline blood pressure 110/65mmHg. After an uneventful inhalational induction, placement of a peripheral IV cannula and an IV bolus of 30 mg of propofol, a laryngeal mask airway is inserted without any problems. Two minutes later, the noninvasive blood pressure reads 65/40 mmHg. The heart rate is 85 bpm. What is the **MOST** appropriate next action?

    A. atropine 0.3 mg IV push
    B. ephedrine 5 mg IV push
    C. epinephrine 0.3 mg IV push
    D. normal saline 300 mL IV

Answer: D
The transplanted heart is dependent on preload and circulating catecholamines to increase the cardiac output. Hypotension is best treated with fluids and careful titration of a direct-acting sympathomimetic. A dose of 0.3 mg of epinephrine (= 10 mcg/kg) is a full-code dose and can result in significant HTN and tachycardia. The denervated heart is "supersensitive" to direct acting sympathomimetic medications due to the lack of presynaptic uptake. Careful titration in small increments is recommended. Atropine is a parasympatholytic and has no effect on the heart rate in the denervated heart. The heart rate is this scenario is 85 bpm and age appropriate. Ephedrine is an indirect acting sympathomimetic. Its effectiveness is dependent on the release of norepinephrine from cardiac nerve endings and therefore reduced in the denervated heart.

6. A 3-year old, 15 kg boy is undergoing a routine surveillance endomyocardial biopsy under general anesthesia with a laryngeal mask airway. Shortly after insertion of the catheter through a sheath in the right internal jugular vein, the heart rate increases suddenly from 110 bpm to 190 bpm. The blood pressure drops from 90/60 mmHg to 70/40 mmHg. The oxygen saturation remains stable at 98%. What is the **MOST** appropriate immediate treatment?

    A. adenosine 1.5mg IV push
    B. catheter manipulation
    C. defibrillation with 30 J
    D. normal saline 300 mL

Answer: B
Episodes of supraventricular tachycardia during endomyocardial biopsies are best treated with initial catheter manipulations (withdrawal of catheter, quick advancement, etc.), cold saline flush, adenosine IV push in reduced dose (0.025–0.05 mg/kg), or synchronized cardioversion with 0.5–1.0 J/kg. Defibrillation with 2 J/kg is the treatment of choice for ventricular fibrillation. Adenosine (0.1mg/kg) is the standard dose and can cause prolonged asystole in the denervated heart. It is recommended to reduce the dose to 25%–50% for patients with transplanted hearts. A fluid bolus will not convert the underlying arrhythmia.

7. After an uneventful routine surveillance biopsy and coronary angiography, a 14-year-old, 50 kg girl is complaining about pain in the right groin. The area is tender to touch but not swollen or bruised. What is the **BEST** treatment option?

    A. acetaminophen 325mg per os
    B. diclofenac 50mg per os
    C. ibuprofen 200 mg per os
    D. ketorolac 15mg IV

Answer: A

For postoperative pain management, nonsteroidal anti-inflammatory drugs are usually avoided due to concerns about renal dysfunction.

8. Six months after heart transplantation for dilated cardiomyopathy, a 5-year-old girl is presenting for a routine surveillance biopsy. Her immunosuppression is currently maintained with tacrolimus. Which of the following side effect is **MOST** typical of tacrolimus?

    A. gingival hyperplasia
    B. glaucoma
    C. nephrotoxicity
    D. osteoporosis

Answer: C

Typical side effects of tacrolimus are nephrotoxicity, HTN, hyperlipidemia, diabetes, and neurotoxicity. Gingival hyperplasia and hypertrichosis are associated with cyclosporine, the other calcineurin inhibitor. Osteoporosis and glaucoma can be seen with glucocorticoid therapy.[19]

9. A 16-year-old boy is presenting for his annual surveillance biopsy and coronary angiography. He receives 50 mcg of fentanyl and 5mg of midazolam intravenously for sedation and is tolerating the procedure well. After the contrast injection into the coronaries, his electrocardiogram tracing suddenly shows massive ST elevations. Heart rate is 60 bpm, and blood pressure 120/70. What medication is **MOST** appropriate to use for the immediate treatment?

    A. epinephrine
    B. nitroglycerine
    C. phenylephrine
    D. vasopressin

Answer: B

ST elevations during contrast injections into the coronaries can be caused by vasospasm, air bubbles, or dissections. Coronary vasospasm can be treated with intra-arterial nitroglycerin injections through the catheter. An appropriate dose should always be prepared. Phenylephrine, epinephrine, and vasopressin are not first-line treatment choices for presumed coronary vasospasm but might be indicated if the ischemia results in hemodynamic instability and cardiac arrest.

10. A 4-year-old girl who received a heart transplant 3 months ago for complex congenital heart disease presented 2 days ago with tachycardia, hypotension, and new onset arrhythmias. Acute rejection was suspected and treatment started. She is now scheduled for an endomyocardial biopsy. On exam she is wheezing but does not have a history of asthma, reactive airway disease or recent upper respiratory infection. Her chest X-ray is clear. The physical finding is **MOST** likely associated with which of her medications?

    A. mycophenolate mofetil
    B. prednisolone
    C. rituximab
    D. tacrolimus

Answer: C

Treatment with rituximab, a monoclonal antibody, can cause infusion related symptoms like bronchospasm or hypotension. As outlined in Table 13.6, tacrolimus, mycophenolate mofetil, and prednisolone, which are mainly used for maintenance therapy, are associated with multiple side effects but usually not bronchospasm or wheezing unless it is caused by an infection or fluid overload.

QUESTIONS AND ANSWERS

This chapter has accompanying questions and answers which are available to subscribers as part of the Oxford eLearning platform. To access the questions, go to ✓ http://oxfordmedicine.com/pediatricanesthesiaPBL

REFERENCES

1. Rossano JW, Dipchand AI, Edwards LB, et al. The Registry of the International Society for Heart and Lung Transplantation: Nineteenth pediatric heart transplantation report 2016: focus theme: primary diagnostic indications for transplant. *J Heart Lung Transplant.* 2016;35(10):1185–1195.

2. Canter CE, Shaddy RE, Bernstein D, et al. Indications for heart transplantation in pediatric heart disease: a scientific statement from the American Heart Association Council on Cardiovascular Disease in the Young; the Councils on Clinical Cardiology, Cardiovascular Nursing, and Cardiovascular Surgery and Anesthesia; and the Quality of Care and Outcomes Research Interdisciplinary Working Group. *Circulation.* 2007;115(5):658–676.

3. Rosenthal D, Chrisant MR, Edens E, et al. International Society for Heart and Lung Transplantation: Practice guidelines for management of heart failure in children. *J Heart Lung Transplant.* 2004;23(12):1313–1333.

4. Assad-Kottner C, Chen D, Jahanyar J, et al. The use of continuous milrinone therapy as bridge to transplant is safe in patients with short waiting times. *J Card Fail.* 2008;14(10):839–843.

5. Birnbaum BF, Simpson KE, Canter CE, et al. Intravenous home inotropic use is safe in pediatric patients awaiting transplantation. *Circ Heart Fail.* 2015;8(1):64–70.

6. Veasy LG, Blalock RC, Orth JL, Boucek MM. Intra-aortic balloon pumping in infants and children. *Circulation.* 1983;68(5):1095–1100.

7. Barbaro RP, Paden ML, Guner YS, et al. Pediatric Extracorporeal Life Support Organization Registry international report 2016. *ASAIO J.* 2017;63(4):456–463.

8. Blume ED, Naftel DC, Bastardi HJ, et al. Outcomes of children bridged to heart transplantation with ventricular assist devices: a multi-institutional study. *Circulation.* 2006;113(19):2313–2319.

9. Davies RR, Russo MJ, Mital S, et al. Predicting survival among high-risk pediatric cardiac transplant recipients: an analysis of the United Network for Organ Sharing database. *J Thorac Cardiovasc Surg.* 2008;135(1):147–155.

10. Pollock-BarZiv SM, den Hollander N, Ngan, B-Y, et al. Pediatric heart transplantation in human leukocyte antigen sensitized patients: evolving management and assessment of intermediate-term outcomes in a high-risk population. *Circulation.* 2007;116(11 Suppl):I172–I178.

11. Morrissey PE, Monaco AP. Donation after circulatory death: current practices, ongoing challenges, and potential improvements. *Transplantation.* 2014;97(3):258–264.

12. Ford MA, Almond CS, Gauvreau K, et al. Association of graft ischemic time with survival after heart transplant among

children in the United States. *J Heart Lung Transplant.* 2011;30(11):1244–1249.

13. Schure AY, Kussman BD. Pediatric heart transplantation: demographics, outcomes, and anesthetic implications. *Paediatr Anaesth.* 2011;21(5):594–603.

14. Schumacher KR, Gajarski RJ. Postoperative care of the transplanted patient. *Curr Cardiol Rev.* 2011;7(2):110–122.

15. Cotts WG, Oren RM. Function of the transplanted heart: unique physiology and therapeutic implications. *Am J Med Sci.* 1997;314:164–172.

16. Awad M, Czer LS, Hou M, et al. Early denervation and later reinnervation of the heart following cardiac transplantation: a review. *J Am Heart Assoc.* 2016;5:1–21.

17. Flyer JN, Zuckerman WA, Richmond ME, et al. Prospective study of adenosine on atrioventricular nodal conduction in pediatric and young adult patients after heart transplant. *Circulation.* 2017;135(25):2485–2493.

18. Ellenbogen KA, Thames MD, DiMarco JP, Sheehan H, Lerman BB. Electrophysiological effects of adenosine in the transplanted human heart: evidence of supersensitivity. *Circulation.* 1990;81:821–828.

19. Singh RK, Humlicek T, Jeewa A, Fester K. Pediatric Cardiac Intensive Care Society 2014 consensus statement: pharmacotherapies in cardiac critical care immune therapy. *Pediatr Crit Care Med.* 2016;17:S69–S76.

20. Kindel SJ, Pahl E. Current therapies for cardiac allograft vasculopathy in children. *Congenit Heart Dis.* 2012;7:324–335.

21. Webber SA, Naftel DC, Fricker FJ, et al. Lymphoproliferative disorders after paediatric heart transplantation: a multi-institutional study. *Lancet.* 2006;367:233–239.

22. Godown J, Harris MT, Burger J, Dodd DA. Variation in the use of surveillance endomyocardial biopsy among pediatric heart transplant centers over time. *Pediatr Transplant.* 2015;19:612–617.

23. Daly KP, Marshall AC, Vincent JA, et al. Endomyocardial biopsy and selective coronary angiography are low-risk procedures in pediatric heart transplant recipients: results of a multicenter experience. *J Heart Lung Transplant.* 2012;31:398–409.

24. Uzark K, Spicer R, Beebe DW. Neurodevelopmental outcomes in pediatric heart transplant recipients. *J Heart Lung Transplant.* 2009;28:1306–1311.

25. Brosig C, Pai A, Fairey E, Krempien J, McBride M, Lefkowitz DS. Child and family adjustment following pediatric solid organ transplantation: factors to consider during the early years post-transplant. *Pediatr Transplant.* 2014;18:559–567.

26. Fredericks EM, Zelikovsky N, Aujoulat I, Hames A, Wray J. Post-transplant adjustment—the later years. *Pediatr Transplant.* 2014;18:675–688.

27. Bertolizio G, Yuki K, Odegard K, Collard V, Dinardo J. Cardiac arrest and neuromuscular blockade reversal agents in the transplanted heart. *J Cardiothorac Vasc Anesth.* 2013;27:1374–1378.

28. Barbara DW, Christensen JM, Mauermann WJ, Dearani JA, Hyder JA. The safety of neuromuscular blockade reversal in patients with cardiac transplantation. *Transplantation.* 2016;100:2723–2728.

14.

TRANSCATHETER CLOSURE OF ATRIAL SEPTAL DEFECTS

Khoa Nguyen and Patrick Callahan

STEM CASE AND KEY QUESTIONS

A 16-year-old otherwise healthy female presents to her primary care physician with shortness of breath and palpitations. She is active and plays soccer but for the last few months states that she is noticing increasing episodes of shortness of breath with self-limiting episodes of palpitations and chest pain. Her review of symptoms is positive for the abdominal pain, diarrhea, and headaches. On physical exam, she has a normal heart rate and blood pressure. The young woman is healthy appearing and in no acute distress. Her lung fields are clear to auscultation bilaterally. She is noted to have a normal S1 and S2 was physiologically split.

WHAT IS THE MOST COMMON REASON FOR CHEST PAIN IN THE CHILDREN AND ADOLESCENTS? IN AN ADOLESCENT WITH AN ATRIAL SEPTAL DEFECTS (ASD), WHAT IS THE MOST COMMON FINDING ON AUSCULTATION OF THE HEART? IF THIS PATIENT HAS AN ASD, WHICH KIND WOULD SHE MOST LIKELY HAVE? IF YOU WERE TO OBTAIN AN ELECTROCARDIOGRAM (EKG), WHAT YOU EXPECT TO SHOW IF SHE HAD AN ASD?

Based on the history and physical exam an EKG and echocardiogram are performed. The EKG shows a normal sinus rhythm with a normal QRS duration of 96 mms, and the QT is top normal as well around 450 mms. There are nonspecific ST-T wave changes. The transthoracic echocardiogram fails to show her coronary artery origins, and there is concern for an atrial level defect with some right-sided volume overload. There is normal ventricular function. She is referred for a cardiac magnetic resonance imaging (MRI) for further evaluation.

The patient's cardiac MRI confirms the presence of an ASD. It is noted to be a large 32 × 18 mm secundum ASD with significant left-to-right shunting. They calculate a Qp:Qs of 2.6:1. There is right-sided volume overload with preserved biventricular systolic function. The coronary artery origins are normal. She is counseled regarding the pathophysiology of ASDs and the possibility for complications including include

right ventricular failure, pulmonary hypertension, and atrial arrhythmias. Closure of her defect is recommended to prevent these complications moving forward. She is referred to the interventional cardiologist by the general cardiologist.

DOES SHE NEED TO RESTRICT HER ACTIVITY LEVEL? DOES SHE REQUIRE SUBACUTE BACTERIAL ENDOCARDITIS FOR DENTAL WORK? THE PATIENT IS WORRIED SHE WILL EXPERIENCE CLAUSTROPHOBIA DURING THE MRI. WOULD OFFER HER SEDATION? IF YES, WHAT KIND OF SEDATION WOULD YOU OFFER? IS SHE AT INCREASED RISK FOR COMPLICATIONS FOR INTRAVENOUS SEDATION? DO CARDIAC MRIS HAVE ANY SPECIAL CONSIDERATIONS?

The interventionalist repeats the transthoracic echocardiogram. It confirms a large posterior secundum ASD with left-to-right atrial shunting. They do not see a posterior rim. The right atrium and right ventricle are both moderately dilated. The lack of a posterior rim is a significant problem in considering her as a candidate for device closure. If there is not adequate tissue surrounding the defect, the device will embolize and not stay in place. While the interventional cardiologist is leaning toward recommending surgical closure, they note that the transthoracic images are limited and the cardiologist recommends a transesophageal echocardiogram to gather more information. Luckily, the transesophageal echocardiogram shows a posterior rim that was not seen on the transthoracic images, and the patient is scheduled for device closure in the cardiac catheterization lab.

DOES THIS PATIENT REQUIRE GENERAL ANESTHESIA FOR THIS CARDIAC CATHETERIZATION LAB PROCEDURE?

Risks of the procedure including infection, arrhythmia, clot formation, stroke, blood loss or transfusion, pulse loss, vessel damage, cardiac arrest, bruising, and device erosion are reviewed with the patient and her family. Two options, the Amplatzer™ septal occluder and the Gore® Cardioform device, are discussed. On the day of the procedure, she has an uneventful induction of anesthesia and the cardiologist gets to work. The patient is prepped and draped and groin access is obtained uneventfully while a transesophageal echocardiogram confirms previous findings. A right and left heart catheterization collects all hemodynamic data from the superior vena cava, right atrium, right ventricle, main pulmonary artery, right pulmonary artery, right pulmonary artery wedge, and descending aorta.

WHAT CATHETERIZATION DATA MOST STRONGLY SUGGEST THE PRESENCE OF AN ASD?

The patient is placed on 100% oxygen, and the intervention portion of the procedure begins. A sizing balloon is advanced and the ASD measures 22–26 mm using the stop-flow technique under transesophageal echocardiography (TEE) guidance (Figure 14.1).

The cardiologist selects a 24 mm Amplatzer™ device based on the balloon occlusion and echo findings. Prior to advancing the device, antibiotics are given intravenously. The device is advanced through the venous sheath across the atrial septum, and this is confirmed on both fluoroscopy and TEE. A residual shunt is seen across the superior portion of the device on TEE. The cardiologist makes the appropriate adjustments, and the shunt is corrected. Shortly after the device is released, the waveform on the end-tidal carbon dioxide slowly but progressively, decreases. No changes in the blood pressure or arterial pressure are appreciated.

HOW DID THE CARDIOLOGIST RESPOND TO THE INITIAL SHUNT SEEN ON TEE? WHAT IS THE EXPLANATION FOR THE CHANGE IN END-TIDAL CARBON DIOXIDE ONCE THE DEVICE IS RELEASED (FIGURE 14.2)?

The transesophageal echocardiogram confirms the anesthesiologist's suspicion that the device had embolized into the pulmonary artery considering the sudden alteration in the end-tidal carbon dioxide tracing. The cardiologist successful retrieves the embolized device and places a slightly larger one in correct position without event.

DISCUSSION

Atrial septal defects make up a significant percentage of congenital heart defects. Most patients with an ASD are asymptomatic from birth until adulthood. They are often found incidentally as a part of a workup for other symptoms. This patient presented with vague complaints of chest pain and shortness of breath. While musculoskeletal sources are the most common source of chest pain in the pediatric population, other sources should be ruled out.[1]

Infants and children with atrial defects may present with slow weight gain, tachypnea, or recurrent respiratory infections.[2,3] Adults with unrepaired ASD can present with fatigue, exercise intolerance, palpitations, syncope, shortness of breath, and peripheral edema. Eisenmenger's syndrome or pulmonary vascular obstructive disease with right to left atrial shunting is uncommon but can be present in 5%–10% of adults with untreated ASD.[4,5]

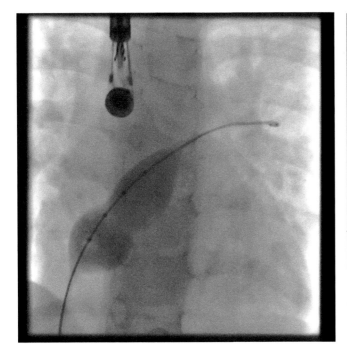

Fig. 14.1

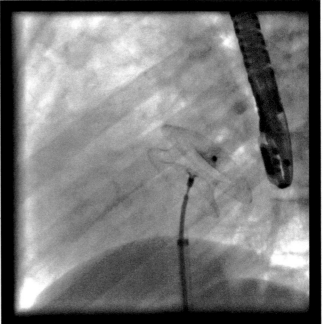

Fig. 14.2

Table 14.1 TYPES OF ATRIAL SEPTAL DEFECTS

TYPE	ANATOMY	ASSOCIATIONS
Patent foramen ovale	Central	Present in 25% of normal adults
Secundum	Central within fossa ovalis	Most common
Primum	Close to right atrial valves	Cleft mitral valve, AV canal defects
Sinus venosus	Near superior vena cava or inferior vena cava orifice	Partial anomalous pulmonary venous return
Coronary sinus	Unroofed coronary sinus	Persistent left superior vena cava

Diagnosis of an ASD starts with physical exam. The precordium is often hyperdynamic to palpation. Auscultation of heart sounds usually reveals a wide fixed split of the second heart (S2) along with a soft systolic ejection murmur. The split second heart sound is due to delayed closure of the pulmonary valve. If pulmonary pressures are high enough the pulmonary component of S2 may be loud. Electrocardiograms of ASD patients usually show tall P waves suggestive of an enlarged atrium, incomplete right bundle branch block, and right axis deviation. Chest radiography may show enlarged right-sided cardiac structures in patients who have defects with significant left to right shunting. Echocardiography is the primary tool used for diagnosis of an ASD. Echocardiogram can detect the presence, location, size, and physiologic characteristics of an ASD.

The majority of the literature lists 5 types of ASDs[6] (Table 14.1). They include patent foramen ovale, secundum, primum, sinus venosus defect, and coronary sinus defect. Patent foramen ovale is a normal intra-atrial communication during fetal circulation. After birth, transitional physiology leads to higher left atrial pressures causing the primum and secundum septums to oppose and eventually narrow. Complete closure of patent foramen ovales occurs in 70%–75% of adults.[7] Secundum ASDs are usually found within the fossa ovalis due to abnormal resorption of septum primum or defective formation of the septum secundum. They are the most common form of ASD. Primum ASDs are due to abnormal formation of the septum primum. Often, primum septal defects are associated with atrioventricular canal defects. Sinus venosus defects make up about 4%–11% of all ASDs.[8] They are due to a communication between the right pulmonary veins and the cardiac end of the superior vena cava or inferior vena cava. The most common location of the sinus venosus defect is between the right upper pulmonary vein and the superior vena cava.[9–11] Coronary sinus defects are relatively uncommon and occur due to partial or complete lack of tissue separating the coronary sinus from the left atrium.

At birth, defects that appear small and demonstrate a mild amount of shunting have a possibility of becoming much worse as the patient ages. Elevated pulmonary vascular resistance and a stiff noncompliant right ventricle delay what may eventually become significant right to left shunting. As the pulmonary vascular resistance drops to normal adult levels over the first few months of life, the ratio of cardiac output traveling to the lungs compared to the cardiac output traveling to the body (Qp:Qs) increases. It is not uncommon for large ASDs to have pulmonary blood flow 3–4 times normal levels.

Over time, left-to-right flow across the atrial septum leads to a variety of consequences. Volume overload to the right side leads to right atrial and right ventricular enlargement. Distention of the heart may lead to rhythm problems. In addition, as the annuli of the tricuspid and pulmonary valves stretch they may become leaky or incompetent. While right-sided enlargement is common, left-sided structures are typically spared in patients with isolated atrial defects. Chronic increases in pulmonary blood flow may lead to pulmonary vascular remodeling and, if allowed to continue long unchecked, severe pulmonary hypertension. The risk of an embolic event across the open atrial septum is yet another real possibility.

Most cardiologists will recommend the closure of any ASD if there is a hemodynamically significant shunt fraction causing enlargement of the right heart structures.[12,13] The definition of a hemodynamically significant shunt was classically a Qp:Qs ratio of 1.5:1. Another indication of closure of an ASD is suspicion of a paradoxical embolism in the absence of another cause. Meanwhile, relative contraindications to closing atrial defects include pulmonary hypertension and severe or restrictive right or left heart lesions that require the ASD to act as a pop off to allow for decompression of a cardiac chamber.

The location of the defect plays a significant role in the treatment approach. Sinus venosus, primum, and coronary sinus septal defects each have open heart surgery as the only legitimate option for closure. Meanwhile secundum defects can be closed surgically, but a significant percentage may also be able to be closed with a transcatheter device in the catheterization lab. Considerations for secundum defects include the size of the defect, the presence of adequate tissue rims for the device to grab on to, and the presences of multiple defects. Holes larger than 36–40 mm in diameter, inadequate margins for device anchoring, and device interference with atrioventricular valves or with pulmonary or systemic venous drainage can interfere with implantation in some patients.[14,15] Another limitation is the size of the patients due to the need for sheaths large enough to allow deployment of the device. Many of the small infants physically do not have veins large enough to accommodate the large sheath needed with possible vascular compromise of the extremity. The American Heart Association has recommended that patients for transcatheter closure be at least 2 year of age and over 15 kgs in weight.[16] If the only option is surgery, cardiologists will typically wait until the age of 3–5 if the patient is asymptomatic.

Transcatheter device closure of ASDs is typically performed under a general anesthetic as transesophageal echocardiography is routinely used to help guide the procedure. Complications that may be encountered include residual shunts, pain or bleeding secondary to the large sheaths required for delivery, embolization of the devices, and thrombus formation. To limit the risks patients are typically started on a dose of baby aspirin 3 days prior to the catheterization, and this would continue for 6 month to prevent clot formation and prevent stroke.

REVIEW QUESTIONS

1. Which of the following is the **MOST** common source of chest pain in the pediatric population?

    A. asthma symptoms
    B. coronary artery disease
    C. gastroesophageal reflux
    D. musculoskeletal pain

Answer: D
Chest pain in children is rarely cardiac in origin. Common causes of chest pain during childhood are idiopathic (52%), musculoskeletal (36%), respiratory (7%), and gastrointestinal (3%). Pain that is cardiac in origin represent less than 1%.

2. What is the **MOST** likely finding on auscultation of the heart in a patient with an ASD?

    A. continuous "machine-like" murmur
    B. crescendo-decrescendo systolic murmur
    C. mid-systolic click with a late murmur
    D. fixed split S2 with soft systolic murmur

Answer: D
Patients with hemodynamically significant ASD usually have a hyperactive precordium, widely split fixed second heart sound, and a soft systolic murmur heard at the left sternal border. A continuous "machine-like" murmur is most likely secondary to a patent ductus arteriosus, a loud systolic crescendo–decrescendo could be secondary to aortic stenosis, and amid-systolic click is typically from mitral valve prolapse.

3. What is the **MOST** common type of ASD?

    A. coronary sinus
    B. secundum
    C. primum
    D. sinus venosus

Answer: B
Ostium secundum ASDs are the most common types of ASDs, representing approximately 70%–80% of all ASD found in children.

4. On EKG, which of the following is the **MOST** likely finding in someone with an ASD?

    A. delta waves
    B. prolonged QT
    C. T wave inversion
    D. tall P waves

Answer: D
Electrocardiograms of ASD patients usually show tall P waves suggestive of an enlarged atrium. Incomplete right bundle branch block and right axis deviation are also frequently seen. Delta waves are seen with Wolff-Parkinson-White syndrome. Prolonged QT can occur in specific syndromes or be secondary to medications. T wave inversion is normal in children but may signify in adult coronary ischemia.

5. Which of the following is the **MOST** likely explanation for an increase in the degree of left to right shunting across an atrial level defect over time?

    A. development of Eisenmenger syndrome
    B. maturation of the heart's sympathetic tone
    C. increased compliance of the right heart
    D. increase in pulmonary vascular resistance

Answer: C
The degree of shunting through the ASD is related to both the size of the defect and the relative compliance of the right and left ventricles. In the fetus, the right ventricle is the dominant ventricle. After birth, with the marked decrease in pulmonary resistance, closure of the patent ductus arteriosus, and systemic output assumed by the left ventricle, the right ventricle's blood volume and pressures decrease. Over time, compliance of the right ventricle increases as its wall becomes less hypertrophic.

6. Which of the following is the **CLEAREST** indication for antibiotic administration to prevent infective endocarditis per the 2007 American Heart Association guidelines (assuming the procedure also meets criteria)?

    A. cardiac transplantation patient, presently using sildenafil.
    B. prosthetic material used in congenital heart disease patient, 10 months postsurgery
    C. staged repair of lesion in congenital heart disease patient, 20 months postsurgery
    D. unrepaired cyanotic congenital heart disease patient, stable on room air

Answer: D
Children who have cyanotic congenital heart disease, prosthetic heart valves, history of endocarditis, or had heart surgery in the past 6 months are at high risk for endocarditis. Antibiotic prophylaxis is indicated in this group of patients. Children who have acyanotic congenital heart defects or had cardiac surgery over 6 months ago do not require subacute bacterial endocarditis prophylaxis.

7. Which of the following is the **MOST** accurate regarding transcatheter device closure of ASDs?

    A. anticoagulation is required after the procedure.
    B. cardiopulmonary bypass is not required.
    C. procedural sedation is sufficient.
    D. recovery and hospital stays are prolonged.

Answer: B
Advantages of transcatheter closure of ASDs include fewer complications, shorter hospitalization, reduced need for blood products, and avoidance of cardiopulmonary bypass. To assure there is no patient movement during device positioning

and deployment, general anesthesia is recommended for these procedures.

8. Which of the following would be the **STRONGEST** indicator from the catheterization data suggesting the presence of an ASD?

    A. left atrial saturation higher than expected
    B. left atrial saturation lower than expected
    C. right atrial saturation higher than expected
    D. right atrial saturation lower than expected

Answer: C

In another wise healthy child with an ASD, oxygenated blood from the pulmonary veins entering into the left atrium will follow the left to right shunt across atrial defect. Venous blood in the right atrium will be oxygen enriched by the shunted blood and have oxygen saturations higher than expected. Left atrial blood saturation should be unaffected by a left to right shunt.

9. Shortly after the ASD device is released, the waveform on the CO_2 slowly decreases with no changes in cuff pressure or arterial pressures. What is the **MOST** likely explanation?

    A. atrial erosion
    B. device embolization
    C. pulmonary vein occlusion
    D. thrombosis formation

Answer: B

Embolization is a well-documented complication of ASD closure device deployment. It occurs in approximately 1% of patients. The devices most often embolize to the main pulmonary artery. Partial occlusion of pulmonary blood flow, with decreased flow to the lung, will decrease opportunity for gas exchange, which will lead to a fall in exhaled CO_2. Atrial wall erosion is a late complication and would result in renewed shunting and conduction abnormalities. Pulmonary vein occlusion would result in pulmonary venous congestion and edema. Thrombosis formation is highly unlikely within the described time course.

10. Of the following periprocedural complications, which is **MOST** commonly seen with device closure of ASDs?

    A. arrhythmias
    B. heart block
    C. transient ST elevations
    D. vascular complications

Answer: A

Arrhythmias are the most common periprocedural complication seen in patients having transcatheter device closure of an ASD. Arrhythmias occur in approximately 2% of patients. Vascular complications occur at rate of approximately 1%, while the occurrence of ST segment elevations and heart block are both about 0.4%. Overall, complication rates are quiet low.

QUESTIONS AND ANSWERS

This chapter has accompanying questions and answers which are available to subscribers as part of the Oxford eLearning platform. To access the questions, go to ✔ http://oxfordmedicine.com/pediatricanesthesiaPBL

REFERENCES

1. Fyfe DA, Moodie DS. Chest pain in pediatric patients presenting to a cardiac clinic. *Clin Pediatrics.* Jun 1984;23(6):321–324.
2. Andrews R, Tulloh R, Magee A, Anderson D. Atrial septal defect with failure to thrive in infancy: hidden pulmonary vascular disease? *Pediatr Cardiol.* Sep-Oct 2002;23(5):528–530.
3. Lammers A, Hager A, Eicken A, Lange R, Hauser M, Hess J. Need for closure of secundum atrial septal defect in infancy. *J Thorac Cardiovasc Surg.* Jun 2005;129(6):1353–1357.
4. Steele PM, Fuster V, Cohen M, Ritter DG, McGoon DC. Isolated atrial septal defect with pulmonary vascular obstructive disease—long-term follow-up and prediction of outcome after surgical correction. *Circulation.* Nov 1987;76(5):1037–1042.
5. Sachweh JS, Daebritz SH, Hermanns B, et al. Hypertensive pulmonary vascular disease in adults with secundum or sinus venosus atrial septal defect. *Ann Thorac Surg.* Jan 2006;81(1):207–213.
6. Geva T, Martins JD, Wald RM. Atrial septal defects. *Lancet.* May 31 2014;383(9932):1921–1932.
7. Schneider B, Zienkiewicz T, Jansen V, Hofmann T, Noltenius H, Meinertz T. Diagnosis of patent foramen ovale by transesophageal echocardiography and correlation with autopsy findings. *Am J Cardiol.* Jun 1 1996;77(14):1202–1209.
8. Attenhofer Jost CH, Connolly HM, Danielson GK, et al. Sinus venosus atrial septal defect: long-term postoperative outcome for 115 patients. *Circulation.* Sep 27 2005;112(13):1953–1958.
9. Wessels A, Anderson RH, Markwald RR, et al. Atrial development in the human heart: an immunohistochemical study with emphasis on the role of mesenchymal tissues. *Anat Rec.* Jul 1 2000;259(3):288–300.
10. Van Praagh S, Carrera ME, Sanders SP, Mayer JE, Van Praagh R. Sinus venosus defects: unroofing of the right pulmonary veins—anatomic and echocardiographic findings and surgical treatment. *Am Heart J.* Aug 1994;128(2):365–379.
11. Blom NA, Gittenberger-de Groot AC, Jongeneel TH, DeRuiter MC, Poelmann RE, Ottenkamp J. Normal development of the pulmonary veins in human embryos and formulation of a morphogenetic concept for sinus venosus defects. *Am J Cardiol.* Feb 1 2001;87(3):305–309.
12. Warnes CA, Williams RG, Bashore TM, et al. ACC/AHA 2008 guidelines for the management of adults with congenital heart disease: a report of the American College of Cardiology/American Heart Association Task Force on Practice Guidelines (Writing Committee to Develop Guidelines on the Management of Adults With Congenital Heart Disease). Developed in collaboration with the American Society of Echocardiography, Heart Rhythm Society, International Society for Adult Congenital Heart Disease, Society for Cardiovascular Angiography and Interventions, and Society of Thoracic Surgeons. *J Am Coll Cardiol.* Dec 2 2008;52(23):e143–e263.
13. Baumgartner H, Bonhoeffer P, De Groot NM, et al. ESC guidelines for the management of grown-up congenital heart disease (new version 2010). *Eur Heart J.* Dec 2010;31(23):2915–2957.
14. Meier B. Percutaneous atrial septal defect closure: pushing the envelope but pushing it gently. *Catheter Cardiovasc Interv.* Nov 2005;66(3):397–399.
15. Marie Valente A, Rhodes JF. Current indications and contraindications for transcatheter atrial septal defect and patent foramen ovale device closure. *Am Heart J.* Apr 2007;153(4 Suppl):81–84.
16. Feltes TF, Bacha E, Beekman RH 3rd, et al. Indications for cardiac catheterization and intervention in pediatric cardiac disease: a scientific statement from the American Heart Association. *Circulation.* Jun 7 2011;123(22):2607–2652.

SECTION 3

THORACIC CONDITIONS

15.

CONGENITAL PULMONARY AIRWAY MALFORMATION

Alina Lazar

STEM CASE AND KEY QUESTIONS

A 2-day old, 3.2 kg term neonate presents with progressive tachypnea, suprasternal and subcostal retractions, and decreased feeding. A large right lung mass was identified on his prenatal ultrasound. After birth, the chest radiograph and computerized tomography (CT) show a large cystic congenital pulmonary airway malformation (CPAM) involving the right lung and mediastinal shift. The patient is scheduled to undergo mass resection via thoracotomy today.

WHAT ARE NORMAL CARDIORESPIRATORY
PARAMETERS IN NEONATES? WHAT
IS THE DIFFERENTIAL DIAGNOSIS
OF RESPIRATORY DISTRESS IN A NEONATE?
WHAT ARE THE MOST COMMON CONGENITAL
LUNG LESIONS, AND HOW AND WHEN DO
THEY TYPICALLY MANIFEST? WHICH
CONGENITAL LESIONS CAN PRESENT
WITH LIFE THREATENING RESPIRATORY
DISTRESS? WHAT CRITERIA DICTATE
THE SURGICAL MANAGEMENT OF THESE
LESIONS IN THE PRE- AND POSTNATAL
PERIOD? WHAT ARE THE ANESTHETIC
IMPLICATIONS FOR INFANTS
WITH CONGENITAL LUNG LESIONS?

The baby's vital signs are: blood pressure 55/31 mmHg, heart rate 167 bpm, respiratory rate 68 breaths per minute, oxygen saturation 93% on 1 L/min oxygen by nasal cannula. Breath sounds are decreased on the right side. His leukocytes are $16 \times 10^3/\times \mu L$, hemoglobin 9 g/dL, and platelets 447,000/mL. There is no blood type and screen.

DO YOU NEED ANY ADDITIONAL
TESTS? DOES THE PATIENT NEED FURTHER
STABILIZATION BEFORE PROCEEDING
WITH SURGERY? SHOULD THE PATIENT
BE INTUBATED PRIOR TO SURGERY?
SHOULD A CHEST TUBE BE PLACED PRIOR
TO INDUCTION?

An echocardiogram shows a patent foramen ovale, patent ductus arteriosus with left to right shunt, a mildly enlarged right atrium and ventricle, and an estimated pulmonary artery pressure of 35/12 mmHg. A sepsis workup is underway and antibiotics are started.

SHOULD SURGERY TAKE PLACE IN THE
OPERATING ROOM OR THE NEONATAL
INTENSIVE CARE UNIT (NICU)? WILL YOU
NEED A NEONATAL VENTILATOR IN THE
OPERATING ROOM? WHAT RISKS AND
POSSIBLE COMPLICATIONS DO YOU DISCUSS
WITH THE PARENTS? WHAT WOULD YOU
LIKE TO DISCUSS WITH THE SURGEON
BEFORE PROCEEDING? WHAT INTRAVASCULAR
ACCESS DO YOU NEED? HOW WILL YOU
MONITOR THE PATIENT?

Consents for general anesthesia and epidural catheter placement are obtained. The surgeon is concerned that the size of the lesion will complicate the procedure and requests lung isolation. The patient is transported to the operating room and regular monitors are attached.

How would you induce anesthesia? Would you paralyze the patient? When? What are the anesthetic options for maintaining spontaneous ventilation? Which patients with congenital pulmonary malformations are more likely to be affected by positive pressure ventilation? Is one-lung ventilation (OLV) necessary for thoracotomy? For thoracoscopy? Which clinical situations make lung isolation desirable for thoracotomy? What methods of lung isolation are available, and what are their limitations? How does OLV affect an infant versus an older child?

As the surgeon is scrubbing, anesthesia is induced with 8% sevoflurane. A few minutes later the vocal cords are sprayed with lidocaine 1% and intubation is attempted—but the patient moves, coughs, and desaturates.

WHAT CAUSED THIS EVENT? WHAT DO
YOU DO NOW? WOULD YOU ADMINISTER
SUCCINYLCHOLINE? HOW COULD COUGHING
AND LARYNGOSPASM BE PREVENTED
WHILE MAINTAINING SPONTANEOUS
VENTILATION?

A dose of propofol is administered and the patient is gently ventilated with 100% oxygen, with improvement in oxygen saturation. A 5F Arndt bronchial blocker is placed fiberoptically with the tip in the right mainstem bronchus alongside a 3.0 microcuff endotracheal tube (ETT) with the tip in the mid-trachea. The bronchial blocker nylon loop is maintained in place to facilitate repositioning the blocker should the need arise, and the cuff is inflated. After placement of an arterial line and an additional intravenous line, the patient is placed in the left lateral decubitus and preparations for thoracic epidural catheter placement begin. A few minutes later, oxygen saturation decreases from 95% to 82%, tidal volume goes from 32 mL to 17 mL, and blood pressure falls from 62/36 to 44/23 mmHg.

WHAT COULD EXPLAIN THESE CHANGES?
WHAT IS THE EFFECT OF LATERAL
POSITIONING AND LUNG ISOLATION
ON RESPIRATORY PHYSIOLOGY IN NEONATES?
COULD THE BRONCHIAL BLOCKER HAVE
CAUSED THE DESATURATION? HAS THE CYST
EXPANDED? WHAT ELSE COULD CAUSE
DIFFICULT OXYGENATION AND VENTILATION
DURING THORACIC ANESTHESIA
IN NEONATES AND SMALL INFANTS? HOW DO
YOU MANAGE HYPOXIA AND HYPERCARBIA?
WAS HYPOTENSION CAUSED BY EXCESSIVE
ANESTHESIA? HOW CAN HYPOTENSION
BE PREVENTED AND TREATED IN SUCH
SITUATIONS?

The epidural placement is aborted, and the bronchial blocker is repositioned. Oxygen saturation improves with oxygen administration. As the surgeon proceeds swiftly with thoracotomy, muscle relaxants are administered and positive pressure ventilation is instituted. The case proceeds uneventfully and with minimal blood loss. At the end of the case, the surgeon requests reinflation of the right lung. You deflate the cuff of the bronchial blocker and hand-ventilate both lungs. Shortly afterward, you notice that the end-tidal CO_2 has increased and oxygen saturation is trending downward. On the arterial blood gas, the pH is 7.10, partial pressure of carbon dioxide 92, partial pressure of oxygen 101, base excess –6, bicarbonate 22. Hand ventilation is becoming difficult and eventually no end-tidal carbon dioxide tracing is obtained; saturation decreases to 61%.

WHAT IS YOUR DIFFERENTIAL?
WHAT DO YOU DO NOW? DO YOU TRY
TO SUCTION THE ETT?

The patient is emergently turned supine, extubated, and reintubated with a new ETT. A large blood clot obstructing the entirety of the old tube lumen is noted. Ventilation and oxygenation return to normal. You reevaluate the pain management options with the surgeon.

DO YOU EXTUBATE THE PATIENT? DO YOU
CONSIDER PLACING AN EPIDURAL CATHETER
NOW? WHAT ALTERNATIVES FOR PAIN
MANAGEMENT DO YOU HAVE? IF YOU OPT
FOR AN EPIDURAL, WOULD YOU INSERT
THE CATHETER AT THE THORACIC LEVEL,
OR THREAD IT UP FROM THE CAUDAL SPACE?
HOW WOULD YOU ENSURE THE CORRECT
PLACEMENT OF THE CATHETER TIP?
WHAT MEDICATION WOULD YOU USE
TO BOLUS THE EPIDURAL CATHETER AND
FOR CONTINUOUS INFUSION? ARE THERE
ANY SPECIAL CONSIDERATIONS PERTAINING
TO THE EPIDURAL ADMINISTRATION
OF ANESTHETICS AND ADJUVANTS
IN NEONATES?

An epidural catheter is placed via the caudal space and its position confirmed at T 5–6. After a negative test dose, the patient is given a 1 mL bolus of 0.1% bupivacaine, and an infusion of 0.6 mL/kg/hour is started. The patient emerges from anesthesia, is extubated, and transported to the NICU in stable condition.

DISCUSSION

RESPIRATORY DISTRESS OF THE NEWBORN

Respiratory distress affects up to 7% of all term newborns.[1] Increased work of breathing manifests as tachypnea (respiratory rate greater than 60 breaths per minute), tachycardia (heart rate >160 bpm), cyanosis, nasal flaring, chest retractions, or grunting. Among the causes of respiratory distress in neonates (see Table 15.1) the most common are transient tachypnea of the newborn (TTN), respiratory distress syndrome (RDS), meconium aspiration syndrome (MAS), neonatal pneumonia, and persistent pulmonary hypertension of the newborn (PPHN). Congenital malformations of the lung are rare causes of respiratory distress in the general population but are a relatively frequent indication for thoracic surgery in children, especially infants and neonates.

Transient tachypnea of the newborn is caused by delayed absorption of fluid in the lungs after birth. TTN is the most common cause of respiratory distress in newborn term infants and is frequently seen in babies born via cesarean section. TTN presents in the first few hours after birth with mild respiratory distress that can persist for up to 48 hours. The chest radiograph shows a "wet silhouette" around the heart with fluid in the horizontal fissures.[1] Some infants require a few days of monitoring and oxygen therapy in the NICU. Antibiotics are routinely used because differentiation from an infective process is difficult. Infants who develop TTN generally recover fully but some may develop asthma later in life.[2]

Table 15.1 CAUSES OF RESPIRATORY DISTRESS IN NEONATES

CAUSE	OUTCOMES
Airway	Nasal obstruction, choanal atresia, micrognathia, macroglossia, laryngomalacia, vocal cord paralysis, subglottic stenosis, laryngeal cyst, web or cleft, laryngeal or tracheal atresia, laryngo- or tracheobronchomalacia, vascular ring, foreign body, tracheoesophageal fistula, airway hemangiomas or papilloma, and external compression from a neck or intrathoracic mass
Thoracic and pulmonary	
Acquired	Respiratory distress syndrome,[a] transient tachypnea of the newborn,[a] meconium aspiration syndrome,[a] pneumonia,[a] pneumothorax,[a] persistent pulmonary hypertension of the newborn,[a] pleural effusion, pulmonary hemorrhage, bronchiolitis, aspiration,[a] intrathoracic tumors, and abdominal distention
Congenital	Bronchopulmonary sequestration, bronchogenic cyst, congenital pulmonary airway malformation, congenital diaphragmatic hernia, pulmonary hypoplasia, congenital lobar emphysema, pulmonary alveolar proteinosis, alveolar capillary dysplasia, congenital pulmonary lymphangiectasis, and surfactant protein deficiency
Cardiovascular	Congenital heart disease,[a] cardiomyopathy, pericardial effusion, fetal arrhythmia with compromised cardiac function, and high-output cardiac failure
Neuromuscular	Central nervous system injury (birth trauma or hemorrhage),[a] hypoxic-ischemic encephalopathy,[a] increased intracranial pressure, Arnold Chiari malformation, brainstem compression, congenital TORCH infections, meningitis, seizure disorder, arthrogryposis, congenital myotonic dystrophy, neonatal myasthenia gravis, spinal muscular atrophy, congenital myopathies, and spinal cord injury
Other	Sepsis,[a] metabolic acidosis,[a] hypoglycemia,[a] hyper- or hyponatremia, inborn errors of metabolism, anemia or polycythemia, hypo- or hyperthermia and medication (neonatal or maternal sedation, antidepressants, or magnesium)

[a]Relatively common causes of respiratory distress.

Respiratory distress syndrome

Respiratory distress syndrome, also called hyaline membrane disease, is caused by deficiency of surfactant commonly seen in preterm infants. The lack of surfactant causes widespread alveolar collapse and decreased lung compliance. Newborns with RDS present with respiratory distress in the first 4–6 hours after birth. The chest radiograph shows air bronchograms and reticulonodular shadowing throughout the lung fields (has "ground glass" appearance).[1] Many affected newborns require respiratory support or mechanical ventilation. Although neonates will quickly produce their own surfactant after birth, in some cases surfactant administration is indicated.[3] Corticosteroids are administered in preterm labor between 24 and 34 weeks gestation to boost fetal lung surfactant production. Newborns with RDS are at high risk of respiratory abnormalities later in infancy and early childhood—including wheezing, asthma, respiratory infections, and pulmonary test abnormalities.[3]

Meconium aspiration syndrome

Meconium aspiration syndrome occurs when the fetus (usually term or postterm) passes and aspirates meconium before or at birth. Of the 13% of births that occur through meconium stained amniotic fluid, 5% will develop MAS.[4] As meconium reaches the small airways, partial obstruction occurs resulting in air trapping and hyperaeration. The acidity of meconium inactivates surfactant and causes chemical pneumonitis. The chest radiograph shows hyperinflated lungs with patchy areas of atelectasis and infiltrates. Common complications of MAS include pneumothorax and PPHN. Management is supportive with oxygen supplementation, continuous positive airway pressure (CPAP), mechanical ventilation, surfactant administration, and, in severe cases, extracorporeal membrane oxygenation (ECMO).

Pneumonia

Pneumonia in neonates is most commonly acquired from inhalation of infected amniotic fluid or, postnatally, from nosocomial infection. It is often difficult to diagnose and differentiate from other causes of respiratory distress because the available laboratory investigations—such as white cell counts, blood cultures, and C-reactive protein—have a low sensitivity and specificity. The chest radiograph shows nonspecific patchy infiltrates with or without pleural effusion. Management is with antibiotics, such as ampicillin and gentamicin, to cover group B Streptococci and E. Coli, and supportive respiratory therapy.

Pulmonary arterial hypertension in neonates

Pulmonary arterial hypertension in neonates occurs in term or late preterm infants when pulmonary vascular resistance remains elevated after birth resulting in a right-to-left shunt across the foramen ovale or ductus arteriosus. This can result from pulmonary vasculature hypoplasia (e.g., congenital diaphragmatic hernia, CPAM), maldevelopment (e.g., increased pulmonary vascular smooth muscle due to chronic fetal hypoxia, total anomalous pulmonary venous return, maternal diabetes), or maladaptation (postnatal elevation in pulmonary vasoconstrictors caused by parenchymal lung disease, such as pneumonia, RDS, or MAS). Preductal and postductal oxygen saturation measurements via pulse oximetry often show a 10% or higher gradient difference (with preductal saturations being higher). The hyperoxia test may help differentiate between persistent pulmonary hypertension and cyanotic heart disease. In response to ventilation with 100% oxygen, partial pressure of oxygen in arterial blood will increase to more than 100 mmHg in infants with PPHN, while it will not rise above 45 mmHg in patients with cyanotic heart defects.

Echocardiography shows raised pulmonary arterial pressure and right-to-left shunting. The diagnosis is confirmed regardless of pulmonary arterial pressure, provided there is right-to-left shunting and an absence of congenital heart disease. A chest radiograph may show an enlarged cardiac silhouette, decreased vascular markings in the lung field, or underlying lung disease. Management consists of oxygen therapy, mechanical ventilation (including high-frequency oscillatory ventilation), nitric oxide, inotrope therapy, and ECMO. Although the mortality rate of infants with PPHN has decreased, in survivors pulmonary hypertension may persist into adulthood.[5] For infants with secondary pulmonary hypertension, the prognosis depends on the underlying condition—that is, good for those with MAS but poor for those with congenital diaphragmatic hernia.

Pneumothorax

Pneumothorax usually occurs secondary to an underlying lung disease such as pneumonia or MAS and is commonly seen in infants mechanically ventilated or vigorously resuscitated. It may also develop spontaneously in 1% of neonates, although only 10% of these are symptomatic.[1] Premature infants have a higher risk for pneumothorax than term infants. The diagnosis can be made by transillumination of the chest and confirmed by chest X-ray. An asymptomatic neonate with a small pneumothorax is treated conservatively, while symptomatic neonates require insertion of a chest tube.

RESPIRATORY DISTRESS CAUSED BY CONGENITAL PULMONARY MALFORMATIONS

Congenital pulmonary airway malformations

Epidemiology. Congenital pulmonary airway malformation is the most common congenital lung defect, with an incidence of 1:7,200 to 1:27,400 newborns.[6] Formerly known as congenital cystic adenomatous malformation,

its nomenclature changed because not all lesions are cystic or adenomatoid. CPAMs represent 25% of congenital pulmonary malformations and can occur in association with bronchopulmonary sequestrations (BPS) and congenital emphysema. They are usually unilobar and unilateral, and have no predilection for sex, race, or side of lung.

Pathogenesis. CPAMs are caused by abnormalities in lung branching occurring at various anatomic levels and stages in the first 20 weeks of gestation. Over-proliferation and dilation of affected airways produce cystic and/or adenomatous areas that maintain communication with the normal tracheobronchial tree, but the connections are not normal. CPAMs retain normal pulmonary arterial supply. They do not participate in air exchange and can restrict the growth and development of adjacent lung tissue. Because cysts have abnormal or absent cartilage, they may become hyperinflated due to air trapping and cause further respiratory distress in the neonatal period. There are 5 types of CPAMs based on their pathologic appearance (primarily cyst size) and area of the tracheobronchial tree involved (see Table 15.2).[7] Because the amount of bronchiolar and alveolar components can vary within the mass, CPAMs can range from solid masses without cysts, to mixed-solid and cystic masses, to cystic masses within the lungs.

Imaging. Almost all CPAMs are detected on the midgestation antenatal ultrasound. Prenatal magnetic resonance imaging helps to distinguish between CPAM and other congenital anomalies. Postnatally, radiography and computer tomography (CT) may show cystic or solid lesions, mediastinal shifts, adjacent lung hypoplasia, and pneumothorax (Figure 15.1). Because thin-walled cystic lesions are difficult to see on a plain radiograph when not infected, a chest CT is needed for a definitive diagnosis. CT scans are able to differentiate between air- and mucus-filled lesions, better distinguish the type of CPAM, and discern type 2 CPAM from BPS, which have systemic arterial supply and no connection to the tracheobronchial tree.

Differential diagnosis. A differential diagnosis includes other space-occupying lesions (e.g., congenital diaphragmatic hernia), and airspace hyperinflation lesions such as congenital lobar emphysema (CLE), bronchogenic cysts, emphysematous lung changes produced by mechanical ventilation, and pneumothorax.

Fetal presentation. Many CPAMs regress in size during the second half of gestation. Only 25% of prenatally diagnosed patients become symptomatic at birth. CPAM volume ratio, a measure of CPAM volume referenced to the fetal head, predicts the risk of hydrops. Large lesions cause polyhydramnios, mediastinal compression, and fetal hydrops. Management of hydropic fetuses consists of cyst drainage or thoracoamniotic shunting for cystic lesions and fetal lobectomy or laser ablation for solid masses. Early delivery and CPAM resection immediately postpartum are indicated for fetuses more than 32 weeks of age. Ex utero intrapartum therapy may be used

TYPE	FREQUENCY	AREA INVOLVED	PATHOLOGY	ONSET OF SYMPTOMS	CLINICAL MANIFESTATIONS
0	1%–3%	Trachea or proximal bronchi	• Diffuse small cysts involving the entire lung; lungs are small, atelectatic	First day of life	Fatal at birth
1	60%–70%	Distal bronchi or proximal bronchioles	• Single or multiloculated, large (2–10 cm), thin-walled air-filled cysts, filled with mucus in 30% of cases • Adjacent alveoli are normal • Wall composed of fibromuscular and elastic tissue and occasional cartilage plate	Birth to adolescence; most cases in first month of life	• Neonatal respiratory distress and mediastinal compression • Later, infection or incidental finding • Good prognosis • Malignant potential
2	15%–20%	Distal bronchioles	• Multiple small 0.5–2.0 cm air-filled cysts with intervening solid areas ("bubbly" appearance) • Similar to bronchopulmonary sequestrations with which they may form hybrid lesions (50% of cases).	First week to first 2 months of life	• Poor prognosis due to frequently associated abnormalities (tracheoesophageal fistula, cardiac, central nervous system, diaphragmatic, intestinal, renal) • Symptoms usually relate to associated abnormalities • Typically no mass effect on adjacent lung or respiratory distress unless lesion is large • Potential for infection
3	5%–10%	Bronchiolar/Alveolar duct	• Very large solid homogenous mass with few small (<0.5 cm) air-filled cystic areas • The original adenomatoid malformation	First week of life	• Mass effect on adjacent lung and severe respiratory distress or death at birth
4	5%–10%	Acini	• Single or multiple large, thin-walled, air-or fluid-filled cysts	Birth to 5 + years	• Wide range of symptoms: asymptomatic, progressive respiratory distress in neonate, pneumothorax • Strongly associated with malignancy

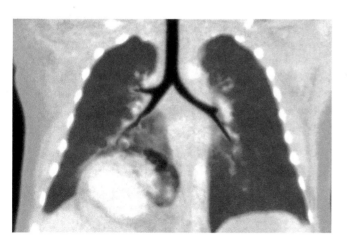

Fig. 15.1 Chest CT shows a bronchopulmonary sequestration and congenital airway malformation within the right lower lobe. The right ectopic kidney is displaced superiorly.

to facilitate lobectomy or ECMO cannulation in fetuses expected to have severe respiratory distress at birth.

Neonatal presentation. Typical symptoms in the neonatal period are tachypnea, grunting, retractions, cyanosis, and difficulty feeding. Half of patients presenting in the neonatal period develop severe respiratory distress.[8] Mediastinal shift, cardiac and caval compression, hemodynamic instability, and pneumo- or hemothorax as a result of cyst rupture may occur. Even a small mass can cause respiratory distress if it compresses the trachea or mediastinum. In symptomatic neonates, an echocardiogram is essential to assess cardiovascular function and guide inotropic support, especially in the case of PPHN.

Patients with mild respiratory distress are managed with noninvasive respiratory support (such as blow-by oxygen, nasal cannula, high-flow cannula, or CPAP). Neonates with large lesions causing severe pulmonary hypoplasia and persistent pulmonary hypertension present with severe respiratory distress and require invasive mechanical ventilation. In patients with cardiac dysfunction, a period of stabilization—high-frequency oscillatory ventilation, nitric oxide, inotropes, or in extreme cases, ECMO—is required before undergoing lobectomy. Neonates with cystic lesions, which communicate with the tracheobronchial tree, will develop progressive expansion of the cysts and rapid worsening of symptoms in the first few days of life, necessitating emergent surgical intervention.[9] Because crying and agitation can cause substantial amounts of air entrapment, these infants are intubated soon after birth, sedated, and mechanically ventilated with low-peak inspiratory pressure, either by conventional ventilation or high-frequency oscillatory ventilation.[10]

Similar to congenital diaphragmatic hernia, the prognosis depends on the degree of associated pulmonary hypoplasia. After a period of improvement following lobectomy, the severely affected infants may deteriorate as a result of worsening pulmonary hypertension and require aggressive interventions, including ECMO.[11]

Childhood presentation . Infants and older children with smaller cysts that do not communicate with the major tracheobronchial system may remain asymptomatic. In these patients, recurrent pulmonary infection is the most frequent complication of CPAM followed by hemo- or pneumothorax, hemoptysis, and chronic cough.[12,13] The association of spontaneous pneumothorax and CPAM type 4 is highly suggestive of pleuropulmonary blastoma. In asymptomatic patients, a thoracoscopic resection can be performed on an elective basis later in infancy to prevent recurrent infections and to eliminate concerns about malignancy.

Special anesthetic considerations . Neonates too unstable to be transported to the operating room may undergo resection in the NICU. A neonatal ventilator may be used to limit the risk of ventilator-induced lung injury in high-risk cases.[14] The use of high-frequency oscillatory ventilation has been reported in the perioperative management of CPAM to promote a still operative field during excision and to minimize peak insufflation pressures.[10,15] By comparison to conventional ventilation, high-frequency oscillatory ventilation can achieve hyperventilation with low inspiratory pressures, which is advantageous in patients with persistent pulmonary hypertension.

In patients with cystic lesions with potential for expansion, spontaneous ventilation or positive ventilation with minimal airway pressure should be continued until the chest is open or OLV of the contralateral lung is achieved. However, hypoxia frequently occurs in spontaneously breathing patients because of hypoventilation, atelectasis, and positioning in lateral decubitus and requires management with controlled ventilation. The surgeon should be present during induction and ready to perform emergent large needle decompression of the hyperinflated lung or thoracotomy should hemodynamic instability occur. OLV is desirable for thoracotomy in patients with rapidly expanding cystic lesions (should time permit), or

to facilitate dissection in large lesions.[16] Because CPAM may contain fluid—varying from clear to purulent in nature—lung isolation decreases the risk of contamination of the healthy lung. However, mucus, pus, or blood from the operated lung may still enter the lumen of the ETT upon resumption of two-lung ventilation and cause ETT obstruction.[17] Nitrous oxide should be avoided to prevent cyst hyperinflation.

Patients without significant pulmonary hypoplasia or complicated surgeries will benefit from extubation following surgery to reduce the risk of barotrauma and air leaks at the resected lobar bronchus stump from positive pressure ventilation. The intraoperative use of short-acting anesthetics and thoracic caudal epidural anesthesia facilitate early extubation.

Beyond the neonatal period, when most patients are asymptomatic or mildly symptomatic, resection is performed as an elective procedure usually via thoracoscopy. A cautious management strategy consists of a smooth inhalational or intravenous induction, gentle positive pressure ventilation, and intubation after muscle relaxation.

Bronchopulmonary sequestration

Bronchopulmonary sequestration, or simply pulmonary sequestration, consists of nonfunctioning lung tissue that receives arterial blood supply from systemic circulation and lacks normal communication with the proximal airway.[18] Venous drainage is usually through a pulmonary vein but occasionally is through azygos, hemiazygos, or portal veins.

Pathophysiology. The formation of BPS occurs in the pseudoglandular stage of lung development (5–17 weeks of gestation) prior to the separation of pulmonary and aortic circulations. An accessory pulmonary bud migrates caudally with the gut and receives vascularization from the systemic vessels that supply the primitive gut. If the lung bud develops before development of pleura, it is incorporated within the pleura and an intralobar BPS develops. If the lung bud arises after pleural formation, it remains extrapleural and an extralobar BPS forms; most form in the lower lobes (frequently, in the posterior basal segment of the left lower lobe) and are usually solitary lesions.

Intralobar sequestrations (75% of BPS) are located within a normal lobe and lack their own visceral pleura. Connections to an adjacent lung or gut may allow bacteria to enter the sequestration and cause recurrent infections. The abnormal tissue is sharply demarcated from adjacent normal tissue and consists of distorted and dilated mucus-filled airspaces and microcystic areas.

Extralobar sequestrations (25% of BPS) are located outside the lung, have their own pleura, consist of normal parenchyma, and do not have connections to the lung which means they are less likely to be complicated by infections. Extralobar sequestrations are more likely to be associated with other congenital anomalies than intralobar sequestrations.

Hybrid BPS/CPAM lesions, which represent up to 40% of all cystic lung lesions, have a systemic arterial blood supply and histologic features of CPAM.[19] In hybrid lesions, the BPS can be either intralobar or extralobar.

Clinical manifestations. Most infants are asymptomatic at birth. A large BPS causes pulmonary hypoplasia and respiratory distress in the neonatal period. If the BPS takes up a large amount of systemic blood flow, high-output heart failure and pulmonary hypertension may ensue. The most frequent presentation after the neonatal period is recurrent pneumonia, primarily in patients with intralobar BPS. Infants may have feeding difficulties if a communication with the gastrointestinal tract is present. Associated congenital abnormalities include congenital diaphragmatic hernia, vertebral anomalies, and congenital heart disease. Patients with bilateral or multifocal cysts and pneumothorax have a high risk for pleuropulmonary blastoma.

Imaging. Many cases are initially detected by prenatal ultrasound. A chest radiograph is done as the first step after birth and shows a uniformly dense mass, usually in the left lower lobe. An air-fluid level may occur in 26% of intralobar BPS.[20] CT scan or magnetic resonance imaging is indicated in the neonatal period for symptomatic infants and later in infancy for asymptomatic patients to confirm the diagnosis, identify the origin of the feeding artery, and assist with surgical planning.

Differential diagnosis. The differential diagnosis includes other cystic lesions such as CPAM, bronchogenic cysts, congenital diaphragmatic hernia, teratoma, and neuroblastoma.

Surgical management. Early surgical resection is indicated for large lesions in symptomatic patients and those at risk for pleuropulmonary blastoma (family history, bilateral and multifocal cysts, and pneumothorax). Management of low-risk, asymptomatic patients is either elective resection or observation with periodic imaging. Because of the moderate risk of infection and malignant degeneration, many authorities recommend elective surgical resection.

Special anesthetic considerations. Because these lesions have no bronchial connections, there is no risk of overexpansion of the lesion with positive pressure ventilation. One-lung ventilation is required to facilitate identification and ligation of the vascular supply, and resection of the mass.

Congenital lobar emphysema

Congenital lobar emphysema, a rare cause of respiratory distress in the neonatal period and early infancy, consists of hyperdistention and air trapping in the distal airways and airspaces that communicate with the bronchial tree.[21] Usually only one lobe, typically the left upper, is affected.

Pathophysiology. CLE is caused by an airway obstruction, either intrinsic (e.g., bronchial cysts or stenosis) or extrinsic (e.g., anomalous pulmonary venous drainage, bronchial cartilage dysplasia, or increased number of alveoli within each acinus). A ball-valve mechanism, in which more air enters the affected lobe during inhalation than leaves during expiration, causes alveolar hyperinflation and not true emphysema.[22] The overdistended lobe compresses normal lung tissue and may herniate into the opposite chest, displacing mediastinum and causing impaired venous return. Because alveolar hyperinflation occurs after birth, there is no pulmonary hypoplasia.

Clinical manifestations. Most patients develop rapidly progressing respiratory distress in the neonatal period. Physical examination reveals asymmetric expansion of the chest, diminished breath and heart sounds, hyperresonance to percussion, wheezing, cyanosis, tachypnea, hypotension, and tachycardia.[23] Recurrent pneumonia and feeding difficulties with failure to thrive are less frequent presentations that may occur in milder forms. A few patients remain asymptomatic for years. Patients with CLE frequently have other congenital abnormalities such as cardiovascular, musculoskeletal, and gastrointestinal defects.

Imaging. A chest radiograph usually confirms a CLE diagnosis (see Figure 15.2). It shows hyperinflation in the affected lobes, mediastinal shift, atelectasis in the nonaffected lobes, and flattened ipsilateral diaphragm. A radiograph can also help differentiate lobar emphysema from pneumothorax or congenital cysts by the presence of faint bronchoalveolar markings extending to the periphery of the affected lobe and herniation of the affected lobe across the midline. At birth, CLE may present as a fluid-filled cyst, until the liquid is fully absorbed from the airspace. A chest CT is indicated in atypical cases. An echocardiogram is useful to rule out associated congenital heart defects (most commonly a ventricular septal defect).

Differential diagnosis. CLE is often misdiagnosed and managed as pneumothorax. Chest tube insertion worsens respiratory distress because it leads to lung contusion and ventilation through the chest tube instead of into the remaining healthy lung.[24] Other conditions in the differential diagnosis include CPAM and congenital diaphragmatic hernia.

Surgical management. Patients with severe symptoms need to undergo emergent resection of the affected lobe, while patients with mild symptoms or who are asymptomatic are managed expectantly. This is because, unlike CPAM, CLE is not associated with an increased risk of infection or malignancy and, in some patients, lung hyperinflation decreases over time. A pre-resection bronchoscopy may diagnose potentially reversible causes of bronchial obstruction.

Special anesthetic considerations. A smooth inhalational induction with sevoflurane and oxygen is often used, and positive-pressure ventilation is minimized until the chest is open to avoid worsening lobar hyperinflation. If hypoventilation and hypoxia ensue, then gentle assisted

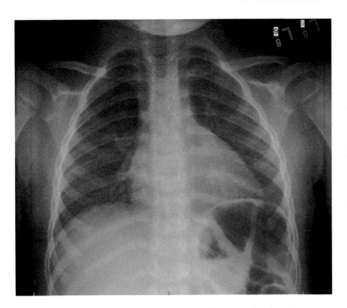

Fig. 15.2 Chest radiograph shows hyperinflated lungs with relatively increased lucency and hyperinflation of the right lung relative to the left.

ventilation with airway pressure less than 20 cm of water may be used.[24] If during induction the diseased lobe expands suddenly, the surgeon should be ready to open the chest immediately to relieve high intrathoracic pressure. Nitrous oxide should be avoided until the chest is open. The administration of a volatile anesthetic along with local anesthetic injected through a thoracic epidural catheter with the tip congruent with the surgical dermatome facilitates the maintenance of spontaneous ventilation.[25] Dexmedetomidine, or ketamine, and sevoflurane maintain hemodynamics while preserving spontaneous ventilation.[26] If the patient is hemodynamically unstable, a careful induction with ketamine alone or in combination with dexmedetomidine, propofol, or fentanyl, and airway topicalization with local anesthetics may be used.[27] The trachea is intubated in a deep plane of anesthesia or after administering a short-acting muscle relaxant and with gentle positive pressure ventilation. The selective endobronchial intubation of the healthy lung is helpful, especially if the resection is done thoracoscopically, but this should not delay start of surgery if the patient is unstable.[28] High-frequency jet ventilation has been used to minimize the risk of hyperinflation.[29]

Other congenital cystic lesions

Bronchogenic cysts result from abnormal branching of the tracheobronchial tree and are differentiated from CPAMs by the presence of bronchial cartilage. They may cause respiratory distress, recurrent pneumonia, and atelectasis due to lung compression. Dermoid cysts are clinically similar to bronchogenic cysts but are lined with keratinized squamous epithelium instead of respiratory epithelium. There are no special anesthetic considerations for surgical resection of these lesions.

GENERAL ANESTHETIC CONSIDERATIONS FOR RESECTION OF CONGENITAL LUNG LESIONS

Preoperative assessment

A review of the chest radiograph and CT offers information about the type of lesion, its cardiovascular impact, potential for dynamic hyperinflation, and the amount of functional lung. Neonates with congenital lung malformations may have associated cardiac, renal, neurologic, and gastrointestinal abnormalities. A preoperative echocardiogram and brain and kidney ultrasounds may be needed. Although blood loss is generally minimal, the potential for injury of the great vessels requires having blood readily available.

Monitoring and anesthetic techniques

For patients with solid lesions, induction of anesthesia may proceed in the usual fashion using either intravenous or inhalational agents, and muscle relaxants. Patients with cystic lesions with potential for hyperinflation should be intubated in a deep plane of anesthesia to avoid coughing, bucking, laryngospasm, and bronchospasm, which may require aggressive positive pressure ventilation. Muscle relaxation is withheld until the institution of OLV or thoracotomy if both lungs are ventilated (see previous for a discussion of anesthetic techniques in specific congenital lung lesions). Large-bore venous access is secured after anesthesia induction. Intra-arterial blood pressure monitoring is generally recommended, especially in complicated cases and for neonates. If central venous access is necessary—because of inadequate peripheral venous access and anticipated need for inotropic agents—the cannulation of the internal jugular or subclavian vein on the side of the procedure is recommended to avoid the possibility of bilateral pneumothorax. A urinary catheter will guide volume replacement and fluid management. Blood glucose levels should be monitored periodically throughout the procedure.

If extubation is planned at the end of surgery, a combination of short-acting volatile anesthetics (e.g., desflurane), opioids (e.g., fentanyl, remifentanil), and regional anesthetic techniques are typically used. If an inhalational anesthetic is used, its expired concentration should be limited to 0.5–1.0 minimal anesthetic concentration to limit its effect on hypoxic pulmonary vasoconstriction. Nitrous oxide is contraindicated because of the risk of cyst hyperinflation. The fraction of inspired oxygen can be decreased to maintain an oxygen saturation of 93%–95%; this is especially important for neonates because of their increased risk of retinopathy of prematurity when exposed to high inhaled oxygen concentrations.

Single-lung ventilation

Thoracoscopy for lung resection has been used successfully in infants, including neonates.[30] However, emergency resection of expanding lung cysts or CLE usually requires an open approach. Surgical access is possible by gently pushing the inflated exposed lung with surgical instruments (thoracotomy), or by insufflating carbon dioxide into the chest cavity (thoracoscopy). However, OLV may be required to facilitate surgical access to large lesions, and decrease bleeding, or to prevent continuous expansion of an overdistended lobe caused by positive pressure ventilation, or spillage of cystic fluid into the healthy lung. Lung isolation is the single most important factor in preventing conversion from thoracoscopy to thoracotomy.[31]

Methods of lung isolation in children younger than 2 years.

Two methods are currently used for provision of OLV in infants: mainstem intubation and the Arndt endobronchial blocker (AEB). Note: The Marraro bilumen tube, consisting of two separate uncuffed tracheal tubes of different lengths attached longitudinally, is currently not available in the United States.[32] The advantages and disadvantages of the two methods are presented in Table 15.3.

Selective mainstem intubation

. This procedure is relatively simple, accomplished either blindly or with fiberoptic or fluoroscopic guidance.[33] Turning the head to the right and rotating the ETT 180 degrees so the bevel of the tube faces the right side of the patient can facilitate intubation of the more steeply angled left-mainstem bronchus.[34] When selecting ETT size, consider that the diameters of the left and right mainstem bronchi are 0.66 and 0.86 fractions of the anteroposterior tracheal diameter.[35] This is the preferred technique of OLV in emergency situations such as airway hemorrhage or contralateral tension pneumothorax.[36] However, there are several limitations with this technique, including an inability to suction or provide oxygen and CPAP to the deflating lung, the need to alternate rapidly between one- and two-lung ventilation, and protecting the healthy lung from aspiration of fluid from the diseased lung. Also, hypoxia may ensue from obstruction of the right upper-lobe bronchus if a cuffed ETT is inserted too far into the right mainstem bronchus. Therefore, when using a cuffed ETT, the distance from the tip of the tube to the proximal end of the cuff must be shorter than the length of the bronchus; this ensures that the entire cuff is within the bronchus and the upper lobe orifice remains unobstructed.

Intraluminal placement of the blocker.

The diameter of the smallest AEB (5F) is 1.7 mm at the shaft and 2.5 mm at the balloon, while the diameter of a fiberoptic bronchoscope (FOB) is 2 mm. This restricts the coaxial endoluminal placement to an ETT 4.5-mm internal diameter (ID) and larger, and thus to children older than 2 years. However, with

Table 15.3 **TECHNIQUES FOR SINGLE-LUNG VENTILATION**

TECHNIQUE	ADVANTAGES	DISADVANTAGES
Selective mainstem intubation	• Relatively easy technique • May be only option in small infants as airway dimensions preclude use of bronchial blocker	• Unable to switch quickly from OLV to TLV • Unable to prevent contamination from diseased lung • Unable to suction, or administer O_2 and CPAP to the operative lung
Balloon-tipped catheters (Fogarty, Swan-Ganz)	• Decreased risk of contamination from the diseased lung • Ability to switch quickly from OLV to TLV	• Unable to suction, or administer O_2 and CPAP to the operative lung through those lacking a central channel • Low-volume, high-pressure cuff increases risk of bronchial trauma • Displacement of blocker cuff into the trachea causes occlusion of the tracheal lumen
Arndt bronchial blocker	• High-volume, low-pressure cuff reduces risk of bronchial trauma • Ability to provide O_2 and CPAP to operative lung • Central channel facilitates operative lung deflation • Internal wire with looped end facilitates positioning	• Small internal channel prevents adequate suctioning of operative lung secretions
Univent*	• Bronchial blocker firmly attaches to the tube, which decreases chance to dislodge • Blocker tube lumen allows suctioning and insufflation of O_2 • Able to switch from OLV to TLV	• Available only for children older than 6 years • Reduced cross-sectional diameter of ventilating lumen
Double-lumen endotracheal tube	• Rapid and easy separation of the lungs • Access to both lungs for suctioning • Ability to administer CPAP or O_2 to the operative lung	• Available only for children older than 8 years

Note. OLV = one-lung ventilation. TLV = two-lung ventilation. CPAP = continuous positive airway pressure.

some modifications, endoluminal placement of the AEB has been reported in neonates.[28,37] The narrowest and most rigid part of the pathway—the connector between the ETT and the breathing circuit—may be enlarged by placing a larger connector outside the 4.0-mm ID ETT and securing it with tape; this increases the maneuvering space of the AEB and FOB. To further facilitate the procedure, the larger sized AEB balloon should be inserted through the ETT before inserting the FOB. Blockers through the ETT can also be placed blindly, fluoroscopically, or via an ETT temporarily inserted into the desired mainstem bronchus and subsequently withdrawn above the carina. But, without a FOB, assessing and correcting blocker position intraoperatively is challenging. A disadvantage of endoluminal AEB placement is the difficulty in suctioning the lumen of the ETT without dislodging the AEB. Alternatively, a 2 or 3F Fogarty embolectomy catheter may be placed either within or external to the ETT.[36] However, there are several disadvantages with the Fogarty catheter: (a) a low-volume, high-pressure cuff, if overinflated, may cause trauma; (b) lack of a guidewire in size 2 and 3F prevents angling the tip into the desired mainstem bronchus; and (c) absence of a central channel delays lung deflation and prevents CPAP administration to the operative lung.

Extraluminal placement of the blocker. Extraluminal placement of the AEB is more common and has the advantage of providing a larger space to maneuver the FOB and ease ETT suctioning. The average neonatal trachea has an anteroposterior diameter of 4.3 mm.[38] The trachea is the shape of an ellipse, with the transverse diameter being larger than the antero-posterior diameter (4.7 mm in a neonate).[39] The extra space laterally allows for the extraluminal insertion of a blocker. In infants younger than 6 months of age, a 3.0 mm ID microcuffed or a 3.5 mm ID uncuffed ETT are commonly used. While the 2.8 mm FOB can pass through the 3.0 mm ID ETT, it is difficult to maneuver and may require the temporary removal of the connector between the ETT and breathing circuit.[40] FOBs with a 2.2 mm diameter are available. A smaller cuffed tube allows easier mobilization of the blocker along the ETT than larger uncuffed ones. If the vertical movement of the blocker is restricted, the ETT cuff may be temporarily deflated to facilitate advancement. A cuffed tube is useful when high inspiratory pressures are required during mechanical ventilation.

The following are several techniques to ensure correct placement of the extraluminal blocker in the desired bronchus:

- Temporarily intubate the mainstem bronchus with an ETT, insert the AEB through the ETT, completely withdraw the ETT, and finally reinsert the ETT in mid-trachea.[41] Prolonged apnea and desaturation may complicate this technique.

- Guide the AEB into the desired mainstem fluoroscopically by rotating the head to the opposite side or by elevating the shoulder on the contralateral side before or after inserting and positioning the ETT in mid-trachea.[42]

- Insert AEB and ETT en bloc with the loop of the blocker wrapped around the tip of the ETT. The loop may dislocate during placement. The FOB is then inserted through the ETT into the mainstem bronchus, and the loop of the AEB is slipped off the tube and advanced over the scope into the bronchus.[43] With this technique, the loop may dislocate during placement, and it may be difficult to reposition the endobronchial blocker after the bronchoscope is withdrawn.

- Place the blocker in mid-trachea initially and then advance it into the desired bronchus, under FOB observation, by twisting the blocker and rotating the patient's head to the opposite side or by twisting the ETT and, indirectly, the blocker.[44]

- Bend either the guide loop or the tip of the blocker 35–45 degrees and twist the blocker clockwise or counterclockwise, under FOB observation, to facilitate endobronchial placement of the blocker without additional interventions.[40,45] Positioning the ETT too close to the carina may impede rotational positioning of the blocker; however, gentle traction on the ETT without removing the tape or neck extension may be enough to increase the distance to the carina.

Leaving the nylon loop in place facilitates maneuvering the blocker should it dislodge during positioning and surgery and does not significantly interfere with lung deflation; however, the loop precludes suctioning, oxygen, and administering positive pressure to the operative lung.[40,44] There is also concern that the wire loop could be inadvertently sutured if the surgeons do not recognize its presence in the field. The wire should be removed prior to removing the blocker to prevent lassoing of the wire around the ETT.

Fiberoptic identification of the tracheal rings and membrane is difficult in infants because of their small airways and equipment limitations. Maintaining oxygenation and ventilation during bronchoscopy are difficult because of the large dead space created by the Arndt multiport airway adaptor, high airflow resistance through the small residual space of the ETT, and air leaks between the small FOB scope and the multiport adaptor. One recommendation is to insert the FOB through the flexible adjustment port, which is intended for insertion of the blocker and can be tightened, or insertion through an adhesive membrane placed over the scope port that has been perforated by a needle. Some experts prefer to insert the FOB directly into the ETT without an intervening adapter.[40] Fluoroscopic guidance of the blocker circumvents the limitations of fiberoptic technology and can be done while the patient is being ventilated; however, it exposes the patient to radiation.

Although dedicated bronchial blockers have high-volume, low-pressure cuffs, the inflation pressure with the recommended amount of air (2 mL) still exceeds systolic arterial pressures.[46] Use of fiberoptic bronchoscopy will ensure that inflation volumes are kept at the minimum levels required to create a seal.

Methods of lung ventilation in children older than 2 years of age. In addition to mainstem intubation and endobronchial blockers, which can be used across all age groups, OLV in older children can be achieved with a Univent® tube or a double lumen tube (DLT).

The Univent® tube . The Univent® tube consists of a standard ETT with an additional lumen attached to its side and through which a balloon-tipped tube is advanced into a bronchus. Because the blocker tube is firmly attached to the main ETT, displacement of the Univent® blocker balloon is less likely to occur than with other techniques. The blocker tube has a small lumen that allows egress of gas and can be used to insufflate oxygen or suction the operative lung. The smallest Univent® tube has an ID of 3.5 mm and an outer diameter of 7.5 mm, which restricts its use to children older than 6 years of age. The large discrepancy between the internal and outer diameters of the tube significantly increases resistance to gas flow.[47]

The double lumen tube. The DLT offers several advantages, including ease of insertion, capacity to suction and oxygenate the operative lung with CPAP, and ability to visualize the operative lung. A left-sided DLT is preferred to a right-sided DLT because of the shorter length of the right main bronchus. A right-sided DLT is more difficult to position accurately because of the greater risk of right upper-lobe obstruction. After the tip of the tube passes through the vocal cords, the stylet is removed, and the tube is rotated 90 degrees to the appropriate side and advanced further into the bronchus until resistance is met. Placement is verified with auscultation and fiberoptic bronchoscopy. Alternatively, the tip of the DLT is inserted in the trachea and then guided fiberoptically into the desired mainstem. The smallest DLT (26 F) can be used in pediatric patients as young as 8 years old. Similar to AEB, DLTs have high-volume, low-pressure balloon cuffs. Although DLT cuffs have a tendency to produce higher "cuff-to-tracheal" pressures than bronchial cuffs, airway damage does not occur unless the cuff is overinflated.

The equation, size = age × 1.5 + 14, can help estimate the correct DLT size.[46] Size selection can be done more precisely by direct measurement of the bronchial width via CT or chest radiography or by computing the width of the left bronchus via known tracheal width using the formula DLB = (0.45 × tracheal width) + 3.3.[48] These techniques are more accurate than relying on age, gender, height, or weight. Ultrasound measurements of the upper trachea have been shown to correlate with left-bronchus sizing and can be used to predict pediatric ETT size.[49,50]

When a tracheal right-upper lobe bronchus is present, deflation of the corresponding lobe may be achieved by inserting a cuffed end-tipped catheter or a bronchial blocker through the tracheal lumen of a left-sided DLT into the aberrant bronchus to block it. Right-sided DLTs are contraindicated in such instances.

A summary of the techniques described above and the tube sizes according to patient age is provided in Table 15.4.

Techniques to deflate the operative lung. Once the bronchial blocker is in the correct bronchus, its depth is

Table 15.4 TYPES AND SIZES OF BREATHING TUBES USED FOR LUNG ISOLATION

AGE (YR)	ETT ID (MM)	BB (F)[A,B]	UNIVENT	DLT (F)
0–0.5	3.0–3.5	2, 3[c] 5 (parallel only)[d]		
0.5–1	3.5–4.0	5 (parallel only)		
1–2	4.0–4.5	5 (parallel only)		
2–4	4.5–5.0	5		
4–6	5.0–5.5	5		
6–8	5.5–6.0	5	3.5	
8–10	6.0 cuffed	5	3.5	26
10–12	6.5 cuffed	5	4.5	26–28
12–14	6.5–7.0 cuffed	5	4.5	32
14–16	7.0 cuffed	5, 7	6.0	35
16–18	7.0–8.0 cuffed	7, 9	7.0	35, 37

[a]The outside diameter in mm can be calculated by dividing the size in French by 3;

[b]BB placement is either coaxial or parallel with the ETT, unless otherwise specified.

[c]Sizes 2 and 3F are available for balloon-tipped catheters only; Arndt endobronchial blockers are available in sizes 5, 7, and 9F.

[d]Some providers prefer mainstem intubation for this age group.

Note. BB = bronchial blocker. DLT = double-lumen tube. F = French size. ID = internal diameter.

adjusted to place the cuff just distal to the carina. The length of the 5F AEB is 1.0 cm, corresponding to the length of the right mainstem bronchus of a 2-year-old child.[51] Consequently, in infants the cuff may block the right-upper lobe bronchus and prevent deflation of the lobe. Deep insertion of the blocker may result in ventilation of the right-upper lobe, whereas a blocker minimally inserted into the mainstem can easily dislodge into the trachea. In the latter scenario, an ETT advanced close to the carina may prevent the herniating blocker from completely blocking the trachea while still ventilating the left lung.[44] Because it is very common for the AEB to change its location after the patient is in lateral decubitus, it is recommended to inflate the cuff after final patient positioning. Avoiding head extension during positioning prevents unintended withdrawal of the blocker from its position. The AEB may be initially advanced until resistance is encountered and then withdrawn to the optimal location after the patient is in lateral decubitus. Upon satisfactory placement of the blocker into the mainstem bronchus, the cuff is inflated until it reaches the bronchial wall but without herniating into the trachea.

Deflation of the operative lung can be achieved passively by reabsorption atelectasis (facilitated by administration of 100% O_2 prior to inflating the blocker cuff) or actively by suctioning the AEB lumen, or extrinsically compressing of the lung. When the lumen of the blocker is occupied by the nylon loop, which is left in place to facilitate repositioning of the blocker during surgery, the surgeon can push down on the lung with the blocker cuff deflated and ETT disconnected from the breathing circuit.

A properly placed AEB can become displaced during surgery because of pulling or traction applied by the surgeons on the operative bronchus. The device can be repositioned under fiberoptic guidance or, in challenging cases, fluoroscopically. Sudden high inspiratory pressures and disappearance of the end-tidal carbon dioxide tracing are highly suggestive of complete airway obstruction by a herniated AEB cuff. The cuff should be immediately deflated and the lungs hand-ventilated with 100% O_2. Inflating the balloon of the bronchial blocker with saline as opposed to air may limit movement and dislodgement during surgical manipulation.[34]

A detailed discussion of the techniques for achieving lung isolation using double-lumen and Univent® tubes can be found elsewhere.[41]

Intraoperative complications

Oxygenation and ventilation problems. In patients with congenital lung disease, hyperinflation of the cystic lesions, the mass effect, and lung hypoplasia can cause intraoperative hypoxia. Rapid cyst expansion or rupture with resultant pneumothorax and severe oxygen desaturation requires immediate needle or surgical lung decompression.

Infants undergoing thoracic surgery in lateral decubitus have impaired lung ventilation and perfusion. Unlike adults, oxygenation in infants does not improve when the diseased lung is in a nondependent position because an infant's easily compressible rib cage cannot fully support the dependent, healthy lung. Airway closure in the dependent lung is more likely to occur as functional residual capacity is reduced and near residual volume. These differences predispose to atelectasis and put the infant at a significantly higher risk of hypoxemia than older children and adults.[41,52] Usually, hypoxemia is limited and improves as hypoxic pulmonary vasoconstriction takes effect. This vasoconstrictive response can be inhibited by volatile anesthetics, other nonspecific vasodilators, and hypocarbia. Hypoxia improves with administration of 100% O_2, recruitment maneuvers, positive end expiratory pressure to the dependent lung, CPAP to the operative lung, and resumption of two-lung ventilation.

Further hypoxia may result from persistent pulmonary hypertension or reopening a previously closed ductus arteriosus in conditions of hypoxemia, hypercarbia, and acidosis. In such instances, a lower O_2 saturation in postductal circulation than in preductal circulation indicates a right to left shunt.

Hypercarbia and respiratory acidosis occur during OLV especially if CO_2 insufflation is used. Additional dead space created by the multiport adapter or the moisture exchange filter worsens hypercarbia. Mucus and blood clots or pus may occlude the ETT lumen, while bronchial blocker cuff migration into the tracheal lumen may completely block it. The occlusion of the right-upper lobe bronchus by the bronchial blocker cuff or a mainstem ETT will restrict ventilation to just two lobes and may cause hypoxia and hypercarbia.

Hemodynamic instability. Large lesions and lung hyperinflation may cause mediastinal shift, compression or kinking of mediastinal vessels, decreased venous return, and, consequently, hypotension. In addition, intrathoracic CO_2 insufflation and traction of mediastinal vessels by maneuvering the operative lung can cause acute episodes of hypotension. A rare but possible cause of acute hypotension is CO_2 embolization into an open blood vessel, more likely in conditions of hypovolemia and low venous pressure. Management consists of the immediate release of the artificial pneumothorax and administration of fluids and inotropic agents. With severe cardiovascular compromise, placing the patient in the head down position may displace the gas into the apex of the right ventricle and restore cardiovascular function. Bleeding, lung edema, and insensitive losses may also cause hypotension.

Postoperative pain management

Postoperative pain management is guided by the type of procedure (thoracoscopy vs thoracotomy), planned duration of postoperative intubation, surgeon preference, and available local resources. Pain management strategies include intravenous opioids, wound infiltration with local anesthetics, intercostal nerve blocks, paravertebral nerve blocks or catheters, and epidural analgesia. Thoracic epidural analgesia is the current gold standard for pain management after thoracotomy. The planned location of both the thoracotomy incision and chest tube should be considered when determining where to position the tip of the catheter for optimal neuraxial analgesia.

The catheter tip should be positioned so that the band of analgesia covers both the thoracotomy and chest tube sites, usually in the T4–T6 intervertebral spaces. Because the risk of neurologic injury is higher in neonates and small infants, direct thoracic insertion of the epidural catheter is reserved for highly experienced anesthesiologists. More commonly, the epidural catheter is inserted caudally and threaded to the thoracic level. Loosely packed epidural fat and lack of lumbar lordosis in nonwalking infants makes advancement of catheters from the caudal to the lumbar and thoracic levels relatively easy. For caudal placement, the recommended needles are Crawford or a regular 18G intravenous catheter. With the latter, there is concern for inadvertent dural, vascular, rectal, or intraosseous puncture. Tuohy needles are not used because it is difficult to align the eye of the needle with the spinal canal. Advancement to the thoracic level is easier with larger catheters (19G or 21G); thinner catheters (23G) are more difficult to thread and tend to coil.[53]

Although blind insertion is said to have a high success rate, numerous reports indicate that catheters threaded from the caudal space do not behave predictably and that placement must be verified. A radiopaque catheter facilitates the placement of the catheter tip at the desired dermatome. Injection of contrast through the catheter may help identify subdural or intravascular placement and predict analgesic coverage.[54] The disadvantages of this technique are cost and radiation and contrast exposure. In the advanced nerve stimulation (Tsui) technique, the operator is able to follow the muscular response.[55] A special kit is now commercially available (although expensive). Placement of the catheter in the subarachnoid space can be detected with this technique. With ultrasound, the epidural puncture and catheter tip advancement can be visualized in real time.[56] Ultrasound-guided placement requires the help of an experienced assistant.

A typical loading dose for epidural catheters is 0.3 mg/kg or 0.03 mg/kg/dermatome. A dose equivalent to half of the initial bolus can be given 90 minutes after the initial dose. Alternatively, a continuous infusion of local anesthetic and adjuvants may be started. Decreased protein binding and immaturity of the hepatic enzymes increase the risk of systemic toxicity with bupivacaine and ropivacaine in neonates and infants and limit their safe infusion rates and duration of administration. Data from the Pediatric Regional Anesthesia Network finds that 31% of neonates receive intra- and postoperative infusions with potentially toxic doses of anesthetics.[57] Bupivacaine infusions have the highest risk of toxicity and in neonates should not be used for more than 48 hours at the maximum acceptable rate.[58] Ropivacaine is safer than bupivacaine because its plasma concentrations are more stable and has less risk of toxicity. Although ropivacaine does not accumulate with prolonged infusions at 0.2 mg/kg/hour in neonates,[59] its potential toxicity risk remains a concern.[60] Lidocaine is less cardiotoxic than bupivacaine, and its plasma concentration can be monitored during infusion. Given its rapid metabolism and wide therapeutic window, 2-chloroprocaine offers an alternative to amide local anesthetics, particularly in patients requiring wide dermatomal coverage. A retrospective study of 52 infants compared the epidural infusion of 1.5% 2-chloroprocaine administered at 0.45 mL/kg/hour and 0.1% ropivacaine administered at 0.25–0.3 mL/kg/hour after lung resection and found a mild reduction of opioid requirements in the 2-chloroprocaine group and no side effects.[61] While 2-chloroprocaine may allow higher infusion rates in infants compared to amino-amide local anesthetics, the larger volumes may cause increased leakage from the epidural insertion site.[62] In neonates, the drugs with the least potential for toxicity and the maximum safe rate of infusion should be selected; this should be clearly communicated to everyone involved in patient care (see Tables 15.5 and 15.6).

The starting infusion rate for catheters with the tip at the operative dermatome is 0.1–0.15 mg/kg/hour. If the tip of the catheter is remote from the optimal location, the infusion rate may be increased, without exceeding the maximum rates listed in Table 15.5. If the anesthetic concentration is decreased to allow for a larger volume administration, adjunctive additives such as opioids and clonidine may be used to improve analgesia. Alternatively, an anesthetic with a better safety profile, such as 2-chloroprocaine may be selected. In a prospective, randomized, double-blind study, the addition of 2 mcg/mL fentanyl to 0.1% bupivacaine administered

Table 15.5 RECOMMENDED RATES (UPPER END) OF LOCAL ANESTHETIC EPIDURAL INFUSION IN PEDIATRIC PATIENTS

DRUG (COMMON CONCENTRATIONS)	RATE (MG/KG/HOUR)		
	0–2 MONTHS	3–6 MONTHS	>6 MONTHS
Bupivacaine (0.05%, 0.1%, 0.125%)	0.25	0.3	0.4
Levobupivacaine (0.1%, 0.125%)	0.25	0.3	0.4
Ropivacaine (0.1%)	0.3	0.4	0.4
Lidocaine (0.1%, 0.3%)	0.8	1	1.5 (not commonly used)
Chloroprocaine (1.5%)	7.5 (mid-thoracic) 9–10.5 (lumbar and low thoracic)	7.5 (mid-thoracic) 9–10.5 (lumbar and low thoracic)	Rarely used

Table 15.6 RECOMMENDED RATES OF ADJUVANTS FOR CONTINUOUS EPIDURAL INFUSION IN PEDIATRIC PATIENTS

| | | TYPICAL CONCENTRATION (MCG/ML) | | |
DRUG	DOSE[A] (MCG/KG/HOUR)	NEONATES (0–2 MONTHS)	INFANTS	CHILDREN
Fentanyl	0.1–0.5	1–2	2 (2–5)	5 (2–5)
Hydromorphone	1.5–2.5	NR	NR	10–20[b]
Morphine	3–5	NR	NR	25–50[b]
Clonidine[c]	0.1–0.2	NR	0.4	0.4–1.0 (lumbar epidural tip) 0.4–0.6 (thoracic epidural tip)

[a]Larger doses of opioids are indicated for opioid-tolerant patients.

[b]Administration of hydrophilic opioids through a thoracic epidural is not recommended in infants younger than 6 months.

[c]When clonidine is added to an epidural solution, the epidural opioid dose should be reduced by 50%.

Note. NR = not recommended.

epidurally provided superior analgesia during the first 24 hours after thoracotomy when compared to bupivacaine alone in infants up to 6 months of age.[63] In addition, patients receiving epidural fentanyl appeared more relaxed, quiet, and comfortable. The authors could not conclude whether the analgesic action of fentanyl (mean dose of 0.5 mcg/kg/hour) was the result of epidural action or systemic absorption. Clonidine has been used as an adjuvant to local anesthetics in thoracic epidural analgesia in infants.[64] However, there is increased concern for apnea and bradycardia in small infants and neonates, particularly with high thoracic epidurals.

Paravertebral block is increasingly being used in thoracic anesthesia, administered both as a single shot and continuous infusion. It may be used in situations when epidural anesthesia is contraindicated such as uncorrected coagulopathy, increased intracranial pressure, or anatomic abnormalities of the spine. In adults, the effectiveness of thoracic paravertebral analgesia is similar to that of epidural analgesia.[65] However, the evidence in the pediatric population is limited.[66] In an observational study of 2,390 thoracic paravertebral nerve blocks in pediatric patients, the most complications were catheter dislodgment (4.9%) and catheter leakage (5.9%).[67]

Morphine and fentanyl are the opioids most commonly used for postoperative pain management after thoracic surgery. Fentanyl is more likely to cause apnea when given as a bolus than as an infusion. Because it is less likely to cause hypotension than morphine, fentanyl administration is particularly advantageous in neonates. Acetaminophen and ketorolac are useful adjuvants to opioids and regional anesthetic techniques. Ketorolac is not recommended in neonates because of its potential complications, which include renal toxicity, necrotizing enterocolitis, platelet dysfunction, and hemorrhage.[68]

CONCLUSIONS

There are 3 main congenital lung abnormalities that may present in infancy and have important anesthesia implications.

First, congenital pulmonary airway malformation consists of solid and/or cystic masses resulting from proliferation of lower airway structures that compromise alveolar development. The cysts have connections with the tracheobronchial tree and may become hyperinflated because of a ball-valve mechanism. They may become infected and are predisposed to malignancy later in life. Second, pulmonary sequestrations lack communication with the tracheobronchial tree and consist of a mass of nonfunctional tissue supplied by aberrant systemic vessels. They may manifest as respiratory distress in neonates, high-output cardiac failure (if large), recurrent pulmonary infections, and have associated congenital abnormalities. Third, CLE consists of overdistended lung that is histologically normal. Positive pressure ventilation may cause lung herniation and hemodynamic instability.

Management of congenital pulmonary abnormalities consists of excision via thoracotomy or thoracoscopy. Lung isolation during thoracic surgery is desirable and may be achieved by advancing the ETT into the nonoperative bronchus, placing an endotracheal blocker (intra- or extra-axially), or inserting a double lumen tube in older children. Pain management strategies after thoracotomy include epidural analgesia, paravertebral block, intercostal block, intrapleural or wound infiltrations with local anesthetics, and systemic opioid administration. When local anesthetics infusions are planned, the hourly rate should not exceed maximum doses to avoid toxicity.

REVIEW QUESTIONS

QUESTIONS

1. A 1-day old neonate is evaluated for respiratory distress, tachypnea, chest retractions, and grunting. Her chest radiograph shows hyperinflated lungs and patchy infiltrates. The **MOST** appropriate treatment for these findings is which of the following intervention?

A. intravenous antibiotics
B. prenatal corticosteroids
C. supplemental oxygen
D. thoracic surgery

Answer: C

Meconium aspiration occurs in term or postterm neonates and causes partial obstruction of small airways with resulting areas of atelectasis and hyperinflation. Lung hyperinflation can be found in other neonatal lung diseases such as congenital emphysema, where it affects only one lobe and causes atelectasis in the adjacent lobes, and in pneumonia, where it occurs because of mechanical ventilation. The neonate described in the question displays lung hyperinflation in the absence of mechanical ventilation, supporting the diagnosis of meconium aspiration. The management of meconium aspiration is supportive and includes oxygen supplementation, mechanical ventilation, and surfactant. In severe cases, which are complicated by persistent pulmonary hypertension, cardiovascular support with vasopressors and inotropes, and EMCO may be needed. Antibiotics (answer A) are indicated in the management of neonatal pneumonia or sepsis but not meconium aspiration. Antibiotics are also routinely administered in infants with transient tachypnea of the newborn, because it is difficult to differentiate between an infective process and delayed absorption of fluid from the lungs after birth. Thoracic surgery (answer D) may be required emergently in the management of respiratory distress of patients with congenital emphysema, or large CPAMs but is not indicated in the management of MAS. Corticosteroids (answer B) is incorrect because the prenatal administration of corticosteroids does not decrease the risk of meconium aspiration. Instead, it increases fetal production of surfactant and decreases the risk of RSD in infants born preterm.

2. A 3-day-old infant born at 34 weeks of gestation is admitted to the NICU for respiratory distress and a blood pressure of 53/20 mmHg. The neonatal radiograph shows a large cystic area in the left lung and mediastinal shift. Pulse oximetry probes placed on the right arm and right foot show an oxygen saturation of 93% and 83%, respectively. What is the **MOST** appropriate next management step?

A. dobutamine at 10 mcg/kg/min
B. emergent left-sided lobectomy
C. high-frequency oscillatory ventilation
D. nitrous oxide at 20 ppm

Answer: C

The infant's presentation suggests severe persistent pulmonary hypertension, likely caused by hypoplasia of the pulmonary vasculature in the cystic lung. High-frequency oscillatory ventilation will correct hypoxia and hypercarbia, decrease pulmonary arterial pressure, and minimize the risk of cyst hyperinflation caused by conventional ventilation. Answer B is incorrect because the patient needs to be stabilized and pulmonary hypertension controlled before resecting the cystic mass. Answer A is incorrect because, although dobutamine decreases pulmonary pressure, it is less effective in neonates and may lower blood pressure. Answer D is incorrect because

nitric oxide, not *nitrous* oxide, is effective in treating pulmonary hypertension. In fact, nitrous oxide will enlarge lung cysts.

3. As compared to intralobar sequestration, which of the following statement is the **MOST** accurate regarding extralobar BPS?

A. greater association with cardiac anomalies
B. higher rate of bacterial infections
C. increased venous return via systemic vessels
D. more frequently occurring

Answer: A

Extralobar BPS are less frequent than intrapulmonary BPS (thus, answer D is incorrect) but are more likely to be associated with other congenital anomalies, such as vertebral anomalies, congenital diaphragmatic hernia, and congenital heart disease (answer A). Because the extrapulmonary BPS lack communication with the lung and have their own pleura, they are less likely to become infected than the intralobar BPS, which are located inside the lung and may be contaminated with bacteria through abnormal communication with distal bronchi, or lung parenchyma via the pores of Kohn (answer B is incorrect). Answer C is incorrect because both intra- and extralobar BPS drain in the pulmonary veins, and occasionally in the systemic circulation via the azygos, hemiazygos, or portal veins.

4. Which of the following chest radiograms findings in an infant with respiratory distress is **LEAST** likely to be associated with pulmonary hypertension in the neonatal period?

A. cystic lesions with air-fluid level in the left hemithorax
B. diffuse "ground-glass" and history of maternal diabetes
C. large cystic mass in the right lung
D. upper lobe hyperinflation with mediastinal shift

Answer: D.

Respiratory distress, lobar hyperinflation, mediastinal shift, and hypotension are features of CLE. In this condition, a ball-valve mechanism, which allows more gas to enter the affected lobe during inspiration and exit during exhalation, causes alveolar hyperinflation. Because hyperinflation occurs after birth, there is no pulmonary hypoplasia or subsequent pulmonary hypertension. Answer A is incorrect because congenital diaphragmatic hernia, as suggested by the infant's respiratory distress, cystic lesions with air-fluid level in the left hemithorax, and a scaphoid abdomen, is likely to cause pulmonary parenchymal, vascular hypoplasia, and pulmonary hypertension. Answer A is incorrect because a large lung mass diagnosed during gestation is likely to compress the adjacent lung and cause pulmonary hypoplasia. Answer B is incorrect because maternal diabetes is a known risk factor for persistent pulmonary hypertension of the neonate. Uncontrolled diabetes mellitus is associated with a high incidence of hyaline membrane disease, hypoglycemia, macrosomia, and fetal distress; all implicated in the etiology of persistent pulmonary hypertension of the neonate.

5. A 1-day old, 3 kg neonate presents for resection of a hyperinflated left-upper lobe. Preinduction, the infant's blood pressure is 51/18 mmHg, heart rate is 183 beats per minute,

respiratory rate is 69 bpm, and oxygen saturation is 92% on room air. Which of the following would be **BEST** for induction of anesthesia in this patient?

    A. dexmedetomidine 3 mcg, intravenous
    B. ketamine 5 mg, intravenous, lidocaine 1% to airway
    C. propofol 10 mg, intravenous
    D. sevoflurane 4%, oxygen 3 L/min, and nitrous oxide 6 L/min

Answer: B

Maintaining spontaneous ventilation until opening the chest is desirable for infants with cystic lung lesions as positive pressure ventilation could worsen alveolar hyperinflation. Modalities to maintain spontaneous breathing during induction of anesthesia and intubation include inhalational and intravenous anesthetics administered in small, titrated doses, alone or in conjunction with lidocaine administered topically over the vocal cords. In this case, the administration of intravenous ketamine and topical lidocaine (answer B) has the additional advantage of a more stable hemodynamic profile. Answer A is incorrect because a 1 mcg/kg bolus of dexmedetomidine will not ensure a deep enough plane of anesthesia for airway instrumentation. Answer C is incorrect because a 3 mg/kg bolus dose of propofol is likely to worsen the already significant hypotension in this infant. Answer D is incorrect because, although the administration of low concentrations of sevoflurane in conjunction with nitrous oxide is likely to maintain hemodynamic stability and spontaneous ventilation, nitrous oxide can further enlarge the cystic lesion and ultimately cause hemodynamic instability and cyst rupture.

6. Using a 3.5-microcuff ETT, which of the following airway management options is **MOST** appropriate for an 8-month old 7 kg infant with pneumonia and right-lower lobe CPAM presenting for lobectomy?

    A. left main bronchus intubation with uninflated cuffed ETT
    B. mid-tracheal intubation with inflated cuffed ETT
    C. mid-tracheal intubation with a 5F AEB placed alongside the ETT with the tip in the right main bronchus
    D. mid-tracheal intubation with a 5F AEB placed coaxial the ETT with the tip in the right main bronchus

Answer: C

Answer A is incorrect because even when advanced into the left mainstem bronchus, an uninflated cuffed ETT may not protect the healthy lung against spillage of pus from the infected right-lung cysts. Answer B is incorrect because an ETT with the tip above the carina does not facilitate OLV and may become occluded with pus from the infected lung. A 3.5 microcuff ETT with an endobronchial blocker placed alongside (answer C) is the best choice because it allows suctioning of the diseased lung while minimizing the risk of bronchial blocker dislodgement. Answer D is incorrect because the coaxial placement of an endobronchial blocker and a small ETT leaves only a small lumen available for suctioning. In addition, suctioning may dislodge the endobronchial blocker.

7. A 6-month old infant presents for resection of a right-upper lobe CPAM. Lung isolation is achieved with a 5F AEB. The proximal end of the blocker cuff can barely be seen in the right bronchus with the fiberoptic scope placed above carina. Upon entering the right hemithorax, the surgeon notices that the upper lobe continues to inflate. Which of the following interventions is **MOST** likely to improve surgical visualization?

    A. suctioning the lumen of the endobronchial blocker
    B. slightly retracting the endobronchial blocker
    C. injecting more air in the cuff of the blocker
    D. increasing the intrathoracic CO_2 insufflation pressure

Answer: D

Because the endobronchial blocker cuff is in the correct position, with the cuff barely visible distal to carina, it is unlikely that the cuff is occluding the take-off of the right-upper lobe bronchus, delaying its collapse. Therefore, answer B is incorrect. Moreover, continuous inflation of the right-upper lobe suggests that the lobe is still ventilated and the possibility of a tracheal right-upper lobe bronchus, with the origin above carina. In this situation, surgical visualization can be improved by retracting the lobe, or by increasing the CO_2 insufflation pressure (answer D). Suctioning the operative lung of secretions that may prevent its deflation (answer A) and adding air to an insufficiently inflated bronchial blocker cuff (answer C) are unlikely to be effective if the blocker is placed distal to the origin of a tracheal bronchus.

8. A 6-month-old infant presents for thoracoscopic resection of a large left-lower lobe BPS. The patient is intubated with a 3.5 microcuff ETT, which is then advanced into the left bronchus. Upon positioning the infant in right-lateral decubitus, his O_2 saturation decreases from 96% to 92%. What is the **MOST** appropriate next management step?

    A. deflation of the bronchial blocker
    B. large bore needle of the left hemithorax
    C. lung recruitment maneuvers
    D. total intravenous anesthesia

Answer: C

Answer A is incorrect because resuming two-lung ventilation is not the first step in managing hypoxia during thoracoscopy. Answer B is incorrect because BPS do not communicate with proximal bronchi; thus, they are unlikely to inflate and rupture (causing a pneumothorax) when instituting positive pressure ventilation. Answer D is incorrect. Although intravenous anesthetics, unlike inhalational anesthetics, do not inhibit hypoxic pulmonary vasoconstriction, switching to total intravenous anesthesia will not improve hypoxia as effectively and immediately as lung recruitment maneuvers (answer C).

9. Following resection of a large thoracic cystic lesion, an epidural catheter was placed in a 3-week-old, 3.2 kg infant. The catheter was placed caudally and could be threaded up only to the T8–T9 level. Which of the following continuous epidural infusions is **MOST** appropriate for postoperative pain management?

    A. bupivacaine 0.1% at 1.2 mL/hour
    B. bupivacaine 0.1% and fentanyl 2 mcg/mL at 0.8 mL/hour

C. 2-chloroprocaine 1.5% at 2 mL/hour

D. 2-chloroprocaine 1.5% and clonidine 0.4 mcg/mL at 2.8 mL/hour

Answer: C

Because of its rapid metabolism, 2-chloroprocaine is an attractive choice for epidural analgesia in neonates, especially when the catheter tip is remote from the optimal location and more anesthetic is required for adequate pain control. Answer A is incorrect because, at the indicated rate, bupivacaine exceeds the upper end of recommended doses for neonates (0.25 mg/kg/hour) and could result in toxicity. Answer B is incorrect because, although the bupivacaine and fentanyl doses are within the recommended limits, the rate of infusion may be insufficient because the tip of the catheter is not in immediate proximity to the surgical dermatomes. Answer D is incorrect because clonidine may cause excessive sedation, apnea, and bradycardia in neonates.

QUESTIONS AND ANSWERS

This chapter has accompanying questions and answers which are available to subscribers as part of the Oxford eLearning platform. To access the questions, go to ✓ http://oxfordmedicine. com/pediatricanesthesiaPBL

REFERENCES

1. Edwards MO, Kotecha SJ, Kotecha S. Respiratory distress of the term newborn infant. *Paediatr Respir Rev.* 2013;14(1):29–36.
2. Yurdakok M. Transient tachypnea of the newborn: what is new? *J Matern Fetal Neonatal Med* .2010;23(Suppl 3):24–26.
3. Engle WA. American Academy of Pediatrics Committee on Fetus and Newborn. Surfactant-replacement therapy for respiratory distress in the preterm and term neonate. *Pediatrics.* 2008;121(2):419–432.
4. Reuter S, Moser C, Baack M. Respiratory distress in the newborn. *Pediatr Rev.* 2014;35(10):417–428.
5. Konduri GG, Kim UO. Advances in the diagnosis and management of persistent pulmonary hypertension of the newborn. *Pediatr Clin North Am.* 2009;56(3):579–600.
6. Durell J, Lakhoo K. Congenital cystic lesions of the lung. *Early Hum Dev.* 2014;90(12):935–939.
7. Stocker JT. The respiratory tract. In: Stocker JT, Dehner LP, eds. *Pediatric pathology.* 2nd ed. Vol. 1. Philadelphia: Lippincott; 1992:466–473.
8. Ruchonnet-Metrailler IE, Leroy-Terquem J, Stirnemann P, et al. Neonatal outcomes of prenatally diagnosed congenital pulmonary malformations. *Pediatrics.* 2014;133(5):e1285–e1291.
9. Nishibayashi, SW, Andrassy RJ, Woolley MM. Congenital cystic adenomatoid malformation: a surgical emergency. *Clin Pediatr.* 1979;18(12):760–761.
10. Nakano S, Tashiro C, Nishimura M, Ueyama H, Uchiyama A. Perioperative use of high-frequency oscillation immediately after birth in two neonates with congenital cystic adenomatoid malformation. *Anesthesiology.* 1991;74(5):939–941.
11. Atkinson JB, Ford EG, Kitagawa H, Lally KP, Humphries B. Persistent pulmonary hypertension complicating cystic adenomatoid malformation in neonates. *J Pediatr Surg.* 1992;27(1):54–56.
12. Gardikis S, Didilis V, Polychronidis A, Mikroulis D, Sividis E, Bougioukas G, Simopoulos C. Spontaneous pneumothorax resulting from congenital cystic adenomatoid malformation in a pre-term infant: case report and literature review. *Eur J Pediatr Surg.* 2002;12(3):195–198.

13. Gornall AS, Budd JLS, Draper ES, Konje JC, Kurinczuk JJ. Congenital cystic adenomatoid malformation: accuracy of prenatal diagnosis, prevalence and outcome in a general population. *Prenat Diagn.* 2003;23(12):997–1002.
14. Bouchut JC, Claris O. Ventilation management during neonatal thoracic surgery. *Anesth Analg.* 2007;104(1):218–219.
15. Bouchut JC, Godard J, Claris O. High-frequency oscillatory ventilation. *Anesthesiology.* 2004;100(4):1007–1012.
16. Guruswamy V, Roberts S, Arnold P, Potter F. Anaesthetic management of a neonate with congenital cyst adenoid malformation. *Br J Anaesth.* 2005;95(2):240–242.
17. Nishimoto C, Inomata S, Kihara S, Miyabe M, Toyooka H. Anesthetic management of four pediatric patients with CCAM for pulmonary lobectomy. *Masui.* 2002;51(2):162–165.
18. DeParedes CG, Pierce WS, Johnson DG, Waldhausen JA. Pulmonary sequestration in infants and children: a 20-year experience and review of the literature. *J Pediatr Surg.* 1970;5(2):136–147.
19. Pumberger W, Hormann M, Deutinger J, Bernaschek G, Bistricky E, Horcher E. Longitudinal observation of antenatally detected congenital lung malformations (CLM): natural history, clinical outcome and long-term follow-up. *Eur J Cardiothorac Surg.* 2003;24(5):703–711.
20. Ko SF, Ng SH, Lee TY, et al. Noninvasive imaging of bronchopulmonary sequestration. *AJR Am J Roentgenol.* 2000;175(4):1005–1012.
21. Leape LL, Longino LA. Infantile lobar emphysema. *Pediatrics.* 1964;34:246–255.
22. Schwartz MZ, Ramachandran P. Congenital malformations of the lung and mediastinum—a quarter century of experience from a single institution. *J Pediatr Surg.* 1997;32(1):44–47.
23. Cote CJ. The anesthetic management of congenital lobar emphysema. *Anesthesiology.* 1978;49(4):296–298.
24. Tempe DK, Virmani S, Javetkar S, Banerjee A, Puri SK, Datt V. Congenital lobar emphysema: pitfalls and management. *Ann Card Anaesth.* 2010;13(1):53–58.
25. Raghavendran S, Diwan R, Shah T, Vas L. Continuous caudal epidural analgesia for congenital lobar emphysema: a report of three cases. *Anesth Analg.* 2001;93(2):348–350.
26. Subramanyam R, Costandi A, Mahmoud M. Congenital lobar emphysema and tension emphysema. *J Clin Anesth.* 2016;29:17–18.
27. Arora MK, Karamchandani K, Bakhta P, and Kumar V. Combination of inhalational, intravenous, and local anesthesia for intubation in neonates with congenital lobar emphysema. *Paediatr Anaesth.* 2006;16(9):998–999.
28. Schmidt C, Rellensmann G, Van Aken H, Semik M, Bruessel T, Enk D. Single-lung ventilation for pulmonary lobe resection in a newborn. *Anesth Analg.* 2005;101(2):362–364.
29. Goto H, Boozalis ST, Benson KT, Arakawa K. High-frequency jet ventilation for resection of congenital lobar emphysema. *Anesth Analg.* 1987;66(7):684–686.
30. Lansdale N, Alam S, Losty PD, Jesudason EC. Neonatal endosurgical congenital diaphragmatic hernia repair: a systematic review and meta-analysis. *Ann Surg.* 2010;252(1):20–26.
31. Mattioli GL, Pio N, Disma M, et al. Congenital lung malformations: shifting from open to thoracoscopic surgery. *Pediatr Neonatol.* 2016;57(6):463–466.
32. Pawar DK, Marraro GA. One lung ventilation in infants and children: experience with Marraro double lumen tube. *Paediatr Anaesth.* 2005;15(3):204–208.
33. Cohen DE, McCloskey JJ, Motas D, Archer J, Flake AW. Fluoroscopic-assisted endobronchial intubation for single-lung ventilation in infants. *Paediatr Anaesth.* 2011;21(6):681–684.
34. Tobias JD. Anaesthesia for neonatal thoracic surgery. *Best Pract Res Clin Anaesthesiol.* 2004;18(2):303–320.
35. Hammer GB, Fitzmaurice BJ, Brodsky JB. Methods for single-lung ventilation in pediatric patients. *Anesth Analg.* 1999;89(6):1426–1429.
36. Golianu B, Hammer GB. Pediatric thoracic anesthesia. *Curr Opin Anaesthesiol.* 2005;18(1):5–11.
37. Disma N, Mameli L, Pini-Prato A, Montobbio G. One lung ventilation with Arndt pediatric bronchial blocker for thoracoscopic

surgery in children: a unicentric experience. *Paediatr Anaesth.* 2011;21(4):465–467.

38. Butz RO Jr. Length and cross-section growth patterns in the human trachea. *Pediatrics.* 1968;42(2):336–341.

39. Griscom NT, Wohl ME. Dimensions of the growing trachea related to age and gender. *AJR Am J Roentgenol.* 1986;146(2):233–237.

40. Templeton TW, Downard MG, Simpson CR, Zeller KA, Templeton LB, Bryan WF. Bending the rules: a novel approach to placement and retrospective experience with the 5 French Arndt endobronchial blocker in children <2 years. *Paediatr Anaesth.* 2016;26(5):512–520.

41. Hammer GB. Single-lung ventilation in infants and children. *Paediatr Anaesth.* 2004;14(1):98–102.

42. Marciniak B, Fayoux P, Hebrard A, Engelhardt T, Weinachter C, Horber RK. Fluoroscopic guidance of Arndt endobronchial blocker placement for single-lung ventilation in small children. *Acta Anaesthesiol Scand.* 2008;52(7):1003–1005.

43. Bastien JL, O'Brien JG, Frantz FW. Extraluminal use of the Arndt pediatric endobronchial blocker in an infant: a case report. *Can J Anaesth.* 2006;53(2):159–161.

44. Stephenson LL, Seefelder C. Routine extraluminal use of the 5F Arndt endobronchial blocker for one-lung ventilation in children up to 24 months of age. *J Cardiothorac Vasc Anesth.* 2011;25(4): 683–686.

45. Hsieh VC, Thompson DR, Haberkern CM pediatric endobronchial blockers in infants: a refinement in technique. *Paediatr Anaesth.* 2015;25(4):438–439.

46. Letal M, Theam M. Paediatric lung isolation. *BJA Educ.* 2017;17:57–62.

47. Slinger PD, Lesiuk L. Flow resistances of disposable double-lumen, single-lumen, and Univent tubes. *J Cardiothorac Vasc Anesth.* 1998;12(2):142–144.

48. Brodsky JB, Lemmens HJ. Tracheal width and left double-lumen tube size: a formula to estimate left-bronchial width. *J Clin Anesth.* 2005;17(4): 267–270.

49. Sustic A, Miletic D, Protic A, Ivancic A, Cicvaric T. Can ultrasound be useful for predicting the size of a left double-lumen bronchial tube? Tracheal width as measured by ultrasonography versus computed tomography. *J Clin Anesth.* 2008;20(4):247–252.

50. Shibasaki M, Nakajima Y, Ishii S, Shimizu F, Shime N, Sessler DI. Prediction of pediatric endotracheal tube size by ultrasonography. *Anesthesiology.* 2010;113(4):819–824.

51. Scammon RE. Dimensions of the respiratory tract at various ages in man. In: Abt IA, ed. *Pediatrics.* Philadelphia, PA: WB Saunders, 1923:257.

52. Cote C, Lerman J, Andersen BJ. *A Practice of Anesthesia for Infants and Children.* 5th ed. Philadelphia, PA: Elsevier Saunders; 2013:277–290.

53. Baidya DK, Pawar DK, Dehran M, Gupta AK. Advancement of epidural catheter from lumbar to thoracic space in children: comparison between 18G and 23G catheters. *J Anaesthesiol Clin Pharmacol.* 2012;28(1):21–27.

54. Taenzer AH, Clark CT, Kovarik WD. Experience with 724 epidurograms for epidural catheter placement in pediatric anesthesia. *Reg Anesth Pain Med.* 2010;35(5):432–435.

55. Tsui BC, Wagner A, Cave D, Kearney R. Thoracic and lumbar epidural analgesia via the caudal approach using electrical stimulation guidance in pediatric patients: a review of 289 patients. *Anesthesiology.* 2004;100(3):683–689.

56. Willschke H, Bosenberg A, Marhofer P, et al. Epidural catheter placement in neonates: sonoanatomy and feasibility of ultrasonographic guidance in term and preterm neonates. *Reg Anesth Pain Med.* 2007;32(1):34–40.

57. Long JB, Joselyn AS, Bhalla T, Tobias J, DeOliveira G, Suresh S. The use of neuraxial catheters for postoperative analgesia in neonates: a multicenter safety analysis from the Pediatric Regional Anesthesia Network. *Anesth Analg.* 2016:122(6):1965–1970.

58. Larsson BA, Lonnqvist PA, Olsson GL. Plasma concentrations of bupivacaine in neonates after continuous epidural infusion. *Anesth Analg.* 1997;84(3):501–505.

59. Bosenberg AT, Thomas J, Cronje L, et al. Pharmacokinetics and efficacy of ropivacaine for continuous epidural infusion in neonates and infants. *Pediatr Anaesth.* 2005;15:739–749.

60. Mazoit JX, Dalens BJ. Ropivacaine in infants and children. *Curr Opin Anaesthesiol.* 2003;16(3):305–307.

61. Muhly WT, Gurnaney HG, Kraemer FW, Ganesh A, Maxwell LG. A retrospective comparison of ropivacaine and 2-chloroprocaine continuous thoracic epidural analgesia for management of postthoracotomy pain in infants. *Paediatr Anaesth.* 2015;25(11):1162–1167.

62. Veneziano G, Tobias JD. Chloroprocaine for epidural anesthesia in infants and children. *Paediatr Anaesth.* 2017;27(6):581–590.

63. Ganesh A, Adzick NS, Foster T, Cucchiaro G. Efficacy of addition of fentanyl to epidural bupivacaine on postoperative analgesia after thoracotomy for lung resection in infants. *Anesthesiology.* 2008;109(5):890–894.

64. Ross EL, Reiter PD, Murphy ME, Bielsky AR. Evaluation of prolonged epidural chloroprocaine for postoperative analgesia in infants. *J Clin Anesth.* 2015;27(6):463–469.

65. El-Morsy GZ, El-Deeb A, El-Desouky T, Elsharkawy AA, Elgamal MA. Can thoracic paravertebral block replace thoracic epidural block in pediatric cardiac surgery? A randomized blinded study. *Ann Card Anaesth.* 2012;15(4):259–263.

66. Bairdain S, Dodson B, Zurakowski D, Waisel DB, Jennings RW, Boretsky KR. Paravertebral nerve block catheters using chloroprocaine in infants with prolonged mechanical ventilation for treatment of long-gap esophageal atresia. *Paediatr Anaesth.* 2015;25(11):1151–1157.

67. Vecchione T, Zurakowski D, Boretsky K. Thoracic paravertebral nerve blocks in pediatric patients: safety and clinical experience. *Anesth Analg.* 2016;123(6):1588–1590.

68. Aldrink JH, Ma M, Wang W, Canianao DA, Wispe J, Puthoff T. Safety of ketorolac in surgical neonates and infants 0 to 3 months old. *J Pediatr Surg.* 2011;46(6):1081–1085.

16.

CONGENITAL DIAPHRAGMATIC HERNIA

Sabina A. Khan and Nitin Wadhwa

STEM CASE AND KEY QUESTIONS

A 36-week-old, 3.1 kg preemie was born with a prenatal diagnosis of a type D right-sided congenital diaphragmatic hernia (CDH). Lung-to-head ratio calculated at 25 weeks of gestation was 1.1. APGARs (appearance, pulse, grimace, activity, and respiration) at 1 and 5 minutes of birth were 3 and 6, respectively. The neonate was cyanotic and in respiratory distress. Physical examination revealed nasal flaring and scaphoid abdomen. Breath sounds on the right were diminished, and bowel sounds were appreciated on the right side of the chest. Vital signs included temperature of 97.0° F, blood pressure of 83/56 (64) mmHg, heart rate of 161 bpm, and respiratory rate of 65 breaths per minute.

WHY IS THIS PATIENT CYANOTIC AND IN RESPIRATORY DISTRESS? WHAT SHOULD BE THE INITIAL MANAGEMENT FOR THIS PATIENT?

First capillary blood gas analysis after birth showed: pH < 6.95, $PaCO_2$ > 95 mmHg, partial pressure of oxygen in arterial blood (PaO_2) of 35 mmHg and bicarbonate (HCO_3) of 22 mEq/L. Due to severe respiratory distress, the baby became hypoxemic and bradycardic shortly after birth and was intubated awake with a 3.5 uncuffed endotracheal tube while maintaining spontaneous respiration. This resulted in improved heart rate and oxygen saturation. An 8 French Replogle tube was placed for gastric decompression. Initial conventional ventilation settings were respiratory rate 60 breaths per minute, pressure control 22, positive end-expiratory pressure 5, and fraction of inspired oxygen (FiO_2) 95%.

HOW DO YOU CONFIRM THE DIAGNOSIS OF CDH POSTNATALLY?

Chest X-ray revealed a right diaphragmatic hernia with bowel, stomach, and liver herniation and leftward mediastinal shift. There was volvulus of stomach appearance without evidence of obstruction along with near complete opacification of bilateral lungs.

WHAT IS HIGH-FREQUENCY OSCILLATORY VENTILATOR (HFOV)? HOW DOES IT WORK?

A preductal, right radial arterial line was placed by the neonatologist for closer hemodynamic monitoring and frequent arterial blood gases (ABGs). Worsening respiratory status along with severe combined respiratory and metabolic acidosis required eventual change to HFOV on 100% FiO_2 with the following settings: mean airway pressure 15, Amplitude 35, hertz 8.

Despite being on HFOV, respiratory acidosis persisted with CO_2 levels >95 mmHg and pH of <6.99. In addition, patient became progressively hypotensive requiring dopamine and milrinone infusions.

HOW DO YOU DETERMINE THE PRESENCE OF PULMONARY HYPERTENSION?

Echocardiogram showed severe pulmonary hypertension (PHTN) with suprasystemic pressures, large patent ductus arteriosus, and patent foramen ovale with right to left shunt. Right atrium and ventricle were markedly enlarged along with mild thickening of the right ventricular wall.

WHEN DO YOU DECIDE TO INITIATE EXTRACORPOREAL MECHANICAL OXYGENATION (ECMO)? DESCRIBE THE TYPES OF ECMO?

An ultrasound of the head performed in anticipation of ECMO demonstrated no intraventricular hemorrhage. Given the lack of improvement and cardiopulmonary interventions exceeding the parameters of conventional management, the ECMO team was mobilized, and the patient was cannulated for veno-arterial ECMO.

ECMO initiation resulted in resolution of hypoxemia, normalization of acid-base status, and hemodynamic stability. Patient was scheduled to undergo CDH repair on day of life. Due to the patient's precarious status and transport to the operating room on ECMO being risky, a bedside surgical repair in the neonatal intensive care unit (NICU) was deemed as the safest option.

Next day, you arrive at the patient's bedside in the NICU. A 24 G peripheral intravenous line is in place, and 50 mL/kg of packed red blood cells) and fresh-frozen plasma is already at the bedside. The perfusionist shows you the most recent ABG, which looks reasonable. Patient's vital signs are stable with good urine output.

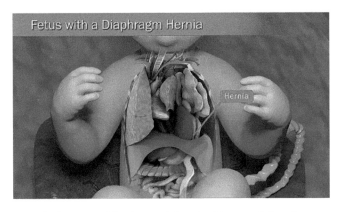

Fig. 16.1 Left congenital diaphragmatic hernia with stomach, intestines, and liver in the thoracic cavity exerting pressure on the heart and great vessels. (Courtesy of Children's Memorial Hermann Hospital/Texas Medical Center, Houston, TX).

WHAT WOULD BE YOUR ANESTHETIC PLAN IN THIS PATIENT? WHAT COMPLICATIONS DO YOU ANTICIPATE?

Surgery on ECMO is initiated after antibiotic administration. Before incision, you administer 15 mcg/kg of fentanyl and 3 mg/kg of rocuronium. During reduction of the hernia, you notice desaturation on the monitor into low 70s on FiO2 of 40%. Arterial waveform dampens, and the patient becomes hypotensive. You notice decreased venous drainage from the

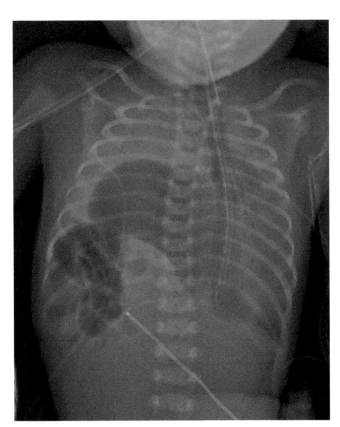

Fig. 16.2 Radiological imaging of a neonate with right congenital diaphragmatic hernia. Liver and air-filled loops of intestines are seen on the right side of the chest.

Fig. 16.3 Illustration of the types of congenital diaphragmatic hernia. Used with permission from Harting, M, Lally K, Congenital Diaphragmatic Hernia Study Group. *J Pediatr Surg.* 2013 Dec;48(12):2408-2415.

ECMO cannula, low pump flows, and high circuit pressures. Mixed venous oxygen saturation is decreased with increased arterial oxygen tension (PaO_2). After communicating with the surgeon and perfusionist, you determine the patient has a contralateral tension pneumothorax after ruling out other potential causes. A chest tube is promptly placed by the surgeon, allowing for hemodynamic stability, and return of baseline ECMO flow. The hernia is reduced using a Gore-Tex® patch, and surgery is completed successfully.

DISCUSSION

PATHOPHYSIOLOGY

Congenital diaphragmatic hernia is a complex congenital syndrome with an incidence between 1:2000 to 1:5000 births.[1] The male to female ratio is 1:1.8.[2] The underlying etiology is an embryological defect in the formation of the diaphragm. During fetal development, a common pleuroperitoneal cavity exists at 4 weeks of gestation. At 8 weeks, the formation of the pleuroperitoneal membrane divides the common cavity into a pleural and peritoneal cavity.[3a] Failure of complete formation of this membrane allows abdominal viscera to extrude into the thoracic cavity, acting as a space-occupying lesion and causing bilateral lung hypoplasia that is more pronounced on the ipsilateral side.

Lung hypoplasia leads to decreased alveolar surface area, decreased bronchopulmonary segments with distal branching, and thicker than normal alveolar walls. It results in suboptimal gas exchange with the capillaries. The pulmonary vasculature is also abnormal, with decreased pulmonary arteries per unit of lung volume and thickened alveolar arterioles and capillaries.[4] The consequential poor pulmonary function and decreased compliance leads to PHTN. PHTN results in persistent fetal

CONGENITAL CIAPHRAGMATIC HERNIA SUMMARY	
Incidence	1:2000–1:5000 live births. Male:female ratio is 1:1.8
Pathogenesis	Embryological defect in pleuroperitoneal membrane. Lung hypoplasia, pulmonary HTN
Classification	Based on location and size of defect. Left more common (80%) than right. Type D has the worst prognosis. (See different types in following table data)
Associated abnormalities[7,19,21]	Chromosomal: Trisomy 13, 18, Turner's CNS: behavioral issues, attention deficit, learning disorders CVS: hypoplastic heart syndrome, excluding PFO and PDA GU: renal dysplasia, cryptorchidism Gastrointestinal: failure to thrive, GERD
Predictors of survival	Mortality predicted prenatally by LHR ratio. A LHR <0.8 predicts 100% mortality, while a LHR >1.4 equates to no mortality
Signs and symptoms	Respiratory distress, hypoxemia, cyanosis, barrel chest, scaphoid abdomen and bowel sounds in the thoracic cavity
Prenatal diagnosis	Maternal ultrasound, fetal magnetic resonance imaging, derum alpha fetoprotein
Perioperative management	Spontaneous ventilation, Intubation, permissive hypercapnia, small tidal volumes for lung protection, HFOV, ECMO
Intraoperative management	Preductal pulse oximetry and arterial line, TIVA, muscle relaxation, prevention of hypertensive crisis and pneumothorax, low ventilation pressures
Postoperative management	Continued intubation; adequate sedation and analgesia
Long-term complications	Developmental and mental delays, sensorineural hearing loss, and GERD

Note. HTN = hypertension. CNS = central nervous system. CVS = chorionic villus sampling. PVO = patent foramen ovale. PDA = patent ductus arteriosus. GU = genitourinary gastric ulcer. GERD = gastroesophageal reflux disease. LHR =lung-to-head ratio. HFOV = high-frequency oscillatory ventilator. ECMO = extracorporeal membrane oxygenation. TIVA = total intravenous anesthesia.

circulation with right-to-left shunting through the foramen ovale and ductus arteriosus, followed by cyanosis, hypoxemia, worsening respiratory status, acidosis, and hypercarbia. A persistent acidotic state leads to a circular pathway of worsening PHTN. PHTN and pulmonary hypoplasia are the 2 underlying factors responsible for the morbidity and mortality of this disease.

In addition, the increased thoracic cavity contents can result in increased intrathoracic pressure leading to mediastinal shift and caval compression causing decreased preload and cardiac output.[1]

CLASSIFICATION

CDH is classified based on the location and size of the defect. Anatomically, a left-sided CDH is the most common form due to later closure of the left side of the pleuroperitoneal membrane and occurs in 80% of cases. The most common defect is a posterolateral defect (Bochdalek's hernia) accounting for 95% of cases. Anteromedial (Morgagni), para-esophageal hernias, and eventrations are extremely rare and account for 5% of cases.[5] Bochdalek's hernia is associated with a higher incidence of congenital heart disease and chromosomal abnormalities.[1] The right-sided hernias with liver herniation are associated with a higher mortality. Bilateral hernias are very rare (2%) and often fatal.[1]

CDH is also classified into types A, B, C, or D, based on the size of the defect with type A being the smallest and type D the largest. This classification helps estimate the length of a patient's hospital stay with type D staying in the NICU for as long as 12 weeks.

DIAGNOSIS AND CLINICAL PRESENTATION

CDH is most commonly diagnosed during a routine prenatal ultrasound. Polyhydramnios, gastric bubble in the thoracic cavity, and mediastinal shift are the suggestive findings. These findings, along with a diagnosis as early as 20 weeks of gestation correlates with poor prognosis.[2] CDH may not be detected by ultrasound in up to 50% of cases. Interestingly, low maternal serum alpha-fetoprotein is also associated with CDH.[1]

Mortality can be predicted prenatally by lung-to-head ratio. At 24–26 weeks, a ratio of the cross-sectional area of the contralateral lung to the head circumference is calculated. A LHR less than 0.8 predicts 100% mortality, while a LHR greater than 1.4 equates to no mortality.[6] In prenatally diagnosed cases, liver herniation along with low LHR decreases the chance of survival by 50%.

Ultrasound and other modalities such as fetal magnetic resonance imaging have improved the early management and clinical course of CDH patients. This provides the opportunity for the mother to be transferred to a tertiary center for expert management of CDH.

Postnatally, respiratory distress, acute hypoxemia, and cyanosis is the classic presentation of CDH. Physical examination includes barrel chest, scaphoid abdomen, and bowel sounds in the thoracic cavity.[1] A plain chest radiograph showing air-filled loops of bowel or abdominal viscera in the chest on the ipsilateral side is confirmatory for CDH. A mediastinal shift with heart and tracheal deviation might also be seen.[6]

FETAL INTERVENTION

In highly select cases, a fetal intervention called fetoscopic endoluminal tracheal occlusion (FETO) procedure can be considered prenatally to prevent lung hypoplasia with definitive CDH repair performed postnatally once the neonate is stabilized.[1]

FETO is a novel technique where the trachea of the fetus is occluded with a balloon placed endoscopically between 26 and 30 weeks of gestation. This occlusion prevents the lung fluid from escaping into the amniotic fluid, thereby increasing airway pressure and promoting lung growth and expansion.

The balloon placement and integrity is monitored at frequent intervals with ultrasounds, and it is ultimately removed via the same fetoscopic approach at 34 weeks. In emergent cases, an ex-utero intrapartum treatment (EXIT) procedure is performed to remove the balloon before delivery.

The EXIT procedure is best described as partial delivery of the baby along with surgical instrumentation or securing of the baby's airway, all while the baby is still attached to the umbilical cord and receiving oxygen from the placenta (maternal "bypass"). Once the balloon is removed from the baby's trachea, the baby can be delivered. FETO is usually reserved for severe CDH cases, and some randomized control trials have shown improved survival in severe isolated CDH cases,[7] while others have not.[8]

SURGICAL VERSUS MEDICAL EMERGENCY

CDH is no longer considered a surgical emergency. Literature has shown improved survival if surgery is performed only once the patient is stabilized. Medical management includes use of sedatives, analgesics, and mechanical ventilation. Serial ABGs are performed to manage hypoventilation, acidosis, and PHTN.[2,3a,6]

PREOPERATIVE MANAGEMENT

The first step of management is to establish adequate oxygenation and ventilation. This is usually achieved by performing endotracheal intubation while keeping the patient spontaneously breathing. It is prudent to avoid positive pressure mask ventilation, as doing so could insufflate the bowel on the side of the hernia and compromise respiratory status further. An orogastric or nasogastric tube should be placed to decompress the stomach. Positive airway pressure after intubation should not exceed 25–30 cm H_2O, as it can result in a contralateral pneumothorax.[2] Serial ABGs are essential to guide therapy. The goal of the ventilation strategy is a preductal oxygen saturation of >85% while maintaining $PaCO_2$ of 45–55 mmHg, pH > 7.3, and peak inspiratory pressure (PIP) of 25 cm H_2O or less.[9]

Neonates requiring PIP greater than 25 cm H_2O are placed on HFOV to improve gas exchange of the hypoplastic lungs.[9] HFOV is intended to prevent ventilator associated lung injury by providing small tidal volumes (less than the anatomic dead space) at a high frequency (300–3,000/min). The oscillatory pump actively provides positive pressure during inspiration and negative pressure during expiration. This alternating pressure change (ΔP) oscillates around the constant mean airway pressure, maintaining lung recruitment and preventing overdistension.[10]

An echocardiogram should be obtained to evaluate cardiac anatomy and function. Pulmonary artery pressures should be measured to estimate the degree of PHTN.

With its role as a selective pulmonary vasodilator, inhaled nitric oxide (iNO) improves oxygenation and ventilation–perfusion mismatch. It has been shown to be beneficial in neonates with persistent PHTN, reducing the need for ECMO and leading to improved neurodevelopmental outcomes.[11] With this mindset, the use of iNO has become widespread for CDH patients with persistent PHTN. However, several reputable studies have shown that iNO does not improve survival or reduce the need for ECMO in patients with CDH. In fact, its use may be associated with higher mortality. iNO use is not standardized, and it is often used in patients that don't have persistent PHTN.[12] In summary, although iNO continues to be used in patients with CDH, its efficacy in improving outcomes has yet to be demonstrated.

Surfactant is another treatment whose efficacy is yet to be proven. According to data from the Congenital Diaphragmatic Hernia (CDH) Registry data group, the use of exogenous surfactant on CDH patients on ECMO did not show any benefit.[13] Its use may be harmful in term infants and is associated with a lower survival rate in preterm infants (<37 weeks).[13,14] Since the use of surfactant has not been proved beneficial in any clinical trial, it must be used judiciously, if at all.

Unresponsiveness to the previously mentioned measures and worsening of hypoxemia and acidosis calls for the use of ECMO.

ECMO is used as a bridge to stabilize the patient's cardiopulmonary status, allowing the lungs to rest and PHTN to

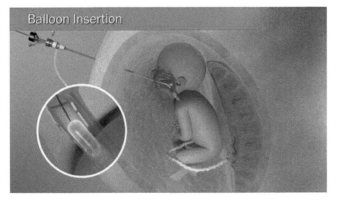

Fig. 16.4 Pictorial illustration of FETO procedure. (Courtesy of Children's Memorial Hermann Hospital/Texas Medical Center, Houston, TX).

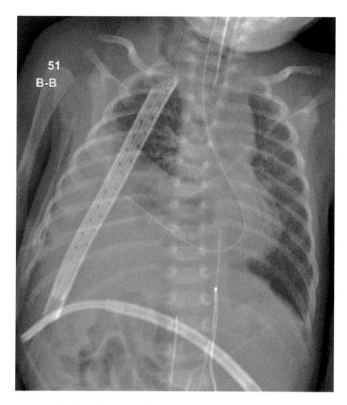

Fig. 16.5 Radiological imaging of a neonate with repaired right congenital diaphragmatic hernia.

improve. Based on the multicenter CDH Registry, ECMO improves the survival rate in CDH patients with a high risk of mortality based on birth weight and 5-minute APGAR scores.[1] Brain ultrasound should be completed to rule out intracranial hemorrhage prior to ECMO initiation.

There are 2 types of ECMO:

1. Veno-arterial ECMO: circuit between the internal jugular vein and the carotid artery. It is used in infants who are unstable and require aggressive cardiopulmonary support.

2. Veno-venous ECMO: circuit with a double lumen catheter in the Internal Jugular Vein. It is used in infants who only need respiratory support.

Although ECMO protocols may be institution specific, the criteria for the initiation of ECMO[15] at our institution is summarized as follows:

1. The inability to maintain preductal saturations above 85% after institution of HFOV and iNO.

2. Mean airway pressure >15 cm H_2O.

3. Oxygenation index consistently ≥40.

4. Inadequate oxygen delivery with metabolic acidosis defined as lactate ≥5 mmol/L and pH <7.20.

5. An increase in $PaCO_2$ >70 resulting in a respiratory acidosis with pH <7.20, despite optimization of ventilator management.

6. Hypotension resistant to fluid therapy and adequate inotropic support, resulting in a urine output <0.5 mL/kg/hour.

The criteria for exclusion of ECMO[9] is as follows:

1. Preterm birth prior to 34 weeks.

2. Weight less than 2,000 grams for veno-arterial and less than 3,000 grams for veno-venous ECMO.

3. Presence of an irreversible disease process.

4. Congenital heart disease.

ANESTHETIC CONSIDERATIONS

1. Patient transport
Stable CDH patients with normal pulmonary artery pressures on conventional ventilators are usually transported to the operating room and transition well to the operating room ventilator. In patients with significant PHTN, low birth weight, or prematurity, it may be safer to use the NICU ventilator to minimize respiratory changes. NICU ventilators are better in these cases as they are equipped to provide smaller tidal volumes with high inspired gas flows.[16] In patients on ECMO, the transport may be hazardous and the surgery should be performed in the NICU.

2. Ventilation goals
The importance of frequent ABGs cannot be emphasized enough as it allows the anesthesiologist to adjust the ventilation settings to prevent acidosis and optimize oxygenation and ventilation.[16]
Pneumothorax is an expected complication if one is not careful with ventilation settings. Gentle ventilation and permissive hypercapnia strategy help prevent this complication, which can occur even while on ECMO. The goal includes pH greater than 7.35 and PIP less than 25 cm H_2O with accepted values of $PaCO_2$ between 55 and 60 mmHg (permissive hypercapnia) and preductal oxygen saturation greater than 85%. Small tidal volumes and high respiratory rates may help achieve this goal.

3. Monitors
   - Pre- and postductal pulse oximetry
   - Capnometry
   - Noninvasive blood pressure
   - Invasive arterial blood pressure, preferentially preductal
   - Electrocardiogram
   - Core body temperature
   - Foley catheter to assess urine output
   - Mixed venous oxygen saturation on ECMO

4. Vascular access
   - Central venous access for fluid resuscitation, frequent blood draws, and inotropic support. Neck veins should be avoided in case ECMO support is indicated.

In the absence of pre-existing umbilical venous catheter, femoral lines are preferred for perioperative management.

- Peripheral intravenous lines are recommended, preferably in the upper extremities for the procedure. Reduction of hernia into the abdominal cavity can result in increased inferior vena-caval pressure resulting in futility of placement.
- Arterial line is indicated for continuous blood pressure monitoring and ABG analysis.
- Placement of invasive lines on ECMO is discouraged due to risk of bleeding secondary to anticoagulation.

5. Anesthetic goals and techniques

To attain best perioperative outcomes, anesthetic goals should include gentle ventilation with small tidal volumes, increased respiratory rate to maintain end-tidal carbon dioxide 45–55 mmHg and low airway pressures.[9] Hypoxia, hypothermia, acidosis, and pain should be avoided as they increase pulmonary vascular resistance. A decrease in systemic vascular resistance leads to hypotension and may increase right to left shunting.[17] Inhaled anesthetics such as sevoflurane can be used carefully along with muscle relaxants since these agents inhibit hypoxic pulmonary vasoconstriction. It may not be tolerated well by premature, unstable neonates due to systemic vasodilation, which may decrease preload and increase right to left shunting. For these patients, high-dose opioids/muscle relaxant combination is a better alternative. Adequate analgesia with opioids helps prevent intraoperative pulmonary hypertensive crisis. The choice of muscle relaxant varies among practitioners, but pancuronium should be avoided due to its sympathomimetic effect. Nitrous oxide should not be used as its diffusion into the bowel may lead to intestinal distension and increased intrathoracic pressure. Nitrous oxide may also expand a pneumothorax.

7. Hemodynamic goals

ABG and blood glucose should be checked periodically. Dextrose containing fluids should be continued throughout the procedure. Anesthetic agents result in changes in preload and afterload. Colloids, blood products, and vasoactive agents should be readily available. Large fluid shifts and blood loss are uncommon during CDH repair, and the main goal is to keep mean arterial pressures appropriate for gestational age. Fluid overload may cause bowel edema resulting in difficult abdominal wall closure. For infants who are consistently hypotensive despite adequate fluid therapy, transthoracic echocardiogram can be utilized to assess left ventricular function and to decide further treatment. A disseminated intravascular coagulation panel and thromboelastogram can be sent for analysis intraoperatively if the patient is bleeding profusely or with severe acidosis. In ECMO patients, platelets should be greater than 50K/μL and hematocrit between 35%–45%.

8. Hypothermia and effects

It is vital to avoid hypothermia as it exacerbates pulmonary vasoconstriction, thereby worsening PHTN and right-to-left shunting. Furthermore, nonshivering thermogenesis in brown adipose tissue in hypothermic neonates results in catecholamine release, which also exacerbates PHTN.[3b]

9. Intraoperative complications

Many complications can arise intraoperatively. Tension pneumothorax and pulmonary hypertensive crisis are the most feared during CDH repair. A pneumothorax should be treated by placement of a chest tube on the affected side. For acute pulmonary hypertensive crisis, it is essential to gently hyperventilate with 100% oxygen, have adequate analgesia and muscle relaxation, and provide adequate inotropic support. ECMO support is recommended if the previously discussed measures fail.[6]

10. Anesthesia on ECMO

CDH is the most common noncardiac surgical procedure performed on ECMO support. Total intravenous anesthesia with fentanyl and muscle relaxants is commonly administered. A significantly higher dose of narcotics and muscle relaxants is needed as the ECMO circuit sequesters significant amounts of the drugs. Vasoactive medications must be readily available to treat acute hemodynamic changes. In addition, packed red blood cells, fresh-frozen plasma, and platelets should be available. The activated clotting time is maintained between 160 and 200 seconds under heparinization.[18] The anesthesiologist should fully understand the intricacies of the ECMO circuit as well as complications that may arise due to anticoagulation, thromboembolic events, renal failure, sepsis, and circuit failure.[1] Constant communication between the anesthesiologist, perfusionist, and surgeon is vital for a safe and successful procedure.

POSTOPERATIVE MANAGEMENT

Patients are left intubated at the end of the procedure due to presence of underlying pulmonary hypoplasia and risk of recurrent PHTN. Adequate sedation and analgesia for pain is required and time is needed for the PHTN to subside.[2]

LONG-TERM EFFECTS/COMPLICATIONS:

Advancements in research and recognition of increased mortality secondary to PHTN has resulted in CDH repair being postponed until optimal conditions are achieved. As a result, most patients do exceptionally well after CDH repair. However, long-term complications may include developmental and mental delays, sensorineural hearing loss, skeletal abnormalities such as pectus excavatum, and gastroesophageal reflux disease.[19]

PROGNOSIS

Although the overall survival rate is 70%, higher rates have been reported in institutions using a protocol driven multidisciplinary plan focused on lung protection strategies (i.e., "gentle ventilation," permissive hypercapnia), treating PHTN, cardiovascular support, implementation of ECMO, and timing the surgical repair after minimizing lung injury.[20]

REVIEW QUESTIONS

1. A neonate was born at 37 weeks with respiratory distress to a 31-year-old female with no prenatal care. Which of the following is **MOST** consistent with the presentation of CDH?

   A. choking and vomiting after feeds
   B. cyanosis that resolves with crying.
   C. diminished left-sided breath sounds.
   D. right-sided rales and choking with feeds.

Answer: C
CDH classically presents with respiratory distress, acute hypoxemia, and cyanosis. Physical examination includes diminished breath sounds, barrel chest, scaphoid abdomen, and bowel sounds in the thoracic cavity.[1] Coughing and choking with feeds are consistent with tracheoesophageal fistula. Respiratory distress and cyanosis will not resolve with crying in CDH. Choking and vomiting after feeds is consistent with reflux.

2. Which of the following statements about the etiology of CDH is **MOST** accurate?

   A. Bilateral hernias are associated with Down syndrome.
   B. Left anterolateral thorax is the most common location.
   C. Maternal history of cocaine has been cited as risk.
   D. Pleuroperitoneal membrane defect is the causative factor.

Answer: D
The underlying etiology of CDH is an embryological defect in the formation of the diaphragm. Failure of complete formation of the pleuroperitoneal membrane allows abdominal viscera to extrude into the thoracic cavity, acting as a space occupying lesion and causing bilateral lung hypoplasia that is more pronounced on the ipsilateral side. The most common defect is a left posterolateral defect. CDH occurs with an incidence of 1:2,000 to 1:5,000 births.[1] The male to female ratio is 1:1.8.[2] While CDH may be associated with chromosomal abnormalities, bilateral hernias are quite rare and often fatal.

3. A 33-year-old G2P1 presents at 21 weeks of gestation for prenatal care. Ultrasound shows left-sided diaphragmatic hernia. She is very nervous and asks you if there are any possible interventions that can be undertaken as soon as possible. She wants to know what are the risks and benefits regarding the FETO procedure. Which of the following is the **MOST** appropriate response to this patient's question?

   A. All effected fetuses can undergo the procedure.
   B. Preventing lung hypoplasia is the aim.
   C. Risk of complications is almost zero
   D. Success rate approaches 100%.

Answer: B
The FETO procedure can be considered prenatally to prevent lung hypoplasia. Definitive CDH repair is performed postnatally.[1] The procedure is performed in select cases only.

4. Which of the following pulmonary alteration is **MOST** likely present in CDH?

   A. increased alveolar surface area
   B. increased bronchopulmonary segments
   C. thickened pulmonary vasculature
   D. thinner alveolar walls

Answer: C
Lung hypoplasia leads to decreased alveolar surface area, decreased bronchopulmonary segments with distal branching, and thicker than normal alveolar walls. It results in suboptimal gas exchange with the capillaries. The pulmonary vasculature is also abnormal, with decreased pulmonary arteries per unit of lung volume and thickened alveolar arterioles and capillaries.[4]

5. A full-term boy was born at 39 weeks with a prenatal diagnosis of CDH. The patient was intubated after birth due to respiratory distress, and a nasogastric tube was placed. What would be the **MOST** appropriate ventilation strategy in this case?

   a. $PaCO_2$ = 25-35 mmHg, pH > 7.5, PIP = 25 cm H_2O
   b. $PaCO_2$ = 45-55 mmHg, pH >7.3, PIP = 25 cm H_2O or less
   c. $PaCO_2$ = 50-60 mmHg, pH > 7.3, PIP >25 cm H_2O
   d. $PaCO_2$ = 60-80 mmHg, pH <7.2, PIP 25 cm H2O or less

Answer: B
The key to preoperative optimization is the establishment of adequate oxygenation and ventilation. Ventilation goals are a preductal oxygen saturation of >85% while maintaining $PaCO_2$ of 45–55 mmHg, pH >7.3, and PIP of 25 cm H_2O or less.[9]

6. Improve oxygenation on HFOV **MOST** likely will occur with an *increase* in which of the following parameters?

   A. amplitude of oscillations
   B. inspiratory time
   C. mean airway pressure
   D. ventilation rate

Answer: C
Neonates requiring peak inspiratory pressure greater than 25 cm H_2O are placed on HFOV to improve gas exchange of the hypoplastic lungs.[9] HFOV is intended to prevent ventilator associated lung injury by providing small tidal volumes (less than the anatomic dead space) at a high frequency (300–3,000/min). The oscillatory pump actively provides positive pressure during inspiration and negative pressure during expiration. This alternating pressure change (ΔP) oscillates around the constant mean airway pressure, maintaining lung recruitment and preventing overdistension.[10] Amplitude, frequency, and inspiratory time affect $PaCO_2$. PaO_2 is determined by mean airway pressure and FiO_2.

7. Which of the following therapeutic interventions will **MOST** likely improve outcomes in patients with CDH?

    A. exogenous surfactant
    B. iNO
    C. HFOV
    D. permissive hypercapnia

Answer: C

A survival rate greater than 70% has been reported in institutions using a protocol driven multidisciplinary plan focused on lung protection strategies (i.e., "gentle ventilation," permissive hypercapnia), treating pulmonary hypertension, cardiovascular support, implementation of ECMO, and timing the surgical repair after minimizing lung injury.[20] Surfactant, iNO, and HFOV have not been shown to improve outcomes.

8. You are called to the NICU bedside to evaluate a 3-day old neonate with a large CDH. He is on HFOV. The baby has an umbilical arterial and venous catheter. Morphine, dopamine, epinephrine, and milrinone are running at high infusion rates. He is hypotensive, cyanotic, and saturating 70% on FiO_2 of 100%. The surgeon is at the bedside and is ready to initiate ECMO support. Which of the following is **MOST** appropriate next step?

    A. echocardiogram
    B. emergent surgical repair
    C. transcranial ultrasound
    D. veno-venous ECMO

Answer: D

Severe cases of CDH may require ECMO as a bridge to stabilize the patient's cardiopulmonary status, allowing the lungs to rest and pulmonary hypertension to improve. Before starting ECMO, echocardiogram should be performed to delineate congenital heart disease, and brain ultrasound should be completed to rule out intracranial hemorrhage. Veno-venous is used in infants who only need respiratory support.

QUESTIONS AND ANSWERS

This chapter has accompanying questions and answers which are available to subscribers as part of the Oxford eLearning platform. To access the questions, go to ✔ http:// oxfordmedicine. com/pediatricanesthesiaPBL

REFERENCES

1. Cote CJ, Lerman J, Todres ID. *A Practice of Anesthesia for Infants and Children.* Philadelphia, PA: Elsevier Health Sciences; 2013:756–758.
2. Lee C, et al. Pediatric diseases. In: Hines RL, Marschall KE, eds. *Stoelting's Anesthesia and Co-Existing Disease.* 5th ed. Philadelphia, PA: Churchill Livingstone/Elsevier; 2008:593–594.
3a. Barash PG, Cullen BF, Stoelting RK eds. Neonatal Anesthesia. *Clinical Anesthesia.* Philadelphia, PA: Lippincott Williams & Wilkins; 2011:1193–1194.
3b. Barash PG, Cullen BF, Stoelting RK eds. Perioperative and Consultative Services. *Clinical Anesthesia.* Philadelphia, PA: Lippincott Williams & Wilkins; 2011:1438–1439.
4. Ameis D, Khoshgoo N, Keijzer R. Abnormal lung development in congenital diaphragmatic hernia. In: *Seminars in Pediatric Surgery.* Philadelphia, PA: WB Saunders; 2017.
5. Brett CM, Davis PJ. Anesthesia for general surgery in the neonate. In: Davis PJ, Cladis FP, eds. *Smith's Anesthesia for Infants and Children.* Philadelphia, PA: Elsevier; 2016:587.
6. In: Gregory GA, Andropoulos DB, eds. *Gregory's Pediatric Anesthesia.* West Sussex, UK: John Wiley; 2012:510–513.
7. Ruano R, Ali RA, Patel P, Cass D, Olutoye O, Belfort MA. (2014). Fetal endoscopic tracheal occlusion for congenital diaphragmatic hernia: indications, outcomes, and future directions. *Obstetr Gynecol Survey.* 2014;69(3):147–158.
8. Harrison MR, Keller RL, Hawgood SB, Kitterman JA, Sandberg PL, Farmer DL, Albanese CT. A randomized trial of fetal endoscopic tracheal occlusion for severe fetal congenital diaphragmatic hernia. *N Engl J Med.* 2003;349(20):1916–1924.
9. Boat AC, Sadhasivam S. Congenital diaphragmatic hernia repair. In: Goldschneider KR, Davidson AJ, Wittkugel EP, Skinner AV, eds. *Clinical Pediatric Anesthesia: A Case-Based Handbook.* Oxford: Oxford University Press; 2012:551–560.
10. Morini F, Capolupo I, van Weteringen W, Reiss I. Ventilation modalities in infants with congenital diaphragmatic hernia. In: *Seminars in Pediatric Surgery.* Philadelphia, PA: WB Saunders; 2017.
11. Campbell BT, Herbst KW, Briden KE, Neff S, Ruscher KA, Hagadorn JI. Inhaled nitric oxide use in neonates with congenital diaphragmatic hernia. *Pediatrics.* 2014;134(2):e420–e426.
12. Putnam LR, Tsao K, Morini F, Lally PA, Miller CC, Lally KP, Harting MT. Evaluation of variability in inhaled nitric oxide use and pulmonary hypertension in patients with congenital diaphragmatic hernia. *JAMA Pediatr.* 2016;170(12):1188–1194.
13. Doyle NM, Lally KP. The CDH Study Group and advances in the clinical care of the patient with congenital diaphragmatic hernia. *Semin Perinatol.* 2004;28(3):174–184.
14. Congenital Diaphragmatic Hernia Study Group. Surfactant does not improve survival rate in preterm infants with congenital diaphragmatic hernia. *J Pediatr Surg.* 2004;39(6):829–833.
15. Harting MT, Davis CF, Lally KP. Congenital diaphragmatic hernia and ECMO. In: Brogan TV, Lequier L, Lorusso R, MacLaren G, Peek G, eds. *Extracorporeal Life Support: The ELSO Red Book.* 5th ed. Ann Arbor, MI: Extracorporeal Life Support Organization; 2017:133.
16. Mendoza JM. Congenital diaphragmatic hernia. In Chu LF, Fuller A, eds. *Manual of Clinical Anesthesiology* (South Asian ed., Kindle ed.) Philadelphia, PA: Wolters-Kluwer; 2012:770–774.
17. Kaparti L, Padmaja R. Anaesthetic management of a neonate with right sided congenital diaphragmatic hernia. *J Clin Diagn Res.* 2013;7(12):3002–3003.
18. In: Jaffe RA, Golianu B, Schmiesing CA, eds. *Anesthesiologist's Manual of Surgical Procedures.* Philadelphia, PA: Lippincott Williams & Wilkins; 2014:1560–1561.
19. Pober BR, Russell MK, Ackerman KG. Congenital diaphragmatic hernia overview. In: *GeneReviews®.* Seattle: University of Washington; 2006.
20. Weems MF, Jancelewicz T, Sandhu HS. Congenital diaphragmatic hernia: maximizing survival. *NeoReviews.* 2016;17(12):e705–e718.
21. Fauza DO, Wilson JM. Congenital diaphragmatic hernia and associated anomalies: their incidence, identification, and impact on prognosis. *J Pediatr Surg.* 1994;29(8):1113–1117.

17.

TRACHEOESOPHAGEAL FISTULA

Michael R. Hernandez

STEM CASE AND KEY QUESTIONS

A 2-day-old term baby presents with respiratory distress and feeding intolerance. The patient is noted to cough and develop respiratory distress during feedings. An attempt is made to pass a nasogastric tube for supplemental feeding, but multiple attempts fail to advance the tube beyond a few centimeters. A "babygram" plain film shows a nasogastric tube coiled high in the esophagus and gas in the stomach and bowel (Figure 17.1). The neonatal intensive care team suspects a diagnosis of tracheoesophageal fistula (TEF) and requests a surgical consultation. Additional findings on exam reveal limb anomalies and the presence of a cardiac murmur.

HOW CAN A DIAGNOSIS OF TEF BE MADE IN A NEWBORN?

The surgical team agrees with a diagnosis of TEF and plans for an operative repair. The attending surgeon feels that the presentation is most consistent with a Gross type C TEF.

WHAT TYPE OF TEF IS MOST COMMON?

She would like to consider a minimally invasive approach (i.e., thoracoscopic), but requests a cardiology consult to rule out congenital heart disease. The patient is suspected to have VACTERL association (i.e., association of vertebral anomalies, anal atresia, cardiac defects, tracheoesophageal fistula, renal anomalies, and limb abnormalities).

WHAT IS VACTERL ASSOCIATION?

The cardiologist performs a transthoracic echocardiogram to further delineate cardiac anatomy. The patient requires escalating respiratory support, and the cardiologist voices concern that a cyanotic cardiac lesion may be present. The neonatal intensive care team places a tracheal tube in the patient due to persistent hypoxemia and increased work of breathing. In the meantime, the cardiologist recommends the initiation of a prostaglandin E1 (PGE1) infusion.

WHAT ROLE DOES A PGE1 INFUSION PLAY IN A NEWBORN WITH SUSPECTED CYANOTIC HEART DISEASE?

The echocardiogram is notable for the presence of hypoplastic left heart syndrome (HLHS) with an associated unrestrictive atrial septal defect (ASD) and a patent ductus arteriosus (PDA). Shunting of blood across the PDA is noted to be right to left with complete mixing at the atrial level due to the large ASD. The great vessels are in their normal position; however, the aortic arch is noted to be hypoplastic. Right ventricular function is qualitatively good, but the left ventricle is markedly hypoplastic.

WHAT IMPACT DOES UNCORRECTED CONGENITAL CARDIAC DISEASE HAVE ON THE SURGICAL/ANESTHETIC PLAN?

Despite endotracheal intubation, the patient requires an acute increase in respiratory support and ventilatory pressures. Although oxygenation initially improves, the patient develops worsening hypoxemia and ventilation. The patient's abdomen is found to be more distended and tympanitic to percussion on exam. An abdominal radiograph is obtained with evidence of a pneumoperitoneum and suspected gastric perforation (Figure 17.2).

WHAT ARE THE RISKS OF POSITIVE PRESSURE VENTILATION IN THE SETTING OF A TEF?

The patient's sudden deterioration forces the surgical team to pursue an emergent surgical intervention. Among other preparations for the operating room, the anesthesia team is alerted and requested for urgent consultation for perioperative management of the patient for planned TEF repair and exploratory laparotomy.

WHAT CAN BE DONE ACUTELY TO TREAT GASTRIC INSUFFLATION AND RESPIRATORY DISTRESS DUE TO VENTILATION OF A TEF?

During transport to the operating room, the child's respiratory status deteriorates further, necessitating a needle

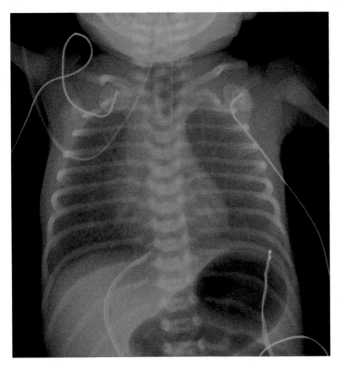

Fig. 17.1 Radiograph showing type C TEF. Note tube coiled in blind pouch esophagus and gas in stomach and bowel from TEF. (Image courtesy of Ramiro J. Hernandez, MD).

decompression of the abdomen. Once in the operating room, the patient is positioned supine, and a laparotomy incision is made. Upon inspection, a gastric perforation is confirmed. The surgical team places an occlusive catheter into the esophagus via the gastric perforation. Ventilation and oxygenation improve after the intervention. A temporary dressing is placed on the abdominal incision, and the patient is positioned for a right thoracotomy. The TEF is ligated, and a primary esophageal anastomosis is performed. The patient is then placed

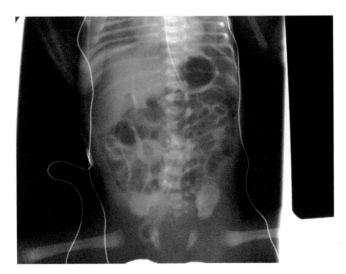

Fig. 17.2 Radiograph showing gastric perforation with free air. Note outline of falciform ligament due to pneumoperitoneum. (Image courtesy of Ramiro J. Hernandez, MD).

supine, and a gastrostomy tube and repair of the gastric perforation are performed.

IS REGIONAL ANALGESIA AN OPTION FOR PATIENTS UNDERGOING NEONATAL TEF REPAIR? IS THIS PATIENT A GOOD CANDIDATE FOR EARLY EXTUBATION IN THE OPERATING ROOM?

The patient is then transported intubated to the intensive care unit. After a prolonged recovery in the intensive care unit, the patient is eventually discharged home.

WHAT ARE THE LONG-TERM OUTCOMES AFTER TEF REPAIR?

Over the next year, the patient is admitted with a series of pneumonias. During the latest admission, the patient's parents describe a several months-long history of chronic cough and occasional wheezing. Upper endoscopy reveals an esophageal stricture with esophageal reflux and likely aspiration. After a series of endoscopic esophageal dilations, the patient's symptoms improve with a marked reduction in medical care in the ensuing years.

DISCUSSION

VACTERL association is a collection of congenital malformations that occur together more frequently than statistically predicted. It is an association rather than a syndrome as there is no unifying causative defect. The association typically requires the presence of at least 3 of the following congenital malformations: vertebral anomalies, anal atresia, cardiac anomalies, TEF, and renal and limb abnormalities (Table 17.1). Estimates of the incidence of VACTERL association place it at approximately 1:10,000 to 1:40,000 of live-born infants.[1]

TRACHEOESOPHAGEAL FISTULA

Tracheoesophageal fistula may exist in several anatomic forms. Despite anatomic variability, several types are more common (Figure 17.3). The most common variant (86%) is esophageal atresia with a blind pouch combined with a distal TEF (Gross type C).[2] The estimated incidence of TEF is 1:2,500 to 1:4,500 live births.[3,4]

DIAGNOSIS

Prenatal diagnosis may be possible in 20%–30% of cases based on the absence of stomach bubble and/or presence of polyhydramnios on ultrasound imaging.[3] Even so, nonspecific ultrasound findings such as polyhydramnios or absent or small stomach bubble only have a positive predictive value of 44%.[5] As a result, the majority of TEF diagnoses occur after birth. Choking and gagging with feeds, copious secretions, and an

Table 17.1 CHARACTERISTICS OF VACTERL ASSOCIATION

FINDING	INCIDENCE	EXAMPLES
Vertebral anomalies	60%–80%	Hemi-vertebrae, fused vertebrae,
Anal atresia	55%–90%	Imperforate anus, anal stenosis
Cardiac anomalies	40%–80%	Range of congenital heart disease from severe to subclinical
Tracheoesophageal fistula	50%–80%	Multiple types possible
Renal anomalies	50%–80%	Renal agenesis, dysplastic or cystic kidneys
Limb anomalies	40%–50%	Radial defects, other limb abnormalities

Source: Solomon BD. VACTERL/VATER association. *Orphanet J Rare Dis.* 2011;6:56.

inability to pass a nasogastric tube beyond a superficial depth suggest a potential TEF. The presence of a TEF in a newborn should also prompt an investigation into other potential associated anomalies.

PATHOPHYSIOLOGY

Care of the newborn with a TEF largely centers on accurate diagnosis of anatomy and prevention of morbidity prior to repair. The anatomic diagnosis is important for proper surgical planning and anticipation of potential complications prior to repair. A Gross type C TEF carries a risk of pulmonary aspiration of pooled secretions from a blind esophageal pouch.

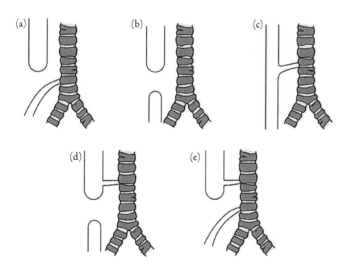

Fig. 17.3 Common types of TEF. Reproduced with permission from Morton NS, Fairgrieve R, Moores A, Wallace E. Anesthesia for the full-term and ex-premature infant. In: Gregory GA, Andropoulos DB, eds. *Gregory's Pediatric Anesthesia.* 5th ed. Oxford: Wiley-Blackwell, 2011:507.

Pooling of secretions can be minimized by continuous suction of secretions via a Replogle tube placed in the esophageal pouch. The patient should be held strictly nil per os to lessen aspiration risk. Intravenous fluid therapy should be initiated to maintain hydration and normoglycemia.

Spontaneous ventilation is ideal for preventing gastric distension in patients with a TEF. Prematurity, congenital heart disease, and/or aspiration may cause respiratory distress in a neonate with a TEF. Positive pressure ventilation may result in significant gas flow through the fistula and the development of gastric distension. Gastric distension may then further compromise the patient's respiratory status due to encroachment on the thoracic domain. In extreme cases, positive pressure ventilation across a TEF can result in gastric perforation. Premature newborns with lung disease may be at higher risk of gastric perforation during positive pressure ventilation due to low lung compliance and preferential ventilation across the fistula.[6]

Newborns with a TEF may require tracheal intubation when diagnosed with lung disease, significant congenital heart disease, or other conditions that may preclude adequate spontaneous ventilation and oxygenation. Positioning of the tracheal tube prior to surgical repair deserves some consideration. Ideally, the tracheal tube should be placed in such a way that the patient may be ventilated with positive pressure without ventilating the fistula and distending the stomach. Excluding the TEF with a tracheal tube can be challenging, particularly if the location and number of fistulas is not known with certainty.

The location of a TEF can vary dramatically. Some may be higher in the trachea, whereas others can be at the level of the carina. Holzki et al.[7] reviewed the bronchoscopic finding of greater than 100 neonates with a diagnosis of TEF. The fistula was noted to be greater than 1 cm above the carina in 67% of cases (Figure 17.4). The fistula was found to be less than 1 cm above the carina in 22% of the patients. The remaining 11% of patients in the cohort had fistulas below the carina. The larger the size of the fistula, the more likely that positive pressure ventilation may result in gastric distension.[8] More distal fistulas increase the likelihood of a tracheal tube sitting above the TEF, or, if beyond the TEF, the tracheal tube may lie in a mainstem bronchus. It is also possible to

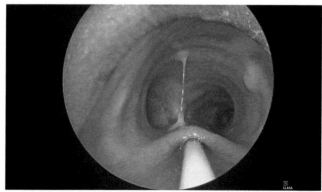

Fig. 17.4 Bronchoscopic view of TEF, catheter in fistula. (Image courtesy of Carlos Munoz-San Julian, MD).

inadvertently intubate the TEF with the tracheal tube, with resulting gastric distension and poor to absent pulmonary ventilation.[9]

TREATMENT

Surgical repair can be approached via both open and minimally invasive techniques. The surgical team may perform a rigid bronchoscopy prior to intubation and incision. Bronchoscopy provides information regarding fistula location, size, and number. It is also possible to attempt isolation of a fistula with a catheter during the bronchoscopy. A well-placed catheter with a balloon can exclude the fistula and allow for positive pressure ventilation without gastric distension.[8] Even if a TEF is not blocked during the bronchoscopy, the location of the fistula(s) can be very useful in planning the optimal position of a tracheal tube prior to surgical ligation of the fistula. The most common operative approach for TEF repair is a right thoracic approach, unless a right aortic arch requires a left-sided approach. Historically, open thoracotomy is the most common approach, but success with thoracoscopic TEF repair has been reported.[10] Open thoracotomy may still be the most expeditious surgical approach but can result in musculoskeletal complications.[10] A thoracoscopic approach may avoid these complications but introduces the physiologic challenges inherent to thoracoscopy in a newborn. These challenges may be greater in the setting of unrepaired congenital heart disease, although reports of success in this patient population do exist.[11,12] Regardless of the surgical plan, the anesthesiology team must be attentive to the challenges of the patient's anatomy, physiology, and impact of surgical technique on the same.

ANESTHETIC CONSIDERATIONS

Induction and airway management

Induction of general anesthesia to facilitate neonatal TEF repair can be approached in a multitude of ways. Knottenbelt et al.[13] performed an audit of anesthetic technique for TEF repair across four hospitals. The authors found two thirds of cases used an inhalational induction with the remaining one third electing an intravenous induction of anesthesia. Neuromuscular blocking agents were administered during induction in one third of cases. The remaining two thirds avoided muscle relaxation and preserved spontaneous ventilation.

Rigid bronchoscopy in the presence of a TEF is an anesthetic challenge. The patient must be deeply anesthetized to allow for airway instrumentation but ideally maintains spontaneous ventilation to avoid gastric distension and to preserve oxygenation during the procedure. Mask induction with a volatile anesthetic may allow preservation of spontaneous ventilation, while additional intravenous anesthetics can be used during bronchoscopy to maintain an adequate depth of anesthesia. In the case of associated esophageal atresia, it is important to continue suction of pooled secretions in the pouch to mitigate aspiration risk.

Many different strategies have been described for optimal tracheal tube placement in the setting of a TEF. If the location of the fistula is known, a tracheal tube with no Murphy eye can be placed at the level of the fistula with the bevel of the tube occluding the fistula orifice. If positioned properly, the tracheal tube would both isolate the TEF and provide a safer means of positive pressure ventilation. In the setting of a distal fistula, some practitioners elect to place the tube in the left mainstem bronchus, assuming a right thoracic approach. This technique can exclude the fistula by ventilating from a more distal location. Mainstem bronchial intubation will result in one-lung ventilation, which may be poorly tolerated. Also, dislodgment of the tube and ventilation or intubation of the TEF is a real possibility. A third strategy involves placing the tracheal tube above the level of the TEF and assessing for fistula ventilation during a careful transition from spontaneous ventilation to positive pressure ventilation. This method is less likely to be useful in cases of large fistulas and in patients with poor lung compliance and need for high airway pressures. Flexible fiberscope guidance can be used as an aid to proper placement of the tracheal tube as well.[4] In cases where isolation of the TEF is not possible and gastric distension results during positive pressure ventilation, an emergent gastrostomy may be necessary. Emergent gastrostomy allows decompression of the stomach, but patients with poor lung compliance may prove difficult to ventilate due to preferential gas flow to the low resistance gastrostomy. Positive pressure ventilation of the TEF can also result in gastric perforation and pneumoperitoneum. Pneumoperitoneum that prevents adequate pulmonary ventilation can be treated with emergent needle decompression. The patient can then be brought to the operating room for exploratory laparotomy followed by TEF ligation.[6]

Analgesia

Analgesia for intraoperative and postoperative surgical pain during TEF repair can be provided by intravenous opioids solely or in combination with regional anesthesia. Neuraxial analgesia has been used successfully in the perioperative management of neonatal TEF. Potential benefits of neuraxial analgesia include avoidance of opioid-related respiratory dysfunction and side effects and the possibility of earlier extubation. Prior to neuraxial interventions, consideration should be given to vertebral anomalies (VACTERL, etc.) and/or coagulation issues that may preclude safe regional analgesia techniques. Epidural catheter placement remains a common regional analgesic technique employed for TEF repair. An epidural catheter can be placed directly into the thoracic epidural space or threaded cephalad from the caudal space. Smaller patients may benefit from a caudally threaded thoracic epidural due to avoidance of direct needle entry proximate to the spinal cord. Caudal catheters threading can result in variability in tip location. Confirmation of tip location allows adjustment of misplaced catheters for optimal results.[14] In addition to epidurogram-based confirmation, additional techniques include the use of stimulating catheters, fluoroscopic guidance, and ultrasound imaging.[15]

Multiple medications can be used for epidural analgesic infusions. In neonatal patients, it is important to be attentive to the possibility of local anesthetic toxicity. Some centers prefer to use chloroprocaine rather than bupivacaine for its more predictable toxicity profile in patients with immature metabolism of bupivacaine. Continuous chloroprocaine epidural infusion appears to be both safe and effective in neonatal patients.[16]

HYPOPLASTIC LEFT HEART SYNDROME

Pathophysiology

Hypoplastic left heart syndrome is a severe form of congenital heart disease. A diagnosis of HLHS includes a hypoplastic aortic arch and left ventricle. A hypoplastic left ventricle cannot effectively contribute to cardiac output given its small size and volume. A hypoplastic aortic arch further limits left ventricular outflow, and left-sided cardiac valves are often stenotic or atretic as well. Patients with HLHS are dependent on their right ventricle for systemic cardiac output; hence, the label "single ventricle" when describing the physiology of patients with HLHS.

Systemic blood flow (i.e., oxygenated blood to the arterial system) does not circulate normally in unrepaired HLHS patients. The majority of blood returning to the heart from the venous system is pumped by the right ventricle to the pulmonary system via the pulmonary artery. The pulmonary system allows for oxygenation of the blood during its transit to the pulmonary veins and subsequently to the left atrium. Newborns with HLHS must have mixing of their deoxygenated and oxygenated blood to provide sufficient oxygenation and perfusion systemically. Systemic cardiac output (oxygenated blood to the arterial side) is dependent on right ventricular output due to a hypoplastic left ventricle and aorta and stenotic or atretic left side cardiac valves. Intracardiac mixing of deoxygenated blood with oxygenated blood returning to left atrium allows for partially oxygenated blood in the systemic right ventricle. This is important in the setting of a PDA, which may be the only path for right ventricular output to the arterial side of the circulation. In simpler terms, the "red" blood and "blue" blood mix to allow for "purple" blood to provide systemic perfusion across a PDA to the rest of the arterial system.

Neonatal management of HLHS

Initial management of the neonate with HLHS requires a thorough understanding of the patient's cardiac anatomy. Neonates with HLHS, who do not have a lesion that allows for total "mixing" of systemic and venous circulations, suffer from poor perfusion with resultant lactic acidosis and hypotension. A patent foramen ovale allows mixing of oxygenated and deoxygenated blood, but it may be insufficient to maintain adequate oxygenation of mixed blood pumped by the right ventricle to both the pulmonary and systemic circulations. In such cases, it is possible to enlarge the patent foramen ovale via a catheter-based balloon atrial septostomy. This can be done at the bedside with echocardiographic guidance. Maintenance of a PDA with a PGE1 infusion is critical to prevent PDA closure and the loss of systemic perfusion from the single right ventricle.

STAGE I NORWOOD PROCEDURE

Although a wide range of congenital heart defects may co-exist with a TEF, this discussion will focus on the example of HLHS. The most common initial palliative surgery for HLHS is the stage I Norwood operation. The stage I Norwood operation is designed to provide stable systemic blood flow via the construction of a neo-aorta using the native pulmonary artery and also to provide stable pulmonary blood flow via a systemic to pulmonary shunt (typically a Blalock-Taussig shunt). Additionally, an atrial septectomy and PDA ligation are performed as well. Neonatal conditions such as TEF often need to be addressed prior to any palliative cardiac surgery.

Prior to the stage I Norwood procedure, an infant with HLHS is often dependent on a PDA for systemic perfusion. The shunt across a PDA can be affected by pulmonary vascular resistance (PVR) and systemic vascular resistance (SVR). If PVR increases, then greater blood flow will be diverted from the single ventricle to the systemic circulation (right-to-left shunt). As a result, decreased pulmonary blood flow may result in hypoxemia. If SVR becomes greater than PVR, then blood may preferentially enter the pulmonary rather than the systemic system. Oxygen saturation may be higher due to increased pulmonary perfusion, but hypotension, acidosis, and poor perfusion are likely due to decreased systemic perfusion. The goal in HLHS patients is to optimize the balance between pulmonary and systemic circulations that allows for adequate oxygenation while maintaining adequate systemic perfusion.

QP:QS

The balance between systemic and pulmonary circulations can be described as a ratio of pulmonary blood flow (Q_P) to systemic blood flow (Q_S). Q_P:Q_S = 1 describes a totally balanced circulation, whereas a Q_P:Q_S >1 favors pulmonary over systemic blood flow, and Q_P:Q_S <1 describes the converse. Although imperfect, arterial oxygen saturation values may be indicative of a patient's Q_P:Q_S. An oxygen saturation of 90% or greater may be indicative of excessive pulmonary circulation (Q_P:Q_S >1), whereas an oxygen saturation lower than 70% may indicate a Q_P:Q_S<1. In general, newborns with HLHS have a goal oxygen saturation of approximately 80%. Room air is the ideal respiratory gas to provide a balanced Q_P:Q_S, but an increased inspired oxygen concentration may be necessary when oxygen saturations remain low despite optimization of other factors.

Beyond the balancing of pulmonary and systemic circulations, patients with HLHS rely on a single ventricle to do all of the "volume-work" done by 2 ventricles in a normal heart. It may be necessary to augment cardiac contractility for HLHS patients with inotropes in the perioperative period.

Optimizing Q_p:Q_s during TEF repair in a patient with unpalliated HLHS can be very challenging. Some surgical teams perform a rigid bronchoscopy prior to TEF repair. Rigid bronchoscopy often leads to periods of hypoventilation, noxious/painful stimuli, hypoxemia, and hypothermia during exposure. Hypercarbia, hypoxemia, pain, cold, and acidosis are all known to raise PVR. In the setting of HLHS, increased PVR relative to SVR (Q_p:Q_s <1) can result in poor pulmonary perfusion and hypoxemia, resulting in an even greater elevation of PVR. Efforts to reduce PVR such as an increased inspired oxygen concentration and hypocarbia can lead to a Q_p:Q_s >1 with hypotension and poor perfusion. The quest for a balanced circulation is a dynamic one. The anesthesia team must be attentive to changes in physiology based on surgical, environmental, and patient factors, while trying to maintain balanced perfusion.

These considerations continue in the setting of one-lung ventilation for TEF ligation. In both open and thoracoscopic approaches, operative lung collapse will increase PVR and complicate ventilation. Thoracoscopic approaches provide the additional challenges of insufflated carbon dioxide and increased intrathoracic pressure. Hypercarbia and decreased venous return should be anticipated prior to insufflation of the chest. The surgeon should take care to minimize insufflation pressure and minimize operative time as much as possible. Despite these challenges, the presence of severe congenital heart disease is not a contraindication to a thoracoscopic approach.[11,12]

In addition to balancing Q_p:Q_s, newborns with HLHS require attention to their intraoperative circulatory volume status. Hypovolemia in the setting of HLHS may be poorly tolerated as cardiac output falls with decreased venous return. Fluid resuscitation may be needed, particularly if the patient is treated with diuretics preoperatively. The early institution of inotropic agents such as dopamine may be useful in periods of decreased cardiac output due to surgical and anesthetic factors.

Adequate oxygenation in HLHS patients is dependent on sufficient hemoglobin oxygen carrying capacity. Even mild blood loss may lower hematocrit sufficiently to cause decreased oxygenation in HLHS patients. Transfusion to maintain a hematocrit above 40% can provide optimal oxygenation with balanced circulation physiology. Over-transfusion resulting in a very high hematocrit increases the risk of red blood cell sludging, thrombosis, and cerebrovascular events.[17] Transfusion thresholds should be adjusted accordingly for HLHS patients to maintain adequate carrying capacity and oxygen saturation.

LONG-TERM OUTCOMES AFTER TEF REPAIR

Survival rates for patients with TEF and esophageal atresia have improved with advances in neonatal, anesthetic, and surgical care. An analysis by Spitz et al.[18] in 1994 resulted in a recommendation for a 3-group risk stratification for esophageal atresia. Group 1 (97% survival) was designated for patients with birth weight greater than or equal to 1,500 grams without major cardiac disease. Group 2 (59% survival) included patients with birth weight less than 1,500 grams, or major cardiac disease. Group 3 (22% survival) included patients with a birth weight less than 1,500 grams and major cardiac disease. The authors concluded that the presence of low birth weight and major cardiac disease predicted the worst outcome for children with esophageal atresia. Subsequent work from Diaz et al.[19] also found low birth weight (<1,500 grams) and an associated cardiac lesion increased the risk of mortality in infants undergoing TEF repair. Their retrospective review also identified the presence of a ductal-dependent cardiac lesion to even further increase the risk of mortality in this patient population. In 2014, Malakounides et al.[20] published their analysis of esophageal atresia outcomes over a 10-year period. The authors used Spitz's[18] 3-group predictive model but found that the survival outcome of Group 2 (low birth weight or major cardiac disease, but not both) had improved relative to the earlier study (82% vs. 59%).[20] Although lower birth weight may be less of an issue for survival than in the past, major cardiac disease remains a threat to survival in this patient population.

Beyond survival, patients can have long-term complications after TEF repair. Recurrent fistulas may occur in an estimated 2.7%–10%.[3] Recurrent fistulas can result in recurrent aspiration pneumonia and the need for additional surgical interventions.

Esophageal strictures may develop after primary esophageal anastomosis for esophageal atresia. Patients may present with dysphagia and gastroesophageal reflux disease. Esophageal strictures may require repeated endoscopies with dilation and/or additional surgical intervention. Tracheomalacia may also be an issue over time.[3,21] Despite improved survival with advances in care, many patients with TEF and esophageal atresia require long-term surveillance and therapy for complications.

MULTIPLE CHOICE QUESTIONS

1. Which of the following clusters of findings are **MOST** likely consistent with VACTERL association?

   A. coloboma, horseshoe kidney, HLHS
   B. imperforate anus, ASD, cystic kidneys
   C. macroglossia, butterfly vertebrae, ventricular septal defect
   D. TEF, thumb aplasia, patent foramen ovale

Answer: B
VACTERL association is not a syndrome but rather a cluster of findings that occur together in a greater frequency than expected by chance. VACTERL association includes vertebral anomalies, anal atresia, cardiac defects, tracheoesophageal fistula, renal anomalies, and limb abnormalities. All of these anomalies are not needed for VACTERL association. Typically, at least 3 characteristic anomalies must be present. Answer B, contains the requisite 3 findings of anal atresia,

cardiac defect, and a renal anomaly. The other choices contain at most 2 of the needed three criteria and therefore are less likely to represent a VACTERL association.

2. Which of the following neonatal characteristics is **MOST** likely to *increase* the risk of mortality in TEF repair?

    A. bronchopulmonary dysplasia
    B. craniofacial abnormality with micrognathia
    C. ductal dependent cyanotic heart lesion
    D. prematurity with a birth weight of 1,700 grams

Answer: C

Although mortality has decreased for newborns with TEF due to advances in care, severe congenital heart disease remains an important risk factor for perioperative mortality. Ductal dependent cardiac lesions are likely to be more severe forms of congenital cardiac disease. Low birth weight has also been shown to be a risk factor, but only for birth weights <1,500 grams. Answer D is greater than 1,500 grams, and answers A and B may complicate management but lack evidence of an increased perioperative mortality for TEF repair.

3. A newborn in no distress is diagnosed with a type C TEF after choking and coughing after feeds. The **BEST** next step is to

    A. order nil per os and place a Replogle tube on suction.
    B. order thickened feeds to prevent aspiration.
    C. pass a nasogastric tube into the stomach to allow feeds.
    D. place a tracheal tube to protect the airway.

Answer: A

A type C TEF consists of esophageal atresia with a TEF to the distal esophagus. The patient in question is at risk of aspiration during feeds and from pooled secretions in the blind esophageal pouch. The best next step is to prohibit oral intake and place a Replogle tube in the esophageal pouch to suction pooled secretions continuously. It is not possible to bypass the esophageal atresia with an orogastric or nasogastric tube, so answer C is incorrect. Similarly, thickened feeds (answer B) is an inappropriate option as aspiration is not a matter of swallowing mechanics but rather the lack of a passage to the stomach from the oropharynx. Placement of a tracheal tube (answer D) may be necessary in cases of respiratory distress and poor lung function but is not ideal given the high likelihood of gastric distension with ventilation of the fistula.

4. Which of the following techniques is **MOST** likely to prevent ventilation of the TEF in a neonate undergoing a right thoracotomy for TEF repair?

    A. bronchial blocker on the operative side
    B. neuromuscular blockade with controlled bag mask ventilation
    C. placement of a gastrostomy tube
    D. tracheal tube with occlusive bevel at the site of the fistula

Answer: D

Isolation of a TEF with a tracheal tube is possible in cases where the fistula is located above the carina. Ideally, a tracheal tube without a Murphy eye can be used to occlude the fistula while still ventilating both lungs. Answer A, placing a bronchial blocker on the operative side, would do nothing to prevent the ventilation of the majority of TEFs that occur above the mainstem bronchi. Answer B would require positive pressure ventilation and increase the risk of ventilation via the fistula. Answer C, the placement of a gastrostomy tube, would allow venting of gastric distension but would not decrease and might even increase ventilation across a TEF.

5. A newborn with HLHS and an oxygen saturation of 98% **MOST** likely indicates a(n)

    A. increased blood flow across a PDA.
    B. decreased mixing of blood across an ASD.
    C. $Q_p:Q_s >1$.
    D. $Q_p:Q_s <1$.

Answer: C

An oxygen saturation of 98% in a patient with HLHS likely indicates excessive pulmonary blood flow at the expense of systemic blood flow. This could be described as a $Q_p:Q_s >1$ or more pulmonary than systemic blood flow. The converse, answer D, would indicate decreased pulmonary blood flow relative to systemic blood flow with likely hypoxemia. Answer A in the setting of HLHS would lead to greater systemic blood flow and likely hypoxemia, not a saturation of 98%. Answer B, decreased mixing of blood across the atria, is also incorrect as it would also tend to result in hypoxemia.

6. A newborn is transferred on day of life 3 from an outside hospital on no medications with hypotension, acidosis, and low urine output and a new diagnosis of HLHS. The **MOST** likely etiology of the patient's decompensation is

    A. adrenal insufficiency with a lack of stress response.
    B. closure of the ductus arteriosus.
    C. failure to administer indomethacin.
    D. hypovolemia due to inadequate resuscitation.

Answer: B

Newborns with HLHS are often dependent on a PDA for systemic blood flow from the single right ventricle. The closure of the PDA that occurs physiologically in the neonatal period threatens systemic perfusion in these patients. Prostaglandin E1 infusion can be used to maintain a PDA until surgical palliation can be accomplished. The patient in this question is likely in shock due to the closure of the ductus arteriosus. Answer A, adrenal insufficiency, is not the most likely etiology of the patient's shock. Answer C, failure to give indomethacin, is incorrect as indomethacin is often administered in an effort to close a PDA in patients who do not benefit from its persistence. Answer D, hypovolemia, is not the most likely etiology of the patients shock.

7. The stage I Norwood procedure for HLHS typically includes

    a. ASD closure.
    b. Blalock-Taussig shunt.
    c. Glenn shunt.
    d. repair of the mitral valve.

Answer: B

The stage I Norwood procedure consists of several steps including, atrial septectomy, creation of a neo-aorta, and a systemic to pulmonary shunt such as a Blalock-Taussig shunt. Answer A, closure of the ASD, is incorrect as it goes contrary to the goal of the procedure in creating complete mixing and a single ventricle system. Answer C, Glenn shunt, is incorrect as this is a later stage palliation (stage II) of the Norwood procedure. It is not applicable to neonates with HLHS. Answer D, repair of the mitral valve, is incorrect as the mitral valve is often atretic or stenotic and attached to a nonfunctional hypoplastic left ventricle. Repair of the mitral valve, if possible, would not provide any benefit in the typical HLHS newborn.

QUESTIONS AND ANSWERS

This chapter has accompanying questions and answers which are available to subscribers as part of the Oxford eLearning platform. To access the questions, go to ✅ http://oxfordmedicine. com/pediatricanesthesiaPBL

REFERENCES

1. Solomon BD. VACTERL/VATER association. *Orphanet J Rare Dis.* 2011;6:56.
2. Ho AMH, Dion JM, Wong JCP. Airway and ventilatory management options in congenital tracheoesophageal fistula repair. *J Cardiothorac Vasc Anesth.* 2016;30(2):515–520.
3. Hunt RW, Perkins EJ, King S. Peri-operative management of neonates with oesophageal atresia and trachea-oesophageal fistula. *Paediatr Respir Rev.* 2016;19:3–9.
4. Broemling N, Campbell F. Anesthetic management of congenital tracheoesophageal fistula. *Pediatr Anesth.* 2011;21:1092–1099.
5. Houben CH, Curry JI. Current status of prenatal diagnosis, operative management and outcome of esophageal atresia/trachea-esophageal fistula. *Prenat Diagn.* 2008;28:667–675.
6. Maoate K, Myers NA, Beasley SW. Gastric perforation in infants with oesophageal atresia and distal trachea-oesophageal fistula. *Pediatr Surg Int.* 1999;15:24–27.
7. Holzki J. Bronchoscopic findings and treatment in congenital trachea-oesophageal fistula. *Paediatr Anaesth.* 1992;2:297–303.
8. Andropoulos DB, Rowe RW, Betts JM. Anaesthetic and surgical airway management during trachea-oesophageal fistula repair. *Pediatr Anesth.* 1998;8:313–319.
9. Alabbad SI, Shaw K, Puligandla PS, Carranza R, Bernard C, Laberge J. The pitfalls of endotracheal intubation beyond the fistula in babies with type C esophageal atresia. *Semin Pediatr Surg.* 2009;18:116–118.
10. Holcomb III GW, Rothenberg SS, Klaas M, et al. Thoracoscopic repair of esophageal atresia and tracheoesophageal fistula: a multi-institutional analysis. *Ann Surg.* 2005;242(3):422–428.
11. Mariano ER, Chu LF, Albanese CT, Ramamoorthy C. Successful thoracoscopic repair of esophageal atresia with tracheoesophageal fistula in a newborn with single ventricle physiology. *Anesth Analg.* 2005;101:1000–1002.
12. Rice-Townsend S, Ramamoorthy C, Dutta S. Thoracoscopic repair of a type D esophageal atresia in a newborn with complex congenital heart disease. *J Pediatr Surg.* 2007;42:1616–1619.
13. Knottenbelt G, Costi D, Stephens P, Beringer R, Davidson A. An audit of anesthetic management and complications of trachea-esophageal fistula and esophageal atresia repair. *Pediatr Anesth.* 2012;22:268–274.
14. Valairucha S, Seefelder C, Houck CS. Thoracic epidural catheters placed by the caudal route in infants: the importance of radiographic confirmation. *Paediatr Anaesth.* 2002;12:424–428.
15. Taenzer AH, Cantwell CV, Kovarik WD. Experience with 724 epidurograms for epidural catheter placement in pediatric anesthesia. *Reg Anesth Pain Med.* 2010;35(5):432–435.
16. Venziano G, Lliev P, Tripi J, et al. Continuous chloroprocaine infusion for thoracic and caudal epidurals as a postoperative analgesia modality in neonates, infants, and children. *Pediatr Anesth.* 2016;26:84–91.
17. Zabala LM, Guzzetta NA. Cyanotic congenital heart disease (CCHD): focus on hypoxemia, secondary erythrocytosis, and coagulation alterations. *Pediatr Anesth.* 2015;25:981–989.
18. Spitz L, Kiely EM, Morecroft JA, Drake DP. Oesophageal atresia: at-risk groups for the 1990s. *J Pediatr Surg.* 1994;29(6):723–725.
19. Diaz LK, Akpek EA, Dinavahi R, Andropoulos DB. Tracheoesophageal fistula and associated congenital heart disease: implication for anesthetic management and survival. *Pediatr Anesth.* 2005;15:862–869.
20. Malakounides G, Lyon P, Cross K, et al. Esophageal atresia: improved outcome in high-risk groups revisited. *Eur J Pediatr Surg.* 2016;26:227–231.
21. Kovesi T, Rubin S. Long-term complications of congenital esophageal atresia and/or tracheoesophageal fistula. *Chest.* 2004;126:915–925.

18.

PECTUS EXCAVATUM

Priti G. Dalal and Meghan Whitley

STEM CASE AND KEY QUESTIONS

A 14-year-old 55 kg, 170 cm male patient presents for pectus excavatum repair. He is otherwise healthy. He has some shortness of breath when he does vigorous exercise. There is a paternal family history of Marfan syndrome.

WHAT IS PECTUS EXCAVATUM? WHAT IS
THE ETIOLOGY OF PECTUS EXCAVATUM?
WHAT SYNDROMES MAY BE ASSOCIATED
WITH PECTUS EXCAVATUM? WHAT SURGICAL
PROCEDURES MAY BE USED FOR CORRECTION
OF THIS DEFORMITY?

He is on no medications other than acetaminophen and ibuprofen for chest pain, as needed. His vital signs are within normal limits. On exam, the patient is thin and tall with an obvious deformity of the anterior chest wall. The heart sounds are displaced.

ARE THERE ANY SPECIAL TESTS THAT ARE
INDICATED PREOPERATIVELY? DO YOU NEED
ANY ADDITIONAL INFORMATION REGARDING
THIS PATIENT? WOULD YOU CONSIDER A
CHEST X-RAY OR COMPUTED TOMOGRAPHY
(CT) SCAN? IS ONE MORE BENEFICIAL THAN
THE OTHER?

The patient's chest X-ray reveals a Haller index of 4.0. His pulmonary function testing reveals an obstructive pattern. Echocardiography reveals mild mitral valve prolapse and normal systolic function of the left ventricle with minimal right ventricular compression.

WHAT IS THE HALLER INDEX? WHAT ARE
THE CARDIOPULMONARY IMPLICATIONS
OF PECTUS EXCAVATUM? SHOULD
PREOPERATIVE PULMONARY FUNCTION TESTS
(PFTS) BE ROUTINELY PERFORMED IN THESE
PATIENTS? DO YOU NEED ANY OTHER
LAB TESTS?

He is scheduled for a Nuss procedure with thoracoscopic assistance. He has a reassuring airway exam and a negative anesthetic history. The surgeon states he will likely require repair using 2 bars given the size of his deformity.

THE PARENTS AND CHILD ARE VERY
CONCERNED ABOUT PERIOPERATIVE
ANALGESIA. WHAT IS YOUR ANALGESIC
MANAGEMENT PLAN? WOULD
AN EPIDURAL BE A GOOD OPTION? IF SO,
AT WHAT THORACIC LEVEL? WHAT ARE
THE COMPLICATIONS OF NEURAXIAL
TECHNIQUES?

There are no contraindications to neuraxial techniques. A thoracic epidural is placed preoperatively with sedation. The patient tolerates the procedure well. The epidural is tested and covers the T4–T8 dermatomes, and an infusion of 0.2% ropivacaine is commenced prior to surgical incision.

WHAT ARE THE INDICATIONS FOR PECTUS
EXCAVATUM REPAIR? WHAT ARE
THE DIFFERENCES WITH AN OPEN VERSUS
MINIMALLY INVASIVE APPROACH?

The patient is transported to the operating room. Standard monitoring is applied. The patient is induced with propofol, fentanyl, and rocuronium. After uneventful tracheal intubation, the surgery commences.

WHAT IS YOUR PLAN FOR ANESTHETIC
MANAGEMENT? DO YOU HAVE ANY
CONCERNS REGARDING POSITIONING
INTRAOPERATIVELY? DOES THE CASE
REQUIRE ONE-LUNG VENTILATION? WHAT
ARE THE POTENTIAL INTRAOPERATIVE
SURGICAL COMPLICATIONS?

The surgery is uneventful. The patient is administered acetaminophen, fentanyl, and morphine intravenously in addition to the continuous epidural infusion of local anesthetic intraoperatively. Ondansetron is administered as antiemetic prophylaxis. The patient is awakened and transported to postanesthesia care unit. Upon arrival, the patient's heart rate is 140 bpm, and rapid shallow breathing is noted. His pain score is 10/10 based on the numeric rating scale.

WHAT IS YOUR PLAN FOR POSTOPERATIVE PAIN MANAGEMENT? WHAT POTENTIAL ANALGESIA TECHNIQUES CAN BE UTILIZED? HOW DOES NEURAXIAL ANALGESIA COMPARE WITH PATIENT-CONTROLLED ANALGESIA (PCA)?

The sensory level of the epidural is checked and found to be at level T10 dermatome bilaterally. A bolus of ropivicaine 0.2% is administered, and the epidural infusion rate is increased. Intravenous opioid PCA is commenced to supplement the epidural.

WHAT ARE THE POSSIBLE POSTOPERATIVE COMPLICATIONS? ARE THERE ANY POSITIONING CONCERNS THAT YOU HAVE IN THE POSTOPERATIVE PERIOD? HOW WILL YOU PREPARE TO TRANSITION THIS PATIENT'S PAIN MEDICATIONS AS HIS HOSPITAL COURSE PROGRESSES?

His postoperative chest X-ray reveals small bilateral pneumothoraces. He denies any symptoms of shortness of breath and is maintaining saturations >94% on room air. The patient is admitted to the floor. He is discharged home after 5 days, once his pain is adequately controlled on oral pain medications.

DISCUSSION

ETIOLOGY AND PATHOGENESIS

Pectus excavatum is the most common congenital chest wall abnormality and is characterized by a funnel-shaped depression of the chest wall[1] (Figure 18.1). Pectus carinatum (pigeon chest) is a chest wall deformity, where the anterior chest wall protrudes outwards. Pectus excavatum accounts for 90% of all chest deformities, followed by 5% for pectus carinatum.[2] Pectus excavatum has an incidence of 1:300 births, with a male prevalence commonly cited as 4:1 or higher.[2]

The exact cause of these deformities is unknown. There is association of pectus excavatum with connective tissue disorders, such as Marfan syndrome and Ehlers-Danlos syndrome, perhaps due to a sternocostal cartilage defect.[1] There also appears to be a dominant inheritance pattern as the deformity may be present in multiple generations in 33%–42% of patients.[1,3]

While the majority of cases are congenital and not associated with a syndrome, some syndromes may have pectus excavatum as a feature.[4] The most common associated syndromes include Marfan syndrome, Noonan syndrome, and Ehlers-Danlos syndrome. Other syndromes noted in the literature include Poland syndrome, Rett syndrome, Turner syndrome, Down syndrome, Osteogenesis imperfecta, homocysteinuria, and camptodactyly.[3] There appears to be an association with decreased bone density and pectus excavatum in Rett syndrome. Patients with Marfan syndrome characteristically have an asymmetric chest wall defect, while patients with Noonan syndrome have a combined defect that is both

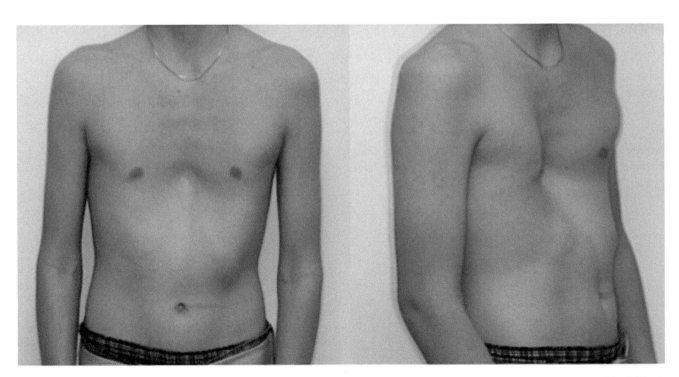

Fig. 18.1 Child with pectus excavatum deformity. (Image courtesy Dr. Kerry Fagelman, MD, Division of Pediatric Surgery, Penn State Health Children's Hospital, Hershey).

a carinatum superiorly and excavatum inferiorly.[1] There is also an association with congenital heart disease (2%), scoliosis (15%–20%), as well as King-Denborough syndrome and spinal muscular atrophy.[3,5,6]

Pectus excavatum is not necessarily a congenital deformity. Patients who underwent congenital diaphragmatic hernia repairs and children with significant upper airway obstruction are at risk for chest wall abnormalities requiring repair[3] due to a combination of malleable chest wall, significant negative intrathoracic pressure requirements, and intercostal muscle use[2].

RETT SYNDROME

Rett syndrome is a progressive neurodevelopmental disorder that occurs almost exclusively in females. The overall incidence is 1 per 10,000. It is linked to a mutation of the MECP2 gene on the X chromosome in the classic variant.[7] However, more than 90% of the cases are sporadic. Development is usually normal for the first 6–18 months of life. This is followed by rapid progressive loss of acquired cognitive, verbal, and motor skills and severe developmental delay. Seizures are a prominent feature and may range from well controlled to intractable.[7] There are stereotyped hand movements with tortuous hand wringing and other automatic hand movements. There is associated weight loss, decreased bone density, osteopenia, and scoliosis with associated deformities of chest, such as pectus excavatum. Respiratory abnormalities occur in a cyclical pattern in the form of hyperventilation followed by hypoventilation and apnea. Cardiac abnormalities include tachycardia, sinus bradycardia, and prolonged corrected QT interval.[7] Associated conditions include spasticity, ataxia, and autonomic dysfunction. These patients may present for repair of scoliosis or other orthopedic procedures. Anesthesia for a patient with Rett syndrome may be challenging.[8] Anesthesia-related problems include hypothermia, gastroesophageal reflux, respiratory abnormalities, risk of apnea, and decreased sensitivity to pain.[8]

CLINICAL MANIFESTATIONS OF PECTUS EXCAVATUM

Pectus excavatum is typically noted at birth but progresses with age and is particularly noticeable at puberty.[1] The characteristic feature is a caved-in or funnel appearance of the chest. The symptoms may range from a vague pain in the chest or back to decreased functional capacity. It is commonly associated with negative body image. It can be associated with psychological disturbances in as many as 75% of children age 11 and older.[3] Many patients may display the classical pectus posture of slumped shoulders, kyphosis, and a large abdomen.[5]

The resting cardiac output may be normal. However, during exercise, there may be a decrease in cardiac output due to the restrictive effect of the chest wall deformity and compression by the sternum. There may be a significant decrease in the cardiac output in the upright versus the supine position (up to 40%) and an inability to increase cardiac output with increasing exercise demands.[9] Patients

with untreated pectus excavatum tend to have lower functional capacity secondary to these reasons and subsequent deconditioning.[10]

DIAGNOSIS AND IMAGING STUDIES

Imaging is utilized to grade the severity of the defect. The Haller index divides the transverse diameter by the most narrow anteroposterior diameter of the chest. A normal Haller index is 2.5.[11] A value >2.5 is considered abnormal, and 3.25 is considered severe enough to warrant surgery. The Haller index can be measured using a CT scan or a two view chest radiograph with strong correlation between the 2 techniques[12] (Figure 18.2). While some recommend chest radiography as the preferred method given its reliable data and lower radiation risk, CT scans also show the degree of mediastinal rotation, cardiopulmonary compression, thoracic asymmetry, or calcification from prior operations. [6,12,13] Severity of the depth of pectus excavatum has also been described using the obstetrical caliper.[14]

Echocardiography is useful in assessing cardiac function in symptomatic patients. Although cardiac compression may occur in the case of severe deformities, routine echocardiography is not indicated unless the patient has cardiac symptoms, such as irregular heart rate, palpitations, or a murmur noted on exam. If the patient has suspected Marfan syndrome, echocardiography should be performed to rule out aortic root dilatation. Mitral valve prolapse can be found in 20% of patients with pectus excavatum. The suspected cause is secondary to cardiac compression and may resolve postoperatively as the cardiac compression is reversed in 50% of patients.[3]

PFTs are useful in determining the severity of the pectus excavatum deformity. The majority of the patients with pectus excavatum deformity demonstrate low lung volumes with an obstructive pattern, while a small percentage demonstrate a restrictive pattern. Further, most patients demonstrate an elevated residual volume, suggesting air trapping and a corresponding decrease in functional residual capacity.[5] A meta-analysis comparing the pulmonary functional recovery after

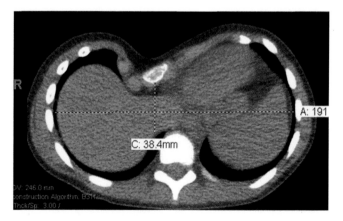

Fig. 18.2 Measurement of the Haller Index. In this example, Haller index = HI = 191/38.4 = 4.97. (Image courtesy of Dr. Kerry Fagelman, MD, Division of Pediatric Surgery, Penn State Health Children's Hospital, Hershey).

Nuss and Ravitch procedures reported some improvements in pulmonary function testing within 1 year with both procedures[16]; however, the Nuss procedure was associated with greater improvements in pulmonary function after bar removal.[16] Another study demonstrated that patients with asymmetric pectus excavatum deformities had lower preoperative total lung capacity, vital capacity, and inspiratory capacity compared to the symmetric subtype. Further reduction in PFT values 4–6 months after the Nuss procedure were also noted in the asymmetric subtype group, suggesting that the smaller hemithorax may not fully compensate for the reduction of the larger hemithorax.[17]

SURGICAL MANAGEMENT

Conservative management has very little role to play in pectus excavatum deformities. In case of mild deformity, deep breathing exercises, posture exercises programs, and the Vacuum Bell may be offered.[18,19] The 2 surgical techniques that have classically been described are the Ravitch and Nuss procedures. The goal of either surgical procedure is to correct the deformity, alleviate the cardiopulmonary symptoms, and improve psychological symptoms by creating cosmetic improvement.

The indications for surgery[14,18] to correct pectus excavatum deformities include:

1. Cardiorespiratory symptoms, including decreased exercise tolerance

2. Pain

3. Rapid progression of the deformity

4. Psychological issues related to body image

5. Haller index >3.25

6. Abnormal PFTs—low forced vital capacity, low forced expiratory volume at 1 second (FEV_1)

7. Compression of the right atrium or right ventricle on the echocardiogram

The Ravitch procedure was described originally in 1949 by Ravitch.[20] Several modifications of this technique have also been described. The procedure entails an anterior submammary chest wall exposure with creation of muscle and skin flaps. It involves extensive resection of the affected rib cartilages and a sternal osteotomy. A modification involving placement of a bar at the lower end of the sternum to prevent recurrence was later described.[21] While the Ravitch procedure was effective in correcting the defect, there was concern about "acquired asphyxiating chondrodystrophy" developing due to rigid, bony scar tissue replacing pliable cartilage and leading to restrictive lung disease.[6] The Ravitch procedure is mainly used for complex pectus excavatum repairs and all pectus carinatum repairs.

The Nuss procedure[13] was described by Dr. Donald Nuss in the 1980s to alleviate the concerns regarding costochondral and sternal resection and offer a minimally invasive alternative. The rationale is that, just as a "barrel chest" occurs in response to chronic obstructive pulmonary disease, similarly, remodeling could occur with internal bracing of the deformity with a bar. With the Nuss procedure, 1 or 2 convex bars (Figure 18.3) are placed posterior to the sternum and anterior to the pericardium through lateral thoracic incisions (Figure 18.4) to provide immediate and continuous support to anteriorly displace the sternum and allow remodeling.[13] The ideal age for the procedure is 7–12 years of age, as the chest wall is malleable, stabilization of the bar is easier, and the child is mature enough to understand post-operative instructions and precautions. The bars are subsequently removed after 2–4 years.[3]

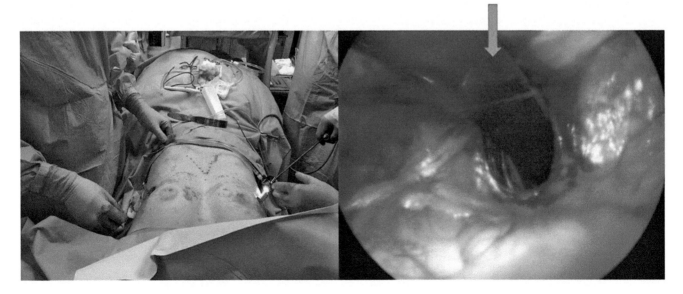

Fig. 18.3 Pectus bar and thoracoscopic view of the pectus excavatum repair (Image courtesy of Dr. Kerry Fagelman, MD, Division of Pediatric Surgery, Penn State Health Children's Hospital, Hershey).

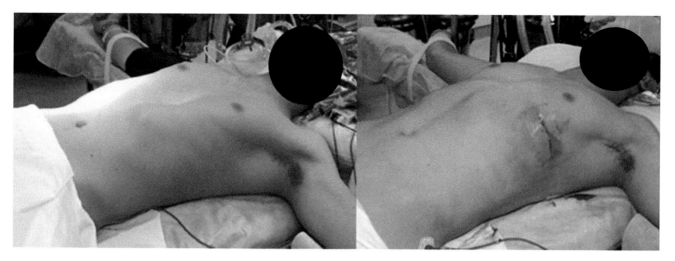

Fig. 18.4 Pre and postoperative appearance of the chest following thoracoscopic placement of pectus bar (Nuss procedure) (Image courtesy of Dr. Kerry Fagelman, MD, Division of Pediatric Surgery, Penn State Health Children's Hospital, Hershey).

SURGICAL COMPLICATIONS

The overall surgical complications include immediate and early complications: pneumothorax, suture site infection, pleural effusion, pericarditis, cardiac tamponade, hemothorax, trauma to mediastinal structures, and cardiac perforation.[22] Delayed complications for the Nuss procedure include sternal erosion, pneumomediastinum, bar displacement, bar over-correction, bar allergy, and recurrence.[22] Use of bar stabilizers, preventing turning motions immediately postoperatively, and performing surgery on older patients have decreased the occurrence of bar related complications.

A meta-analysis comparing the complications of the Ravitch and Nuss procedures reported that while the Ravitch procedure was associated with a longer operative time, the Nuss procedure was associated with a higher rate of reoperation for bar migration or deformity as well as a higher risk of pneumothorax and hemothorax.[23] Patients, who underwent a Nuss procedure, described less postoperative discomfort or concern regarding their appearance. There was no difference in length of stay, time to ambulation, or need for blood transfusion between the two surgical procedures, despite one being open and the other minimally invasive. A recent meta-analysis also revealed no difference in complication rate with both these procedures in pediatric patients, although in adults the Ravitch procedure resulted in fewer complication.[24]

PNEUMOTHORAX

Pneumothorax may occur in up to 59% of the patients, who have a minimally invasive repair of pectus excavatum.[22,25] The mechanism of pneumothorax is primarily due to manipulation of the interpleural space during surgical repair with the scope or bar placement and is not due to air leak from damage to the lungs. Suctioning of pleural spaces and a Valsalva maneuver are used to alleviate the pneumothorax. A chest radiograph is recommended in the recovery unit. The majority of pneumothoraces are small and resolve spontaneously. Hence, they are usually managed conservatively and resolve in 24 hours.[22]

ANESTHETIC MANAGEMENT

General endotracheal anesthesia is commonly utilized for this procedure. Standard monitors are typically utilized unless the patient's history warrants further monitoring. Following either intravenous or inhalational induction, a nondepolarizing neuromuscular blockade is utilized to facilitate intubation. A single lumen endotracheal tube is sufficient, as carbon dioxide can be utilized to allow thoracoscopic visualization for dissection. Nitrous oxide should be avoided in these cases given the risk of worsening a likely pneumothorax. The patient is positioned with arms greater than 90 degrees, which may be achieved by placing a vertical roll between the shoulder blades to increase surgical exposure. Hence, there is increased risk of brachial plexus injuries. Postoperatively, the patient is advised to keep the back straight with the bed flexed at the level of the hips. Any rotation of the trunk or flexing of the thoracic spine is to be avoided due to concern for migration of the pectus bar and its associated complications.

POSTOPERATIVE ANALGESIA

Both surgical procedures are associated with significant pain. Currently, the Nuss procedure is by far the more commonly performed procedure. Complaints of pain can be secondary to the incisions, pressure from the bar, inflammatory mediators, or muscle spasms. Depending on the comfort level of the provider, a combination of regional techniques, intravenous narcotic medications, and muscle relaxants may be utilized.[26,27] Additionally, the patient may receive benzodiazepines in the postoperative period for muscle spasms or anxiety. Other intravenous medications including ketamine have also been used as a rescue analgesic in those with insufficient pain control postoperatively.

The options for regional techniques include epidural catheters, paravertebral catheters, intercostal nerve blocks, and wound infusion catheters. Most commonly, the epidural technique is used. A preoperatively placed thoracic epidural with catheter tip located at the T5–T7 level should provide adequate analgesia.[28] Epidural solutions include 0.1% bupivavaine or 0.2% ropivacaine with additives such as fentanyl, hydromorphone, or clonidine. Plain local anesthetic solutions (without opioids) can also be utilized concomitantly with an intravenous opioid PCA to improve quality of analgesia. Table 18 shows a suggested analgesic regimen for postoperative analgesia management[28].

In a recent report, the amount of morphine equivalents utilized for patients undergoing Nuss procedures in the first 24 hours correlated with age and was highest in patients under 12 years old.[26] Perhaps, this is related to mechanical stress and growth zones in the rib cage in the pediatric population, where pain is primarily reported in the anterior part of the thorax compared to the posterior part in the adult population.[26] Whether epidural or intravenous PCA is superior is still a matter of debate, and many centers use a combination of epidural analgesia with the intravenous PCA. Based on a meta-analysis, epidural and PCA appear to have equivalent pain control; however, epidurals seem to have a higher failure rate.[29] Paravertebral catheters have the advantage of being an effective nonneuraxial alternative with equivalent analgesic benefit and a favorable side-effect profile.[30,31] They are usually placed utilizing an ultrasound-guided technique. Epidural or paravertebral catheters may be placed before or after induction of anesthesia based on provider and patient comfort. Reports of permanent neurological injury in patients has raised some concerns regarding utilization of thoracic epidurals for repair of pectus excavatum.[32,33] There has, therefore, been a shift in paradigm toward the use of paravertebral catheters and/or intravenous opioid PCA[22] in recent years.

Intercostal nerve blocks are another alternative to epidural analgesia. This involves use of multiple bilateral injections under general anesthesia. A randomized study demonstrated superior analgesia, decreased postoperative pain scores, and reduced opioid consumption in those children, who received ultrasound guided intercostal nerve blocks versus the intravenous PCA group.[34] Application of cryotherapy to the intercostal nerve blocks under direct thoracoscopic visualization prior to pectus bar placement has demonstrated analgesia for two months or even longer.[35] Wound infusion catheters or chest wall catheters are multiorifice catheters placed bilaterally below the costal margin, in the posterior axillary line deep to the latissimus dorsi and close to rib cage and surgical incision.[27] This technique appears to be comparable to epidural infusion and concomitant intravenous PCA and has the advantages of reduced nausea and vomiting, shorter operating room times, and shorter hospital stay.[27,36]

Postoperatively, narcotics may be required for 1–3 weeks; children <12 years may need narcotics for less than a week.

Table 18. 1 ANALGESIC MANAGEMENT FOR PECTUS EXCAVATUM REPAIR

TIMING IN RELATION TO SURGERY	ANALGESIC REGIMEN	COMMENTS
Preoperative	• Thoracic epidural catheter *or* • Bilateral paravertebral catheters	• Preinduction + sedation *or* • Postinduction + general anesthesia
Intraoperative	• LA infusion via catheter throughout the procedure • IV low-dose ketamine infusion • IV acetaminophen • IV ketorolac	• May need bolus with infusion • LA solution may have additives like clonidine or opioids • Caution with parenteral opioids if used in LA solution • Use ketorolac once bleeding is controlled
PACU/ Postoperative Day 0	• Continue LA infusion • Rescue PRN opioids or IV opioid PCA	• Consider PRN benzodiazepines (diazepam or lorazepam) for muscle spasms • PRN antiemetics
Postoperative Day1	• Continue LA infusion • Rescue PRN opioids or IV opioid PCA • Start oral opioids • Start oral acetaminophen	• Consider PRN benzodiazepines (diazepam or lorazepam) for muscle spasms • PRN antiemetics
Postoperative Day 2	• Continue LA infusion • Rescue PRN parental opioids • Wean parental opioids • Continue oral opioids + acetaminophen	• PRN benzodiazepines (diazepam or lorazepam) for muscle spasms • PRN antiemetics
Postoperative Day 3	• Discontinue LA infusion and PCA • Continue oral opioids + acetaminophen • Start oral ibuprofen • Remove catheters after adequate pain control confirmed with oral medications	Continue oral opioids after day 3, discussion about oral "take-home medications" should take place after day 3

Note. LA = local anesthetic. IV = intravenous. PRN = "when necessary." PCA = patient-controlled analgesia.

While in the hospital, incentive spirometry and breathing exercises are encouraged, while heavy lifting is avoided for a minimum of 6 weeks.[22]

ANESTHESIA FOR REMOVAL OF PECTUS BAR

Bar removal is usually performed after 2–4 years. This is done under general endotracheal anesthesia. The technique involves mobilizing the bar at both ends, straightening, and then sliding the bar out. The anesthesiologist should watch for changes in electrocardiography during the manipulation and removal.[18] The anesthesiologist should also be prepared for massive hemorrhage during removal due to the potential for trauma to surrounding structures from bar migration or erosion.[37]

CONCLUSION

- Pectus excavatum is the most common type of congenital chest wall deformity.

- The Ravitch or Nuss procedure is utilized for surgical repair.

- Preoperative evaluation includes assessment of the extent of the deformity, Haller index value, clinical symptoms, or cardiopulmonary effects.

- Acute postoperative pain management may be challenging. A combination of analgesic techniques and a multimodal pain management strategy is recommended.

- Preoperative preparation should include a discussion with the child and parents regarding a pain management strategy and the expected postoperative course.

- Intraoperative vigilance is paramount due to potential for catastrophic events.

REVIEW QUESTIONS

1. A 12-year-old presents for evaluation of a chest wall deformity. He has noticed a worsening in the deformity over the last few years and is interested in surgical repair. Which of following is **MOST** accurate regarding pectus excavatum?

   A. associated with Marfan syndrome
   B. characterized by protrusion of the sternum
   C. more common in females
   D. prevalence is 1:5,000 live births

Answer: A
Pectus excavatum is associated with a number of syndromes. The most commonly associated syndromes include Marfan syndrome, Ehlers-Danlos syndrome, and Turner syndrome.[1] Answer B is incorrect as pectus excavatum is the most common chest wall deformity and has a higher incidence of 1:300 births. It is more commonly seen in males with a prevalence of at least 4:1[2]; therefore, Answer C is incorrect. Pectus excavatum is characterized by depression of the sternum and

the adjacent ribs while pectus carinatum is characterized by protrusion of the sternum and anterior ribs (answer D)[15]. While there may be asymmetry in pectus excavatum, pectus carinatum consists of symmetric protrusion of the sternum.

2. A 13-year-old boy presents with pectus excavatum. He is a soccer player and is keen to continue playing sports; however, he has noted difficulty keeping up with his teammates lately. Which of the following statements is **MOST** likely to be an indication for surgical repair in this patient?

   A. Haller index 2.5
   B. negative echocardiography
   C. normal exercise tolerance
   D. psychosocial issues

Answer D.
The Haller index provides objective assessment of the severity of the pectus excavatum deformity.[11,12] The Haller index is the ratio of the transverse diameter of the thorax to the anteroposterior diameter at its narrowest part. A normal Haller index is less than 2.5. A value >3.25 may be an indication of surgery. Occurrence of cardiorespiratory symptoms is also an indication for surgery (answer C). Echocardiography is not warranted in all cases, but cardiac compression secondary to a severe defect may be an indication for surgery (answer D). Poor body image, psychological issues, and social maladjustment are all reasonable indications for surgery.[22]

3. You see a patient in the preoperative clinic, who is scheduled for a Nuss procedure. He complains of shortness of breath with activity, and his pediatrician has previously ordered PFTs. Which of the following measurement is the **MOST** likely increased given his deformity?

   A. forced expiratory flow between 25% and 75% (FEF 25%–75%).
   B. FEV_1
   C. maximal voluntary ventilation (MVV)
   D. residual volume

Answer: D
The majority of patients who have pulmonary function testing done show an obstructive pattern; however, a restrictive pattern can also be seen.[15] The hallmark signs of compression include low lung volumes and elevated residual volumes. Given the high likelihood of an obstructive pattern, one would expect this patient to have a low FEV_1 as well as FEF (25%–75%); therefore, answers B and D are incorrect. MVV is normally calculated to be $FEV_1 \times 40$; however, MVVs are low in patients with obstruction (answer C).

4. A 14-year-old patient is having minimally invasive repair of pectus excavatum utilizing the Nuss procedure. The parents and patient have concerns regarding postoperative pain. Which of the following is the **MOST** reasonable option for acute postoperative pain management in this patient?

   A. intravenous PCA
   B. multimodal approach
   C. paravertebral blocks
   D. thoracic epidural

Answer: B

Either thoracic epidural or paravertebral catheters are suitable options for postoperative analgesia management in patients undergoing a Nuss procedure; however, a multimodal approach utilizing multiple analgesia techniques is best given the multiple components of pain, including incisional pain, pressure from the bars, and muscle spasms and anxiety. In one retrospective study [38] both paravertebral catheters (answer A) and thoracic epidurals (answer B) resulted in equivalent opioid consumption. Similarly in a meta-analysis,[29] opioid PCA (answer D) and thoracic epidural blocks were also found to be comparable. Of note, the site of insertion of the epidural needle may be anywhere from T6–T7 to T10–T11; however, the goal should be to have the catheter tip at the level of T5–T7[28].

5. You are anesthetizing a 13-year-old male with Marfan syndrome for a Nuss procedure. The surgeon has just made incision and is using blunt finger dissection prior to thoracoscopic insertion. Which of the following is the **MOST** accurate regarding the Nuss procedure?

    A. Costal cartilage is resection.
    B. Hemorrhage risk is present.
    C. Significant pain is rare.
    D. Single bar is always sufficient.

Answer: B

The Nuss procedure involves insertion of a substernal bar to correct the pectus deformity. The bar is inserted via two lateral thoracic incisions, and the bar is guided substernally through the mediastinum using a thoracoscope.[13,18] Although minimally invasive, there is a risk of hemorrhage with the Nuss procedure due to the proximity of the surgical site to the heart and major blood vessels[39].Unlike the Nuss procedure, the Ravitch procedure involves complete resection of the costochondral cartilages and mobilization of the sternum (answer A).[20] Both procedures, however, are associated with significant pain (answer D), warranting a multimodal pain strategy. Patients with significant deformities may require two bars to be placed to correct the deformity. These patients typically have associated syndromes, including Marfan syndrome (answer C).

6. Following successful placement of one pectus bar, a 12-year-old female, with a thoracic epidural, complains of severe chest pain and shortness of breath in the recovery unit. The **BEST** treatment strategy, following examination, includes

    A. ensuring sensory block level of thoracic epidural.
    B. instituting an ultralow dose ketamine infusion.
    C. providing additional intravenous pain medications.
    D. reassuring the patient this pain is expected.

Answer: B

Pain following pectus bar insertion may be due to the incision, conformational changes in the thoracic cage due to presence of the bar, muscle spasms, and/or inflammatory mediators. For this reason, a multimodal strategy is very important in pain control in this group of patients.[28] While intravenous medications (answer C) and ketamine infusions (answer D) may be utilized for rescue techniques, it is important to assess appropriate sensory

blockade for whatever regional technique is utilized. Untreated pain can be associated with worsening shortness of breath, atelectasis, pneumonia, and respiratory decompensation, and all efforts should be made to adequately manage pain control in these patients (answer A) to avoid these complications.

7. Bilateral pneumothoraces are noted in a teenager following a Nuss procedure. Which of the following is the **MOST** appropriate statement regarding the management of pneumothorax?

    A. bilaterally needle aspiration
    B. conservative management
    C. immediate chest tube placement
    D. return to the operating room

Answer: B

Pneumothorax is commonly seen following pectus repair with the Nuss procedure. It is usually due to incomplete evacuation of carbon dioxide used during thoracoscopic visualization[18] and is not secondary to lung injury (answer C). The majority of these are managed conservatively and resolve spontaneously within 24 hours.[25] Therefore, routine insertion of chest tube is not recommended (answer A). While certain strategies are utilized to limit the size of pneumothoraces, including avoiding nitrous oxide, chest radiographs are routinely ordered, and the patient is clinically followed for worsening of symptoms (answer D).

8. A patient with a severe deformity with a Haller index of 3.6 is scheduled for a Nuss procedure. Which of the following statements is **MOST** accurate regarding the anesthetic management of this patient?

    A. lateral decubitus positioning for surgery
    B. Arterial line placement is typically indicated.
    C. Central line placement is typically indicated.
    D. smooth extubation without coughing

Answer: D

It is important to avoid coughing or straining (answer D) at extubation as there is a potential risk of displacement of the bar or subcutaneous emphysema from the residual pneumothorax.[28] The intraoperative positioning is supine with the arms abducted bilaterally for midaxillary incisions; therefore, answer A is incorrect. An arterial line (answer B) is not necessary unless the echocardiography findings suggest significant derangement of cardiopulmonary function. While central line monitoring (answer C) is not mandated unless the patient has pre-existing clinical comorbidities, a second large bore intravenous access is reasonable in case of inadvertent injury to mediastinal structures during insertion of the pectus bar.[28]

9. An 18-year-old presents for removal of his pectus bar. His initial surgery was uncomplicated, but he is now having pain at the site of the bar. Which of the following is the **MOST** appropriate statement regarding removal of the pectus bar?

    A. Chest X-ray following procedure is not necessary.
    B. Effect on the electrocardiogram should be noted before bar removal.
    C. Performed typically 6–8 years after insertion.
    D. Risk of hemorrhage with this procedure is minimal.

Answer: B

Bar removal is usually performed 2–4 years (answer A) after the initial surgery. This time period balances the risk of recurrence if the bar is removed too early with the risk of pain or outgrowing the bar. Although the surgical procedure is generally safe, removal of the pectus bar has potential risk for massive hemorrhage due to adhesions, erosion into the mediastinum, and proximity to major mediastinal structures.[37] After removal, a chest X-ray is indicated in the recovery unit to check for pneumothoraces.

QUESTIONS AND ANSWERS

This chapter has accompanying questions and answers which are available to subscribers as part of the Oxford eLearning platform. To access the questions, go to ✓ http://oxfordmedicine. com/pediatricanesthesiaPBL

REFERENCES

1. Cobben JM, Oostra RJ, van Dijk FS. Pectus excavatum and carinatum. *Eur J Med Genet.* 2014;57(8):414–417.
2. Koumbourlis AC. Pectus excavatum: pathophysiology and clinical characteristics. *Paediatr Respir Rev.* 2009;10(1):3–6.
3. Williams AM, Crabbe DC. Pectus deformities of the anterior chest wall. *Paediatr Respir Rev.* 2003;4(3):237–242.
4. Kotzot D, Schwabegger AH. Etiology of chest wall deformities—a genetic review for the treating physician. *J Pediatr Surg.* 2009;44(10):2004–2011.
5. Goretsky MJ, Kelly RE Jr, Croitoru D, Nuss D. Chest wall anomalies: pectus excavatum and pectus carinatum. *Adolesc Med Clin.* 2004;15(3):455–471.
6. Kelly RE Jr. Pectus excavatum: historical background, clinical picture, preoperative evaluation and criteria for operation. *Semin Pediatr Surg.* 2008;17(3):181–193.
7. Chahrour M, Zoghbi HY. The story of Rett syndrome: from clinic to neurobiology. *Neuron.* 2007;56(3):422–437.
8. Dearlove OR, Walker RW. Anaesthesia for Rett syndrome. *Paediatr Anaesth.* 1996;6(2):155–158.
9. Beiser GD, Epstein SE, Stampfer M, Goldstein RE, Noland SP, Levitsky S. Impairment of cardiac function in patients with pectus excavatum, with improvement after operative correction. *N Engl J Med.* 1972;287(6):267–272.
10. Mocchegiani R, Badano L, Lestuzzi C, Nicolosi GL, Zanuttini D. Relation of right ventricular morphology and function in pectus excavatum to the severity of the chest wall deformity. *Am J Cardiol.* 1995;76(12):941–946.
11. Haller JA, Jr., Kramer SS, Lietman SA. Use of CT scans in selection of patients for pectus excavatum surgery: a preliminary report. *J Pediatr Surg.* 1987;22(10):904–906.
12. Khanna G, Jaju A, Don S, Keys T, Hildebolt CF. Comparison of Haller index values calculated with chest radiographs versus CT for pectus excavatum evaluation. *Pediatr Radiol.* 2010;40(11):1763–1767.
13. Nuss D, Kelly RE Jr., Croitoru DP, Katz ME. A 10-year review of a minimally invasive technique for the correction of pectus excavatum. *J Pediatr Surg.* 1998;33(4):545–552.
14. Colombani PM. Preoperative assessment of chest wall deformities. *Semin Thorac Cardiovasc Surg.* 2009;21(1):58–63.
15. Koumbourlis AC. Pectus deformities and their impact on pulmonary physiology. *Paediatr Respir Rev.* 2015;16(1):18–24.
16. Chen Z, Amos EB, Luo H, et al. Comparative pulmonary functional recovery after Nuss and Ravitch procedures for pectus excavatum repair: a meta-analysis. *J Cardiothorac Surg.* 2012;7:101.
17. Jeong JY, Ahn JH, Kim SY, et al. Pulmonary function before and after the Nuss procedure in adolescents with pectus excavatum: correlation with morphological subtypes. *J Cardiothorac Surg.* 2015;10:37.
18. Nuss D, Obermeyer RJ, Kelly RE Jr. Pectus excavatum from a pediatric surgeon's perspective. *Ann Cardiothorac Surg.* 2016;5(5):493–500.
19. Schier F, Bahr M, Klobe E. The vacuum chest wall lifter: an innovative, nonsurgical addition to the management of pectus excavatum. *J Pediatr Surg.* 2005;40(3):496–500.
20. Ravitch MM. The operative treatment of pectus excavatum. *Ann Surg.* 1949;129(4):429–444.
21. Adkins PC, Blades B. A stainless steel strut for correction of pectus escavatum. *Surg Gynecol Obstet.* 1961;113:111–113.
22. Nuss D, Obermeyer RJ, Kelly RE. Nuss bar procedure: past, present and future. *Ann Cardiothorac Surg.* 2016;5(5):422–433.
23. Nasr A, Fecteau A, Wales PW. Comparison of the Nuss and the Ravitch procedure for pectus excavatum repair: a meta-analysis. *J Pediatr Surg.* 2010;45(5):880–886.
24. Kanagaratnam A, Phan S, Tchantchaleishvili V, Phan K. Ravitch versus Nuss procedure for pectus excavatum: systematic review and meta-analysis. *Ann Cardiothorac Surg.* 2016;5(5):409–421.
25. Knudsen MR, Nyboe C, Hjortdal VE, Pilegaard HK. Routine postoperative chest X-ray is unnecessary following the Nuss procedure for pectus excavatum. *Interact Cardiovasc Thorac Surg.* 2013;16(6):830–833.
26. Frawley G, Frawley J, Crameri J. A review of anesthetic techniques and outcomes following minimally invasive repair of pectus excavatum (Nuss procedure). *Paediatr Anaesth.* 2016;26(11):1082–1090.
27. Choudhry DK, Brenn BR, Sacks K, Reichard K. Continuous chest wall ropivacaine infusion for analgesia in children undergoing Nuss procedure: a comparison with thoracic epidural. *Paediatr Anaesth.* 2016;26(6):582–589.
28. Mavi J, Moore DL. Anesthesia and analgesia for pectus excavatum surgery. *Anesthesiol Clin.* 2014;32(1):175–184.
29. Stroud AM, Tulanont DD, Coates TE, Goodney PP, Croitoru DP. Epidural analgesia versus intravenous patient-controlled analgesia following minimally invasive pectus excavatum repair: a systematic review and meta-analysis. *J Pediatr Surg.* 2014;49(5):798–806.
30. Davies RG, Myles PS, Graham JM. A comparison of the analgesic efficacy and side-effects of paravertebral vs epidural blockade for thoracotomy—a systematic review and meta-analysis of randomized trials. *Br J Anaesth.* 2006;96(4):418–426.
31. Scarci M, Joshi A, Attia R. In patients undergoing thoracic surgery is paravertebral block as effective as epidural analgesia for pain management? *Interact Cardiovasc Thorac Surg.* 2010;10(1):92–96.
32. Kelly RE, Goretsky MJ, Obermeyer R, et al. Twenty-one years of experience with minimally invasive repair of pectus excavatum by the Nuss procedure in 1215 patients. *Ann Surg.* 2010;252(6):1072–1081.
33. Meyer MJ, Krane EJ, Goldschneider KR, Klein NJ. Case report: neurological complications associated with epidural analgesia in children: a report of 4 cases of ambiguous etiologies. *Anesth Analg.* 2012;115(6):1365–1370.
34. Luo M, Liu X, Ning L, Sun Y, Cai Y, Shen S. Comparison of ultrasonography-guided bilateral intercostal nerve blocks and conventional patient-controlled intravenous analgesia for pain control after the Nuss procedure in children: a prospective randomized study. *Clin J Pain.* 2017;33(7):604–610.
35. Graves C, Idowu O, Lee S, Padilla B, Kim S. Intraoperative cryoanalgesia for managing pain after the Nuss procedure. *J Pediatr Surg.* 2017;52(6):920–924.
36. Jaroszewski DE, Temkit M, Ewais MM, et al. Randomized trial of epidural vs. subcutaneous catheters for managing pain after modified Nuss in adults. *J Thorac Dis.* 2016;8(8):2102–2110.
37. Notrica DM, McMahon LE, Johnson KN, Velez DA, McGill LC, Jaroszewski DE. Life-threatening hemorrhage during removal of a Nuss bar associated with sternal erosion. *Ann Thorac Surg.* 2014;98(3):1104–1106.
38. Hall Burton DM, Boretsky KR. A comparison of paravertebral nerve block catheters and thoracic epidural catheters for postoperative analgesia following the Nuss procedure for pectus excavatum repair. *Paediatr Anaesth.* 2014;24(5):516–520.
39. Jeong JY, Suh JH, Yoon JS, Park CB. Delayed-onset hypovolemic shock after the Nuss procedure for pectus excavatum. *J Cardiothorac Surg.* 2014;9:15.

SECTION 4

HEAD, NECK, AND RESPIRATORY SYSTEMS

19.

TONSILLECTOMY AND ADENOIDECTOMY IN THE PEDIATRIC PATIENT WITH DOWN SYNDROME

Ellen Y. Choi

STEM CASE AND KEY QUESTIONS

A 9-year-old boy with Down syndrome (DS) presents for tonsillectomy and adenoidectomy for severe obstructive sleep apnea (OSA).

WHAT IS DS? WHAT ARE COMMON AND IMPORTANT FEATURES OF DS? HOW IS DS DIAGNOSED? WHAT ARE ASSOCIATED CONGENITAL CONDITIONS AND COMORBIDITIES?

He was born at 37 5/7 weeks gestation by planned cesarean section to a 39-year-old G2P1 diabetic mother and was admitted to the neonatal intensive care unit for further monitoring. Prenatal ultrasound showed features consistent with DS, and the diagnosis was confirmed with amniocentesis. Fetal echocardiogram showed complete atrioventricular septal defect (AVSD), which was confirmed after birth. In the early neonatal period, he was diagnosed with duodenal atresia and underwent laparotomy and duodenoduodenostomy. His heart condition was managed with captopril, furosemide, and digoxin until he underwent complete biventricular repair of his AVSD at 3 months of age without complications.

WHAT FURTHER INFORMATION DO YOU REQUIRE FOR YOUR PREOPERATIVE EVALUATION OF THIS PATIENT? WHAT CARDIAC STUDIES, IF ANY, ARE NEEDED? WILL YOU CHECK LABS? WHAT INFORMATION WOULD YOU LOOK FOR ON PAST ANESTHETIC RECORDS?

The patient has regular, annual, follow-up visits with his cardiologist. His last echocardiogram was performed almost 6 months ago and showed no residual patch leak, good biventricular function, and moderate regurgitation across the mitral and tricuspid valves. There was no comment on right ventricular enlargement or overload. He is a "difficult stick" according to his parents, and it is hard to draw blood, partially due to his phobia of needles. In addition to his duodenal atresia repair and his cardiac surgery, he has had bilateral myringotomy and ear tubes placed, as well as strabismus surgery. Two years ago, he had general anesthesia for dental rehabilitation for severe caries and extractions, wherein the endotracheal tube (ETT) needed to be downsized to achieve an appropriate air leak. Afterwards, his mouth was also noted to be "oozy" according to his parents.

WHAT TYPE OF NEUROLOGIC ASSESSMENT, IF ANY, WILL YOU PERFORM? HOW WILL YOU ASSESS HIS COGNITIVE AND DEVELOPMENTAL LEVEL? WHAT IS ATLANTOAXIAL INSTABILITY (AAI), HOW IS IT DIAGNOSED, AND WHAT IS ITS SIGNIFICANCE FOR THE ANESTHESIA PROVIDER? WOULD YOU SCREEN FOR AAI PREOPERATIVELY IN THIS PATIENT?

His medical chart notes a history of motor, developmental, and cognitive delay. He attends special school and participates in sports. He does not have any neck pain or focal neurologic symptoms. Flexion and extension cervical spine X-rays taken 3 years ago, as a school requirement, are negative for AAI.

HOW IS OSA DIAGNOSED IN THE PEDIATRIC POPULATION? WHAT ARE ASSOCIATED COMORBIDITIES OF SLEEP APNEA? HOW IS OSA TREATED IN CHILDREN WITH DS?

His parents report that he snores heavily with apneic pauses during sleep. He had a polysomnogram (PSG) with an apnea-hypopnea index of 15 and a room air oxygen saturation nadir of 80%. He has chronic nasal congestion and rhinorrhea and typically breathes noisily through his mouth. On exam, he has typical Down's facies, midface hypoplasia, a small mouth opening, relative macroglossia, and a Mallampati Class 3 airway. The otolaryngologist's preoperative visit note reports bilateral + 2–3 tonsillar and adenoid hypertrophy. Vital signs in the preoperative area are as follows: blood pressure 101/79 mmHg, heart rate 90 bpm, respiratory rate 22 breaths/minute, oxygen saturation by pulse oximetry 97%, temperature 36.7°C, weight 40 kg, and height 120 cm. He has been nil per os (NPO) for greater than 8 hours for food, and last drank water 3 hours prior to surgery.

HOW WOULD YOU MANAGE PERIOPERATIVE
ANXIETY? WHAT TYPE OF PREMEDICATION,
IF ANY, WOULD YOU ADMINISTER TO THIS
PATIENT? WHAT IS YOUR RATIONALE
TO PREMEDICATE OR NOT PREMEDICATE
THE PATIENT? WHAT ASSISTANCE COULD A
CHILD LIFE SPECIALIST OFFER?

He appears nervous in the preoperative area, and his parents inquire about an oral sedative for anxiolysis prior to going to the operating room (OR). He is cooperative with elements of your exam, but his manner is withdrawn. He responds, however, to the child life specialist and is readily engaged by her iPad tablet.

WHAT ARE YOUR GOALS FOR INDUCTION?
WOULD YOU PLACE A PERIPHERAL
INTRAVENOUS CATHETER (PIV) WHILE THE
PATIENT IS AWAKE AND PERFORM
AN INTRAVENOUS (IV) INDUCTION OR
PROCEED WITH A MASK INDUCTION?
HOW WOULD YOU SECURE TIMELY
INTRAVENOUS ACCESS GIVEN THAT HE IS A
"DIFFICULT STICK?" HOW WILL YOU TREAT
BRADYCARDIA IF IT OCCURS? WHAT IS
YOUR AIRWAY MANAGEMENT PLAN? HOW
WOULD YOU MANAGE SEVERE OBSTRUCTION
DURING INDUCTION? WHAT TYPE AND SIZE
OF ETT WOULD YOU CHOOSE?

In the OR, he is induced by sevoflurane mask anesthesia. He has severe upper airway obstruction that is relieved by placement of an oral airway along with head tilt. He becomes bradycardic, which resolves when the inhaled sevoflurane concentration is decreased. Several attempts for IV access are made by multiple providers. Ultimately, one 22G PIV was placed with the use of point-of-care ultrasound. Direct laryngoscopy with careful extension of the neck yields a grade II view and extremely large tonsils. He is intubated with a cuffed oral Ring-Adair-Elwyn ETT. The first attempt at ETT placement is aborted because of resistance to passage of the tube past the vocal cords. An ETT that is one size smaller is placed on the second attempt, and the cuff is inflated to a minimal occlusion pressure of 20 cm water.

HOW WOULD YOU POSITION THE PATIENT?
WOULD POSITIONING BE DIFFERENT IF THE
PATIENT HAS AAI? WHAT PRECAUTIONS
WOULD YOU TAKE FOR THE PREVENTION
OF AIRWAY FIRE DURING SURGERY? HOW
WOULD YOU COMMUNICATE WITH THE
OTOLARYNGOLOGIST ABOUT PATIENT
POSITION AND FIRE PREVENTION
DURING THE CASE? HOW WOULD YOU
MAINTAIN ANESTHESIA? WHAT IS YOUR
INTRAOPERATIVE ANALGESIC PLAN? ARE
PROPHYLACTIC ANTIBIOTICS FOR THE
PREVENTION OF ENDOCARDITIS INDICATED?

The bed is turned 90 degrees away from the anesthesia provider. During the surgical time out, precautions for airway fire prevention and patient positioning concerns are addressed. The mouth gag is placed, and the patient is placed in careful suspension with the minimum extension necessary for adequate visualization of the surgical field. Heart rate and blood pressure climb with positioning and with incision. Maintenance is achieved with volatile inhaled anesthetic in 21% fraction of inspired oxygen (FiO_2), which provides adequate oxygenation. The patient receives IV ampicillin 50 mg/kg, dexamethasone, glycopyrrolate, and ondansetron. Analgesic medications and adjuncts include small doses of morphine, IV acetaminophen, and dexmedetomidine. Constant communication is maintained with the surgeon regarding FiO_2 and the progress of the case.

WHAT ARE YOUR GOALS FOR EMERGENCE?
HOW WOULD YOU MANAGE EMERGENCE
DELIRIUM IF IT PRESENTS? WHAT IS YOUR
POSTOPERATIVE ANALGESIC PLAN? WHAT
COMPLICATIONS ARE YOU CONCERNED
ABOUT IN THE POSTANESTHETIC RECOVERY
PERIOD? SHOULD THIS PATIENT BE
ADMITTED OVERNIGHT? IF SO, WHAT
LEVEL OF MONITORING DOES HE REQUIRE
POSTOPERATIVELY?

The patient is awakened and extubated in the OR. Upon extubation, he is coughing, with significantly noisy breathing and upper airway obstruction that improves with jaw thrust. He is still somnolent and is taken to the postanesthesia care unit in the lateral recovery position. One hour later, he is more alert and requires multiple boluses of morphine for pain control. He continues to have bloody oral secretions and nausea. Two hours into the recovery period, he throws up a large number of bloody clots.

HOW WOULD YOU MANAGE
POSTTONSILLECTOMY HEMORRHAGE?
WOULD YOU SEND LABS? HOW WOULD
YOU ASSESS THE AMOUNT OF BLOOD LOSS?
WHAT IS YOUR TRANSFUSION TRIGGER?
SHOULD THIS PATIENT BE REINTUBATED
PRIOR TO PROCEEDING TO THE OR? HOW
WOULD YOU SECURE THE AIRWAY? WHERE
SHOULD THIS PATIENT BE ADMITTED NOW
(E.G., INTENSIVE CARE UNIT, PEDIATRIC
WARD)? HOW WOULD YOU DISCUSS THIS
COMPLICATION WITH THE PARENTS?

The OR staff and otolaryngologist are notified, and the patient is taken to the OR for coagulation of the tonsillar bleed. During transfer, with administration of a 20 mL/kg IV fluid bolus, the PIV is found to be infiltrated. The PIV is replaced with ultrasound and volume resuscitation is continued. Labs, including complete blood count, coagulation profile, and blood type are sent, as well as venous blood gas for quicker results. Two units of O-negative blood are available. The patient undergoes a rapid sequence intubation. Two suction canisters with two Yankauer suction tips are readily available.

Direct visualization of the vocal cords is poor due to blood in the oropharynx, but intubation is successful. The bleeding is cauterized. Prior to extubation, an orogastric tube is placed under direct visualization, and the stomach is suctioned. The patient is extubated at the end of the surgery and taken to the postanesthesia care unit. After an uneventful recovery period, he is admitted overnight to a monitored bed.

DISCUSSION

DS, or Trisomy 21, was first characterized by John Langdon Down in 1866, and is the most common chromosomal abnormality with an incidence of 1:600–800 live births.[1] There are currently approximately 250,000 people living with DS in the United States.[2] It is a genetic disorder, caused by an extra copy of all or part of chromosome 21 in utero. The syndrome is typically not inherited; most parents of children with DS do not have trisomy 21. Female DS patients will transmit the chromosomal abnormality to their offspring, but they have reduced fertility. Women of advanced maternal age carry a greater risk of giving birth to babies with DS than those who are younger.[3] Prenatal screening by lab tests, chromosomal analysis, and ultrasound can identify the disease. After birth, the syndrome is diagnosed by clinical features and confirmatory genetic testing. Overall life expectancy for patients with DS is currently well into the fifth decade of life, due to improvements in medical care, compared with 25 years in the 1980s.[2] As such, the anesthesia practitioner will most likely care for multiple patients with DS during the course of their career.

Patients with DS have characteristic facial features.[4] They typically have a flat face, short neck, epicanthal folds, brachycephaly, a small nose, a flat nasal bridge, and upward slanted palpebral fissures. They have a small mouth and relative macroglossia. Other physical characteristics include obesity, increased nuchal skin, single palmar crease, joint laxity, and widened gap between the first and second toes.

DS affects multiple organ systems, including the neurologic, cardiac, respiratory/airway, gastrointestinal, endocrine, musculoskeletal, hematologic, and immunologic systems (Table 19.1).[4–7] The spectrum of disease severity can vary. The American Academy of Pediatrics (AAP) practice guidelines recommend regularly screening individuals with DS for associated diseases (Table 19.2).[8] Conditions of particular significance to the anesthesia provider include abnormalities of the airway and respiratory tract, congenital heart disease (CHD), sleep apnea, AAI, and neurologic disability.

All patients with DS exhibit intellectual disability with an average IQ of approximately 50 points.[7] They have delayed myelination of neuronal fibers and take longer to reach developmental milestones than patients without DS.[7] Language skills and behavior can be variable. Early childhood intervention, education, socialization, speech and occupational therapy help improve quality of life.

The DS patient may have multiple abnormalities of the upper and lower airway tracts. They have midface and mandibular hypoplasia, leading to the typical flattened midface, small mouth, and narrow palate, which may make mask fit

Table 19.1 CLINICAL CONDITIONS ASSOCIATED WITH DOWN SYNDROME

ORGAN SYSTEM	ASSOCIATED CONDITIONS
Neurologic	Hypotonia, developmental delay, autism spectrum disorder, seizures, MoyaMoya/strokes, depression, Alzheimer's, hearing loss, vision abnormalities, strabismus
Respiratory	Airway abnormalities, obstructive sleep apnea, pulmonary hypoplasia, recurrent pneumonia
Musculoskeletal	Ligamentous laxity (atlantoaxial instability), hip dislocations, slipped capital femoral epiphysis, scoliosis
Cardiac	Congenital heart disease, pulmonary hypertension, arrhythmias
Endocrine	Hypothyroidism, diabetes
Gastrointestinal	Gastroesophageal reflux disease, obesity, duodenal atresia, tracheoesophageal fistula, Hirschsprung's, imperforate anus, celiac disease
Genitourinary	Cryptorchidism (testicular cancer), posterior urethral valves
Hematologic	Myeloproliferative disorder, leukemia

and laryngoscopy difficult. They have adenoid, tonsillar, and lingual tonsillar hypertrophy. They have glossoptosis, leading to a relative macroglossia in the setting of a small mouth, and pharyngomalacia with hypopharyngeal collapse. Both of these elements can exacerbate symptoms of OSA, particularly in DS patients with poor muscle tone. Abnormalities of the lower airway include laryngomalacia, subglottic stenosis, and tracheal stenosis. Current otolaryngology literature recommends downsizing the expected ETT diameter by 2 sizes when intubating a patient with DS.[4,9,10] It is also prudent to ensure an appropriate air leak of 15–25 cm water.

Obstructive sleep apnea is defined as a "disorder of breathing during sleep characterized by prolonged partial upper airway obstruction and/or intermittent complete obstruction (obstructive apnea) that disrupts normal ventilation during sleep and normal sleep patterns."[11] While various methods exist to diagnose OSA in children, including history and questionnaire, the gold standard is the PSG. While specific criteria for the interpretation of sleep studies may vary by institution, most practitioners define diagnostic criteria for OSA in pediatrics to include an apnea-hypopnea index >1 (Table 19.3).[12]

OSA occurs more frequently and with greater severity in pediatric patients with DS than in the general population, with an incidence of 30%–75%.[6,8] By adulthood, greater than 90% of DS patients will have sleep apnea.[6] They have increased sensitivity to the effects of sedatives and opioids and are at increased risk of acute obstruction and respiratory depression.[6] Pretreatment with sedating antianxiolytics should be considered with caution. Family members may report

Table 19.2 SUMMARY OF SELECTED AMERICAN ACADEMY OF PEDIATRICS SCREENING GUIDELINES FOR PATIENTS WITH DOWN SYNDROME

PATIENT AGE	RECOMMENDED TESTING
Birth—1 month	Electrocardiogram, echocardiogram, hearing screen, complete blood count, TSH
1 month—1 year	Eye exam, TSH at 6 and 12 months Audiology evaluation at 6 months
>1 year	Hemoglobin, TSH annually Sleep study by 4 years

Note. TSH = thyroid stimulating hormone.

that the patient has heavy snoring, fatigue, and restless sleep. Daytime sleepiness is not common. There may be failure to thrive and behavior changes such as hyperactivity and poor school performance. When left untreated, chronic obstruction may lead to the development of pulmonary hypertension and congestive heart failure. There is a greater association between DS and pulmonary hypertension, thought secondary to multiple factors, including chronic obstruction, CHD, abnormal pulmonary architecture, and increased incidence of gastroesophageal reflux disease.[13,14]

Sleep apnea is an indication for tonsillectomy and adenoidectomy in children and often leads to complete resolution of symptoms with normalization of the PSG in 75%–100% of patients.[11] Despite surgery, 50% of patients with DS will not have their sleep apnea resolve, and 73% of patients will still have an abnormal PSG.[4,6,15] General risk factors for postoperative respiratory complications in pediatric adenotonsillectomy patients include age <3 years, severe OSA, cor pulmonale, failure to thrive, obesity, prematurity, recent respiratory infection, craniofacial abnormalities, and neuromuscular disorders.[11] DS patients are known to have a higher rate of postoperative respiratory complications, including postoperative obstruction, and take a longer time to return to normal per os intake. Current guidelines recommend that patients with DS who undergo tonsillectomy be admitted to the hospital overnight for monitoring.[11,15]

Congenital heart disease occurs in 45%–60% of patients with DS.[8,16,17] Put another way, 10% of children with DS have CHD.[16,17] It is the most common cause of death for patients with DS in the first 2 years of life.[16,18] The most common type of congenital heart lesion in DS is the AVSD, or endocardial

Table 19.3 PEDIATRIC POLYSOMNOGRAM CRITERIA FOR OBSTRUCTIVE SLEEP APNEA

APNEA-HYPOPNEA INDEX	GRADING OF OBSTRUCTIVE SLEEP APNEA
1.5–5	Mild
>5–10	Moderate
>10	Severe

cushion defect, which occurs 45%–50% of the time.[16,19] Other common lesions include atrial septal defect, ventricular septal defect, patent ductus arteriosus, and Tetralogy of Fallot.[16,19] Patients with untreated AVSD have pulmonary overcirculation, which can manifest with symptoms of congestive heart failure, failure to thrive, and pulmonary hypertension. Patients with DS and untreated CHD are known to have a greater risk of and faster time course to the development of pulmonary hypertension, and most lesions are repaired early in life to prevent the development of serious sequelae. Depending on the timing, type, and success of the repair, patients may have residual intracardiac shunt(s), pulmonary hypertension, and/or mitral or tricuspid valvular insufficiency.[20] These patients generally have regular evaluation of their cardiac structure and function by a cardiologist, and preoperative cardiac assessment should include a recent echocardiogram.

Patients for whom prophylaxis for infective endocarditis (IE) is indicated include those who are considered high-risk and are undergoing certain types of surgical procedures.[21,22] High-risk patients are those with (a) prosthetic cardiac valve or repair; (b) history of previous IE; (c) unrepaired cyanotic CHD including shunts or conduits; (d) completely repaired CHD with prosthetic material or device within 6 months (incomplete endothelialization); (e) repaired CHD with residual defects at or near the prosthetic material or device (inhibits endothelialization); and (f) heart transplant recipients with valvulopathy. Surgical indications for IE prophylaxis include (a) all dental procedures that manipulate gingival tissue or perforate oral mucosa; (b) invasive respiratory tract procedures with disruption of mucosa such as tonsillectomy and adenoidectomy; and (c) procedures involving infected tissue of the skin, musculoskeletal tissue, respiratory tree, gastrointestinal, or genitourinary tracts.[21,22]

Patients with DS also have abnormal autonomic regulation and can have blunted activation of the sympathetic system with excitatory stimuli. Bradycardia has been described during induction with inhaled volatile anesthetic. In 2 retrospective studies, approximately half the patients with DS, with or without CHD, exhibited bradycardia during sevoflurane induction, which resolved with direct laryngoscopy or decreasing the inhaled sevoflurane concentration. Pretreatment with anticholinergic did not preclude the development of bradycardia.[23,24]

Obesity, hypotonia, joint laxity, and doughy skin may make vascular access difficult in the DS patient.[25] Ligamentous laxity also contributes to the development of AAI. Approximately 15% of patients with DS have AAI, and almost all are asymptomatic.[8,26] AAI denotes increased mobility at the articulation of the first and second cervical vertebrae (atlantoaxial joint). Evaluation of AAI includes lateral cervical spine X-rays in the neutral, flexion, and extension positions. The atlantoaxial distance, also known as the anterior atlantodental interval, is measured from the anterior surface of the dens and the posterior surface of the anterior arch of C1. Measurements >5 mm on lateral X-ray is considered abnormal.[27,28] Movement of the cervical spine, such as flexion, extension, and lifting motions (i.e., laryngoscopy), can cause subluxation and injury to the spinal cord. Rotation has been reported to kink the vertebral arteries and cause syncope.[29]

There are limitations to the diagnostic ability of cervical spine X-rays. Some asymptomatic individuals who have normal cervical spine X-rays initially may have abnormal X-rays later, and others with initially abnormal X-rays will have normal follow-up X-rays. Currently, the AAP does not recommend routine radiographic screening of the cervical spine in asymptomatic patients.[8]

Guidelines encourage providers to discuss with families the importance of cervical spine positioning precautions for protection of the cervical spine during any anesthetic, surgical, or radiographic procedure. Patients who play sports or require clearance for physical activity generally have X-rays.

Symptomatic AAI results from subluxation (excessive slippage) that is severe enough to injure the spinal cord or from dislocation at the atlantoaxial joint. Symptoms may be difficult to elicit from the patient with DS due to developmental and cognitive delay (Box 19.1). Those patients who are symptomatic for AAI should have cervical spine X-rays in the neutral position. If these are normal, flexion and extension X-rays may be taken. It is important to keep in mind that X-rays are useful only in patients who are greater than 3 years old and have sufficient bone mineralization for the exam. Patients should also be referred to a neurosurgeon or orthopedic spine surgeon for consultation.[8,26]

There does not appear to be a high rate of complications related to AAI and anesthesia for DS patients. Review of the ASA closed claims database revealed 1 report of cervical injury in a DS patient.[30] The case involved a cervical nerve root injury from disc herniation, and the anesthesiologist was eventually dropped from the suit. Medline reports from 1966 to 2003 revealed only 2 reports of cervical injury related to direct laryngoscopy.[30]

The practitioner should continue to keep in mind general considerations for adenotonsillectomy in the patient with DS. Adenotonsillectomy is considered a procedure that is high risk for airway fire given the close proximity of a fuel source, an oxygen-enriched environment, and heat. Steps should be taken to minimize this risk, including close communication with the surgeon throughout the procedure, use of the lowest possible oxygen concentration to prevent hypoxia, avoidance of nitrous oxide, use of a cuffed ETT, and most of all, vigilance by all personnel.[31]

Postoperatively, the patient should be monitored for complications, which include uncontrolled pain, poor oral intake, hemorrhage, acute obstruction, and pulmonary edema. Patients should receive aggressive prophylaxis for postoperative nausea and vomiting and should be well hydrated with IV fluids. Dexamethasone has long been used to decrease postoperative nausea and vomiting, decrease airway edema, improve pain control, and has not been associated with clinically significant bleeding.[32] Small doses of IV opioids as needed for pain may be necessary in the early postoperative period. Recent Food and Drug Administration black box warnings for codeine and tramadol have limited their use for postoperative analgesia.[33,34] Acetaminophen and nonsteroidal antiinflammatory drugs, with the exception of ketorolac, have not been definitively shown to increase the risk of surgical bleeding in adenotonsillectomy and are, therefore, an acceptable choice for pain control without respiratory depression.[35,36] Intraoperative dexmedetomidine may be used as an analgesic adjunct and has also been shown to help with emergence delirium.[37] Some surgeons will also inject local anesthetic into the tonsillar beds, which has been shown to reduce pain.[38]

Posttonsillectomy bleeding can be categorized as primary (occurs within 24 hours of surgery) or secondary (within the first postoperative week when the eschar separates from the tonsillar fossa). Bleeding is typically venous in origin but may be brisk, and estimates of blood loss are often inaccurate as large amounts of blood can be swallowed.[39] Important anesthetic considerations include (a) assessment for hypovolemia and adequate volume resuscitation prior to induction; (b) a potentially difficult airway that is obscured by bleeding in the oropharynx; and (c) a high aspiration risk from blood in the stomach, and possibly food if NPO times are inadequate.[40] Laboratory hematologic evaluation as well as possible transfusion with type-specific or with O-negative blood in emergency situations should be considered. The anesthesia provider should be prepared to perform a rapid sequence intubation with a cuffed ETT and have multiple suction set-ups in case of clots. Adequate IV access is imperative. Even if the patient has a lull in bleeding, clots may destabilize at any point and bleeding resume prior to surgical cauterization; OR staff should be scrubbed and ready to go with all instruments.[40]

REVIEW QUESTIONS

1. A 5-year-old, 13 kg, patient with DS presents for strabismus surgery. She has a history of atrial septal defect, severe developmental delay, and heavy snoring. There are no records available for her. Of the following, the **MOST** appropriate next step in her preoperative evaluation is:

A. Order a complete blood count.
B. Obtain an echocardiogram.
C. Perform a visual exam.
D. Schedule a hearing test.

Answer: B
Preoperative echocardiogram is indicated to assess her atrial septal defect and cardiac function, as well as look for evidence

---

Box 19.1 **SYMPTOMS OF ATLANTOAXIAL INSTABILITY**

Syncope
Head tilt, torticollis
Neck pain, radicular pain
Sensory deficit
Change in muscle tone, weakness, spasticity
Gait abnormality, clumsiness, fatigability
Change in bowel or bladder function
Hyperreflexia, clonus, Babinski

of pulmonary hypertension or right ventricular overload from chronic left-to-right shunting through her septal defect. Visual exam, hearing test, and hematologic assessment, while part of recommended preventative screening tests for patients with DS, are not indicated as routine preoperative testing.

2. A 2-year-old patient with achondroplasia and a history of closed ventricular septal defect presents for adenotonsillectomy for severe OSA. Of the following factors, which contributes the **LEAST** to an increased risk of postoperative respiratory complications?

  A. achondroplasia
  B. age at the time of surgery
  C. ventricular septal defect
  D. severe OSA

Answer: C
Age <3 years, craniofacial abnormalities, and severe sleep apnea all increase the risk of postoperative respiratory complications.

3. You are scheduled to deliver the anesthetic for an otherwise healthy 7-year-old patient getting an adenotonsillectomy. An OR fire happened recently at your hospital. Your surgeon approaches you about decreasing the risk of airway fire during the case. Of the following, the **MOST** appropriate action would be:

  A. limiting the inspired oxygen concentration to 21%.
  B. limiting fresh gas flow of oxygen to 2 L/min.
  C. limiting the inspired nitrous oxide concentration to less than 30%.
  D. placing an uncuffed ETT that is sized to achieve no air leak above 30 cm H_2O.

Answer: A
Operating room fires require the triad of heat, fuel, and an oxygen-enriched environment. Adenotonsillectomy cases pose an increased risk of airway fire, given the close proximity to each other of all three elements. Limiting the inspired oxygen concentration to the minimum necessary to prevent hypoxia, close communication with the surgical and OR staff, draping the patient to prevent pockets of oxygen-enriched air, avoidance of nitrous oxide, and complete drying of surgical prep solutions are all steps in the prevention of OR fires. Limiting the fresh gas flow of oxygen to 2 L/min is not relevant without knowing the concentration of oxygen. While minimizing air leak may prevent oxygen escaping to the surgical field, placing an uncuffed ETT with no leak above 30 cm H_2O may lead to tracheal ischemia.

4. A 10-year-old, 40 kg patient presents to the emergency room with oral bleeding. He had his tonsils removed 5 days ago. The surgeons want to take him urgently to the OR for cauterization of the tonsillar beds. The **MOST** appropriate next management step would be:

  A. assessment of NPO status to determine a safe start time.
  B. empiric transfusion of 1 unit O-negative packed red blood cells.

  C. examination of the oropharynx to assess level of bleeding.
  D. volume resuscitation with 20 mL/kg of isotonic crystalloid solution.

Answer: D
The patient requires volume resuscitation prior to induction of anesthesia. There may be a large amount of occult blood loss as patients can swallow large amounts of blood. The patient is considered to have a full stomach and consideration of NPO times is irrelevant. While the patient may eventually require blood transfusion, empiric transfusion in the absence of further information, such as vital signs and labs, potentially exposes the patient unnecessarily to the risks of transfusion.

5. You are seeing a 6-year-old patient with DS in the preoperative clinic. She is scheduled for neck dissection for excision of a mass. Which of the following is the **MOST** appropriate initial step for assessment of her cervical spine?

  A. screening for cervical pain and radiculopathy
  B. consultation with a neurologist
  C. electromyographic studies
  D. flexion-extension cervical spine X-rays

Answer: A
Current AAP guidelines do not recommend routine cervical spine X-rays to screen for atlantoaxial stability in asymptomatic patients with DS. Consultation with a neurologist and electromyographic studies are not part of initial workup.

6. A 3-year-old patient with a history of tricuspid atresia and bidirectional Glenn shunt at 5 months of age is scheduled for adenotonsillectomy for recurrent streptococcus pharyngitis. Which of the following factors **MOST** determines the need for prophylaxis for IE in this patient?

  A. diagnosis of tricuspid atresia
  B. cardiac surgery less than 6 years ago
  C. history of bacterial infections
  D. otolaryngology procedure

Answer: A
American Heart Association guidelines recommend antibiotic prophylaxis for IE only when high risk patients undergo high-risk surgical procedures. This patient has unrepaired cyanotic CHD with a palliative shunt and is undergoing adenotonsillectomy.

7. A full-term baby is born via vaginal delivery. After birth, he is noted to have physical features consistent with DS, and genetic analysis confirms the diagnosis. The **MOST** appropriate next step for screening for comorbid conditions is:

  A. abdominal contrast study to evaluate for duodenal atresia.
  B. bone marrow biopsy to evaluate for myeloproliferative disease.
  C. cervical spine X-rays for evaluation of AAI.
  D. echocardiogram to evaluate for CHD.

Answer: D
AAP guidelines for DS patients recommend an echocardiogram at birth to assess for CHD. Cervical spine X-rays at this age will not provide an evaluation for AAI. Duodenal atresia typically presents with vomiting within hours of life. Bone marrow biopsy is inappropriate without a clinical suspicion for myeloproliferative disease.

QUESTIONS AND ANSWERS

This chapter has accompanying questions and answers which are available to subscribers as part of the Oxford eLearning platform. To access the questions, go to ✓ http://oxfordmedicine. com/pediatricanesthesiaPBL

REFERENCES

1. Parker SE, Mai CT, Canfield MA, et al. Updated National Birth Prevalence estimates for selected birth defects in the United States, 2004–2006. *Birth Defects Res A Clin Mol Teratol.* 2010;88(12):1008–1016. doi:10.1002/bdra.20735
2. Presson AP, Partyka G, Jensen KM, et al. Current estimate of Down syndrome population prevalence in the United States. *J Pediatr.* 2013;163(4):1163–1168. doi:10.1016/j.jpeds.2013.06.013
3. Mai CT, Kucik JE, Isenburg J, et al. Selected birth defects data from population-based birth defects surveillance programs in the United States, 2006 to 2010: featuring trisomy conditions. *Birt Defects Res A Clin Mol Teratol.* 2013;97(11):709–725. doi:10.1002/bdra.23198
4. Chin CJ, Khami MM, Husein M. A general review of the otolaryngologic manifestations of Down syndrome. *Int J Pediatr Otorhinolaryngol.* 2014;78(6):899–904. doi:10.1016/j.ijporl.2014.03.012
5. King K, O'Gorman C, Gallagher S. Thyroid dysfunction in children with Down syndrome: a literature review. *Ir J Med Sci.* 2013;183(1):1–6. doi:10.1007/s11845-013-0994-y
6. Watts R, Vyas H. An overview of respiratory problems in children with Down's syndrome. *Arch Dis Child.* 2013;98(10):812–817. doi:10.1136/archdischild-2013-304611
7. Hwang SW, Jea A. A review of the neurological and neurosurgical implications of Down syndrome in children. *Clin Pediatr.* 2013;52(9):845–856. doi:10.1177/0009922813491311
8. Bull MJ. Health supervision for children with Down syndrome. *Pediatrics.* 2011;128(2):393–406. doi:10.1542/peds.2011-1605
9. Shott SR. Down syndrome: analysis of airway size and a guide for appropriate intubation. *Laryngoscope.* 2000;110(4):585–592. doi:10.1097/00005537-200004000-00010
10. Shott SR. Down syndrome: common otolaryngologic manifestations. *Am J Med Genet C Semin Med Genet.* 2006;142C(3):131–140. doi:10.1002/ajmg.c.30095
11. Marcus CL, Brooks LJ, Draper KA, et al. Diagnosis and management of childhood obstructive sleep apnea syndrome. *Pediatrics.* 2012;130(3):576–584. doi:10.1542/peds.2012-1671
12. Beck SE, Marcus CL. Pediatric polysomnography. *Sleep Med Clin.* 2009;4(3):393–406. doi:10.1016/j.jsmc.2009.04.007
13. King P, Tulloh R. Management of pulmonary hypertension and Down syndrome. *Int J Clin Pract Suppl.* 2011;(174):8–13. doi:10.1111/j.1742-1241.2011.02823.x
14. McDowell KM, Craven DI. Pulmonary complications of Down syndrome during childhood. *J Pediatr.* 2011;158(2):319–325. doi:10.1016/j.jpeds.2010.07.023
15. Lal C, White DR, Joseph JE, van Bakergem K, LaRosa A. Sleep-disordered breathing in Down syndrome. *Chest.* 2015;147(2):570–579. doi:10.1378/chest.14-0266
16. Freeman SB, Taft LF, Dooley KJ, et al. Population-based study of congenital heart defects in Down syndrome. *Am J Med Genet.* 1998;80(3):213–217.doi:10.1002/(SICI)1096-8628(19981116)80:3<213::AID-AJMG6>3.0.CO;2-8
17. Hoffman JIE, Kaplan S. The incidence of congenital heart disease. *J Am Coll Cardiol.* 2002;39(12):1890–1900. doi:10.1016/S0735-1097(02)01886-7
18. Kucik JE, Shin M, Siffel C, Marengo LK, Correa A. Trends in survival among children with Down syndrome in 10 regions of the United States. *Pediatrics.* 2013;131(1):e27–e36.
19. Al-Biltagi MA. Echocardiography in children with Down syndrome. *World J Clin Pediatr.* 2013;2(4):36–45. doi:10.5409/wjcp.v2.i4.36
20. Atz AM, Hawkins JA, Lu M, et al. Surgical management of complete atrioventricular septal defect: associations with surgical technique, age, and trisomy 21. *J Thorac Cardiovasc Surg.* 2011;141(6):1371–1379. doi:10.1016/j.jtcvs.2010.08.093
21. Wilson W, Taubert KA, Gewitz M, et al. Prevention of infective endocarditis: guidelines from the American Heart Association: a guideline from the American Heart Association Rheumatic Fever, Endocarditis, and Kawasaki Disease Committee, Council on Cardiovascular Disease in the Young, and the Council on Clinical Cardiology, Council on Cardiovascular Surgery and Anesthesia, and the Quality of Care and Outcomes Research Interdisciplinary Working Group. *Circulation.* 2007;116(15):1736–1754. doi:10.1161/CIRCULATIONAHA.106.183095
22. Allen U. Infective endocarditis: updated guidelines. *Can J Infect Dis Med Microbiol.* 2010;21(2):74–77.
23. Bai W, Voepel-Lewis T, Malviya S. Hemodynamic changes in children with Down syndrome during and following inhalation induction of anesthesia with sevoflurane. *J Clin Anesth.* 2010;22(8):592–597. doi:10.1016/j.jclinane.2010.05.002
24. Kraemer FW, Stricker PA, Gurnaney HG, et al. Bradycardia during induction of anesthesia with sevoflurane in children with Down syndrome: *Anesth Analg.* 2010;111(5):1259–1263. doi:10.1213/ANE.0b013e3181f2eacf
25. Sulemanji DS, Donmez A, Akpek EA, Alic Y. Vascular catheterization is difficult in infants with Down syndrome. *Acta Anaesthesiol Scand.* 2009;53(1):98–100. doi:10.1111/j.1399-6576.2008.01804.x
26. Fitness C on SM and. Atlantoaxial instability in Down syndrome: subject review. *Pediatrics.* 1995;96(1):151–154.
27. Cremers MJ, Ramos L, Bol E, van Gijn J. Radiological assessment of the atlantoaxial distance in Down's syndrome. *Arch Dis Child.* 1993;69(3):347–350.
28. Radhakrishnan R, Towbin AJ. Imaging findings in Down syndrome. *Pediatr Radiol.* 2014;44(5):506–521.doi:10.1007/s00247-013-2859-y
29. Hata T, Todd MM. Cervical spine considerations when anesthetizing patients with Down syndrome. *J Am Soc Anesthesiol.* 2005;102(3):680–685.
30. Hindman BJ, Palecek JP, Posner KL, et al. Cervical spinal cord, root, and bony spine injuries: a closed claims analysis. *Anesthesiology.* 2011;114(4):782–795. doi:10.1097/ALN.0b013e3182104859
31. Apfelbaum JL, Caplan RA, Barker SJ, et al. Practice advisory for the prevention and management of operating room fires: an updated report by the American Society of Anesthesiologists Task Force on Operating Room Fires. *Anesthesiology.* 2013;118(2):271–290. doi:10.1097/ALN.0b013e31827773d2
32. Gallagher TQ, Hill C, Ojha S, et al. Perioperative dexamethasone administration and risk of bleeding following tonsillectomy in children: a randomized controlled trial. *JAMA.* 2012;308(12):1221–1226. doi:10.1001/2012.jama.11575
33. Weaver JM. New FDA Black Box warning for codeine: how will this affect dentists? *Anesth Prog.* 2013;60(2):35–36. doi:10.2344/0003-3006-60.2.35
34. FDA Drug Safety Communication. FDA restricts use of prescription codeine pain and cough medicines and tramadol pain medicines in children; recommends against use in breastfeeding women. https://www.fda.gov/Drugs/DrugSafety/ucm549679.htm. Accessed February 19, 2018.

35. Riggin L, Ramakrishna J, Sommer DD, Koren G. A 2013 updated systematic review and meta-analysis of 36 randomized controlled trials; no apparent effects of non steroidal anti-inflammatory agents on the risk of bleeding after tonsillectomy. *Clin Otolaryngol Off J ENT-UK Off J Neth Soc Oto-Rhino-Laryngol Cervico-Facial Surg.* 2013;38(2):115–129. doi:10.1111/coa.12106

36. Lewis SR, Nicholson A, Cardwell ME, Siviter G, Smith AF. Nonsteroidal anti-inflammatory drugs and perioperative bleeding in paediatric tonsillectomy. *Cochrane Database Syst Rev.* 2013;7:CD003591. doi:10.1002/14651858.CD003591.pub3

37. Zhang C, Hu J, Liu X, Yan J. Effects of intravenous dexmedetomidine on emergence agitation in children under sevoflurane anesthesia: a meta-analysis of randomized controlled trials. *PloS One.* 2014;9(6):e99718. doi:10.1371/journal.pone.0099718

38. Grainger J, Saravanappa N. Local anaesthetic for post-tonsillectomy pain: a systematic review and meta-analysis. *Clin Otolaryngol Off J ENT-UK Off J Neth Soc Oto-Rhino-Laryngol Cervico-Facial Surg.* 2008;33(5):411–419. doi:10.1111/j.1749–4486.2008.01815.x

39. Windfuhr JP, Chen Y-S. Incidence of post-tonsillectomy hemorrhage in children and adults: a study of 4,848 patients. *Ear Nose Throat J.* 2002;81(9):626–628, 630, 632.

40. Fields RG, Gencorelli FJ, Litman RS. Anesthetic management of the pediatric bleeding tonsil. *Paediatr Anaesth.* 2010;20(11):982–986. doi:10.1111/j.1460-9592.2010.03426.x

20.

CLEFT PALATE, CLEFT LIP, AND PIERRE ROBIN SEQUENCE

Michelle Keese Harvey and Ihab Ayad

STEM CASE AND KEY QUESTIONS

A 10-month old, 8 kg male with Pierre Robin Sequence presents for cleft palate repair. He was born full term at 39 weeks and had respiratory distress and feeding difficulties in the neonatal period.

WHAT IS PIERRE ROBIN SEQUENCE (PRS)? HOW IS NEONATAL AIRWAY OBSTRUCTION IN PRS MANAGED?

In the neonatal intensive care unit, frequent desaturations during sleep did not resolve with lateral or prone positioning, but placement of a nasopharyngeal airway did decrease the frequency of airway obstruction.

WHAT ARE THE TREATMENT OPTIONS FOR PRS PATIENTS? HOW WOULD YOU APPROACH AIRWAY MANAGEMENT FOR SURGERY IN THE NEONATE WITH PRS?

He underwent bilateral mandibular distraction osteogenesis at 4 weeks of age. An otolaryngologic surgeon was present for induction of anesthesia and performed a direct laryngoscopy and bronchoscopy with the patient spontaneously ventilating to rule out laryngotracheomalacia. The trachea was intubated by the otolaryngologic surgeon with a 3.5 uncuffed oral Ring-Adair-Elwyn (RAE) endotracheal tube (ETT) with a grade 3 view of the glottis with the Parsons laryngoscope. He was successfully extubated on postoperative day 6, and mandibular distraction continued through postoperative day 14.

WHAT IS CLEFT PALATE? HOW WOULD YOU ASSESS THE AIRWAY PREOPERATIVELY FOR REPAIR OF THE CLEFT?

At 3 months of age, he returned for removal of the distractors. At that time, the patient was kept spontaneously ventilating through an intravenous (IV) induction, and a grade 2b view of the glottis was obtained with a Miller 1 blade. Since discharge, he has been doing well with some noisy breathing during sleep but no signs of sleep apnea or desaturations. He currently has clear rhinorrhea.

HOW WOULD YOU EVALUATE THIS PATIENT'S RHINORRHEA? WOULD YOU POSTPONE SURGERY FOR POSSIBLE UPPER RESPIRATORY TRACT INFECTION (URI)?

He has no fever, cough, or evidence of ear discomfort. He has had no sick contacts and often has rhinorrhea per parents' report. Prior to entering the operating suite, the patient is premedicated with oral midazolam for anxiolysis with good effect.

HOW WOULD YOU INDUCE ANESTHESIA? WHAT IS YOUR PLAN FOR AIRWAY MANAGEMENT?

He is induced by mask with sevoflurane and oxygen and is kept spontaneously ventilating until an IV line is established. Manual ventilation is easily achieved. He is intubated with a 4.0 uncuffed oral RAE ETT using video laryngoscopy with a grade 2 view. The ETT is sutured in place by the surgeon, as well as securely taped to the lower jaw using liquid adhesive and tape. The bed is turned 90 degrees to the right away from the anesthesia machine.

WHAT NERVE BLOCKS CAN BE USED FOR PAIN MANAGEMENT FOR CLEFT PALATE REPAIR?

The patient receives rectal acetaminophen as well as IV dexamethasone. A suprazygomatic maxillary nerve block is performed. The face is prepped. An oral retractor is placed along with a throat pack.

WHAT ARE YOUR INTRAOPERATIVE CONCERNS FOR THE PATIENT HAVING CLEFT PALATE REPAIR?

During placement of the retractor, tidal volumes acutely decrease. The retractor is readjusted to relieve kinking of the ETT. Maintenance of anesthesia proceeds with sevoflurane in air/oxygen and morphine boluses. Halfway during the case, there is sudden loss of airway pressure and end-tidal carbon dioxide due to inadvertent extubation.

WHAT IS YOUR AIRWAY MANAGEMENT PLAN FOR EMERGENT REINTUBATION?

The patient is emergently reintubated after several attempts using video laryngoscopy and a fresh ETT with intermittent mask ventilation. The case proceeds quickly. At the end of the case, a tongue stitch is placed by the surgeon. The throat pack is removed, and the stomach is suctioned with an orogastric tube. The bed is turned back 90 degrees toward the anesthesia machine.

WHAT IS YOUR PLAN FOR EMERGENCE? WHAT ARE YOUR POSTOPERATIVE CONCERNS IN THIS PATIENT?

After a smooth emergence and extubation, the patient has noisy breathing and stertor. Upper airway obstruction is improved with pulling on the tongue stitch and with careful lateral positioning of the patient. The patient has an uneventful recovery in the postanesthesia care unit and is admitted to a monitored pediatric bed overnight.

DISCUSSION

PIERRE-ROBIN SEQUENCE

Etiology and clinical manifestation

Pierre Robin sequence is characterized by the triad of micrognathia, glossoptosis, and airway obstruction and is often associated with cleft palate. It is referred to as a sequence and not a syndrome because there is one inciting feature but multiple possible causes of that inciting feature. The abnormalities in PRS stem from mandibular hypoplasia in the ninth week of gestation that leads to posterior displacement of the tongue with improper retraction from between the palatal shelves as the palate is fusing (glossoptosis). This can occur spontaneously or as a result of oligohydramnios, genetic disorders, myotonia, or connective tissue disease. Pierre Robin sequence is usually an isolated finding, but one third of the time is associated with a syndrome, the most common being Stickler syndrome, velocardiofacial syndrome, Treacher-Collins syndrome, and fetal alcohol syndrome.[1]

The micrognathia and glossoptosis lead to airway obstruction and respiratory compromise, especially in the neonate. As they grow and the mandibular disproportion improves, the obstruction may improve, but this can take several months to a couple of years. Feeding difficulties are not uncommon, and many patients require a feeding tube or gastrostomy tube. Prolonged and repeated airway obstruction and respiratory distress can lead to failure to thrive, hypoxemia, pulmonary hypertension, cardiac arrest, and death if left untreated. Mortality rates increase significantly in PRS patients with other comorbid anomalies or syndromes.

Therapies for PRS

There are several treatment options for management of airway obstruction in PRS for the neonate. The choice of treatment depends on the severity of obstruction, comorbidities, and institutional preference. Conservative measures include lateral or prone positioning, nasopharyngeal airway placement, and nasal continuous positive airway pressure or intermittent mandatory ventilation. These are often used for mild to moderate obstruction and can temporize until the patient grows and obstruction improves. More invasive measures are sometimes needed for more severe obstruction. A flexible nasolaryngoscopy may be performed by an otolaryngologic surgeon to evaluate the severity and location of obstruction. It can also rule out other causes of obstruction such as laryngomalacia, vocal cord abnormalities, and choanal atresia. A direct laryngoscopy and bronchoscopy would need to be done to rule out tracheomalacia or other tracheal anomalies.[1] PRS patients may require intubation at or soon after birth. Longer lasting interventions include tongue–lip adhesion (TLA), mandibular distraction osteogenesis, and tracheostomy.

Tongue-lip adhesion is performed in some patients to alleviate airway obstruction from the posteriorly displaced tongue. The ventral tongue is sutured to the lower lip, including not just mucosa but also the genioglossus and orbicularis oris muscles. TLA is performed under general anesthesia with the patient often remaining intubated, sedated, and paralyzed during initial healing in the postoperative period. Extubation is performed days later in the operating room and another general anesthetic is required to take down the TLA, usually before the patient reaches 1 year of age.[1] Glossopexy is slightly different, with the base of the tongue being sutured to the mandible. Both of these interventions are reversible but seem to be less effective or definitive than distraction osteogenesis or tracheostomy.

Mandibular distraction osteogenesis is gaining popularity in infants with severe obstruction and in syndromic PRS. It can be used as an alternative to tracheostomy or as a means of facilitating decannulation in a child with a tracheostomy. An osteotomy is made near the angle of the mandible with a distraction device inserted between two portions of the mandible. Turning arms expand this section over a period of 2–3 weeks, allowing for new bone formation and a gradual elongation of the mandible. Mandibular distraction osteogenesis allows patients to avoid tracheostomy, usually resolves sleep apnea, and may even improve the ability to feed orally and help patients avoid gastrostomy tube placement. Like TLA, mandibular distraction osteogenesis also carries the risk of 2 general anesthetics, 1 to place the distractors and 1 to remove them after 12–16 weeks. Other risks include tooth loss or malformation, nerve damage, blood loss, and hypertrophic scarring.[2]

Tracheostomy is an option for patients with severe obstruction, especially when combined with a syndrome or neurologic deficits. It bypasses the supraglottic obstruction and provides a secure airway. Risks of tracheostomy include accidental decannulation, mucous plugging, recurrent infection, and bleeding at the stoma, as well as long-term effects on proper speech and swallowing development.

Airway management in PRS

In a patient with PRS, the possibility of difficult mask ventilation and/or intubation should always be considered. For the stable patient with anticipated difficult airway, adequate supplies, backup equipment, and personnel should always be made available.

During an elective intubation in the operating room, neonates or infants with an anticipated difficult airway should have an IV line placed, positioning optimized, and IV or inhaled anesthetics given with the goal of maintaining spontaneous ventilation. After preoxygenation, several different agents can be used for induction as long as they are carefully titrated. Common choices include sevoflurane in 100% oxygen, dexmedetomidine, ketamine, and propofol. Once the patient is adequately sedated/anesthetized, the ability to give positive pressure ventilation needs to be determined. If there is difficulty with mask ventilation, possible interventions include lateral or prone positioning, an oral or nasopharyngeal airway, and a two-handed jaw thrust. If there is still difficulty with mask ventilation, consider placement of a laryngeal mask airway (LMA). The LMA can then be used to facilitate fiberoptic bronchoscopy.

Muscle relaxation may be considered once the ability to ventilate with positive pressure has been established. Next, an attempt may be made with an appropriately sized straight blade. If this is unsuccessful, attention should be directed toward optimizing laryngoscopy conditions if this has not yet been achieved, with the most experienced anesthesiologist attempting laryngoscopy. Serious consideration should be given toward using a video laryngoscope such as the Storz DCI, Storz CMAC, or Glidescope. As long as ventilation can be maintained between attempts, a fiberoptic intubation could also be attempted. If mask ventilation cannot be established, options include LMA placement for the duration of the procedure, waking the patient up, or proceeding with fiberoptic intubation (with or without LMA) while the patient is spontaneously ventilating. Success with awake LMA placement in the patient with PRS, followed by induction of anesthesia has been described.[3,4] If the previously discussed techniques fail, a pediatric otolaryngologic surgeon could perform rigid bronchoscopy. Emergency cricothyrotomy and surgical tracheostomy is very difficult in neonates and would be a last resort.

For the unstable patient or emergent intubation, there may not be time or resources for the previous sequence of events. Help should be requested as soon as possible. Any technique to temporize, including non-invasive positive pressure ventilation, hand mask ventilation, or LMA, is valuable while making a plan and obtaining resources. Nonsedated or non-premedicated direct laryngoscopy and tracheal intubation may be indicated in the apneic or unconscious patient but is more controversial in awake patients.

CLEFT LIP AND PALATE

Classification

Cleft lips are small gaps or indentations of the lips. They may be partial and only affect the lip or may be complete and extend to the nose. They may be unilateral or bilateral. Lips form during the fourth to seventh week of gestation, and clefts occur when there is failure of fusion of the maxillary and medial nasal processes.

Cleft palates are defects in the hard and/or soft palate that can be partial or complete and unilateral or bilateral. The primary palate, located anterior to the incisive foramen, forms during the fifth to sixth week of gestation from the fusion of the medial nasal, lateral nasal, and maxillary processes. The secondary palate is formed from the palatal shelves which fuse around 7–12 weeks gestational age. Around this time, with extension of the head and mandibular growth, the tongue is withdrawn from between the shelves, and they can then fuse in the midline forming the hard and soft palate. Incomplete cleft palates involve the secondary palate, while complete cleft palates involve the primary and secondary palates.

The incidence of orofacial clefts is about 1 in every 500–750 births. Cleft lips are more common in males, whereas isolated cleft palates are more common in females. Cleft lip is involved in two thirds of patients with a cleft; the other one third of patients have isolated cleft palates. Orofacial clefts may be associated with a syndrome, such as PRS, Treacher Collins syndrome, velocardiofacial syndrome, or Stickler syndrome. Orofacial clefts can cause problems with feeding, ear infections, hearing, and speech.

Surgical repair and management

The goal of cleft lip repair is to achieve good function and aesthetics. Cleft lips are generally repaired around 2–3 months. Some institutions use the rule of 10s, waiting until the infant is 10 weeks old, 10 pounds, and has a hemoglobin level of 10 g/dL. One common technique used is a Millard repair, which involves rotation advancement and closure of a unilateral defect. Patients usually stay in the hospital overnight, and elbow restraints may be used for a week to prevent disruption of the sutures.

The goal of cleft palate repair is to obtain good palatal function, normal hearing, normal speech and swallowing, and optimal dental and jaw growth. The repair is generally done between 6 and 12 months. Earlier repair allowing for intact function of the velum and palate before speech development is ideal. However, in younger patients, surgical repair is more difficult, and the negative effects on facial growth are more pronounced. Common techniques include two-flap palatoplasty or Furlow Z-plasty. Many patients only require 1 surgery, but sometimes it is staged into 2 procedures. Patients can develop oronasal fistulas or velopharyngeal insufficiency, requiring corrective surgery later in life as well. Patients are admitted after surgery, take a soft diet, and elbow restraints are often used postoperatively.

Preoperative considerations

A thorough history and physical examination should be performed preoperatively. Patients with isolated cleft lip are usually otherwise healthy, but a standard evaluation for URI symptoms, nil per os times, and family history of anesthetic complications should be done. Even with large or bilateral cleft lips, airway management is usually not difficult. In particular, a good seal with a face mask is not usually difficult to obtain.

For nonsyndromic patients presenting for cleft palate repair, there are a few more specific preoperative considerations. Anxious patients and parents are not uncommon. These patients interface frequently with medical professionals and may have more surgeries as well, so ensuring as positive an experience as possible is important. One should be sensitive to speech and hearing difficulties when communicating with the older patient. Chronic serous otitis and clear rhinorrhea are common due to eustachian tube dysfunction; however, any acute ear infection should be treated prior to surgery. Due to difficulty with feeding, nutritional status should be assessed. Patients should be evaluated for symptoms of airway obstruction, sleep apnea, congenital heart disease, and association with known syndromes. Syndromes associated with cleft palate include PRS, Treacher Collins syndrome, and Klippel Feil syndrome. Difficulty with the airway is more likely in syndromic patients, those with severe obstructive sleep apnea, right-sided clefts, and retrognathia.

The main concern in the case stem is the patient's his-tory of a difficult airway. Assessment of any patient with PRS should include a detailed history of any airway obstruction, noisy breathing, apneic episodes, and feeding difficulties. A thorough airway exam should be done if possible, paying close attention to the degree of retrognathia post-mandibular advancement. Prior anesthetic records should be carefully reviewed. Given that this patient has now grown, had a mandibular distraction, and was intubated recently without too much difficulty, one would expect intubation to be easier than prior. Based on prior anesthesia records, this does seem to be the case; however, it remains prudent to perform a thorough review and be prepared should difficulties arise.

Given the patient's rhinorrhea, another concern would be for a possible URI. Upper respiratory tract infection is associated with an increased risk of perioperative pulmonary complications such as apnea, bronchospasm, laryngospasm, prolonged coughing, and desaturation. Most of these complications can be easily recognized and treated. However, in the setting of cleft palate repair with possible postoperative swelling of the tongue and oropharynx, increased secretions, and bleeding, the risk may be somewhat higher. Also, if the patient's airway is challenging at baseline, treatment of these complications may be more difficult. Further, prolonged coughing is not ideal for wound healing after cleft palate repair.

A thorough evaluation of a possible URI including physical examination should be performed to determine the etiology of the symptoms, the severity of illness, and the risk of perioperative pulmonary complications. For example, presence of fever, sick contacts, eating/sleeping behavior, and copious or colored sputum can help determine if the etiology is infectious versus noninfectious (allergic rhinitis, vasomotor rhinitis, congestive heart failure, etc.). Clinical predictors of perioperative complications in children with URI include a history of prematurity, history of reactive airway disease, copious secretions, nasal congestion, and parental smoking.

Airway surgery and use of an ETT is also associated with increased risk, as is the parent's assessment of whether or not the patient has a "cold." In various studies, children with URIs were 2–11 times more likely to have perioperative pulmonary complications. In otherwise healthy patients, these seem to be easily recognized and treated and do not cause significant morbidity.[5]

The patient's entire clinical picture should be considered when determining whether to proceed with surgery in the setting of a URI. Of course, emergency surgery should not be postponed. In many patients with mild symptoms and minimal comorbidities, it is likely safe to proceed with appropriate anesthetic management and vigilance. In this particular patient, clear rhinorrhea without other symptoms of a URI is likely due to his cleft lip/palate and difficulty with handling secretions, so, after a thorough evaluation, proceeding with surgery would be reasonable.

Intraoperative considerations

Approaches to induction of anesthesia may vary. For this patient, we do not know if it was easy to mask ventilate him since he was kept spontaneously ventilating during induction in his previous anesthetic. One reasonable approach would be to mask induce him with sevoflurane, obtain an IV once he is in a deep plane of anesthesia, take over breathing to prove that he can be manually ventilated with positive pressure, paralyze, and then proceed with laryngoscopy. A Miller 1 blade could be used initially, but a video laryngoscope, LMA, and fiberoptic should be available for backup. An appropriately sized curved oral ETT (RAE) should be placed, if possible, to optimize surgical exposure and minimize the chances of the tube kinking with retractor placement.

Once the patient is induced and the airway is secured, airway complications can still occur. Close attention should be paid to the end-tidal carbon dioxide and peak airway pressures along with other vital signs since accidental extubation, disconnection of the circuit, and kinking of the ETT are common. This can happen throughout the procedure since the surgeons are working in the airway but especially during placement of the Dingman retractor and throat pack placement. Tidal volumes and peak pressures should be closely monitored. Since accidental extubation is always possible with surgery in such close quarters to the airway, appropriate equipment and a new styletted ETT should be prepared and easily accessible throughout the case.

Maintenance of anesthesia in these cases is usually a combination of oxygen, air, and sevoflurane with or without opioid boluses. Continued muscle relaxation is not usually necessary. Consider giving dexamethasone 0.5 mg/kg to decrease airway and palatal edema. Rectal acetaminophen 20–40 mg/kg can be administered at the beginning of the case. Temperature may be managed with a forced air warmer as long as the patient is kept well covered, though attention should be paid to not overwarming the patient. Fluid management with crystalloid is usually adequate; blood transfusion is rarely required.

Prior to emergence, the airway should be inspected for adequate hemostasis and for edema. A problem with either would warrant further intervention and/or keeping the patient intubated. A tongue stitch may be placed in those patients with anticipated airway obstruction during emergence and the immediate postoperative period. If the patient obstructs, gentle traction on the suture will lift the tongue off the back of the oropharynx. Placement of an oropharyngeal or nasopharyngeal airway should be avoided if possible. Once the throat pack is removed, orogastric suctioning is often done to remove any blood or gastric fluids from the stomach. Any additional suctioning should be done with a soft suction catheter, avoiding the suture lines. Elbow restraints may be placed prior to emergence to prevent the patient from reaching into the mouth and disrupting any sutures.

A smooth emergence is ideal to minimize hypertension, coughing, and gagging which can increase bleeding and disruption of sutures. This can be accomplished with opioids, small doses of ketamine, dexmedetomidine, or nitrous oxide, allowing for a smooth awake extubation with the patient breathing spontaneously and protecting his airway. A deep extubation may not be ideal in any difficult airway but also because of possible swelling of the tongue and airway as well as blood in the airway. Further, if any lip or nose repair has been done, a face mask may damage it, making the first line for rescue of an inadequate airway difficult.

Postoperative considerations

Concerns after a cleft palate repair include airway edema and obstruction, bleeding, prevention of palate dehiscence, and pain management. Airway edema can occur secondary to surgical manipulation, laryngoscopy and traumatic intubation, and fluid administration. This can lead to the airway being easily obstructed, especially in the presence of sedation and respiratory depression from pain medication, sedatives, and residual anesthetics. The patient should be closely observed and monitored. Possible interventions include supplemental oxygen, chin lift/jaw thrust, pulling on the tongue stitch, racemic epinephrine, dexamethasone if not given already, reversal of narcotics, and reintubation.

Multiple measures may be taken to prevent palate dehiscence. These include avoiding things like spoons, oral and nasal airways, and inflexible suction catheters that can physically disrupt sutures. Elbow restraints or "no-nos" can be used when the patient is unsupervised so they cannot reach into the mouth. On emergence from anesthesia and into the postoperative period, keeping pain and agitation to a minimum will help avoid excessive crying and coughing. The approach to feeding varies but usually includes only liquids and soft foods for a period of time.

Postoperative analgesia is important not only for patient comfort but also to prevent excessive agitation that can impair wound healing. This must be carefully balanced against the side effects of sedation and respiratory depression that can occur in these young patients who are prone to airway obstruction. A reasonable approach would include local anesthesia infiltration of the incision by the surgeon, rectal

acetaminophen around the clock, along with a long acting opioid, such as morphine as needed or via nurse-controlled analgesia. A multimodal approach could include nonsteroidal anti-inflammatory drugs, but their use is often delayed until 12–24 hours postoperatively to avoid possible bleeding complications. Some studies also suggest that intraoperative dexmedetomidine and/or ketamine administration can decrease postoperative opioid requirements.[6] Peripheral nerve blocks are also a good option for providing analgesia without the side effects of opioids.

Nerve blocks

For cleft lip repair, bilateral infraorbital nerve block has been shown in some studies to reduce postoperative pain, reduce opioid requirements, and even reduce emergence agitation.[7] A Cochrane review[8] of the literature in 2016 concluded that an infraorbital nerve block may reduce postoperative pain compared with placebo or other analgesics but stated that the quality of evidence is low given small sample sizes and heterogeneity of the studies' interventions and measured outcomes. The infraorbital nerve supplies the upper lip, lateral nose, medial cheek, and lower eyelid. This nerve is blocked as it exits the infraorbital foramen. Based on a cadaver study of infants by Bosenberg and Kimble,[9] this is located halfway between the midpoint of the palpebral fissure and the angle of the mouth, about 7.5 mm from the base of the nasal ala. A needle is inserted perpendicular to the skin, advanced until bone is felt, then local anesthetic is injected. A potential complication of the infraorbital nerve block is globe injury if the orbit is entered by the needle. Two studies found decreased time to first feeding after surgery, but, in one of these studies, the patients who received the block had more difficulty feeding though no decrease in the volume consumed.[10]

An external nasal nerve block may be needed for complete analgesia after a cleft lip repair. The external nasal nerve supplies the nasal ala and tip of the nose. It is blocked by injecting local anesthetic at the junction of the nasal bone and cartilage, about 5–7 mm off midline.

Multiple nerve blocks have been used for cleft palate repair including the suprazygomatic maxillary nerve block, greater and lesser palatine nerve block, and the nasopalatine nerve block. The suprazygomatic maxillary nerve block has gained popularity for being easy, reliable, and efficacious. This block anesthetizes the anterior and posterior palate, the dental arch, and the upper lip. A needle is inserted perpendicular to where the upper edge of the zygomatic arch and the posterior side of the orbital rim meet. The needle is then redirected toward the nasolabial fold and local anesthetic injected in the pterygopalatine fossa. This may be done under ultrasound guidance. Chiono et al.[11] found reduced morphine consumption at 48 hours in patients who received the block versus those who received a sham block. They also found a possible decrease in desaturation events requiring oxygen in those with the block.

The greater palatine nerve block anesthetizes the mucosa of the hard palate from its posterior end to the first premolar, while the lesser palatine nerve block anesthetizes the soft palate. Local anesthetic is injected about 1 cm medial to the junction of the second and third molar and will usually cover both nerves. The nasopalatine nerve block (incisive nerve block or sphenopalatine nerve block) anesthetizes the palate in the region of the upper front 6 teeth. It is blocked by injecting at the incisive foramen, so it cannot be performed in patients with a complete cleft palate.[12]

The choice of the previously discussed blocks will depend on patient anatomy, extent of surgery, and the anesthesiologist's preference and level of comfort. As with any regional technique in pediatric patients, local anesthetic toxicity is a potential risk. Not only should the dose be carefully considered, but the local anesthetic given by the surgeon for infiltration of the surgical site, whether at the beginning or end of the case, should be considered as well.

MULTIPLE-CHOICE QUESTIONS

1. An otherwise healthy 3-month-old male presents with bilateral cleft lip and palate and is scheduled for cleft lip repair. The exam is notable for a large cleft, retrognathia, and a nasoalveolar molding device in place. Which of the following findings is **LEAST** predictive of a difficult intubation?

    A. age of 3 months
    B. bilateral cleft lip
    C. bilateral cleft palate
    D. retrognathia

Answer: B
In nonsyndromic patients with cleft lip and/or palate, difficult intubation is associated with age less than 6 months, retrognathia, and large bilateral or right sided cleft palates. Right-sided cleft palates may cause more difficulty because the tip of the laryngoscope can fall into the cleft.[13]

2. Which of the following features is **LEAST** associated with PRS?

    A. airway obstruction
    B. cleft palate
    C. glossoptosis
    D. micrognathia

Answer: B
Cleft palate is common in PRS but is not part of the diagnostic triad. All patients must have airway obstruction to be diagnosed with PRS. Although the cause of the micrognathia varies, it is thought that the micrognathia leads to abnormal positioning of the tongue and both then contribute to airway obstruction.[1]

3. What is the **MOST** optimal age for repair of a cleft palate in an otherwise healthy full-term patient?

    A. 3 months
    B. 12 months
    C. 24 months
    D. 36 months

Answer: B
Of the choices, 12 months is most ideal. Timing of cleft palate repair is somewhat controversial. Most institutions perform repair between 6–12 months. Repair before language development is preferred so that speech may develop normally. However, there are concerns that earlier repair is associated with more inhibition of maxillary growth, which may affect facial appearance.[14]

4. One hour into a primary repair of a cleft palate in a patient who is intubated with a 3.5 mm oral RAE, the end-tidal carbon dioxide tracing is abruptly lost. Which of the following is **MOST** likely to have occurred?

    A. accidental extubation
    B. air embolism
    C. fat embolism
    D. mainstem intubation

Answer: A
During surgery on the airway in a small infant or child, there is a significant risk of accidental extubation, kinking of the ETT or circuit, advancement of the ETT causing mainstem intubation, mucous plugging, and disconnection of the ETT from the circuit. The patient should be closely monitored with backup airway equipment readily available. Air embolism and fat embolism are very unlikely in this age group undergoing this procedure. Mainstem intubation would not cause a loss of the end-tidal carbon dioxide tracing.

5. A neonate who has PRS suffers obstruction and failed conservative treatment. Which of the following procedures would **LEAST** likely be the next step in his management?

    A. TLA
    B. tracheostomy
    C. mandibular distraction
    D. Le Fort 1

Answer: D
Conservative management of airway obstruction in the neonate includes lateral or prone positioning, nasopharyngeal airway placement, and nasal continuous positive airway pressure or intermittent mandatory ventilation. When these interventions are not adequate, more invasive, long lasting intervention is often the next step. These include TLA, glossopexy, mandibular distraction osteogenesis, and tracheostomy. The Le Fort 1 procedure is used to correct midface deformities, including maxillary hypoplasia.[1]

6. Of the following possible surgical complications, which is **LEAST** likely to occur following mandibular distraction?

    A. hypertrophic scarring
    B. mandibular overgrowth
    C. nerve damage
    D. tooth loss

Answer: B
Complications of mandibular distraction osteogenesis include tooth loss or damage, damage to the marginal mandibular

branch of the facial nerve, and hypertrophic scarring. Other possible complications are temporomandibular joint ankylosis, infection, premature consolidation of the bone, instability of the distraction device, and failure of distraction.[2]

7. Which of the following nerve blocks would be **MOST** effective for a cleft lip repair?

    A. greater palatine nerve block
    B. infraorbital nerve block
    C. nasopalatine nerve block
    D. suprazygomatic maxillary nerve block

Answer: B
A bilateral infraorbital nerve block anesthetizes the upper lip, lateral nose, medial cheek, and lower eyelid. It will cover most of the area involved in a cleft lip repair. Depending on the extent of surgery, it can be supplemented by an external nasal nerve block that covers the nasal ala and tip of the nose. The other 3 blocks would be useful for cleft palate surgery.[12]

8. A 12-month-old who had an uneventful cleft palate repair arrives in the postanesthesia care unit. Ten minutes after arrival, he has obstructed breathing and hypoxemia despite being on face mask oxygen with an adequate respiratory rate. Which of the following would be the **MOST** appropriate next step?

    A. bag mask ventilate
    B. call the surgeon to the bedside
    C. pull on the tongue stitch
    D. reintubate

Answer: C
Many patients undergoing cleft palate repair, especially those with airway anomalies, will have a tongue stitch placed by the surgeon prior to emergence. The ends of the sutures are then taped to the cheek for easy access. If the patient obstructs and has respiratory distress as a result, a simple intervention is to pull on the tongue stitch to alleviate a possible etiology of the obstruction. The other interventions would all be helpful, but the quickest, least invasive next step would be to pull on the tongue stitch.

QUESTIONS AND ANSWERS

This chapter has accompanying questions and answers which are available to subscribers as part of the Oxford eLearning platform. To access the questions, go to ✓ http://oxfordmedicine.com/pediatricanesthesiaPBL

REFERENCES

1. Cladis F, Kumar A, Grunwaldt L, Otteson T, Ford M, Losee JE. Pierre Robin sequence: a perioperative review. *Anesth Analg.* 2014;119(2):400–412.
2. Scott AR, Tibesar RJ, Lander TA, Sampson DE, Sidman JD. Mandibular distraction osteogenesis in infants younger than 3 months. *Arch Facial Plast Surg.* 2011;13(3):173–179.
3. Stricker, PA, Budac, S, Fiadjoe, JE, Rehman, MA. Awake laryngeal mask insertion followed by induction of anesthesia in infants with the Pierre Robin sequence. *Acta Anaesthesiol Scand.* 2008;52:1307–1308.
4. Templeton TW, Bryan YF. A two-stage approach to induction and intubation of two infants with Pierre Robin sequence using a LMA Classic and Air-Q: two cases report. *Korean J Anesthesiol.* 2016;69(4):390–394.
5. Tait AR, Malviya S. Anesthesia for the child with an upper respiratory tract infection: still a dilemma? *Anesth Analg.* 2005;100:59–65.
6. Kayyal TA, Wolfswinkel EM, Weathers WM, et al. Treatment effects of dexmedetomidine and ketamine on postoperative analgesia after cleft palate repair. *Craniomaxillofac Trauma Reconstr.* 2014;7(2)131–138.
7. Wang H, Liu G, Fu W, Li, S-T. The effect of infraorbital nerve block on emergence agitation in children undergoing cleft lip surgery under general anesthesia with sevoflurane. *Pediatr Anesth.* 2015;25:906–910.
8. Feriani G, Hatanaka E, Torloni MR, da Silva EMK. Infraorbital nerve block for postoperative pain following cleft lip repair in children. *Cochrane Database Sys Rev.* 2016;4:CD011131.
9. Bosenberg AT, Kimble FW. Infraorbital nerve block in children: a computerized tomographic measurement of the location of the infraorbital foramen. *Reg Anesth Pain Med.* 2006;31:211–214.
10. Simion C, Corcoran, J, Iyer A, Suresh S. Postoperative pain control for primary cleft lip repair in infants: is there an advantage in performing peripheral nerve blocks? *Pediatr Anesth.* 2008;18:1060–1065.
11. Chiono J, Raux O, Bringuier S, et al. Bilateral suprazygomatic maxillary nerve block for cleft palate repair in children: a prospective, randomized, double-blind study versus placebo. *Anesthesiology.* 2014;120(6):1362–1369.
12. Reena, Bandyopadhyay KH, Paul A. Postoperative analgesia for cleft lip and palate repair in children. *J Anaesthesiol Clin Pharmacol.* 2016;32:5–11.
13. Gregory GA, Andropoulos DB. *Gregory's Pediatric Anesthesia.* 5th Ed. Sussex, UK: Wiley-Blackwell; 2012.
14. Colbert SD, Green B, Brennan PA, Mercer N. Contemporary management of cleft lip and palate in the United Kingdom. Have we reached the turning point? *Brit J Oral Max Surg.* 2015;53:594–598.

21.

CRANIOSYNOSTOSIS AND APERT SYNDROME

Petra M. Meier and Thomas O. Erb

STEM CASE AND KEY QUESTIONS

In a male fetus, craniofacial malformations are diagnosed by prenatal ultrasound. The parents are told that their unborn baby does not have fingers or toes and also has frontal protrusion. The baby is delivered via cesarean section at 37 weeks gestational age, with a weight of 2.9 kg, to a 36-year-old G1P0 mother and 33-year-old father. After delivery, the baby is clinically diagnosed with Apert syndrome based on apparent craniofacial malformations associated with finger and toe syndactyly. The physical examination reveals a brachycephalic head shape, large anterior fontanelle, prominent high broad forehead, retrusive midface hypoplasia, and protruding, down-slanting eyes with shallow orbits. He has a depressed nasal bridge. The ears are low set and posteriorly rotated but well formed. The mouth has a high-arched palate. The neck is normal. There is cutaneous and bony fusion of all 5 digits, including thumbs and the great toes. Neurologic examination is within normal range. Genetic testing confirms Apert syndrome.

WHAT IS CRANIOSYNOSTOSIS? WHAT ARE THE MOST IMPORTANT ASSOCIATED SYNDROMES? WHAT IS APERT SYNDROME? WHAT ARE THE ASSOCIATED ABNORMALITIES?

He is admitted to the neonatal intensive care unit for 2 weeks and requires continuous positive airway pressure (CPAP) because of recurrent desaturations (peripheral capillary oxygen saturation down to 60s), grunting, and retractions. He has frequent premature atrial contractions and short runs of wide complex tachycardia at rates of over 200 bpm of unclear etiology. He is treated with propranolol, and the arrhythmias resolve. There is no family history of craniofacial malformations. A family meeting is scheduled by the Craniofacial Clinic and Plastics Clinic to discuss a treatment plan for feeding management as well as sequencing of surgical procedures for the craniofacial malformation and the complex pan-syndactyly type III.

PRESENT A TREATMENT ALGORITHM FOR APERT SYNDROME.

Because of problems with suction and swallowing, he requires a gastrostomy tube as a neonate. At 6 weeks of age,

computed tomography (CT) scans confirms bilateral coronal synostosis.

WHAT ARE THE SURGICAL TREATMENT OPTIONS FOR CRANIOSYNOSTOSIS?

At 8 weeks of age and a weight of 4.2 kg, the first-stage procedure, a bilateral coronal endoscopic strip craniectomy (ESC), is performed, followed by helmet therapy, to mitigate the progression of turricephaly. During the following 2 years, he does well, including an excellent correction of his skull shape, and his neurological exams are within normal range. Multiple hand and feet syndactyly releases are performed, ear tubes are placed twice, and his severe V-pattern strabismus is corrected. At 2 years of age, his head circumference is approximately at the 60th percentile. The CT shows no sign of Chiari malformation; however, the majority of sutures start to fuse except those where the coronal sutures have been released. The brain is judged to still have enough space for development. During a regular follow-up visit at 2.5 years of age, eye examination reveals mild exorbitism and disk edema with progressive tortuosity of veins, indicative of the development of increased ICP. His head circumference is at the 50th percentile. Fusions are diagnosed: both lambdoid sutures and the metopic suture are affected, and there is partial fusion of one of the coronal sutures. Based on these findings, the child has been scheduled for fronto-orbital advancement (bilateral frontal craniectomy, orbital bandeau removal and parietal temporal barrel stave osteotomies), ear tubes, and adenoidectomy. The child and his parents are evaluated in the preoperative anesthesia clinic.

WHAT WORKUP WOULD YOU REQUEST DURING EVALUATION IN THE PREOPERATIVE ANESTHESIA CLINIC?

He weighs 14.2 kg, measures 94 cm in height, and is in no acute distress. His parents state that he is snoring with witnessed apneic pauses every night. He is waking frequently and is a restless sleeper. He struggles with chronic nasal congestion and mouth breathing. He is noted to have a crowded oropharynx with a grooved palate, and it is difficult to visualize the back of his throat. He has very tight nasal cavities and approximately 2–3+ obstructing adenoids.

HOW WOULD YOU PLAN HIS ANESTHESIA AND INTRAOPERATIVE MANAGEMENT? WHAT MONITORS ARE INDICATED FOR MONITORING?

On the day of surgery, the patient presents unchanged from his preoperative evaluation. The patient is taken to the operating room. Monitors and lines (3 peripheral venous catheters, radial arterial line catheter) are placed, and the child is placed in a supine position. Maintenance of anesthesia includes fentanyl, a non-depolarizing muscle relaxant, and an inhalational agent in an oxygen/air mixture. The vital signs are blood pressure 92/55 mmHg, heart rate 145 beats per minute, oxygen saturation 99%, esophageal temperature 36.2°C, and the baseline arterial blood gas analysis shows, pH = 7.38, partial pressure of carbon dioxide = 38 mmHg, partial pressure of oxygen = 218 mmHg, hematocrit (HCT) = 35.9%, platelets = 177 x10^9/L, sodium = 135 mmol/l, potassium = 4.6 mmol/l, base excess = –3.5 mmol/l, and lactate = 0.8 mmol/l. Fibrinogen is 2.52 g/L (platelet fibrinogen product 446). The airway is successfully secured. The examination of the ears and adenoidectomy are performed by otolaryngologic surgeon. Thereafter, the surgical team starts the preparation of the skull. During the bicoronal scalp incision, there is continuous blood loss, which is substituted with crystalloids and albumin 5%. Twenty minutes into the bilateral frontal craniectomy, there is increased blood loss. A dopamine infusion is started at 5–10 μg/kg/min to treat hypotension, and blood is transfused. There is a significant amount of bleeding. HCT drops to 22%.

WHAT IS YOUR PLAN FOR FLUID MANAGEMENT AND BLOOD PRODUCT TRANSFUSION MANAGEMENT?

Multiple osteotomies are performed, including the use of a saw in the midline to ultimately remove the entire orbital bandeau. Thereafter, multiple barrel stave osteotomies are necessary to gain more space for the brain in the lateral axis. There is continuous brisk blood loss, and the massive transfusion protocol is activated. The blood pressure falls to 48/25 mmHg, heart rate increases to 180 beats per minute, and capnography drops from 35 to 26 mmHg. Blood and coagulation products are given rapidly. Suddenly, there are changes in the electrocardiogram (EKG), and there is a slight change in the Doppler sound. The patient is placed on 100% oxygen. The arterial line fails to provide an arterial trace. EKG shows ventricular tachycardia. Help is requested.

The rapidly drawn new arterial blood gas analysis shows: pH = 7.199, partial pressure of carbon dioxide in arterial blood = 31 mmHg, partial pressure of oxygen in arterial blood = 219 mmHg, HCT = 34%, platelets 157 x 10^9/L, sodium = 135 mmol/l, potassium = 7.23 mmol/l, calcium = 0.85 mmol/l, glucose = 154 mg/dL, lactate = 2.6 mmol/l, base excess = –10.4 mmol/l. Coagulopathy has not been corrected: prothrombin time (PT) = 19.3 sec (normal range 11.7–14.4 sec), partial thromboplastin time (PTT) = 31.7 (normal range 25–37 sec), international normalized ratio (INR) 1.7, and fibrinogen 0.96 g/L (platelet fibrinogen product 151).

WHAT IS YOUR DIAGNOSIS AND NEXT STEPS FOR MANAGEMENT?

After appropriate treatment, the patient is in sinus rhythm and blood pressure is now 83/35 mmHg. HCT is 24%. During calvarial remodeling, in which bone grafts are used, the patient is successfully stabilized, and the coagulopathy and metabolic acidosis are corrected. After placement of two drains, the scalp incision is closed, and the surgeon would like to perform a neurological examination at the conclusion of the surgery.

WHAT ARE YOUR POSTOPERATIVE CONSIDERATIONS?

Based on the stable course over the last hours you decide to extubate the patient in the operating room. With the patient fully awake this is achieved within a quarter of an hour. The airway is best stabilized with the patient in the lateral position when the patient is transferred to the Intensive Care Unit. Ongoing respiratory, hemodynamic and metabolic monitoring is needed in order to safeguard initial postoperative recovery.

DISCUSSION

CRANIOSYNOSTOSIS AND ASSOCIATED SYNDROMES

The estimate of prevalence of craniosynostosis ranges from 0.4 to 1 per 1,000 live births.[1,2] It is defined as a premature closure of 1 or more calvarial sutures with failure of normal growth perpendicular to the suture and compensatory overgrowth parallel to the affected suture. The abnormal cranial shape is determined by the specific sutures involved (Figure 21.1). The clinical diagnosis is confirmed by plain skull roentgenogram or CT scan. If left unrepaired, the resulting cranial defect may lead to intracranial hypertension, cerebral compression, impaired brain growth, auditory impairment,[3] visual loss,[4] and thus can have lifelong effects on neurocognitive development and appearance for the affected child.[5]

Classification

Craniosynostosis occurs as either an isolated single suture fusion (80%) or as multiple fusions (20%) that can be syndromic or non-syndromic. Sagittal craniosynostosis is the most common form (sagittal: 50%–60%, coronal 20%, metopic 10%–20%). Increased intracranial pressure (ICP) can occur in 14%–24% of infants with single sutural synostosis and in 40%–70% of those with syndromic craniosynostoses.[6-8] The etiology of most cases is sporadic. Genetic mutations described to be responsible for the syndromic craniosynostoses include mutations in the fibroblast growth factors receptor (FGFR1, FGFR2, FGFR3), TWIST, and MSX2 genes. Multiple suture closure is often associated with premature closure of the base skull sutures.

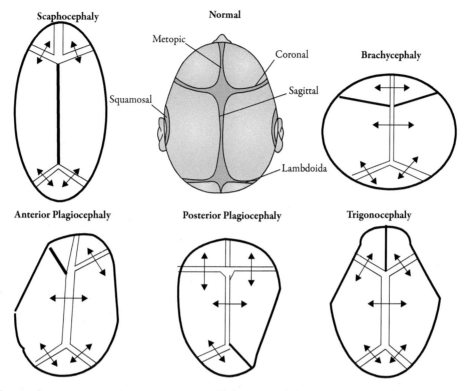

Fig. 21.1 Morphological types of craniosynostosis. Diagrammatic views of different morphological types of craniosynostosis. The premature closed suture is marked as a bold line. The resulting skull shape is determined by the sutures involved. Reprinted with permission: Meier PM, Goobie SM. Craniofacial surgery. In: Morgan PD, Soriano S, Sloan T, eds. *A Practical Approach to Neuroanesthesia*. 1st ed. Philadelphia, PA: Lippincott Williams & Wilkins. 2013.

These are called complex craniofacial synostoses and are often syndromic in nature, such as Apert and Crouzon syndrome.

Progressive postnatal craniosynostosis, a rare presentation, is characterized by a normal cranial shape and normal radiological images at birth. Later in childhood there is slow development of ICP, with signs/symptoms such as headaches, vomiting, irritability, papilledema, progressive optic atrophy, seizures, and bulging fontanelles.[9]

Positional plagiocephaly, known as deformational plagiocephaly, is extremely common and can be confused with craniosynostosis, particularly lambdoid fusion. There is characteristic unilateral occipital flattening and anterior displacement of the ipsilateral ear. This harmless condition is treated nonsurgically by an orthotic helmet in early life.[10,11]

Apert syndrome and associated abnormalities

Craniosynostosis is associated with numerous syndromes. The most frequent ones are detailed in Table 21.1.

Apert Syndrome (acrocephalosyndactyly type 1 (Figure 21.2) is a congenital condition characterized by primary craniosynostosis, midface malformations, and complex symmetric syndactyly malformations of the hands and feet (Table 21.1). It can present with varying degrees of developmental delay and intellectual disability.

Apert syndrome is inherited in an autosomal dominant manner and belongs to the FGFR related craniosynostosis spectrum. Along the spectrum, there are Pfeiffer syndrome, Crouzon syndrome, Beare-Stevenson syndrome, FGFR2-related isolated coronal synostosis, Jackson-Weiss syndrome, Crouzon syndrome with acanthosis nigricans, and Muenke syndrome. The coronal sutures are most commonly involved in Apert syndrome, resulting in a high forehead and flat facies. A horizontal groove above the supraorbital ridge and break in the continuity of eyebrows are common. Most of these infants will present with splayed metopic and anterior sagittal sutures, which appears to allow for some degree of cranial decompression. However, with increasing number of sutural fusions, there is increasing risk of elevated ICP. Rarely, children with Apert syndrome will present with pansutural fusion (including both lambdoid sutures) which creates a Kleeblattschaedel-like towering skull (turribrachycephaly) identical to the more severe presentations of Pfeiffer syndrome.

Example treatment algorithm for Apert syndrome

Many different treatment algorithms are used in different centers.[12] As an example, the treatment algorithm used for this child is outlined and includes the treatment plan of hand, feet, and cranial malformations, as well as feeding management, along with the sequencing of these procedures:

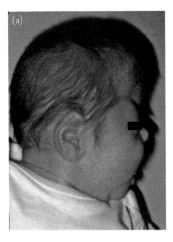 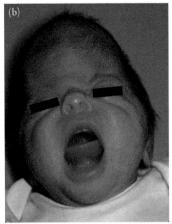 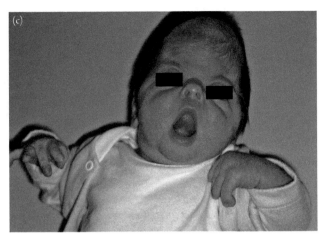

Fig. 21.2 Pfeiffer/Apert syndrome (FGFR2 mutation) and a "clover-leaf" cranial deformity (coronal, posterior sagittal, and lambdoid synostosis), orbital hypertelorbitism, proptosis, midfacial hypopoplasia, high arched-palate, choanal stenosis, Chiari I malformation, obstructive sleep apnea, scoliosis and hand abnormalities (radial clinodactyly of both thumbs, bilateral fourth-fifth metacarpal synostosis) as well as simple syndactyly of both feet. (Image courtesy of Dr. John B. Mulliken.) Adapted and reprinted with permission: Meier PM. Anesthesia for Plastic Surgery. In McCann ME, Greco C, Matthes K, eds. *Essentials of Anesthesia for Infants and Neonates* © Cambridge University Press; 2018.

Table 21.1 CRANIOSYNOSTOSIS AND FREQUENTLY ASSOCIATED SYNDROMES

SYNDROME	DESCRIPTION	ANESTHESIA IMPLICATIONS
Apert (sporadic defect; autosomal dominant)	Most common coronal synostosis, exorbitism, midface hypoplasia, choanal stenosis, possible increased ICP; airway anomalies (2%) syndactyly of hands and feet, synphalangism, partial cervical spine fusion C5/6 (70%); CHD (10%); genitourinary anomalies; cognitive impairment	Obstructive sleep apnea; possible difficult intubation; possible increased ICP; evaluation for CHD
Carpenter syndrome (autosomal recessive)	Wide towering skull (oxycephaly), premature closure of all cranial sutures, hypoplastic mandible, short neck, short upper extremities, syndactyly of hands and feet, variety of cardiac anomalies, omphalocele, mental retardation	Hypoplastic mandible may make intubation difficult, evaluation for CHD
Crouzon (craniofacial dysostosis) (autosomal dominant)	Multiple suture synostosis (coronal, sagittal), possible increased ICP resulting from progressive hydrocephalus, intracranial abnormalities (Chiari); exorbitism; midface hypoplasia, choanal atresia, airway obstruction; low set ears; rare cardiac anomaly; vertebral anomalies C2/3; mental retardation	Difficult airway, elective tracheostomy might be indicated; possible increased ICP; ocular protection
Muenke (autosomal dominant)	Most common craniosynostosis syndrome; coronal synostosis; midface hypoplasia rare	Possible mild obstructive sleep apnea
Pfeiffer (sporadic defect; autosomal dominant)	Multiple suture synostosis (brachycephaly, turricephaly, most common cause of trilobar cranial deformity (Kleeblattschädel); possible increased ICP, Chiari malformation; ocular proptosis; midface hypoplasia; CHD; cervical vertebral fusions, mild syndactyly, short broad thumbs and toes	Possible difficult airway; obstructive apnea; possible seizures (interaction anticonvulsants with anesthetic drugs); evaluation for CHD
Saethre Chotzen (autosomal dominant)	Unilateral or bilateral coronal suture synostosis (brachycephaly, plagiocephaly); possible increased ICP; maxillary hypoplasia; CHD; syndactyly, cervical spine abnormalities, clavicular anomalies	Possible difficult intubation due to cervical vertebral fusion; possible increased ICP

Note. ICP = intracranial pressure. CHD = congenital heart disease.

Source. Modified from Meier PM. Anesthesia for plastic surgery. In: McCann ME, Greco C, Matthes K, eds., *Essentials of Anesthesia for Infants and Neonates.* Cambridge, UK: Cambridge University Press; 2018. © Cambridge University Press 2018. Reprinted with permission.

1. Head CT at 6–10 weeks.

2. Endoscopic strip craniectomy within the first 3 months of life may often mitigate the progression of turricephaly. It does not eliminate the need for cranial vault remodeling. However, it can correct the dysmorphology to some degree, which makes later cranial vault remodeling procedures easier and more successful.

3. The syndactyly procedures of the upper and lower extremities will be multiple stage procedures beginning at approximately 9 months of age.

4. The potentially more extensive cranial vault remodeling, performed at a later time point as determined by the neurosurgical and plastic surgical treatment teams. Surgery is coordinated with the hand surgeons to minimize separate trips to the operating room.

Treatment goals focus on (a) prevention of avoidable developmental delays (from raised ICP and sleep apnea), (b) normalization of physical appearance, and (c) coordination of care and reducing operative interventions, which may potentially improve developmental outcome. Frequent assessments for raised ICP and sleep apnea are critical components of the care for children with Apert syndrome.

SURGICAL TREATMENT OPTIONS FOR CRANIOSYNOSTOSIS

Traditionally, craniosynostosis repair has involved extensive cranial vault remodeling characterized by significant blood loss and lengthy hospital stays. The treatment of craniosynostosis continues to evolve with the use of minimally invasive techniques. Most common among these techniques is endoscopic-assisted repair in conjunction with postoperative orthotic molding therapy.[13] This technique can be applied to most types of craniosynostosis, but it is generally reserved for small infants (less than 3 months of age) because of the thinness of the cranial bone and the subsequent rapid brain growth that allows for correction and normalization of the craniofacial skeleton.[14] A recent study of ESC versus open craniosynostosis repair using propensity-score matching from the North American Pediatric Craniofacial Collaborative Group[15] confirmed the advantages of ESC for young infants, including lower morbidity, mortality, and hospital costs, as well as shorter hospital stays.[16–21] This multicenter analysis, including 1,382 infants, reported significantly reduced utilization of blood and coagulation products in the ESC group compared to the open repair group. Median blood donor exposure, median administered volume of red blood cells, anesthesia and surgical duration, days in intensive care unit (ICU), and hospital length of stay were all significantly lower in infants undergoing ESC. The incidence of complications requiring treatment with vasoactive agents, venous air embolism (VAE), and hypothermia were similar, whereas postoperative intubation was significantly higher in the open repair group.

There are important anesthetic implications in the assessment of infants with syndromic craniosynostoses. The history, physical exam, and past anesthetic records need to be integrated to anticipate problems and formulate a workup plan. A history of mouth breathing, snoring, or sleep apnea suggests obstructive breathing. Drowsiness and poor attention span during the day might also be symptoms of sleep disturbances. An examination for ankyloses of the joints and reduced mobility of the head and neck that can make intubation difficult should be performed.

Airway comorbidity

Children with craniosynostosis, especially those associated with a syndrome, may present with a compromised airway.[22,23] Major upper airway obstruction is more prevalent in craniosynostosis patients with Crouzon, Pfeiffer, and Apert syndromes.[24] The anatomic features, maxillary hypoplasia, hypertelorism, and proptosis result from dysostosis of the cranial bones composing the cranial fossa. Maxillary hypoplasia with impaired anterior–posterior and downward growth of the maxilla results in a narrowed nasopharyngeal airway. Choanal stenosis is most common. Therefore, most of these children are mouth breathers, and obstruction of the oropharyngeal airway results in significant obstruction of ventilation. Consequently, the incidence of patients with sleep disorder and obstructive sleep apnea syndrome (OSAS) is exceedingly high, though often unrecognized.[25,26] Exacerbation of obstructive sleep apnea symptoms occur in almost half of the children during episodes of upper respiratory tract infections. Ideally, preoperative evaluation should include sleep studies.

Lower airway anomalies, such as tracheal cartilaginous sleeve, is a rare congenital cartilage malformation reported only in children with craniosynostosis syndromes (characterized by fusion of the tracheal arches of various extension).[27]

It is important to reflect on the potential effect of chronic airway obstruction on the cardiovascular system and the central nervous system. For example, chronic hypoventilation and hypoxia can potentially lead to pulmonary hypertension, and subsequently, cor pulmonale. Increased ICP can lead to decreased cerebral perfusion pressure with potentially negative effects on neurological and cognitive development.[28]

Central versus obstructive sleep apnea

The risk of sleep disordered breathing in children with craniofacial syndromes is high.[29] Scoring of respiratory abnormalities in children with sleep apnea distinguish obstructive, central and mixed apneas, and hypopneas and periodic breathing. These abnormalities range from complete cessation of airflow (apneas) to apparent reductions in airflow (hypopneas) to breath sequences with simple flow limitation recovery. Polysomnographic analyses are well described and allow distinct classification in most cases.

Central and obstructive features may coexist in many children with sleep apnea. However, in children with syndromic craniosynostosis, central apnea has been shown to be rare even if central nervous anatomic abnormalities are detected.

Of note, there is some natural improvement in sleep apnea, particularly during the first 3 years of life. However, children with Apert, Crouzon, or Pfeiffer syndrome show the least improvement. In the absence of other comorbid risk factors, it is highly unlikely that, if severe OSAS is not present early in life, it will develop during childhood. Ongoing clinical surveillance is important, and asking parents whether their child has breathing abnormalities during sleep can exclude the presence of clinically significant OSAS with a high probability.

Cardiac comorbidity

Craniosynostosis syndromes can occasionally be associated with cardiac anomalies. Congenital heart disease (e.g., patent ductus arteriosus, atrial septal defect, ventricular septal defect, pulmonary stenosis, tetralogy of Fallot, and coarctation of the aorta), both repaired and unrepaired, has been shown to increase the risk for anesthesia. Here, children with patent foramen ovale or ductus arteriosus are at risk for paradoxical air emboli (coronary or cerebral air embolism).

Children with craniosynostosis syndromes, history of cardiac symptoms, and/or severe sleep apnea should be carefully evaluated for further work up (chest X-ray, recent cardiologic assessment). In the presented case stem, cardiac arrhythmia was noted postnatally, including premature atrial contractions. The echocardiographic examination of this child showed a structurally normal heart with a patent foramen ovale. He was treated briefly with propranolol and a holter monitoring examination at 6 months of age showed only premature atrial contractions.

Neurological comorbidity

Several factors contribute to the risk of developing increased ICP, including decreased intracranial volume and an increased number and location of sutural fusion.[30] Although it is well known that increased ICP is commonly associated with multiple suture craniosynostosis,[24] ICP monitoring has demonstrated that 14%–24% of infants with single suture craniosynostosis also have raised ICP.[7] Thompson et al.[8] reported that, in single suture synostosis, an additional 38% of patients had borderline increased ICP, and normal ICP was observed in only 45% of children. Positron emission tomography scans have shown reduced cortical blood flow in the vicinity of sagittal synostosis in 70% of cases, which can be corrected by early release.[31]

Hydrocephalus is seen occasionally in patients with craniosynostosis, particularly associated with Crouzon, Pfeiffer, and Kleeblattschädel. Multisuture craniosynostoses, particularly with lambdoid involvement, are associated with a higher incidence of acquired Chiari deformation, requiring multiple operative procedures, and may result in increased developmental delay, compared with isolated single suture synostosis.[32] Evidence of jugular foraminal stenosis or atresia and dilated collateral emissary veins in children with syndromic craniosynostosis are associated with venous outflow obstruction and elevated intracranial venous hypertension.[33,34] Enlarged basal emissary foramina, which transmit enlarged emissary veins, result from stenosis or atresia of the jugular foramen. Disruption of emissary veins during an operation can produce massive hemorrhage. Bilateral basilar venous atresia can be found in patients with crouzonoid features and acanthosis nigrans (FGFR3 ala391glu mutation) and in patients with Apert syndrome (FGFR2 mutations).[33] Therefore, preoperative assessment of patients with syndromic craniosynostosis and enlarged emissary foramina should include skull base vascular imaging of the basilar venous drainage.[33] Significant increased intracranial bleeding is to be expected in these patients during craniectomy.

Ophthalmologic comorbidities

Ophthalmologic examinations may reveal papilledema and optic atrophy in children with chronically raised ICP.[35] Syndromic craniosynostoses with shallow, deformed orbits, and exorbitism increases the risk of corneal abrasion and ocular trauma during surgical interventions.

Evaluation and coordination with otolaryngologist

Consultation with an otolaryngologist is recommended because of the ubiquitous need for myringotomy tube placement.

Cervical vertebral anomalies

Neck motion (flexion and extension) may be limited, particularly in Apert, Pfeiffer, and Crouzon syndromes, and can increase the difficulty of intubation and positioning for the operation.

ICU admission

It is best to plan for an ICU bed in the postoperative period for hemodynamic and respiratory management, neurological observation, and optimization of the coagulation profile.

PLAN FOR ANESTHESIA

The anesthetic management of children with Apert syndrome must consider the problems associated with the syndrome itself as well as the surgical reconstruction.

Potentially difficult airway management

Children with syndromic craniosynostosis can present with difficult airway management[22,23] as they have some degree of midface hypoplasia, hypertelorism, and proptosis. The temporomandibular joints are normal. The mandible is of normal size but appears to be relatively prognathic because of midface hypoplasia. The palate is high-arched, and the nasal passages are small (choanal stenosis), resulting in mouth breathing. The midface hypoplasia and proptosis may cause problems with mask fit, making the management of the airway by mask difficult. Closure of the mouth occludes the airway as the tongue fills the smaller oral cavity, while the small nares and choanal stenosis cause resistance to nasal air flow. This can be overcome by holding the mouth open during induction and pressing down with the mask to obtain a good seal.[36] Alternatively, an oral airway can be used. In cases with severe obstruction, topicalizing the mouth with lidocaine spray prior to induction can be helpful to allow placement of an oral airway at a light depth of anesthesia. In most cases, tracheal intubation is not difficult unless there are major vertebral abnormalities and reduced cervical mobility. However, it is advisable to use a slightly smaller cuffed endotracheal tube than expected because of tracheal abnormalities. In case of anticipated difficult intubation, having the difficult airway cart (e.g., laryngeal mask airway, fiberoptic bronchoscope, and videolaryngoscopy) and the otolaryngologist in the operating room is advisable. A recent analysis from the multicenter Pediatric Difficult Intubation Registry[37] showed that in infants with difficult airway, fiberoptic intubation via supraglottic airway is associated with a higher first-attempt success rate than videolaryngoscopy (54% vs 36%, odds ratio, 2.12, P = 0.042), while in older children, first-attempt success rate with fiberoptic intubation showed a trend to be more successful but did not reach statistical significance (59% vs 51%, odds ratio, 1.35, P = 0.16). Patients with severe airway problems often have obstructive apnea and may require perioperative CPAP, but rarely require tracheostomy unless there is marked facial dysmorphism.[38] Meticulous attention to mid-deep tracheal tube placement and secure fixation is essential because the child's head is constantly rotated and extended during these cranial procedures.[39] Intraoperative access to the airway is limited, and the loss of the airway during the procedure is life threatening. Most experienced surgical teams do not rely on taping the endotracheal tube to the nose or chin. If a nasotracheal tube is necessary, it should be secured with a transseptal suture, and an orotracheal tube should be secured with a circum-mandibular wire for cranial vault remodeling procedures.

Protection of the eyes must be provided by the anesthesia/surgical teams (i.e., lubrication and tarsorrhaphy sutures) to prevent corneal damage, especially in children with ocular proptosis.

Anesthesia and monitoring

In a comprehensive evaluation, the Pediatric Craniofacial Collaborative Group,[40] composed of 31 North American institutions, reported perioperative management and outcomes in pediatric complex cranial vault remodeling in 1,223 children. The group identified significant variability for both perioperative management and in-hospital outcomes. Nearly all patients were managed with an inhaled anesthetic-opioid technique, at least 2 peripheral intravenous catheters sufficient for rapid massive transfusion, and an arterial line for invasive arterial blood pressure monitoring and blood sampling. A central venous catheter or peripherally inserted central catheter was placed in 13% of infants and 14% of older children, for which inadequate peripheral venous access was the most common rationale.

A Foley catheter is necessary for long procedures, due to the high fluid requirements and for monitoring urinary output. Warming the operating room during the induction period, forced-air warming, and fluid warmers are essential to keep the patient normothermic. If rapid blood transfusion is anticipated, it is prudent to use a device to detect and remove air from the infusion line.

Anticipation of significant blood loss is of paramount importance. The vascularity of the head and the numerous osteotomies of the skull may make hemostasis extremely difficult. It is not uncommon to lose 1 or more circulating blood volumes, especially in small infants. Substantial blood loss may be hidden in the surgical drapes. Therefore, rapid laboratory assessment of blood gases, electrolytes, metabolic status, and coagulative status needs to be readily available. Standard laboratory tests of coagulation have a limited ability to predict clinical bleeding.[41] Viscoelastic point of care tests, such as thromboelastometry (ROTEM) and thromboelastography (TEG), have been purported to be a means to assess specific components of coagulation function and guide hemostatic therapy,[42,43] and their use has demonstrated efficacy in cranial vault remodeling.[44] Meier et al.[45] reported a predictive algorithm in children undergoing cranial vault reconstruction for substantial intraoperative blood loss (defined as >60 mL/kg) and need for coagulation products with cut-off values: platelet fibrinogen product <343, α-angle <62 degrees, maximum amplitude <55 mm, and K time >2.1 min. The best prognostic combination included at least 2 of these 4 predictors. However, in the Pediatric Craniofacial Collaborative Group data set,[40] thromboelastography TEG® (Haemonetics Corporation) was utilized in only a minority of patients.

Venous air embolism occurs frequently in children undergoing open craniofacial surgical procedures,[46,47] and a variety of different monitors are used for detection of VAE well before cardiovascular collapse occurs—for example, precordial Doppler ultrasonography (characteristic change of signal, second highest sensitivity). Routine use of precordial Doppler has been suggested; however, Doppler monitoring is sensitive but nonspecific, with the vast majority of episodes being clinically insignificant. Other monitors include end-tidal carbon dioxide monitoring (precipitous decrease in carbon dioxide tension), end-tidal nitrogen monitoring (sudden increase in the nitrogen concentration in the exhaled breath), and transesophageal echocardiography (presence of air in the right ventricular outflow tract, highest sensitivity).[48,49] Insertion of central catheters for withdrawal of air is limited to a 33% success rate by the small size of the infant and the catheter because the ability to rapidly aspirate air decreases with the size of the catheter.[50]

Blood conservation

A comprehensive multimodal blood management strategy is essential in optimizing patient care, minimizing blood product transfusion, and consequently limiting transfusion-related complications.[51,52] The goal is to maintain fluid homeostasis for hemodynamic stability, oxygen carrying capacity, and adequate perfusion of vital organs, (i.e., kidneys and brain in the presence of increased ICP).

There are several intraoperative options for blood management to be used in combination:

1. Careful fluid administration should maintain normovolemia, including the use of Ringers Lactate (273 mOsm) and Plasmalyte (294 mOsm) in the United States and acetate solutions in Europe for replacement of maintenance fluid, which are associated with less acidosis than isotonic saline.[53,54] Blood loss is replaced with additional crystalloid solution in a ratio 1:3 for the first 10%–20% of estimated blood volume that is lost and then 1:1 with colloids for the next 20% of estimated blood volume lost. Thereafter, packed red blood cell and coagulation products are used, if needed. In a meta-analysis,[55] it was concluded that colloids and crystalloids can be similarly used for fluid resuscitation.

2. Normothermia should be maintained, since hypothermia, especially in combination with acidosis, leads to impaired coagulation.

3. Surgical techniques can help control bleeding, for example, using tissue infiltration of a dilute vasoconstrictor solution (epinephrine) to decrease blood loss and incision through the scalp with a Colorado needle.

4. Preoperative administration of recombinant human erythropoietin can be used to increase preoperative HCT.[56] Erythropoietin is also used as dual therapy with cell saver[57,58] or in combination with iron substitution.

5. Intraoperative blood cell salvage involves collecting autologous blood from the surgical site, processing it, and retransfusing it to the patient during the surgery.[59,60] Contraindications include tumor surgery, the use of agents that would result in red blood cell lysis (sterile water, alcohol, hydrogen peroxide), the use of clotting agents (surgical and gelfoam), the presence of contaminants (urine, bone, infection), and the use of irrigating solutions.

6. Intraoperative prophylactic antifibrinolytics are efficacious in decreasing blood loss and transfusion.[61] Rationale for the use of the antifibrinolytic agent, tranexamic acid (TXA), was derived from 2 randomized, double-blinded, placebo-controlled studies[62,63] that demonstrated its effectiveness in reducing blood loss and perioperative transfusion requirements in children with extensive craniofacial procedures. Several dosing regimens have been described. The lowest effective intraoperative dosing regimen of TXA as well as the effective therapeutic plasma concentration of TXA to inhibit fibrinolysis are uncertain.[64] On the basis of pharmacokinetic data and modeling, a TXA loading dose of 10–30 mg/kg over 30 minutes followed by a 5–10 mg/kg/hour maintenance infusion may be sufficient to maintain adequate TXA plasma concentrations during craniosynostosis surgery, based on a presumed minimal TXA plasma concentration of 20 µg/mL. For epsilon aminocaproic acid, a loading dose of 100 mg/kg followed by an infusion of 40 mg/

kg/hour has been shown to maintain therapeutic plasma concentrations.[65]

7. In an otherwise healthy patient, who is in the ICU and hemodynamically stable, with corrected coagulation parameters and minimal drain output, a lower transfusion target of a hemoglobin of 7 g/dL instead of 9 g/dL can be tolerated to avoid further exposure to blood products. Restrictive transfusion practice has been shown to be safe in the pediatric ICU setting.[66,67]

Preoperative autologous blood donation, normovolemic hemodilution, and deliberate induced hypotension are not suitable techniques for infants.

BLOOD/COAGULATION TRANSFUSION MANAGEMENT

Perioperative bleeding management should be individualized, avoiding a single transfusion trigger and using, instead, a transfusion target that considers age, weight, comorbidities, and type of surgical procedure and its course and utilizing point-of-care testing for specific coagulation products. Decisions regarding maintenance of intravascular volume and blood product transfusion are guided by monitoring arterial blood pressure and arterial blood gas measurements, including HCT, with an individualized transfusion target. Packed red blood cells are transfused in increments of 10–15 mL/kg to increase the HCT by approximately 10–12 HCT points. Blood product management is guided by the recommendations of the American Society of Anesthesiologists Task Force on Blood Component Therapy[42]; however, no specific pediatric guidelines have been put forth. Traditionally, fresh frozen plasma is intraoperatively transfused in 10–15 mL/kg increments if INR/PT/PTT measurements are prolonged to 1.5 times of normal. In the acute setting of substantial bleeding during extensive cranial vault remodeling procedures, the clinical utility of the traditional coagulation tests (PT, PTT, INR) is limited due to lengthy laboratory turnaround times (in our institution 45–60 minutes). Furthermore, PT/PTT testing is performed on centrifuged plasma fractions and provide information only on isolated portions of the coagulation cascade and are poor predictors of increased bleeding.[68] On the other hand, TEG and ROTEM as point-of-care tests provide quickly available, comprehensive information about the coagulation process by real-time observation of evolving clot formation using a bedside remote graphical display. The question arises if goal-directed TEG or ROTEM–based hemostatic resuscitation with specific component therapy could reduce the amount of blood loss by early treatment and specific targeting of a developing coagulopathy.[44,45,51] A practical recommendation could be to perform baseline TEG or ROTEM analysis following induction of anesthesia with subsequent reanalysis after scalp dissection and during craniotomy before blood transfusion. During time periods of excessive blood loss, arterial blood gas and TEG/ROTEM analyses might be indicated every 30–60 minutes to guide specific component blood product administration. The platelet fibrinogen product, defined as platelet count (10^9/L) × fibrinogen concentration (g/L) is a clinically useful indicator of bleeding and reduced clot strength in circumstances where TEG/ROTEM is unavailable.[45,69] Current guidelines support the substitution of fibrinogen if below 1.5–2.0 g/L or if maximum clot firmness in the ROTEM fibrin-based thromboelastometry assay is less than 8 mm.[43,70] Treatment of acquired fibrinogen deficiency traditionally consists of transfusion of fresh frozen plasma or cryoprecipitate (increments of 1U/5 kg) or administration of purified fibrinogen concentrate (calculated dose based on ROTEM measurements). Cryoprecipitate contains higher concentrations of fibrinogen as compared with fresh frozen plasma but has been withdrawn in European countries because of the risk of immunologic reactions and the potential transmission of infectious agents.[71] Alternatively, intraoperative substitution with fibrinogen concentrate, currently only available in Europe, can be safely and effectively used to treat fibrinogen deficiency.[72] General consensus is that a minimal platelet count of 50–100 × 10^9/L should be maintained for patients with ongoing bleeding. Platelet count can be expected to rise by approximately 50–100 × 10^9/L after transfusion of 5–10 mL/kg of an apheresis platelet unit.

Massive hemorrhage is defined as blood loss exceeding one circulating blood volume within a 24-hour period, blood loss of 50% of the circulating blood volume within a 3-hour period, or transfusion rate equal to 10% of the circulating blood volume every 10 minutes. The goal of a massive transfusion protocol is to avoid coagulopathy as a consequence of platelet and clotting factor depletion secondary to high packed red blood cell administration caused by massive hemorrhage. Such a protocol helps to optimize resources in the operating room and blood bank.

COMPLICATIONS

Perioperative complications

Perioperative complications can occur from numerous sources and may result in significant morbidity or mortality. Cardiac arrest has been reported from massive blood loss and coagulopathy, electrolyte and metabolic disturbances, VAE, cerebral edema and airway problems.

Complications of blood transfusion

Although the safety of blood transfusion has greatly improved in recent decades, there remain potentially serious hazards to the patient. Since the infectious risks of red-cell transfusion have become very low, the noninfectious risks are the primary transfusion complications in frequency and severity.[73,74]

1. The noninfectious transfusion reactions can be separated into nonimmune- and immune-mediated categories.
   - The majority of pediatric reports include nonimmune-mediated complications: human error, (e.g., over-/undertransfusion, incorrect blood component transfusion), transfusion-associated circulatory overload (TACO), metabolic derangements (hyperkalemia, hypocalcemia), and coagulopathic complications.
   - Immune-mediated complications include acute transfusion reactions, most of them allergic/urticarial/anaphylactic in nature, transfusion-related acute lung injury (TRALI), hemolytic transfusion reactions, febrile nonhemolytic transfusion reactions, and transfusion-related immunomodulation.

2. In developed countries, the risk of a transfusion-transmitted disease has become very small (less than 1:1,000,000) for the pathogens of greatest concern, HIV and hepatitis C virus.[75] The increased mobility of populations may result in increasing rates of, at present, very rare pathogens. Bacterial infections are a predominant problem in platelets, which are stored at room temperature.

Hyperkalemia is caused by rapid transfusion of blood and has been associated with fatal hyperkalemia and cardiac arrest in small infants and children.[76] The Wake Up Safe initiative from the Society of Pediatric Anesthesia recommends that packed red blood cell transfusions should be fresh (less than 1-week old) or washed if the patient is below 1 year old or weighs less than 10 kg to avoid hyperkalemia. Citrate, a component in the storage of packed red cells, is metabolized in the liver. In the presence of liver failure or when transfused rapidly in sufficient quantity, citrate can bind to divalent cations, resulting in hypocalcemia and hypomagnesemia, with resultant hypotension, tetany, and arrhythmias. Hypothermia may increase the cardiac toxicity of hypocalcemia and hyperkalemia and contribute to coagulopathy. The triad of acidosis, hypothermia, and coagulopathy needs to be diagnosed early and treated aggressively.

With improvement in the recognition and reporting of complications, TACO is now the most common reported risk of transfusion.[74] TACO is characterized by cardiogenic pulmonary edema and occurs most commonly in patients with an underlying hypervolemic state.

TRALI is a less common cause of respiratory distress (1 case per 12,000 units across all blood components). TRALI is a noncardiogenic pulmonary edema occurring within 6 hours after transfusion, characterized by hypoxemia and bilateral pulmonary infiltrates[77] in the absence of other risk factors for an acute respiratory distress syndrome. The pathogenesis is primarily mediated by leukoagglutinating antibodies in donor plasma, and in most cases, is reversible with supportive care within 24–96 hours after cessation of transfusion.

Venous air embolism

Venous air embolism may occur during any operative procedure in which the surgical site is above the level of the heart and noncollapsible veins are exposed to air.[48] The development of a pressure gradient between the surgical site and the right atrium increases the potential to entrain air via dural sinuses or bony venous sinusoids. The risk of venous air emboli can be reduced by maintaining euvolemia. A precordial Doppler ultrasound can detect minute VAE by a change in the character and intensity of the emitting sound. Clinical signs include sudden drops in end-tidal CO_2, hypotension, dysrhythmias, and/or ischemic changes in the EKG. Several therapeutic maneuvers should be instituted simultaneously in the case of VAE: (a) administration of 100% oxygen and fluid, (b) application of bone wax or direct pressure to seal the sites of egress, (c) flooding of the surgical field with warm saline, (d) lowering the surgical field or placing the patient in Trendelenburg position, (e) positive pressure ventilation with end-expiratory pressure of 5 cm water, and (f) attempting to aspirate air from a right atrial catheter if a catheter is in place. Further entrainment of intravascular air might be prevented by compression of the jugular veins, which increases ICP and reduces cerebral perfusion, a severe limitation of this technique. For catastrophic VAE with cardiovascular collapse, use of inotropic support and cardiopulmonary resuscitation, if necessary, are standard measures. Extracorporeal membrane oxygenation may be used to clear out air trapped in the heart. Open remodeling procedures are associated with large blood losses and a risk of hypotensive episodes. Consequently, VAE might be overlooked as a possible cause of intraoperative hypotension.

POSTOPERATIVE CONSIDERATIONS

The majority of patients require admission to the ICU for continued management of their respiratory, neurologic, and overall physiologic status. Patients who have an uneventful intraoperative course are extubated fully awake after the surgical procedure in the operating room. Postoperative intubation and admission to the ICU or postanesthesia care unit/ward depends on the duration of the operation, hemodynamic stability, pre-existing comorbidities (preoperative respiratory compromise, obstructive sleep apnea, difficult intubation), and complications during the procedure such as hypothermia, massive fluid resuscitation, electrolyte disturbances, and coagulopathy. Since the surgical procedure is focused on the cranium, the airway rarely becomes edematous, except by mechanical irritation of the vocal cords caused by the endotracheal tube secondary to frequent head repositioning. In select cases, if facial morphology permits noninvasive ventilatory support, CPAP or bilevel positive airway pressure may be a postoperative option. The initial management centers upon airway monitoring, sedation, pain management, thermoregulation, and correction of any residual volume deficits, acidosis, and coagulopathy. Isotonic solutions are maintained until fluid shifts are complete. Of particular importance is the risk of hyponatremia. The cause of hyponatremia is likely to be related to antidiuretic syndrome or administration of hypotonic intravenous fluids. Close hemodynamic and neurologic monitoring is provided until the risk of bleeding has passed. Coagulopathy may be consumptive, dilutional, or mixed in nature and requires specific correction. Continued blood loss via surgical drains needs to be monitored and replaced appropriately, while vigilance should be maintained for additional concealed losses.

ACKNOWLEDGMENT

The authors thank John B. Mulliken, MD, Department of Plastic and Oral Surgery, Boston Children's Hospital, Harvard Medical School, Boston, MA, USA for discussion and photographic images.

REVIEW QUESTIONS

1. Which of the following statements about the airway in a child with Apert syndrome is **LEAST** accurate?

A. Neck mobility may be limited, compromising intubation.
B. Temporomandibular joints and the mandibular size are normal.
C. Choanal atresia results in a high incidence of mouth breathing.
D. Central sleep apnea syndrome is frequently encountered.

Answer: D
Choanal stenosis is most common. Most of these children are mouth breathers and obstruction of the oropharyngeal airway results in significant obstruction of ventilation. The incidence of patients with sleep disorder and OSAS is exceedingly high but is often unrecognized.

2. Which of the following statements with respect to syndromes associated with craniosynostosis is **LEAST** accurate?

A. Apert syndrome is frequently associated limb abnormalities.
B. Crouzon syndrome has an increased incidence for elective tracheostomy.
C. Muenke syndrome results in the most severe forms of craniosynostosis.
D. Syndromes most frequently show autosomal dominant inheritance.

Answer: C
See Table 21.1 about craniosynostosis and frequently associated syndromes.

3. Which of the following statements about intraoperative blood conservation in infants undergoing cranial vault remodeling is **LEAST** effective?

A. antifibrinolytics prophylaxis
B. blood cell salvage and transfusion
C. deliberate induced hypotension
D. vasoconstrictor infiltration

Answer: C
Deliberate induced hypotension is not a suitable technique for infants due to concerns of maintaining adequate perfusion of vital organs, that is, kidneys and particularly the brain in the presence of potentially increased ICP.

4. Which of the following statements regarding complications of massive blood transfusion is **MOST** accurate?

A. Infectious complications are more frequently seen with platelets transfusion
B. Transfusion-related acute lung injury is the most common complication in children.
C. Hypocalcemia and hypomagnesemia may be caused by citrate metabolism.
D. Hypothermia may mitigate the cardiac toxicity of hypocalcemia and hyperkalemia.

Answer: A

Because platelets are stored at room temperature, the risk of bacterial infections is higher compared with all other blood products.

5. Which of the following statements about VAE is **LEAST** accurate?

A. Bony venous sinusoids and dural sinuses can entrain air.
B. Cardiovascular collapse necessitates cardiopulmonary resuscitation.
C. Maintenance of euvolemia significantly reduces risk.
D. Sudden increase in end-tidal CO_2 is a clinical sign.

Answer: B

Clinical signs of VAE include a sudden drop in end-tidal CO_2.

6. Which of the following approaches to perioperative bleeding management in children undergoing cranial vault remodeling is the **LEAST** recommended?

A. goal-directed TEG or ROTEM-based with specific component therapy
B. fibrinogen levels, PT, PTT and INR to predict increased bleeding
C. individualization without using a single transfusion trigger
D. platelet fibrinogen product to assess the reduction of clot strength

Answer: B

In the acute setting of substantial bleeding during extensive cranial vault remodeling procedures, the clinical utility of the traditional coagulation tests (PT, PTT, INR) is limited because of lengthy laboratory turnaround times. Furthermore, PT/PTT are performed on centrifuged plasma fractions and provide information of only isolated portions of the coagulation cascade and are poor predictors of increased bleeding.

7. Which of the following statements regarding intraoperative monitoring in children undergoing cranial vault reconstruction is **LEAST** accurate?

A. Central venous catheter air withdrawal has a low success rate in children.
B. Devices for monitoring air are indicated, if rapid blood transfusion is anticipated.
C. Precordial Doppler detection of venous air embolus is sensitive and specific.
D. Transesophageal echocardiography detects air in the right ventricular outflow tract.

Answer: C

Precordial Doppler monitoring is sensitive but nonspecific, with the vast majority of episodes being clinically insignificant.

QUESTIONS AND ANSWERS

This chapter has accompanying questions and answers which are available to subscribers as part of the Oxford eLearning platform. To access the questions, go to ✓ http:// oxfordmedicine. com/pediatricanesthesiaPBL

REFERENCES

1. Flores-Sarnat L. New insights into craniosynostosis. *Semin Pediatr Neurol.* Dec 2002;9(4):274–291.
2. Cohen MM Jr, MacLean RE. *Craniosynostosis: diagnosis, evaluation, and management.* 2nd ed. New York; Oxford: Oxford University Press; 2000.
3. Church MW, Parent-Jenkins L, Rozzelle AA, Eldis FE, Kazzi SN. Auditory brainstem response abnormalities and hearing loss in children with craniosynostosis. *Pediatrics.* Jun 2007;119(6):e1351–1360.
4. Hertle RW, Quinn GE, Minguini N, Katowitz JA. Visual loss in patients with craniofacial synostosis. *J Pediatr Ophthalmol Strabismus.* Nov-Dec 1991;28(6):344–349.
5. Koh JL, Gries H. Perioperative management of pediatric patients with craniosynostosis. *Anesthesiol Clin.* Sep 2007;25(3):465–481.
6. Tamburrini G, Caldarelli M, Massimi L, Santini P, Di Rocco C. Intracranial pressure monitoring in children with single suture and complex craniosynostosis: a review. *Childs Nerv Syst.* Oct 2005;21(10):913–921.
7. Renier D, Sainte-Rose C, Marchac D, Hirsch JF. Intracranial pressure in craniostenosis. *J Neurosurg.* Sep 1982;57(3):370–377.
8. Thompson DN, Malcolm GP, Jones BM, Harkness WJ, Hayward RD. Intracranial pressure in single-suture craniosynostosis. *Pediatr Neurosurg.* 1995;22(5):235–240.
9. Connolly JP, Gruss J, Seto ML, et al. Progressive postnatal craniosynostosis and increased intracranial pressure. *Plast Reconstr Surg.* Apr 15 2004;113(5):1313–1323.
10. Mulliken JB, Vander Woude DL, Hansen M, LaBrie RA, Scott RM. Analysis of posterior plagiocephaly: deformational versus synostotic. *Plast Reconstr Surg.* Feb 1999;103(2):371–380.
11. Laughlin J, Luerssen TG, Dias MS. Prevention and management of positional skull deformities in infants. *Pediatrics.* Jul 2011;112(1 Pt 1):199–202.
12. Fearon JA, Podner C. Apert syndrome: evaluation of a treatment algorithm. *Plast Reconstr Surg.* Jan 2013;131(1):132–142.
13. Barone CM, Jimenez DF. Endoscopic craniectomy for early correction of craniosynostosis. *Plast Reconstr Surg.* Dec 1999;104(7):1965–1973.
14. Jimenez DF, Barone CM. Endoscopic technique for sagittal synostosis. *Childs Nerv Syst.* Sep 2012;28(9):1333–1339.
15. Thompson DR, Zurakowski D, Haberkern CM, et al. Endoscopic versus open repair for craniosynostosis in infants using propensity score matching to compare outcomes: a multicenter study from the Pediatric Craniofacial Collaborative Group. *Anesth Analg.* Mar 2018;126(3):968–975.
16. Jimenez DF, Barone CM, Cartwright CC, Baker L. Early management of craniosynostosis using endoscopic-assisted strip craniectomies and cranial orthotic molding therapy. *Pediatrics.* Jul 2002;110(1 Pt 1):97–104.
17. Clayman MA, Murad GJ, Steele MH, Seagle MB, Pincus DW. History of craniosynostosis surgery and the evolution of minimally invasive endoscopic techniques: the University of Florida experience. *Ann Plast Surg.* Mar 2007;58(3):285–287.
18. Shah MN, Kane AA, Petersen JD, Woo AS, Naidoo SD, Smyth MD. Endoscopically assisted versus open repair of sagittal craniosynostosis: the St. Louis Children's Hospital experience. *J Neurosurg Pediatr.* Aug 2011;8(2):165–170.
19. Meier PM, Goobie SM, DiNardo JA, Proctor MR, Zurakowski D, Soriano SG. Endoscopic strip craniectomy in early infancy: the

initial five years of anesthesia experience. *Anesth Analg.* Feb 2011;112(2):407–414.

20. Abbott MM, Rogers GF, Proctor MR, Busa K, Meara JG. Cost of treating sagittal synostosis in the first year of life. *J Craniofac Surg.* Jan 2012;23(1):88–93.

21. Chan JW, Stewart CL, Stalder MW, St Hilaire H, McBride L, Moses MH. Endoscope-assisted versus open repair of craniosynostosis: a comparison of perioperative cost and risk. *J Craniofac Surg.* Jan 2013;24(1):170–174.

22. Nargozian C. The airway in patients with craniofacial abnormalities. *Paediatr Anaesth.* Jan 2004;14(1):53–59.

23. Nargozian C. Apert syndrome: anesthetic management. *Clin Plast Surg.* Apr 1991;18(2):227–230.

24. De Jong T, Bannink N, Bredero-Boelhouwer HH, et al. Long-term functional outcome in 167 patients with syndromic craniosynostosis; defining a syndrome-specific risk profile. *J Plast Reconstr Aesthet Surg.* Oct 2010;63(10):1635–1641.

25. Hoeve LJ, Pijpers M, Joosten KF. OSAS in craniofacial syndromes: an unsolved problem. *Int J Pediatr Otorhinolaryngol.* Dec 2003;67(Suppl 1):S111–S113.

26. Pijpers M, Poels PJ, Vaandrager JM, et al. Undiagnosed obstructive sleep apnea syndrome in children with syndromal craniofacial synostosis. *J Craniofac Surg.* Jul 2004;15(4):670–674.

27. Scheid SC, Spector AR, Luft JD. Tracheal cartilaginous sleeve in Crouzon syndrome. *Int J Pediatr Otorhinolaryngol.* Sep 2 2002;65(2):147–152.

28. Hayward R, Gonsalez S. How low can you go? Intracranial pressure, cerebral perfusion pressure, and respiratory obstruction in children with complex craniosynostosis. *J Neurosurg.* Jan 2005;102(1 Suppl):16–22.

29. Tan HL, Kheirandish-Gozal L, Abel F, Gozal D. Craniofacial syndromes and sleep-related breathing disorders. *Sleep Med Rev.* Jun 2016;27:74–88.

30. Bristol RE, Lekovic GP, Rekate HL. The effects of craniosynostosis on the brain with respect to intracranial pressure. *Semin Pediatr Neurol.* Dec 2004;11(4):262–267.

31. David LR, Genecov DG, Camastra AA, Wilson JA, Argenta LC. Positron emission tomography studies confirm the need for early surgical intervention in patients with single-suture craniosynostosis. *J Craniofac Surg.* Jan 1999;10(1):38–42.

32. Czerwinski M, Kolar JC, Fearon JA. Complex craniosynostosis. *Plast Reconstr Surg.* Oct 2011;128(4):955–961.

33. Robson CD, Mulliken JB, Robertson RL, et al. Prominent basal emissary foramina in syndromic craniosynostosis: correlation with phenotypic and molecular diagnoses. *AJNR Am J Neuroradiol.* Oct 2000;21(9):1707–1717.

34. Rich PM, Cox TC, Hayward RD. The jugular foramen in complex and syndromic craniosynostosis and its relationship to raised intracranial pressure. *AJNR Am J Neuroradiol.* Jan 2003;24(1):45–51.

35. Tuite GF, Chong WK, Evanson J, et al. The effectiveness of papilledema as an indicator of raised intracranial pressure in children with craniosynostosis. *Neurosurgery.* Feb 1996;38(2):272–278.

36. Bruppacher H, Reber A, Keller JP, Geiduschek J, Erb TO, Frei FJ. The effects of common airway maneuvers on airway pressure and flow in children undergoing adenoidectomies. *Anesth Analg.* Jul 2003;97(1):29–34.

37. Burjek NE, Nishisaki A, Fiadjoe JE, et al. Videolaryngoscopy versus fiber-optic intubation through a supraglottic airway in children with a difficult airway: an analysis from the Multicenter Pediatric Difficult Intubation Registry. *Anesthesiology.* Sep 2017;127(3):432–440.

38. Sculerati N, Gottlieb MD, Zimbler MS, Chibbaro PD, McCarthy JG. Airway management in children with major craniofacial anomalies. *Laryngoscope.* Dec 1998;108(12):1806–1812.

39. Moll J, Erb TO, Frei FJ. Assessment of three placement techniques for individualized positioning of the tip of the tracheal tube in children under the age of 4 years. *Paediatr Anaesth.* Apr 2015;25(4):379–385.

40. Stricker PA, Goobie SM, Cladis FP, et al. Perioperative outcomes and management in pediatric complex cranial vault reconstruction: a multicenter study from the Pediatric Craniofacial Collaborative Group. *Anesthesiology.* Feb 2017;126(2):276–287.

41. Goobie SM, Haas T. Bleeding management for pediatric craniotomies and craniofacial surgery. *Paediatr Anaesth.* Jul 2014;24(7):678–689.

42. American Society of Anesthesiologists Task Force on Perioperative Blood Management. Practice guidelines for perioperative blood management: an updated report by the American Society of Anesthesiologists Task Force on Perioperative Blood Management. *Anesthesiology.* Feb 2015;122(2):241–275.

43. Kozek-Langenecker SA, Afshari A, Albaladejo P, et al. Management of severe perioperative bleeding: guidelines from the European Society of Anaesthesiology. *Eur J Anaesthesiol.* Jun 2013;30(6):270–382.

44. Haas T, Goobie S, Spielmann N, Weiss M, Schmugge M. Improvements in patient blood management for pediatric craniosynostosis surgery using a ROTEM(R)-assisted strategy—feasibility and costs. *Paediatr Anaesth.* Jul 2014;24(7):774–780.

45. Meier PM, Zurakowski D, Goobie SM, et al. Multivariable predictors of substantial blood loss in children undergoing craniosynostosis repair: implications for risk stratification. *Paediatr Anaesth.* Oct 2016;26(10):960–969.

46. Harris MM, Yemen TA, Davidson A, et al. Venous embolism during craniectomy in supine infants. *Anesthesiology.* Nov 1987;67(5):816–819.

47. Faberowski LW, Black S, Mickle JP. Incidence of venous air embolism during craniectomy for craniosynostosis repair. *Anesthesiology.* Jan 2000;92(1):20–23.

48. Mirski MA, Lele AV, Fitzsimmons L, Toung TJ. Diagnosis and treatment of vascular air embolism. *Anesthesiology.* Jan 2007;106(1):164–177.

49. Meyer PG, Renier D, Orliaguet G, Blanot S, Carli P. Venous air embolism in craniosynostosis surgery: what do we want to detect? *Anesthesiology.* Oct 2000;93(4):1157–1158.

50. Soriano SG, McManus ML, Sullivan LJ, Scott RM, Rockoff MA. Doppler sensor placement during neurosurgical procedures for children in the prone position. *J Neurosurg Anesthesiol.* Jul 1994;6(3):153–155.

51. Goobie SM, Haas T. Perioperative bleeding management in pediatric patients. *Curr Opin Anaesthesiol.* Jun 2016;29(3):352–358.

52. Di Rocco C, Tamburrini G, Pietrini D. Blood sparing in craniosynostosis surgery. *Semin Pediatr Neurol.* Dec 2004;11(4):278–287.

53. Zunini GS, Rando KA, Cox RG. Fluid replacement in craniofacial pediatric surgery: normal saline or ringer's lactate? *J Craniofac Surg.* Jul 2011;22(4):1370–1374.

54. Butterworth JFt, Mythen MG. Should "normal" saline be our usual choice in normal surgical patients? *Anesth Analg.* Aug 2013;117(2):290–291.

55. Perel P, Roberts I. Colloids versus crystalloids for fluid resuscitation in critically ill patients. *Cochrane Database Syst Rev.* Mar 16 2011;3:CD000567.

56. Fearon JA, Weinthal J. The use of recombinant erythropoietin in the reduction of blood transfusion rates in craniosynostosis repair in infants and children. *Plast Reconstr Surg.* Jun 2002;109(7):2190–2196.

57. Krajewski K, Ashley RK, Pung N, et al. Successful blood conservation during craniosynostotic correction with dual therapy using procrit and cell saver. *J Craniofac Surg.* Jan 2008;19(1):101–105.

58. Helfaer MA, Carson BS, James CS, Gates J, Della-Lana D, Vander Kolk C. Increased hematocrit and decreased transfusion requirements in children given erythropoietin before undergoing craniofacial surgery. *J Neurosurg.* Apr 1998;88(4):704–708.

59. Fearon JA. Reducing allogenic blood transfusions during pediatric cranial vault surgical procedures: a prospective analysis of blood recycling. *Plast Reconstr Surg.* Apr 1 2004;113(4):1126–1130.

60. Baumann C, Lamesic G, Weiss M, Cushing MM, Haas T. Evaluation of the minimum volume of salvage blood required for the successful use of two different autotransfusion devices. *Paediatr Anaesth.* Mar 2015;25(3):258–264.

61. Goobie SM, Cladis FP, Glover CD, et al. Safety of antifibrinolytics in cranial vault reconstructive surgery: a report from the pediatric craniofacial collaborative group. *Paediatr Anaesth*. Mar 2017;27(3):271–281.

62. Dadure C, Sauter M, Bringuier S, et al. Intraoperative tranexamic acid reduces blood transfusion in children undergoing craniosynostosis surgery: a randomized double-blind study. *Anesthesiology*. Apr 2011;114(4):856–861.

63. Goobie SM, Meier PM, Pereira LM, et al. Efficacy of tranexamic acid in pediatric craniosynostosis surgery: a double-blind, placebo-controlled trial. *Anesthesiology*. Apr 2011;114(4):862–871.

64. Goobie SM, Meier PM, Sethna NF, et al. Population pharmacokinetics of tranexamic acid in paediatric patients undergoing craniosynostosis surgery. *Clin Pharmacokinet*. Apr 2013;52(4):267–276.

65. Stricker PA, Zuppa AF, Fiadjoe JE, et al. Population pharmacokinetics of epsilon-aminocaproic acid in infants undergoing craniofacial reconstruction surgery. *Br J Anaesth*. May 2013;110(5):788–799.

66. Lacroix J, Hebert PC, Hutchison JS, et al. Transfusion strategies for patients in pediatric intensive care units. *N Engl J Med*. Apr 19 2007;356(16):1609–1619.

67. Secher EL, Stensballe J, Afshari A. Transfusion in critically ill children: an ongoing dilemma. *Acta Anaesthesiol Scand*. Jul 2013;57(6):684–691.

68. Haas T, Fries D, Tanaka KA, Asmis L, Curry NS, Schochl H. Usefulness of standard plasma coagulation tests in the management of perioperative coagulopathic bleeding: is there any evidence? *Br J Anaesth*. Feb 2015;114(2):217–224.

69. Moganasundram S, Hunt BJ, Sykes K, et al. The relationship among thromboelastography, hemostatic variables, and bleeding after cardiopulmonary bypass surgery in children. *Anesth Analg*. Apr 1 2010;110(4):995–1002.

70. Spahn DR, Bouillon B, Cerny V, et al. Management of bleeding and coagulopathy following major trauma: an updated European guideline. *Crit Care*. Apr 19 2013;17(2):R76.

71. Stanworth SJ, Brunskill SJ, Hyde CJ, McClelland DB, Murphy MF. Is fresh frozen plasma clinically effective? A systematic review of randomized controlled trials. *Br J Haematol*. Jul 2004;126(1):139–152.

72. Haas T, Spielmann N, Restin T, et al. Higher fibrinogen concentrations for reduction of transfusion requirements during major paediatric surgery: a prospective randomised controlled trial. *Br J Anaesth*. Aug 2015;115(2):234–243.

73. Lavoie J. Blood transfusion risks and alternative strategies in pediatric patients. *Paediatr Anaesth*. Jan 2011;21(1):14–24.

74. Carson JL, Triulzi DJ, Ness PM. Indications for and adverse effects of red-cell transfusion. *N Engl J Med*. Sep 28 2017;377(13):1261–1272.

75. Zou S, Dorsey KA, Notari EP, et al. Prevalence, incidence, and residual risk of human immunodeficiency virus and hepatitis C virus infections among United States blood donors since the introduction of nucleic acid testing. *Transfusion*. Jul 2010;50(7):1495–1504.

76. Lee AC, Reduque LL, Luban NL, Ness PM, Anton B, Heitmiller ES. Transfusion-associated hyperkalemic cardiac arrest in pediatric patients receiving massive transfusion. *Transfusion*. Jan 2014;54(1):244–254.

77. Kleinman S, Caulfield T, Chan P, et al. Toward an understanding of transfusion-related acute lung injury: statement of a consensus panel. *Transfusion*. Dec 2004;44(12):1774–1789.

22.

LARYNGOTRACHEAL RECONSTRUCTION

Annery Garcia-Marcinkiewicz and John E. Fiadjoe

STEM CASE AND KEY QUESTIONS

A 30-month-old female with grade 3 subglottic stenosis (SGS) presents for microlaryngoscopy, bronchoscopy (MLB) and laryngotracheal reconstruction with anterior and posterior costal cartilage graft. Her past medical history is notable for prematurity (gestational age of 29 weeks at birth), tracheomalacia, and chronic respiratory failure requiring tracheostomy. She previously required mechanical ventilation during sleep; however, she is currently on a heat moisture exchanger during the day and T-piece overnight. Her mother reports that she is at her baseline, requiring suctioning every few hours for thin white secretions. Her tracheostomy tube is changed every week without problems.

WHAT IS LARYNGOTRACHEAL RECONSTRUCTION (LTR)? WHAT PATIENT POPULATION CAN BENEFIT FROM LTR? WHAT ARE SOME RISK FACTORS FOR SGS?

Born at 29 weeks gestational age, the patient experienced respiratory distress and was intubated at birth. She received surfactant at 17 hours of life, was extubated on day of life (DOL) 1 and reintubated on DOL 3 for pulmonary hemorrhage. She was placed on high frequency oscillatory ventilation and was transitioned to conventional ventilation on DOL 27. She was extubated on DOL 33 to noninvasive mechanical ventilation. She received a course of dexamethasone and was placed on heliox on DOL 40 for 3 days due to airway edema. She was gradually weaned from noninvasive mechanical ventilation to continuous positive airway pressure and eventually transitioned to high-flow nasal cannula. She subsequently experienced severe respiratory failure with significant desaturation and was intubated. A tracheostomy was then performed with a 4.0 uncuffed BivonaÒ tube.

WHAT ARE SOME CAUSES OF ACQUIRED SGS? HOW IS SGS GRADED? WHAT ARE SOME STRATEGIES FOR PREVENTION?

A follow-up visit with otolaryngology reveals an oral aversion, increased episodes of coughing, gagging, and arching after feeds with poor weight gain. Results from upper endoscopy, microlaryngoscopy, and bronchoscopy demonstrate squamous cells with abundant pale cytoplasm, numerous intraepithelial eosinophils, and posterior laryngeal

inflammation. Omeprazole is started, and she is scheduled for follow-up in 3 months.

WHAT IS THE ROLE OF UNTREATED GASTROESOPHAGEAL REFLUX DISEASE (GERD) IN THE MANAGEMENT OF SGS AND OUTCOMES AFTER LTR?

The patient's GERD symptoms improve, and a recent esophagogastroduodenoscopy (EGD) is normal. She presents on the morning of her scheduled LTR, and, on evaluation, her preoperative nurse notes copious, thick, white and yellow secretions from her tracheostomy tube. Her temperature is 38.5°C with oxygen hemoglobin saturations of 92%–93%.

WOULD YOU PROCEED WITH HER CASE TODAY? WHAT ARE THE IMPLICATIONS OF RESPIRATORY SYNCYTIAL VIRUS BRONCHIOLITIS AND RECONSTRUCTION OUTCOMES?

The patient is admitted to the intensive care unit (ICU) for treatment of respiratory syncytial virus bronchiolitis. After stabilizing from her hospital admission, she presents for a follow-up appointment with otolaryngology. Her mother reports she is at her baseline, requiring suctioning every few hours for thin white secretions. She continues on heat moisture exchanger during the day and T-piece at night, and her weekly tracheostomy tube changes remain uncomplicated. At present, she walks, signs, and vocalizes a little bit around the tracheostomy tube, although with no words. Although she eats some foods by mouth, her primary calorie intake is via her gastrostomy tube. A recent microlaryngoscopy continues to demonstrate grade 3 SGS. Bronchoscopy shows no evidence of bronchitis. EGD is within normal limits, and an impedance probe study is normal. She continues to do well on omeprazole.

WHAT ARE THE TREATMENT OPTIONS FOR SGS? WHAT ARE SOME FACTORS THAT MIGHT MAKE A MULTISTAGE PROCEDURE MORE SUITABLE THAN A SINGLE-STAGE PROCEDURE?

The patient presents on the day of her procedure for a two-stage LTR with anterior and posterior cartilage graft. Her preoperative examination on the morning of surgery is unremarkable from her baseline. Anesthesia is induced with a combination of nitrous oxide, oxygen, and sevoflurane via the patient's tracheostomy. A 22-gauge peripheral intravenous (IV) line is secured in the left upper arm, and anesthesia is maintained with a propofol infusion at 300 mcg/kg/min and vecuronium. Ceftazidime is administered as prophylaxis, and 1 mcg/kg of fentanyl is provided for pain control.

WHAT ARE THE STEPS FOR CLASSIC (MULTISTAGE) LTR? WHAT POTENTIAL COMPLICATIONS CAN OCCUR DURING THESE STEPS?

After induction of anesthesia, the airway is visualized using a laryngoscope. The larynx is visualized without notable inflammation, but a grade 3 elliptical shaped SGS is noted. Bronchoscopy is next performed, and again a grade 3 SGS is visualized necessitating a neonatal endoscope (2.7 mm) to traverse the lumen. Distally, large granulation tissue obstructs the airway. The distal trachea, carina, and mainstem bronchi appear normal.

Next, the patient's 4.0 cuffless tracheostomy is replaced with a cuffed 4.0 anode tube. This is secured to the chest wall with sutures.

The neck is then extended on a shoulder roll in preparation for the rest of the procedure. After cricoid palpation, a horizontal incision is marked near the cricoid. Additionally, a horizontal incision is marked on the right chest near the inferior border of the pectoralis major. The incisions are injected with 1% lidocaine with 1:100,000 of epinephrine. The neck and chest are then prepped and draped. Approximately 30 minutes after induction of general anesthesia, the patient's oxygen saturation decreases to 88%. Tidal volumes decrease to approximately 2 mL/kg and peak inspiratory pressures have increased to 37 cm H_2O.

WHAT HAS OCCURRED? HOW SHOULD THIS SITUATION BE MANAGED?

The patient's breathing tube is withdrawn to the correct position with improvement in her ventilatory status. The surgery proceeds. An incision is made in the neck and superior and inferior subplatysmal flaps are elevated. The strap muscles are identified in the midline and bisected laterally. The soft tissue overlying the laryngotracheal complex is gently elevated. The cricothyroid muscles are identified and preserved.

The airway is visualized under bronchoscopy and entered under direct visualization by incision in the midline at the level of the cricoid. Proximal scar lysis is performed under guidance of a bronchoscope with caution to minimize injury to the vocal folds. The vocal folds are distracted to identify the anterior commissure and care is made to avoid them. The posterior cricoid plate is found to be scarred and stenosed. Next, 1% lidocaine with 1:100,000 of epinephrine is infiltrated into the posterior cricoid plate. An incision is made in the posterior cricoid plate in the midline, and the incision

is extended submucosally into the interarytenoid area to lyse the interarytenoid muscles and avoid creation of a cleft. The deeper perichondrium is kept intact, and a small pocket is elevated deep to the posterior cricoid plate. A cut endotracheal tube (ETT) is used to size the airway (Figure 22.1).

A T-tube is used as a suprastomal stent and placed into the airway. A suture is placed through-and-through the strap muscle/trachea/stent/trachea/strap muscle. The proximal end of the stent is sutured closed with the knot placed intraluminally in the stent.

The rib cartilage graft is next harvested. The muscle overlying the inframammary area of the right fifth rib is incised, exposing the cartilaginous rib. The superior and inferior edges are skeletonized, and a blade is used to score the perichondrium. A caudal elevator is used to lift the inner perichondrium off of the cartilage, maintaining it intact. The wound is irrigated, and Valsalva maneuvers are performed to 30 cm H_2O.

The patient is now noted to have slowly progressive hypotension and a heart rate of 144 bpm. Her heart rate increases to 150 bpm, and a 20 mL/kg fluid bolus is administered. Blood pressure is now 50/45 mmHg, oxygen saturation drops from 93% to 85%, and peak airway pressure is now 34 cm H_2O.

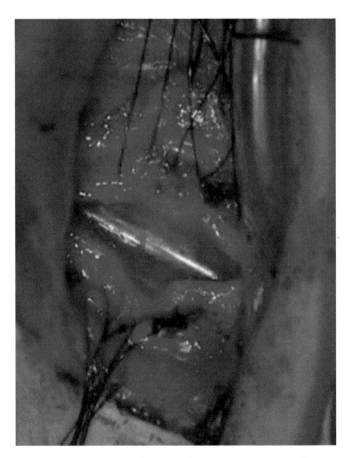

Fig. 22.1 Intraoperative view of an inserted stent. From Bitar MA, Al Barazi R, Barakeh R. Airway reconstruction: review of an approach to the advanced stage laryngotracheal stenosis. *Braz J Otorhinolaryngol.* 2017;83(3):299–312.

WHAT IS IN YOUR TOP DIFFERENTIAL DIAGNOSIS? HOW WOULD YOU MANAGE THE DESCRIBED CONDITION?

Auscultation reveals reduced air entry on the right side. Needle aspiration of the pleural space is performed in the right second intercostal space at the midclavicular line with initially good physiologic response but no audible decompression. A second-needle thoracostomy is performed resulting in an audible hiss and improved hemodynamics. A chest drain is placed, the patient remains in stable condition, and the surgery proceeds.

The graft is split into 2 properly sized portions to accommodate the dimensions of the anterior and posterior cartilage defects. A stent is positioned into the airway, and the anterior split is sutured closed. The strap muscles and cricothyroid muscles are reapproximated, and the platysmal layer is also reapproximated. The skin is sutured. The pediatric 4.0 mm cuffed tracheostomy tube is replaced. The patient is transferred to the pediatric intensive care unit for continued management.

WHAT ARE IMPORTANT POST-OPERATIVE MANAGEMENT GOALS AFTER LTR? WHAT POSTOPERATIVE SEDATION OPTIONS ARE THERE FOR SINGLE-STAGE LTR (SS-LTR), AND WHAT ARE ADVANTAGES AND DISADVANTAGES OF EACH?

The patient is transferred to the ICU in stable condition recovering from sedation. The ICU team is made aware that the patient has a critical airway and cannot be intubated or mask ventilated from above her tracheostomy site. A postoperative chest X-ray is obtained, demonstrating improvement in the pneumothorax, and she is continued on perioperative antibiotic coverage for another 72 hours. The rest of her postoperative course in the hospital is uneventful. The patient's tracheostomy site is deccanulated 6 months later. On follow-up visit, the patient is noted to be doing well without concerns regarding her breathing. It is noted that her stoma site fully closed, and she has no drainage. She is now cleared for water exposure and swimming activities.

DISCUSSION

Fearon and Cotton[1] first described LTR in 1972 and are noted to have said "there isn't anything more devastating than having a child who has fully recovered from a critical illness requiring prolonged intubation die from complications of a long term tracheotomy that is required due to iatrogenic SGS." Prior to this, severe SGS had a 25% mortality rate.[1] Since its popularization, LTR has become the standard of care to manage pediatric laryngotracheal stenosis.[2]

ETIOLOGY AND PATHOGENESIS

Laryngotracheal stenosis can be congenital or acquired. Although the exact pathogenesis is unknown, 90% of patients with acquired SGS have a history of tracheal intubation.[3] Stenosis can also occur after other internal or external airway injury (Figure 22.2).

Histologic studies show that injury is inevitable when the infant larynx is intubated.[4] Pressure necrosis and mucocillary stasis occur due to pressure caused by the ETT.[4] Edema and ulceration in subglottic tissues can deepen and expose cartilage eventually leading to the formation of granulation tissue. (Figure 22.3).

Ulcer healing starts after a few days, rapidly progresses from day 10 and is usually complete in 30 days.[4] Repeated movement of an ETT and multiple instrumentation attempts increase the risk of airway trauma. Risk factors, such as low birth weight, and systemic factors, such as bacterial infection, chronic illness, dehydration, immunosuppression and GERD, contribute to laryngeal mucosal injury.[2] There is a high association between SGS and GERD. GERD is not only a pathogenic factor in the formation of SGS but can negatively impact outcomes in SGS and, therefore, is aggressively treated.[5]

CLINICAL MANIFESTATIONS AND DIAGNOSIS OF SGS

Signs of SGS include stridor, respiratory distress, recurring croup, multiple extubation failures, and inability to breathe without a tracheostomy tube. Further evaluation includes radiographs of the neck, which can demonstrate subglottic narrowing or subglottic masses, and evaluation of the trachea for narrowing, stenosis or near complete rings. Microlaryngoscopy and/or bronchoscopy establishes the definitive diagnosis (Figure 22.4). Patients will also typically undergo a functional endoscopic evaluation of swallowing to identify any dysfunctional feeding, as this may complicate airway reconstruction by increasing the risk of postoperative aspiration and consequent inflammation.

TREATMENT OPTIONS OF SGS

Treatment options for SGS depends on the degree of the lesion, patient factors, and comorbidities (Table 22.1).

Internal trauma
  Intubation injury
External trauma
  Blunt
  Penetrating
Other
  Trauma
    After laryngeal surgery: high tracheostomy, glottic web, supraglottic collapse
    Burns
  Chronic infection (eg, tuberculosis, syphilis)
  Chronic inflammation
  Systemic: sarcoidosis, systemic lupus erythematosus, pemphigus, Wegener's reflux
  Laryngeal neoplasm
    Primary lesion: chondroma, fibroma, carcinoma
    Secondary involvement: tumor infiltration, radionecrosis, postoperative scarring

Fig. 22.2 Causes of acquired laryngotracheal stenosis. Reproduced with permission from Boardman SJ, Albert DM. Single stage and multistage pediatric laryngotracheal reconstruction. *Otolaryngol Clin North Am.* 2008;41(5):947–958.

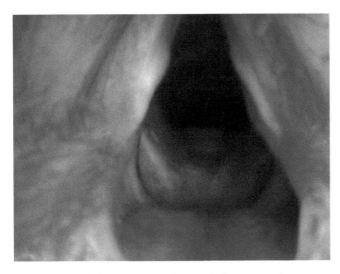

Fig. 22.3 Loss of subglottic mucosa and exposed subglottic cartilage following intubation of neonatal airway. Reproduced with permission from Boardman SJ, Albert DM. Single stage and multistage pediatric laryngotracheal reconstruction. *Otolaryngol Clin North Am.* 2008;41(5):947–958.

Patients undergo a comprehensive assessment to formulate an individualized treatment plan. Pertinent history includes the severity of SGS, degree of respiratory compromise, systemic diseases, and other coexisting conditions that affect the airway at other levels such as craniofacial anomalies, and chronic lung disease. Infants weighing >4 kg with gestational age >30 weeks have been found to have a greater chance of success with achieving airway patency and eventual extubation after LTR. This may be due to comorbidities in younger and smaller

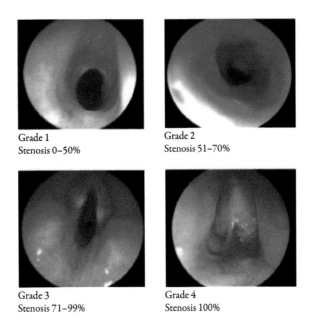

Grade 1
Stenosis 0–50%

Grade 2
Stenosis 51–70%

Grade 3
Stenosis 71–99%

Grade 4
Stenosis 100%

Fig. 22.4 Myer-Cotton grading system of laryngeal stenosis. (Courtesy of Dr. Ian Jacobs, MD, Director of the Center for Pediatric Airway Disorders, Division of Otolaryngology at The Children's Hospital of Philadelphia. The Children's Hospital of Philadelphia subglottic stenosis website http://www.chop.edu/conditions-diseases/subglottic-stenosis#. Accessed June 20, 2017).

infants, and a small margin of tolerance for airway compromise in this group.[6] In general, earlier lesions may respond to medical or endoscopic therapy or anterior cricoid split.[2] More advanced lesions are considered for LTR.

Cricotracheal resection (CTR) has become an important alternative approach in the management of laryngotracheal stenosis in children.[7] The goal of CTR for the management of SGS is to remove the cartilaginous segment leading to the stenosis. This approach differs from LTR, in which the goal is to widen the subglottic airway without removing the underlying lesion.[8] Until more recently, CTR was not typically accepted as a treatment modality for severe SGS in pediatric patients[9] and was utilized mainly as "salvage CTR"[7] for patients who previously had LTR and failed to achieve decannulation. CTR was not considered first choice treatment for severe SGS due to concerns for the risk of possible dehiscence at the site of anastomosis, possibility of injury to the recurrent laryngeal nerves, and interference of normal growth of the larynx.[9] Monnier et al.[9] conducted a study of 38 infants and children with severe SGS who underwent partial cricoid resection with primary thyromental anastomosis and found decannulation rates similar to that of LTR. All patients showed normal growth of the larynx and trachea.[9] The choice between LTR or CTR as a treatment modality for patients with severe SGS is multifactorial. Important considerations include factors related to the anatomy of the stenosis and factors related to the patient. CTR involves extensive tracheal mobilization and resection of a variable amount of trachea, which may be an excessive process for mild stenosis (Myer-Cotton grade 1).[7] CTR is given more consideration for complete (grade 4) stenosis. The best treatment modality for patients with grade 2 and 3 stenosis is not as clearly defined. Additional factors to consider include the length of the stenosis (with longer stenosis requiring more extensive resections) and the level of the stenosis (resections that are too close to the vocal cords have greater potential to affect vocal cord mobility and can lead to aspiration and voice problems).[7] Precise selection criteria for CTR versus LTR remain unclear, and the choice of management is based on careful considerations that are unique to each case.

SINGLE VERSUS DOUBLE STAGE LTR

Laryngotracheal reconstruction has traditionally been performed as a multistage procedure with a tracheostomy in place.[2] The goals of the surgery are to safely create a stable airway that is age appropriate with conservation of laryngeal function. The main components of the surgical technique for LTR involve division of the narrow segment of the airway, followed by placement of anterior and/or posterior cartilage interposition graft to widen the airway lumen (Figure 22.5). In the single-stage procedure, the reconstructed airway is stented by an ETT postoperatively. In ds-LTR, the patient's tracheostomy tube is kept in situ, and the patient is decannulated at a later time.[2] Single-stage LTR has the advantage of immediate decannulation of tracheostomy or avoiding a tracheostomy all together. The stages of airway stabilization, healing, and decannulation, which typically take several months, are compressed into a shorter period of time with ss-LTR. Prolonged stenting is required in ds-LTR, whereas the

Table 22.1 SELECTION OF TREATMENT MODALITY FOR SGS

SELECTION OF TREATMENT MODALITY

TREATMENT MODALITY	CRITERIA/PATIENT FACTORS
Larynageal rest/elective period of intubation	Early stenosis: ederna only/no fibrosis "Small" babies—age and weight laryngeal compoenl (e.g., reflux infection)
Endoscopic treatment of granualations and early stenosi: cold steel rather thatn CO_2 laser, balloon dilatation milomycin C, endoscopic cricoid split	Early/"soft" stenosis/granualation tissue/primarily ederna without fibrosis Limited/isolated pathology: grade 1 stenosis
	"Seal flipper" granulations
	In patients not suitable for open surgical intervention because of oxygen requirements, neurologic comorbidities, crniofacial anomalies
	Repeated failure of extubation in neeonate with isolated subglottic stenosis
	Paient weight >1,500 g
	No active respiratory/cardiac comorbidities
Laryngotracheal reconstruction with cartilage augmentation	Symptomatic laryngotracheal stenosis Most appropriate for grades 2 and 3 stenosis patient weight > 2000 g
Cricotracheal resection	Severe grade 3 or grade 4 stenosis
	At least 2 mm from cords
	Long segment stenosis extending into trachea
	Salvage after failed laryngotrachel reconstruction
Tracheostomy	Mediaclly unsitable for other techniques
	Failure of other techniques

Source. Reproduced with permission from Boardman SJ, Albert DM. Single stage and multistage pediatric laryngotracheal reconstruction. *Otolaryngol Clin North Am.* 2008;41(5):947–958.

ETT serves as a stent in ss-LTR, as the patient typically remains intubated for a period of 7 days.[2] The choice between ss-LTR and ds-LTR is based on careful assessment of preoperative disease severity and overall medical status.[10] Patients with higher grades of stenosis and complex multilevel stenosis, significant neurologic deficits, and/or significant lung disease or anatomy that makes reintubation technically difficult (craniofacial or vertebral anomalies) are deemed more suitable for a double stage reconstruction.[10] Single-stage reconstruction is usually reserved for patients who could tolerate compressing the various stages of healing, airway stabilization, and decannulation into a short period of time.[2] Despite there being only a single open procedure with ss-LTR, multiple subsequent endoscopic procedures may be required to further optimize the airway while healing occurs. Since there is no tracheostomy left in place, patients that have undergone ss-LTR have greater reliance on the newly reconstructed airway, and respiratory compromise caused by planned or unplanned extubation can lead to significant morbidity in this patient group. Therefore, the choice of performing ss-LTR requires careful patient selection.

COMPLICATIONS OF LTR

Complications of LTR can be classified based on the type of LTR performed and the time point in the perioperative period: intraoperative or early, intermediate, or late postoperative.[11] Intraoperative complications include pneumothorax, which can occur during rib harvest or distal tracheal mobilization. Air leaks, hematomas, wound infections, pneumonias, or excessive granulation tissue can develop postoperatively. Restenosis is also a complication that can develop over time. It is worth noting that respiratory syncytial virus bronchiolitis and pseudomonal wound abscess were found to prolong the duration of intubation and increased the rates of LTR failure.[12] It is of extreme importance that the ICU team be made aware of the structure of the patient's airway and what to do if inadvertent extubation occurs. This is of particular significance with ss-LTR, as the patient does not have a tracheostomy and the reconstructed airway is stented by an ETT.

POSTOPERATIVE SEDATION

A matter that requires dedicated attention with ss-LTR is adequate sedation. Postoperatively, after ss-LTR, the immediate goal is to keep the patient safe and calm in order to tolerate the ETT. Children typically undergo microlaryngoscopy and downsizing of the ETT under steroid coverage after 7 days, along with a trial of extubation the following day as long as the reconstructed airway appears adequate.[2] Postoperative sedation management is an integral part of the perioperative care of patients after ss-LTR and requires a multidisciplinary team. Sedation practices differ from center to center and can include a spectrum of levels of sedation either alone or in combination with muscle relaxants.[2] The purpose of sedation is to

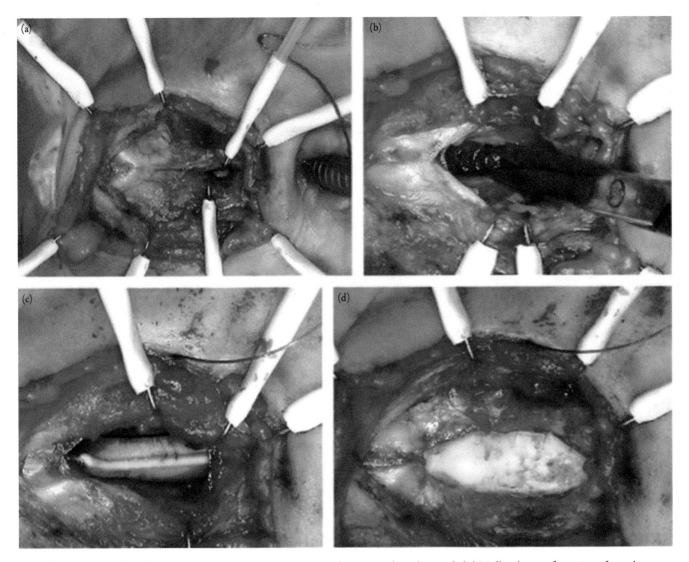

Fig. 22.5 Operative procedure for laryngotracheal reconstruction using autologous costal cartilage graft. (A) Midline laryngofissure is performed. (B) Posterior cricoid split may be required. (C) Stent is positioned appropriately. (D) Boat-shaped anterior cartilaginous graft is fashioned and sutured in place. Reproduced with permission from Boardman SJ, Albert DM. Single stage and multistage pediatric laryngotracheal reconstruction. *Otolaryngol Clin North Am.* 2008;41(5):947–958.

minimize excessive neck movement that could place tension on the newly reconstructed airway thereby causing repeated trauma to the airway mucosa and disrupting cartilage grafts and suture lines. Sedation is typically used for 3–7 days, and the focus is then shifted to weaning off the sedative agents.[13] A quality improvement study by Kozin et al.[13] found that use of a daily assessment tool with a recommended sedation wean plan visible to all members of the multidisciplinary team favorably impacted sedation related outcomes with a 50% decrease in duration of sedation and fewer patients discharged requiring narcotic prescriptions. A retrospective review by Powers et al.[14] of 34 patients treated with ss-LTR reported no significant differences in a sedation (with or without muscle paralysis) and an awake with narcotic pain medicine as needed group. There were, however, significant increases in rates of withdrawal, nursing concerns of withdrawal, sedation level, pulmonary complications, and prolonged hospital stay due to withdrawal in the group that received sedation.[14]

The authors suggest that avoiding sedation for postoperative management after ss-LTR can lead to decreased risk of morbidity without increasing mortality. As noted by the authors, these findings should be interpreted with caution as patients in the nonsedated group were older (median age 39 months vs. 16 months in the sedated group). The authors conclude that minimal sedation may be beneficial in children that are old enough to understand instructions regarding minimization of movement after airway surgery and cooperation with keeping the ETT in place.[14] Optimal postoperative sedation techniques after ss-LTR remain an area of ongoing research.

CONCLUSIONS

- Subglottic stenosis in pediatric patients is most commonly acquired. Of children with acquired SGS, 90% have a history of tracheal intubation.

- The pathogenesis of acquired SGS typically involves the following: intubation→pressure injury→mucosal edema→ulceration and perichondral injury→fibroblasts and granulation tissue→circumferential scarring.

- GERD and systemic factors, such as chronic illness, immunosuppression, and dehydration, increased the susceptibility of the laryngeal mucosa to injury.

- The Myer-Cotton grading system of laryngeal stenosis is the most commonly used classification system with grade 1, 0%–50% obstruction; grade 2, 51%–70%; grade 3, 71%–99%; and grade 4, no detectable lumen.

- Numerous techniques may be used to treat patients with SGS, including medical management to address any reversible components such as reflux and infection, endoscopic treatment of granulations, anterior cricoid split, LTR with cartilage augmentation (single and double stage), cricotracheal resection, and permanent tracheostomy if the patient is medically unsuitable or has failed other techniques.

- Treatment of SGS depends on the degree of the lesion as well as patient factors and other comorbid conditions.

- The choice between ss-LTR and ds-LTR is based on careful assessment of preoperative disease severity and overall medical status. Patients with higher grades of stenosis and with complex systemic disease generally are deemed more suitable for a double-stage reconstruction.

- The operative technique of ss-LTR is very similar to ds-LTR with the exception that the reconstructed airway is stented by an ETT.

- Single-stage LTR has the advantage of immediate deccanulation of tracheostomy or avoiding a tracheostomy completely. The stages of airway stabilization, healing, and decannulation, which typically take several months are compressed into a shorter period of time with ss-LTR.

- Decannulation outcomes after ss-LTR and ds-LTR have been found to be similar.

- Optimal postoperative sedation technique after ss-LTR remains elusive; however, a good communication and sedation wean plan visible to all members of the multidisciplinary team has been found to favorably impact sedation related outcomes.

REVIEW QUESTIONS

1. A 4-month-old infant is transferred to the ICU from an outside hospital for further management of multiple extubation failures. The patient has been intubated since birth due to respiratory failure. He currently has a 2.0 ETT. Microlaryngoscopy and bronchoscopy demonstrates nearly no detectable lumen. The patient's Myer-Cotton grade of laryngeal stenosis can be **BEST** described as:

A. 69%
B. Grade IV
C. 70%
D. Grade 3

Answer: D

The patient has near complete SGS, leading to inability to tolerate extubation attempts. Answer A, 69% occlusion, is not

Table 22.2. **PERCENTAGE OBSTRUCTION BY ACTUAL ENDOTRACHEAL TUBE SIZE**

PATIENT AGE	NORMAL ID (MM)	NORMAL OD (MM)	OBSTRUCTION WITH ACTUAL ENDOTRACHEAL TUBE SIZE (%)								
			ID = 2.0	ID = 2.5	ID = 3.0	ID = 3.5	ID = 4.0	ID = 4.5	ID = 5.0	ID = 5.5	ID = 60
Premature	2.0	2.8	0								
	2.5	3.6	40	0							
	3.0	4.3	58	30	0						
0–3 mo	3.5	5.0	68	48	26	0					
3–9 mo	4.0	5.6	75	59	41	22	0				
9 mo–2 y	4.5	6.2	80	67	53	38	20	0			
2 y	5.0	7.0	84	74	62	50	35	19	0		
4 y	5.5	7.6	86	78	68	57	45	32	17	0	
6 y	6.0	8.2	89	81	73	67	54	43	30	16	0

Note. ID = inside diameter. OD = outside diameter. Percentage of obstruction by actual endotracheal tube size.

Source. Reproduced with permission from Myer CM, O'Connor DM, Cotton RT. Proposed grading system for subglottic stenosis based on endotracheal tube sizes. *Ann Otol Rhinol Laryngol.* 1994;103(4 pt.1):319–323.

correct because the patient's stenosis is more severe than grade 2. The patient still has some subglottic lumen through which a 2.0 ETT passes (Table 22.2), and, therefore answer B, grade 4 SGS, is not correct. Answer C is also within the realm of grade 2 SGS.

Myer-Cotton grading system of laryngeal stenosis.[15]

2. Which of the following patients would be **LEAST** appropriate for treatment with ss-LTR?

    A. a 3-year-old female with trisomy 21, grade 2 SGS, and tracheostomy dependence

    B. a 2-year-old female with Pierre-Robin, grade 3 SGS, and tracheostomy dependence

    C. a 3-year-old female with congenital grade 3 SGS and tracheostomy with multiple failed balloon dilatation procedures

    D. a 3-year-old female with trisomy 21, grade 3 SGS, and tracheostomy dependence

Answer: B

Although not specified in the description, this patient likely has a difficult airway along with a higher severity of SGS. This patient is unlikely to tolerate the compression of the stages of airway stabilization, healing, and decannulation, which typically take several months, into the shorter period of time allowed by ss-LTR. Patients with higher grade of stenosis and anatomy that makes reintubation technically difficult are deemed more suitable for a double stage reconstruction. The patients described in answer choices C and D have high, grade 3 SGS and can certainly also be considered appropriate for ds-LTR; however, there is no additional history mentioned that places them at risk for being a difficult airway, possibly making them suitable candidates for a single-stage procedure.

3. A 30-month old female is undergoing ds-LTR. The procedure begins with a MLB, which confirms grade 3 SGS. In preparation for the rest of the procedure, the patient's neck is extended on a shoulder roll. Thirty minutes after induction of anesthesia, the patient's oxygen saturation decreases to 88%, tidal volumes decrease to approximately 1 mL/kg, and a leak is noted in the breathing circuit. What is the next **BEST** course of action?

    A. Perform immediate needle thoracostomy below the right fifth rib.

    B. Ask the surgeon to advance the anode tube slightly.

    C. Replace the anode tube with the patient's original tracheostomy tube.

    D. Ask the surgeon to withdraw the anode tube slightly.

Answer: B

Complications of LTR can be classified as intraoperative or early, intermediate, or late postoperative. Careful vigilance must be maintained during all parts of the surgery as displacement of exchanged airway devices can occur, particularly during positioning. Many of the patients presenting for LTR can have various comorbid conditions and may not be the most straightforward airways. Answer A is incorrect because the patient does not have a pneumothorax. Answer D is incorrect because the tip of the ETT is not in a mainstem bronchus

or distal airway. Answer C is not the best course in this situation and will only consume time.

4. A 16-month-old male is undergoing ds-LTR. The laryngotracheal skeleton is exposed, and the decision is made to proceed with the laryngotracheal expansion procedure. The previously prepped chest is exposed, and a costal cartilage graft is harvested from the right fifth rib. As the wound is being irrigated, the patient is noted to have slowly progressive hypotension and heart rate of 174 beats per minute. Oxygen saturation drops from 93% to 85%, and peak airway pressure is now 40 cm H_2O. What is the next **BEST** course of action?

    A. Ask the surgeon to advance the anode tube slightly.

    B. Replace the anode tube with the patient's original tracheostomy tube.

    C. Obtain a chest X-ray.

    D. Perform needle thoracostomy below the right fifth rib.

Answer: D

The patient has a life-threatening pneumothorax and needs immediate needle decompression followed by a chest tube. Pneumothorax is a potential intraoperative complication of LTR that can occur during rib harvest or distal tracheal mobilization. Answers A and B will not help manage the pneumothorax. It is unnecessary to obtain a chest X-ray prior to treating a life threating pneumothorax (answer C).

5. A 27-month-old female with grade 3 SGS scheduled for MLB and ds-LTR presents for anesthesia consultation in the preoperative evaluation clinic. Her past medical history is notable for gestational age of 27 weeks at birth and chronic respiratory failure requiring tracheostomy. The patient is at her baseline at present, although her mother notes increased secretions and some episodes of coughing and gagging after meals. Which of the following is **MOST** likely upon further evaluation?

    A. EGD biopsy results demonstrate abundant pale cytoplasm and numerous intraepithelial eosinophils, and, therefore, omeprazole is not required.

    B. EGD biopsy results are within normal limits, and omeprazole is prescribed.

    C. EGD biopsy results are within normal limits, and omeprazole is not required.

    D. No further workup is necessary at this time, and the patient can proceed with surgery.

Answer: B

This patient has symptoms consistent with GERD and requires treatment for reflux. There is a high association between SGS and GERD. GERD not only is a pathogenic factor in the formation of SGS but can negatively impact outcomes with LTR and is therefore aggressively treated. An upper endoscopy might not necessarily be diagnostic of GERD, even when clinically present. Answer A describes EGD biopsy results consistent with GERD but does not include treatment, which is required for best outcomes in this patient. Answers C and D are incorrect as they do not involve treatment.

6. A 1-month-old, former 26-week gestational age, 2.6 kg male has been unable to be extubated since birth. Echocardiogram demonstrates a small VSD with left to right shunt. An MLB

demonstrates grade 3 SGS. Which of the following is the **LEAST** appropriate treatment option at this time?

    A. double-stage LTR
    B. laryngeal rest/elective period of intubation
    C. omeprazole
    D. endoscopic balloon dilatation

Answer: A

Infants weighing <4 kg with gestational age <30 weeks have been found to have a lower chance of success with achieving airway patency and eventual extubation after LTR. This may be due to compromise posed by their various other comorbidities and a small margin of tolerance for airway compromise in this group. Answers B–D are all appropriate considerations at this time.

7. A 30-month-old male is recovering in the ICU after ss-LTR performed 5 days prior. Past medical history includes trisomy 21, stage 2 SGS, and previous tracheostomy, which has now been removed. The patient is nasotracheally intubated and mechanically ventilated. He is maintained on morphine and midazolam infusions. This morning, the patient's bedside nurse reports increased tachycardia, hypertension, and overall irritability in the patient. He reports that some changes were made with the patient's infusions overnight. Which of the following would be the **LEAST** appropriate action at this time?

    A. Increase the patient's midazolam infusion rate.
    B. Check ETT position.
    C. Discontinue the patient's morphine infusion.
    D. Start a dexmedetomidine infusion.

Answer: C

This patient is likely experiencing signs of medication withdrawal. Sedative medication withdrawal is a significant concern after ss-LTR. The goal of sedation after ss-LTR is to minimize excessive neck movements that place tension on the newly reconstructed airway. Sedation practices vary from center to center and can include sedative agents alone or sedatives in combination with muscle relaxants. Answers A, B, and D would all be appropriate steps.

QUESTIONS AND ANSWERS

This chapter has accompanying questions and answers which are available to subscribers as part of the Oxford eLearning platform. To access the questions, go to ✔ http:// oxfordmedicine. com/pediatricanesthesiaPBL

REFERENCES

1. Fearon B, Cotton RT. Surgical correction of subglottic stenosis of the larynx. preliminary report of an experimental surgical technique. *Ann Otol Rhinol Laryngol.* 1972;81(4):508–513.
2. Boardman SJ, Albert DM. Single-stage and multistage pediatric laryngotracheal reconstruction. *Otolaryngol Clin North Am.* 2008;41(5):947–958.
3. Cotton RT, Evans JN. Laryngotracheal reconstruction in children: five-year follow up. *Ann Otol Rhinol Laryngol.* 1981;90(5):516–520.
4. Gould SJ, Young M. Subglottic ulceration and healing following endotracheal intubation in the neonate: a morphometric study. *Ann Otol Rhinol Laryngol.* 1992;101(10):815–820.
5. Meier JD. White DR. Multisystem disease and pediatric laryngotracheal reconstruction. *Otolaryngol Clin North Am.* 2012;45(3):643–651.
6. McQueen CT, Shapiro NL, Leighton S, et al. Single-stage laryngotracheal reconstruction: the Great Ormond Street experience and guidelines for patient selection. *Arch Otolaryngol Head Neck Surg.* 1999;125:320–322.
7. Hartley BE, Rutter MJ, Cotton RT. Cricotracheal resection as a primary procedure for laryngotracheal stenosis in children. *Int J Pediatr Otorhinolaryngol.* 2000;54(2–3):133–136.
8. Triglia JM, Nicollas R, Roman S. Primary cricotracheal resection in children: indications, technique and outcome. *Int J Pediatr Otorhinolaryngol.* 2001;58(1):17–25.
9. Monnier P, Lang F, Marcel S. Cricotracheal resection for pediatric subglottic stenosis. *Int J Pediatr Otorhinolaryngol.* 1999;49 (Suppl 1):S283–S286.
10. Smith LP, Zur KB, Jacobs IN. Single-vs double stage LTR. *Arch Otolaryngol Head Neck Surg.* 2010;136(1):60–65.
11. Cotton RT. Management of subglottic stenosis. *Otolaryngol Clin North Am.* 2000;33(1):111–130.
12. Ludemann JP. Hughes CA. Noah Z, et al. Complications of pediatric laryngotracheal reconstruction: prevention strategies. *Ann Otol Rhinol Laryngol.* 1999;108(11):1019–1026.
13. Kozin ED, Cummings BM, Roger DJ, et al. System wide change of sedation wean protocol following pediatric laryngotracheal reconstruction. *JAMA Otolaryngol Head Neck Surg.* 2015;141(1) 27–33.
14. Powers MA, Mudd P, Gralla J, et al. Sedation-related outcomes in postoperative management of pediatric laryngotracheal reconstruction. *Int J Pediatr Otorhinolaryngol.* 2013;77(9):1567–1574.
15. Jacobs I. Subglottic stenosis. The Children's Hospital of Philadelphia SGS website. http://www.chop.edu/conditions-diseases/subglottic-stenosis#. Accessed June 20, 2017

23.

CYSTIC FIBROSIS

Jamey Snell and Thomas J. Mancuso

STEM CASE AND KEY QUESTIONS

A 13-year-old girl is scheduled for a gastric fundoplication. She carries the diagnosis of cystic fibrosis (CF) and gastroesophageal reflux disease (GERD). The diagnosis of GERD is based on her symptoms of epigastric and chest pain and dysphagia. She has been hospitalized twice in the past year for pulmonary exacerbations, and the most recent hospitalization included time in the intensive care unit, receiving noninvasive ventilatory support. She is chronically colonized in her lungs with *Aspergillus*.

Her medications are

- Inhaled deoxyribonuclease
- Nebulized tobramycin
- Nebulized hypertonic saline
- Levalbuterol
- Inhaled steroids
- Omeprazole
- Supplemental O_2 via nasal cannula, 1–2 LPM at night for peripheral capillary oxygen saturation (SpO_2) <92% (family and primary pediatrician are considering starting noninvasive ventilation at night)

WHAT DIAGNOSTIC STUDIES WOULD GENERALLY HAVE BEEN USED TO CONFIRM THE CLINICAL DIAGNOSIS OF GERD IN THIS PATIENT?

In all patients, GERD can be confirmed with clinical signs and symptoms but these are nonspecific and many are present in patients with CF in the absence of GERD (Table 23.1).

Diagnostic studies that can confirm the clinical suspicion of GERD include a contrast esophagogram, esophageal pH testing, upper endoscopy, and laryngotracheal endoscopy. A contrast esophagogram is not specific or sensitive for GERD but can reveal an esophageal stricture, stenosis, hiatal hernia, or gastric outlet obstruction. Esophageal pH monitoring of the distal esophagus provides a quantitative record of acid reflux episodes. There are established normal values for exposure of the esophagus to acid, generally less than 8% of the time. This study can be used to help make the diagnosis and also to assess the adequacy of acid suppression treatment. Upper endoscopy can be used to diagnose esophagitis or strictures. Biopsies can be taken that can demonstrate allergic or infectious causes for esophagitis. Laryngotracheobronchoscopy evaluates the airway for signs that are seen in patients with symptomatic GERD, such as inflammation or nodules on the vocal cords. Bronchoalveolar lavage samples can be analyzed for pepsin or lipid-laden macrophages.

WHAT WOULD PULMONARY FUNCTION TESTS LIKELY SHOW IN THE PATIENT?

Early: obstructive disease

- Increased residual volume and functional residual capacity
- Little response to bronchodilators
- Increased alveolar-arterial O_2 difference

Late: restrictive disease

- Decreased vital capacity
- Decreased total lung capacity

WHAT OTHER LABORATORY TESTS WOULD YOU WANT TO REVIEW PRIOR TO GOING TO THE OPERATING ROOM (OR)?

Electrolytes and glucose: Up to 20% of adolescents with CF develop diabetes mellitus (DM). Even in the absence of the typical signs and symptoms, such as polyuria, polydipsia, and weight loss, it is possible that the first early sign of DM will be a random glucose that is elevated above the normal range. A hyponatremic, hypochloremic metabolic alkalosis may be seen in patients with CF, particularly in the setting of gastroenteritis or in warm climate. For severe cases, liver function tests may be abnormal as well.

Complete blood count: The most common abnormality seen in the complete blood count of CF patients is an iron deficiency anemia. This hypochromic, microcytic anemia is seen

Table 23.1 CLINICAL SIGNS AND SYMPTOMS OF GASTROESOPHAGEAL REFLUX DISEASE

Symptoms of GERD

- **Weight loss**
- **Recurrent emesis**
- **Dysphagia**
- **Chest pain**
- **Cough/Hoarseness**

Signs of GERD

- **Esophagitis**
- **Esophageal stricture**
- **Recurrent pneumonia**
- **Anemia**

Note. GERD = gastroesophageal reflux disease

particularly in patients with poor gastrointestinal (GI) function and vitamin deficiencies.

HOW WOULD YOU PREPARE THIS PATIENT FOR THE SURGERY AND ANESTHETIC?

- Pulmonary toilet

- Antibiotics

- Review imaging studies

- Inquire about exercise tolerance

- Consult with their outpatient pulmonologist for perioperative recommendations

- Approach the patient with a keen sensitivity to the psychosocial challenges common for adolescents living with chronic diseases, such as anxiety and depression

- Inform patient, family, and postoperative personnel for the possibility of noninvasive ventilation or intubation following surgery

WOULD YOU PREMEDICATE THIS PATIENT? IF SO, WHEN? HOW?

For the anxious child, a conservative weight-appropriate dose of oral or intravenous (IV) midazolam is appropriate. Simple face mask oxygen should be given prior to any medications that will affect respiratory drive and/or pulmonary function. Consideration should be given to administration of nebulizer treatments prior to going to the OR. The patient might benefit from treatment with her usual hypertonic saline by nebulizer. In addition, she may be aware that nebulized bronchodilators have been beneficial for prior exacerbations. If so, treatments with albuterol or levalbuterol should be considered to reduce the risk of bronchospasm. The role of glycopyrrolate is somewhat controversial due to the risk of inspissating secretions, making them more difficult to mobilize and clear.

HOW WOULD YOU PLAN TO MONITOR THIS PATIENT DURING THIS CASE?

- Standard American Society of Anesthesiologists monitors and arterial line.

- Arterial blood gases followed during the case: significant increase in dead space to tidal volume ratio (V_d/V_t) as CF progresses; therefore, end-tidal CO_2 will not reflect arterial partial pressure of CO_2 in arterial blood ($PaCO_2$).

WHAT IS YOUR INDUCTION PLAN?

Given the indication for the surgery, it can be assumed that the patient has an incompetent lower esophageal sphincter. This may lead to passive passage of acidic gastric fluid into the oropharynx, and potentially the airway, during an inhalational induction or prolonged IV induction, especially while supine. Options to mitigate pulmonary aspiration risks include slight head-up positioning, rapid sequence induction, or modified rapid sequence induction employing the use of cricoid-pressure with small tidal volume ventilation to optimize preoxygenation prior to laryngoscopy. Medication dosing should take into account alterations in drug metabolism due to lower body mass and volume of distribution, hepatic function, and possible renal dysfunction from chronic aminoglycoside use.

IF THE SURGICAL PLAN IS TO PERFORM THE PROCEDURE VIA A LAPAROSCOPIC APPROACH, WOULD YOU INCLUDE REGIONAL ANALGESIA AS PART OF THE ANESTHETIC? IF AN OPEN APPROACH?

Though abdominal wall blocks, such as transversus abdominis plane and rectus sheath blocks, may be employed for laparoscopic surgery, typically infiltration of the trocar sites with local anesthetic by the surgeon provides similar results. For an open approach, however, the use of regional or neuraxial anesthesia can provide significant benefits for postoperative recovery. Breathing can aggravate pain at the surgical incision, leading to splinting and hypoventilation. Subsequent atelectasis and impaired ability to clear secretions can not only increase supplemental oxygen requirements and the need for respiratory support but also increase the risk for pneumonia. A midthoracic epidural can reduce the amount of intraoperative opioids required and facilitate postoperative recovery by allowing for full participation in incentive spirometry, respiratory therapy, and early ambulation.

WHAT SPECIAL PREPARATIONS WOULD YOU MAKE REGARDING INTUBATION OF THIS PATIENT?

Although utilization of a laryngeal mask airway has the advantage of causing less irritation to the airway, gastric fundoplication requires controlled ventilation for surgical purposes and, therefore, endotracheal intubation. Laryngoscopy does not typically present unique challenges in this population. Endotracheal tube size should take into consideration the advantages of larger tubes, which allow for better pulmonary toilet, versus smaller tubes, which may be preferred to reduce compression on the laryngotracheal mucosa, causing less subsequent edema. Finally, warming the tube prior to intubation helps to reduce the risk of bronchospasm.

HOW WILL YOU VENTILATE THIS PATIENT ONCE INTUBATION IS ACCOMPLISHED?

In general, mechanical ventilation can have deleterious effects on the fragile lungs of CF patients. Warm, moist air is replaced with cold, dry air, leading to inspissated secretions, mucociliary dysfunction, and loss of protective epithelial surface fluid. Use of a filter or heat–moisture exchanger between the anesthesia circuit and endotracheal tube (ETT) should be employed to reduce the potential for insult. When possible, use of spontaneous negative-pressure ventilation is superior to controlled positive-pressure ventilation due to the former's ability to utilize the diaphragm and more efficiently provide ventilation and perfusion to the bases of the lungs, where the majority of gas-exchange takes place. Positive-pressure ventilation also has the theoretical risk of forcing secretions more distally down the tracheobronchial tree into the alveoli and bronchioles. However, when muscle paralysis is required for surgical purposes, the following steps can be taken to optimize mechanical ventilation:

- Higher positive end-expiratory pressure (PEEP; 8–10 cm H_2O) to prevent airway collapse

- A 1:1 inspiratory:expiratory time ratio for patients with pulmonary function tests suggestive of restrictive physiology

- A 1:3 inspiratory:expiratory time ratio for patients with pulmonary function tests suggestive of obstructive physiology

- Volume-controlled, pressure-limited controlled ventilation mode during laparoscopic procedures, where pneumoperitoneum can dynamically alter intrathoracic compliance.

Rarely, patients with severe CF may require anesthesia for pulmonary hygiene to reduce mucus burden or bronchoalveolar lavage for sputum samples to guide antibiotic therapy. One should be aware that the ability to completely clear all secretions is not a reasonable goal. Repeated, aggressive suctioning can within itself lead to trauma to the tracheobronchial mucosa and induce inflammation and edema. When possible, consult with pulmonology for a comprehensive perioperative plan for elective cases, when time permits.

DISCUSSION

Cystic fibrosis is an inherited, autosomal recessive, multisystem disease. Dysfunction of the CF transmembrane conductance regulator protein (CFTR) in epithelial cells is the primary defect in CF and is responsible for the clinical presentations of CF. Defects in CFTR are the cause for lung disease, exocrine pancreatic insufficiency and failure, male infertility, and liver disease. Though most often diagnosed by newborn screening, the condition can present with a variety of respiratory and GI signs, including meconium ileus in the newborn period, hypernatremic dehydration, pulmonary insufficiency, nasal polyps, and insulin-dependent DM. As affected children grow, dysfunction in CFTR leads to chronic and progressive lung disease, characterized by suppurative infection and the development of bronchiectasis. CFTR dysfunction also affects exocrine function, leading to pancreatic insufficiency, malabsorption, and growth failure.

Cystic fibrosis transmembrane conductance regulator protein regulates sodium and chloride transport through the epithelial sodium channel and promotes bicarbonate secretion. The CFTR gene, located on chromosome band 7q31.2, is composed of more than 1,800 amino acids. More than 1,500 mutations have been identified, and the majority have been classified into 1 of 5 classes based on the specific effect on CFTR (Figure 23.1). The most common CFTR mutation, ΔF508, accounts for 70% of the CF alleles in northern European and North American populations. Surprisingly, an individual patient's genotype may not correlate with the severity of their phenotype, reflecting an effect of secondary modifiers.

In the past, history and physical exam with sweat chloride testing were the cornerstones of diagnosis. Diagnosis is now made with the newborn screening test for immunoreactive trypsinogen.[1] High levels found in this test prompt a repeat to rule out a spurious result, followed by a diagnostic sweat chloride test.

DEMOGRAPHICS AND LIFE EXPECTANCY

Cystic fibrosis occurs in all ethnic and geographic groups but is seen most commonly in Caucasians of northern European descent. In this group, the prevalence is 1 in 3,000 Caucasian Americans, 1 in 10,000 Latin Americans, and 1 in 15,000 African Americans.

Advances in newborn screening, respiratory therapy, nutrition, and medical interventions have led to significant increases in survival and quality of life for patients with CF over the past decades. According to the Cystic Fibrosis Foundation Patient Registry, when comparing data from 2015 to 2000, nearly 29,000 persons were living in the United States with CF in 2015 versus 22,000 in 2000; adults comprise 51.6% of the living CF population versus 38.7%; mortality rates has decreased from 1.9 to 1.5 per 100 persons, annually; predicted median survival has increased from 33.3 to 41.7 years of age, with a small number of patients reaching 60+ years of age.[2] In fact, for newborns born and diagnosed in 2015, the life expectancy is estimated at 45 years.[1] Leading causes of death continue to be cardiopulmonary in nature (64.5%), followed by lung transplant-related complications (19.2%), and liver failure (3.3%).[1] As a result, these improvements in survival have also led to an increase in patients with CF presenting to

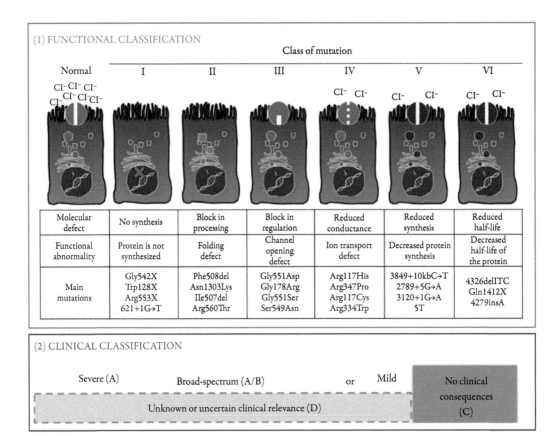

(1) FUNCTIONAL CLASSIFICATION

Class of mutation

	Normal	I	II	III	IV	V	VI
Molecular defect		No synthesis	Block in processing	Block in regulation	Reduced conductance	Reduced synthesis	Reduced half-life
Functional abnormality		Protein is not synthesized	Folding defect	Channel opening defect	Ion transport defect	Decreased protein synthesis	Decreased half-life of the protein
Main mutations		Gly542X Trp128X Arg553X 621+1G→T	Phe508del Asn1303Lys Ile507del Arg560Thr	Gly551Asp Gly178Arg Gly551Ser Ser549Asn	Arg117His Arg347Pro Arg117Cys Arg334Trp	3849+10kbC→T 2789+5G→A 3120+1G→A 5T	4326delITC Gln1412X 4279insA

(2) CLINICAL CLASSIFICATION

Severe (A)   Broad-spectrum (A/B)   or   Mild   No clinical consequences (C)

Unknown or uncertain clinical relevance (D)

Fig. 23.1 Classification models for CF based upon CFTR function (1) and clinical manifestations (2). ©2015 Anne Bergougnoux, Magali Taulan-Cadars, Mireille Claustres, and Caroline Raynal. Originally published in *New Molecular Diagnosis Approaches—From the Identification of Mutations to their Characterization, Cystic Fibrosis in the Light of New Research*, Dr. Dennis Wat (Ed.), InTech, under Creative Commons Attribution 3.0 Unported license. Available from: 10.5772/60679

the OR. Common procedures for which CF patients present are listed in Table 23.2, and a more detailed description of less common manifestations can be found in O'Sullivan and Freedman's[2] review article published in the *Lancet* in 2009.

DIAGNOSIS AND NATURAL HISTORY

Early diagnosis and intervention has played an essential role in improving the health care of patients living with CF. The

Table 23.2 **COMMON SURGERIES IN CYSTIC FIBROSIS PATIENTS**

NEONATES	CHILDREN/TEENAGERS	ADULTS
Meconium ileus	Nasal polpectomy	Esophageal varices
Meconium peritonitis	Vascular access	Recurrent pneumothorax
Intestinal atresia/ obstruction	Ear/nose/throat surgery	Cholecystectomy
Intussusception	Bronchoalveolar lavage	Lung or liver transplantation
	Nissen fundoplication	
	Rectal prolapse repair	
	Appendectomy	

Note. Modified from Della Rocca G. Anaesthesia in patients with cystic fibrosis. *Curr Opin Anaesthesiol.* 2002;15:95–101.

Center for Disease Control[3] recommends all newborns be screened for immunoreactive trypsinogen as part of a standard panel. A positive screening test is confirmed by either diagnostic sweat chloride testing or nasal potential difference test. Still other patients, with a high index of suspicion, are diagnosed prenatally (chorionic villus sampling, amniocentesis, etc.), by DNA analysis or by family history. Over the past 15 years, the number of patients diagnosed by newborn screening has increased dramatically from 8.1% to 59.6%.[2] Given that a significant number of newborns may be asymptomatic during infancy, this important trend reduces the likelihood of a delayed or missed diagnosis. A Cochrane review, based upon two large randomized controlled trials inclusive of over 2 million neonates, concluded that CF diagnosed in screened populations had improved nutritional and, perhaps also, pulmonary outcomes.[4]

The variability in genetic mutations and CFTR function associated with CF results in a wide range of clinical manifestations, from nearly asymptomatic to severe multisystem dysfunction due to exocrinopathies (Table 23.3). Presentations for which one should suspect CF in the undiagnosed patient includes those with chronic sinopulmonary infection, GI and nutritional abnormalities, dehydration with hyponatremic hypochloremic metabolic alkalosis, or reproductive abnormalities in males. Manifestations during the neonatal period include conditions, such as meconium ileus

Table 23.3 CLINICAL MANIFESTATIONS OF CYSTIC FIBROSIS

RESPIRATORY/CARDIAC

- Chronic productive cough
- Lower airways bacterial colonization
- Endobronchial infection
- Exercise intolerance
- Hypoxemia
- Bronchiectasis
- Pneumothorax
- Hemoptysis
- Digital clubbing
- Pleuritis
- Rib fractures
- Pulmonary hypertension/heart failure

Upper airway

- Chronic pansinusitis
- Nasal polyposis

Gastrointestinal/Nutritional

- Vitamin A, D, E, and K deficiencies
- Zinc deficiency dermatitis
- Protein and fat malabsorption
- Malnutrition/failure to thrive
- Meconium ileus
- Distal intestinal obstruction syndrome
- Obstructive jaundice
- Focal biliary cirrhosis
- Portal hypertension
- Rectal prolapse
- Recurrent pancreatitis
- Diabetes mellitus

Other systemic conditions

- Anxiety/depression
- Hyponatremic dehydration
- Hypochloremic alkalosis
- Male infertility

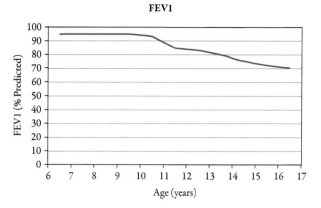

Fig. 23.2 FEV_1, % predicted according to age, demonstrating onset of decline during adolescence. ©2012 Iara Maria Sequeiros and Nabil A. Jarad. *Radiological Features of Cystic Fibrosis, Cystic Fibrosis—Renewed Hopes Through Research,* Dr. Dinesh Sriramulu (Ed.), InTech, under Creative Commons Attribution 3.0 Unported license. Available from: doi:10.5772/29614.

and prolonged jaundice[3]. During infancy and childhood, complications include malnutrition, fat-soluble vitamin deficiency, hypoproteinemia, failure to thrive, and growth restriction. Respiratory conditions become more apparent and may include nasal polyposis and sinus infections, chronic cough and sputum production, chronic infection—typically by *Staphylococcus aureus, Haemophilus influenzae,* or *Pseudomonas aeruginosa,* and less commonly by *Burkholderia cepacia* complex, *Stenotrophomonas maltophilia, Mycobacterium,* and *Aspergillus*—leading to inflammation, bronchiectasis, air trapping, and obstructive physiology. In adulthood, infertility, recurrent pancreatitis leading to diabetes, digital clubbing, liver failure, pulmonary hypertension, and right heart failure from chronic hypercapnia and hypoxia may ensue.[3,2]

Throughout the lifetime of CF patients, pulmonary function progressively declines and remains the most significant source of morbidity and mortality. Pulmonary dysfunction, most frequently assessed by trending forced expiratory volume in the first second (FEV_1) as a relative percentage of predicted normal values, is considered mild when >70%, moderate when between 70% and 40%, and severe when <40%.[1] Although FEV_1 declines progressively throughout life, the rate of decline is not uniform and, within itself, can be more predictive of long-term outcomes than viewing an individual's FEV_1 in isolation at a single time point.[2] In fact, the majority of young children have only mild respiratory disease, as determined by pulmonary function tests, until adolescence, when a precipitous decline in function is seen on the population-level (Figure 23.2).[2]

TREATMENT

The well understood pathophysiology of CF makes the condition an ideal candidate for targeted molecular therapy. Though the mainstay of medical treatment focuses on symptom management, these targeted therapies specifically aim to normalize function of the CFTR protein itself. Ivacaftor, a drug that works by binding to CFTR and potentiating its ability to conduct chloride ions, was approved in 2012 for children and adults with specific gene mutations. A second drug, Lumacaftor, a chaperone drug that facilitates proper protein folding and trafficking to the cell surface membrane, was approved in 2015 for select patients with other gene mutations. Despite the myriad of genetic mutations implicated in patients with CF, those potentially treatable by CFTR modulator therapies represent approximately half of affected individuals, and there are more in the clinical trial pipeline.[1,2,5]

The majority of medical therapy in CF focuses primarily on addressing respiratory, GI, and endocrine dysfunction. In the lungs, impaired mucociliary function hampers the ability of the airway to clear secretions and pathogens. This leads to mucus plugging, atelectasis, recurrent bacterial infection (pneumonia and bronchitis), and subsequent chronic inflammatory damage. Persistent inflammation evolves to bronchiectasis, impaired gas exchange, ventilation/perfusion mismatch, bronchial hyperreactivity, pneumothorax from emphysema with bullae, and hemoptysis from vascular proliferation.

Chronic therapies aim to improve airway clearance by mechanical and pharmacologic means and to treat infections. Mechanical airway clearance techniques include manual chest percussion, postural drainage, positive expiratory pressure devices, chest wall oscillation vests, vibratory expiration devices, and forced expiration combined with induced coughing exercises.[3,6] Drugs that facilitate hydration and clearance of secretions include inhaled hypertonic (7%) saline and nebulized deoxyribonuclease, which cleaves accumulated nuclear debris from neutrophils.[6] With regard to reducing inflammation, extended use of ibuprofen has been shown to decrease the rate of decline of lung function in some patients; however, chronic steroid use either systemic or inhaled has no proven efficacy outside of treatment of concomitant asthma.[7] For managing chronic bacterial colonization, regular cycled use of inhaled antibiotics, such as tobramycin, colistin, and aztreonam, and oral azithromycin, have all been demonstrated to improve lung function and reduce exacerbations.[4] It is important to note that these treatment modalities represent patient-specific recommendations, taking into account age, lung function, and bacterial flora.

Pulmonary exacerbations represent an acute on chronic disease presentation, which has significant implications for morbidity and mortality.[3] They are characterized by increased cough, change in sputum, fever, decreased appetite, weight loss, increased work of breathing, and/or new onset of crackles or wheezes on exam. Further workup can reveal radiographic changes on chest X-ray (Figure 23.3), leukocytosis, and decrease in FEV_1.[3] In addition to maintaining chronic therapies, treatment of acute exacerbations also incorporate IV antibiotics, typically aimed at pseudomonas. Inhaled bronchodilators also have a role for those presenting with airway hyperresponsiveness.[5]

Despite improvements in medical therapies, progression of the disease process toward end-stage disease and respiratory failure leads to over 200 bilateral lung transplants annually.[2] Indications include progressive loss of FEV_1 to <30%–40% predicted, persistent hypoxemia and hypercapnia, and increased frequency of acute exacerbations refractory to medical treatment. Efforts to optimize the risk–benefit ratio of such a limited supply of donor organs requires careful selection of patients deemed sick enough to require surgical intervention but with the greatest likelihood of survival posttransplant. That often excludes children who, by potentially qualifying for being listed for transplant early in life, can be inferred to have more aggressive disease and will either die while on the waiting list or not be listed at all.[3]

In addition to pulmonary function, optimizing nutrition is the second most important health objective to improve outcomes and quality of the care in patients with CF. In children, goal body mass index is >50th percentile, which is associated with improved survival and pulmonary function testing.[1] Guidelines support the use of pancreatic enzymes and fat-soluble vitamin supplements in those with pancreatic insufficiency, and acid blockers are prescribed to over half of patients to treat GERD.[1] Other GI complications requiring therapy include CF-related diabetes, occurring in about 8% of children, and hepatobiliary disease, which may progress to cirrhosis and liver failure in a fraction of patients, necessitating transplantation.[6]

CONCLUSIONS

1. As medical therapy continues to increase the life expectancy of patients with CF, their presentation for anesthesia and surgery is becoming more frequent.

2. Neonatal screening has significantly decreased the incidence of missed diagnoses; however, the presence of a CF-related condition should raise the index of suspicion for those without the diagnosis and even those with a negative sweat-chloride test.

3. Anesthetic goals include preoperative utilization of pulmonary exercises to clear secretions, minimizing any impairment to respiratory function with a balanced anesthetic and multimodal analgesia, and dosing medications with an awareness to alterations in drug metabolism.

4. In addition to respiratory and GI dysfunction, nutritional deficits, exocrinopathies, and psychosocial conditions can also have implications for their perioperative care.

5. Though FEV_1 is the most common objective parameter used to trend CF disease progression, exercise tolerance, rate of decline of FEV_1, frequency and severity of

Fig. 23.3 Chest radiograph of a CF patient with hyperinflated lungs and severe bilateral and diffuse bronchiectasis. Note the port-a-cath device used for the administration of IV antibiotics (arrows). ©2012 Iara Maria Sequeiros and Nabil A. Jarad. *Radiological Features of Cystic Fibrosis, Cystic Fibrosis–Renewed Hopes Through Research*, Dr. Dinesh Sriramulu (Ed.), InTech, under Creative Commons Attribution 3.0 Unported license. Available from: doi:10.5772/29614.

exacerbations, nutritional status, and other CF-related diseases should all be taken to account for a comprehensive preoperative assessment.

6. Consult with pulmonology when possible to develop a comprehensive perioperative plan.

REVIEW QUESTIONS

1. A 10-year-old girl with a known history of CF presents to the OR for surgical repair of a fractured distal radius, sustained from a sports-related injury ~24 hours ago. Though pulses in the affected limb are strong, she does report mild paresthesias in her fingers. While in the emergency room, her pain has been reasonably controlled with acetaminophen and ibuprofen. While assessing the patient's past medical history, you are informed that she is known to the pulmonology service at your hospital, and her baseline FEV_1 is 68%; however, she has had increased cough and sputum production within the past few days. She is afebrile, and her SpO_2 is 94% on room air, from a baseline of 98%. She does not appear in respiratory distress. She has been nil per os for >12 hours and denies GI-related co-morbidities other than pancreatic insufficiency. Which of the following would be **BEST** to obtain prior to proceeding with surgery?

A. arterial blood gas
B. chest radiography
C. pulmonary consult
D. pulmonary function tests

Answer: B

This is an urgent case given the risk for neurovascular compromise from her fracture. Though the patient's FEV_1 suggests only mild to moderate respiratory dysfunction, her symptoms could reflect the early stages of a pulmonary exacerbation, which could require further treatment during this admission. Although the repair of her fracture should not be significantly delayed, a quick portable chest X-ray could help obtain useful radiographic information about her current pulmonary status prior to introducing the confounding element of general anesthesia. This may not change her anesthetic plan per se but would certainly be useful for a pulmonary consult, which would be more appropriately obtained postoperatively. Given the time-sensitive nature of the procedure, pulmonary function tests, or a nutritional consult would also cause an unnecessary delay. Since the patient is not in respiratory distress, an arterial blood gases is also not indicated at this time.[8]

2. Which of the following, with general anesthesia, is the **MOST** appropriate plan?

A. endotracheal intubation with rapid sequence induction
B. endotracheal intubation with standard IV induction
C. endotracheal intubation with standard IV induction, and regional anesthesia
D. laryngeal mask airway with standard IV induction, and regional anesthesia

Answer: D

Preservation of normal respiratory function is of utmost importance in the perioperative setting. Although spontaneous ventilation can also be achieved with endotracheal airway management, the ability to avoid muscle relaxant optimizes diaphragmatic function and gas exchange at the lung bases throughout the anesthetic, reducing atelectasis and V/Q mismatch. This is best achieved via laryngeal mask airway. Due to the time frame of the patient's injury, adequate pain control, and lack of preoperative opioid administration, the likelihood of gastroparesis, and risk for aspiration with induction is low. Finally, if surgically acceptable, regional anesthesia provides pain control without the side effects of opioids that are particularly deleterious to patients with CF, namely respiratory depression and constipation.[9]

3. A 28-year-old man with CF was recently admitted to the hospital for IV antibiotics and supportive care due to a pulmonary exacerbation. His presentation is complicated by significant pleuritic chest pain due to 2 right-sided rib fractures from violent coughing episodes. He reports fairly constant 8/10 pain. Prior to this admission, he was in a reasonable state of health and could tolerate mild to moderate exercise. You are consulted as part of the acute pain service to provide recommendations for managing his pain. With addition of scheduled ibuprofen and acetaminophen, which option represents the **MOST** ideal analgesic plan?

A. lidocaine (5%) patches
B. morphine patient-controlled analgesia
C. paravertebral catheter for local anesthesia infusion
D. regularly scheduled doses of oxycodone

Answer: C

Ibuprofen and acetaminophen present no enhanced risks to CF patients compared with healthy patients. In fact, ibuprofen is often prescribed for chronic use in some individuals for its anti-inflammatory effects in the lungs; although, clinical evidence proving its efficacy is mixed. In the setting of acute chest wall pain, use of nonsteroidal anti-inflammatory drugs and acetaminophen can be beneficial as adjuncts but will likely be inadequate alone to prevent the respiratory splinting that would put this patient at risk for decline in pulmonary function. A stronger analgesic is therefore indicated. Oxycodone and morphine are not ideal due to their side effects. Choices C and D both offer nonopioid alternatives; however, given the possible duration of the patient's stay and the ability of a paravertebral catheter to offer a more extensive nerve block, it would be a more effective approach.[3,8]

4. A 15-year-old boy with a history of moderate CF based upon FEV_1, and moderate, persistent asthma presented to the hospital 3 days ago with a pulmonary exacerbation. Coincidentally, he was scheduled to undergo elective surgery around this same time for tonsillectomy due to recurrent infection and mild sleep disordered breathing. His parents have requested that he get the tonsillectomy during this admission, so he does not miss his appointment. At home, he only had a nocturnal oxygen requirement of 1–2 L/min. In the hospital, he now requires the same flow rate while awake to maintain

an SpO_2 >95%. He is mildly tachypneic, has a frequent and productive cough, and is anxious about receiving general anesthesia. Which option represents the **MOST** appropriate postoperative plan?

A. Encourage delay of procedure until his exacerbation has passed.
B. Extubate in OR, high-flow nasal cannula in postanesthesia care unit, transfer to the floor.
C. Extubate in OR, bilevel positive airway pressure in postanesthesia care unit, transfer to the floor.
D. Remain intubated, transfer directly to the intensive care unit from the OR.

Answer: A

Extubation should always be the goal, when possible, in the postoperative setting for patients with CF. For many older children, adults, and their families, there is a keen awareness and anxiety of the possibility of a prolonged intubation. In the setting of an acute exacerbation, the introduction of endotracheal intubation and general anesthesia are almost guaranteed to worsen symptoms and possibly preclude postoperative extubation. Even bronchoscopy for diagnostic and therapeutic purposes should be carefully considered for the risks and benefits in the setting of an acute exacerbation. Elective procedures requiring general anesthesia should be avoided whenever possible in the acute period and delayed until at least 2–4 weeks after the exacerbation has been treated. Consultation with the patient's pulmonologist can provide even greater insight into the appropriate timing and perioperative plan for elective surgery.[3,8]

5. Which of the following controlled, mechanical ventilation goals would be **MOST** reasonable for an intubated child with moderate to severe CF undergoing a 2-hour operation?

A. high fresh gas flows
B. low lung volumes
C. minimal PEEP settings
D. normal to elevated end-tidal CO_2

Answer: D

Patients with mild to moderate disease may have low to normal $PaCO_2$ due to compensatory hyperventilation accompanying their obstructive respiratory physiology. As the disease process worsens, a more restrictive pattern is seen, along with a decline in pulmonary compliance and less efficient gas exchange. This can lead to CO_2 retention, chronic hypercarbia, respiratory acidosis, and even cor pulmonale. Ventilation goals should seek to maintain the patient's baseline. In the absence of an arterial blood gas, examining the bicarbonate level on a basic metabolic panel may provide clues into the patient's preoperative acid-base status. Answer choice A is correct given that this patient has moderate to severe disease. Other goals during controlled ventilation include minimizing atelectasis by avoiding low lung volumes and utilizing normal to high PEEP, increasing the inspiratory time if restrictive physiology is present, and lower flows of dry gases to reduce dehydration of the airways and inspissation of secretions.[8,9]

6. Which of the following is the **MOST** likely lab value in a 2-day-old newborn scheduled for an exploratory laparotomy for meconium ileus?

A. eosinophil count > 1000 (1.0×10^9/L)
B. hemoglobin = 17 g/dL
C. platelet count < 90,000
D. Prolonged PT/activated PTT

Answer: B

Normal newborn hemoglobin is 19 gm/dL +/−2 gm/dL, and newborns with CF will fall within this normal range.[9] Some patients with CF develop allergic bronchopulmonary aspergillosis, and part of the presentation of this entity includes the presence of eosinophils in the sputum and also may include increased eosinophils in the peripheral blood; however, this tends to occur later in life and not in the immediate postnatal period, so answer A is not correct. Platelet count is normal in patients with CF, so answer C is not correct. Infants who receive IM vitamin K at birth only very rarely exhibit bleeding disorders and significant abnormalities of coagulation studies, so D is not correct.[10,11]

7. A 3 kg newborn with a diagnosis of CF and intestinal obstruction is presumed to have meconium ileus. Attempts to relieve the obstruction with hypertonic enemas have led to a bowel perforation, and the child is coming emergently to the OR for an exploratory laparotomy. In addition to continuing the patient's usual maintenance fluids, what is the **MOST** appropriate perioperative fluid management for the patient?

A. dextrose 10% in water, 10 mL/kg
B. dextrose 5%/0.2 normal saline, 30 mL IV bolus, then 12 mL/hr
C. 0.9 normal saline, 60 mL
D. dextrose 5% in lactated Ringer's injection, 12 mL/hr

Answer: C

The enemas, often diatrizoate (Gastrografin®) or N-acetylcysteine (Mucomyst®), work by absorbing fluid from the bowel wall into the intestinal lumen, decreasing intravascular volume. Replenishment of that lost volume with isotonic fluid is the most appropriate management. Of course, as mentioned, glucose containing fluids should be continued at the preoperative rate. Answer B is not correct since dextrose 5%/0.2 normal saline is hypotonic, and answer D is not correct, both because additional glucose is not needed and because the rate of infusion is insufficient.[12]

8. An anxious 16-year-old young lady with CF is scheduled for extensive dental restorations with general anesthesia. In her preanesthetic laboratory evaluation, the values are all within normal limits except for a glucose of 190 mg/dL. Repeat is 188 mg/dL. What is the **MOST** likely explanation for the high glucose value?

A. daily inhaled steroid use
B. not fasting prior to the phlebotomy
C. preoperative anxiety
D. undiagnosed CF-related DM

Answer: D

In addition to exocrine dysfunction, patients with CF may develop DM. This occurs in the second or third decade of life, and the diabetes has features of both type 1 and type 2. Progressive damage to the pancreas leads to diminishing secretion of insulin by the islet cells—mimicking the presentation of type 2, but eventually the deficiency of insulin is complete. As in type 1, children with CF-related DM have yet another reason for poor weight gain and perhaps worsened pulmonary function. Patients with CF-related DM also develop the microvascular complications typically associated with DM but at a slower rate. Inhaled steroids do not have the systemic effect of increased serum glucose, so answer A is not correct. Prior food intake will not lead to hyperglycemia in a nondiabetic patient, so answer B is not correct. Anxiety may lead to secretion of stress hormones and higher heart rate and blood pressure but not hyperglycemia, so answer C is not correct.[13]

9. A 6-year-old male with known CF is scheduled for colonoscopy to evaluate new bloody diarrhea. He has had 1 recent pulmonary exacerbation and has not been compliant with pancreatic enzymes, resulting in poor nutrition. The bloody diarrhea has been ongoing for 3–4 days. He is in mild respiratory distress and appears tired. Vitals: heart rate 110 bpm, respiratory rate 32 breaths per minute, blood pressure 98/70 mmHg, room air SpO_2= 95%. Labs: white blood cells $10 \times 10^3/\mu L$ with normal differential, hemoglobin 9 g/dL, platelets 225 K/μL, prolonged PT, normal activated PTT. What is the **MOST** likely explanation for these laboratory values?

  A. disseminated intravascular coagulation
  B. liver failure
  C. sepsis
  D. vitamin K deficiency

Answer: D

Prolongation of PT results from deficiency of factor VII, a vitamin K dependent factor. Vitamin K is a fat-soluble vitamin, and children with CF, especially those not compliant with enzyme replacement therapy, may not absorb sufficient vitamin K. Liver failure would also include abnormal electrolytes and abnormal PTT, so answer B is not correct. Disseminated intravascular coagulation, from sepsis or other causes, includes low platelet count as well as abnormal PTT, so answers A and C are not correct.[14]

10. A 19-year-old woman with CF, who underwent bilateral lung transplantation 3 months ago, is scheduled for flexible bronchoscopy for biopsy/bronchoalveolar lavage. She has had increased dyspnea and developed a requirement for night time supplemental oxygen over the past month. The **LEAST** important anesthetic consideration(s) for the care of this patient is

  A. possible damage to the anastomosis site by the ETT or bronchoscope.
  B. increased chance of pulmonary edema with excessive IV fluid administration.

  C. decreased pulmonary compliance.
  D. increased risk for infection secondary to immunosuppressives

Answer: D

All complications are possible in this clinical setting, and actions should be taken to mitigate them. Review of postoperative imaging, operative reports, or past bronchoscopies can provide information about the location of the anastomosis and indicate an appropriate ETT depth. Intravenous fluid administration should be guided by nil per os status, maintenance requirements, and an awareness of the opposing vulnerability to dehydration. Bronchoalveolar lavage procedures will always leave a residual volume of the diluent used for the lavage. Asking the pulmonologist for the volume difference between the amounts administered and the amount suctioned in return will provide some objective information to anticipate the potential implications this has for affecting gas exchange, compliance, and respiratory function. Risk of infection, although always a concern, is not increased by general anesthesia in this patient.

QUESTIONS AND ANSWERS

This chapter has accompanying questions and answers which are available to subscribers as part of the Oxford eLearning platform. To access the questions, go to ✔ http:// oxfordmedicine. com/pediatricanesthesiaPBL

REFERENCES

1. Egan ME, Green DM, Voynow JA. Cystic fibrosis. In: Kliegman RM, Stanton B, eds. *Nelson Textbook of Pediatrics.* 20th ed. Philadelphia, PA: Elsevier; 2017:2098–2113. Chapter 403.
2. Cystic Fibrosis Foundation. *Cystic Fibrosis Foundation Patient Registry: 2015 Annual Data Report.* Bethesda, MD: Cystic Fibrosis Foundation; 2016. https://www.cff.org/Our-Research/CF-Patient-Registry/2015-Patient-Registry-Annual-Data-Report.pdf. Accessed April 1, 2017.
3. O'Sullivan BP, Freedman SD. Cystic fibrosis. *Lancet.* 2009;373:1891–1904.
4. Kriegel D, Shanahan J. Cystic fibrosis. In: *Essential Evidence Plus.* Hoboken, NJ: John Wiley; 2017. http://www.essentialevidenceplus. com/content/eee/671. Accessed June 1, 2017.
5. Paranjape SM, Mogayzel Jr PJ. Cystic fibrosis in the era of precision medicine. *Paediatr Respir Rev.* 2018;25:64–72. http://dx.doi.org/ 10.1016/j.prrv.2017.03.001
6. Montgomery GS, Howenstine M. Cystic fibrosis. *Pediatr Rev.* 2009;30:302–310.
7. Smyth AR, Bell SC, Bojcin S, et al. European cystic fibrosis society standards of care: best practice guidelines. *J Cyst Fibros.* 2014;13(Suppl 1):S23–S42
8. Firth PG, Kinane TB. Essentials of pulmonology. In: Cote CJ, Lerman J Anderson BJ eds. *A Practice of Anesthesia for Infants and Children.* 5th ed. Philadelphia, PA: Elsevier; 2017:233–234.
9. Trivedi PM, Glass N. Cystic fibrosis. In: Davis PJ, Cladis FP, eds. *Smith's Anesthesia for Infants and Children.* 9th ed. Philadelphia, PA: Elsevier; 2017:1121–1124.
10. Bizzarro MJ, Ehrenkranz RA, Colson E. Differential diagnosis and management of anemia in the newborn. *Pediatr Clin North Am.* 2004;51(4):1087–1107

11. Maheshwari A, Carlo, W. Blood disorders. In: *Nelson Textbook of Pediatrics* 20th ed. Philadelphia, PA: Elsevier; 2016:888–889. Chapter 103.4.

12. Hackam DJ, Grikscheit T, Wang, J et al. Pediatric surgery. In: Brunicardi FC, ed. *Schwartz's Principles of Pediatric Surgery*. 10th ed. New York: McGraw-Hill; 2010:1618–1619.

13. Svoren, BM, Jospe N. Diabetes mellitus. In: *Nelson Textbook of Pediatrics*. 20th ed. Philadelphia, PA: Elsevier; 2016:2789–2790. Chapter 589.3.

14. Mehta N. Nutrition in the critically ill child. In: *Pediatric Critical Medicine*, 5th ed. Philadelphia, PA: Elsevier; 2017:1205–1206.

24.

AIRWAY FOREIGN BODY ASPIRATION

Sarah Nizamuddin and Caitlin Aveyard

STEM CASE AND KEY QUESTIONS

A 2-year-old boy presents to the emergency department with a 3-hour history of coughing and noisy breathing. He and his family were at a neighborhood party when his parents noticed him choking and vigorously coughing after helping himself to a handful of food from a table full of snacks. After a few minutes, he stopped coughing and seemed to be breathing normally while sitting on his mother's lap. However, when he got up and started playing, he began coughing and breathing noisily. The symptoms did not resolve, so his parents presented to the emergency department. A chest X-ray does not clearly demonstrate a foreign body, but the patient has expiratory wheezing greater in the right than left lung fields. The parents state that several types of food were within reach of the patient, including raw vegetables, peanuts, popcorn, and potato chips.

WHAT IS THE DIFFERENTIAL DIAGNOSIS FOR FOREIGN BODY ASPIRATION?

Although this child presents with a strong history to support aspiration of a foreign body, it is important to consider alternative diagnosis. Infections such as an upper respiratory infection or bronchitis can present with a vigorous cough. Laryngitis or epiglottitis frequently have noisy breathing as a sign and may resemble a laryngeal foreign body. Croup, tracheomalacia, and tracheal stenosis may also present with noisy breathing. An asthma exacerbation frequently involves coughing and noisy breathing as well. Obstruction of the bronchi or bronchioles may have symptoms similar to congenital cystic adenomatoid malformations, bronchitis, bronchiolitis, or bronchiectasis, to name a few.[1] Given the patient's lack of noisy breathing and cough prior to his current presentation, congenital malformation, laryngomalacia, tracheomalacia, tracheal stenosis, bronchiolitis, or bronchiectasis are unlikely. This patient does not have a fever, sick contacts, or other signs/symptoms of an infection. While this could be an initial presentation of asthma, the history of him coughing and choking while eating is strongly indicative of foreign body aspiration.

WHAT DIAGNOSTIC TESTS ARE INDICATED?

If the patient is stable, a chest X-ray is often performed. While only radio-opaque objects will be readily seen on X-ray, other findings may be present. Some of these findings include distal hyperinflation if the foreign body creates a ball-valve effect, opacification of the distal lung, mediastinal shift, and atelectasis.

Our patient's chest radiograph does not clearly show a foreign body, but lack of such a finding does not rule out a foreign body aspiration.

WHAT IS THE TREATMENT?

The definitive treatment is to remove the foreign body, usually with rigid or flexible bronchoscopy. If bronchoscopy fails, thoracotomy may be necessary for removal of the foreign body. Close communication with the proceduralist/surgeon is necessary for optimal planning and safety. For our patient, the pediatric otolaryngologist plans to perform rigid bronchoscopy to evaluate the patient's airway and remove the foreign body. Although it is not apparent on the chest X-ray, the object is likely a piece of aspirated food. Given the right-sided wheezing and anatomy of the bronchi, the foreign body is likely in the right main-stem bronchus.

IS THIS AN EMERGENCY? DO WE WAIT FOR THE PATIENT TO BE APPROPRIATELY NIL PER OS (NPO)?

While any foreign body in the airway is a worrisome condition, the nature of the aspirated material and the clinical presentation of the patient determine the urgency of removal of the foreign body. If the patient has signs of respiratory or cardiac instability or impending respiratory failure, the foreign body must be removed emergently. Nonorganic materials commonly aspirated include straight pins, coins, and batteries. Aspirated sharp objects carry a risk of perforation and damage to airway structures and necessitate urgent removal. Alkaline batteries can release corrosive electrolyte solutions (such as sodium or potassium hydroxide) leading to serious tissue damage. Lithium batteries can produce an electrical current that can also lead to serious tissue damage. Consequently, aspirated batteries need to be removed urgently. Organic materials such as nuts and seeds can cause significant mucosal inflammation, eventually leading to granulation tissue and lung infection if not removed in a timely manner. Peanuts in particular can lead to a significant inflammatory reaction. While we do not know what material our patient aspirated, peanuts are a possibility given his access to them. Since our patient is not clinically unstable, we have time to plan and proceed to the operating room in an urgent rather than emergent fashion. Because there is a good chance that the aspirated material will set up an inflammatory reaction, it is not advised to wait 8 hours for appropriate NPO time.

SHOULD WE OBTAIN A PREINDUCTION INTRAVENOUS (IV) LINE? SHOULD WE PROVIDE AN INHALATIONAL OR AN IV INDUCTION?

Some patients with foreign body aspiration who present to the emergency department have a peripheral IV catheter placed prior to anesthetic evaluation. If the patient does not have a previously placed IV, the decision whether to place one prior to induction is up to the anesthesiologist and often depends on the situation (age of the patient, ability to cooperate, urgency, respiratory status, etc.). If the patient has worsening respiratory distress with agitation, performing an inhalational induction and placing an IV after induction is reasonable. Another consideration is NPO status. As with our patient, aspiration frequently occurs with eating, so the patient is not optimally NPO. Further aspiration could worsen the clinical situation. However, known respiratory distress must be weighed against possible aspiration. Our patient exhibits worsening respiratory distress when he is upset and agitated, so we will proceed with an inhalational induction.

IS SPONTANEOUS VENTILATION OR POSITIVE PRESSURE VENTILATION BETTER? SHOULD WE INTUBATE?

The choice of spontaneous ventilation or positive pressure ventilation as well as the plan to intubate or not is influenced by the surgeon's plan/method of foreign body removal. A benefit of spontaneous ventilation is the ability to maintain ventilation during rigid bronchoscopy, thus allowing more time for the surgeon to manipulate the airway and retrieve the foreign body before significant desaturations occur. However, the airway is not secured while the rigid bronchoscope is in the airway, so there is potentially increased risk of aspiration and laryngospasm. Positive pressure ventilation has the advantage of controlling ventilation and greater ease in maintaining a deep level of anesthesia with volatile agents, thereby decreasing the risk of coughing and laryngospasm. While positive pressure ventilation allows for the use of paralytic agents, it may increase the risk of aspiration in a patient who is not ideally NPO, thus necessitating intubation. Another disadvantage of positive pressure ventilation is the risk of pushing the foreign body further into the airway, perhaps causing worsening obstruction.

Intubating the patient is advantageous if the proceduralist or surgeon plans to remove the foreign body with a flexible bronchoscope. However, if the surgeon plans to use rigid bronchoscopy or if the foreign body is larger than the inner diameter of the endotracheal tube (ETT), intubation may be disadvantageous. It may be acceptable to intubate the patient for part of the procedure, but the ETT may need to be removed at times during the procedure.

For our patient, the otolaryngologist plans to use rigid bronchoscopy for the removal of the foreign body. We maintain spontaneous ventilation during induction and peripheral IV placement, but have several sizes of ETT immediately available if intubation becomes necessary.

SHOULD WE MAINTAIN ANESTHESIA WITH VOLATILE AGENT OR WITH A TOTAL IV ANESTHETIC (TIVA)?

While it is possible to maintain anesthesia with either volatile agents or TIVA in these cases, there are advantages and disadvantages to each method. Advantages to using volatile agents to maintain anesthesia for the removal of airway foreign bodies include ease of monitoring the depth of anesthesia and bronchodilation (especially if the patient has reactive airways). However, a large disadvantage is leakage of the volatile agent to the operating room environment. This leakage may make maintaining a deep anesthetic level difficult and exposes operating room personnel to the volatile agent. Use of a TIVA (propofol, narcotics, ketamine, dexmedetomidine) technique has the advantage of a lack of operating room contamination with volatile agents. Disadvantages of using TIVA include expense and increased difficulty in evaluating depth of anesthesia. A combination of both volatile agents and IV agents is possible as well.

We will use a combination of volatile and IV agents for our patient. We have used volatile agents to induce our patient but will convert to a TIVA to reduce exposure of operating room staff to volatile agents. Prior to insertion of the rigid bronchoscope, we will also administer topical lidocaine to the patient's vocal cords and trachea as an adjunct to our systemic anesthetic. Despite a high level of vigilance and excellent communication with our surgical colleagues, the patient coughs during placement of the rigid bronchoscope. A bolus of propofol settles the patient down, but he is now not maintaining adequate ventilation with spontaneous respiration, and he begins to desaturate. Thanks to good communication with our surgical colleagues as well as preparedness, the patient is quickly intubated, and oxygen saturation returns to normal. After 2–3 minutes of ventilation with 100% oxygen, the surgeon removes the ETT and proceeds with the rigid bronchoscopy. Food-like material (likely a nut) is identified and grasped. Unfortunately, the foreign material slips out of the surgeon's grasp as it is withdrawn into the trachea. The patient desaturates and the ETT is replaced, but ventilation is difficult (increased peak airway pressures and decreased tidal volumes). The foreign material is likely causing increased obstruction now that it is in the trachea. The surgeon pushed the foreign body back onto the right mainstem bronchus, and we are able to adequately ventilate. After again ventilating the patient with 100% oxygen, the surgeon removes the ETT, inserts the rigid bronchoscope, and uses a different grasper to grab the foreign material. The object is successfully removed from the patient's airway, the ETT is inserted into the trachea, and adequate ventilation is resumed.

IS EXTUBATION APPROPRIATE?

The decision to extubate a child after airway foreign body retrieval depends on the patient's ability to adequately ventilate, oxygenate, and protect his airway. If concern for significant airway edema from trauma and/or irritation exists, it may be appropriate to keep the patient intubated following the procedure.

For our patient, the otolaryngologist uses a flexible bronchoscope to evaluate the airway after retrieval of the foreign body. She does not observe a significant amount of trauma or edema. We administer dexamethasone to decrease the likelihood of additional edema of the airway. By this time, our patient has regained spontaneous ventilation and is oxygenating well on 21% inspired oxygen, so we extubate the child after he has sufficiently emerged from our anesthetic.

DISCUSSION

INTRODUCTION

Aspiration of a foreign body has the potential to be life threatening and must be managed promptly and appropriately. The incidence of foreign airway body obstruction is estimated at 0.66 per 100,000,[2] and it is one of the leading causes for accidental infantile death.[3] The incidence is the highest for children between 1 and 4 years of age.[4] Children at this age often walk, laugh, or talk while eating, which may increase chances of aspiration. However, it is important to understand that, while children under the age of 1 are less mobile, they still can aspirate and should be carefully monitored. Children under 4 years of age lack molar teeth and a well-coordinated swallow reflex, which may also contribute to increased incidence of aspiration.[5,6] Males are more likely to experience an aspiration event, with male to female ratios ranging from 1.4–1.7:1.[2,7,8] Aspirated foreign bodies vary from common foods to nonedible objects. Symptoms may range from immediate total airway obstruction to a slight nagging cough. All possible aspirations require a thorough history, physical exam, and possible diagnostic tests to properly diagnose and treat a potentially fatal aspiration event.

CLINICAL SIGNS AND SYMPTOMS

A thorough history is necessary when evaluating a child for aspiration, as some patients may have a completely normal examination.[9,10] Preoperative assessment should aim to establish what was aspirated, when the event occurred, and where the object currently lies. However, these details are not always elucidated.

Symptoms concerning for an aspiration event include choking, prolonged cough, difficulty breathing, stridor, wheezing, and nonresolving pneumonia. Cough is considered very sensitive for aspiration but lacks specificity. On the other hand, stridor and cyanosis are very specific but not sensitive.[11] On physical examination, there may be unilateral or bilateral decreased breath sounds, wheezing, or stridor. Location of the

Table 24.1 **CLINICAL SIGNS AND SYMPTOMS OF AIRWAY FOREIGN BODIES**

CLINICAL SYMPTOMS AND PHYSICAL EXAM FINDINGS CONCERNING FOR FOREIGN BODY ASPIRATION
Cough
Choking
Difficulty breathing or respiratory distress
Nonresolving pneumonia
Wheezing
Stridor
Decreased breath sounds
Cyanosis
Cardiac arrest

foreign body can affect the symptoms that a child exhibits. A foreign body in the upper airway (extrathoracic) may lead to inspiratory stridor or, if completely occluding, cardiac arrest. On the other hand, a foreign body in the lower airway (intrathoracic) is more likely to lead to wheezing or expiratory stridor. (Table 24.1)

DIFFERENTIAL DIAGNOSIS

When considering airway foreign body obstruction, it is necessary to also consider other diagnoses, which may present with similar signs and symptoms. Infections, such as laryngitis or epiglottitis, may resemble a laryngeal foreign body. Objects, which are partially occluding the trachea, may mimic croup, tracheomalacia, or tracheal stenosis. Obstruction of the bronchi or bronchioles may have symptoms similar to congenital cystic adenomatoid malformations, bronchitis, bronchiolitis, or bronchiectasis, to name a few.[1] The patient's past medical history, the narrative of the inciting event, and further diagnostic studies should be considered when narrowing a diagnosis (Table 24.2).

Table 24.2 **OHER POSSIBLE DIAGNOSES**

DIFFERENTIAL DIAGNOSES
Laryngitis
Epiglottis
Tracheomalacia
Congenital cystic adenomatoid malformation
Bronchitis
Bronchiolitis
Bronchiectasis

Chest radiograph

Workup of a possible airway aspiration should be tailored to the urgency of the situation at hand. If there are any concerns for impending respiratory failure, one should not delay treatment for imaging. For patients with a questionable aspiration, a chest radiograph is commonly performed. However, 1 study found only 11% of aspirated objects to be radio opaque on chest X-ray[11] (Figure 24.1). If the foreign body creates a ball-valve effect, air trapping from distal hyperinflation may be seen. Other signs on a chest radiograph that may point to an aspirated foreign body include mediastinal shift, atelectasis, or opacification of the distal lung.[10,11]

Bronchoscopy

Both rigid and flexible bronchoscopies are used for definite diagnosis and retrieval of aspirated objects (Figure 24.2). Although rigid bronchoscopy has been known to be the "gold standard" for treatment, flexible bronchoscopy is increasingly used.[11] Benefits of flexible bronchoscopy use as a treatment method include ability to perform through a laryngeal mask airway, increased access to smaller distal airways, and ability to more effectively ventilate around a flexible fiberoptic scope.[12] However, even when the plan for extraction involves a flexible fiberoptic scope, rigid scopes should be available as back up. In the rare case that bronchoscopy is not successful in removal of the foreign body, thoracotomy may be necessary.

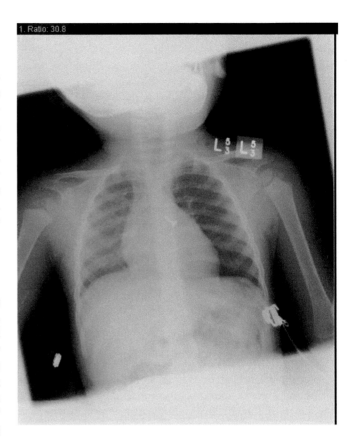

Fig. 24.1 Radio opaque objects can make the diagnosis of airway foreign body clearer on chest x-ray; however, many foreign bodies do not show up on x-ray. (Photo courtesy of Fuad Baroody, MD).

MANAGEMENT

Urgency

Management of a patient with an aspirated foreign body is dependent on several factors. Most important, the urgency of the situation at hand is critical and will determine the initial steps when evaluating these patients. If there are signs of respiratory or cardiac collapse or impending respiratory failure, then immediate resuscitation or retrieval of the foreign body, whether through bronchoscopy or invasively, will be necessary. This may occur either in the emergency department or, if time allows, in the operating room. It is vital for the surgery

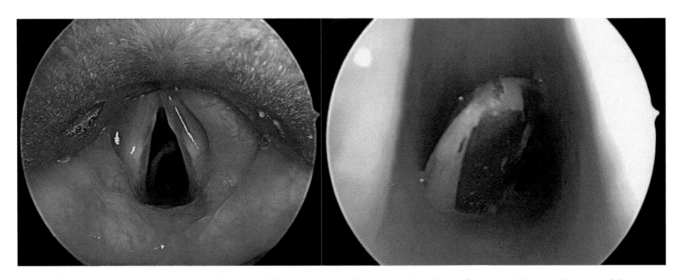

Fig. 24.2 A bronchoscope is most commonly used to retrieval foreign objects in the airway, such as the sunflower seed shown in this image. (Photo courtesy of Fuad Baroody, MD).

and anesthesia teams to discuss the plan for securing the foreign body and airway management.

If time allows for a more thorough workup and history, then this should be performed prior to definitive treatment so that the appropriate steps are taken for the current situation. Information that is helpful to know prior to surgical management include the type of aspirated object, the location, and the surgeon's plan for retrieval.

Type of aspirated object

In a review of over 12,000 cases by Fidkowski et al.[11] in 2010, 81% of foreign bodies aspirated were organic materials, including nuts, seeds, dried fruit, and vegetable matter.[4] Organic materials such as nuts and seeds can cause significant mucosal inflammation, eventually leading to granulation tissue and lung infection if not removed in a timely manner. Nonorganic materials commonly aspirated include straight pins, coins, and batteries. Aspirated sharp objects carry a risk of perforation and damage to airway structures (Figure 24.3).

Knowledge of the type of foreign body aspirated can be helpful, as it may direct the urgency and need for removal. Alkaline batteries may leak an electrolyte solution, usually sodium or potassium hydroxide. Leakage of this solution can quickly lead to liquefaction necrosis and serious injury to tissues.[13] Lithium batteries can also lead to corrosion by generating a small electrical current and also need to be urgently removed. During removal, the mucosa around the object should be carefully inspected for damage.

Location

The majority of foreign bodies lodge in the bronchial tree, with the remainder in the trachea or larynx.[11] The right main bronchus is more vertical, shorter, and wider than the left, leading to a larger proportion of foreign bodies going down the right side.[14]

Anesthesia for retrieval of airway foreign body

Intravenous access. Patients who present with airway foreign bodies often come from the emergency department with an IV catheter already in place. For those who come without IV access, it is up to the anesthesiologist to determine whether one is necessary prior to induction. Placing an IV in an upset patient that has a foreign body in the airway may worsen respiratory distress. Factors to consider include the age of the patient, ability to cooperate, urgency, and current respiratory status.

Induction, breathing, and airway . When planning a method for induction and airway access, it is important to consider whether the patient's airway will be maintained with a mask, supraglottic airway, or ETT, as well as whether the patient will have spontaneous or controlled ventilation. This largely depends on the surgeon's planned method for foreign body retrieval. Converting a patient from negative to positive pressure ventilation carries the risk of causing complete airway obstruction due to dislodging of the foreign body to a location further

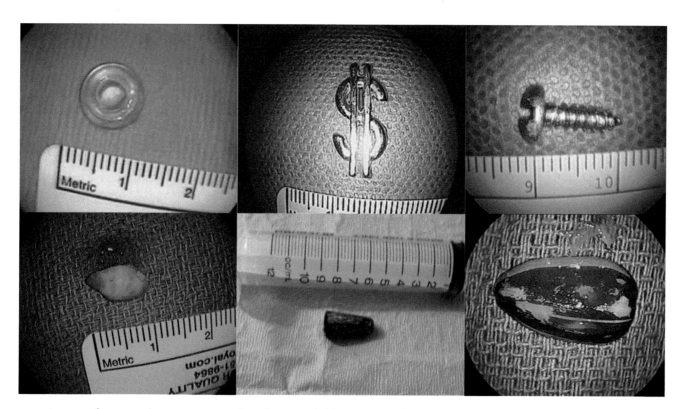

Fig. 24.3 A variety of organic and nonorganic materials can be aspirated. (Photo courtesy of Fuad Baroody, MD).

down the bronchial tree. Some choose to keep patients spontaneously ventilating through an inhalational or gentle IV induction. This is especially helpful during rigid bronchoscopy when the patient cannot be ventilated mechanically while the scope is in airway. The ability of the patient to maintain spontaneous ventilation during attempts at retrieval of the foreign airway body can provide additional time for the surgeon prior to desaturations requiring removal of the scope. However, when the airway is not secured, there remains a risk of laryngospasm or aspiration from the patient not maintaining an adequate level of anesthesia. Therefore, the anesthesiologist must remain vigilant about the patient's depth of anesthesia.

If the decision is made to proceed with positive pressure ventilation, a benefit is the ability to deepen the patient further to decrease chances of coughing or laryngospasm during airway manipulation. Some situations may warrant the use of paralysis to further ensure the patient will not move during stimulating points in the procedure. However, maintaining positive pressure ventilation in a population that may not be appropriately NPO may require securing the airway with an ETT. With the increasing use of flexible fiberoptic scopes for diagnosis and therapeutic management of airway foreign bodies, this may still be acceptable. On the other hand, if the plan for retrieval involves a rigid bronchoscope or if the foreign body is larger than the inner diameter of the ETT, then use of an ETT for an airway would not be appropriate. Jet ventilation is an alternative technique that allows for ventilation during bronchoscopy without an ETT if the appropriate equipment and trained personnel are involved.

Maintenance of anesthesia. Anesthesia may be maintained with volatile agents, TIVA, or a combination of both. Benefits of using volatile agents for anesthesia maintenance include quicker set up time, which can be beneficial in urgent situations, as well as clearer ability to monitor a patient's anesthetic levels. However, due to the presence of scopes in the airway, there will be a significant leak into the environment, as well as times when the patient is not receiving any anesthetic and may lighten more than desired. A TIVA technique, using propofol, remifentanil, dexmedetomidine, and/or ketamine, eliminates the risk of gas pollution and lightening of the patient when the surgeon is in the airway. However, TIVA is often more expensive, and it is harder to evaluate the anesthetic levels in these patient than with volatile agents. An adjunct to either inhalational or IV anesthesia maintenance includes topical lidocaine to the vocal cords and trachea. Regardless of the anesthetic technique used, a high level of vigilance is necessary to ensure proper depths of anesthesia and ideal conditions for appropriate retrieval or treatment.

Extubation. The decision on whether to extubate a child after retrieval of foreign body should be made on a case-by-case basis. A large majority of patients can be successfully extubated without signs of further respiratory distress.

However, if the patient is unable to maintain satisfactory oxygen saturations at the end of the case or if there are concerns about significant airway swelling and irritation from the foreign body, keeping the patient intubated postoperatively may be most appropriate.

COMPLICATIONS

Depending on the type of foreign body aspirated and the location of the object, risks of damage to the airway structures include severe edema, bronchospasm, perforation causing fistulas, pneumothorax or pneumomediastinum, or severe hypoxia leading to cardiac arrest or brain damage.[11]

During retrieval of a foreign body from a distal airway, dropping of the object in the trachea, leading to complete airway occlusion, remains a risk. If this were to happen, the surgeon may try to expeditiously retrieve the object or, if that is not possible, push it down the airway into a mainstem bronchus to allow for some ventilation. Once ventilation is reestablished, the surgeon may then reattempt retrieval.

POSTOPERATIVE MANAGEMENT

Careful monitoring in the postanesthesia recovery unit (PACU) is necessary following retrieval of airway foreign bodies. Inflammation and irritation of the airway can lead to postoperative pulmonary complications and desaturations. Racemic epinephrine, steroids, and humidified oxygen may be helpful in these situations. If the patient remains in respiratory distress, then intubation may be necessary until the edema and inflammation subsides. If there are any concerns about the patient's respiratory status, consider admission into an intensive care unit for closer monitoring and potential interventions.

CONCLUSION

Airway foreign body aspiration in pediatric patients can lead to significant morbidity, if not promptly diagnosed and appropriately managed. A thorough history and physical are vital as imaging is not always diagnostic. The most commonly aspirated foreign bodies include organic materials, such as nuts and seeds. Treatment usually involves bronchoscopy in the operating room with clear communication and coordination with the entire team, so that the appropriate anesthesia is administered. Children should be closely monitored in either the PACU or intensive care unit postoperatively with the providers remaining vigilant for signs of impending respiratory distress or failure.

REVIEW QUESTIONS

1. A 2-year-old male presents to the emergency department with his mother for concern of foreign body aspiration. Per

his mother, he was eating peanuts when he began coughing. In the emergency department bay, the patient's vitals are heart rate 132 beats per minutes, peripheral capillary oxygen saturation (SpO_2) 82%, blood pressure 78/50 mmHg, and temperature 37.2°C. The patient has labored breathing. What is the **MOST** appropriate immediate next step in the management of this patient?

A. Administer antibiotics.
B. Administer oxygen.
C. Obtain IV access.
D. Order a chest V-ray.

Answer: B

It is imperative to first stabilize a patient prior to pursuing additional work up for concern of airway foreign body. This patient's SpO_2 of 82% is concerning. Supplemental O_2 support would be beneficial while assessing the patient's airway.

2. Workup is underway for a 4-year-old female who presented with respiratory distress and unilateral breath sounds. Her father states she was playing alone in her room with Lego' toys while eating candy when she began crying and has been inconsolable since. A chest X-ray is performed, which shows no visual foreign objects and slight hyperinflation of the right lungs. Vital signs are currently stable. What is the **MOST** appropriate next step?

A. Consider other diagnoses.
B. Consult with pediatric otolaryngology.
C. Emergently intubate.
D. Order a computed tomography.

Answer: B

Discussion: Only a small proportion of airway foreign bodies will show up as radiopaque on X-ray. Other signs of possible foreign body include hyperinflation of lungs due to air trapping, mediastinal shift, atelectasis, and opacification of the distal lung, to name a few. If the patient's history and physical exam suggest airway foreign body, do not be persuaded by a normal chest X-ray. Confirmation of an airway foreign body by computed tomography is usually not necessary and delays treatment. If the patient is relatively stable, intubation should be delayed until the otolaryngology team is readily available and the plan for retrieval has been discussed.

3. A 1-year-old male is going emergently to the operating room for direct laryngoscopy, bronchoscopy, and retrieval of an aspirated coin, which is visible in the right main stem bronchus on chest X-ray. He appears to be in mild respiratory distress, but SpO_2 is 97%. He last had formula 1 hour ago. What is the **MOST** appropriate next step in management?

A. Delay the case until the patient is appropriately NPO.
B. Determine the type and amount of formula ingested.
C. Go ahead with induction of anesthesia with the otolaryngology team in the operating room.
D. Suggest the otolaryngology team create a surgical airway.

Answer: C

Urgent and emergent cases may need to be performed without appropriate NPO status, depending on the patient's status. In this situation, retrieval of an airway foreign body in a patient who is in respiratory distress is warranted despite recent formula ingestion.

4. Following a bronchoscopy and retrieval of peanut fragments in an 8-year-old child's distal airway, the patient is extubated and taken to the PACU. After 15 minutes, the patient becomes progressively stridulous, with labored breathing and SpO_2 of 89%. The nurse administered supplemental O_2. What is the next **MOST** appropriate step?

A. Administer racemic epinephrine.
B. Call otolaryngology for a surgical airway.
C. Continue monitoring.
D. Give IV antibiotics.

Answer: A

Inflammation and irritation of the airway from foreign objects and instrumentation can lead to postextubation stridor and respiratory distress, if severe enough. Supplemental O_2, racemic epinephrine, steroids, and humidified oxygen can help alleviate these symptoms. If the symptoms do not improve or more significant and concerning respiratory distress is present, consider reintubation with otolaryngology readily available.

5. You receive a call from a pulmonologist regarding an 18-month-old boy with persistent cough for 1 week and wheezing in the right lower lung field. He has had no fever, nasal discharge, or sick contacts. His chest X-ray did not reveal a foreign body, but some overinflation of the right lower lung is appreciated. His vital signs are within normal limits, including a SpO_2 of 98% on room air. The pulmonologist wants to perform a flexible bronchoscopy to evaluate for a foreign body. The patient last ate pancakes and milk 3 hours ago. However, she requests a supraglottic airway because the bronchoscope she needs to remove a possible foreign body will not fit through an appropriately sized ETT. What is the **MOST** appropriate management plan?

A. Administer antibiotics.
B. Proceed immediately to the operating room.
C. Inform pulmonology that the case must be with ETT.
D. Wait for the patient to be appropriately NPO.

Answer: D

Due to the size of a small child, an appropriately sized ETT is often too narrow for a pulmonologist's bronchoscope while an appropriately sized supraglottic airway often is large enough for the scope and provides a conduit for oxygen and inhaled agents. Because the child has a subacute process (this cough has been present for a week) and is stable with good oxygenation, it is reasonable to wait until he is appropriately NPO to reduce the risk of aspiration.

6. A 3-year-old-girl is undergoing a direct laryngoscopy and rigid bronchoscopy for removal of a coin from the right mainstem bronchus. The otolaryngologic surgeon has removed the ETT, so he can fit his rigid scope and grasper

into the airway to retrieve the coin. While pulling the coin back into the trachea, it slips from the grasper. The patient is starting to desaturate, so he replaces the ETT. You are having difficulty ventilating the patient with higher peak pressures. What is the **MOST** appropriate next step?

A. Ask the surgeon to perform an emergent surgical airway.
B. Ask the surgeon to remove the tube and reposition of the coin.
C. Keep attempting positive pressure ventilation with greater peak pressures.
D. Perform a direct laryngoscopy to ensure ETT position.

Answer: B

Airway foreign bodies are often slippery due to secretions, and it is not uncommon for the object to slip out of the graspers during removal. Unfortunately, when this happens, the object may be oriented in a fashion that causes occlusion of the airway. The best action is for the proceduralist to adjust the orientation or position of the foreign body to allow better airflow and then attempt ventilation again. These moments are often tense, but good communication with your otolaryngology colleague is essential!

7. After a technically difficult rigid bronchoscopy to remove a large airway foreign body, you notice that the patient's airway is inflamed and edematous. The patient is saturating well on 21% inspired oxygen and has maintained stable blood pressure and heart rate throughout the procedure. What is the next **MOST** appropriate management step?

A. Administer dexamethasone, then extubate the patient.
B. Extubate, but be prepared to re-intubate, if necessary.
C. Leave the patient intubated and go to the pediatric intensive care unit.
D. Suggest the surgeon perform a tracheostomy.

Answer: C

While the patient may have been easy to intubate prior to the procedure, the trauma caused by removal of the foreign body is likely to lead to airway edema causing increased difficulty with intubation. While dexamethasone will help decrease the inflammation caused by airway trauma, it does not work immediately, so keeping the patient intubated until the edema subsides is the safest way to proceed. The edema will subside over hours to days, so there is no need to perform a surgical airway.

QUESTIONS AND ANSWERS

This chapter has accompanying questions and answers which are available to subscribers as part of the Oxford eLearning platform. To access the questions, go to ✓ http://oxfordmedicine. com/pediatricanesthesiaPBL

REFERENCES

1. Salih AM, Alfaki M, Alam-Elhuda DM. Airway foreign bodies: A critical review for a common pediatric emergency. *World J Emerg Med*. 2016;7(1):5–12.
2. Hughes CA, Baroody FM, Marsh BR. Pediatric tracheobronchial foreign bodies: historical review from the Johns Hopkins Hospital. *Ann Otol Rhinol Laryngol*. 1996;105(7):555–561.
3. Borse N, Sleet DA. CDC childhood injury report: patterns of unintentional injuries among 0- to 19-year olds in the United States, 2000–2006. *Fam Community Health*. 2009;32(2):189.
4. Berdan EA, Sato TT. Pediatric airway and esophageal foreign bodies. *Surg Clin North Am*. 2017;97(1):85–91.
5. Reilly JS, Cook SP, Stool D, Rider G. Prevention and management of aerodigestive foreign body injuries in childhood. *Pediatr Clin North Am*. 1996;43(6):1403–1411.
6. Rybojad B, Aftyka A, Rudnicka-Drozak E. Nursing activities in the prevention and treatment of perioperative complications after airway foreign body removal in pediatric patients. *J Perianesth Nurs*. 2016;31(1):49–55.
7. Cohen SR, Herbert WI, Lewis GB Jr., Geller KA. Foreign bodies in the airway. five-year retrospective study with special reference to management. *Ann Otol Rhinol Laryngol*. 1980;89(5 Pt 1):437–442.
8. Kaur K, Sonkhya N, Bapna AS. Foreign bodies in the tracheobronchial tree: a prospective study of fifty cases. *Indian J Otolaryngol Head Neck Surg*. 2002;54(1):30–34.
9. Even L, Heno N, Talmon Y, Samet E, Zonis Z, Kugelman A. Diagnostic evaluation of foreign body aspiration in children: a prospective study. *J Pediatr Surg*. 2005;40(7):1122–1127.
10. Richards AM. Pediatric respiratory emergencies. *Emerg Med Clin North Am*. 2016;34(1):77–96.
11. Fidkowski CW, Zheng H, Firth PG. The anesthetic considerations of tracheobronchial foreign bodies in children: a literature review of 12,979 cases. *Anesth Analg*. 2010;111(4):1016–1025.
12. Tenenbaum T, Kahler G, Janke C, Schroten H, Demirakca S. Management of foreign body removal in children by flexible bronchoscopy. *J Bronchology Interv Pulmonol*. 2017;24(1):21–28.
13. Louie MC, Bradin S. Foreign body ingestion and aspiration. *Pediatr Rev*. 2009;30(8):295–301, quiz 301.
14. Limper AH, Prakash UB. Tracheobronchial foreign bodies in adults. *Ann Intern Med*. 1990;112(8):604–609.

SECTION 5

NEUROMUSCULAR SYSTEM AND SPINE

25.

NEURAL TUBE DEFECTS

Jimmy Hoang and Samuel David Yanofsky

STEM CASE

An ex 39-week old baby with a known neural tube defect diagnosed on antenatal ultrasound was born via cesarean section to a G1P1 mother. The infant weighed 3.4 kg and her APGAR (appearance, pulse, grimace, activity, and respiration) scores were 8 and 9. Upon examination, she was found to have a 4 × 4 cm membranous sac protruding from her lumbosacral area. She was diagnosed with a myelomeningocele. The sac was covered with saline soaked gauze and the infant was positioned slight laterally. She has spontaneous movement of her lower extremities and has voided and passed meconium within the first few hours of life. Vital signs are stable, and she is saturating 97% on room air.

WHAT ARE NEURAL TUBE DEFECTS (NTDS)? HOW ARE THEY CLASSIFIED? WHAT ARE THE MOST COMMON ONES?

Upon further questioning, it was discovered that the mother had received poor prenatal care. She had gestational diabetes and reports a history of smoking during her first trimester. She did not take any medications or supplements during her antenatal period. The mother denied having any relatives with a known history of NTDs.

ARE THERE ANY ENVIRONMENTAL OR MATERNAL RISK FACTORS THAT CONTRIBUTE TOWARD THE DEVELOPMENT OF NTDS? HOW CAN EXPECTANT MOTHERS MINIMIZE THAT RISK?

There was concern about the infant's head looking large, so it was measured and found to be at the 99th percentile. She underwent a cranial ultrasound for further assessment and was diagnosed with hydrocephalus. Neurosurgery is planning a concurrent repair of the myelomeningocele along with ventriculoperitoneal shunting to address the hydrocephalus. The infant is stable and showing no signs of vomiting, excessive somnolence, respiratory depression, or abnormal arrhythmias.

IS HYDROCEPHALUS COMMONLY ASSOCIATED WITH MYELOMENINGOCELE? WHAT IMAGING MODALITIES CAN BE USED TO DETECT IT, AND WHAT RADIOGRAPHIC FINDINGS ARE PRESENT? WHEN IS SURGICAL REPAIR INDICATED?

The infant is transported to the operating room with 1 peripheral intravenous line on room air. She is placed in a slight left lateral decubitus position to offload any pressure from the myelomeningocele. Intravenous induction with propofol and vecuronium is uneventful. The patient is easily masked in the lateral position and subsequently intubated without issue. A second peripheral intravenous line is obtained. An arterial line is not attained after discussion with the surgeon.

WHY IS THE PATIENT PLACED IN A LATERAL DECUBITUS POSITION? DOES IT MATTER LEFT VERSUS RIGHT LATERAL DECUBITUS? WHAT ARE SOME CONSIDERATIONS FOR INTUBATION? ARE THERE OTHER POSITIONS THE PATIENT CAN BE INTUBATED IN? WHAT LINES ARE NECESSARY FOR THIS TYPE OF SURGERY?

Surgical repair of the neural tube defect and placement of the ventriculoperitoneal shunt proceeds uneventfully. The infant receives one 0.05 mg/kg dose of morphine during the case and has spontaneous ventilation by skin closure. After administering reversal, she has adequate tidal volumes with a regular respiratory pattern and no breath holds. She maintains an end-tidal CO_2 of less than 50 mmHg and moves vigorously. She is extubated and transferred to the neonatal intensive care unit.

HOW MUCH PAIN MEDICINE DO THESE PATIENTS REQUIRE? WHAT ARE THE EXTUBATION CRITERIA? ARE THERE ANY CONCERNS THAT WOULD MAKE ONE MORE INCLINED TO LEAVE THEM INTUBATED?

After spending a week in the hospital, the patient is stable enough to be discharged home. She has regular follow-up with her pediatrician and neurosurgeon in 2 weeks. There are no residual neurologic deficits of her lower extremities. She has an uneventful life until 3 years of age when she suddenly develops restlessness associated with nausea, vomiting, and lethargy. The symptoms continue to progress over the period of 1 day so she is brought to the emergency department for further evaluation. A head computed tomography shows enlargement of her ventricles concerning for ventriculoperitoneal shunt malfunction. She is taken to the operating room urgently for ventriculoperitoneal shunt revision.

DO THESE PATIENTS DEVELOP ANY COMPLICATIONS AFTER REPAIR? WHAT ARE SOME WARNING SIGNS AND SYMPTOMS?

The patient does well and is discharged 2 days later from the hospital. She hits all of her age appropriate milestones as expected while her doctors continue to monitor her closely for any signs of ventriculoperitoneal shunt malfunction.

DISCUSSION

CLASSIFICATION

Neural tube defects are classified into 3 main types: anencephaly, encephalocele, and spina bifida. Anencephaly is a failure of a large portion of brain and skull development. Encephalocele is a protrusion of membranous covered brain and cerebrospinal fluid through a defect in the skull. Craniorachischisis is an extremely rare NTD in which there is failure of neural tube fusion over the entire body. Spina bifida is a result of aberrations in the fusion of the posterior arch resulting in spinal defects and possible herniation of neural contents. Spina bifida can be further classified as open where contents are exposed versus closed where there is the presence of skin covering the defect.[2,4] Myelomeningocele is a type of spina bifida cystica where a membranous sac containing neural tissue protrudes through an opening in the back. Spina bifida occulta is a closed spinal lesion and considered to be a milder NTD where there is no herniation of neural contents (see Figure 25.1).[4]

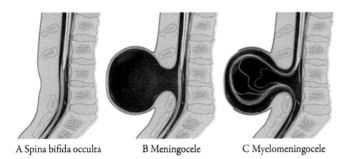

A Spina bifida occulta   B Meningocele   C Myelomeningocele

Fig 25.1 A. Vertebral defect without herniation of meninges. The dura and skin are intact. There may be a dimple, birthmark or tuft of hair overlying the skin surface. B. Protusion of meninges through the vertebral defect. C. Protrusion of spinal cord and nerves through the vertebral defect.

Neural tube defects are believed to have both genetic and environmental influences. There are more than 200 genes known to cause NTDs in mice but progress in identifying the genes that play a role in NTDs in humans has been limited.[1,5] The prevalence of NTDs is highest in Ireland and Scotland where the frequency approaches 10 per 1,000 births compared to 1 in 1,000 births in the United States.[6] There is a 2%–5% risk of recurrence in subsequent pregnancies for those with 1 affected sibling.[7]

A key environmental factor centers on nutrition and its implications on the development of NTDs. Folate is a water-soluble B-complex vitamin that is found naturally in certain foods. It functions as an essential coenzyme in the metabolism of nucleic and amino acids. Folic acid is the oxidized and most active form of folate. It is generally found in vitamin preparations and has twice the bioavailability of folate.[8]

Several retrospective studies[6,9,10] have been done on the relationship between maternal folic acid supplementation and the occurrence of NTDs. They showed significant risk reductions between 35%–75%. Prospective trials have also examined this relationship, but most assessed risk of recurrence. A notable study by Czeizel and Dudas[11] in 1992 looked at primary occurrence. In this study, Hungarian women were randomly assigned to a study group who took a supplement of 0.8mg of folic acid daily versus a control group. None of the 2104 women in the study group had children with NTDs compared to 6 out of 2,052 women in the control group who had children with NTDs.[11] In light of all the compelling evidence in support of folic acid supplementation for pregnant women to prevent NTDs, the United States Preventive Services Task Force[12] released a recommendation that all women considering pregnancy take 0.4 to 0.8 mg of folic acid daily.

Other environmental factors that may affect the risk for NTDs include maternal diabetes, maternal cigarette smoking, hyperthermia during early development, arsenic exposure, and valproate consumption.[8,13,14]

PATHOPHYSIOLOGY

The neural plate is formed by a plate of thickened ectoderm that appears in the third week of gestation. Invagination along the midline of the neural plate forms the neural groove whilst an elevation of the groove's lateral edges creates the neural folds. The folds continue to elevate and eventually converge and fuse to become the neural tube.[15] As shown in Figure 25.2 fusion starts in the cervical region and continues both cephalad and caudally. The 2 ends are referred to as neuropores. The cranial neuropore closes first at around 24 days followed by the caudal neuropore 2 days after. Mesenchyme covers the dorsal aspect of the neural tube. Failure of any point along the neural tube to close results in NTDs.[1,2,15,16] Exposure of the open NTD to amniotic fluid hinders neuronal differentiation leading to neuroepithelial degeneration.[1] Defects that occur in the brain

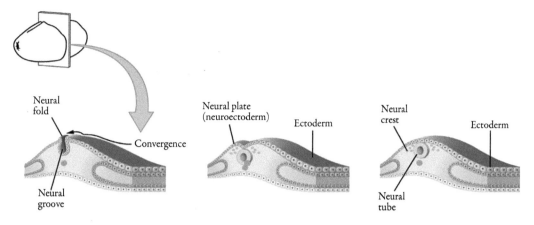

Fig 25.2 The lateral edges of the neural groove fold upwards and converge to form the neural tube.

include anencephaly and encephalocele while those that occur along the spine are known as spina bifida. NTDs can be classified as open versus closed. Myelomeningocele is the most common open NTD in which meninges and spinal cord are exposed. In contrast, closed defects are covered by skin at the site of defect and may have an overlying dimple, tuft of hair, or birthmark.[17]

SCREENING

The American College of Obstetricians and Gynecologists supports universal screening for all expectant mothers. Early detection will allow for timely preparation and counseling.[18] Families and health providers are able to facilitate in utero intervention, postnatal care, or termination.

Alpha-fetoprotein (AFP) is the primary serum protein in early embryonic development. Open NTDs result in leakage of AFP into the amniotic fluid.[2,16] It will not detect closed NTDs such as spina bifida occulta. AFP levels can be checked invasively by amniocentesis or noninvasively via maternal blood sample commonly drawn during the second trimester as part of the "quad screen" which checks for AFP, human chorionic gonadotropin, estriol, and inhibin A levels. Amniotic AFP peaks between 12 and 14 weeks and then decreases exponentially to the point of being indiscernible during term. Maternal AFP peaks between 28 and 32 weeks before finally declining. Timing of the screening is important due to the variable concentrations depending on the gestational age. Elevated maternal serum AFP levels can be up to 80% sensitive in the detection of NTD. Consider that other fetal anomalies can also be associated with elevated AFP levels such as abdominal wall defects. [18,19]

Second trimester ultrasound can be used to detect NTDs with an increased sensitivity of 90% compared to maternal serum AFP testing. It can be utilized as a solo test or in conjunction with an elevated AFP screening. Accurate detection is contingent upon several factors including the location and size of the defect, maternal size, fetus position, volume of amniotic fluid, skill of the sonographer, and type of equipment.[19] In addition to the presence of spine anomalies, ventriculomegaly, microcephaly, and Chiari II, malformation can furthermore be seen on ultrasound. Two sonographic findings that may manifest as a result of Chiari II malformation are the banana and lemon signs. The banana sign depicts the distinct posterior convexity of the cerebellum, and lemon sign represents the concave shape of the frontal calvarium (see Figure 25.3).[20,21]

ASSOCIATED ABNORMALITIES

Chiari II malformation

Herniation of the cerebellum and brain stem through the foramen magnum is commonly diagnosed on magnetic resonance imaging in patients afflicted with myelomeningocele. As a result of brainstem compression, affected individuals may develop a constellation of symptoms including dysphagia, vocal cord paresis, weakness of upper and/or lower extremities, neurologic deficits, hydrocephalus, and even apnea.[16,22] Depending on the severity of symptoms, some infants may require decompression surgery to help relieve pressure on the posterior fossa structures.

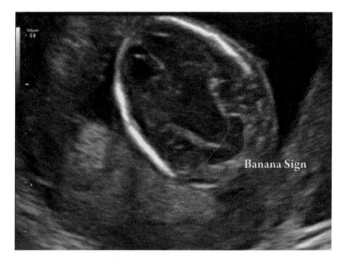

Fig 25.3 In Chiari II malformation, there is downward displacement of the posterior fossa through the foramen magnum. The cerebellum becomes compressed and resembles the shape of a banana.

Hydrocephalus

Chiari malformations can obstruct the normal flow of cerebrospinal fluid causing hydrocephalus. A large percentage of infants will continue to develop hydrocephalus even after repair of myelomeningocele. Close surveillance of head circumference and head imaging are utilized to track the degree of hydrocephalus. Gradual increases in otherwise asymptomatic infants can be managed conservatively with surveillance. If neurologic deterioration is present, acute excessive cerebrospinal fluid buildup can result in an emergency. Those children generally present with lethargy, altered mental status, seizures, nausea, vomiting, poor feeding, and or apnea.[16,23,24] They require immediate surgical intervention to shunt the flow of cerebrospinal fluid. Although most infants who have undergone ventriculoperitoneal shunting thrive, they still need to be monitored closely for the development of shunt malfunction later in life.

Concern for obstructive sleep apnea versus central apnea

The presence of apnea should prompt a thorough investigation. These individuals need closer monitoring especially in the perioperative period where they are at higher risk for respiratory failure. Polysomnography can help distinguish between obstructive versus central sleep apnea. Findings consistent with central apnea point to the involvement of the respiratory center and pathways located within the brainstem. Consultation with a pulmonologist and neurosurgeon can determine the need for surgical intervention.[3,16,25,26]

PREOPERATIVE ASSESSMENT

Following delivery, the defect should be examined paying particular attention to its size, location, and the presence of an outer membrane or cerebrospinal fluid. Latex precautions should be employed because of the possible risk for the development of an allergic sensitization to latex.[19,27] The infant should be positioned in either a prone or semilateral position to minimize pressure burden on the lesion.[28] In addition, the defect should also be covered with sterile and damp dressing to reduce the evaporative heat loss and to prevent the infection. Prophylactic broad spectrum antibiotics have also been shown to lower central nervous system infection.[3]

The location of the defect will determine the spinal cord level that is affected. Sacral lesions tend to spare motor function of the lower extremities whereas higher lesions may be accompanied with motor and or sensory deficits.[29] Providers should assess spontaneous movement, muscle tone, deep tendon reflexes, and response to painful stimuli. Other important considerations include genitourinary and gastrointestinal function. It is imperative to monitor voiding and stooling patterns as a decrease in anticipated frequency can indicate bladder dysfunction or fecal incontinence requiring a surgical intervention. The infant may present with other congenital anomalies including but not limited to: heart defects, airway abnormalities, solitary kidney, scoliosis, hip dysplasia, lower extremity contractures, and clubfeet.[30] The presence of

cyanosis and pathologic murmurs may warrant the need for an echocardiogram and further cardiac consultation for preoperative management.

As discussed earlier, the presence and symptomatology of hydrocephalus and Chiari II malformation need to be examined. This will serve as a neurologic baseline for future comparison. If not detected early, complications from hydrocephalus or a Chiari II malformation can lead to serious morbidity and neurologic dysfunction.

To minimize infection risk, surgical repair of the myelomeningocele usually occurs within 72 hours of birth. It may be done singly or in conjunction with a ventriculoperitoneal shunt or craniocervical decompression if there is an urgent need to address the hydrocephalus or Chiari malformation.

A minimum of 1 peripheral intravenous line should be present for induction. Infants typically undergo line placement shortly after delivery for the administration of antibiotics and dextrose containing maintenance fluids. Occasionally, an umbilical vein line may be placed in lieu of difficult peripheral intravenous access.

INTRAOPERATIVE CONSIDERATIONS

Positioning

Careful transport of the patient to the operating room and transfer to the operating table is crucial to ensure there is no disruption of the lesion. Depending on the location and size of the lesion, the lesion may be placed inside of a donut pillow, while maintaining a supine position. If the lesion is too large or cephalad not allowing for optimal supine positioning, the patient may be turned semilateral, preferably left-side down, with the aid of gel rolls or linens.[28] The patient in left side down position will facilitate the intubating process because the laryngoscope and endotracheal tube are typically entered on the right side of the mouth.

Induction

After placement of standard American Society of Anesthesiologists monitors and adequate preoxygenation, intravenous induction can take place with the aid of a nondepolarizing neuromuscular blocking agent. Ventilation can be difficult in a lateral position and may require using the right hand to obtain a better seal. Use of an oral airway may improve ventilation. Intubating in a semilateral position is more challenging than the conventional supine position. A second provider can help to assist with head stabilization to prevent rocking of the head side to side. The paraglossal intubation approach with a straight blade can be utilized if there is difficulty with obtaining an optimal view using a traditional midline approach. Proper positioning is obtained by directing the blade to the right of the tongue, over the molar region, toward the tonsil. The distal portion of the blade can be directed medially but the proximal portion of the blade should remain lateral to the central incisor region. Once the epiglottis is visualized, the blade tip is passed under the epiglottis.[31,32] The tube is inserted through the far right corner of the mouth. The improved view often comes at the expense of the limited amount of space there is for tube insertion and manipulation.

Once the endotracheal tube is secured, one can consider placing a second peripheral intravenous line if the defect is large and significant fluid losses are expected. An arterial line may be placed if there is need for hemodynamic support, concern for rapid hemodynamic shifts, or if underlying associated cardiac abnormalities are present in which a continuous pressure waveform is necessitated. Otherwise, surgical repair is minimally invasive and entails approximation of the lateral edges of the neural plate.

Maintenance

The use of volatile anesthetics is appropriate for myelomeningocele repair. The infant may only require a small dose of opiates if sensory deficits are present. If there is a concern for central apnea as a result of brainstem involvement, providers should use opiates judiciously.

Extubation

The decision to extubate at the termination of the procedure will be determined by the stability of the patient. Most infants are able to be extubated at the completion of the case, assuming that they were otherwise hemodynamically stable and not requiring respiratory support preoperatively. Specific considerations when determining whether or not to extubate include, Is the patient ventilating with appropriate tidal volumes? Maintaining adequate oxygenation? Are they vigorous? Hemodynamically stable? Appear to be at their neurologic baseline? If the infant required preoperative respiratory support or exhibited signs of apnea, the decision may be for the infant to remain intubated postoperatively.

POSTOPERATIVE CONCERNS

Hydrocephalus

Many infants may develop hydrocephalus after myelomeningocele repair. Routine surveillance of head circumference is imperative, and if neurologic deterioration occurs, the need for ventriculoperitoneal shunt placement should be considered. If the patient has an existing shunt, acute neurologic deterioration may signify shunt malfunction or infection. Patients can present with new onset seizures and will require a ventriculoperitoneal shunt revision to prevent further deterioration potentially leading to serious morbidity.

Tethered cord

Symptomatic retethering is a common event after myelomeningocele repair.[33] Adhesions of the spinal cord to the surrounding dura from scar tissue can lead to abnormal stretching of the cord resulting in lower extremity deficits, urinary dysfunction, and pain.[3,17] Magnetic resonance imaging can aid to exclude other causes for acute deterioration.

Surgical repair involves releasing the scar tissue to allow the cord to untether.

FETAL SURGERY

Several specialized centers throughout the United States and Europe offer fetal surgery to repair the defect in utero. The basis for early repair is to prevent the development of sequelae such as hydrocephalus or Chiari II malformations.[3] However, there is an associated increased risk for preterm delivery and obstetrical complications such as placental abruption so patients must be selected carefully. Generally, fetuses with a normal karyotype and free of any other associated abnormalities, such as underlying cardiac conditions, are the best candidates to undergo fetal surgery. The Management of Myelomeningocele Study was conducted from 2003–2010 to compare outcomes for fetuses who underwent early repair at 18–25 weeks gestation versus infants who had early postnatal repair. The results showed that the need for early cerebrospinal fluid shunting during the first year of life was lower in the early repair group contrasted to the early postnatal group. In addition, motor function at 30 months of age was better in the early repair group.[3,34]

CONCLUSIONS

- Neural tube defects can be classified as closed or open.

- Myelomeningocele is the most common neural tube defect and is comprised of a membranous sac containing neural tissue, which protrudes out of a defect along the spine.

- Screening can be done via maternal blood tests or antenatal imaging for early in utero detection.

- There are several associated abnormalities including hydrocephalus and Chiari II malformation. Close surveillance and/or imaging modalities may be necessitated to determine the need for intervention.

- Careful positioning is indicated to avoid disruption of the membranous sac and facilitate intubation.

- Patients will need to be monitored carefully in the perioperative period if there is any concern for apnea.

- Complications such as the development of hydrocephalus, need for a ventriculoperitoneal shunt revision or a tethered cord can develop at any time following NTD repair.

REVIEW QUESTIONS

1. A 22-year-old mother with no prenatal care delivers a baby boy at 37 weeks who is found to have anencephaly. Which of the following **MOST** accurately describes this condition's clinical features?

A. Bony skull absence with intact brainstem and cerebellum
B. Neural tube defect over the entire body axis
C. Skull defect with protruding brain and meninges
D. Vertebral defect with exposed spinal cord and meninges

Answer: A
Anencephaly is failure of the cephalic folds to fuse into a neural tube leading to the absence of a bony skull. The brainstem, cerebellum and spinal cord are present. Most if not all of the diencephalon is absent. This condition is generally lethal within hours but some have survived for a few days to weeks. Answer B describes craniorachischisis, answer C describes encephalocele, and answer D describes myelomeningocele.[2,24]

2. A 6-year-old boy with spina bifida and a chronic indwelling urinary catheter has severe hypotension and hypoxemia during augmentation cystoplasty. Which of the following is the **MOST** likely cause?

A. autonomic neuropathy
B. latex allergy
C. disseminated intravascular coagulopathy
D. urinary sepsis

Answer: B
Latex allergy can produce anaphylaxis. It presents as severe hypotension, rash, or hives and hypoxemia due to bronchoconstriction. Previous reports indicate a prevalence of latex allergy in patients with spina bifida ranging between 10% and 73%. From the initial surgical repair of the myelomeningocele, children with spina bifida are submitted to multiple surgeries due to the neurologic, orthopedic, and urologic problems they may present. Consequently, these children are exposed to several latex-containing products during their multiple interventions and they get sensitized. Accordingly, latex allergy manifestations can be prevented. Latex-containing products should be avoid using since the birth of children with spina bifida. In children already operated on for myelomeningocele but without evidence of latex allergy, one should avoid the use of latex materials during their successive admissions to hospital and during further surgeries. In children known to have developed latex allergy, one should require a latex-free operating room. Autonomic neuropathy is a disorder affecting the autonomic nerves. Causes include diabetes, amyloidosis, and autoimmune disorders. Patients can present with hypotension but usually not hypoxemia. Disseminated intravascular coagulation can cause abnormal bleeding, and hypovolemia can cause hypotension, but hypoxemia is unlikely. Urinary sepsis would present with hypotension; again, hypoxemia is unlikely.[35,36]

3. A 4-month old baby presents to the operating room for hydrocephalus and myelomeningocele repair. Which of the following is the **MOST** important consideration for myelomeningocele during anesthesia management?

A. horseshoe kidney associated with hydronephrosis

B. hyperkalemia associated with succinylcholine administration
C. restrictive lung disease associated with kyphoscoliosis
D. sleep disorder associated with apnea and vocal paralysis

Answer: D
Myelomeningocele is the most common open neural tube defect in which meninges and spinal cord are exposed. The spinal cord and meninges protrudes through the spinal column with no skin protective covering. The disease process is usually associated with apnea and vocal cord paralysis with compression of the posterior fossa causing sleep disorders and prolonged intubation postoperatively. Other associated diseases are horseshoe shaped kidneys, club feet, hip dislocation, and kyphoscoliosis. The defect occurs early during embryologic development and not associated with muscle denervation.[37pp530-531]

4. What is the **most important** prenatal environmental factor associated with NTDs?

A. cigarette smoking
B. gestational diabetes
C. hyperthermia
D. poor nutrition

Answer: D
One of the most important environmental factors centers on nutrition and its implications on the development of NTDs. Folate is a water-soluble, B-complex vitamin that is found naturally in certain foods. It functions as an essential coenzyme in the metabolism of nucleic and amino acids. Folic acid is the oxidized and most active form of folate. It is generally found in vitamin preparations and has twice the bioavailability of folate. Other environmental factors include maternal diabetes, maternal cigarette smoking, hyperthermia during early development, arsenic exposure, and valproate consumption.[8,13,14]

5. Which of the following conditions is **MOST** likely associated with a 1-day-old neonate born with a myelomeningocele presenting to the operating for neurosurgical repair?

A. Arnold-Chiari Type II malformation
B. double collecting duct system
C. hypoplastic left heart syndrome
D. increased intracranial pressure

Answer: A
Primary closure of a myelomeningocele usually occurs within the first day of life to minimize infection. In addition, a ventriculoperitoneal shunt is placed since most patients will have associated hydrocephalus. Type II Chiari malformations are almost associated myelomeningocele. Other associated congenital conditions include bladder exstrophy, prolapsed uterus, and Klippel-Feil syndrome. There are congenital cardiac defects associated with myelomeningocele such as atrial septal defects, but hypoplastic left heart syndrome is typically not common. In addition, since it is an open neural tube defect, these neonates rarely present with an increased intracranial pressure.[38,39]

6. Which week of developmental life is **MOST** closely related to failure of neural tube closure which causes anencephaly and spina bifida?

A. 3 weeks
B. 5 weeks
C. 7 weeks
D. 8 weeks

Answer: A

The neural plate is formed by a plate of thickened ectoderm that appears in the third week of gestation. Invagination along the midline of the neural plate forms the neural groove while an elevation of the groove's lateral edges creates the neural folds. The folds continue to elevate and eventually converge and fuse to become the neural tube. Fusion starts in the cervical region and continues both cephalad and caudally. The 2 ends are referred to as neuropores. The cranial neuropore closes first at around 24 days, followed by the caudal neuropore 2 days after. Mesenchyme covers the dorsal aspect of the neural tube. Failure of any point along the neural tube to close results in NTDs. Exposure of the open NTD to amniotic fluid hinders neuronal differentiation leading to neuroepithelial degeneration. Defects that occur in the brain include anencephaly and encephalocele while those that occur along the spine are known as spina bifida.[15,16]

7. The **GREATEST** benefit from an ex intrapartum treatment procedure for fetuses/infants with myelomeningocele disease is a **decreased** incidence of which of following complications?

A. fetal morbidity due to pulmonary edema
B. mild to moderate hindbrain herniation
C. neonatal infectious meningomyelitis
D. ventriculoperitoneal shunt requirements

Answer: D

The Management of Myelomeningocele Study was conducted from 2003 to 2010 to compare outcomes for fetuses who underwent early repair at 18–25 weeks gestation versus infants who had early postnatal repair. The results showed that the need for early cerebrospinal fluid shunting during the first year of life was lower in the early repair and moderate to severe brain herniation group contrasted to the early postnatal group. In addition, mental and motor function at 30 months of age was better in the early repair group. The prenatal group, however, had a higher fetal and maternal morbidity rate including placental abruption and pulmonary edema.[3,34]

QUESTIONS AND ANSWERS

This chapter has accompanying questions and answers which are available to subscribers as part of the Oxford eLearning platform. To access the questions, go to ✓ http:// oxfordmedicine. com/pediatricanesthesiaPBL

REFERENCES

1. Copp AJ, Greene NDE. Genetics and development of neural tube defects. *J Pathol*. 2010;220(2):217–230.
2. Salih MA, Murshid WR, Seidahmed MZ. Classification, clinical features, and genetics of neural tube defects. *Saudi Med J*. 2014;35(Suppl 1):S5–S14.
3. McLone DG, Bowman RM. Overview of the management of myelomeningocele (spina bifida). In: Post T, ed. *UpToDate*. Waltham, MA: UpToDate; 2016. www.uptodate.com. Accessed April 10, 2017.
4. Copp AJ, Stanier P, Greene NDE. Neural tube defects—recent advances, unsolved questions and controversies. *Lancet Neurol*. 2013;12(8):799–810.
5. Greene NDE, Stanier P, Copp AJ. Genetics of human neural tube defects. *Hum Mol Genet*. 2009;18(R2):R113–R129.
6. Murphy M, Whiteman D, Stone D, Botting B, Schorah C, Wild J. Dietary folate and the prevalence of neural tube defects in the British Isles: the past two decades. *BJOG*. 2000;107:885–889.
7. Sebold CD, Melvin EC, Siegel D, et al. Recurrence risks for neural tube defects in siblings of patients with lipomyelomeningocele. *Genet Med*. 2005;7:64–67.
8. Goeltz LM. Folic acid supplementation in pregnancy. In: Post T, ed. *UpToDate*. Waltham, MA: UpToDate; 2017. www.uptodate.com. Accessed June 1, 2017.
9. Blencowe H, Cousens S, Modell B, Lawn J. Folic acid to reduce neonatal mortality from neural tube disorders. *Int J Epidemiol*. 2010;39(Suppl 1):i110–i121.
10. Werler MM, Shapiro S., Mitchell AA. Periconceptual folic acid exposure and risk of occurent neural tube defects. *JAMA*. 1993;269(10):1257–1261.
11. Czeizel AE, Dudas I. Prevention of the first occurrence if neural-tube defects by periconceptual vitamin supplementation. *N Engl J Med*. 1992;327:1832–1835.
12. U.S. Preventive Services Task Force. Folic acid for the prevention of neural tube defects: U.S. Preventive Services Task Force Recommendation Statement. *Ann Intern Med*. 2009;150:626–631
13. Mitchell L. Epidemiology of neural tube defects. *Am J Med Genet*. 2005;135C:88–94.
14. Sarmah W, Muralidharan P, Marrs J. Common congenital anomalies: environmental causes and prevention with folic acid containing multivitamins. *Birth Defects Res C Embryo Today*. 2016;108:274–286.
15. Wallingford JB, Niswander LA, Shaw GM, Finnell RH. The continuing challenge of understanding, preventing, and treating neural tube defects. *Science*. 2013;339:1222002.
16. McLone DG, Bowman RM. Pathophysiology and clinical manifestations of myelomeningocele (spina bifida). In: Post T, ed. *UpToDate*. Waltham, MA: UpToDate; 2017. www.uptodate.com. Accessed June 1, 2017.
17. Khoury C. Closed spinal dysraphism: clinical manifestations, diagnosis and management. In: Post T, ed. *UpToDate*. Waltham, MA: UpToDate; 2015. www.uptodate.com. Accessed April 17, 2017.
18. Driscoll DA, Gross S, Professional Practice Guidelines Committee. Screening for fetal aneuploidy and neural tube defects. *Genet Med*. 2009;11(11):818–821.
19. Dukhovny S, Wilkins-Haug L. Open neural tube defects: risk factors, prenatal screening and diagnosis, and pregnancy management. In: Post T, ed. *UpToDate*. Waltham, MA: UpToDate; 2017. www.uptodate.com. Accessed April 17, 2017.
20. Nicolaides KH, Campbell S, Gabbe SG, Guidetti R. Ultrasound screening for spina bifida: cranial and cerebellar signs. *Lancet*. 1986;2:72.
21. Monteagudo A, Timor-Tritsch IE. Ultrasound diagnosis of neural tube defects. In: Post T, ed. *UpToDate*. Waltham, MA: UpToDate; 2016. www.uptodate.com. Accessed June 1, 2017.
22. Ganesh D, Sagayaraj BM, Barua RK, Sharma N, Ranga U. Arnold Chiari malformation with spina bifida: a lost opportunity of folic acid supplementation. *J Clin Diagn Res*. 2014;8(12).OD01–OD03.
23. Chance A, Sandberg D, Hydrocephalus in patients with closed neural tube defects. *Child's Nerv Syst*. 2015;31:329–332.
24. Haridas A, Tomita T. Hydrocephalus in children: physiology, pathogenesis, and etiology. In: Post T, ed. *UpToDate*. Waltham, MA: UpToDate; 2017. www.uptodate.com. Accessed June 1, 2017.
25. Verity C, Firth H, Ffrench-Constant C. Congenital abnormalities of the central nervous system. *J Neurol Neurosurg Psychiatry*. 2003;74:i3–i8.

26. Dauvilliers Y, Stal V, Abril B, et al. Chiari malformation and sleep related breathing disorders. *J Neurol Neurosurg Psychiatry*. 2007;78(12):1344–1348.

27. Pearson ML, Cole JS, Jarvis WR. How common is latex allergy? A survey of children with myelodysplasia. *Dev Med Child Neurol*. 1994;36:64–69.

28. Holland CE, Mansoor S, Butt AL, de Armendi AJ. Novel approach to supine positioning for infants with spina; neural tube defects. *Pediatr Anesth*. 2017;27:211–212.

29. Copp AJ, Greene NDE. Neural tube defects-disorders of neuralation and related embryonic processes. *Wiley Interdiscip Rev Dev Biol*. 2013;2(2):213–227

30. Swaroop VT, Dias L. Orthopedic issues in myelomeningocele(spina bifida). In: Post T, ed. *UpToDate*. Waltham, MA: UpToDate; 2017. www.uptodate.com. Accessed June 1, 2017.

31. Henderson JJ. The use of paraglossal straight blade laryngoscopy in difficult tracheal intubation. *Anaesthesia*. 1997;52:552–560.

32. Anderson P, Espinaco Valdes J, Vorster JG. Successful difficult airway intubation using the Miller laryngoscope blade and paraglossal technique. *S Afr J Anaesth Analg*.2015;21:46–48.

33. Mehta VA, Bettegowda C, Ahmadi SA, et al. Spinal cord tethering following myelomeningocele repair. *J Neurosurg Pediatrics*. 2010;6(5):498–505.

34. Adzick NS, Thom EA, Spong CY, et al. A randomized trial of prenatal versus postnatal repair of myelomeningocele. *N Engl J Med*. 2011;364(11):993–1004.

35. Cremer R Lobarcher M, Hering F, Englskirchen R. Natural rubber latex sensitisation and allergy in patients with spina bifida, urogenital disorders and oesophageal atresia compared with a normal paediatric population. *Eur J Pediatric Surg*. 2007;17(3):194–198.

36. Martinez-Lage JF. Moltó MA, Pagán JA. Latex allergy in patients with spina bifida: prevention and treatment. *Neurocirugia (Astur)*. 2001;12(1):36–42.

37. Cote CJ, Lerman J, Todres ID, eds. *A Practice of Anesthesia for Infants and Children*. 4th ed Philadelphia PA: Saunders Elsevier; 2009.

38. Davis PJ, Cladis FP, Motoyama EK, eds. *Anesthesthesia for Infants and Children*. 8th sd. St Louis, MO: Elsivier Mosby; 2011.

39. Koçak G, Önal C, Koçak A, et al. Prevalence and outcome of congenital heart disease in patients with neural tube defect. *J Child Neurol*. 2008;23:526–530.

26.

INTRACRANIAL TUMOR

Rebecca S. Isserman and Justin L. Lockman

STEM CASE AND KEY QUESTIONS

A 15-month-old, 13 kg, previously healthy full-term female child was referred to the emergency department by her pediatrician because of 2 weeks of almost daily vomiting and 3 days of vomiting all oral intake. Since yesterday, she has had increased irritability, and she is unable to stand unassisted (previously was ambulatory). She was seen by her pediatrician 1 week ago for nonbloody/nonbilious vomiting but was otherwise well-appearing and well-hydrated. Head circumference was measured earlier today at the pediatrician's office and was at the 75th percentile for age, compared to 25th percentile at her 9-month well visit.

WHAT IS THE DIFFERENTIAL DIAGNOSIS IN A CHILD PRESENTING WITH VOMITING, IRRITABILITY, AND LOSS OF MILESTONES?

Laboratory results, including a complete blood count, electrolytes, serum ammonia, and toxicology screen, are all within normal limits.

On exam, the patient is fussy but consolable by her mother and has photophobia. She is afebrile with heart rate of 108 bpm, is breathing 20 times per minute with oxygen saturation of 99% in air, and has a blood pressure of 105/70 mmHg. She has a full and tense anterior fontanelle and no motor deficits on neurologic examination.

A noncontrasted head computed tomography (CT) is obtained in the emergency department and shows a hyperdense mass in the posterior fossa with enlarged lateral and third ventricles, consistent with hydrocephalus. Subsequent magnetic resonance imaging (MRI) demonstrates a nonhomogenous lesion with solid and cystic components, located off midline to the left, displacing and compressing the fourth ventricle.

GIVEN THE IMAGING AND PRESENTATION, WHAT TYPES OF TUMORS ARE MOST LIKELY IN THIS PATIENT?

The patient is scheduled for a craniotomy with tumor biopsy and debulking for the following day; however while awaiting admission, she becomes lethargic and, when examined again, remains immobile on the stretcher. Her fontanelle in this position feels tense and is bulging. She is breathing without distress but her respiratory rate has decreased to 12 breaths per minute. Her heart rate is 89 bpm, and blood pressure is 116/71 mmHg.

WHAT DETERMINES INTRACRANIAL PRESSURE (ICP)?

Due to this change in clinical status, the decision is made to proceed urgently to the operating room for placement of an external ventricular drain (EVD), as well as tumor debulking. A blood type and screen is sent, and the patient is crossmatched for 1 unit of packed red blood cells.

WHAT ARE SOME WAYS TO MANAGE THIS PATIENT'S INCREASED ICP WHILE MOBILIZING FOR THE OPERATING ROOM?

The patient arrives to the operating room with a 24-gauge peripheral intravenous (IV) line in her left hand. She last ate breakfast approximately 5 hours ago, although she vomited after eating. She is listless, with no protest of monitor placement or preoxygenation. Her HR is 67 beats per minute, and her BP is 138/84.

HOW WOULD YOU INDUCE ANESTHESIA?

Induction of anesthesia proceeds without issue. After you secure the endotracheal tube, the surgeon places an EVD and notes high-pressure cerebrospinal fluid (CSF) drainage. You note a heart rate increase to 120 bpm and normalization of blood pressure for age with CSF drainage. A left radial arterial line is placed under ultrasound guidance. A 20-gauge IV is placed in the right saphenous, a 22-gauge IV is placed in the right hand, and a double lumen 4 French, 12-cm long central venous catheter is placed in the left subclavian vein. The patient is then positioned in the prone position for tumor debulking.

With surgical incision, the patient's hemodynamics remains unchanged. About 2 hours into a difficult resection, the patient's heart rate acutely drops from 125 to 54 beats per minute, and her blood pressure also decreases from a mean arterial pressure of 60 mmHg to a mean of 45 mmHg. All other vital signs, including peripheral capillary oxygen saturation (SpO_2) and end-tidal carbon dioxide ($EtCO_2$) remain the same.

WHAT IS THE LIKELY CAUSE OF THIS OCCURRENCE AND WHAT IS THE ACUTE MANAGEMENT?

The patient's vitals return to her baseline, and the surgeon resumes the resection without further vital sign changes. An intraoperative hemoglobin is measured and is 12 g/dL. The partial pressure of carbon dioxide in arterial blood ($PaCO_2$) on an arterial blood gas is 34 mmHg, which correlates with an $EtCO_2$ of 31 mmHg. Suddenly, the arterial blood pressure once again acutely drops to 50/30, with an increase in heart rate to 165. The $EtCO_2$ on the ventilator is now reading 12 mmHg.

WHAT IS THE LIKELY CAUSE OF THIS HEMODYNAMIC INSTABILITY AND WHAT IS THE MANAGEMENT?

This episode resolves and after normalization of vital signs, the surgeon is ready to resume the operation.

WHAT ADDITIONAL NONINVASIVE MONITOR MAY BE PLACED BEFORE RESUMPTION?

Frozen pathological sections reveal likely pilocytic astrocytoma (PA). The surgeon completes the resection, and the patient is positioned supine for emergence from anesthesia and extubation. The patient opens her eyes, intermittently cries around the endotracheal tube, and reaches for the tube but does not have consistent respiratory effort, even after a prolonged observation period in the operating room. The patient remains intubated and is transported to the intensive care unit for neurological monitoring and respiratory support. She requires invasive ventilation for 3 days, despite wakefulness, due to lack of spontaneous respiratory effort and poor gag reflex.

WHAT IS THE LIKELY CAUSE OF THIS PATIENT'S POSTOPERATIVE RESPIRATORY DEFICIT?

On postoperative day 4, the patient is successfully extubated. Despite adequate respiratory status, she had persistent ataxia, irritability, complete mutism, and severe apathy.

WHAT MIGHT BE THE CAUSE OF THESE SYMPTOMS, AND WHEN WOULD RESOLUTION BE EXPECTED?

The patient is discharged to home with outpatient rehab and oncology follow-up on postoperative day 10. At this time she has had resolution of irritability and apathy, with only mild ataxia. Her speech had returned to her baseline number of words but is notable for apraxia. Final pathology showed a Grade 1 PA and follow-up imaging demonstrated complete resection.

DISCUSSION

Intracranial tumors are the second most common childhood malignancy, secondary to leukemia, and the most common solid organ tumor in children. They are also the leading cause of cancer death in children.[1] Almost half of pediatric brain tumors are located in the posterior fossa.[2]

SIGNS AND SYMPTOMS AND DIFFERENTIAL DIAGNOSIS

Evidence of increased ICP is common at presentation, seen in up to 80% of posterior fossa tumors. In small infants with unfused cranial sutures, abnormal CSF flow and/or intracranial hypertension may be tolerated for some time before neurological changes become evident. A bulging fontanelle and increasing head circumference would be earlier signs in this case. Headaches, nausea and vomiting, and papilledema are also common presentations of increased ICP.[3]

In addition to signs of intracranial hypertension, ataxia and incoordination strongly suggests a posterior fossa lesion. Specific cranial nerve palsies, including abnormal eye movements, hearing loss or vertigo, and facial palsy may also be present at presentation.[3]

Often initial symptoms of an intracranial tumor, including headache, vomiting, lethargy, incoordination, and developmental delay, are nonspecific with a broad differential diagnosis. Infectious etiologies (including bacterial and viral gastroenteritis or meningitis,) toxic ingestion, trauma, and metabolic derangements may all present with similar signs and symptoms.[4]

TUMOR CLASSIFICATION

The majority of all pediatric brain tumors are gliomas (arising from glial cells), with PAs and other low-grade gliomas being the most common within this histological category. Central nervous system (CNS) embryonal tumors are a heterogeneous group of neoplasms that arise from embryonic cells remaining in the CNS after birth and include medulloblastomas (MBs), atypical teratoid/rhabdoid tumors (AT/RT), and primitive neuroectodermal tumors. The incidence of CNS embryonal tumors approaches that of gliomas in infants, less than 1 year.[1,5]

Specifically in the posterior fossa, MBs and cerebellar PA (CPA) account for the majority of the tumors. Differential diagnosis between these 2 tumor types is crucial, as MB has a much poorer prognosis. MB is often located in the midline vermis and on T2-weighted MRI images is isointense to hypointense compared with gray matter, while CPA lesions are often found in the cerebellar hemisphere and are hyperintense on comparable MRI images. Tissue diagnosis, however, is necessary for definitive diagnosis and to guide therapy.[6]

TUMOR-ASSOCIATED ICP AND ITS MANAGEMENT

Tumors in the posterior fossa frequently lead to increased ICP. Assuming a fixed intracranial volume, the determinants of ICP include the volumes of blood, CSF, and brain tissue. The Monro-Kellie hypothesis states that these cranial components are in state of volume equilibrium and that any increase in volume of one of these components must be compensated by a decrease in volume of another to maintain normal ICP. A tumor, in this case, may act as a space-occupying lesion, increasing the volume of the brain tissue compartment. In addition, a tumor in the posterior fossa often causes obstruction of cerebral spinal fluid (CSF) outflow, increasing the volume of intracranial CSF as well. Due to the relative plasticity of the skull of a young child, macrocephaly will form as the volume of CSF increases, delaying the development of increased ICP.[2,7]

Definitive management of increased ICP due to a posterior fossa tumor requires CSF drainage. This can be accomplished either by tumor resection/relief of outflow obstruction, by an alternative pathway for drainage via ventriculoperitoneal shunt or endoscopic third ventriculostomy, or both. Temporizing measures may be necessary to decrease ICP and prevent tonsillar/downward brain herniation prior to definitive management of intracranial hypertension. Vital signs indicating an urgent need to treat elevated ICP include hypertension for age and relative bradycardia, as well as irregular respirations (Cushing's Triad). Deterioration, or lateralization, of neurologic exam are concerning signs and require prompt treatment of elevated ICP.[8–10]

Acute management of increased ICP includes elevating the head of the bed to a maximum of 30 degrees and maintaining a midline position to promote venous drainage.[7,9] There is current Class II evidence supporting the use of hypertonic saline (3%) in intracranial hypertension associated with severe pediatric traumatic brain injury (TBI) and significant clinical experience demonstrating the safety of mannitol in the same setting.[10,11] While dexamethasone therapy is specifically not recommended following TBI, it is an effective treatment in tumor-associated vasogenic cerebral edema.[8]

In an intubated patient, mild hyperventilation to a $PaCO_2$ of no less than 30 mmHg may be used to temporary decrease cerebral blood flow and ICP; however, severe hyperventilation may cause cerebral ischemia, worsening outcomes. Sedation and neuromuscular blockade in these patients can also be used to decrease cerebral metabolic demand associated with agitation; however, hemodynamic stability is paramount and much be maintained during sedation.[10,11]

ANESTHETIC INDUCTION

Anesthesia management of a patient with elevated ICP should be tailored to avoid increases in ICP; however, it is also critical to maintain hemodynamic stability and, therefore, cerebral perfusion throughout all phases of anesthesia. While a number of induction techniques can achieve these goals, high-dose fentanyl (5–10 mcg/kg) usually helps to maintain hemodynamic stability, while blunting the sympathetic response to laryngoscopy.

Ketamine increases cerebral blood flow and has historically been avoided in cases of intracranial hypertension but has been shown to be a reasonable induction agent in patients with TBI and elevated ICP due to its effectiveness at maintaining blood pressure.[12] Similarly, succinylcholine, traditionally contraindicated in patients with ICP concerns,

should be considered when pulmonary aspiration is a real risk; the hypothetical adverse outcomes of further increasing ICP with succinylcholine is outweighed by the need to quickly secure the airway.[13]

Etomidate might be considered an ideal induction agent, as it, unlike ketamine, does not increase cerebral blood flow, while still providing hemodynamic stability. However the risk of adrenal suppression from even a single dose in pediatric patients should be weighed in the decision to use this agent.[11,14]

INTRAOPERATIVE COMPLICATIONS DURING SURGERY FOR A POSTERIOR FOSSA TUMOR

Hemodynamic instability during surgical procedures in the posterior fossa should be anticipated and can have multiple etiologies. Prompt recognition of an intraoperative event and quick determination of potential causes is critical to allow for immediate treatment.

The trigeminocardiac reflex (TCR) is a brainstem reflex defined by a decrease in heart rate and arterial blood pressure of more than 20% from baseline, coinciding with surgical manipulation of the trigeminal nerve.[15,16] Central TCR occurs with stimulation of the intracranial trigeminal nerve, as in the case of posterior fossa surgery, while peripheral TCR is triggered by trigeminal nerve stimulation outside the cranium and encompasses the well-described oculocardiac reflex.[16]

Cessation of surgical manipulation is frequently sufficient to restore heart rate and blood pressure to normal values. However, if this does not occur, the anesthesiologist should administer an anticholinergic agent (atropine or glycopyrrolate) intravenously, followed by epinephrine if still no improvement in the vital signs. Cardiopulmonary resuscitation may be required if pharmacological intervention does not ameliorate the physiological derangements. Bradycardia can result in a reduction of cardiac output and must be normalized to prevent cerebral ischemia due to decreased perfusion.[16,17]

A more frequently described cause of hemodynamic instability in posterior fossa surgery is venous air embolism (VAE). While a common occurrence in the sitting position, VAE is still a risk in small children during craniotomies regardless of positioning, as their relatively large head often rests at or above the level of the heart.[2] Small amounts of air may travel to the distal pulmonary vasculature and cause increased pulmonary vascular resistance and increased pulmonary arterial pressure, as well hypoxemia from ventilation/perfusion mismatch. When a significant amount of air enters the circulation, right ventricular output may become obstructed, leading to cardiopulmonary collapse. The risk of an arterial air embolism also exists if air crosses through a patent foramen ovale or a patent ductus arteriosus.[2,18,19]

Early recognition of venous air allows for early intervention and likely prevention of hemodynamic instability. Precordial Doppler ultrasonography is a noninvasive and sensitive monitor that provides early detection of intravenous air, often prior to any physiological change. The probe should be positioned over the fourth intercostal space at the right sternal border. The position can be tested by forceful injection of 5 mL of agitated normal saline, which should produce a change in the Doppler sound.[20] When a similar change is noted during surgery, immediate action by the anesthesiologist (converting to 100% inspired oxygen, performing Valsalva maneuver via hand ventilation, lowering the head of the bed, and attempting to aspirate air through a central venous catheter) and the surgeon (identifying and occluding the site of air entry by flooding the exposed area with saline or applying bone wax to exposed edges) may prevent further air entrainment.[2]

A sudden decrease in $EtCO_2$ occurs with more air entrainment and often coincides with hemodynamic evidence of VAE, such as hypotension. In this setting of low cardiac output with concern for VAE, the anesthesiologist should provide fluid resuscitation and vasopressor support (1–10 mcg/kg of epinephrine), and direct initiation of chest compressions with a rate of 100 to 120/minute to maintain cardiac output and to force intracardiac air through the ensuing air lock, even if there is not a cardiac arrest.[21] Of note, acute massive blood loss may also present similarly, and communication is essential to determine the need for blood transfusion as well.

POSTOPERATIVE COMPLICATIONS FOLLOWING SURGERY IN THE POSTERIOR FOSSA

Surgical injury to, or postoperative edema around, respiratory centers in the brainstem (dorsal respiratory group, ventral respiratory group, and apneustic center) or to the lower cranial nerve nuclei or tracts (CN IX–XII) may lead to respiratory failure and/or dysphagia, with unplanned intubation and ventilation requirements following surgery.[17,22] Duration of these problems depends on mechanism of injury; resolution is often quick and complete when due to transient postoperative edema, but cranial neuropathy often persists following direct nerve injury and may necessitate gastrostomy and/or tracheostomy placement.[22]

While not apparent immediately after surgery, posterior fossa syndrome (PFS), a neurological complication, can develop in up to 25% of children following posterior fossa surgery. The development of symptoms is typically delayed up to 5 days postoperatively, with mutism or other speech changes being the most prominent finding. Changes in speech are also accompanied by ataxia, behavioral symptoms (such as physical agitation), and emotional liability.[22–24]

Multiple theories have been proposed regarding the etiology of PFS, including aggressive surgery of the cerebellum, transient impairment of the afferent and efferent pathways of the dentate nuclei of the cerebellar hemisphere, vermis involvement, or vascular injury, without a consensus among researchers.[22–26] Most successful treatment for these patients focuses on multimodal therapy (behavioral, physical, occupational, and speech) tailored to the individual patient and focused on recovery of function.[23]

While the mutism tends to be transient in this syndrome, averaging 8 weeks in duration, persistent deficits are almost universal.[26] Speech often remains slow and dysarthric, and ataxia commonly remains. Deficits in processing speed, attention, and memory may all persist and may be permanent.[25,26] As such, multidisciplinary evaluation and treatment is essential of optimize function and quality of life of patients recovering from PFS. Further research into the mechanism of this disorder may allow for focused treatment and even prevention in the future.[26]

CONCLUSION

- Pediatric brain tumors commonly occur in the posterior fossa, where signs and symptoms of increased ICP are often evident at presentation.

- Temporizing measures to manage intracranial hypertension are often required prior to surgical intervention.

- Anesthetic management must be tailored to avoid further increases in ICP.

- Hemodynamic instability during posterior fossa surgery is common and may have multiple etiologies.

- Postoperative nerve palsies and the PFS can occur following posterior fossa surgery, with variable recovery in the short- and long-term.

REVIEW QUESTIONS

1. Which of the following is **MOST** likely diagnosis for a 24-month-old child with morning vomiting (without diarrhea), irritability, and loss of developmental milestones?

    A. abdominal migraine
    B. gastroenteritis
    C. intracranial tumor
    D. normal toddler

Answer: C
While vomiting may be a presenting sign of gastroenteritis or abdominal migraine, the loss of developmental milestones is a concerning finding that would not be present in either of these diagnoses, and makes an intracranial tumor a more likely diagnosis.[3]

2. For the routine evaluation of a toddler with altered mental status, which of the following assessments is the **LEAST** important?

    A. glucose level
    B. toxicology screening
    C. MRI of the brain
    D. psychological evaluation

Answer: D
There is a broad differential diagnosis of altered mental status in a toddler, including an intracranial process, as well as infectious, toxic, traumatic, and metabolic etiologies. Initial assessment should focus on these acute abnormalities. The incidence of psychological disease is extremely low in this demographic.[4]

3. Evidence of severe intracranial hypertension in a 15-month-old child is **MOST** likely to present as which of the following phenotypes?

    A. hypertension, bradycardia, and irregular respirations
    B. hypertension, tachycardia, and tachypnea
    C. hypotension, bradycardia, and tachypnea
    D. seizure and hypoventilation

Answer: A

Cushing's Triad describes the cardiopulmonary changes that occur in the setting of increased ICP and includes hypertension, bradycardia, and irregular respirations. While not all three findings are always present in this setting, Cushing's Triad is more common than other variants such as hypertension with tachycardia and irregular respirations.[27]

4. Assuming a fixed intracranial space, the **MOST** important determinants of ICP are which of the following?

    A. brain, cerebrospinal fluid, and intracranial blood volumes
    B. cerebral metabolic rate ($CMRO_2$) and blood flow to the brain
    C. presence or absence of seizure activity
    D. venous, arterial, and capillary blood volumes

Answer: A

The Monro-Kellie Doctrine states that the volumes of venous and arterial blood, CSF, and brain tissue (including edema and/or tumor) are the most important determinants of ICP. While changes in blood volume due to seizure activity and increased cerebral metabolism may increase ICP, CSF and brain tissue volumes also influence this relationship.[7]

5. Which of the following induced states is the **MOST** effective for lowering ICP in the child with intracranial hypertension?

    A. hyperthermia
    B. hypocarbia
    C. hyposmolarity
    D. hypoxemia

Answer: B

There is Class II evidence for the use of hypertonic (hyperosmolar) saline for intracranial hypertension. Uncertainty exists regarding the use of hypothermia to control intracranial hypertension, but hyperthermia should be avoided. Hyperventilation continues to be a common practice to manage increased ICP, although there is a lack of published evidence in the pediatric literature. Level III recommendations from the adult literature include hyperventilation to reduce $EtCO_2$ as a temporizing measure with measurements of brain oxygen delivery. Hypoxemia and hyposmolarity would be expected to raise ICP.[11]

6. Of the following changes, which is the **LEAST** likely to be a sign of VAE?

    a. acute reduction of $EtCO_2$
    b. appearance of end-tidal nitrogen
    c. precordial Doppler detection of turbulence
    d. sudden and unexplained hypertension

Answer: D

Depending on monitoring devices used, VAE may be detected via gas sampling (presence of end-tidal nitrogen or reduction in $EtCO_2$) or noninvasively via precordial Doppler ultrasound. Hypotension (not hypertension) would be expected with decreased cardiac output in the setting of VAE.[28]

7. The **MOST** critical, lifesaving maneuvers for a child with massive VAE are

    A. central venous catheter placement and air aspiration from the right atrium.
    B. chest compressions and elimination of the source of air entrainment.
    C. electrical cardioversion and epinephrine administration.
    D. hyperbaric oxygen therapy and reduction of embolus size.

Answer: B

The most critical management goals of a massive VAE include prevention of further air entry, hemodynamic support, and a reduction in the volume of air entrained, if possible. Eliminating the source of entrainment by covering/flooding the surgical field and lowering it to the level of the heart is critical. Chest compression can relieve an airlock in the right heart, forcing air out into the smaller pulmonary vessels, improving blood flow even in the absence of cardiac arrest. The success rate of significant air aspiration is low, especially in children.[17,28]

8. Regarding prognosis, the **MOST** important difference between CPA and MB is which of the following?

    a. Long-term survival following diagnosis is poorer with MB.
    b. Risk of preoperative intracranial hypertension is lower with MB.
    c. Severe intraoperative bleeding is more likely with CPA tumors.
    d. Short-term neurologic dysfunction more likely with CPA tumors.

Answer: A

CPA and MB together make up over 70% of all posterior fossa masses in children. While CPA is a low-grade tumor with excellent prognosis after surgical resection, MB is highly malignant with poorer prognosis. Typically, treatment for MB requires resection, radiation, and chemotherapy.[6]

9. In a patient following posterior fossa surgery, which of the following criteria is the **LEAST** important for assuring safe endotracheal extubation conditions?

    a. ability to follow commands
    b. adequate tidal volumes
    c. intact airway protective reflexes
    d. spontaneous respirations

Answer: A

Surgical manipulation of the posterior fossa may cause cranial nerve dysfunction and disruption of respiratory centers by direct stimulation/disruption or compromise due to edema or a vascular event. Dysphagia/bulbar nerve palsy may result in loss of airway protection, while damage to respiratory centers may result in hypoventilation or complete central apnea. It is critical to ascertain that these functions are intact prior to extubation.[17,22]

QUESTIONS AND ANSWERS

This chapter has accompanying questions and answers which are available to subscribers as part of the Oxford eLearning platform. To access the questions, go to ✔ http:// oxfordmedicine. com/pediatricanesthesiaPBL

REFERENCES

1. Ostrom QT, de Blank PM, Kruchko C, et al. Alex's Lemonade Stand Foundation infant and childhood primary brain and central nervous system tumors diagnosed in the United States in 2007–2011. *Neuro Oncol.* 2015;17:x1–x35.
2. Vavilala MS, Soriano SG, Krane EJ. Anesthesia or neurosurgery. In Davis PJ, Cladis FP, eds. *Smith's Anesthesia for Infants and Children.* 9th ed. Philadelphia, PA: Elsevier; 2017:744–772.
3. Wilne, S, Collier J, Kennedy C, Koller K, Grundy R, Walker D. Presentation of childhood CNS tumours: a systematic review and meta-analysis. *Lancet Oncol.* 2007;8:685–695.
4. Hayashi N, Kidokoro H, Miyajima Y, et al. How do the clinical features of brain tumours in childhood progress before diagnosis? *Brain Dev.* 2010;32: 636–641.
5. Fisher PG. Embryonal tumors. In Gupta N, Banerjee A, Haas-Kogan DA, eds. *Pediatric CNS Tumors.* Berlin, Heidelburg: Springer; 2004:83–105.
6. Brandão, LA Poussaint, TY. Posterior fossa tumors. *Neuroimag Clin N Am.* 2017;27:1–37.
7. Czosnyka, M, Pickard JD, Steiner LA. Principles of intracranial pressure monitoring and treatment. In Wijdicks EFM, Kramer AH, eds. *Handbook of Clinical Neurology, Vol. 140: Critical Care Neurology, Part I.* Philadelphia, PA: Elsevier; 2017:67–89.
8. Horvat, CM, Mtaweh H, Bell MJ. Management of the pediatric neurocritical care patient. *Semin Neurol.* 2016;36:492–501.
9. Pitfield, AF, Carroll AB, Kissoon N. Emergency management of increased intracranial pressure. *Pediatr Emerg Care.* 2012;28: 200–204.
10. Carney N, Totten AN, O'Reilly C, et al. *Guidelines for the Management of Severe Traumatic Brain Injury.* 4th ed. Brain Trauma Foundation; 2016. https://braintrauma.org/uploads/03/12/Guidelines_for_Management_of_Severe_TBI_4th_Edition.pdf. Accessed July 4, 2017.
11. Kochanek PM, Carney N, Adelson PD, et al. Guidelines for the acute medical management of severe traumatic brain injury in infants, children, and adolescents—second edition. *Pediatr Crit Care Med.* 2012;13:s1–s82.
12. Chang LC, Raty SR, Ortiz J, Bailard NS, Mathew SJ. The emerging use of ketamine for anesthesia and sedation in traumatic brain injuries. *CNS Neurosci Ther.* 2013;19:390–395.
13. May N, Anderson K. Towards evidence based emergency medicine: best BETs from the Manchester Royal Infirmary. BET 3: Suxamethonium (succinylcholine) for RSI and intubation in head injury. *Emerg Med J.* 2012;29:511–514.
14. Lundy JB, Slane ML, Frizzi JD. Acute adrenal insufficiency after a single dose of etomidate. *J Intensive Care Med.* 2007;22:111–117.
15. Schaller B, Probst R, Strebel S, Gratzl O. Trigeminocardiac reflex during surgery in the cerebellopontine angle. *J Neurosurg.* 1999;90(2):215–220.
16. Abdulazim A, Stienen MN, Sadr-Eshkevari P, et al. trigeminocardiac reflex in neurosurgery—current knowledge and prospects. In Signorelli, F. ed. *Explicative Cases of Controversial Issues in Neurosurgery.* InTech; 2012. https://www.intechopen.com/books/explicative-cases-of-controversial-issues-in-neurosurgery/the-trigeminocardiac-reflex-in-neurosurgery-current-knowledge-and-prospects. Accessed June 19, 2017.
17. Artru AA, Cucchiara RF, Messick JM. Cardiorespiratory and cranial-nerve sequelae of surgical procedures involving the posterior fossa. *Anesthesiology.* 1980;52:83–86.
18. Porter SS, Albin MS. Venous air embolism in a child undergoing posterior fossa craniotomy: a case report. *Can Aesth Soc J.* 1984;31:86–90.
19. Orebaugh SL. Venous air embolism: clinical and experimental considerations. *Crit Care Med.* 1992;20:1169.
20. Tinker JH, Gronert GA, Messick JM, Michenfelder JD. Detection of air embolism, a test for positioning of right artrial catheter and doppler probe. *Anesthesiology.* 1975;43(1):104–106.
21. Society for Pediatric Anesthesia. *Critical Events Checklist.* http://www.pedsanesthesia.org/critical-events-checklists/. Accessed July 13, 2017.
22. Kumar R, Mallucci C. Surgical complications. In Özek MM, Cinalli G, Maixner W, Sainte-Rose C, eds. *Posterior Fossa Tumors in Children.* Cham, Switzerland: Springer International; 2015:861–884.
23. Lanier JC, Abrams AN. Posterior fossa syndrome: review of the behavioral and emotional aspects in pediatric cancer patients. *Cancer.* 2017;123:551–559.
24. Catsman-Berrevoets CE, Aarsen FK. The spectrum of neurobehavioural deficits in the posterior fossa syndrome in children after cerebellar tumour surgery. *Cortex.* 2010;46:933–946.
25. Steinbok P, Cochrane DD, Perrin R, Price A. Mutism after posterior fossa tumour resection in children: incomplete recovery on long-term follow-up. *Pediatr Neurosurg.* 2003;39:179–183.
26. Gadgil N, Hansen D, Barry J, Change R, Lam S. Posterior fossa syndrome in children following tumor resection: knowledge update. *Surg Neurol Int.* 2016,7:s179–s183.
27. Fodstad H, Kelly PJ, Buchfelder M. History of the Cushing reflex. *Neurosurgery.* 2006;59:1132–1137.
28. Mirski MA, Lele AV, Fitzsimmons L, Toung TJ. Diagnosis and treatment of vascular air embolism. *Anesthesiology.* 2007;106:164–177.

27.

SEIZURE SURGERY

Caroll N. Vazquez-Colon and Srijaya K. Reddy

STEM CASE AND KEY QUESTIONS

A 7-year-old girl with intractable epilepsy is scheduled for a craniotomy with resection of her seizure focus. Her past medical history is significant for seizure disorder refractory to medical therapy and global developmental delay. She is on a ketogenic diet, and her medications include levetiracetam, topiramate, clonazepam, and fosphenytoin.

WHAT IS EPILEPSY? WHAT ARE THE UNDERLYING CAUSES OF EPILEPSY? WHAT TREATMENT OPTIONS ARE AVAILABLE FOR PATIENTS WITH SEVERE EPILEPSY?

The night before surgery, the patient's mother asks the neurosurgeon if her daughter should take her seizure medications before coming into the hospital for her procedure. She usually takes all of her medications with water when she wakes up in the morning around 8:00 AM; however, surgery is scheduled for 7:30 AM. The neurosurgeon asks you to respond to the mother.

HOW WOULD YOU INSTRUCT THE MOTHER TO ADMINISTER THIS PATIENT'S ANTIEPILEPTIC MEDICATIONS? WHAT ARE THE POTENTIAL EFFECTS OF HER ANTIEPILEPTIC MEDICATIONS ON THE PHARMACOLOGY OF ANESTHETIC MEDICATIONS TYPICALLY USED DURING SURGERY?

In the preoperative holding area, your evaluation of the patient reveals a very anxious child who is terrified about having surgery. The parents tell you that they strictly follow a ketogenic diet for their daughter because they have seen a slight decrease in seizure frequency ever since she was placed on the special diet.

WHAT IS A KETOGENIC DIET, AND HOW DOES IT WORK TO SUPPRESS SEIZURE ACTIVITY? IS THERE ANYTHING YOU WOULD WANT TO AVOID USING IN A PATIENT ON A KETOGENIC DIET? WHY? WOULD YOU CONSIDER A PREMEDICATION? WHAT METHOD OF ANXIOLYSIS WOULD YOU USE FOR THIS PATIENT?

After discussing the risks of anesthesia and your plan with the parents, the neurosurgeon alerts you that they would like to use electrocorticography (ECoG) as well as intraoperative electroencephalogram (EEG) during the case. He also gives you a perioperative seizure plan for the patient that was given to him by the neurologist. You review the neurologist's plan to make sure you have all medications available in the event of an intraoperative seizure.

HOW WOULD YOU INDUCE THIS PATIENT? WHAT ANESTHETIC OPTIONS ARE AVAILABLE TO YOU FOR MAINTENANCE OF ANESTHESIA GIVEN THE INTRAOPERATIVE NEUROMONITORING THAT WILL OCCUR? WHICH ANESTHETIC AGENTS ARE PROCONVULSANT, AND WHICH ONES ARE CONSIDERED ANTICONVULSANTS? WOULD YOU PLACE AN ARTERIAL LINE IN THE PATIENT FOR THIS CASE?

After an uneventful induction, intubation, and placement of lines, the patient is positioned on a horseshoe headrest and prepped for surgery. You begin your chosen anesthetic maintenance technique. About 45 minutes into the procedure, the patient's heart rate increases to 178 bpm, and oxygen saturation decreases acutely to 92%. You also notice that the patient's hand is twitching.

WHAT IS YOUR DIFFERENTIAL DIAGNOSIS?

You speak with the neurophysiologist who confirms that he is not running motor-evoked potentials during this case. You suspect that the patient is having a seizure given the abrupt change in hemodynamics.

HOW WOULD YOU ADDRESS THIS ISSUE? HOW WOULD YOU MODIFY YOUR ANESTHETIC, IF AT ALL?

The rest of the operation progresses without incident. The patient is extubated at the end, and you take her to the pediatric intensive care unit (PICU) for further management. On arrival to the PICU, the patient is tachycardic, moaning, and seems to be experiencing pain despite your generous administration of opioids intraoperatively. The PICU attending is concerned that her pain will result in a breakthrough seizure if not treated immediately.

DISCUSSION

BACKGROUND/EPIDEMIOLOGY

The World Health Organization estimates that approximately 50 million people currently live with epilepsy worldwide and estimates that 2.4 million people are diagnosed with epilepsy each year.[1] Epilepsy is a disease more commonly seen in the pediatric population with an incidence of 700 cases per 100,000 children less than 16 years of age.[2] Seizures can develop secondary to brain tumors, trauma, infection, stroke, or due to unspecified causes.

PHYSIOLOGIC CONSIDERATIONS

Epilepsy is a chronic disorder of the brain causing seizures. Epilepsy is one of the most common disorders of childhood. It is defined as the tendency to recurrent spontaneous seizures. A seizure is a sudden, excessive, uncontrolled electrical discharge of cortical neurons.[3]

The International League Against Epilepsy has developed new terms to classify and describe seizures. The new classification lists three major groups of seizures: generalized onset seizures, focal onset seizures, and unknown onset seizures. Generalized onset seizures describe seizures that occur in both sides of the brain (this term includes tonic–clonic or absence). Focal onset seizures describe a group of seizures that originate in one side of the brain. The term "focal" replaced the previous designation of partial onset seizures. Focal onset seizures are further classified into either focal onset awake or focal onset impaired seizures. Unknown onset seizure is used to describe seizures where the onset is unknown.[4] Recently, it has been suggested that the term "refractory" be replaced by drug-resistant epilepsy.

Drug-resistant epilepsy may be defined as failure of adequate trials of 2 tolerated and appropriately chosen and used antiepileptic drug (AED) schedules (whether as monotherapies or in combination) to achieve sustained seizure freedom.[5] This group also includes patients who cannot tolerate the negative side effects of AEDs even though the medications provide adequate seizure control. Studies have identified anatomic abnormalities associated with drug-resistant seizures. These anatomic abnormalities are known as cortical dysplasia or abnormal cortical migration. Drug-resistant epilepsy can have a significant negative impact on cognitive development in children.

Physiologic differences in pediatrics

In the first month of life, children are more predisposed to seizures or seizure-like activity. This is mostly due to the immaturity of the brain, which has a lower seizure threshold. Full-term infants have the ability to autoregulate their cerebral circulation, but because their head has a higher surface area than the body as compared to adults, a larger percentage of cardiac output is directed to the brain, resulting in higher cerebral blood volume.[6] This increases the risk of hemodynamic instability during neurosurgical interventions in infants and children as compared to adults. As opposed to adults, infants have immaturity of the renal system, predisposing them to fluid overload and electrolyte abnormalities during cases that require large fluid and blood administration. Infants also have immaturity of the hepatic system, which must be taken into consideration as this might lead to altered metabolism of certain drugs.[7]

The increased neuroplasticity of the developing brain makes pediatric patients better candidates for surgical intervention. In children, seizure control is of utmost importance due to the risk of cognitive dysfunction in a developing brain. Additionally, there are potential negative side effects of AEDs on cognitive and social development, so each case needs to be thoroughly evaluated. Studies have shown that patients with drug-resistant epilepsy who undergo successful surgical treatment exhibit improved cognition and learning capabilities.[8]

Pediatric patients presenting for seizure surgery could have associated comorbidities. A complete evaluation should be performed, focusing on possible side effects of AEDs that may affect the anesthetic plan.

IMAGING TECHNIQUES

The use of imaging techniques in children for diagnostic purposes can be challenging. In adults, these studies can be performed without sedation even though most of these studies require significant periods of immobility and cooperation. For obvious reasons, children might require sedation to obtain quality images. The level of sedation can range from anxiolysis to general anesthesia. To ensure that there is no interference with certain imaging modalities, the choice of anesthetic agent should be discussed with the radiologist prior to sedation. The development of new imaging technology provides accurate diagnostic data that can be entered in the surgical navigation system for exact intraoperative guided resection of localized seizure focus.

Electroencephalography

Electroencephalography has been the gold standard for evaluating and diagnosing epilepsy. It consists of evaluating abnormal electrical activity in the brain by placing leads along the scalp and recording brain wave patterns. The placement of leads in children with or without cognitive impairment might require some sedation to ensure optimum results. Invasive EEG monitoring is another diagnostic method that can identify areas in the brain that can be surgically resected. This method consists of surgically placing cortical grids under general anesthesia and then monitoring brain activity in the postoperative period. This is usually the first part of a staged surgical resection.

Magnetic resonance imaging

Magnetic resonance imaging is routinely ordered during initial workup for new onset of seizures. MRI evaluates structural abnormalities of the brain. Certain types of MRI like magnetic resonance angiography (MRA) and functional MRI (fMRI) provide more anatomical definition and language lateralization, which can be useful for surgical resection. In adults, MRI is primary done without sedation, but in the case of young children or highly anxious patients, some level of sedation might be needed to ensure better image quality.

Single photon emission-CT and positron emission tomography

Single photon emission-computed tomography (SPECT) and positron emission tomography (PET) are diagnostic modalities that have decreased the time to diagnosis and enhanced structural evaluation and identification of the seizure focus relationship with functional areas of the brain. SPECT can identify areas of increased perfusion that correlate with seizure focus, making it very useful during the ictal period when compared with the interictal period (shows hypoperfusion). In patients who require sedation, the timing of radionucleotide injection during seizure onset is important and should be coordinated with the anesthesiologist. PET scan identifies areas of metabolic activity in the brain. When perform in the interictal period, PET can localize seizure focus by showing areas of decreased metabolism. If performed during a seizure, it can demonstrate areas of increased metabolism.

Magnetoencephalography

Magnetoencephalography (MEG) is a noninvasive functional neuroimaging technique that identifies magnetic fields produced by electrical currents in the brain, and when combined with MRI, MEG can provide better localization of areas of the brain that generate seizures. Information obtained from MEG can guide the neurosurgeon in placing invasive EEG grids. MEG is a relatively newer technology, so there is paucity of data and experience in the literature for use in the pediatric population.

SURGICAL TREATMENT

The choice of surgical treatment largely depends on preoperative evaluation, imaging, and on the type of seizure. The most common surgical interventions are vagal nerve stimulator (VNS) placement and focal resection of seizure foci. Other surgical modalities seen in patients with seizure disorders include subdural grid placement and nonfocal surgical resection. Hemispheric resection can be done in case of intractable seizures or patients with specific diagnosis.

Vagal nerve stimulator

The placement of a VNS is the most common surgical intervention for intractable epilepsy in children. The mechanism of action is not clear, but it is believed that vagal nerve stimulation leads to activation of the nucleus tractus solitarius and other brainstem centers, which then transmits signals that modulate cerebral neuronal excitability.[9]

The procedure involves exposure of the left vagal nerve and attaching a stimulating electrode in the sternocleidomastoid muscle. The generator is placed in the pectoralis muscle fascia, and the electrode is then connected via tunneling. During this procedure, the anesthesiologist should be aware of possible damage to the surrounding structures including the trachea and major vessels. In the immediate postoperative period, patients may complain of hoarseness and sore throat.

Focal resection

Focal resection is undertaken when identified seizures foci are unilateral and not near any motor or language areas of the brain. A craniotomy is performed to expose the identified affected areas of the brain (previously identified with MRI and SPECT); a neuronavigation system and stereotactic guidance allow for precise resection. Resection with intraoperative MRI allows for a more accurate localization and complete resection of previously identified lesions. Anesthetic considerations for this procedure include the use of MRI-safe technology and monitoring. Protocols for intraoperative MRI should be present to ensure patient safety and desirable outcomes. Some cases may require a two-step approach in which the first phase involves the craniotomy for EEG grid placement directly in the affected brain areas. The patient is usually transferred to PICU for ongoing monitoring and identification of seizure foci. Once the foci are identified, the patient then undergoes another craniotomy for surgical resection.

Awake craniotomy

The most reliable monitor for neural function is an awake cooperative patient. An awake craniotomy can be achieved with mature, highly motivated patients. Most pediatric patients will not tolerate awake craniotomies, so anesthesia will be required. Sedative adjuvants such as dexmedetomidine, remifentanil, and propofol have all been used in awake craniotomies. Intraoperative techniques such as "asleep–awake–asleep" have been successfully tolerated in mature patients. Children with high levels of anxiety or any developmental delay are probably not ideal candidates for this type of procedure. Patient positioning is very importance during awake craniotomies, as patients should be comfortable with easy access to the airway.

Nonfocal surgical resection

Newer minimally invasive neurosurgical techniques have been developed and implemented successfully in pediatric patients. One of these advancements is the Visualase® procedure, which incorporates advanced MRI-guided laser ablation technology with thermal ablation. Laser energy is delivered to the target area using a laser applicator. As light is delivered through the laser applicator, temperatures in the target area begin to rise, destroying the unwanted tissue.[10] Visualase® is done under general anesthesia and is usually shorter in operative duration and less invasive than other neurosurgical procedures. The beginning Visualase® procedures are done in the operating room to facilitate a smooth induction, intubation, and placement of lines, while the laser ablation portion of the procedure is done while in the MRI suite. For this minimally invasive procedure, MRI-safe standard American Society of Anesthesiologists (ASA) monitors and 2 peripheral intravenous lines (IVs) are recommended. More invasive monitoring will vary depending on the individual patient. MRI safety protocols and standards should be in place for all intraoperative MRI procedures.

ANESTHETIC CONSIDERATIONS

Preoperative evaluation

During the preoperative evaluation, anesthesiologists will need to review the intraoperative and postoperative plan for the procedure with the parents and patients. This evaluation is vital in establishing a rapport with families and patients and to decrease preoperative anxiety. During this time, is also important to review AED treatment plan with the neurosurgeon, neurologist, and neurophysiologist to discuss possible interactions of anesthetic drugs, clarify the type of monitoring that will be used for the case, and review desired medication plan for the procedure. Furthermore, consultation with the intensivist who will manage the patient in the postoperative period should include postoperative antiseizure medical management.

History and physical. The preoperative evaluation should focus on a detailed neurological history in which the onset of seizures, type, duration, and quality of seizures should be disclosed. It is important to consider existing comorbidities such as metabolic derangements, brain tumors, or genetic syndromes associated with seizures. The level of cognitive impairment, if present, should be established. Use of preoperative anxiolytics might affect the recording of seizures intraoperatively, so use of these medications should be discussed with the neurology team prior to surgery. For cases in which premedication with benzodiazepines is contraindicated, alternative options such as distraction techniques, parental presence induction, and child life specialist assistance should be considered. Medication history, including current medications and possible side effects should also be obtained. It is important to note the timing and dose of medications in order to avoid gaps in treatment or possible overdosing. Physical examination should note any neurological injury including, but not limited to, weakness and decreased sensation.

Laboratory tests. Prior to surgery patients should obtain basic laboratory work including complete blood count, comprehensive metabolic panel, PT, INR, and PTT. Type and crossmatched red blood cells should be considered for invasive procedures with the potential for blood loss.

Antiepileptic drugs. AEDs have potential anesthetic-related side effects, so it is important for the anesthesiologist to understand how to address these issues in the perioperative period. The mechanism of action of these drugs typically involves the potentiation of GABA pathways or the inhibition of ion channels ($Na+$ or $Ca2+$) in the central nervous system. AEDs can be divided into first generation (phenytoin, primidone, carbamazempine, and phenobarbital) and second generation (vigabatrin, lamotrigine, and zonisaminde, levetiracetam, pregabalin) drugs. The first-generation AEDs have effects on cytochrome p450 (induce or inhibit), which can affect the metabolism of many anesthetic drugs. Second-generation AEDs have fewer interactions since they have no hepatic effects. AEDs that affect coagulation or impair the metabolism of drugs administered as part of the anesthetic are of particular concern for the anesthesiologist. The most well-known side effect of AEDs seen is the resistance to non-depolarizing muscle relaxants. The mechanism of action at the molecular level involves a decrease in acetylcholine release (NMDR) at the neuromuscular junction, which causes an acute sensitivity to NMDRs but causes upregulation of acetylcholine receptors leading to resistance with chronic use of AEDs. Of importance, topiramate can lead to normal anion gap metabolic acidosis; sodium valproate is associated with platelets abnormalities that can lead to increased bleeding during surgery; lancozamide has been shown to cause PR prolongation; and patients on carbamazepine may present with hyponatremia.[11]

Metabolic abnormalities secondary to AED administration should be considered in the event of intraoperative electrolytes abnormalities. Recognizing the effects of AEDs on medications used during anesthesia is paramount to the anesthesiologist during epilepsy surgery. Direct effects of AEDs and anesthetic medications can be seen with propofol and neuromuscular blocking agents. Studies have suggested reduced propofol dose requirement and increased time to emergence in patients on chronic AEDs.[12] Patients on chronic phenytoin and carbamazepine medications show an increased clearance and decreased duration of action of commonly used neuromuscular blocking agents such as rocuronium, pancuronium, and vecuronium.

Ketogenic diet. A ketogenic diet is a high-fat, low-carbohydrate diet that promotes ketosis and is often used for patients with intractable seizures.[13] The proposed mechanism of action is not completely understood, but it has been thought that acidosis in the brain due to chronic ketosis reduces neuronal excitability, thus reducing seizure activity. Patients on a ketogenic diet will most likely have metabolic acidosis, which will be evident on an arterial blood gas. In the event a patient on a ketogenic diet requires anxiolysis prior to surgery, alternate forms will need to be considered since the oral (PO) formulation of midazolam contains considerable amounts of carbohydrates. Due to the nature of this diet, anesthesiologists should also avoid dextrose-containing IV fluids in the perioperative period.[14]

Intraoperative management

Positioning. Patient positioning should be discussed with the surgeon in advance of surgery. Access to the patient's airway during awake craniotomies is crucial for intraoperative management. If a seizure is to be elicited during surgery, either an arm or leg of the patient should be easily visualized. If the head of the bed will be elevated for the surgery, monitoring for venous air embolism should be considered.

Induction and maintenance. Most pediatric patients will not have an IV catheter present prior to induction. Smooth controlled inhalational induction should be considered. Maintenance of anesthesia can be achieved with a combination of narcotic and inhaled anesthesia agents. Volatile anesthetics decrease the cerebral metabolic rate and are potent cerebral vasodilators and should not be used as sole anesthetic agents. Volatile anesthetics can also interfere with neuromonitoring, so their use should be limited for cases in which neuromonitoring, especially ECoG, will be used.

Intracranial hypertension. In the event of intracranial hypertension, brain swelling can be treated with elevation of head of the bed, mannitol, and increasing ventilation. Furosemide and/or 3% sodium chloride can also be used. Monitoring of electrolytes and acid-base status is encouraged to avoid severe electrolyte abnormalities.

IV access. In view of the possible rapid blood loss during craniotomies, it is recommended that 2 large bore peripheral intravenous catheters are placed. In case of difficult IV placement, a central line should be considered, but they are not routinely necessary for these cases.

Monitoring. Patients presenting for seizure surgery will need standard ASA monitors, and most of them, depending on the complexity of case, will likely benefit from having invasive blood pressure monitoring. Continuous blood pressure monitoring is often warranted since any acute changes in hemodynamics can result in impending brain injury. The use of a precordial Doppler and end-tidal carbon dioxide analyzer should be considered in cases where the risk of venous air embolism is high.[15] Serum glucose levels and acid-base status should be monitored during cases, especially for patients on a ketogenic diet. The use of neuromonitoring will vary among cases and should be discussed prior to the induction of anesthesia.

In cases of seizure mapping and the use of ECoG, it is important to know the acceptable drugs that do not interfere with microelectrode recording. Although many anesthetic agents have anticonvulsant properties, several medications have shown to have proconvulsant properties, such as sevoflurane, enflurane, methohexital, and etomidate. It is imperative that while ECoG is being used, these medications are minimized or avoided altogether. Dexmedetomidine and propofol have been used successfully in this setting, and both medications are acceptable during seizure mapping.[16]

POSTOPERATIVE CONSIDERATIONS

Unless contraindicated, an awake extubation should be prioritized after seizure surgery, as this will allow for a complete neurological evaluation to rule out any possible intraoperative central nervous system trauma. Motor function and ability to follow commands should be evaluated prior to extubation. Pain control can be accomplished using multimodal therapeutic agents, which include local anesthetics administered by surgeon, IV narcotics, IV acetaminophen, and dexmedetomidine if needed. Most patients will go to the PICU postoperatively for close monitoring. Seizures in the postoperative period may occur, so a postoperative seizure plan should be discussed with the PICU team. Monitoring of serum electrolytes should be done since syndrome of inappropriate antidiuretic hormone secretion, cerebral salt wasting, and diabetes insipidus may occur.

During seizure surgery, most patients will receive a loading dose of an AED, so this should be communicated with the PICU team as well to ensure adequate timing and dosing of scheduled AEDs. Unlike in the adult population, pediatric patients may need adjuvant sedative agents in the PICU. In the PICU, sedation with dexmedetomidine is recommended as it will not mask a seizure event, and it will not cause significant respiratory depression.

REVIEW QUESTIONS

1. The **MOST** appropriate timing for seizure surgery is when a patient has intractable epilepsy despite combination therapy with at least 2 AEDs over which of the following periods?

   A. 6–2 months
   B. 12–18 months
   C. 18–24 months

D. 24–30 months
E. 30–36 months

Answer: **C**

Indications for epilepsy surgery include intractable seizures over a period of 18 to 24 months despite combination therapy with at least 2 antiepileptic medications at maximally tolerated doses.[4] Patients who have adequate seizure control with medications, yet experience significant side effects from AEDs, may also be considered for surgical management.

2. A patient with which of the following conditions would benefit the **LEAST** if placed on a ketogenic diet?

   A. acute pancreatitis
   B. diabetes mellitus
   C. Dravet syndrome
   D. hyperlipidemia
   E. morbid obesity

Answer A:

Ketogenic diets are not recommended for patients with pancreatitis, hepatic failure, metabolic disorders with a defect in fat metabolism, and mitochondrial disorders.[7]

3. Which of the following is the **MOST** common side effect seen after placement of a VNS?

   A. bradycardia
   B. excessive coughing
   C. hoarseness
   D. surgical site infection
   E. vocal cord paralysis

Answer: **C**

After VNS placement, the most common side effect seen is hoarseness, often with alteration of voice quality. While all of the other answers listed are possible adverse effects related to VNS surgery, they are seen less commonly.[4]

4. Which of the following AEDs **MOST** commonly leads to platelet abnormalities after chronic use?

   A. diazepam
   B. keppra
   C. lacosamide
   D. topiramate
   E. valproate

Answer: **E**

Topiramate can lead to normal anion gap metabolic acidosis; sodium valproate is associated with platelets abnormalities that can lead to increased bleeding during surgery; Lacosamide has been shown to cause PR prolongation, and patients on carbamazepine may present with hyponatremia.[6]

5. Which of the following medications that should be **MOST** avoided in patients on Ketogenic diet?

   A. acetaminophen ER
   B. dexmedetomidine IN
   C. glycerin PR
   D. midazolam PO
   E. oxycodone IR

Answer: **D**

The proposed mechanism of action of ketogenic diet is not completely understood, but it has been thought that acidosis in the brain due to chronic ketosis reduces neuronal excitability, thus reducing seizure activity. In the event a patient on a ketogenic diet requires anxiolysis prior to surgery, alternate forms will need to be considered since the PO formulation of midazolam contains considerable amounts of carbohydrates.

6. Which inhalational agent should be avoided the **MOST** for patients returning to the OR for cortical grid removal?

   A. desflurane
   B. halothane
   C. isoflurane
   D. nitrous oxide
   E. sevoflurane

Answer: **D**

In patients presenting to the operating room for repeat craniotomy for removal of intracranial grid and strip electrodes, nitrous oxide should be avoided. It is important to avoid administration of nitrous oxide until the dura is opened since intracranial air can persist for up to 3 weeks after a craniotomy. Nitrous oxide can cause expansion of air cavities and result in tension pneumocephalus.[16]

QUESTIONS AND ANSWERS

This chapter has accompanying questions and answers which are available to subscribers as part of the Oxford eLearning platform. To access the questions, go to ✔ http://oxfordmedicine. com/pediatricanesthesiaPBL

REFERENCES

1. World Health Organization. *Epilepsy Fact Sheet*. http://www.who.int/mediacentre/factsheets/fs999/en/ Accessed November 20, 2017.
2. *The Epilepsies: The Diagnosis and Management of the Epilepsies in Adults and Children in Primary and Secondary Care*. NICE Clinical Guideline 137. London: Royal College of Physicians; 2012.
3. Peter M, Crean, ST. Essentials of neurology and neuromuscular disease. In: Cote C, Lerman J, Todres D, eds. *A Practice of Anesthesia for Infants and Children*. 4th ed. Philadelphia, PA: Saunders; 2009:491–507.
4. Scheffer IE, Berkovic S, Capovilla G, et al. ILAE classification of the epilepsies: position paper of the ILAE Commission for Classification and Terminology. *Epilepsia*. 2017;58:512–521. doi:10.1111/epi.1370
5. Kwan P, Arzimanoglou A, Berg AT, et al. Definition of drug resistant epilepsy: consensus proposal by the ad hoc Task Force of the ILAE Commission on Therapeutic Strategies. *Epilepsia*. 2010;51:1069–1077. doi:10.1111/j.1528-1167.2009.02397.
6. Vavilala MS, Lee LA, Lam AM. The lower limit of cerebral autoregulation in children during sevoflurane anesthesia. *J Neurosurg Anesthesiol*. 2003;15(4):307–312.

7. Soriano SG, Bozza P. Anesthesia for epilepsy surgery in children. *Child Nerv Syst.* 2006;22:834–843.
8. Noachtar S, Borggraefe I. Epilepsy surgery: a critical review. *Epilepsy Behav.* 2009;15:66–72.
9. Koh, J, Egan B, McGraw T. Pediatric epilepsy surgery: anesthetic considerations. *Anesthesiology Clin.* 2012;30:191–206.
10. Hawasli A, Bagade S, Shimony JS, Miller-Thomas M, Leuthardt EC. Magnetic resonance imaging-guided focused laser interstitial thermal therapy for intracranial lesions: single-institution series. *Neurosurgery.* Dec 2013;73(6):1007–1017.
11. Halasz P, Kalviainen R, Mazurkiewicz-Beldzinska M, et al. Adjunctive lancosamide for partial-onset seizures: efficacy and safety results from a randomized control trial. *Epilepsy.* 2009;50: 443–453.
12. Ouchi K, Suglyama K. Required propofol dose for anesthesia and time to emerge are affected by the use of antiepileptics: prospective cohort study. *BMC Anesthesiol.* 2015;1(Suppl):34.
13. Wilder RM. The effects of ketonemia on the course of epilepsy. *Mayo Clin Proc.* 1921;2:307–308.
14. Kossoff EH, Zupec-Kania BA, Amark PE, et al. Optimal clinical management of children receiving the ketogenic diet: recommendations of the International Ketogenic Diet Study Group. *Epilepsia.* 2009;50:304–317. doi:10.1111/j.1528-1167.2008.01765
15. Reasoner DK, Todd MM, Scamman Fl, Warner DS. The incidence of pneumocephalus after supratentorial craniotomy: observations on the disappearance of intracranial air. *Anesthesiology.* 1994;80(5):1008–1012.
16. Kofke AW. Anesthetic management of the patient with epilepsy or prior seizures. *Curr Opin Anaesthesiol.* 2010;23:391–399.

28.

ANESTHETIC MANAGEMENT OF CHIARI DECOMPRESSION

Eric Boudreau and Brian Egan

STEM CASE AND KEY QUESTIONS

A previously healthy 13-year-old girl was being followed by a neurologist for concussion-like symptoms characterized by worsening chronic occipital headaches following a closed head injury sustained while playing lacrosse. She presented to the emergency department at an outside hospital several months after the accident with headache and emesis accompanied by right arm weakness and numbness of her face, lips, and tongue. A noncontrast head computerized tomography (CT) scan was obtained, which showed Chiari type I malformation with herniation of the tonsils below the level of the foramen magnum. With the stroke-like symptoms on presentation, a magnetic resonance arteriogram and venogram (MRA/MRV) were obtained to evaluate for vascular malformations or dissection. Imaging showed a type I Chiari malformation with 11 mm of tonsillar herniation below the foramen magnum and partial flow obstruction of cerebrospinal fluid, but no additional abnormalities. She was started on amitriptyline and topiramate to assist with her headache symptoms as this was affecting her performance in school and extracurricular activities. She was then referred to neurosurgery where she was scheduled for Chiari decompression. She now presents in your preoperative care clinic for evaluation and preparation for surgery.

WHAT IS A CHIARI MALFORMATION, AND HOW COMMON IS IT? HOW DOES A PATIENT WITH CHIARI MALFORMATION TYPICALLY PRESENT? WOULD THE PRESENTATION BE DIFFERENT, IF YOUR PATIENT WAS 3 YEARS OLD? ON WHAT SPECIFIC ASPECTS OF HER MEDICAL HISTORY AND PHYSICAL EXAM WOULD YOU FOCUS? WOULD YOU RECOMMEND ANY MEDICATIONS TO BE USED AT HOME PREOPERATIVELY?

You met your patient in the preoperative area, and after revisiting your focused history and physical, she was brought to the operating room (OR). Standard American Society of Anesthesiologists (ASA) monitors were placed and general anesthesia was induced via inhalation of sevoflurane and oxygen. After induction, intravenous (IV) access was obtained and endotracheal intubation was accomplished via direct laryngoscopy. Additional peripheral access and arterial cannulation was obtained after the airway was secured. Prior to placing the patient in Mayfield pins, 3 mcg/kg of fentanyl was administered. The patient was then flipped prone, and all pressure points were padded. After the functionality of all IVs was insured and bilateral breath sounds were confirmed, the patient was prepped and draped.

SHOULD YOU HAVE GIVEN YOUR PATIENT AN ANXIOLYTIC OR AN ANTACID PRIOR TO BRINGING HER TO THE OR? WAS AN INHALATION INDUCTION AND DIRECT LARYNGOSCOPY THE SAFEST WAY TO START YOUR ANESTHETIC? IS AN ARTERIAL NECESSARY FOR THIS SURGERY?

Decompression of the posterior fossa was accomplished via a midline incision. A portion of the occipital bone was removed, as was a portion of the first cervical vertebrae. Following the bony work, the dura was opened to further decompress the posterior fossa. Once the surgeon was satisfied with the decompression, the dura was closed with a patch. The patient was flipped supine, additional fentanyl was titrated to achieve a stable, comfortable respiratory rate, ondansetron was administered, resolution of neuromuscular blockade was confirmed, and the patient was extubated when criteria were met. The patient was transported to the postanesthesia care unit (PACU) with standard monitors and sign out was given.

WHAT RISKS TO YOUR PATIENT ARE INCREASED DURING POSITIONING HER HEAD FOR OPTIMIZATION OF SURGICAL ACCESS? WHAT POSTOPERATIVE COMPLICATIONS SHOULD BE CONSIDERED WHEN EXTUBATING YOU PATIENT? ARE THERE OTHER AVAILABLE TREATMENTS TO MINIMIZE POSTOPERATIVE PAIN FOR YOUR PATIENT, BESIDES SYSTEMIC ANALGESICS?

The anesthesiologist should work with the neurosurgeon during the positioning to avoid excessive flexion of the head to prevent additional kinking of the medulla due to pressure from the Chiari malformation.

DISCUSSION

Chiari malformation represents a congenital neurodevelopmental abnormality resulting in a spectrum of herniation of cerebellar and/or midbrain tissue below the foramen magnum. In 1881, Theodor Langerhans described anatomic findings of hindbrain herniation in the absence of any myelodysplastic syndrome. He labeled this finding "pyramidal tumors" during his gross dissection. Further, Langerhans hypothesized that tonsillar herniations were responsible for impeding the flow of blood and cerebrospinal fluid (CSF), as well as likely displacing and affecting ventral spinal cord function. Ten years later, Austrian pathologist Hans Chiari published his first paper, which described varying displacement of cerebellar and brainstem tissue through the foramen magnum. He hypothesized that these pathologic changes stemmed from congenital hydrocephalus, as they were not observed in patients with late-onset or acute hydrocephalus. Chiari detailed four types of malformation. His classification provided the foundation with which we describe the disease process carrying his eponym today.[1] Current evidence suggests that Chiari malformations may stem from an underdevelopment of the germ layers resulting in a posterior fossa that is too small for the mature hindbrain. This facilitates downward displacement of neural tissue obstructing CSF flow at the level of the foramen magnum.[2]

The type I malformation involves caudal displacement of the cerebellar tonsils below the foramen magnum without involvement of the brainstem or spinal dysraphism. From a radiologic perspective, 5 mm tonsillar displacement is considered diagnostic of a type I malformation (Figures 28.1 and 28.2). Type II patients almost wholly are associated with spinal dysraphism and will demonstrate downward displacement of the cerebellar vermis, as well as portions of the brainstem and fourth ventricle. Both types I and II may present with hydrocephalus. Type III involves cervical spina bifida with partial absence of the tentorium cerebelli facilitating downward displacement of the entire cerebellum and fourth ventricle (myelocerebellomeningocele). Type IV does not have any downward displacement of the cerebellum; rather, it results from hypoplasia of the cerebellum.[3] Syringomyelia, dilation of the substance of the spinal cord, may be present in association with types I and II and occasionally with type III malformations. While estimates vary, upwards of 70% to 80% of Type I patients will present with concomitant syringomyelia.[4] Likely, alterations to the normal flow of CSF result in the abnormal dilatation of the spinal canal or cord (Figure 28.3). In fact, Chiari type II patients with syringomyelia can see resolution with adequate shunting of the lateral ventricles. Chiari malformation patients may also have accompanying scoliosis, and oftentimes otherwise asymptomatic patients will be incidentally diagnosed during scoliosis workup.[5]

Syringomyelia occurs when a fluid-filled cyst (syrinx) forms within the spinal cord. The condition is thought to be due to abnormal CSF flow. The degree of enlargement and location within the cord will determine the accompanying symptoms as well as degree of severity. Classically, patients with syringomyelia will present with weakness and atrophy of the hands and arms with accompanying loss of deep-tendon reflexes. Pain and temperature sensation will be impaired in the upper extremities, neck, and torso, classically described as a "cape-like distribution."[3,6] Proprioception and light touch, carried through the dorsal columns, will be preserved. Patients may experience hypertonia and increased deep-tendon reflexes in their lower extremities. The exact mechanism of syrinx formation is unclear with no consensus.[6]

Type I Chiari malformation is the most common presentation, and prevalence is estimated between 1:1,000 to 5,000 individuals. This is likely underestimating the true prevalence due to the numerous asymptomatic, undiagnosed individuals.[7] There tends to be a slight female preponderance among patients diagnosed with a Chiari malfomation.[8] It is estimated that as many as 57% of patients with diagnosed Chiari will be asymptomatic at the time of diagnosis.[9]

PRESENTING SYMPTOMS

The most common presenting complaint of symptomatic Chiari malformation is headache, which is classically described as an occipitocervical headache with intermittent, short-duration pain.[10] Headaches are exacerbated by activities that trigger a Valsalva-type response including sneezing, coughing, defecating, yelling, or physical activity.[6,8] Other common symptoms include neck pain, ataxia, and vertigo.[10] Many children with Chiari malformations will present with scoliosis that may or may not be accompanied by syringomyelia, although there does appears to be an association between the two.[6,11,12] While less common, symptoms of brainstem or cervical cord compression can produce much more serious symptoms: respiratory dysfunction resulting in hypoventilation or sleep apnea, sensorimotor deficits ranging from hemiparesis to quadriparesis, spasticity, and bladder dysfunction. Occasionally, lower cranial nerves may be involved. Up

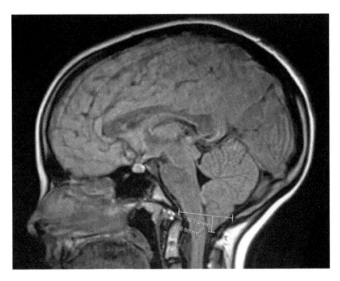

Fig. 28.1 Sagittal MRI of Chiari malformation demonstrating tonsillar herniation (vertical line) below foramen magnum (horizontal line).

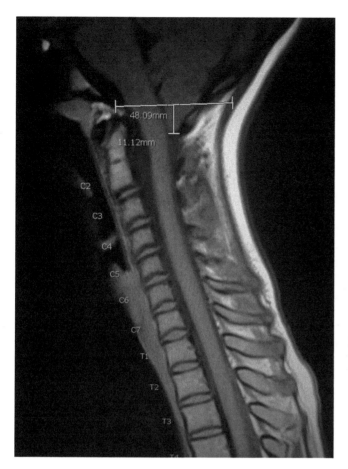

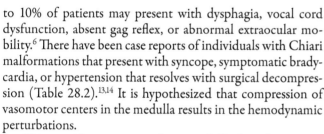

Fig. 28.2 T1 MRI of C-spine.

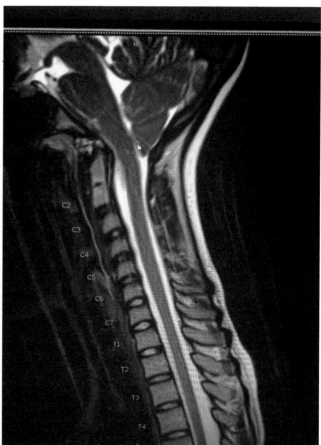

Fig. 28.3 T2 MRI of C-spine (white arrow denoting obstruction of CSF flow).

to 10% of patients may present with dysphagia, vocal cord dysfunction, absent gag reflex, or abnormal extraocular mobility.[6] There have been case reports of individuals with Chiari malformations that present with syncope, symptomatic bradycardia, or hypertension that resolves with surgical decompression (Table 28.2).[13,14] It is hypothesized that compression of vasomotor centers in the medulla results in the hemodynamic perturbations.

Chiari malformations may be more difficult to diagnose in younger patients partially due to their inability to adequately describe the symptoms of headache. The practitioner can be guided by behavioral clues (e.g., situational exacerbating factors) as well as associated symptoms (e.g., oropharyngeal dysfunction). In fact, one case series found that a majority of children less than 3 years old with Chiari malformations presented initially for oropharyngeal dysfunction. Twenty percent of them had previously undergone fundoplication and/or gastrostomy prior to diagnosis. Polysomnography study may be helpful in patients with Chiari malformations. Central sleep apnea may be indicative of brainstem compression. If the decision is made to not intervene surgically, then the patient will be followed over time to assess for any worsening symptoms. Regardless of neuroimaging, most neurosurgeons will intervene if symptoms thought to be due to a Chiari malformation are affecting the patient's activities of daily living.

TREATMENT

Initial conservative management derives from addressing presenting symptoms, as Chiari malformations are often not diagnosed until neuroimaging is obtained. This may involve nonsteroidal anti-inflammatory drugs, opioids, antiepileptics, transcutaneous electrical nerve stimulation, physical therapy, or occipital nerve blocks. The latter 2 treatments are aimed at addressing occipital neuralgia as the cause of headache.

Table 28.1 **CLASSIFICATION OF CHIARI MALFORMATIONS**

TYPE OF MALFORMATION	ANATOMY
Type I	Caudal displacement of cerebellar tonsils (>5 mm on radiology studies)
Type II	Caudal displacement of cerebellar vermis, medulla +/- pons; may see kinking of medulla
Type III	Caudal displacement of the entire cerebellum and fourth ventricle into external sac
Type IV	Hypoplasia of the cerebellum

Table 28.2 **SYMPTOMS OF CHIARI MALFORMATION**

BRAINSTEM-MEDIATED	SYRINGOMYELIA-MEDIATED	OTHER SYMPTOMS
• Respiratory dysfunction (sleep apnea, hypoventilation) • Dysphagia/oropharyngeal dysfunction • Vocal cord dysfunction • Abnormal extraocular movements • Vasomotor instability	• Weakness and atrophy in upper extremities • Loss of deep-tendon reflexes • Loss of pain and temperature sensation in "cape-like distribution" with preservation of light touch and proprioception	• Headache (occipitocervical location) • Ataxia • Vertigo • Scoliosis • Sensorimotor deficits (hemiparesis to quadriparesis)

The only definitive management is surgical decompression of the posterior fossa by craniectomy. Cerebellar tonsil displacement up to 2 mm below the foramen magnum is considered normal, whereas 5 mm caudal displacement of the tonsils is considered diagnostic. Patients with radiographic Chiari malformations may be asymptomatic at diagnosis while other patients may be symptomatic with tonsillar displacement between 2 and 4 mm. The surgical goal for patients with headache as the primary symptom is to decrease severity and frequency of headaches. In patients with syringomyelia, the goal is to prevent future neurologic deficit from occurring.[15] Currently, there are no consensus guidelines for surgical intervention exist.[5] In patients presenting with symptomatic Chiari, decompressive surgery will often stabilize or improve the presenting symptoms. Concomitant syringomyelia will normally decrease in size or completely resolve after decompressive surgery.[2] An international survey of neurosurgeons regarding their decision to intervene returned a consensus that no operation should be undertaken in an asymptomatic patient unless there was concurrent syringomyelia present, as this was felt to ultimately progress to symptomatic over time. Similarly, there was also a consensus that decompression of the malformation should be performed in patients presenting with scoliosis as well as syringomyelia.[6]

Posterior fossa decompression is the typical surgical treatment for Chiari malformation. With the patient in a prone position, likely in surgical pins, a small piece of the occipital bone is removed in hopes of decompressing the posterior fossa to prevent progressive herniation of the cerebellum. Some surgeons will also perform a cervical laminectomy. There is a lack of consensus on whether or not to open the dura mater for further decompression, as well as whether or not to perform a duraplasty to close the dura when satisfactory decompression is achieved.[6] Shunting of the syrinx is not recommended as a primary treatment for syringomyelia and usually employed in patients who fail to respond to surgical decompression.[8] It is the practice of neurosurgeons at our institution to open the dura during decompression. Following duraplasty, a positive pressure breath of 30 to 40 mmHg is delivered to assess the integrity of the duraplasty and check for residual cerebrospinal fluid (CSF) leak prior to completing the closure. After closure, the patient is returned to a supine position and extubated when appropriate criteria are met.

PREOPERATIVE CONSIDERATIONS

Planning for decompressive craniectomy for Chiari malformation involves adequately assessing the individual patient.

This may seem intuitive; however, the great heterogeneity in presentation of the Chiari patient requires a thorough and focused history and physical. A detailed neurological exam should be performed by the anesthesiologist delivering the anesthetic to establish a baseline from which the patient may be assessed following emergence. The anesthesiologist should assess range of motion of the neck in the preoperative area. Cervical spine instability or compression of cervical nerve roots may be elicited by flexion and extension of the neck. Range of motion may also be limited. If signs or symptoms are present, the anesthesiologist should take steps to avoid excessive extension during intubation whether it is an awake or asleep fiberoptic intubation or intubation with in-line stabilization using a conventional or video laryngoscope.

Care should be taken to assess for any history of gastroesophageal dysmotility as this may necessitate the need for a rapid sequence induction to minimize the risk of aspiration. One must also consider long-standing myopathy when deciding to use depolarizing neuromuscular blockade due to risks of hyperkalemic arrest.

Preoperative respiratory status should be investigated to assess for any signs of hypoventilation, sleep apnea, or any airway disease stemming from chronic aspiration. This is helpful to establish a baseline, as well as optimizing any potentially correctable conditions prior to undergoing anesthesia.

Finally, in any patient with a history of type II Chiari malformation, it should be investigated whether or not he or she has a latex allergy. As stated previously, the vast majority of type II patients have a coexisting history of spinal dysraphism, which has a strong association with latex allergy.

INTRAOPERATIVE CONSIDERATIONS

Choice of induction largely depends on the individual patient and provider comfort level. It is our institution's practice to utilize a mask induction, barring any contraindications, with additional intravenous anesthetic and neuromuscular blocker given after an IV is started. We recommend providing an anesthetic that maintains a mean arterial pressure within 10% of baseline to maintain an adequate cerebral perfusion to what is most likely a chronically injured cerebellum and/or brainstem.

In addition to the ASA standard monitors, it is our practice to routinely use invasive arterial blood pressure monitoring for Chiari decompressions. This not only facilitates continuous measurement of perfusion pressures, it also allows for periodic monitoring of laboratory.

Following induction and obtaining additional venous and arterial access, the patient is placed in Mayfield pins and flipped to a prone position. Care must be taken to adequately pad all pressure points and make certain that all IV catheters are functional prior to draping as the patient's arms will likely be tucked to allow the surgeons maximal access to the posterior fossa. The anesthesiologist should work with the neurosurgeon during positioning to avoid excessive flexion of the head to prevent additional kinking of the medulla due to pressure from the Chiari malformation. Finally, the endotracheal tube position should be confirmed via auscultation or fiberoptic visualization once the surgeons have finished positioning the patient in pins as varying degrees of neck flexion may result in the endotracheal tube potentially migrating to a mainstem position.

POTENTIAL COMPLICATIONS

Reported complications from Chiari decompression include, but are not limited to, aseptic meningitis, CSF leak, hydrocephalus, swallowing dysfunction, respiratory failure, pseudomeningocele, dysesthesia, craniocervical instability, brainstem compression, and cerebellar signs such as worsening ataxia[4] (Table 28.3). Another potential complication from posterior fossa decompression is persistent pain ranging in caliber from incisional to generalized headache. Postcraniotomy pain is well-established for posterior fossa procedures and may persist for many months with varying degrees of severity.[17] It is hypothesized that injuries to greater and lesser occipital nerves occur during incision or retraction. This can result in an entrapment syndrome or a traumatic neuroma resulting in chronic pain.[18] Occipital nerve block can be used to treat the postoperative incision-related pain, and prophylactic perioperative occipital nerve blocks may prevent this outcome, though no large studies have investigated this hypothesis.

POSTOPERATIVE CONSIDERATIONS

It is our institution's practice to send this patient population to a monitored floor after meeting discharge criteria from the PACU. There they will be able to receive regular neurological examinations. Any changes from baseline examination could merit immediate neuroimaging.

The anesthesiologist must evaluate for signs or symptoms of sleep apnea as this issue would not be expected to resolve

Table 28.3 **COMPLICATIONS FOLLOWING CHIARI DECOMPRESSION**

COMPLICATIONS	
• Aseptic meningitis	• Dysesthesia
• Cerebrospinal fluid leak	• Craniocervical instability
• Hydrocephalus	• Brainstem compression
• Swallowing dysfunction	• Cerebellar signs
• Respiratory failure	• Incisional/occipital pain
• Pseudomeningocele	

immediately following decompression. Arrangements should be made preoperatively to have continuous positive airway pressure (CPAP) or other noninvasive positive pressure ventilation available to the patient postoperatively.

Postoperatively, we employ a multimodal approach to pain management. Depending on any coexisting sleep apnea, varying degrees of opiate-sparing analgesics will be utilized at our institution. All patients, barring a contraindication, will be started on a dexmedetomidine infusion during emergence and this will be continued through the PACU course to the inpatient ward.

Following surgical correction of Chiari malformation, rehabilitation will be a large component of the patient's care. This involves physical therapy, speech therapy, and others depending on the extent of the preoperative dysfunction.

REVIEW QUESTIONS

1. A patient is booked for decompressive craniotomy for type I Chiari malformation. Considering the anatomy of the malformation and criteria on neuroimaging, what structure will **MOST** likely be seen 5cm below the foramen magnum?

    A. crus of the cerebellum
    B. lingula of the cerebellum
    C. tonsils of the cerebellum
    D. vermis of the cerebellum

Answer: C
Diagnostic imaging will demonstrate at least 5 mm of caudal or downward displacement of the cerebellar tonsils below the foramen magnum. The most common imaging modalities are CT and MRI scans.

2. On CT scan, following a motor vehicle collision, a 14-year-old female is found to have downward displacement of her cerebellar tonsils 3 mm below the foramen magnum and cervical syringomyelia. Other than a bruised forehead, she has no injuries from the accident. Her history indicates no signs or symptoms consistent with a Chiari malformation. What is the **MOST** appropriate treatment plan?

    A. decompressive posterior fossa craniectomy to address syringomyelia
    B. immediate surgical intervention for emergency drainage of the syrinx
    C. monitor via serial imaging of syrinx size and tonsillar protrusion
    D. no intervention or monitoring necessary; the patient is asymptomatic

Answer: A
Asymptomatic, caudal displacement of the cerebellar tonsils may not require surgery. However, there is consensus among neurosurgeons that in the presence of concomitant syringomyelia, the patient should be recommended for decompressive surgery. It is felt that these will all become symptomatic over time.

3. In the preoperative exam room, you obtain a thorough history and physical on your next patient—scheduled for

a posterior fossa craniectomy. He is 5 years old, with a type I malformation, but otherwise he is a healthy, thin child. What symptom, related by the parents, would be **MOST** concerning for brainstem compression?

A. ataxia
B. headache
C. sleep apnea
D. weakness

Answer: C
Other symptoms related to brainstem compression include oropharyngeal dysfunction, vocal cord dysfunction, abnormal extraocular movements, and vasomotor instability. If sleep apnea is a concern preoperatively, then it will be after the surgery as well. Since immediate correction of the sleep apnea is not anticipated, an opioid-sparing technique and postoperative use of CPAP may be indicated.

4. You are reviewing the next patient's chart prior to entering the preoperative exam room. The 11-year-old girl is scheduled to undergo decompressive craniectomy for type I Chiari malformation with concomitant syringomyelia. The syrinx is located in the cervical spine and has become symptomatic with weakness in her arms and hands. On your exam, what sensory/motor function would you **MOST** likely find to be preserved?

A. deep tendon reflexes of the upper extremities
B. pain sensation of the upper extremities
C. proprioception of the upper extremities
D. temperature sensation of the upper extremities

Answer: C
Proprioception and light touch are carried by the dorsal columns of the spinal cord and are normally preserved in the presence of syringomyelia. The expected deficits include weakness and atrophy of the upper extremities (possibly lower), loss of deep tendon reflexes, and loss of pain and temperature in a "cape-like" distribution.

5. A neurosurgeon refers her patient to you for debilitating occipital headaches. The child is 13 years old and recently diagnosed with a Chiari malformation. Her surgery is scheduled next month. Headaches are keeping the patient home from school, and she does not like how she feels after taking "pain meds." The family is interested in trying an occipital nerve block. What should you advise the family and patient as the **MOST** likely outcome of the block?

A. complete resolution of headache and other symptoms
B. improvement in pain that might last until her surgery
C. no relief from headache until definitive surgery is performed
D. worsening of pain associated with her occipital headache

Answer: B
Patients may experience partial or complete relief of an occipital headache via a nerve block. The duration of relief for any patient may vary and can be influenced by which local anesthetic and if any adjuvants are used in the injection.

6. Young children can be difficult to diagnose, and this can be especially true with respect to Chiari malformations. The correct diagnosis may take years to arrive at, and in the meantime, some children undergo additional procedures to treat symptoms attributable to a Chiari malformation. Which of the following symptoms is **LEAST** likely to be attributable to a type of Chiari malformation?

A. bladder dysfunction
B. central sleep apnea
C. chronic otitis media
D. oropharyngeal dysfunction

Answer: C
Although, children with Chiari malformations may certainly get ear infections like other children, the ear infections are not associated with the Chiari. On the other hand, oropharyngeal dysfunction and central sleep apnea can result from brainstem compression with a Chiari. Moreover, spinal dysraphism is seen with type II malformations, which often results in bladder and/or bowel dysfunction.

7. Chiari malformations can be associated with other diagnoses. Which of the following diagnoses is **MOST** likely to occur in conjunction with a Type I malformation?

A. hydrocephalus
B. scoliosis
C. spinal dysraphism
D. syringomyelia

Answer: D
The incidence of concomitant syringomyelia in type I malformations might be upwards of 70% to 80%.

QUESTIONS AND ANSWERS

This chapter has accompanying questions and answers which are available to subscribers as part of the Oxford eLearning platform. To access the questions, go to ✓ http://oxfordmedicine. com/pediatricanesthesiaPBL

REFERENCES

1. Tubbs RS, Oakes WJ. The Chiari malformations: a historical context. In: Tubbs RS, Oakes WJ, eds. *The Chiari Malformations.* New York: Springer; 2013:5–11.
2. Aitken LA, Lindan CE, Sidney S, et al. Chiari type I malformation in a pediatric population. *Pediatr Neurol.* 2009;40:449–454.
3. Graham A, Davis JE, Gouvernayre AJ, Thomas JA. An unusual cause of neck pain: acquired Chiari malformation leading to brainstem herniation and death. *J Emerg Med.* 2012;43:1000–1003.
4. Zhao J, Li M, Meng W, Wang C, Meng, W. A systematic review of Chiari I malformation: techniques and outcomes. *World Neurosurg.* 2016;88:7–14.
5. Pomeraniec IJ, Ksendzvosky A, Awad AJ, Fezeu F, Jane JA. Natural and surgical history of Chiari malformation type I in the pediatric population. *J Neurosurg Pediatr.* 2016;17:343–352.

6. Pindrik J, Johnston JM. Clinical presentation of Chiari I malformation and syringomyelia in children. *Neurosurg Clin N Am.* 2015;26:509–514.

7. Milhorat TH, Bolognese PA, Nishikawa M, et al. Syndrome of occipitoatlantoaxial hypermobility, cranial settling, and Chiari malformation type I in patients with hereditary disorders of connective tissue. *J Neurosurg.* 2007;7:601–609.

8. Dones J, De Jesus O, Colen CB, Toledo MM, Delgado M. Clinical outcomes in patients with Chiari I malformation: a review of 27 cases. *Surg Neurol.* 2003;60:142–147.

9. Bengalis D, Covington D, Bhatia R, et al. Outcomes in pediatric patients with Chiari malformation type I followed up without surgery. *J Neurosurg Pediatrics.* 2011;7:375–379.

10. Toldo I, Tangari M, Mardari R, et al. Headache in children with Chiari I malformation. *Headache.* 2014;54:899–908.

11. Victorio MC, Khoury CK. Headache and Chiari I malformation in children and adolescents. *Semin Pediatr Neurol.* 2016;23:35–39.

12. Greenlee JDW, Donovan KA, Hasan DM, Menezes AH. Chiari I malformation in the very young child: the spectrum of presentations and experience in 31 children under age 6 years. *Pediatrics.* 2002;110:1212–1219.

13. Selmi F, Davies KG, Weeks RD. Type I Chiari deformity presenting with profound sinus bradycardia: case report and literature review. *Br J Neurosurg.* 1995;9:543–545.

14. Ghasemi M, Golabchi K, Shaygannejad V, Rezvani M. Is Chiari malformation a cause of systemic hypertension and sinus bradycardia? A case report and literature review. *J Res Med Sci.* 2011;16:115–118.

15. Rocque BG, Oakes WJ. Surgical treatment of Chiari I malformation. *Neurosurg Clin N Am.* 2015;26:527–531.

16. Schijman E, Steinbok P. International survey on the management of Chiari I malformation and syringomyelia. *Childs Nerv Syst.* 2004;20:341–348.

17. Papangelou A, Radzik BR, Smith T, Gottschalk A. A review of scalp blockade for cranial surgery. *J Clin Anesth.* 2013;25(2):150–159.

18. Silverman DA, Hughes GB, Kinney SE, Lee JH. Technical modifications of suboccipital craniectomy for prevention of postoperative headache. *Skull Base.* 2004;14:77–84.

29.

ANESTHETIC MANAGEMENT OF SCOLIOSIS SURGERY IN CHILDREN

Arati Patil and Sophie R. Pestieau

STEM CASE AND KEY QUESTIONS

A 15-year-old female with a history of mild intermittent asthma and idiopathic scoliosis presented for posterior spinal fusion (PSF). Her scoliosis extended from T4–L1 with a curvature of 66 degrees. She had donated a unit of blood 1 month prior, at the time of her preoperative clinic visit. In the operating room, standard American Society of Anesthesiologists (ASA) monitors were placed and a peripheral intravenous (IV) line was inserted. She underwent a smooth IV induction, and her airway was secured with an endotracheal tube without difficulty. An additional large-bore peripheral IV and an arterial line were placed immediately following intubation, as well as an intrathecal (spinal) injection of morphine. After positioning on the Jackson spinal table, initial neuromonitoring testing was performed and showed normal sensory and motor signals. The surgical procedure went smoothly, including placement of multiple screws until insertion of the rods when the neuromonitoring technician encountered a loss of signal. The technician promptly alerted the surgeon and anesthesiologist to determine an immediate plan of action.

WHAT IS SCOLIOSIS, AND HOW IS IT MEASURED?

Scoliosis is an abnormal spinal curve measuring 10 degrees or greater and is typically diagnosed by a child's parent or pediatrician. There is no specific known cause for idiopathic scoliosis; however, there may be an associated genetic component as a positive family history can be found in some patients. The incidence of scoliosis is about 1%–3% of patients less than 16 years of age and is more common in females than males (7:1).[1]

As scoliosis develops, the spine may rotate or twist along with the ribs, leading to a multidimensional curve. Patients may present with pain in the lower back, uneven shoulders and hips, and an asymmetric back when bending forward. Once scoliosis is suspected, a radiographic image of the entire spine is used to confirm the diagnosis and to determine the severity of scoliosis. In 0.25% of cases, the scoliosis will require treatment including bracing or surgery.[2] The location of the scoliotic curve varies and can be thoracic, lumbar, or thoracolumbar.

The Cobb angle assesses the degree of scoliosis or lateral curvature of the spine and was first described in 1948 by Dr. John Cobb.[3] An anterior–posterior or posterior–anterior radiograph is needed to assess the Cobb angle. It is measured between the superior surface of the proximal most tilted vertebra and the inferior surface of the distal most tilted vertebra.[4] A parallel line is drawn from the most superior tilted vertebra and from the most inferior tilted vertebra. The intersecting perpendicular lines from these parallel lines form the Cobb angle (Figure 29.1). The Cobb angle is then used to determine the severity of the scoliosis and whether monitoring or intervention is indicated. A Cobb angle greater than 40 degrees can impair pulmonary function and can lead to restrictive lung disease. The Cobb angle can also be used to determine a patient's postoperative cardiac or respiratory function.

WHAT IS THE TREATMENT FOR SCOLIOSIS AND HOW IS THAT DETERMINED?

The Risser sign was first described by John Risser in 1958. Risser observed that the patient's spinal skeletal maturity is closely associated with the state of ossification of the iliac apophysis.[5] Based on a pelvic radiograph, the growth plate at the top of the pelvis is rated on a scale of 0–5 with 0 indicating skeletal immaturity with no ossification and 5 indicating skeletally maturity with fusion of the apophyseal ring to the ilium.[6] Typically, the spinal curve is at risk for progressing during rapid growth phases such as prior to menses in females. However, even after skeletal maturity, certain curvatures can progress with age. Spinal curves from 10–25 degrees are monitored with radiographs until a Risser scale of 5 is reached. Braces are used in curves ranging from 25–45 degrees to prevent progression of the curve.[7] The timing of surgery depends on the Cobb angle, the Risser sign, and the size and progression of the curve. Typically, surgical intervention is indicated in patients with a curve greater than 45 degrees.

WHAT ARE THE DIFFERENT TYPES OF SCOLIOSIS?

There are 3 types of scoliosis: idiopathic, neuromuscular, and congenital. Idiopathic scoliosis occurs in previously healthy patients and is usually categorized by age: infantile (birth–3 years of age), juvenile scoliosis (3–9 years of age); and

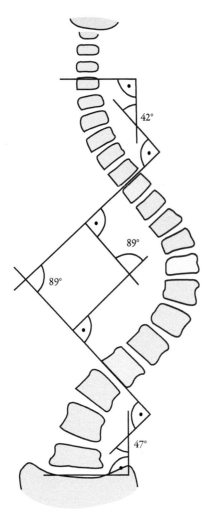

Fig. 29.1 Cobb angle measurement of scoliosis. (http://www.gnu.org/copyleft/fdl.html; http://creativecommons.org/licenses/by-sa/3.0/)

these patients have thoracolumbar scoliosis with pelvic obliquity, which can lead to pelvic malpositioning, which, in turn, may worsen the scoliosis.[9] These patients may be mobile or wheelchair bound at baseline. Their respiratory function must be assessed preoperatively as it can impact their ventilation and postoperative management. Cardiac function can be affected in muscular dystrophy and should also be evaluated preoperatively.

Congenital scoliosis develops in utero and is a rare occurrence. The true etiology of congenital scoliosis is unknown but is thought to be due to genetics, environmental factors, vitamin deficiencies, or medication use.[10] The scoliosis develops in the early embryologic period and may be associated with other congenital syndromes. A vertical expandable prosthetic titanium rib (VEPTR) device can be used to correct spine and chest wall abnormalities while allowing the spine to grow.[11] It allows the patient to have a functional thorax and optimize ventilation. Early-onset scoliosis is a challenge as it can cause thoracic insufficiency syndrome due to cardiac and respiratory constriction. Early spinal fusion is avoided as this can prevent future growth. Types of treatment include serial casting, bracing, VEPTR, and growing rods. Growing rods are attached to proximal and distal anchors that can be lengthened through surgical exposure. Magnetically controlled systems use similar spinal anchors, but the rods can be lengthened through magnetic stimulation, avoiding additional operative procedures and associated anesthetics.[12]

WHAT IS THE GOAL OF THE PERIOPERATIVE SURGICAL HOME?

The perioperative surgical home is a patient-centered, team-based approach to care that has been shown to decrease length of stay, intensive care use, perioperative blood transfusion, time in the operating room, and opioid consumption in patients with AIS undergoing PSF.[13] The perioperative surgical home includes the different phases of transition in care of surgical patients: the preoperative, intraoperative, postoperative, and postdischarge phases.

The preoperative phase focuses on laboratory work, imaging, autologous blood donation, patient education, and a preoperative anesthesia consult. Typical laboratory work includes a complete blood count, coagulation factors, urine culture, and radiograph imaging. Autologous blood donation is done 1 month before surgery and can decrease allogenic transfusion. Patients are often prescribed iron supplements prior to the procedure. The preoperative anesthesia consult allows an anesthesiologist to discuss the patient's history, perform a physical exam, and discuss the plan of care with the patient and his or her guardians. As constipation and postoperative ileus are common after PSF surgery, patients may be prescribed bowel prep.

The intraoperative phase focuses on standardized prewarming measures (i.e., warming blankets with forced-air warmer), decreased time for patient positioning, and standardized anesthesia protocols as well as workflow of surgical staff. The entire team is familiar with the intraoperative events as they often staff these procedures, which decreases

adolescent (10–18 years of age), with adolescent idiopathic scoliosis (AIS) being the most common. Idiopathic scoliosis has 2 types of curves: a C-shaped curve and an S-shaped curve. The etiology for idiopathic scoliosis is likely multifactorial. Multiple studies have evaluated the role of genetics in idiopathic scoliosis with variable conclusions. It is possible there is a multiple gene inheritance or sex-linked dominant inheritance associated with variable expression. The exact mode of genetic inheritance is still not yet known.[8] It is also believed that upright posture is related to idiopathic scoliosis. Spinal loading conditions are altered in the upright posture due to dorsally directed shear loads and facet joints aiding with spinal stability

Neuromuscular scoliosis (NMS) can be present in various types of neuromuscular disease. These cases are typically more complex than idiopathic scoliosis. Knowledge and understanding of the associated neuromuscular disease is important as this can alter the treatment and anesthesia required. The etiology of NMS can be neurologic (i.e., cerebral palsy, neuropathy, myelomeningocele, myasthenia, etc.) or muscular (Duchenne muscular dystrophy or other muscular dystrophies). NMS has a higher prevalence in these pathologies than idiopathic scoliosis in the general population. Many of variability in the operating room setting. The postoperative phase includes standardized postoperative care and postoperative pain management. The postdischarge team follows up on wound care, patient mobility, pain management, and patient satisfaction. These phases and respective teams encompass the entirety of the perioperative surgical home and play a large role in improving the care of these patients.

HOW IS THE PATIENT MONITORED IN THE OPERATING ROOM?

Operating room monitoring includes standard ASA monitors, 2 large-bore peripheral intravenous IV lines, an arterial line, a Foley catheter, an esophageal temperature probe, and neuromonitoring. Standard ASA monitors allow the anesthesiologist to evaluate the patient's heart rate and rhythm, pulse oximetry, blood pressure, and ventilation. The peripheral IV lines allow medication administration, fluid management, and blood transfusion if needed. The arterial line allows for invasive blood pressure monitoring and blood gas sampling. The arterial line is especially important to ensure adequate spinal cord perfusion during rod placement and derotation of the scoliotic curve. The Foley catheter allows for urine output monitoring, end organ perfusion, and guides intraoperative fluid management.

Temperature monitoring is vital as intraoperative hypothermia can result in various complications. Hypothermia occurs when the core temperature is less than 36°C. This can lead to impaired platelet function, coagulopathy, increased bleeding, and increased transfusion requirements. Impaired wound healing as well as increased surgical site infections may also result from hypothermia. In addition, hypothermia can delay drug metabolism and prolong the effect of anesthetics and opioids, which, in turn, may delay emergence from anesthesia. Lastly, intraoperative hypothermia can increase oxygen consumption and impair neuromonitoring.[14,15] Patients undergoing spinal fusion are at risk for intraoperative hypothermia due to the length of the procedure and large exposure. Prone positioning may also limit the effectiveness of underbody forced-air warmers. Warming techniques to avoid intraoperative hypothermia include use of preoperative and intraoperative forced air warmers, increasing operating room temperatures prior to draping, and warming IV and surgical fluids.

WHAT ARE THE DIFFERENT TYPES OF NEUROMONITORING, AND HOW ARE THEY AFFECTED BY THE ANESTHETIC MANAGEMENT?

Neuromonitoring is used to detect and prevent neurological deficit after PSF. It is performed by neuromonitoring technicians and consists of somatosensory-evoked potentials (SSEPs), transcranial motor-evoked potentials (TcMEPs), and electromyography (EMG). SSEPs monitor the somatosensory pathway whereas TcMEPs monitor the corticospinal tract or motor activity. A decrease in amplitude of 50% and increase in latency of more than 10% with SSEPs are considered

significant changes that may require intervention.[16] Volatile anesthetics reduce the amplitude and prolong the latency of SSEPs and should be used at less than half the minimum alveolar concentration (MAC). TcMEPs are also sensitive to inhalational anesthetics. Neuromuscular blockade affects TcMEPs and can be used for induction but should be avoided thereafter. TcMEPs are also sensitive to changes in spinal blood perfusion which may indicate impairment to the spinal cord. EMG evaluates nerve root injury and is frequently used for testing pedicle screw placement. It is sensitive to neuromuscular blocking agents but is not affected by volatile anesthetics.

DISCUSSION

PAIN MANAGEMENT

Spinal fusion surgery can lead to extensive postoperative pain. Multimodal pain management is the mainstay of therapy and consists of opioid and nonopioid medications. Opioids can be a mixture of long- and short-acting and may be given IV, intrathecally, via the epidural route and orally. Nonopioid pain management can include muscle relaxants, acetaminophen, nonsteroidal anti-inflammatory drugs (NSAIDs), and gabapentin.

Intrathecal morphine is a long-acting opioid that can be used as the main modality for intraoperative analgesia. It is given via a single shot spinal injection by the anesthesiologist prior to the start of surgery or by the surgeon after surgical exposure of the meninges. The morphine directly affects the opioid receptors in the dorsal horn and remains in the cerebral spinal fluid while migrating cephalad.[17] The effects may last up to 24 hours and do not interfere with neuromonitoring. Pain scores have been shown to be significantly lower in patients who received intrathecal morphine supplemented by patient-controlled analgesia (PCA) morphine compared to patients receiving PCA alone, along with a significant decrease in opioid consumption.[18] A similar study showed that intrathecal morphine significantly improved analgesia (by evidence of lower pain scores and opioid consumption) when compared to placebo.[19] In addition to improving pain control, studies have shown a decrease in blood loss and transfusion requirements in patients receiving intrathecal morphine.[18,19] Side effects of intrathecal morphine include pruritus, respiratory depression, nausea and vomiting.[17,20]

Methadone is an alternative long-acting opioid that can be given intraoperatively. Methadone, which is a μ-opioid receptor agonist and NMDA antagonist, inhibits the reuptake of serotonin and norepinephrine. It has been shown to improve postoperative pain control and reduce opioid consumption in complex spine surgery patients.[21] A more recent randomized, double-blinded control trial has shown that methadone reduced postoperative opioid requirements, improved pain scores, and increased patient satisfaction after PSF.[22] Methadone can be given IV intraoperatively as an alternative to intrathecal morphine.

Nonopioid pain medications are used as adjuncts for pain control. Ketorolac is a NSAID that is given IV and specifically targets pain caused by inflammation or edema in tissues affected by the surgery. One study showed that ketorolac decreases postoperative pain scores and opioid consumption.[23] Ketorolac can affect platelet function, which may lead to bleeding so it is important to evaluate if it is appropriate for each patient. A previous concern regarding ketorolac was the risk for pseudoarthrosis or nonunion. A retrospective review showed no difference in the rate of pseudoarthrosis in patients who received ketorolac versus those who did not.[24] Acetaminophen can also be given IV or orally and has shown to reduce pain scores but not opioid consumption.[25] Diazepam is a benzodiazepine that treats muscle spasms near the surgical incision and can be given IV or orally. Other nonbenzodiazepine muscle relaxants may also be given as needed. Gabapentin or pregabalin has been used for postoperative pain management. Preoperative gabapentin with continued administration has been shown to reduce postoperative morphine consumption and pain scores after scoliosis surgery.[26] Ketamine is an NMDA antagonist that has not been shown to decrease opioid use after PSF when given as a low dose infusion[27]. In addition, ketamine has not been shown to prevent remifentanil-induced hyperalgesia during pediatric spinal surgery.[28]

FLUID MANAGEMENT

Goal directed therapy is used for perioperative fluid management of patients undergoing spinal fusion. Crystalloids, in the form of Lactated Ringer's or normal saline, are administered for fluid maintenance and are restricted to 5 cc/kg/hr or less. Additional fluids are given in the setting of an increasing base deficit or lactate, decreasing urine output or pulse pressure variation. Colloid can be given for volume replacement if indicated. In otherwise healthy patients, the hemoglobin should be maintained above 7 mg/dL in the perioperative period and higher in the setting of associated cardiopulmonary comorbidity. Blood transfused as indicated by hemoglobin level, hemodynamics, or acute blood loss. Autologous blood products can be given to increase oxygen delivery and support intravascular volume if needed. Intraoperative cell salvage can be returned to increase hemoglobin and decrease allogenic blood transfusion requirements.

COMPLICATIONS

There are a multitude of complications that can occur with spinal fusion surgery.

Massive bleeding

Intraoperative massive bleeding and hemorrhage can ultimately lead to cardiac arrest if not treated emergently. There are patient specific and surgery specific factors that can affect blood loss and lead to massive intraoperative hemorrhage. Degree of Cobb angle, type of spinal deformity, thoracic kyphosis, and male sex are patient specific factors that can increase the risk of intraoperative bleeding. Surgery specific factors include operative time, surgical technique, number of vertebrae fused, number of screws, mean arterial pressure during surgery, blood salvage techniques, and use of antifibrinolytics.[28] Large databases report an overall transfusion rate of 25% to 30%.[29] Preoperative autologous blood donation has helped decrease the need for allogenic transfusion.[30,31] Intraoperative cell salvage is also commonly used as it reduces the rate of transfusion. Patients undergoing PSF with intraoperative cell salvage have been shown to receive fewer transfusions during the perioperative period.[32] Acute normovolemic hemodilution has not been supported in the literature for children and adolescents undergoing PSF although it could be considered in patients refusing blood transfusion.[33] Although studies are conflicting, a recent meta-analysis of randomized controlled trials indicates that mean blood loss, mean volume of blood transfused, and transfusion rate are decreased in patients with perioperative use of antifibrinolytics.[34] ε-aminocaproic acid (EACA) is an antifibrinolytic which inhibits fibrin degradation by binding to plasminogen which has recently been studied in children. Pediatric pharmacokinetic (PK) data have shown that EACA PK behavior is influenced by weight and age. The recommended infusion rate is 3 times what has been used in prior EACA efficacy studies.[35] Tranexamic acid (TXA) is a synthetic antifibrinolytic that inhibits fibrinolysis and the activation of plasminogen. A recent retrospective study showed that patients receiving TXA had a significant decrease in transfusion requirements with an associated reduced intraoperative blood loss.[36] Controlled hypotension is another method that has been used to decrease intraoperative blood loss; however, there is a risk of decreased spinal cord perfusion as well as a rare occurrence of blindness.[31] If controlled hypotension is being used, the mean arterial pressure should be no less than 20% below baseline. Additionally, the mean arterial pressure should be above 65 mmHg during periods of spinal cord compromise or manipulation to ensure adequate spinal cord and organ perfusion. Surgical hemostatic agents include bipolar sealant devices, fibrin sealant, and gelatin matrix with human thrombin. They have not been validated thus far but are commonly used because they work locally, quickly, and improve visibility of the surgical field. Despite the use of intraoperative cell salvage, antifibrinolytics, and surgical hemostatic agents to decrease surgical bleeding, if massive bleeding occurs it needs to be addressed emergently and may require use of a rapid transfuser and activation of massive transfusion protocol.

Blindness

Visual loss after spinal fusion surgery is an uncommon but devastating complication. According to the ASA's Postoperative Visual Loss Registry (POVL), the most common causes of perioperative vision loss in spine procedures are anterior and posterior ischemic optic neuropathy (ION), accounting for 89% of the cases.[37,38] Other known causes include retinal ischemia, cortical blindness, and posterior reversible encephalopathy. In 2012, the POVL Study Group performed a multicenter study comparing 80 patients with ION to 315 unaffected controls, and identified the following risk factors associated with ION for patients undergoing prone spinal fusion surgery: obesity, male sex, the use of a Wilson frame, longer anesthetic duration, increased blood loss, and decreased colloid administration.[37] With the exception of gender, these risk factors are thought to promote a rise in venous pressure and interstitial edema limiting optic nerve perfusion. A more recent review of the Nationwide Inpatient Sample for spine surgery showed perioperative ION is estimated to develop in 1:10,000 adult patients (0.01%) undergoing spinal fusion.[39] There are fewer reports focusing on visual loss after spine surgery in children. In 2016, De la Garza-Ramos[40] performed a retrospective study of 42,339 children under the age of 18 undergoing surgery for AIS. The incidence of visual loss was 1.6 per 1,000 procedures (0.16%). Patients with visual loss were significantly more likely to be younger and male, have Medicaid insurance, a history of anemia, and undergo fusion of eight or more spinal levels. Cortical blindness accounted for all cases of visual loss.

Loss of neuromonitoring signals

Neuromonitoring is crucial in spinal fusion surgery to detect and to prevent new neurological deficits. It is important to have a plan of action in place when changes in neuromonitoring occur (Figure 29.2). The anesthesiologist will need to quickly optimize mean arterial pressure to improve spinal cord perfusion, increase the hematocrit via blood transfusion to maximize oxygen delivery, optimize pH and partial pressure of carbon dioxide, avoid hypothermia, and communicate with the rest of the team members regarding a potential wake-up test. The neuromonitoring technician needs to promptly review the anesthetic agents used, including non-depolarizing muscle relaxants, check electrode and connections, as well as neck and limb positioning, and determine the pattern and timing of signal changes. The surgeon needs to review the events that occurred prior to signal loss and consider removing traction, decrease distraction, remove rods and/or screws, and evaluate for spinal cord compression.[41] Imaging can be used to evaluate placement of the rods and screws.

Infection

The incidence of surgical site infections that can occur from spinal fusion surgery in patients with idiopathic and non-idiopathic scoliosis varies from 3.7% to 8.5%.[42] Surgical site infections can lead to repeat surgeries, prolonged antibiotic treatments, and hospital readmissions, which can, in turn, significantly increase hospital cost. Standardized infection prevention protocols have been created to decrease infection rates. This includes preoperative preparation such as chlorhexidine gluconate wipes to the surgical area, IV antibiotic use, wound irrigation, limited operating room access, and minimization of dressing changes.

Checklist for the response to intraoperative neuromonitoring changes in patients with a stable spine

GAIN CONTROL OF ROOM	ANESTHETIC/SYSTEMIC	TECHNICAL NEUROPHYSIOLOGIC	SURGICAL
☐ Intraoperative pause: stop case and announce to the room	☐ Optimize mean arterial pressure (MAP)	☐ Discuss status of anesthetic agents	☐ Discuss events and actions just prior to signal loss and consider reversing actions:
☐ Eliminate extraneous stimuli (e.g. music, conversations, etc.)	☐ Optimize hematocrit	☐ Check extent of neuromuscular blockade and degree of paralysis	☐ Remove traction(if applicable)
☐ Summon ATTENDING anesthesiologist, SENIOR neurologist or neurophysiologist, and EXPERIENCED nurse	☐ Optimize blood pH and pCO2	☐ Check electrodes and connections	☐ Decrease/remove distraction or other corrective forces
	☐ Seek normothermia	☐ Determine pattern and timing of signal changes	☐ Remove rods
☐ Anticipate need for intraoperative and/or perioperative imaging if not readily available	☐ Discuss POTENTIAL need for wake-up test with ATTENDING anesthesiologist	☐ Check neck and limb positioning; check limb position on table especially if unilateral loss	☐ Remove screws and probe for breach
			☐ Evaluate for spinal cord compression, examine osteotomy and laminotomy sites
			☐ Intraoperative and/or perioperative imaging (e.g. O-arm, fluoroscopy, x-ray) to evaluate implant placement

ONGOING CONSIDERATIONS
☐ REVISIT anesthetic/systemic considerations and confirm that they are optimized
☐ Wake-up test
☐ Consultation with a colleague
☐ Continue surgical procedure versus staging procedure
☐ IV steroid protocol: Methylprednisolone 30 mg/kg in first hr, then 5.4 mg/kg/hr for next 23 hrs

Fig. 29.2 Reproduced with permission from Vitale MG, Skaggs DL, Pace DL, et al. Best practices in intraoperative neuromonitoring in spine deformity surgery: development of an intraoperative checklist to optimize response. *Spine Deform.* 2014:2(5):333–339.

POSTOPERATIVE MANAGEMENT

Postoperative management includes fluid management, pain management, avoidance of early complications, and patient disposition. Early complications include hypotension, anemia, atelectasis, systemic inflammatory response syndrome (SIRS), nausea, vomiting, decreased urine output, and constipation. Hypotension may be caused by anemia or hypovolemia and is treated with fluid management and a transfusion of red blood cells if needed. Anemia is caused by acute blood loss during the surgery and is monitored by checking laboratory levels and hemodynamics to determine if a transfusion is necessary. Atelectasis occurs from collapse of alveoli, which can occur during the surgery or postoperatively due to decreased lung compliance or splinting from pain. It can lead to hypoxia or tachypnea and is treated with deep breathing, incentive spirometry, physical activity, and postoperative pain management. SIRS may result from the systemic inflammation developed during the surgery. Signs of SIRS include tachycardia, fever, tachypnea, and an elevated white blood cell count. Common postoperative complications are nausea, vomiting, and constipation, which may be caused by opioid medications or the anesthesia. Constipation is also caused by decreased mobility and dehydration, and can be treated with physical activity, hydration, and stool softeners. Decreased urine output may occur from hypovolemia. Urinary retention after Foley catheter removal can be caused by opioid pain medication and is treated by decreasing opioid use, encouraging physical activity, and hydration. More severe complications include deep vein thrombosis, pulmonary embolism, and blindness (see the discussion on complications).

Postoperative pain management includes multimodal pain medication as discussed previously as well as patient controlled analgesia with a transition to oral medication when tolerated. Patient disposition includes the postanesthesia care unit, the intensive care unit, or the standard postoperative surgical floor. The disposition is determined by the patient's comorbidities and intraoperative surgical and anesthetic events.

CONCLUSIONS

- Scoliosis surgery in pediatric patients is determined by the type of scoliosis (idiopathic, neuromuscular, or congenital) and the severity of the Cobb angle. The timing of surgery depends on the Cobb angle, the Risser sign, and the size and progression of the curve.

- Neuromonitoring using SSEPs, TcMEPs, and EMGs is routinely used to prevent neurological injury after PSF.

- Intraoperative blood loss can be managed by preoperative autologous blood donation, intraoperative cell salvage, and the use of antifibrinolytics and surgical hemostatic agents.

- Intraoperative and postoperative pain control can be managed with long acting opioids (intrathecal morphine or IV methadone), IV opioids, and nonopioid pain medications.

- The perioperative surgical home is a patient centered, team-based approach to care that has shown to decrease hospital length of stay, the need for intensive care, perioperative blood transfusion, and postoperative opioid use after PSF.

REVIEW QUESTIONS

1. What is the **BEST** explanation for the mechanism of action of aminocaproic acid?

   A. Enhances the activity of plasminogen.
   B. Enhances the conversion of prothrombin to thrombin.
   C. Increases fibrinolysis.
   D. Inhibits fibrin degradation.
   E. Inhibits protein C and S.

Answer: D
Aminocaproic acid binds to plasminogen and blocks the binding of plasminogen to fibrin. This prevents the conversion of plasminogen to plasmin, which leads to the inhibition of fibrin degradation. Answer A is incorrect as it decreases the activity of plasminogen. Answer C is incorrect as aminocaproic acid is an antifibrinolytic agent, which decreases the breakdown of clot. Answers B and E are incorrect as aminocaproic acid binds to plasminogen and does not inhibit protein C and S or affect the conversion of prothrombin.[43]

2. Which of these patients is the **MOST** appropriate to undergo a spinal fusion surgery?

   A. 12-year-old female with a Cobb angle of 35 degrees and Risser scale of 5
   B. 13-year-old female with a Cobb angle of 35 degrees and a Risser scale of 3
   C. 13-year-old male with a Cobb angle of 40 degrees and a Risser scale of 5
   D. 15-year-old male with a Cobb angle of 48 degrees and a Risser scale of 3
   E. 16-year-old female with a Cobb angle of 40 degrees and a Risser scale of 5

Answer: D
Surgery is recommended for a Cobb angle of 40 to 50 degrees to stop progression. The Cobb angle of 48 degrees with a Risser scale of 3 indicates the potential for progression to a more severe Cobb angle. Risser scale is rated on a scale of 0 to 5 with 0 indicating skeletally immature with no ossification of the pelvis on a pelvic radiograph and 5 indicating skeletally mature with fusion of the apophyseal ring to the ilium. Answers A, B, C, and E are incorrect. The patients in answer A, C, and E have a Cobb angle of 40 degrees or less and a Risser scale of 5, indicating that skeletal maturity has been reached. The patient in answer B has the possibility of progression to a higher Cobb angle than the current 35 degrees; however, other modalities may be used such as bracing. There are surgical and nonsurgical treatments for pediatric scoliosis

that depend on the Cobb angle, Risser sign, the size and progression of the curve, comorbidities, pulmonary function, and cardiac function. If the scoliosis is severe enough, it can affect the rib cage and consequently affect pulmonary function and development. Patients with severe scoliosis can develop restrictive lung disease, which should be evaluated by pulmonary function tests. The vital capacity is diminished in patients with a Cobb angle of greater than 60 degrees.[44]

3. A 13-year-old female with AIS is scheduled to have a PSF performed for a COBB angle of 55 degrees. Neuromonitoring of SSEPs and MEPs are to be performed. What anesthetic agents will affect the neuromonitoring the **GREATEST** during the case?

    A. morphine intrathecally
    B. propofol infusion
    C. remifentanil bolus
    D. rocuronium at induction
    E. volatile agent increase

Answer: E
Volatile agents at greater than 0.5 MAC affect SSEPs and at greater than 0.3 MAC affect TcMEP). Answer A and C are incorrect because remifentanil and narcotics do not affect SSEP or TcMEPs. Answer B is incorrect as a propofol infusion increases latency for SSEPs in a dose-dependent fashion but does not affect neuromonitoring more than volatile anesthetics.[45] Answer D is incorrect as small doses of neuromuscular blockade ort a short acting muscle relaxant can be given during induction to facilitate intubation.

4. The patient in question 3 is undergoing her PSF. The surgical procedure went smoothly until insertion of the rods when the neuromonitoring technician encountered a loss of signal. What is the **MOST** appropriate first step for the anesthesiologist?

    A. bolus intravenous fluids
    B. increase mean arterial pressure
    C. increase volatile anesthetic
    D. perform a wake up test
    E. produce hypothermia

Answer: B
If there are intraoperative neuromonitoring changes in a patient with a stable spine, the anesthesiologist should immediately optimize mean arterial pressure to improve spinal perfusion. Answer A is a possible option to increase mean arterial pressure; however, that can be done with pressor medications. A transfusion of red blood cells should be considered to optimize hematocrit. Answer C is incorrect as volatile anesthetics prolong the latency and reduce the amplitude of SSEPs and also affect MEPs.[41] Answer D should be considered in a patient with a loss of signal but is not the first step that should be undertaken. Answer E is incorrect as normothermia is the goal.

5. What is the **MOST** likely side effect of intrathecal morphine?

    A. decreased sensory signals

    B. headache
    C. increased blood loss
    D. loss of motor signals
    E. nausea

Answer: E
Common side effects from intrathecal morphine include nausea, vomiting, pruritus, respiratory depression, and urinary retention. Answers A and D are incorrect as intrathecal morphine does not affect neuromonitoring. Intrathecal morphine is a central opioid injection as opposed to a local anesthetic injection. Answer C is incorrect as intrathecal morphine has been shown to decrease blood loss and transfusion requirements. Answer B is incorrect as it is not the most likely side effect of intrathecal morphine. Headache can occur due to intentional dural puncture.[46]

6. What is the **MOST** likely mechanism for blindness in children undergoing PSF?

    A. anterior ischemic optic neuropathy
    B. central retinal artery occlusion
    C. corneal abrasion
    D. cortical blindness
    E. posterior ischemic optic neuropathy

Answer: D
Cortical blindness has been shown to be the most likely cause of blindness after PSF surgery in children. It occurs from injury to the striate cortex, which may be due to hypoperfusion or ischemic injury. Answers A, B, and E are incorrect as cortical blindness is the most common etiology for postoperative vision loss in pediatric patients. Ischemic optic neuropathy, the most common cause of perioperative vision loss after spinal surgery in adults, develops from decreased perfusion of the optic nerve head.[37] Central retinal artery occlusion occurs most often from direct pressure on the globe however it is not as common. Answer C is incorrect as corneal abrasion is not a cause of postoperative vision loss in PSF patients.[40]

7. What is the **LEAST** favored blood salvaging technique in scoliosis repair?

    A. antifibrinolytic therapy
    B. autologous blood donation
    C. controlled hypotension
    D. intraoperative cell salvage
    E. surgical hemostatic agents

Answer: C
Controlled hypotension has been used to decrease intraoperative blood loss; however, there is a risk of decreased spinal cord perfusion and blindness and is therefore not routinely used.[31] Answer A is incorrect as antifibrinolytic therapy has been shown to decrease mean blood loss, volume transfused, and transfusion rate. Answer B is incorrect as preoperative autologous blood donation has helped decrease the need for allogenic transfusion in spinal fusion cases. Answer D is incorrect as intraoperative cell salvage is commonly used to decrease the need for allogenic transfusion. Answer E is incorrect as surgical hemostatic agents are commonly used because they work locally, efficiently, and improve visibility for the surgeon.[34]

QUESTIONS AND ANSWERS

This chapter has accompanying questions and answers which are available to subscribers as part of the Oxford eLearning platform. To access the questions, go to ✅ http://oxfordmedicine.com/pediatricanesthesiaPBL

REFERENCES

1. Borden TC, Bellaire LL, Fletcher ND. Improving perioperative care for adolescent idiopathic scoliosis patients: the impact of a multidisciplinary care approach. *J Multidiscip Healthc.* 2016;9:435–445. https://www.ncbi.nlm.nih.gov/pubmed/27695340

2. Asher MA, Burton DC. Adolescent idiopathic scoliosis: natural history and long term treatment effects. *Scoliosis.* 2006;1(1):2. https://www.ncbi.nlm.nih.gov/pubmed/16759428

3. Langensiepen S, Semler O, Sobottke R, et al. Measuring procedures to determine the Cobb angle in idiopathic scoliosis: a systematic review. *Eur Spine J.* 2013;22(11):2360–2371. https://www.ncbi.nlm.nih.gov/pubmed/23443679

4. Sud A, Tsirikos AI. Current concepts and controversies on adolescent idiopathic scoliosis: part I. *Indian J Orthop.* 2013;47(2):117–128. https://www.ncbi.nlm.nih.gov/pubmed/23682172

5. Risser JC. The Iliac apophysis: an invaluable sign in the management of scoliosis. *Clin Orthop.* 1958;11:111–119. https://www.ncbi.nlm.nih.gov/pubmed/13561591

6. Yang JH, Bhandarkar AW, Suh SW, Hong JY, Hwang JH, Ham CH. Evaluation of accuracy of plain radiography in determining the Risser stage and identification of common sources of errors. *J Orthop Surg Res.* 2014;9:101. https://www.ncbi.nlm.nih.gov/pubmed/25407253

7. Greiner KA. Adolescent idiopathic scoliosis: radiologic decision-making. *Am Fam Physician.* 2002;65(9):1817–1822. https://www.ncbi.nlm.nih.gov/pubmed/12018804

8. Kouwenhoven JW, Castelein RM. The pathogenesis of adolescent idiopathic scoliosis: review of the literature. *Spine.* 2008;33(26):2898–2908. https://www.ncbi.nlm.nih.gov/pubmed/19092622

9. Vialle R, Thévenin-Lemoine C, Mary P. Neuromuscular scoliosis. *Orthop Traumatol Surg Res.* 2013;99(1 Suppl):S124–S139. https://www.ncbi.nlm.nih.gov/pubmed/23337438

10. Hensinger RN. Congenital scoliosis: etiology and associations. *Spine.* 2009;34(17):1745–1750. https://www.ncbi.nlm.nih.gov/pubmed/19602997

11. Campbell RM. VEPTR: past experience and the future of VEPTR principles. *Eur Spine J.* 2013;22(Suppl 2):S106–S117. https://www.ncbi.nlm.nih.gov/pubmed/23354777

12. Bekmez S, Dede O, Yazici M. Advances in growing rods treatment for early onset scoliosis. *Curr Opin Pediatr.* 2017;29(1):87–93. https://www.ncbi.nlm.nih.gov/pubmed/27798426

13. Thomson K, Pestieau SR, Patel JJ, et al. Perioperative surgical home in pediatric settings: preliminary results. *Anesth Analg.* 2016;123(5):1193–1200. https://www.ncbi.nlm.nih.gov/pubmed/27749348

14. Horn EP, Bein B, Böhm R, Steinfath M, Sahili N, Höcker J. The effect of short time periods of pre-operative warming in the prevention of peri-operative hypothermia. *Anaesthesia.* 2012;67(6):612–617. https://www.ncbi.nlm.nih.gov/pubmed/22376088

15. Görges M, Ansermino JM, Whyte SD. A retrospective audit to examine the effectiveness of preoperative warming on hypothermia in spine deformity surgery patients. *Paediatr Anaesth.* 2013;23(11):1054–1061. https://www.ncbi.nlm.nih.gov/pubmed/23738627

16. Neira VM, Ghaffari K, Bulusu S, et al. Diagnostic accuracy of neuromonitoring for identification of new neurologic deficits in pediatric spinal fusion surgery. *Anesth Analg.* 2016;123(6):1556–1566. https://www.ncbi.nlm.nih.gov/pubmed/27861447

17. Tripi PA, Poe-Kochert C, Potzman J, Son-Hing JP, Thompson GH. Intrathecal morphine for postoperative analgesia in patients with idiopathic scoliosis undergoing posterior spinal fusion. *Spine.* 2008;33(20):2248–2251. https://www.ncbi.nlm.nih.gov/pubmed/18794769

18. Eschertzhuber S, Hohlrieder M, Keller C, Oswald E, Kuehbacher G, Innerhofer P. Comparison of high- and low-dose intrathecal morphine for spinal fusion in children. *Br J Anaesth.* 2008;100(4):538–543. https://www.ncbi.nlm.nih.gov/pubmed/18305080

19. Gall O, Aubineau JV, Bernière J, Desjeux L, Murat I. Analgesic effect of low-dose intrathecal morphine after spinal fusion in children. *Anesthesiology.* 2001;94(3):447–452. http://www.ncbi.nlm.nih.gov/pubmed/11374604

20. Urban MK, Jules-Elysee K, Urquhart B, Cammisa FP, Boachie-Adjei O. Reduction in postoperative pain after spinal fusion with instrumentation using intrathecal morphine. *Spine.* 2002;27(5):535–537. http://www.ncbi.nlm.nih.gov/pubmed/11880840

21. Gottschalk A, Durieux ME, Nemergut EC. Intraoperative methadone improves postoperative pain control in patients undergoing complex spine surgery. *Anesth Analg.* 2011;112(1):218–223. https://www.ncbi.nlm.nih.gov/pubmed/20418538

22. Murphy GS, Szokol JW, Avram MJ, et al. Clinical effectiveness and safety of intraoperative methadone in patients undergoing posterior spinal fusion surgery: a randomized, double-blinded, controlled trial. *Anesthesiology.* 2017;126(5):822–833. https://www.ncbi.nlm.nih.gov/pubmed/28418966

23. Munro HM, Walton SR, Malviya S, et al. Low-dose ketorolac improves analgesia and reduces morphine requirements following posterior spinal fusion in adolescents. *Can J Anaesth.* 2002;49(5):461–466. https://www.ncbi.nlm.nih.gov/pubmed/11983659

24. Sucato DJ, Lovejoy JF, Agrawal S, Elerson E, Nelson T, McClung A. Postoperative ketorolac does not predispose to pseudoarthrosis following posterior spinal fusion and instrumentation for adolescent idiopathic scoliosis. *Spine.* 2008;33(10):1119–1124. https://www.ncbi.nlm.nih.gov/pubmed/18449047

25. Hiller A, Helenius, I, Nurmi E, et al. Acetaminophen improves analgesia but does not reduce opioid requirement after major spine surgery in children and adolescents. *Spine.* 2012;37(20):E1225–E1231. https://www.ncbi.nlm.nih.gov/pubmed/22691917

26. Mayell A, Srinivasan I, Campbell F, Peliowski A. Analgesic effects of gabapentin after scoliosis surgery in children: a randomized controlled trial. *Paediatr Anaesth.* 2014;24(12):1239–1244. https://www.ncbi.nlm.nih.gov/pubmed/25230144

27. Pestieau SR, Finkel JC, Junqueira MM, et al. Prolonged perioperative infusion of low-dose ketamine does not alter opioid use after pediatric scoliosis surgery. *Paediatr Anaesth* 2014;24:582–590.

28. Engelhardt T, Zaarour C, Naser B, et al. Intraoperative low-dose ketamine does not prevent a remifentanil-induced increase in morphine requirement after pediatric scoliosis surgery. *Anesth Analg.* 2008;107(4):1170–1175. https://www.ncbi.nlm.nih.gov/pubmed/18806023

29. Ialenti MN, Lonner BS, Verma K, Dean L, Valdevit A, Errico T. Predicting operative blood loss during spinal fusion for adolescent idiopathic scoliosis. *J Pediatr Orthop.* 2013;33(4):372–376. https://www.ncbi.nlm.nih.gov/pubmed/23653024

30. Yoshihara H, Yoneoka D. Predictors of allogeneic blood transfusion in spinal fusion for pediatric patients with idiopathic scoliosis in the United States, 2004–2009. *Spine.* 2014;39(22):1860–1867. https://www.ncbi.nlm.nih.gov/pubmed/25077907

31. Murray DJ, Forbes RB, Titone MB, Weinstein SL. Transfusion management in pediatric and adolescent scoliosis surgery: efficacy of autologous blood. *Spine.* 1997;22(23):2735–2740. https://www.ncbi.nlm.nih.gov/pubmed/9431607

32. Oetgen ME, Litrenta J. Perioperative blood management in pediatric spine surgery. *J Am Acad Orthop Surg.* 2017;25(7):480–488. https://www.ncbi.nlm.nih.gov/pubmed/28644187

33. Bowen RE, Gardner S, Scaduto AA, Eagan M, Beckstead J. Efficacy of intraoperative cell salvage systems in pediatric idiopathic scoliosis patients undergoing posterior spinal fusion with segmental spinal instrumentation. *Spine.* 2010;35(2):246–251. https://www.ncbi.nlm.nih.gov/pubmed/20081521

34. Joseph SA Jr, Berekashvili K, Mariller MM, et al. Blood conservation techniques in spinal deformity surgery: a retrospective review of patients refusing blood transfusion. *Spine*. 2008;33(21): 2310–2315. https://www.ncbi.nlm.nih.gov/pubmed/18827697

35. Wang M, Zheng XF, Jiang LS. Efficacy and safety of antifibrinolytic agents in reducing perioperative blood loss and transfusion requirements in scoliosis surgery: a systematic review and meta-analysis. *PLoS One*. 2015;10(9):e0137886. https://www.ncbi.nlm.nih.gov/pubmed/26382761

36. Stricker PA, Gastonguay MR, Singh D, et al. Population pharmacokinetics of ε-aminocaproic acid in adolescents undergoing posterior spinal fusion surgery. *Br J Anaesth*. 2015;114(4):689–699. https://www.ncbi.nlm.nih.gov/pubmed/25586726

37. Sui WY, Ye F, Yang JL. Efficacy of tranexamic acid in reducing allogeneic blood products in adolescent idiopathic scoliosis surgery. *BMC Musculoskelet Disord*. 2016;17:187. https://www.ncbi.nlm.nih.gov/pubmed/27117696

38. American Society of Anesthesiologists Task Force on Perioperative Visual Loss. Practice advisory for perioperative visual loss associated with spine surgery: an updated report by the American Society of Anesthesiologists Task Force on Perioperative Visual Loss. *Anesthesiology*. 2012;116(2):274–285. http://www.ncbi.nlm.nih.gov/pubmed/22227790

39. Ho VT, Newman NJ, Song S, Ksiazek S, Roth S. Ischemic optic neuropathy following spine surgery. *J Neurosurg Anesthesiol*. 2005;17(1):38–44. http://www.ncbi.nlm.nih.gov/pubmed/15632541

40. Rubin DS, Parakati I, Lee LA, Moss HE, Joslin CE, Roth S. Perioperative visual loss in spine fusion surgery: ischemic optic neuropathy in the United States from 1998 to 2012 in the Nationwide Inpatient Sample. *Anesthesiology*. 2016;125(3):457–464. http://www.ncbi.nlm.nih.gov/pubmed/27362870

41. De la Garza-Ramos R, Samdani AF, Sponseller PD, et al. Visual loss after corrective surgery for pediatric scoliosis: incidence and risk factors from a nationwide database. *Spine J*. 2016;16(4):516–522. http://www.ncbi.nlm.nih.gov/pubmed/26769351

42. Vitale MG, Skaggs DL, Pace GI, et al. Best practices in intraoperative neuromonitoring in spine deformity surgery: development of an intraoperative checklist to optimize response. *Spine Deform*. 2014;2(5):333–339. https://www.ncbi.nlm.nih.gov/pubmed/27927330

43. Ryan SL, Sen A, Staggers K, et al. A standardized protocol to reduce pediatric spine surgery infection: a quality improvement initiative. *J Neurosurg Pediatr*. 2014;14(3):259–265. https://www.ncbi.nlm.nih.gov/pubmed/24971606

44. Lexi-Drugs. Aminocaproic acid. Lexicomp. http://online.lexi.com

45. Bettany-Saltikov J, Weiss H-R, Chockalingam N, Kandasamy G, Arnell T. A comparison of patient-reported outcome measures following different treatment approaches for adolescents with severe idiopathic scoliosis: a systematic review. *Asian Spine J*. 2016;10(6):1170–1194. https://www.ncbi.nlm.nih.gov/pubmed/27994796

46. Strike SA, Hassanzadeh H, Jain A, et al. Intraoperative neuromonitoring in pediatric and adult spine deformity surgery. *Clin Spine Surg*. 2017;30(9):E1174–E1181. https://www.ncbi.nlm.nih.gov/pubmed/27231831

47. Gehling M, Tryba M. Risks and side-effects of intrathecal morphine combined with spinal anaesthesia: a meta-analysis. *Anaesthesia*. 2009;64(6):643–651. https://www.ncbi.nlm.nih.gov/pubmed/19462494

30.

ACHONDROPLASIA

Andrew J. Costandi and Lydia Andras

STEM CASE AND KEY QUESTIONS

A 10-year-old girl diagnosed with achondroplasia presents to the anesthesia perioperative area in preparation for a right proximal tibia and fibular osteotomies.

> WHAT IS ACHONDROPLASIA? DISCUSS THE PATHOPHYSIOLOGY. WHAT ARE THE CLINICAL FEATURES ASSOCIATED WITH ACHONDROPLASIA? WHAT ARE THE COMPLICATIONS SEEN WITH ACHONDROPLASIA? FOR WHICH SURGERIES DO PATIENTS WITH ACHONDROPLASIA COMMONLY PRESENT?

Preoperative anesthetic evaluation revealed an obese 36 kg girl of short stature with a large head circumference, a large protruding forehead, and a large tongue. Patient was also noted to have leg bowing. Past surgical history was significant for adenotonsillectomy at the age of 5 years due to obstructive sleep apnea (OSA).

> WHAT ARE THE DIFFERENT TYPES OF SLEEP APNEA? WHAT PREDISPOSES THIS PATIENT TO SLEEP APNEA? IS ADENO-TONSILLECTOMY EFFECTIVE IN TREATING OSA IN CHILDREN? WHAT ABOUT CHILDREN WITH ACHONDROPLASIA? WHAT ARE THE PERIOPERATIVE ANESTHETIC CONSIDERATIONS OF ACHONDROPLASIA?

Vital signs during preoperative evaluation were heart rate 91 bpm, respiratory rate 20 breaths per minute, blood pressure 109/56 mmHg, and O_2 saturation on room air 98%. Airway evaluation revealed a short neck, adequate mouth opening, adequate neck mobility, and a Mallampati Class III. A recent chest X-ray showed a slightly enlarged cardiac silhouette with normal lung fields and mild kyphoscoliosis. Electrocardiogram (EKG) showed a normal sinus rhythm with a heart rate of 91 bpm. Intravenous (IV) access was difficult to obtain.

> IS AN ECHOCARDIOGRAM NEEDED PREOPERATIVELY? WHAT ABOUT PULMONARY FUNCTION TESTS? WOULD YOU REQUEST ANY OTHER TESTS? ARE YOU GOING TO PROCEED WITHOUT IV ACCESS? WHAT ARE YOUR GOALS FOR INDUCTION? HOW ARE YOU GOING TO INDUCE THIS PATIENT? ARE YOU EXPECTING DIFFICULT VENTILATION? WHAT ABOUT DIFFICULT INTUBATION? HOW ARE YOU GOING TO SECURE IV ACCESS?

The decision was made to undergo inhalational mask induction with 8% sevoflurane in a 50:50 admixture of N_2O and O_2 in an attempt to keep the patient spontaneously breathing. Upper airway obstruction was noted, and an 80 French oral airway was inserted resulting in improvement in ventilation with gentle assistance. A 22G IV was obtained using ultrasound after multiple failed attempts, but patient began to obstruct and ventilation became more difficult. Oxygen saturation dropped to 85%

> WHAT WOULD BE YOUR NEXT STEP? HOW ARE YOU GOING TO VENTILATE AND EVENTUALLY INTUBATE THE PATIENT? DOES THE SIZE SELECTION OF THE ENDOTRACHEAL TUBE MATTER IN CHILDREN WITH ACHONDROPLASIA? ARE YOU CONCERNED ABOUT POSITIONING DURING THE CASE? WHY?

Patient was eventually intubated with a 6 mm cuffed endotracheal tube using a fiberoptic bronchoscope (FOB) through an intubating laryngeal mask airway (LMA). Anesthesia was maintained with 2% sevoflurane and intermittent fentanyl doses of 0.5 mcg/kg. Single-shot sciatic nerve block was performed.

WOULD YOU CONSIDER NEURAXIAL
ANALGESIA TO DECREASE POSTOPERATIVE
OPIOID REQUIREMENT? WHY? WHY NOT?
WHAT ABOUT PERIPHERAL NERVE BLOCK?
WHAT IS YOUR VENTILATION STRATEGY?
JUSTIFY.

Surgery was completed uneventfully; the patient was extubated and then transferred to the postanesthesia care unit (PACU). Within a few minutes, the nurse called you for bedside assistance due to patient's desaturation to 85%.

IN CHILDREN, WHAT ARE THE COMMON
CAUSES OF UPPER AIRWAY
OBSTRUCTION IN PACU? IN CHILDREN
WITH ACHONDROPLASIA, WHAT IS THE MOST
COMMON PROBLEM ENCOUNTERED IN PACU?
WHY? HOW ARE YOU GOING TO MANAGE
THE UPPER AIRWAY OBSTRUCTION?

Patient was placed in left lateral position, oral airway inserted and 6 L of oxygen administered via face mask. Oxygen saturation improved with no desaturations and stable vital signs. Patient was then transferred to the floor.

DISCUSSION

Achondroplasia is a rare genetic skeletal dysplasia occurring in 0.5 to 1.5 of 10,000 live births and affecting over 250,000 individuals worldwide.[1,2] It is the most common cause of short stature or "dwarfism," with an average adulthood height of 4 feet. The earliest biological evidence of this type of skeletal dysplasia dates back to ancient Egypt around 2700 BC.[3] The word Achondroplasia is derived from the Greek word akhondrosplasisia, which means "no cartilage growth," but inaccurately describes the actual pathophysiology of the condition.

PATHOPHYSIOLOGY

Achondroplasia is inherited in an autosomal dominant fashion. However, most achondroplastic children will have parents of normal height because 80% to 90% of cases are a result of a new point mutation in the fibroblast growth factor receptor 3 (FGFR3) gene.[4] Glycine is substituted with arginine in the amino acid 380 position leading to overexpression of FGFR3 at the growth plate of long bones.[5] Physiologically, FGFR3 regulates bone growth by inhibiting endochondral ossification in the long bones. With the point mutation, overactivation of the FGFR3 receptor expressed in chondrocytes and mature osteoblasts occurs. As a result, growth plate size and cartilage proliferation are inhibited in association with premature ossification of epiphyseal cartilage, leading to impaired bone growth during childhood.[6] Homozygous achondroplasia is a lethal condition that leads to still birth or mortality in early infancy due to pulmonary hypoplasia and severe respiratory insufficiency resulting from deformed rib cage.[7]

CLINICAL PRESENTATION

The diagnosis of achondroplasia is usually made prenatally with an ultrasound or upon clinical and radiographic findings when the baby is born. If confirmation is required, molecular testing is completed to detect the mutant variant in FGFR3.[8]

Clinically, achondroplasia presents with unique craniofacial features including large head, frontal bossing, midface hypoplasia, and large tongue. Disproportionate short stature with shortening of the upper arms and thighs leads to an altered trunk to limb ratio. Other clinical features include narrow chest, brachydactyly, genu varum, thoracolumbar kyphoscoliosis, and worsening lumbar lordosis (see Figure 30.1). Affected children may show delay in motor developmental milestones like crawling and walking due to global hypotonia, but this improves as they grow and regain muscle tone.[9,10] Most individuals with achondroplasia have normal intelligence and life expectancy but may face many psychosocial problems. These features, while not life-threatening, make 5% to 10% of individuals with achondroplasia more prone to serious medical complications.[11]

COMPLICATIONS

Central nervous system

Abnormal bone growth at the level of the foramen magnum and premature fusion at the base of the skull result in progressive narrowing of the foramen and cervical canal, leading to

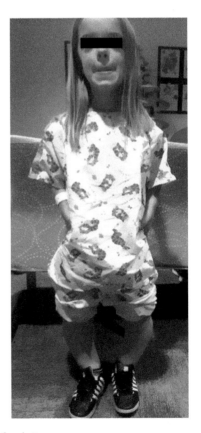

Fig. 30.1 Achondroplasia.

cervical medullary compression and cervical myelopathy.[12] Although rare, the coexistence of os odontoideum can lead to atlantoaxial instability and worsen the cervical medullary compression.[13] Ten percent of affected individuals suffer from true cervical medullary compression requiring surgical decompression, and 2% to 5% unfortunately experience sudden infant death in the absence of aggressive evaluation, most likely from central sleep apnea (CSA)[14]. Moreover, narrowing of the subarachnoid space leads to increased intracranial venous hypertension and may increase the risk of hydrocephalus during the first 2 years of life.[15] The American Academy of Pediatrics recommends careful neurologic history and examination, polysomnography, and surveillance neuroimaging of the head and neck in the form of computed tomography scan or magnetic resonance imaging for all infants with achondroplasia.[16]

Ear, nose, and throat

Short eustachian canals, midface hypoplasia, and adenoidal hypertrophy have been attributed to recurrent otitis media, increasing the risk of hearing loss, problems with language and speech, and learning disabilities.[10,11] Prevention and aggressive treatment, including ventilatory myringotomy tube placement during childhood, is essential to avert these problems.[17]

Respiratory

Sleep disordered breathing is very common among children with achondroplasia. Both CSA and OSA have been reported with incidences ranging between 30% and 75%, especially in early childhood. CSA is thought to be caused by compression of the medullary respiratory center at the level of the foramen magnum while OSA is due to compression of the lower motor neurons [18] Moreover, the altered craniofacial features such as a disproportionately large head with prominent forehead, flattened nasal bridge (saddle nose), midfacial hypoplasia, large tongue in addition to a small upper airway, physiologic adenoidal hypertrophy, and hypotonia of nasopharyngeal airway muscles may worsen OSA.[19] Polysomnography is helpful in predicting the presence of CSA and/or OSA in up to 60% of children with achondroplasia.[20] Though adenotonsillectomy has a high success rate in treating children with OSA, this rate is much less (60%) in children with achondroplasia.[21] These patients may require continuous positive airway pressure (CPAP) therapy following adenotonsillectomy due to persistent airway obstruction.

Restrictive pulmonary disease occurs in less than 5% of children with achondroplasia who are younger than 3 years of age.[22] Recurrent pneumonias from reduced chest circumference and rib hypoplasia, abnormal spine curvature, and obesity alter respiratory mechanics resulting in decreased functional residual capacity, increased closing volume, atelectasis and chronic respiratory insufficiency.[23]

While failure to gain weight during childhood can occur due to restrictive lung disease, obesity is also very common later in life and may worsen OSA as well as the genu vara, arthritis, and lumbar lordosis that often plague achondroplastic patients.[24]

Cardiovascular

Pulmonary hypertension and cor pulmonale may develop as a result of chronic respiratory insufficiency, sleep apnea, kyphoscoliosis, and the associated chronic hypoxemia and hypercarbia. A 42-year follow-up study looking at premature death rates in patients with achondroplasia showed a tenfold increase of heart disease related mortality between ages 25 and 35 years compared to general population.[25]

Gastrointestinal

A subcategory of patients present with severe gastroesophageal reflux with tendency for hyper salivation. This is usually more common in children with neurorespiratory complications and may lead to chronic aspirations and worsen their respiratory problems.[26]

Musculoskeletal

Spinal abnormalities include thoracolumbar kyphoscoliosis, which appears to be worst during infancy due to poor muscle tone and unsupported sitting. This should resolve with age as muscle tone improves and the child starts walking. On the other hand, lumbar lordosis becomes more pronounced as the child grows and commonly leads to lumbar spine stenosis in adulthood presenting as weakness and altered deep tendon reflexes in the lower extremities. Contracted hip joints along with hypermobile knee joints have been reported frequently and may exaggerate the lumbar lordosis and contribute to back pain. Disproportionate proximal shortening of both upper and lower extremities, also called rhizomelic shortening, results in limited elbow mobility and lower extremity axis deviation. Forty percent of affected individuals present with bowing of both lower legs (genu varum). This is usually a result of lax joints early in childhood and tibial bowing and fibular overgrowth later in life.[27]

PERIOPERATIVE ANESTHETIC EVALUATION

Children affected with achondroplasia usually present to the operating room for numerous procedures. This may include decompressive suboccipital craniectomy, cerebrospinal fluid shunting procedures, adenotonsillectomy, myringotomy tube placement, and various orthopedic procedures including limb lengthening, laminectomies, and scoliosis correction.[28]

Patients with achondroplasia should be thoroughly evaluated with an emphasis on the airway, as difficulties associated with airway management have been reported and should be anticipated. Clinical craniofacial features suggestive of potentially difficult mask ventilation and intubation include obesity, large head, maxillary hypoplasia, saddle nose, nasopharyngeal hypotonia, and odontoid hypoplasia with atlantoaxial instability.[28]

Thorough preoperative evaluation and complete assessment of cardiopulmonary status should include detailed history, physical exam, routine chest X-ray, and EKG in all patients. Preoperative pulmonary function tests, blood gas analysis, and echocardiogram are reserved for those with chronic restrictive lung disease and OSA to assess the degree of pulmonary hypertension and right heart function.[29]

History of loud snoring, glottal stops, observed episodes of obstructive apnea, neck hyperextension in sleep, and self-awakenings with daytime irritability are clinically predictive of OSA. These symptoms necessitate polysomnography to assess the degree and type of sleep apnea for possible corrective measures preoperatively.[29,30]

The increased prevalence of foramen magnum stenosis and atlantoaxial instability, especially in children less than 1 year of age, mandates neuroimaging of the head and neck as well as neurosurgical clearance.

Extended PACU stay, postoperative overnight hospital admission, and intensive care unit stay should be scheduled appropriately depending on patient's existing medical condition and surgical intervention.

INTRAOPERATIVE ANESTHETIC MANAGEMENT

Premedication

Emotional and physical stress, due to multiple surgical procedures, contribute to heightened anxiety.[31] Proper counseling and the involvement of distraction techniques, such as the use of an iPad, and child life services is encouraged. Anxiolysis may be beneficial but should be used judiciously, especially with those at risk of difficult airway management and sleep apnea. Antisialagogues may be considered in patients with excessive salivation to minimize aspiration and help with fiberoptic visualization during intubation. Histamine H_2 antagonists should also be considered in the subcategory of patients experiencing severe gastroesophageal reflux.

Monitoring

American Society of Anesthesiologists (ASA) standard monitoring should be utilized in all patients. The choice of the right size blood pressure cuff could be challenging. Additional invasive monitoring such as arterial cannulation, central venous pressure, or transesophageal echocardiogram is determined on a case-by-case basis depending on surgical procedure and patient's baseline cardiopulmonary function.

Vascular access

Short proximal extremities associated with redundant soft tissue, increased subcutaneous fat, and contracted joints make venous access and arterial cannulation difficult.[29,33] The use of vessel visualization equipment (like vein viewer) and ultrasound have been reported and should be utilized to minimize the number of sticks and increase the likelihood of success. The need for a central venous line should be anticipated in major surgeries. Ultrasound guidance is encouraged as the short neck, narrow deformed chest, and contracted hips may

complicate accessing the internal jugular vein, subclavian vein, and femoral vein, respectively.[28] The use of intraosseous route in achondroplasia is not reported in literature. However, it is a fast, reliable, and safe approach to obtain vascular access via the bone marrow and should be used in emergency cases if all else fails.

Positioning

Care and proper positioning should be exercised while positioning patients on operating tables as joints present with a mixed pattern. Exaggerated lax knee joints are prone to accidental injuries under anesthesia, while the limited mobility and contractures in the hip and elbow joints will necessitate adequate padding. The head is relatively big compared to the body so there is a good chance of a significant drop in body temperature especially in children. Adjusting the ambient room temperature and covering the head is recommended.

Induction and airway management

Previous records of anesthetics and airway management should be obtained when possible. A difficult airway cart with appropriate sized facemasks, oral airways, nasal trumpets, endotracheal tubes, LMAs, intubating LMAs, and an FOB should be prepared for possible difficult airway management. Preoxygenation is beneficial as vital capacity and functional residual capacity are often reduced.

In children, it is preferable to establish preoperative IV access prior to anesthesia induction when feasible. If not, inhalational induction is acceptable. In both cases, maintaining spontaneous ventilation with titrated doses of ketamine, dexmedetomidine, and sevoflurane is encouraged. Establishing mask ventilation is imperative before administering neuromuscular blockade. Endotracheal intubation with in line stabilization using FOB or video laryngoscope (i.e., GlideScope) is recommended. Conventional direct laryngoscopy for tracheal intubation may be difficult, especially in the presence of cervical kyphosis or prior cervical neck fusion. Endotracheal tube size in children should be based on weight rather than age, as a smaller endotracheal tube is often required due to laryngeal hypoplasia and arytenoid hypertrophy.[19,28,32] At all times, caution should be exercised while manipulating the neck during intubation, as unintentional spinal cord compression at the level of the foramen magnum can occur with neck hyperextension.

In adults with preoperative suspected difficult airway, an "awake" FOB is the safest way to secure the airway.

In cases of unanticipated difficult airway, the ASA difficult airway algorithm should be followed. Utilization of an LMA, in rescue situations, can be effective in reestablishing ventilation and serving as a conduit for endotracheal intubation. However, restrictive lung disease may cause increased ventilatory difficulty, and the distorted craniofacial anatomy may complicate an optimal fit for LMA. While not Food and Drug Administration–approved for use in children, sugammadex has been reported in the literature as a successful agent in immediate reversal of the effects of rocuronium and vecuronium in children and should be used if difficulty with intubation is encountered after muscle relaxant administration.

Multiple studies in the literature reported difficult mask ventilation and intubation in only 5%–10% of achondroplastic children.[32] Regardless, the possibility of difficult airway management should always be kept in mind. Care and caution should always be exercised when intubating these patients to avoid unnecessary airway complications.

Maintenance of anesthesia

Intravenous anesthetics and inhalational agents have both been used without issues. Medication dosages should be based according to weight. A multimodal analgesic approach is preferred especially in the presence of sleep apnea. For patients with cardiopulmonary compromise, all efforts should be taken to maintain adequate tidal volume, avoid hypoxia and hypercarbia, both of which worsen pulmonary hypertension.

Regional anesthesia

The use of regional anesthesia is controversial, though it has been reported multiple times in the literature. While the use of neuraxial analgesia is associated with overall less opioid requirement, the deformed spine anatomy and hip contractures could make spinal and epidural techniques more challenging. Conducting a full neurological exam to establish baseline neurological function and reviewing spine imaging is of extreme importance before proceeding with any neuraxial blocks. Their narrow epidural space with engorged veins increase the incidence of inadvertent dural or venous puncture, as well as difficulty in placing epidural catheters and reliability of local anesthetic spread. However, in children, injection of local anesthetic into the caudal canal is easier and more predictable.[28,33] Needle placement and catheter insertion for peripheral nerve blocks could sometimes prove challenging especially in the presence of joint contracture.

POSTOPERATIVE CARE

Assuming the patient is maintaining oxygenation, adequate ventilation hemodynamically stable, and not requiring respiratory support, extubation awake in the operating room is feasible. Patients with OSA managed by CPAP therapy should be initiated on CPAP immediately postoperatively. Postoperative mechanical ventilation in intensive care is not mandatory but may be necessary in certain cases depending on patient's age, the severity of sleep apnea, and nature of the surgical procedure. Extended stay in PACU or overnight hospital stay is reasonable for those with sleep apnea especially the ones requiring CPAP or oxygen supplementation.

Achondroplasia has a higher than usual rate of postoperative upper airway obstruction and respiratory complications, thus vigilant monitoring of ventilation and oxygenation in PACU, bronchopulmonary toilet, incentive spirometry, and early ambulation are important to prevent atelectasis. This is mainly due to reduction of airway tone from general anesthesia in already narrowed nasopharyngeal passages and

flexion of disproportionate large head. Auscultating for bilateral breath sounds and administering supplemental oxygen are recommended, as are placing the patient in lateral position, while avoiding head flexion, applying jaw thrust, and inserting oral or nasal airway to help alleviate this problem. If obstruction persists, consider CPAP and possible endotracheal intubation with mechanical ventilation in refractory cases. Differential diagnosis of upper airway obstruction in children should include OSA, laryngospasm, inflammatory etiology (croup), airway lesions, and foreign body.

CONCLUSION

- Achondroplasia is an autosomal dominant disorder caused by mutations in the FGFR3 gene.

- Achondroplasia presents with unique craniofacial features including macrocephaly with frontal bossing, saddle nose, short stature with disproportionate trunk to limb ratio, and rhizomelic shortening of the upper and lower extremities.

- Life-threatening complications like cervical medullary compression, sudden infant death syndrome, and restrictive lung disease occur in 5%–10% of individuals affected with achondroplasia and not aggressively evaluated.

- Children affected with achondroplasia usually present to the operating room for numerous procedures including suboccipital craniectomy, adeno-tonsillectomy, myringotomy tube placement, and limb-lengthening orthopedic procedures.

- Preoperative anesthetic evaluation should focus on assessment of airway and cardiopulmonary function.

- The pathophysiology of achondroplasia presents several challenges to anesthesiologists; however, with appropriate care and knowledge, care can be delivered safely.

REVIEW QUESTIONS

1. When electing preparing to intubate achondroplastic patient, which of the following methods is the **MOST** reliable way to determine endotracheal tube size?

    A. body surface area
    B. chronological age
    C. measured weight
    D. neck circumference

Answer: C

Choosing an endotracheal tube size for a child with achondroplasia, based on age, will likely lead to overestimation of appropriate size. Due to the smaller size of facial structures and potential laryngeal hypoplasia and arytenoid hypertrophy, choosing a size based on weight is a more appropriate technique.

2. A 15-year-old achondroplastic patient is coming to your operating room for bilateral femoral osteotomies and limb lengthening. The patient and his family are concerned about postoperative pain. They ask about regional for postoperative pain control. What is the **MOST** accurate statement to give the patient and his family regarding regional anesthesia for postoperative pain control in achondroplastic patients?

  A. Caudal blocks are avoided to prevent injury to the low lying conus medullaris.
  B. Epidural catheter insertion is made challenging by skeletal abnormalities.
  C. Neuraxial dosing of opioids is similar to that in the general population.
  D. Peripheral nerve blocks are straightforward to obtain with ultrasound guidance.

Answer: B
Neuraxial analgesia is often technically challenging due to abnormal spinal anatomy. Additionally, positioning can be complicated by hip contractures. A narrow epidural space with engorged veins can also increase chance of dural or venous puncture. If the opioid-sparing and pain-control benefits warrant attempting neuraxial technique, a thorough baseline neurological exam should be documented.

3. Of the following, which is the **MOST** common spinal abnormality found achondroplastic pediatric patients?

  A. lumber hypolordosis
  B. os odontoideum
  C. spondylolisthesis
  D. thoracolumbar kyphosis

Answer: D
Thoracolumbar kyphosis and lumbar hyperlordosis are both extremely common in achondroplastic patients. Lumbar lordosis worsens later in life and can lead to spinal stenosis.

4. Temperature regulation is important in all patients while under anesthesia. In addition to the normal factors that affect all patients, which of the following causes is the **MOST** significant contributing factor in achondroplastic patients developing hypothermia?

  A. head proportional size
  B. circulatory abnormalities
  C. hypothalamus dysfunction
  D. subcutaneous fat paucity

Answer: A
While other types of skeletal dysplasia have been associated with temperature regulation challenges, the most likely challenge faced by the anesthesiologist in an achondroplastic patient is hypothermia due to disproportionate head size.

5. An 8-year-old achondroplastic patient is involved in a car accident and must be taken to the operating room emergently to gain control of internal bleeding. The emergency room was only able to obtain a positional 24 gauge IV in the wrist. Of the following explanation, which is the **MOST** accurate reason that achondroplastic patients often pose a challenge for vascular access?

  A. chronic state of low hydration
  B. short proximal extremities with contractures
  C. thick skin with decreased subcutaneous visibility
  D. vessels of smaller caliber with thin walls

Answer: B
Limb contractures, along with fat pads and redundant soft tissue, can make venous access difficult. Adjuvant technologies such as vein viewers and ultrasound machines can be helpful.

6. A 7-month-old achondroplastic male presents to the pre-operative clinic prior to an inguinal hernia repair for a reducible left inguinal hernia. While they may all be reasonable, which of the following is **MOST** essential to complete prior to undergoing anesthesia for a nonemergent case?

  A. cardiac evaluation of EKG and echocardiogram
  B. neurosurgical evaluation of cervical and foraminal anatomy
  C. pulmonary evaluation for chronic obstructive pulmonary disease
  D. orthopedic evaluation for scoliosis and kyphoscoliosis

Answer: B
The potential for central apnea is high in these infants, and, as such, all patients under 1 year of age should be evaluated thoroughly with physical exam and history, polysomnography, and neuroimaging.

7. A 5-year-old achondroplastic patient presents to your operating room for adenotonsillectomy due to OSA symptoms. The child is extremely anxious, and the decision to proceed with mask induction is made. Shortly after induction, you are unable to ventilate the patient despite oral airway and 2-hand mask attempts; additionally, you can't obtain a view with direct laryngoscopy. The **BEST** next step is:

  A. FOB with intermittent masking
  B. LMA that is appropriately sized
  C. standard laryngoscopy with reattempt by senior staff
  D. nasal airway with reattempts at masking

Answer: B
Placing an LMA can be challenging and may not provide the best fit to provide adequate pressures to ventilate these patients especially in patients with severe restrictive lung disease. However, in can't intubate/can't ventilate situations, the ASA difficult airway algorithm should always be followed.

8. What is the **MOST** common cause of achondroplasia?

  A. autosomal dominant inheritance
  B. autosomal recessive inheritance
  C. sporadic genetic mutation
  D. teratogen gestation exposure

Answer: C
Despite being inherited in an autosomal dominant fashion, approximately 80% of achondroplasia cases are the result of a sporadic mutation in children of parents who are normal height.

9. CSA and OSA are very common in patients with achondroplasia. Which statement is **MOST** accurate about sleep apnea in these patients?

    A. Adenotonsillectomy OSA cure rate is similar to that in the general population.

    B. CSA is common later in life but not in infancy.

    C. Medulla compression causes central and OSA.

    D. Polysomnography can detect OSA and CSA.

Answer: D

Foramen magnum stenosis and resultant cervicomedullary compression can lead to central apnea, and OSA is common due to compression of lower motor neurons and altered craniofacial anatomy.

10. Which of the following is **LEAST** common reason for children with achondroplasia to undergoing surgery?

    A. adenoidectomy

    B. spinal stenosis

    C. suboccipital craniectomy

    D. ventricular peritoneal shunt

Answer: B

The most common procedures that achondroplastic patients undergo include otolaryngologic, neurosurgical, and orthopedic, in addition to neuroimaging. Spinal stenosis typically develops when these patients are adults.

QUESTIONS AND ANSWERS

This chapter has accompanying questions and answers which are available to subscribers as part of the Oxford eLearning platform. To access the questions, go to ✓ http:// oxfordmedicine. com/pediatricanesthesiaPBL

REFERENCES

1. Horton WA, Hall JG, Hecht JT. Achondroplasia. *Lancet.* 2007;370(9582):162–172.
2. Waller DK, Correa A, Vo TM, et al. The population-based prevalence of achondroplasia and thanatophoric dysplasia in selected regions of the US. *Am J Med Genet A.* 2008;146A(18):2385–2389.
3. Kozma C. Skeletal dysplasia in ancient Egypt. *Am J Med Genet A.* Dec 1 2008;146A(23):3104–3112.
4. Shiang R, Thompson LM, Zhu YZ, et al. Mutations in the transmembrane domain of FGFR3 cause the most common genetic form of dwarfism, achondroplasia. *Cell.* 1994;78:335–342.
5. Francomano CA. The genetic basis of dwarfism. *N Engl J Med.* 1995;332:58–59.
6. Sahni M, Ambrosetti DC, Mansukhani A, Gertner R, Levy D, Basilico C. FGF signaling inhibits chondrocyte proliferation and regulates bone development through the STAT-1 pathway. *Genes Dev.* Jun 1 1999;13(11):1361–1366.
7. Pauli RM, Conroy MM, Langer LO Jr, et al. Homozygous achondroplasia with survival beyond infancy. *Am J Med Genet.* Dec 1983;16(4):459–473.
8. Boulet S, Althuser M, Nugues F, Schaal JP, Jouk PS. Prenatal diagnosis of achondroplasia: new specific signs. *Prenat Diagn.* 2009;29:697–702.
9. Shirley ED, Ain MC. Achondroplasia: manifestations and treatment. *J Am Acad Orthop Surg.* 2009;17:231–241.
10. Hunter AG, Bankier A, Rogers JG, Sillence D, Scott CI Jr. Medical complications of achondroplasia: a multicentre patient review. *J Med Genet.* Sep 1998;35(9):705–712.
11. Trotter TL, Hall JG. Health supervision for children with achondroplasia. *Pediatrics* 2005;116(3):771–783.
12. Rimoin DL. Cervicomedullary junction compression in infants with achondroplasia: when to perform neurosurgical decompression. *Am J Hum Genet.* 1995;56(4):824–827.
13. Rahimizadeh A, Soufiani HF, Hassani V, Rahimizadeh A. Atlantoaxial subluxation due to an Os odontoideum in an achondroplastic adult: report of a case and review of the literature. *Case Rep Orthop.* 2015:142586.
14. Pauli RM, Scott CI, Wassman ER Jr, et al. Apnea and sudden unexpected death in infants with achondroplasia. *J Pediatr.* 1984;104(3):342–348.
15. Steinbok P, Hall J, Flodmark O. Hydrocephalus in achondroplasia: the possible role of intracranial venous hypertension. *J Neurosurg.* 1989;71(1):42–48.
16. American Academy of Pediatrics Committee on Genetics. Health supervision for children with achondroplasia. *Pediatrics.* 1995;95(3):443–451.
17. Collins WO, Choi SS. Otolaryngologic manifestations of achondroplasia. *Arch Otolaryngol Head Neck Surg.* 2007;133(3):237–244.
18. White KK, Parnell SE, Kifle Y, Blackledge M, Bompadre V. Is there a correlation between sleep disordered breathing and foramen magnum stenosis in children with achondroplasia? *Am J Med Genet A.* Jan 2016;170A(1):32–41.
19. Sisk EA, Heatley DG, Borowski BJ, Leverson GE, Pauli RM. Obstructive sleep apnea in children with achondroplasia: surgical and anesthetic considerations. *Otolaryngol Head Neck Surg.* 1999;120:248–254.
20. Waters KA, Everett F, Sillence D, Fagan E, Sullivan CE. Breathing abnormalities in sleep in achondroplasia. *Arch Dis Child.* 1993;69:191–196.
21. Waters KA, Everett F, Sillence DO, et al. Treatment of obstructive sleep apnea in achondroplasia. *Am J Med Genet.* 1995;59:460–466.
22. Stokes DC, Phillips JA, Leonard CO, et al. Respiratory complications of achondroplasia. *J Pediatr.* Apr 1983;102(4):534–541.
23. Stokes DC, Pyeritz, RE, Wise, RA, Fairclough, D, Murphy EA. Spirometry and chest wall dimensions in achondroplasia. *Chest.* 1988;93:364–369.
24. Hoover-Fong JE, McGready J, Schulze KJ, Barnes H, Scott CI. Weight for age charts for children with achondroplasia. *Am J Med Genet A.* Oct 1 2007;143A(19):2227–2235.
25. Wynn J, King TM, Gambello MJ;, Waller DK, Hecht JT. Mortality in achondroplasia study: a 42-year follow-up. *Am J Med Genet A.* 2007;143A(21):2502–2511.
26. Tasker RC, Dundas I, Laverty A, Fletcher M, Lane R, Stocks J. Distinct patterns of respiratory difficulty in young children with achondroplasia: a clinical, sleep, and lung function study. *Arch Dis Child.* Aug 1998;79(2):99–108.
27. Lee ST, Song HR, Mahajan R, Makwana V, Suh SW, Lee SH. Development of genu varum in achondroplasia: relation to fibular overgrowth. *J Bone Joint Surg Br.* Jan 2007;89(1):57–61.
28. Jain A, Jain K, Makkar JK, Mangal K. Anaesthetic management of an achondroplastic dwarf undergoing radical nephrectomy. *S Afr J Anaesthesiol Analg.* 2010;16:77–79.
29. Krishnan BS, Eipe N, Korula G. Anaesthetic management of a patient with achondroplasia. *Paediatr Anaesth.* Jul 2003;13(6):547–549.
30. Tenconi R, Khirani S, Amaddeo A, et al. Sleep-disordered breathing and its management in children with achondroplasia. *Am J Med Genet A.* Apr 2017;173(4):868–878.
31. Kalla GN, Fening E, Obiaya MO. Anaesthetic management of achondroplasia. *Br J Anaesth.* Jan 1986;58(1):117–119.
32. Mayhew JF, Katz J, Miner M, Leiman BC, Hall ID. Anaesthesia for the achondroplastic dwarf. *Can Anaesth Soc J.* Mar 1986;33(2):216–221.
33. Di Nardo SK. Anesthetic consideration for the achondroplastic dwarf. *AANA J.* Feb 1988;56(1):42–48.

31.

VEIN OF GALEN MALFORMATION

Elizabeth C. Eastburn and Mary Landrigan-Ossar

STEM CASE AND KEY QUESTIONS

Patient was prenatally diagnosed at 33 weeks' gestation with a vein of Galen intracranial arteriovenous malformation (VGM) measuring 3 × 2 × 2.5 cm. Fetal echocardiography demonstrated cardiomegaly with dilation of the right atrium, right ventricle, and the main pulmonary artery. As a result of the diagnosis, her parents elected to transfer prenatal care and plan for delivery at a tertiary care center with expertise in this disease process.

WHAT IS VGM? HOW IS IT DIAGNOSED? ARE THERE ANY DIFFERENTIAL DIAGNOSES?

The patient was born at 38 weeks gestation by normal spontaneous vaginal delivery. The infant's initial appearance at delivery was reassuring with 1- and 5-minute APGAR (appearance, pulse, grimace, activity, and respiration) scores of 7 and 8, but on arrival in the neonatal intensive care unit (NICU), she required intubation for a pronounced respiratory acidosis; preintubation arterial pH was 7.1 with a partial pressure of carbon dioxide in arterial blood ($PaCO_2$) of 81. Initial echocardiography showed right ventricular (RV) pressures likely equal to systemic pressure. Initial management goals were to treat the pulmonary hypertension with O_2, sedation and inhaled nitric oxide (iNO) in the hope that as pulmonary vascular resistance fell in the postdelivery period, her condition would stabilize. She continued over the next 24 hours to have difficulty oxygenating, and the decision was made to attempt urgent endovascular embolization of the VGM in interventional neuroradiology (INR) on day of life 3.

IS PRIMARY TREATMENT OF THIS CONDITION MEDICAL OR INTERVENTIONAL? WHEN IS THE IDEAL TIME TO BEGIN ENDOVASCULAR TREATMENT OF A VGM? ARE THERE CRITERIA THAT HELP DETERMINE TREATMENT? WHAT ARE THE POSSIBLE COMPLICATIONS OF ENDOVASCULAR TREATMENT OF VGM? WHAT ARE THE ANESTHETIC GOALS FOR THIS CASE?

The patient tolerated the first embolization, which lasted 8 hours. After the INR physician embolized some of the feeding arteries to reduce flow through the malformation,

the anesthesia team was able to wean off her dopamine infusion. However, significant flow through the malformation remained at the end of the procedure, and this hemodynamic improvement proved to be temporary. Four days later a second embolization was performed over 6.5 hours, again with temporary resolution of the need for pressors.

The patient's NICU course was notable for persistent pulmonary hypertension treated with iNO that could not be weaned off and ongoing difficulty with oxygenation. Pressor requirements waxed and waned over the course of her stay, with nonsustained improvements following further rounds of neuroembolization. Serial echocardiograms showed persistent RV dysfunction, persistent suprasystemic RV pressures, and worsening left ventricular dysfunction over time. Serial magnetic resonance imaging (MRI) demonstrated continued accumulation of parenchymal injury to the brain, and the patient developed seizures. Over 3 months, a total of 5 attempts each lasting 6 to 9 hours were made in INR to embolize the VGM via a transarterial approach, with no success in maintaining decreased flow through the malformation and its network of feeding vessels and no sustainable improvement in the patient's condition.

ARE THERE TREATMENT OPTIONS OTHER THAN ENDOVASCULAR EMBOLIZATION? IS SURGICAL EXCISION A POSSIBILITY?

A final attempt at embolization via the transvenous approach was made despite the known higher procedural risk with this method. This attempt was preceded by a long discussion involving the attending anesthesiologist, the NICU attending, the INR attending, and the parents about the risks of intracranial hemorrhage and the parent's goals for resuscitation in that scenario. While the procedure was a success in terms of safely placing coils into the venous portion of the malformation, flow was not reduced, and the patient's clinical situation continued to deteriorate.

A family meeting was held with the parents, the NICU team, cardiology, and the INR physician. The INR physician explained that there were no further neurointerventional options for treatment of the malformation and that surgical treatment had been considered but was not an option. In light of the patient's poor clinical status with no options for improvement, the family elected to withdraw care, and the patient died peacefully in her parent's arms.

DISCUSSION

EPIDEMIOLOGY

VGM is the most common intracranial arteriovenous malformation that is detected on prenatal imaging.[1] Nevertheless, it is a very rare condition, estimated to occur in 1:25,000 births. It develops in the 6th to 11th weeks of embryonic life as an abnormal connection between the primitive arteries of the choroid plexus and the median prosencephalic vein of Markowski. The formation of this abnormal shunt prevents the process of invagination of this embryonic vein and its replacement by the normal vein of Galen. Blood flow through the abnormal connections results in significant ectasia of the vessels involved, particularly on the venous side, resulting in a characteristic angiographic appearance (Figures 31.1 and 31.2).Various schemes for classification of this malformation have been proposed, one of the most commonly referenced is that of Lasjaunias et al.[2] This classification depends on the angioarchitecture of the malformations, dividing them into mural or choroidal types.[2] Mural-type malformations have direct arteriovenous fistulas within the wall of the venous pouch and tend to result in a less severe presentation. Choroidal-type malformations are characterized by a network of feeding arteries that originate from the choroidal arteries; this network of feeders empties directly into the dilated venous pouch. These patients have an earlier presentation and a more severe phenotype.

No single causative gene has been identified for this malformation. There are case reports of VGM patients with defects in a variety of genes that have been associated with other vascular malformations. These genes include RASA1, mutations in which have been found in various arteriovenous malformation syndromes,[3] and endoglin, which has been implicated in hereditary hemorrhagic telangiectasia.[4] Based on these limited data, it is likely that defects in several points in the early control of angiogenesis will result in a common final pathway of a VGM, and it is conceivable that the different phenotypes of malformation result from disruption of different genes or steps in the pathway.

DIAGNOSIS AND PRESENTATION

In the developed world, diagnosis of VGM is often accomplished *in utero*. It is readily identified in the third trimester of pregnancy, although there are isolated reports of diagnosis in the late second trimester.[5] On ultrasound, it is apparent as a hypoechoic structure midline in the posterior third ventricle, which can be proven on Doppler ultrasonography to have intraluminal arterial-type flow consistent with a vascular structure. Fetal MRI and fetal echocardiography are increasingly being utilized to further characterize the lesion, as well as to evaluate for any associated abnormalities.

If a patient's lesion is not identified before birth, clinical presentation varies markedly depending on the age at which symptoms manifest. Those patients with choroidal-type malformations most often present in the neonatal period in high output cardiac failure and potentially with multiorgan dysfunction. The malformation acts as a low-resistance, high-volume shunt that increases work for the left heart ventricle. The high volume of blood returning to the right side of the heart then causes pulmonary edema; increased work on the right ventricle can then lead to RV dysfunction, pulmonary hypertension, and eventually failure. Increased intracardiac pressure can impair coronary artery perfusion and can lead to myocardial ischemia. It is estimated that 80% of a patient's cardiac output may be directed to the VGM. This results in decreased blood flow to the remaining brain and to the rest of the body, putting patients at risk for hypoperfusion and

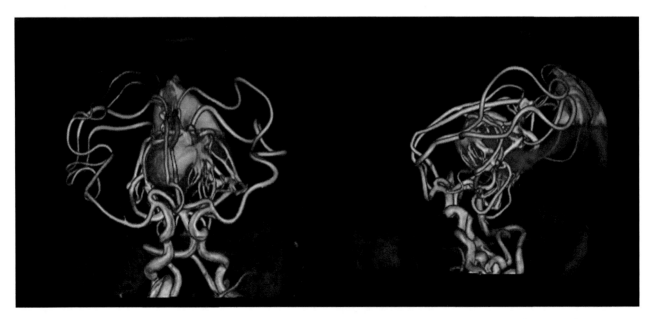

Fig. 31.1 Three dimensional reconstruction of MRI angiography; coronal (left) and sagittal (right) views of patient's vein of Galen malformation prior to any treatment.

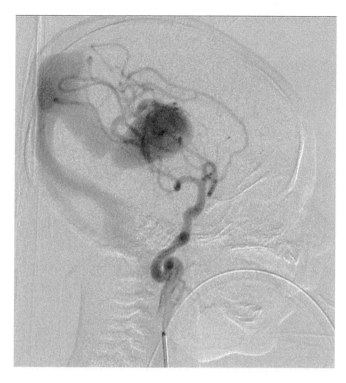

Fig. 31.2 Catheter angiography of vein of Galen malformation; sagittal view of injection into the carotid artery.

organ failure. Hydrocephalus occurs most likely secondary to intracranial venous hypertension. Myocardial and cerebral ischemia cause the significant morbidity and mortality that is associated with significant choroidal-type malformations. Mortality for this severe presentation, if untreated, has been reported to approach 100%.[6,7]

Older infants and children have a less severe presentation, which tends to be more closely associated with a mural-type malformation. These patients present in infancy with macrocephaly, asymptomatic cardiomegaly, or neurologic symptoms such as developmental delay. Older children and occasionally adults present with developmental delay, seizures, cerebrovascular hemorrhage, or nonspecific symptoms such as headache. Despite an initially more benign presentation in older children, mortality in untreated patients is estimated to be 68% for infants and 45% for older children and adults.

WORKUP AND DECISION TO TREAT

Fetal MRI is increasingly being performed for confirmation of the initial ultrasound diagnosis and to allow identification of associated brain damage, which is important for determining degree of disease severity.[1] Workup for a child not diagnosed until after birth is similar, with MRI and echocardiography being standard. Diagnostic catheter angiography has been considered the gold standard to characterize intracranial arteriovenous lesions,[8] but as MRI angiography becomes increasingly high resolution, a separate catheter angiogram may not always be indicated prior to treatment.

In addition to characterizing the arteriovenous malformation itself, preprocedure workup and risk stratification

requires consideration of the patient and their overall clinical situation. Lasjaunias et al.[2] developed the now widely accepted Bicetre neonatal evaluation score to stratify patient prognosis and medical decision-making. This scoring system requires evaluation of the neurologic, cardiac, and respiratory systems and also evaluates end-organ performance by determining hepatic and renal function, assigning points based on their function (Table 31.1). A combined score of less than 8 is associated with a very poor prognosis, and intervention may not be offered due to futility. With a score of 8 to 12, the patient is considered to be demonstrating significant systemic effects of the fistula, and emergent endovascular intervention should be considered. With a score greater than 12, the neonatal patient can be managed medically until they are at least 5 months of age, unless their clinical condition deteriorates and requires earlier treatment. Five months was determined by this group to represent the ideal window for beginning treatment in stable babies before more deterioration began to develop.[2]

TREATMENT

With severe presentation of VGMs, the immediate goal of initial medical management in the NICU is support of cardiac function to maximize brain and end-organ perfusion. Some centers have reported successful treatment of patients with a Bicetre score of less than 8, stating that a key component of their success is aggressive and carefully calibrated perioperative treatment of heart failure.[9]

In addition to ongoing NICU management, consultation with cardiology and neurology helps to guide initial stabilization. Inhaled nitric oxide can be a helpful in reducing RV afterload. Infusions of vasoactive medications such as dopamine or dobutamine may be needed for hemodynamic support and to maintain end organ perfusion. An echocardiogram and lab tests are necessary prior to intervention to assist with prognostication and to guide immediate management. In severe disease states, echocardiography may show that both ventricles are dysfunctional, and the patient may have significant pulmonary hypertension. Echocardiogram findings may include right to left shunting at the foramen ovale or through an atrial septal defect. Echocardiography may show reversal of flow in the aorta during diastole indicating a steal phenomenon as most of the cardiac output is directed toward the head. Lab tests should also be done specifically to evaluate kidney (blood urea nitrogen/creatinine) and liver function (liver function tests, prothrombin time/partial thromboplastin time/international normalized ratio).[10] Neurologic workup including MRI may reveal encephalomalacia and seizures.[7]

As much as possible, the patient should be medically optimized by the NICU before coming for neuroembolization. On occasion, the need for intervention will be deemed emergent, and the desire for medical optimization must be weighed against the potential improvement in hemodynamics if flow through the malformation can be slowed.[11,12] When the decision is made that the patient requires neuroembolization, the anesthetic management of these interventions should in large part be a continuation of the ongoing medical management in the NICU. Prior to starting anesthetic care, the patient's

Table 31.1 BICETRE NEONATAL EVALUATION SCALE

BICÊTRE NEONATAL EVALUATION SCORE

POINTS	CARDIAC FUNCTION	CEREBRAL FUNCTION	RESPIRATORY FUNCTION	HEPATIC FUNCTION	RENAL FUNCTION
5	Normal	Normal	Normal		
4	Overload, no medical treatment	Subclinical, isolated EEG abnormalities	Tachypnea, finishes bottle		
3	Failure, stable with medical treatment	Nonconvulsive intermittent neurologic signs	Tachypnea, doesn't finish bottle	No hepatomegaly, normal hepatic function	Normal
2	Failure, not stable with medical treatment	Isolated convulsion	Assisted ventilation, normal saturation FiO_2 <25%	Hepatomegaly, normal hepatic function	Transient anuria
1	Ventilation necessary	Seizure	Assisted ventilation, normal saturation FiO_2 >25%	Moderate or transient hepatic insufficiency	Unstable diuresis with treatment
0	Resistant to medical therapy	Permanent neurological signs	Assisted ventilation, desaturation	Abnormal coagulation, elevated enzymes	Anuria

Note. EEG = electroencephalogram, FiO_2 = fraction inspired oxygen, Maximal score = 5 (cardiac) + 5 (cerebral) + 5 (respiratory) + 3 (hepatic) + 3 (renal) = 21

Source. Adapted from Lasjaunias PL, Chng SM, Sachet M, Alvarez H, Rodesch G, Garcia-Monaco R. The management of vein of Galen aneurysmal malformations. Neurosurgery. 2006;59(5 Suppl 3):S184–S194. Used with permission.

current clinical status should be carefully reviewed and a sign-out of recent significant clinical events should be given to the anesthesia team by the NICU team. Supportive measures and medications such as iNO and vasopressors should be continued during the perioperative period and titrated as clinically indicated. Usually the patient is intubated and sedated in the NICU so sedating infusions can be continued. Patients may require the addition of muscle relaxants and intermittent boluses of narcotics, although once arterial access is obtained the procedure is not painful. Muscle relaxation is recommended to remove the chance of patient movement while catheters are deployed in the cerebral vasculature. Due to their labile cardiovascular status, inhaled anesthetics may be poorly tolerated. An arterial line greatly improves beat-to-beat management of blood pressure; this should be separate from the arterial access used for the procedure as that will be largely unavailable for transducing pressures. In the hands of an experienced pediatric neurointerventionalist, the risk of blood loss is very low. It is important to bear in mind that an ongoing fluid burden of heparinized saline will, by necessity, be delivered through the intracranial catheter to reduce the chance of clot on the catheter tip; this should be factored into fluid management for the case and may be significant for small infants.[13]

Transcatheter neuroembolization is the current standard treatment for VGM. The goal of the initial embolization is to partially embolize the malformation to reduce flow through the arteriovenous shunt by one third to one half. The goal of this partial embolization is to reduce the stress on the right side of the heart while allowing for its gradual exposure to the increases in systemic vascular resistance that results as the channels are coiled. It is important to note that complete cessation of flow through the malformation in one session has been associated with catastrophic intracranial venous thrombosis.[7] One final reason staged closure may be necessary in small neonates is the limitation placed on the neurointerventionalist by restrictions on contrast dosing.

In older children, treatment of VGM is similarly staged to decrease the risk of thrombosis. Anesthetic management of these patients is more straightforward as they tend to be more clinically stable. Mask or IV induction may be used, and an arterial line may be deferred if the patient's clinical situation does not require it. Good peripheral intravenous (IV) access to allow for adequate hydration in the setting of the osmotic effect of IV contrast is essential.[14] Patients can usually be extubated postprocedure, although some consideration must be given to the need for a calm, still patient in the immediate postoperative period to allow for femoral artery hemostasis. Observation in the ICU is recommended for close neurological monitoring. Postoperative anticoagulation may be initiated to decrease risk of intracranial venous thrombosis.

The surgical approach to VGM control has been described, with several variations and techniques attempted over the middle to latter part of the last century.[6] However, this method has been nearly universally supplanted in the past 20 years by the progressive evolution of endovascular methods, aided by the development of an increasing range of catheters suitable for pediatric patients. Surgery is now by far the more risky procedure and is reserved for cases that have failed endovascular methods. Surgical management of acute hydrocephalus may be necessary, although there is evidence that ventriculoperitoneal shunts in the setting of unpalliated VGM incurs a large risk of hemorrhage and should only be attempted after careful consideration of the risks and benefits.[15]

COMPLICATIONS

Complications from neurointerventional embolization of a VGM can be separated into issues common to any cerebral neurodiagnostic procedure and those specific to embolization of VGM. The overall complication rate for cerebral angiography in children is estimated at less than 0.4%.[16] The most common complication is femoral hematoma or bleeding. Vascular or neurologic injury after pediatric diagnostic angiography is very rare. Embolization of an intracranial vascular lesion carries some specific risks. These include inadvertent embolization of neighboring normal blood vessels resulting in loss of perfusion to normal brain tissue, and vascular injury including vessel perforation or rupture.[13] Analysis of case series from high-volume centers has suggested that endovascular treatment by the transvenous approach may result in up to a 10% risk in intracranial hemorrhage,[2] and it is thus not generally used as a first-line treatment.

A significant contrast load is an inevitable part of neuroembolization. This presents several potential challenges for the anesthesiologist. All patients will experience an osmotic diuresis as a result of contrast administration,[17] and perioperative hydration strategies must take this into consideration. A more dangerous issue that the anesthesiologist must be cognizant of is an acute contrast reaction. Approximately 0.2% to 0.7% of patients will have an acute reaction to IV contrast, a reaction that can range from nausea and flushing to full cardiorespiratory collapse reaction.[18] This reaction is most commonly seen in the hour immediately following contrast administration, although a delayed-onset reaction is also described. Treatment for this reaction is that which is standard for anaphylaxis, although the reaction itself is anaphylactoid. Risk factors for contrast reaction include a previous reaction to contrast, asthma, and atopy. The assumed association between shellfish allergy and contrast reaction has been disproven, and there is no cross-reaction between IV noniodinated contrast and gadolinium used for MRI contrast. For patients with a high likelihood of contrast reaction who nevertheless require it, premedication with steroid and antihistamine has been utilized.

When extubating a neonate, it is important to bear in mind the risk of postanesthetic apnea. This phenomenon has been well characterized, with many pertinent risk factors for the VGM population.[19] Infants, particularly those born preterm, have an increased risk of apnea after the administration of general anesthetics. This is exacerbated by anemia, infection, central nervous system pathology and other comorbidities. While the risk of apnea in infants is less after spinal anesthetics compared to general anesthesia,[20] this technique with its limited duration of action would not be amenable to a lengthy embolization. Consequently, care must be taken to monitor infants for apnea after these lengthy anesthetics. While the exact age at which the increased risk of apnea declines, is unclear, most institutions mandate inpatient admission for monitoring for infants up to the age of 48 to 60 weeks postgestational age.

PROGNOSIS

The outcome for patients with untreated VGM is grim, with estimates of 45% to 100% mortality, depending on the patient's age and severity of presenting symptoms. Those patients who survive without treatment will nearly always suffer significant neurologic compromise.[7] Historical attempts at surgical control of the malformation were extremely risky, with some case series showing greater than 90% mortality for infants and 50% mortality for older children. Endovascular management has revolutionized the prognosis for this disease, and continues to improve. Patient series from high-volume centers now report up to 90% survival for patients who undergo neurointerventional treatment.[2] The cognitive and functional status of these patients after treatment is generally quite high.[21]

However, it is important to recognize that this auspicious-seeming situation is based on the careful selection of patients for treatment. Neonates who present in heart failure, particularly those with associated anomalies, still have a very high risk of death or, if they survive, an significant risk of poor neurologic outcome. One study that looked at all patients prenatally diagnosed with VGM at their center found that 17 of 21 had a "poor" outcome that included intellectual disability, elective termination of pregnancy for poor prognosis, and death.[22] Those patients without associated anomalies who did survive to treatment had a 75% chance of a good neurologic outcome. This indicates the importance of careful patient selection and equally careful counseling of parents about the still-significant risks of this disease process.

CONCLUSIONS

The case presented in this chapter represents an extreme presentation of VGM with associated heart failure, which unfortunately was not survivable. Advances in endovascular treatment for appropriately selected patients have in many cases lifted the almost inevitable death sentence associated with this diagnosis, although a there remains a significant subset of patients for whom treatment is not successful. This extremely rare congenital malformation requires treatment by experienced neurointerventional radiologists in the setting of an institution with knowledgeable pediatric anesthesiologists and an intensive care unit with expertise in the stabilization of neonates in heart failure and the care of patients after neuroembolization. It is to be hoped that with continued advances in the treatment of the associated heart failure and in endovascular techniques, the survivability of this malformation will continue to increase.

1. A 12-hour-old neonate with a prenatal diagnosis of a VGM was admitted to the NICU from the delivery room. He was intubated on arrival to the NICU due to tachypnea and desaturation. His blood pressure is stable and within normal range on a high-dose dopamine infusion. He is requiring 70% fraction of inspired oxygen (FiO_2) to maintain oxygen saturation >92%. The NICU is considering starting iNO. His EEG shows abnormal activity, but no clinical seizures are present. Liver and kidney function tests are currently within normal limits. What be the **BEST** way to counsel the family regarding treatment of the VGM?

    A. Medical optimization will allow him to grow and gain weight.
    B. Transition from fetal to normal circulation will improve his status.
    C. Treatment will most likely be futile, and care should be redirected.
    D. Urgent neurointerventional embolization will most likely be needed.

Answer: D
Timing of the initial neurointerventional treatment for neonates presenting with VGM depends on several patient factors. Lasjaunias et al.[2] developed the widely accepted Bicetre neonatal evaluation score to help with patient prognosis and medical decision making based on evaluation of several organ systems' function Table 31.1). A combined score of less than 8 is associated with a very poor prognosis, and intervention may not be offered due to futility. With a score of 8 to 12, the patient is considered to be demonstrating significant systemic effects of the fistula, and emergent endovascular intervention should be considered. With a score greater than 12, the neonatal patient can be managed medically until they are at least 5 months of age, unless their clinical condition deteriorates and requires earlier treatment. This patient has a score of 13, but in the context of deteriorating clinical status this places him in need of urgent embolization.

2. A 2-week-old patient with a history of a VGM has undergone 2 rounds of endovascular embolization and is scheduled for a third. Her most recent echocardiogram was prior to the second treatment. She is currently on stable ventilator settings and stable doses of IV dopamine and iNO. She does have occasional desaturations with suctioning. Which of the following is **MOST** accurate regarding her preparation for general anesthesia?

    A. Anesthesiology services should not be needed for future procedures.
    B. Echocardiography should be repeated just prior to the procedure.
    C. Inhaled nitric oxide should be weaned off prior to the procedure.
    D. Vasopressors should be increased in anticipation of procedural exsanguination.

Answer: B
Periprocedure medical optimization of patients for neurointerventional procedures requires close communication between the NICU and anesthesia teams. In general, the length of a procedure combined with rapid ongoing changes in the patient's physiology as the malformation is closed requires ongoing care by a knowledgeable anesthesia team. It is not recommended that the teams try to wean patients off IV pressor medications or iNO unless the patient's condition warrants that; preprocedure medications can and should be continued into the operative setting to maintain patient stability. Blood loss in the hands of an experienced neurointerventional radiologist is rarely a problem.

3. The **MOST** likely mechanism by which a patient with a VGM develops renal and hepatic dysfunction is

    A. hepatorenal vasculature abnormalities associated with VGM.
    B. hypotension and hypoxia associated with general anesthesia.
    C. nephrotoxicity and hepatotoxicity associated with embolization materials.
    D. poor organ perfusion associated with steal phenomena and ventricular dysfunction.

Answer: D
It is estimated that up to 80% of a patient's cardiac output can be directed to the VGM. This causes a number of problems. Most obvious is the high volume of blood returning to the right side of the heart, causing pulmonary edema. The increased work on the right ventricle can then lead to RV dysfunction, pulmonary hypertension, and eventually failure. Increased intracardiac pressure can impair coronary artery perfusion and can lead to myocardial ischemia. Decreased blood flow is also a problem for the remaining brain and the rest of the body, putting patients at risk for hypoperfusion ultimately leading to organ failure.

4. A 16-month-old has successfully undergone treatment of a VGM. Which of the following would be **LEAST** likely be present and contribute to his need for ongoing medical care?

    A. diuretics for prevention of pulmonary edema
    B. opioid tolerance secondary to prenatal exposure
    C. seizure activity secondary to tissue injury
    D. subglottic stenosis secondary to prolonged intubation

Answer: B
Ongoing treatment of heart failure may be necessary for some time after successful treatment of a VGM, and patients should be followed closely by cardiologists to wean their cardiac medications, including diuretics, as their clinical situation warrants. Steal phenomena resulting in brain hypoperfusion may result in long-term brain damage and seizure activity, which will require ongoing management. Depending on the length of time that a patient was intubated in the periprocedure period, there may be resultant subglottic stenosis. While opioid tolerance as a result of exposure in the perioperative period may be an issue, prenatal exposure for medical reasons is not indicated and thus least likely to be an issue.

5. A 6-month-old develops new onset seizures. On MRI, a mural type VGM is found. The **BEST** treatment course would be which of the following:

A. endovascular embolization

B. observation with serial imaging

C. cerebrospinal fluid shunting to prevent hydrocephalus

D. surgical clipping of malformation

Answer: A

The natural history of a VGM is to continue to expand; an untreated malformation will result in the eventual development of intractable seizures, widespread neurologic and hemodynamic dysfunction, and even death, making observation an unacceptable choice. Cerebrospinal fluid shunting and surgical management of a VGM have both been shown to have very high rates of serious complications and death and should be considered only if neuroembolization has failed and with full understanding of the inherent risks.

6. A 4-month-old presents for elective hernia repair. Of the following conditions, which one would increase the risk of postoperative apnea the **LEAST**?

A. gestational diabetes

B. hematocrit of 28%

C. history of prematurity

D. intraoperative opioids

Answer: A

Apnea after general anesthesia is a recognized risk for infants. Risk factors for postoperative apnea include young age (less than 45–60 weeks postmenstrual age), prematurity, anemia, and presence of comorbidities including central nervous system pathology. Administration of general anesthesia increases risk versus spinal anesthetics, and administration of opioids increases apnea risk.

7. A 3-year-old patient with a history of an intracranial arteriovenous malformation requires an MRI and magnetic resonance angiogram (MRA) scans to assess disease progression. During her coiling procedure done 1 year ago, under general anesthesia, she developed wheezing and a diffuse rash. She was treated at that time with albuterol, IV diphenhydramine, and IV steroids for presumptive reaction to IV contrast. She had rapid improvement in her symptoms and no hemodynamic instability, and the procedure was completed uneventfully. Which of the following plans, would be **BEST** plan for this patient?

A. alternative imaging technique(s) that require no contrast

B. MRI as long as no contrast is needed or given

C. MRI/MRA with contrast and no pretreatment

D. MRI/MRA with steroid/antihistamine pre-treatment

Answer: C

Acute reaction to iodinated IV contrast is seen in 0.2% to 0.7% of patients. Its presentation can range from nausea and flushing to full cardiorespiratory collapse. This is most commonly seen in the hour immediately following contrast administration, although a delayed-onset reaction is also described. Treatment for this reaction is that which is standard for anaphylaxis, although the reaction itself is anaphylactoid. Risk factors for contrast reaction include a previous reaction to contrast, asthma, and atopy. There is no cross-reaction

between IV noniodinated contrast and gadolinium used for MRI contrast. For patients with a high likelihood of contrast reaction who nevertheless require it, premedication with steroid and antihistamine has been described.

QUESTIONS AND ANSWERS

This chapter has accompanying questions and answers which are available to subscribers as part of the Oxford eLearning platform. To access the questions, go to ✔ http://oxfordmedicine. com/pediatricanesthesiaPBL

REFERENCES

1. Deloison B, Chalouhi GE, Sonigo P, et al. Hidden mortality of prenatally diagnosed vein of Galen aneurysmal malformation: retrospective study and review of the literature. *Ultrasound Obstet Gynecol.* 2012;40(6):652–658.

2. Lasjaunias PL, Chng SM, Sachet M, Alvarez H, Rodesch G, Garcia-Monaco R. The management of vein of Galen aneurysmal malformations. *Neurosurgery.* 2006;59(5 Suppl 3):S184–S194; discussion S3-13.

3. Grillner P, Soderman M, Holmin S, Rodesch G. A spectrum of intracranial vascular high-flow arteriovenous shunts in RASA1 mutations. *Childs Nerv Syst.* 2016;32(4):709–715.

4. Tsutsumi Y, Kosaki R, Itoh Y, et al. Vein of Galen aneurysmal malformation associated with an endoglin gene mutation. *Pediatrics.* 2011;128(5):e1307–e1310.

5. Bohiltea RE, Turcan N, Mihalea C, et al. Ultrasound prenatal diagnosis and emergency interventional radiologic therapy of Galen aneurysmal malformation in a newborn. *Maedica.* 2016;11(4):334–340.

6. Blount JP, Oakes WJ, Tubbs RS, Humphreys RP. History of surgery for cerebrovascular disease in children. Part II: vein of Galen malformations. *Neurosurg Focus.* 2006;20(6):E10.

7. Gailloud P, O'Riordan DP, Burger I, et al. Diagnosis and management of vein of galen aneurysmal malformations. *J Perinatol.* 2005;25(8):542–551.

8. Kaufman TJ, Kallmes DF. Diagnostic cerebral angiography: archaic and complication-prone or here to stay for another 80 years? *Am J Roentgenol.* 2008;190:1435–1437.

9. Frawley GP, Dargaville PA, Mitchell PJ, Tress BM, Loughnan P. Clinical course and medical management of neonates with severe cardiac failure related to vein of Galen malformation. *Arch Dis Child Fetal Neonatal Ed.* 2002;87(2):F144–F149.

10. Hansen D, Kan PT, Reddy GD, Mohan AC, Jea A, Lam S. Pediatric knowledge update: approach to the management of vein of Galen aneurysmal malformations in neonates. *Surg Neurol Int.* 2016;7(Suppl 12):S317–S321.

11. Theix R, Williams A, Smith E, Scott R, Orbach D. the use of onyx for embolization of central nervous system arteriovenous lesions in pediatric patients. *Am J Neuroradiol.* 2010;31:112–120.

12. Ashida Y, Miyahara H, Sawada H, Mitani Y, Maruyama K. Anesthetic management of a neonate with vein of Galen aneurysmal malformations and severe pulmonary hypertension. *Paediatr Anaesth.* 2005;15(6):525–528.

13. Landrigan-Ossar M, McClain CD. Anesthesia for interventional radiology. *Paediatr Anaesth.* 2014;24(7):698–702.

14. McClain CD, Landrigan-Ossar M. Challenges in pediatric neuroanesthesia: awake craniotomy, intraoperative magnetic resonance imaging, and interventional neuroradiology. *Anesthesiol Clin.* 2014;32(1):83–100.

15. Jea A, Bradshaw TJ, Whitehead WE, Curry DJ, Dauser RC, Luerssen TG. The high risks of ventriculoperitoneal shunt procedures for hydrocephalus associated with vein of Galen malformations in

childhood: case report and literature review. *Pediatr Neurosurg.* 2010;46(2):141–145.

16. Burger I, Murphy KJ, Jordan LC, Tamargo RJ, Gailloud P. Safety of digital subtraction angiography in children: complication rate analysis in 241 consecutive diagnostic angiograms. *Stroke.* 2006;37:2535–2539.

17. Lenhard DC, Pietsch H, Sieber MA, et al. The osmolality of nonionic, iodinated contrast agents as an important factor for renal safety. *Invest Radiol.* 2012;47(9):503–510.

18. Beckett KR, Moriarity AK, Langer JM. safe use of contrast media: what the radiologist needs to know. *Radiographics.* 2015;35(6):1738–1750.

19. Cote CJ, Zaslavsky A, Downes JJ, et al. Postoperative apnea in former preterm infants after inguinal herniorrhaphy: a combined analysis. *Anesthesiology.* 1995;82(4):809–822.

20. Davidson AJ, Morton NS, Arnup SJ, et al. Apnea after awake regional and general anesthesia in infants: the general anesthesia compared to spinal anesthesia study—comparing apnea and neurodevelopmental outcomes, a randomized controlled trial. *Anesthesiology.* 2015;123(1):38–54.

21. Ellis JA, Orr L, Ii PC, Anderson RC, Feldstein NA, Meyers PM. Cognitive and functional status after vein of Galen aneurysmal malformation endovascular occlusion. *World J Radiol.* 2012;4(3):83–89.

22. Deloison B, Chalouhi GE, Sonigo P, et al. Hidden mortality of prenatally diagnosed vein of Galen aneurysmal malformation: retrospective study and review of the literature. *Ultrasound Obstet Gynecol.* 2012;40(6):652–658.

32.

MOYAMOYA DISEASE

Christina Brown and Jamie E. Rubin

STEM CASE AND KEY QUESTIONS

A previously healthy 16 kg 4-year-old Japanese-American girl presents with transient right-sided facial drooping. Her birth and development up to this point have been unremarkable. History reveals that the patient experienced several episodes of unexplained falls in the last year, as well as intermittent headaches. She was previously healthy with no history of seizures, chronic medical conditions, recent illnesses, or traumatic injury. Family history was also negative for seizures or other neurological disorders.

On exam, she is shy and clinging to her mother. Vital signs are appropriate for age with blood pressure 94/55 mmHg and heart rate 91 bpm. Her right face appears slightly drooped compared to her left face. Strength is 3/5 throughout her right arm and 5/5 in her left arm. Leg strength is 5/5 bilaterally. Deep tendon reflexes in right elbow and right wrist are decreased. All other deep tendon reflexes are normal. Gait assessment is deferred secondary to her refusal to leave her mother's arms. Complete blood count, basic metabolic panel, and routine coagulation studies are within normal limits.

WHAT IMAGING STUDIES SHOULD WE ORDER FOR THIS PATIENT? WHAT CONDITIONS SHOULD WE CONSIDER IN THE DIFFERENTIAL DIAGNOSIS?

Computerized tomography (CT) of the brain shows a small hypodense area in the left temporal lobe. CT angiography of the brain reveals bilateral narrowing of the distal internal carotid arteries (ICAs) and partial segments of the middle cerebral arteries (MCA) and anterior cerebral arteries (ACA) with development of collateral circulation of the MCA and ACA regions. Magnetic resonance imaging (MRI) demonstrates increased fluid attenuated inversion recovery signal intensity along fissures and gyri of bilateral cerebral hemispheres. Magnetic resonance angiography (MRA) shows similar narrowing and collateral development to computed tomography angiography. Perfusion MRI demonstrates decreased blood flow through bilateral ICAs, bilateral MCAs, and bilateral ACAs. A probable diagnosis of Moyamoya is made based on the patient's history and imaging findings (Figure 32.1).

WHAT IS MOYAMOYA DISEASE, AND HOW IS IT DIAGNOSED? WHAT ARE THE SURGICAL AND NONSURGICAL MANAGEMENT OPTIONS FOR MOYAMOYA?

The surgical team schedules the patient for encephalo-duro-arterio-synangiosis (EDAS) to provide indirect revascularization. The morning of the procedure, after the risks and benefits of anesthetic care were explained, the patient's mother expresses concerns over her daughter's potential postoperative pain and how that will affect her recovery.

WHY IS PAIN CONTROL PARTICULARLY IMPORTANT IN THIS PATIENT? WHAT ARE THE OPTIONS FOR PAIN MANAGEMENT IN THIS CASE? WHAT OTHER PREOPERATIVE CONCERNS DO YOU HAVE FOR THIS PATIENT?

After discussion with the surgical team, the patient's mother consents for a scalp block at the end of surgery. Inhalational induction is achieved with sevoflurane via mask followed by placement of a peripheral intravenous line. The patient is intubated after receiving rocuronium, fentanyl, and propofol. An additional peripheral intravenous line and a left radial arterial line are inserted after intubation.

WHAT ARE THE OPTIONS FOR NEUROMONITORING IN THIS PATIENT? WHAT SHOULD WE USE FOR MAINTENANCE OF ANESTHESIA?

Anesthesia is maintained with 50% nitrous oxide in oxygen, 0.5 minimal anesthetic concentration of isoflurane, and a remifentanil infusion. Continuous electroencephalogram (EEG) is performed throughout the case. As the case progresses, a brisk bleed develops from the dura. As the surgical team attempts to control the bleeding, the patient becomes hypotensive, and the neuromonitoring technician reports EEG slowing. Vasopressors are administered as well as blood and fluids, which increases the patient's blood pressure and improves the EEG. The surgical team successfully achieves hemostasis and the remainder of the procedure is completed uneventfully.

WHAT ARE YOUR HEMODYNAMIC GOALS FOR THIS PATIENT?

Isoflurane, nitrous oxide, and remifentanil are discontinued during skin closure. A scalp block is placed at the end of the procedure for pain management. However, 45 minutes after anesthetic discontinuation, the patient remains unresponsive. She is spontaneously breathing at a rate of 20 breaths per minute with 8 mL/kg tidal volumes, and she is hemodynamically stable without vasoactive support.

WHAT IS THE DIFFERENTIAL DIAGNOSIS FOR HER DELAYED EMERGENCE, CONSIDERING HER KNOWN NEUROVASCULAR DISEASE? WHAT SHOULD BE OUR NEXT STEPS IN THE MANAGEMENT OF THIS PATIENT?

The decision is made to keep the patient intubated. Train-of-four monitoring demonstrates four twitches with no visible fade. Her pupils are 3 mm and reactive to light, and her esophageal temperature is 36.7°C. Finger stick blood glucose is 97 mg/dL. Emergent head CT is then obtained, which shows increased size of the hypodense area in the temporal lobe compared to her preoperative study.

WHAT ARE THE KEY POSTOPERATIVE CONCERNS FOR THIS PATIENT? WHEN SHOULD WE EXPECT IMPROVEMENTS IN HER CEREBROVASCULAR FLOW?

The patient was transported to the pediatric intensive care unit for postoperative mechanical ventilation as well as blood pressure monitoring and frequent neurologic assessment. Her mental status improved the morning after surgery, and she was extubated uneventfully. She continued to have weakness in her right arm postoperatively and worked with physical and occupational therapy during her hospital stay. She was discharged home on postoperative day 8.

DISCUSSION

Moyamoya is a cerebrovascular disorder characterized by progressive stenosis of the ICA and its proximal branches. Collateral vessels from the leptomeningeal vessels and the external and intracranial ICAs develop to perfuse the segments of the brain distal to the stenosis, leading to the characteristic angiographic appearance of "a puff of smoke" for which the disease is named.[1] Diagnostic criteria specific to children based on guidelines from the Research Committee on Moyamoya Disease are shown in Figure 32.2. The Suzuki criteria define severity of disease by angiographic appearance as shown in Figure 32.3. Moyamoya disease excludes a syndromic cause of the vascular abnormality.[2,3] Those patients with Moyamoya-type vascular abnormalities arising from a syndrome are said to have Moyamoya syndrome rather than Moyamoya disease. Some commonly associated syndromes giving rise to Moyamoya syndrome include PHACE syndrome, cardio-facio-cutaneous syndrome/Noonan, neurofibromatosis type 1, sickle cell disease, Fanconi's anemia, type 1 glycogenesis, congenital heart disease, radiation vasculitis, renovascular hypertension, renal artery stenosis, persistent primitive trigeminal artery variant, Ito's hypomelanosis, Hageman factor deficiency, and Trisomy 21.[1,2,4,5]

DIAGNOSIS AND IMAGING STUDIES

Moyamoya disease is usually diagnosed based on cerebrovascular imaging. Traditional angiography has been supplemented and in some instances replaced by newer imaging modalities, particularly in pediatric patients.

1. **Digital subtraction angiography:** The gold standard for diagnosis of Moyamoya disease is digital subtraction angiography, but this method is not commonly used in the pediatric population given the degree of radiation, the risk of contrast-related nephrotoxicity, and the potential stress caused to the patient.[6,7] If other imaging modalities demonstrate the necessary criteria discussed in Figure 32.2, then conventional angiography is not necessary in the pediatric population for diagnosis.[7]

2. **Computed tomography:** CT has become the most commonly used imaging modality for quick differentiation of multiple causes of neurological symptoms. This imaging technique can quickly evaluate for hemorrhage, large infarction, tumor, or elevated intracranial pressure. Once Moyamoya is suspected, imaging limitations and radiation exposure have prevented CT angiography from coming to the forefront of pediatric evaluation. While this technique can often discern narrowing of vasculature and some collateral circulation formation, additional techniques are often still required to fully qualify the severity of disease.[7,8]

3. **Magnetic resonance imaging/angiography:** MRI/ MRA have become commonly used imaging modalities for the pediatric population. The absence of ionizing radiation with this technique makes it amenable to serial studies which are often desired both for surgical planning and for postoperative surveillance. Imaging findings include those related to ischemia, specifically low signals on T1-weighted imaging with high signals in similar locations on T2-weighted imaging. The "ivy sign," or leptomeningeal enhancement related to leptomeningeal vascular engorgement, has been reported as particularly indicative of Moyamoya disease, although it has now been observed in several other conditions including subarachnoid hemorrhage, meningitis, and Sturge-Weber syndrome.[7] While MRA has not yet reached the imaging precision of cerebral angiography, as imaging techniques improve, better discernment of small caliber vessels has become achievable and MRA can now be used in place of angiography to officially diagnose Moyamoya.[4,6,7] In particular, MRA may overestimate stenoses and may be

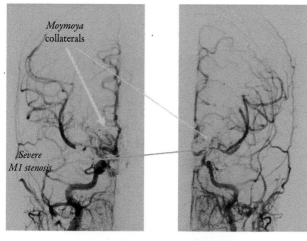

Moymoya collaterals

Severe M1 stenosis

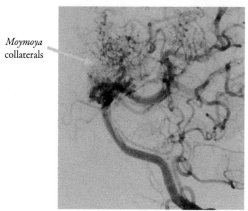

Moymoya collaterals

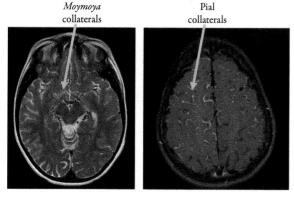

Moymoya collaterals

Pial collaterals

Fig. 32.1 Images courtesy of Manu S. Goyal, MD, MSc, Assistant Professor in Neuroradiology, Mallinckrodt Institute of Radiology, Washington University School of Medicine, St. Louis, MO.

less reliable for discerning small vessel occlusions when compared with angiography.[7]

4. **Cerebral perfusion imaging:** Despite advances in anatomic imaging capabilities, the patient's clinical presentation does not always mirror the findings on radiographic studies. For these cases, further evaluation with cerebral perfusion imaging is commonly used to evaluate blood flow before and after surgery for both diagnosis and postoperative follow-up.[6,7] Multiple modalities for this type of imaging exist including single-photon emission computed tomography, positron emission tomography, CT perfusion, and MR perfusion.[6]

These techniques may employ the use of a cerebral vasodilator to better compare low-flow and high-flow states. Results of these studies may help to define surgical outcomes for these patients.[7]

5. **Transcranial ultrasound:** Some studies have shown promising results using transcranial Doppler ultrasound for diagnosis and surgical follow-up in the pediatric population.[4,7] Doppler imaging can determine blood flow velocity in the branches of the ICA, which correlates with blood flow in the same cerebral hemisphere. These measurements thereby help identify patients with decreased cerebral blood flow who are at risk for stroke; however, this method provides no information regarding the distribution of blood flow or the location of narrowed arteries.[7] Transcranial ultrasound has not yet become mainstream as it has variable sensitivity depending on operator technique and often generates spurious results.[4,7]

CLINICAL MANIFESTATIONS OF MOYAMOYA

Cerebral ischemia is the most common clinical manifestation of Moyamoya in the pediatric population as opposed to cerebral hemorrhage, which is the more common presentation in adults. This difference may be related to the higher cerebral metabolic demand in childhood.[9,10] In Moyamoya patients under 10 years of age, transient ischemic attack (TIA) occurs in 40% of patients while infarct is seen in 30%.[11] Common symptoms include headache, hypertension, blindness, and developmental delay, with headache being the most commonly observed (approximately 30% of patients).[6,11] These symptoms can be precipitated by crying, playing, or activities causing hyperventilation such as playing the flute, blowing up a balloon, or eating hot foods.[10] Developmental delay and disturbances in activities of daily living worsen with duration of disease and younger onset.[12] Kawabori et al.[11] showed a relationship between headache and changes in cerebral hemodynamics.

DIFFERENTIAL DIAGNOSIS

A broad differential should be considered when evaluating a child with new neurologic symptoms. Seizures may cause transient postictal paralysis, called Todd's paresis, but prolonged duration of symptoms should prompt investigation for other causes. Intracranial neoplasms can present with worsening neurological deficits as the tumor grows. Intracerebral infections, such as meningitis, cerebellitis, intracranial abscess, or subdural empyema should also be considered in the differential.[13] Complicated migraines may cause focal neurologic deficits that may take up to 24 hours to resolve; this diagnosis is more likely if the patient has a family history of migraines. Thrombotic strokes may arise from inherited clotting disorders, sickle cell disease, or congenital cardiac defects, and hemorrhagic strokes may be related to arteriovenous malformations or hereditary coagulopathies.[14] Stroke-like episodes may be caused by numerous metabolic

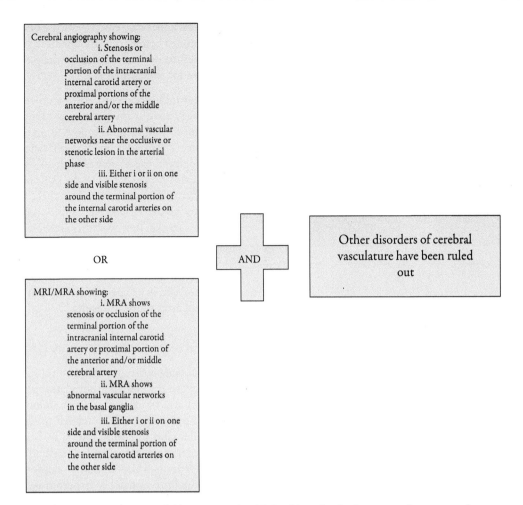

Cerebral angiography showing:

i. Stenosis or occlusion of the terminal portion of the intracranial internal carotid artery or proximal portions of the anterior and/or the middle cerebral artery

ii. Abnormal vascular networks near the occlusive or stenotic lesion in the arterial phase

iii. Either i or ii on one side and visible stenosis around the terminal portion of the internal carotid arteries on the other side

OR

MRI/MRA showing:

i. MRA shows stenosis or occlusion of the terminal portion of the intracranial internal carotid artery or proximal portion of the anterior and/or middle cerebral artery

ii. MRA shows abnormal vascular networks in the basal ganglia

iii. Either i or ii on one side and visible stenosis around the terminal portion of the internal carotid arteries on the other side

AND

Other disorders of cerebral vasculature have been ruled out

Fig. 32.2 Diagnostic criteria for Moyamoya disease in children. From Fukui M. Guidelines for the diagnosis and treatment of spontaneous occlusion of the circle of Willis ("Moyamoya" disease). Research Committee on Spontaneous Occlusion of the Circle of Willis (Moyamoya Disease) of the Ministry of Health and Welfare, Japan. *Clin Neurol Neurosurg.* 1997;99(Suppl 2):S238–S240.

Grade	Definition
I	Narrowing of ICA bifurcation
II	Appearance of characteristic Moyamoya collateral vessels
III	Increase in ICA stenosis, intensification of Moyamoya vessels
IV	Appearance of ECA collateral vessels
V	Intensification of ECA vessels, reduction in Moyamoya vessels
VI	Occlusion of ICA, disappearance of Moyamoya vessels, brain supplied only by ECA

Fig. 32.3 Suzuki criteria adapted from Suzuki J, Takaku A. Cerebrovascular "Moyamoya" disease: disease showing abnormal net-like vessels in base of brain. *Arch Neurol.* 1969;20(3):288-299. ICA: internal carotid artery. ECA: external carotid artery.

disorders such as mitochondrial encephalomyopathy, lactic acidosis, and stroke-like episodes, Leigh syndrome, and myoclonic epilepsy and ragged red fiber (MERRF) syndrome.[15] Recreational drug use, particularly in the adolescent population, may cause cerebral vasculopathies or intracranial hemorrhage.[14] Imaging studies have greatly improved over the years and are now the primary means to narrow the differential in these patients.

PATHOPHYSIOLOGY

The pathophysiology of Moyamoya remains to be fully elucidated, but increasing evidence suggests that the classic arteriopathy with development of lenticulostriate collaterals is the common end-stage of a variety of abnormalities. While the exact mechanism of the progressive stenosis has not been determined, histological studies have shown fibrointimal hyperplasia, impairment of the medial elastic layer, and proliferation of vascular smooth muscle cells. A genetic basis for Moyamoya disease is strongly suspected, given the observation of familial patterns of inheritance as well as increased incidence in certain ethnic groups, but multiple genes have been implicated. Further complicating the picture is the possibility of a relationship between infectious factors, specifically Propionibacterium acnes and HIV, and the development of the disease. Four types of Moyamoya disease have been characterized based on clinical findings at presentation, including bleeding, epileptic, infarction, and TIA types. Approximately 70% to 80% of children present with either infarction or TIA type, with the infarction type being more common than the TIA type.[6]

TREATMENT OF MOYAMOYA

Three main modalities exist for the treatment of Moyamoya disease: conservative management, direct surgery, and indirect surgery. The goal of both direct and indirect surgery is the establishment of collateral circulation through the external carotid artery (ECA) in an attempt to prevent further brain ischemia.[6]

1. **Conservative therapy:** Conservative therapies such as steroids, vasodilators, antiplatelet agents, and surgical sympathectomies have not been shown to offer long-term improvement. Typically, conservative treatment is not the primary treatment chosen for children with this disease, although some aspects can be combined with either of the surgical modalities.[1,6]

2. **Direct revascularization:** The most common direct surgical technique is the superficial temporal artery (STA) to MCA (STA–MCA) bypass.[6,11] Direct revascularization has been shown to be superior to indirect techniques in adults with Moyamoya disease[9]. However, the efficacy of direct revascularization may be limited in children secondary to the small caliber and fragility of the superficial cerebral vasculature. The direct approach may be better in emergent situations as it allows for shorter time to formation of the collateral circulation.[6,16]

3. **Indirect revascularization:** Some indirect surgical procedures include EDAS, encephalomyosynangiosis, encephalo-duro-myo-synangiosis, encephalo-duro-arterio-myo-synangiosis, cranial-omental transposition, indirect cerebral revascularization with multiple burr holes, and burr holes combined with indirect or direct revascularization.[1,6,17,18] It remains unclear which of these indirect techniques is more effective, but early surgical

treatment provides better outcomes than conservative management alone. Children achieve better results than adults after indirect procedures.[6] Headache symptoms may be best improved with a combined indirect and direct technique, which may be an indication that there are improved cerebral hemodynamics with a combined approach.[11]

PREOPERATIVE ASSESSMENT

As with any patient, preoperative assessment of the patient with Moyamoya disease is vital to the decision to proceed with surgery. As previously discussed, multiple systemic disorders can be associated with this disease and should be ruled out prior to proceeding to the operating room. A thorough history and physical examination should be sufficient to rule out most associated disorders. If any associated condition is suspected, further workup to rule out other systemic manifestations should be performed. Children often present with history of multiple preoperative TIA, which increases the patient's risk perioperatively. Even in healthy children, intracerebral vascular surgery can cause rapid shifts in fluid status. Therefore, baseline hemoglobin and hematocrit along with antibody screening should be assessed. Aggressive preoperative hydration may prevent decreases in cerebral blood flow associated with dehydration.[19]

INTRAOPERATIVE MANAGEMENT

1. **Maintenance of cerebral perfusion pressure:** Intraoperative management of the Moyamoya patient should emphasize maintenance of cerebral perfusion. Both hypertension and hypotension can lead to neurologic deficits following surgery. While a short duration of hypotension in the perioperative period is not known to be associated with clinically significant ischemia, care must be taken to minimize any hypotensive episodes during the perioperative period.[16,20] Adequate access for the administration of vasoactive agents is vital to maintain hemodynamic stability. Techniques such as near-infrared spectroscopy have been used to evaluate blood pressure ranges in children with Moyamoya disease to determine limits of autoregulation. This research suggests that for children ages 2 to 16 years, the optimal mean arterial pressure (MAP) for cerebral perfusion lies between 60 and 80 mmHg.[21] For patients younger than 2 years, preoperative MAP may be a good starting point for the lower limit of acceptable intraoperative blood pressure. Studies in adults and children suggest that an individualized approach to MAP goals based on cerebral autoregulation may improve outcomes.[22]

2. **Maintenance of normocapnia:** Both hypercapnia and hypocapnia have been shown to result in cerebral ischemia for the patient with Moyamoya disease. Hypocapnia reduces cerebral blood flow, and even a small decrement resulting from mild hyperventilation may reduce blood

flow enough to compromise ischemic areas of the brain. Hypercapnia, which often results from overzealous attempts to avoid hyperventilation may also reduce cerebral perfusion as the result of cerebrovascular steal phenomenon. Because the diseased vasculature may not dilate normally in response to hypercapnia, the unaffected areas of the brain may divert blood flow from the ischemic areas. Furthermore, sudden changes in end-tidal carbon dioxide in either direction have been associated with decreased perfusion.[16]

3. **Choice of anesthetic agent:** The literature has not demonstrated superiority of either inhalation-based anesthetics versus total intravenous anesthesia. While some studies have shown improvements in cerebral blood flow with propofol-based technique, studies have not shown a difference in postoperative complications.[23–25] A small retrospective study found no difference in postoperative neurological deficit between children who received nitrous oxide during indirect revascularization procedures and those who did not receive nitrous oxide.[16]

4. **Monitoring:** Given the risk of fluid shifts, blood loss and hemodynamic instability, invasive monitoring including arterial line and central venous pressure should be considered in addition to standard American Society of Anesthesiologists monitors. Urine output should also be followed for the duration of the case.[19] Newer noninvasive monitoring of fluid status may be utilized, but these monitors have not yet been well-studied in children. Use of cerebral monitoring with a bispectral index monitor or auditory-evoked potentials may allow lower concentration of anesthetic agents to be used, thereby promoting quicker extubation.[26] Monitors of cerebral perfusion may be used including invasive intracranial pressure monitors, EEG, cerebral oximetry, transcranial Doppler, somatosensory-evoked potentials, and near infrared spectroscopy. As newer technologies emerge, options for tailoring perfusion goals to the individual patient will likely improve.[19,22]

5. **Temperature:** Studies generally agree that hyperthermia is detrimental to patients with Moyamoya disease secondary to the cerebral ischemia that is potentially caused by increased cerebral metabolic rate and oxygen consumption. Controversy remains regarding the benefit or detriment of hypothermia, particularly during temporary occlusion of the cerebral vessels. Current practices follow the brain trauma guidelines and recommend maintenance of normothermia.[19]

6. **Fluid maintenance:** Maintenance of relative hypervolemia is often recommended for the patient with Moyamoya disease. This goal not only assists with maintaining blood pressure but also helps to prevent polycythemia, which has been shown to be a risk factor for cerebral ischemia. Caution must be used to strike a balance between adequate volume and preventing hemodilution as this has also been shown to contribute to

ischemia.[19] One study showed that a urine output around 4 mL/kg/hr led to fewer ischemic complications than a urine output of 2 mL/kg/hr.[27]

7. **Pain management:** A good pain management plan is helpful in avoiding hyperventilation related to discomfort, which in turn aids the maintenance of hemodynamic stability in these patients. Continuous infusions of short acting opioids, such as fentanyl, remifentanil, or sufentanil, are often utilized to achieve stability during these procedures. Pain management with regional techniques may improve hemodynamic stability and may be associated with decreased rates of delirium and morbidity as well as fewer cerebral infarcts and reversible ischemic neurologic deficits.[28] Other multimodal pain management techniques may also be employed including the use of adjuvants such as acetaminophen.

POSTOPERATIVE COMPLICATIONS

Postoperative concerns for the patient with Moyamoya after revascularization include cerebral ischemia, cerebral edema, hyperperfusion syndrome, epidural hematoma, and scalp ischemia.[29] Epidural hematoma requiring surgical intervention is more likely after craniotomy in the pediatric patient with Moyamoya than in patients without Moyamoya (4.8% vs. 0.8%, respectively).[29] CT has limited sensitivity to detect ischemia during the first few hours after the initial insult; therefore, traction on the brain tissue or ischemia will likely not be evident on early postoperative CT. Frequent preoperative TIA and preoperative cerebral infarction are associated with postoperative cerebral ischemia in the pediatric Moyamoya patient after STA–MCA bypass.[30] Hyperperfusion syndrome is suspected to occur when there is a sudden increase in blood flow to an area of brain which was previously hypoperfused. This leads to cerebral edema and a constellation of symptoms including headache, seizures, altered mentation, and focal neurological deficits. Intraoperative MRI may be of use in predicting which patients are at risks for hyperperfusion syndrome.[31] Older age at presentation is associated with postoperative edema after STA–MCA bypass, possibly related to postoperative hyperperfusion syndrome.[30] Hyperperfusion syndrome is absent in patients after indirect revascularization, but symptom improvement is typically delayed one to two weeks while new blood vessels grow into the cerebral tissue. Hyperventilation should be avoided since it may cause cerebral ischemia in the postoperative period; careful management of pain and anxiety is key in avoiding this complication.[32]

DIFFERENTIAL DIAGNOSIS OF DELAYED EMERGENCE

Delayed emergence is not well defined in the literature, but it is generally defined as failure to regain consciousness for a longer than anticipated time after the cessation of general anesthesia. Common causes of delayed emergence include use of benzodiazepines or barbiturates, residual anesthetic agent, residual neuromuscular blockade, opioid overdose, hypothermia, electrolyte imbalance, hypoglycemia, hypoxia, hypercarbia, cerebral ischemia, intracranial hemorrhage, and extensive surgical resection. Causes related to the surgery must be high on the differential after intracranial surgical procedures, and clinicians should have a low threshold for obtaining a CT scan.[33,34] Pharmacologic causes should be ruled out including possible interactions with medications or herbal remedies. While less commonly used in children than adults, psychotropic, anticonvulsant, and antidepressant medications may all interact with anesthetic agents leading to longer than expected duration of sedative effects.[35] Acute administration of anticonvulsants may lead to prolongation of neuromuscular blockade.[36] While delirium in pediatric patients is most often associated with symptoms of agitation and combativeness, a hypoactive variant has been described and may be a less common cause of delayed emergence from anesthesia.[35] Genetic variations in propofol metabolism have been described in older patients, although not in children.[37]

LONG-TERM OUTLOOK

The incidence of stroke recurrence and disturbed activities of daily living is reduced after surgical intervention. The frequency of postsurgical ischemic events is higher in children under 3 years of age than in older children. Patients who have undergone early surgery have an improved long-term intellectual outcome compared with those patients treated conservatively or with late-stage surgery. Unfortunately, a substantial portion of pediatric patients still experience social and cognitive delay despite intervention, particularly children under 3 years old at the time of diagnosis. Age of onset seems to be correlated with worsened cognitive impairment and increased risk of postoperative infarction regardless of surgical intervention. Independent predictors of worsened intellectual outcomes in pediatric patients include completed stroke and small craniotomy.[32,38]

BILATERAL VERSUS UNILATERAL SURGERY

Moyamoya is a bilateral disease of the cerebral arteries, and therefore revascularization is often completed for both cerebral hemispheres either during the same surgery or staged with a short interval between the two sides. However, ischemic symptoms may not appear on both sides simultaneously. When a patient presents with only unilateral symptoms, controversy exists with regards to timing of a revascularization procedure on the contralateral side. Some experts suggest waiting until development of ischemic symptoms such as TIAs on the contralateral side, or at least delaying surgery until imaging demonstrates evidence of progression of the cerebrovascular stenosis. Patients who have had known unilateral disease should likely undergo imaging at regular intervals to monitor for advancement of disease.[39]

CONCLUSIONS

- Moyamoya disease is a rare disorder characterized by narrowing of the large cerebral arteries, most commonly the internal carotid and middle meningeal arteries.

- In recent years, diagnosis has been made using less invasive neuroangiographic imaging modalities.

- Children typically are better candidates for indirect revascularization procedures rather than direct revascularization procedures because of the smaller caliber of their vasculature.

- Maintenance of cerebral perfusion pressure is one of the primary goals of the anesthesiologist.

- Despite improvements in intellectual functioning after early surgical intervention, patients often still have some level of long-term cognitive or social impairment.

- Cerebral ischemia must be high on the differential for the patient undergoing revascularization for Moyamoya disease with delayed emergence.

REVIEW QUESTIONS

1. A 4 year-old male with Moyamoya presents for EDAS. Which of the following interventions are **MOST** likely to improve postoperative neurological outcome?

    A. hypotension (controlled)
    B. hypothermia (moderate)
    C. hypovolemia (mild)
    D. scalp blocks (bupivacaine)

Answer: D
Scalp blocks after surgery may improve hemodynamic stability after surgery and is associated with improved neurological outcomes including decreased cerebral ischemia.[28] One possible mechanism is reduction in postoperative hyperventilation related to poorly controlled pain. Maintaining adequate cerebral perfusion pressure is essential for a good neurological outcome after surgery, and therefore hypovolemia (answer A) should be avoided. Mild hypothermia (33–35°C) has been proposed to improve neurological outcome during occlusion of the cerebral vessels during surgery, but moderate or deep hypothermia (answer B) is not recommended. Hypovolemia (answer C) may worsen cerebral ischemia by decreasing cerebral blood flow.

2. Which of the following preoperative patient characteristics is correlated with increased cognitive impairment following EDAS in a child with Moyamoya disease?

    A. age greater than 3 years
    B. early surgical intervention
    C. large craniotomy surgery
    D. preoperative completed stroke

Answer: D

Pediatric patients with a completed stroke prior to surgical intervention are at increased risk of cognitive impairment after revascularization surgery. The remainder of the answer choices (answers A, B, C) are all associated with improved postoperative outcomes and decreased risk of postoperative infarction.[38]

3. In contrast to adults, children with Moyamoya disease are **MOST** likely to present with which of the following?

    A. headache, severe
    B. hypertensive crisis
    C. cerebral ischemia
    D. cerebral hemorrhage

Answer: C

Cerebral ischemia is the most common clinical manifestation in the pediatric population as opposed to cerebral hemorrhage, which is the more common presentation in adults, possibly related to the higher cerebral metabolic demand in childhood.[9,10] In patients under 10 years of age, TIA occurs in 40% while infarct is seen in 30%.[9]

4. In patients who require emergent surgical intervention, which of the follow procedures will **MOST** likely be performed?

    A. burr holes
    B. encephalo-duro-arterio-myo-synangiosis
    C. pial synangiosis
    D. STA–MCA bypass

Answer: D

STA–MCA bypass provides the most rapid improvement in patients with current ischemia secondary to Moyamoya disease. The rest of the procedures listed (answers A, B, C) take anywhere from 2 to several weeks to increase cerebral blood flow to ischemic areas.

5. The **MOST** accurate imaging method for diagnosing Moyamoya disease is

    A. CT angiography.
    B. digital subtraction angiography.
    C. MRI/MRA.
    D. transcranial Doppler ultrasound.

Answer: B

Digital subtraction angiography is the gold standard imaging modality for diagnosis of Moyamoya disease. Although MRI and MRA (answer C) are being increasingly used for diagnosis particularly in the pediatric population, this modality has decreased sensitivity for detecting small vessel occlusions. Transcranial Doppler ultrasound (answer D) can detect overall decreased blood flow to either cerebral hemisphere, but it lacks the ability to locate specific lesions and is dependent on the skill of the ultrasonographer. CT angiography (answer A) is not routinely used for diagnosis in children since it supplies similar information to MRI/MRA and poses additional risk from radiation exposure.[7]

6. In a 6-year-old female patient with Moyamoya disease undergoing indirect revascularization surgery, which of the

following represents the best intraoperative ventilation goal for partial pressure of carbon dioxide in arterial blood ($PaCO_2$)?

    A. 30 mmHg
    B. 35 mmHg
    C. 40 mmHg
    D. 45 mmHg

Answer: C

Multiple studies have emphasized the maintenance of normocarbia to avoid cerebral ischemia. Hyperventilation (answers A, B) and the resulting hypocapnia may reduce blood flow to already compromised areas of the brain. Hypoventilation (answer D) can also result in reduction of blood flow to ischemic areas, since the diseased vasculature may not dilate normally in response to hypercapnia and therefore result in diversion of blood to unaffected areas of the brain.[17]

7. A 14-year-old male patient with Trisomy 21 presents with progressively worsening neurological deficits over a 4-year period. MRI/MRA suggests vessel pathology of grade V/VI by Suzuki criteria, and he is diagnosed with late-stage Moyamoya disease. Which of the following findings are **MOST** likely to be found on imaging?

    A. cerebral blood flow, to ischemic areas, improved with acetazolamide
    B. ECA predominantly supplying left cerebral hemisphere
    C. internal carotid arteries are dilated at their bifurcation, bilaterally
    D. leptomeningeal vessels not visible on MRA

Answer: B

According to the staging system initially established by Suzuki, grade V and VI Moyamoya vasculature are characterized by reduction in the classic Moyamoya collaterals and appearance of collaterals from the ECA. In the end stages of Moyamoya, the brain is fed almost exclusively by the ECA, and the branches of the ICA have been completely obliterated. Because the affected vessels are either maximally dilated or abnormally response to cerebral dilation, administration of a cerebrovascular dilator (answer A) would likely cause a "steal" phenomenon and result in diversion of blood to other less-affected areas of the brain. Moyamoya disease results in stenosis at the bifurcation of the ICA (answer C). The "ivy sign," or enhancement of the leptomeningeal vessels (answer D) has been found to be indicative of Moyamoya disease on MRA.

QUESTIONS AND ANSWERS

This chapter has accompanying questions and answers which are available to subscribers as part of the Oxford eLearning platform. To access the questions, go to ✓ http:// oxfordmedicine. com/pediatricanesthesiaPBL

REFERENCES

1. Setzen G, Cacace AT, Eames F, et al. Central deafness in a young child with Moyamoya disease: paternal linkage in a Caucasian

family: two case reports and a review of the literature. *Int J Pediatr Otorhinolaryngol.* 1999;48:53–76.

2. Ishiguro Y, Kubota T, Takenaka J, et al. Cardio-facio-cutaneous syndrome and moyamoya syndrome. *Brain Dev.* 2002;24:245–249.

3. Fukui M. Guidelines for the diagnosis and treatment of spontaneous occlusion of the circle of Willis ("moyamoya" disease). Research Committee on Spontaneous Occlusion of the Circle of Willis (Moyamoya Disease) of the Ministry of Health and Welfare, Japan. *Clin Neurol Neurosurg.* 1997;99(Suppl 2):S238–S240.

4. Ipsiroglu OS, Eichler F, Stöckler-Ipsiroglu S, Trattnig S. Cerebral blood flow velocities in an infant with moyamoya disease. *Pediatr Neurol.* 1999;21:739–741.

5. Loddenkemper T, Friedman NR, Ruggieri PM, Marcotty A, Sears J, Traboulsi EI. Pituitary stalk duplication in association with moyamoya disease and bilateral morning glory disc anomaly—broadening the clinical spectrum of midline defects. *J Neurol.* 2008;255:885–890.

6. Piao J, Wu W, Yang Z, Yu J. Research progress of moyamoya disease in children. *Int J Med Sci.* 2015;12:566–575.

7. Currie S, Raghavan A, Batty R, Connolly DJ, Griffiths PD. Childhood moyamoya disease and moyamoya syndrome: a pictorial review. *Pediatr Neurol.* 2011;44:401–413.

8. Smith ER, Scott RM. Spontaneous occlusion of the circle of Willis in children: pediatric moyamoya summary with proposed evidence-based practice guidelines: a review. *J Neurosurg Pediatr.* 2012;9:353–360.

9. Arias EJ, Dunn GP, Washington CW, et al. Surgical revascularization in North American adults with moyamoya phenomenon: long-term angiographic follow-up. *J Stroke Cerebrovasc Dis.* 2015;24:1597–1608.

10. Tagawa T, Naritomi H, Mimaki T, Yabuuchi H, Sawada T. Regional cerebral blood flow, clinical manifestations, and age in children with moyamoya disease. *Stroke.* 1987;18:906–910.

11. Kawabori M, Kuroda S, Nakayama N, et al. Effective surgical revascularization improves cerebral hemodynamics and resolves headache in pediatric moyamoya disease. *World Neurosurg.* 2013;80:612–619.

12. Kurokawa T, Tomita S, Ueda K, et al. Prognosis of occlusive disease of the circle of Willis (moyamoya disease) in children. *Pediatr Neurol.* 1985;1:274–277.

13. Shellhaas RA, Smith SE, O'Tool E, Licht DJ, Ichord RN. Mimics of childhood stroke: characteristics of a prospective cohort. *Pediatrics.* 2006;118:704–709.

14. Tsze DS, Valente JH. Pediatric stroke: a review. *Emerg Med Int.* 2011;2011:734506.

15. Pavlakis SG, Kingsley PB, Bialer MG. Stroke in children: genetic and metabolic issues. *J Child Neurol.* 2000;15:308–315.

16. Jagdevan S, Sriganesh K, Pandey P, Reddy M, Umamaheswara Rao GS. Anesthetic factors and outcome in children undergoing indirect revascularization procedure for moyamoya disease: an Indian perspective. *Neurol India.* 2015;63:702–706.

17. Navarro R, Chao K, Gooderham PA, Bruzoni M, Dutta S, Steinberg GK. Less invasive pedicled omental-cranial transposition in pediatric patients with moyamoya disease and failed prior revascularization. *Neurosurgery.* 2014;10(Suppl 1):1–14.

18. McLaughlin N, Martin NA. Effectiveness of burr holes for indirect revascularization in patients with moyamoya disease—a review of the literature. *World Neurosurg.* 2014;81:91–98.

19. Parray T, Martin TW, Siddiqui S. Moyamoya disease: a review of the disease and anesthetic management. *J Neurosurg Anesthesiol.* 2011;23:100–109.

20. Martino JD, Werner LO. Hypocarbia during anaesthesia in children with moyamoya disease. *Can J Anaesth.* 1991;38:942–943.

21. Lee JK, Williams M, Jennings JM, et al. Cerebrovascular autoregulation in pediatric moyamoya disease. *Paediatr Anaesth.* 2013;23:547–556.

22. Rivera-Lara L, Zorrilla-Vaca A, Geocadin RG, Healy RJ, Ziai W, Mirski MA. Cerebral autoregulation-oriented therapy at the bedside: a comprehensive review. *Anesthesiology.* 2017;126:1187–1199.

23. Adachi K, Yamamoto Y, Kameyama E, Suzuki H, Horinouchi T. [Early postoperative complications in patients with Moyamoya disease--a comparison of inhaled anesthesia with total intravenous anesthesia (TIVA)]. *Masui.* 2005;54:653–657.

24. Kikuta K, Takagi Y, Nozaki K, et al. Hashimoto N: effects of intravenous anesthesia with propofol on regional cortical blood flow and intracranial pressure in surgery for moyamoya disease. *Surg Neurol.* 2007;68:421–424.

25. Sato K, Shirane R, Kato M, Yoshimoto T. Effect of inhalational anesthesia on cerebral circulation in moyamoya disease. *J Neurosurg Anesthesiol.* 1999;11:25–30.

26. Recart A, Gasanova I, White PF, et al. The effect of cerebral monitoring on recovery after general anesthesia: a comparison of the auditory evoked potential and bispectral index devices with standard clinical practice. *Anesth Analg.* 2003;97:1667–1674.

27. Sato K, Shirane R, Yoshimoto T. Perioperative factors related to the development of ischemic complications in patients with moyamoya disease. *Childs Nerv Syst.* 1997;13:68–72.

28. Ahn HJ, Kim JA, Lee JJ, et al. Effect of preoperative skull block on pediatric moyamoya disease. *J Neurosurg Pediatr.* 2008;2:37–41.

29. Kim T, Oh CW, Bang JS, Kim JE, Cho WS. Moyamoya disease: treatment and outcomes. *J Stroke.* 2016;18:21–30.

30. Hayashi T, Shirane R, Fujimura M, Tominaga T. Postoperative neurological deterioration in pediatric moyamoya disease: watershed shift and hyperperfusion. *J Neurosurg Pediatr.* 2010;6:73–81.

31. Wang D, Zhu F, Fung KM, et al. Predicting cerebral hyperperfusion syndrome following superficial temporal artery to middle cerebral artery bypass based on intraoperative perfusion-weighted magnetic resonance imaging. *Sci Rep.* 2015;5:14140.

32. Wang KC, Phi JH, Lee JY, Kim SK, Cho BK. Indirect revascularization surgery for moyamoya disease in children and its special considerations. *Korean J Pediatr.* 2012;55:408–413.

33. Winn HR, ed. *Youmans and Winn Neurological Surgery.* 7th ed. Philadelphia, PA: Elsevier; 2017.

34. Black S, Enneking FK, Cucchiara RF. Failure to awaken after general anesthesia due to cerebrovascular events. *J Neurosurg Anesthesiol.* 1998;10:10–15.

35. Tzabazis A, Miller C, Dobrow MF, Zheng K, Brock-Utne JG. Delayed emergence after anesthesia. *J Clin Anesth.* 2015;27:353–360.

36. Sahoo S, Kaur M, Sawhney C, Mishra A. An unusual cause of delayed recovery from anesthesia. *J Anaesthesiol Clin Pharmacol.* 2012;28:415–416.

37. Yonekura H, Murayama N, Yamazaki H, Sobue K. A case of delayed emergence after propofol anesthesia: genetic analysis. *A Case Rep.* 2016;7:243–246.

38. Shim KW, Park EK, Kim JS, Kim DS. Cognitive outcome of pediatric moyamoya disease. *J Korean Neurosurg Soc.* 2015;57:440–444.

39. Nagata S, Matsushima T, Morioka T, et al. Unilaterally symptomatic moyamoya disease in children: long-term follow-up of 20 patients. *Neurosurgery.* 2006;59:830–836; discussion 836–837.

33.

NEUROBLASTOMA

Christina Brown and Meredith Kato

STEM CASE AND KEY QUESTIONS

A 19-month-old, 12 kg male child presents for resection of a neuroblastoma arising from his right adrenal gland. Biopsy revealed favorable histology without *MYCN* amplification. His tumor had initially encased his inferior vena cava, crossed the midline and was unresectable. He began treatment with chemotherapy. After 2 cycles, his computed tomography images suggest that the tumor is now amenable to resection. The surgeon wishes to attempt the resection laparoscopically.

WHAT EFFECTS CAN NEOADJUVANT CHEMOTHERAPY HAVE? WHAT SIDE EFFECTS HAVE ANESTHETIC IMPLICATIONS?

Intermediate risk, stage 3 neuroblastoma is commonly treated with a 4-drug regimen including cisplatin, cyclophosphamide, etoposide, and doxorubicin.[1] Each of the 4 drugs causes bone marrow suppression, malaise, anorexia, nausea and vomiting, and alopecia. In addition, cisplatin can cause renal toxicity. This is related to cumulative dose and can be severe. Cyclophosphamide is a plasma cholinesterase inhibitor, which can prolong the duration of succinylcholine. Doxorubicin, an anthracycline, can cause dose-related cardiotoxicity. In the acute phase, this can manifest as arrhythmias, heart block, myocarditis, and pericarditis. With chronic toxicity, it can cause cardiomyopathy with reduced ejection fraction. Both etoposide and cisplatin can cause significant peripheral neuropathy.[2]

The anesthesia plan for a patient with recent chemotherapy must take into consideration the adverse effects of these powerful medications. These children are often neutropenic and are at risk of severe infection. They struggle to maintain nutrition and can be dehydrated from vomiting. The more serious adverse effects require more in-depth review of cardiac and renal function. Underlying pain from peripheral neuropathy can complicate the postoperative pain management strategy.

WHAT PREOPERATIVE INFORMATION WOULD YOU LIKE PRIOR TO STARTING THE CASE?

Taking care of a child with serious systemic disease and receiving oncologic treatment with chemotherapeutic drugs requires careful consideration and planning. It is important to remember that these children might also have common childhood diseases, such as asthma, in addition to their cancer.

As with any anesthetic, start with a careful chart review, history, and physical. Look for problems unrelated to their cancer, allergies, and any information about their developmental milestones and behavior in the healthcare setting.

Determine the location of the tumor and the extent of surgery. Discuss positioning, approach, and likelihood of converting to an open procedure with the surgeon.

As a neuroendocrine tumor, a neuroblastoma can over secrete active substances. Ascertain whether the child is dehydrated as a result of watery diarrhea from over secretion of vasoactive intestinal peptide (VIP). These tumors can also secrete catecholamines causing sweating or hypertension. Children should get urine vanillylmandelic acid and homovanillic acid. While treatment for these disturbances is surgical resection, knowing these effects can modify the anesthetic plan.

Ask about their cancer treatment. How have they done with the treatment protocol? Any neutropenic fever or sepsis? Have they gotten transfusions, and if so, were there any adverse reactions to them? These surgeries can be bloody and an intraoperative transfusion of blood products might be necessary. It is important to know their nutritional status; some kids require supplemental feeding via a nasogastric tube, and some even require parenteral nutrition. Similarly, assess for dehydration. Many kids are dehydrated from vomiting or anorexia; this can be compounded by being nil per os.

It is important to know their baseline pain status. Some children experience pain as a consequence of their chemotherapy and some from the tumor itself. Keep their baseline narcotic usage and preoperative pain in mind when planning intraoperative and postoperative pain management.

Some preoperative laboratory testing is essential to do these cases safely. A hematocrit will help set a maximum allowable blood loss and guide transfusion intraoperatively. Similarly platelet levels are helpful and cannot be obtained quickly from point of care testing in the operating room (OR). While it is rare for an anesthesiologist to diagnose tumor lysis syndrome, a devastating set of metabolic abnormalities from the massive lysis of tumor cells in the setting of chemotherapy, it is nonetheless important to check electrolytes. Abnormalities in potassium, phosphate, and calcium can have serious hemodynamic effects complicating both the intraoperative and postoperative course. Knowing the creatinine can help assess the degree of renal insufficiency due to chemotherapy or, in some cases, from tumor obstruction of the urinary tract.

Finally, a cardiac assessment is useful as a baseline before commencing therapy. Children generally get an electrocardiogram and echocardiogram prior to chemotherapy, but come to the OR during or after treatment. It is important to look at these studies, but it is vital to understand that conduction irregularities and cardiomyopathy may be afoot even with recent reassuring cardiac evaluations. This must be kept in mind throughout the case and postoperative period as transfusions and fluid shifts may unmask previously subtle or subclinical manifestations of cardiac compromise.

WHAT ARE THE POSTOPERATIVE PAIN MANAGEMENT OPTIONS YOU DISCUSS WITH THE PARENTS?

In preparing a postoperative pain management plan following major abdominal surgery, the importance of a multimodal approach cannot be overstated.[3] This is true of any patient, but especially so in the pediatric population, where patients' discomfort may be difficult to ascertain and interpret. It is important to discuss with the family options for regional anesthesia, adjuvant medications such as acetaminophen and nonsteroidal anti-inflammatory drugs and opioid-based therapies. Given the extent of surgery often necessary for resection of neuroblastoma, most patients will need all available modalities to achieve the best outcomes: early extubation, early mobilization, early return to bowel function, reduced length of stay in the intensive care unit, and in the hospital in general. While postoperative pain is generally less following laparoscopic procedures, one must always prepare for the possibility of a conversion to open procedure, especially in surgical oncology where tumors can create a less than totally predictable operative course.

Epidural analgesia combined with general anesthesia carries many benefits for major abdominal surgery in children, even laparoscopic surgery. An epidural decreases the requirement for volatile agent, neuromuscular blockade and intraoperative opioids; it also decreases the stress response to surgery.[4] In the postoperative period, an indwelling epidural catheter can completely obviate the need for intravenous (IV) opiate analgesia. This decrease in the need for narcotics shortens the time to extubation[5,6] and return to bowel function.[7]

It is now considered standard of care to place epidurals in pediatric patients after the induction of general anesthesia. This avoids not only the challenge of placement in a squirming, unhappy child but also avoids the stressful experience, which can do lasting damage to the child's emotional health and trust in the medical establishment. Safety data from the Pediatric Regional Anesthesia Network demonstrates that placement of regional blocks, including neuraxial, is as safe in a patient under general anesthesia as awake.[8]

The rate of complications for regional anesthesia in pediatrics is quite low (0.7%). The complications to keep in mind and to discuss with parents include superficial infection (11%), failed block (2%), vascular puncture (2%), dural puncture (0.9%) with or without a postdural puncture headache,

short-term neurologic sequelae, such as Horner's (0.6%) or paresthesiae (1%) and respiratory complications (0.2%).[9] In general, the complication rate is higher for neonates and infants than for older children.[10] While it is difficult to ascertain the true incidence of rare and devastating events such as epidural hematoma or abscess, it is important to keep them in mind and to include them in conversations about risk with the parents.

The incisions for resection of neuroblastoma, regardless of whether it is a laparoscopic or open procedure, depends upon the size and location of the tumor, additional structures involved in tumor growth, and surgeon preference. There are generally 4 port sites for laparoscopic adrenalectomy, three 5 mm and one 10 mm in the lateral abdomen with the patient in the lateral decubitus position.[11] Preferred open approach can include midline, transverse, bilateral subcostal (chevron), and thoracoabdominal incisions.[11] When planning analgesia for the case and postoperative period, it is important to communicate with the surgeon and ascertain the planned approach. Generally, a midthoracic (T7) epidural will cover the port sites and incision should the case be converted to open.

Occasionally, very large incisions cannot be completely covered by an epidural catheter. It is preferable to get as much benefit from a working epidural even if it is incomplete. One way to handle this situation is to remove any narcotic from the epidural infusion and supplement with IV narcotics. The rationale is that less narcotic is necessary to cover the areas of the incision that are out of reach of the epidural than if IV narcotic was the sole modality.

Contraindications to epidural catheter placement might be relevant in this population. It is important to check platelets and to inquire about coagulopathy. A physical exam will reveal any anatomic abnormality such as a sacral dimple or local infection.

If a narcotic-based strategy is preferred, it is important to take the age and development of the child into consideration as well as the degree of pain expected from the surgery. Patient-controlled analgesia (PCA) is a great way to empower patients to manage their own pain with a safe delivery method. A recent paper demonstrated that even children as young as 5 years of age can safely use a PCA.[12] With toddlers and infants, nurse-controlled analgesia is a safe and effective mode, with or without a basal continuous basal rate.[13] One study looked at nurse-controlled analgesia in infants and found it safe and effective but suggested that fentanyl and hydromorphone might be safer than morphine.[14]

On exam, the patient is thin and pale and has alopecia. He is hysterically anxious. You give a 0.5 mg/kg midazolam oral premedication, and he eventually allows you to pick him up and examine him, but he is still whimpering. You take him back to the OR with the plan for an inhalational induction.

WHAT MONITORS ARE INDICATED FOR THIS PROCEDURE?

These cases tend to be longer, potentially can have high blood loss with incumbent fluid shifts, and can require extensive incisions. As such, they require an endotracheal tube, two large bore IVs, and an arterial line, in addition to standard American Society of Anesthesiologists monitors. Often these children come with a central line placed for chemotherapy administration. This can be used for induction, and the IVs and arterial line can be placed when asleep. Central access is not necessarily required as children rarely need pressors, but they do often need blood transfusions and rapid resuscitation.

The patient is intubated, two 22g IVs, a 22g arterial line, and a midthoracic epidural are placed. The belly is prepped and draped, and after a team pause and antibiotic administration, the abdomen is entered and insufflated.

WHAT ARE THE RISKS OF LAPAROSCOPIC SURGERY IN THE PEDIATRIC POPULATION?

Although laparoscopic surgery offers many potential benefits, including smaller incisions, less pain, and shorter hospital stays,[15] there are several challenges in the pediatric population. The pediatric patient's small size creates unique technical challenges for surgeons attempting to navigate a field already reduced by tumor bulk. Damage to surrounding tissues is more likely given the proximity of other tissues and the relative fragility in the developing patient. These can lead to longer surgical times and increased exposure to general anesthesia.[16] Complications of laparoscopy in children can be as high as 5.8%, but serious complications including bowel, bladder, or great vessel injury are, thankfully, much less frequent at 0.38%.[17] The rates of complications are inversely proportional to operator experience.

Abdominal insufflation causes elevation of intra-abdominal pressure, which results in compression of the thoracic cavity. This leads to higher peak inspiratory pressures, collapse of small airways, ventilation/perfusion mismatch, and potentially hypoxemia. Adequate positive end expiratory pressure along with mild increases in inspired oxygen concentration are typically sufficient to facilitate these procedures.[18]

The cardiovascular effects of abdominal insufflation increase as intra-abdominal pressure increases.[18,19] Low insufflation pressure (5 mmHg) can increase cardiac index, while higher pressures decrease it.[19] Typical recommendations are to maintain intra-abdominal pressure below 10 to 12 mmHg.[18] Higher pressures lead to reduced cardiac output, increased afterload, decreased venous return secondary to inferior vena cava compression, increased systemic vascular resistance, and increased pulmonary vascular resistance.[18] In infants specifically, pneumoperitoneum with an intra-abdominal pressure of 10 mmHg reduced aortic blood flow and stroke volume, although it did not reduce mean arterial pressure.[20] If intra-abdominal pressures above 15 mmHg are required to facilitate surgery, it is generally recommended to convert to an open approach. For patients under 4 months old, intra-abdominal pressure should not exceed 6 mmHg.[20]

Carbon dioxide is the gas of choice for most laparoscopic procedures as it decreases the risk of combustion and of gas embolism. However, CO_2 insufflation increases partial pressure of CO_2 in arterial blood through reduction in minute ventilation and increase in CO_2 absorption.[16,21,22] To compensate, infants, particularly those less than 10 kg, need a disproportionately larger increase in minute ventilation than adults.[16,23] This is limited by concerns for barotrauma and volutrauma, given the higher pressures necessary to compensate for the increased intraperitoneal pressure.[16]

Insufflation of CO_2 leads to high flows of dry, cold CO_2 into the peritoneum, which can lead to hypothermia through evaporative heat loss.[16,24] Smaller patients are far more sensitive to this heat loss than their adult counterparts.[16]

Abdominal insufflation can increase intracranial pressure.[18] It can also lead to decreased renal blood flow, renal function, and urine output through direct pressure on the renal parenchyma and reductions in cardiac output. Direct compression and resultant decreased blood flow leads to compensatory upregulation of the renin-angiotensin-aldosterone system, which further contributes to oliguria in these patients despite adequate fluid resuscitation. For this reason, careful attention must be paid to fluid balance in these procedures.[25]

WHAT IS THE CONTROVERSY OF LAPAROSCOPIC RESECTION IN NEUROBLASTOMA?

Many high-quality studies demonstrate the surgical benefits and oncologic safety of laparoscopy in a variety of abdominal malignancies in adults.[26–29] In contrast, there is a relative paucity of data for a laparoscopic approach to abdominal or retroperitoneal malignancies in children.[30] There has been some headway in the laparoscopic resection of well-encapsulated tumors such as Wilm's tumors.[31] However, neuroblastomas are generally not well encapsulated and are thus less amenable,[32] especially if they are invasive into vital structures. The International Neuroblastoma Risk Group classification identifies image-defined risk factors that aid in pretreatment risk stratification and surgical planning.[33] With this classification in mind, Shirota et al.[34] compare open versus laparoscopic approach in 16 patients without image-defined risk factors. Patients receiving a laparoscopic approach have a significantly shorter time to meal consumption and less blood loss but see no differences in operative time, disease recurrence, or survival. While this is encouraging, laparoscopy for neuroblastoma remains controversial and, as such, is surgeon and institution dependent.

After an hour of careful dissection, the surgeon says, "I'm in the cava." He is handed a scalpel, and he opens and packs the abdomen.

WHAT ARE SOME GUIDELINES FOR BLOOD TRANSFUSION DURING PEDIATRIC SURGERY?

Surgical bleeding in the pediatric population can be a challenge. Children begin with smaller blood volumes and can reach a critical blood loss very quickly. The maximum allowable blood loss can be calculated ahead of time, which can guide the decision to administer products. However, if the surgeon communicates a situation of immediate and significant blood loss, it is better to transfuse rather than wait for a predetermined threshold to be reached.

A suggested dose for a transfusion of blood for a pediatric patient starts with 10 mL/kg of packed red cells per dose. This can be expected to raise the hematocrit by 3% to 6%. If multiple doses are expected to be given, it is recommended to administer plasma and platelets in a 1:1:1 ratio to prevent a dilutional coagulopathy. Doses should be administered through tubing that includes a 170 to 260 micron filter to eliminate small clots and should be flushed in with normal saline. Citrate used to prevent coagulation in stored blood binds calcium[35] and should not be given with calcium containing fluids, such as lactated Ringer's, in the same line. Warming the blood is very important if the blood is to be given rapidly. Chilled blood can cause hypothermia, which can, in turn, worsen a coagulopathy.

Rapid or high-volume transfusion can have significant metabolic effects. Chilled blood contains a high proportion of potassium, which can reach dangerous levels rapidly.[36] During a resuscitation, blood and fluids should be run through a warmer. Hypocalcemia resulting from citrate in blood should be monitored and replaced as needed. Citrate metabolism also results in the production of CO_2, which can result in a metabolic acidosis if minute volume is not increased to compensate.[37]

Transfusion in immunocompromised patients does put them at increased risk of graft versus host disease (GVHD), where donor leukocytes proliferate within and attack the recipient. It is usually fatal. This risk can be mitigated by the use of irradiated blood. Irradiation prevents the proliferation of donor leukocytes within the recipient and drastically reduces the incidence of GVHD.[38,39]

The surgeon obtains control of the bleeding quickly; you give only 1 dose of 10 mL/kg of packed red cells. The rest of the case goes uneventfully. The surgeons feel that they have gotten all of the tumor (R0 resection). They close. The case lasted 4 hours.

DO YOU EXTUBATE? WHAT ARE THE FACTORS THAT GO INTO YOUR DECISION?

The risk of airway complications is higher in the pediatric population, especially during induction and emergence from anesthesia and increases with decreasing age.[40–43] The adult literature suggests multiple explanations for the increased risk surrounding extubation after emergence from general anesthesia including exaggerated, reduced, or dysfunctional airway reflexes; reduced oxygen stores after extubation; airway injury; and human factors, all of which apply to the pediatric patient. It is important to have a postextubation plan in place, should the patient need assistance or reintubation.[44]

As with any patient, assessment of airway risk, adequate oxygenation, adequate ventilation, sufficient reversal of neuromuscular blockade, cardiovascular stability, and normothermia must all be completed. For patients who have had long, open abdominal surgery and received large volume resuscitation, third spacing of fluids may lead to laryngeal edema. This must be taken into account along with ongoing resuscitation needs in the postoperative period. In addition, the endotracheal tube should be checked for a cuff leak prior to removal.

You extubate and take the patient to the recovery area. Upon arrival he is thrashing around, you struggle to prevent him from pulling out all of his lines.

WHAT ARE THE RISK FACTORS FOR EMERGENCE DELIRIUM?

Emergence delirium is characterized as hypersensitivity, disorientation, averted or closed eyes, and nonresponsivity in a patient who is acutely recovering from the effects of general anesthesia.[45] The incidence is not well characterized and ranges from 10% to 80% depending on the type of anesthetic and the metric used.[45,46] The cause of emergence delirium remains unclear. Risk factors include exposure to volatile anesthetics, particularly sevoflurane and desflurane, pain, male sex, preschool age, previous emergence delirium, preoperative anxiety, and ophthalmologic or otolaryngology surgery.[46,47]

WHAT ARE THE OPTIONS FOR TREATMENT?

Small boluses of propofol (1mg/kg), fentanyl (1 mcg/kg), or dexmedetomidine (0.5mcg/kg) have been used successfully to treat emergence delirium in children.[48–52] Minimizing risk factors can help to prevent emergence delirium. This includes decreasing preoperative anxiety and ensuring adequate pain control. In addition, propofol and dexmedetomidine given prior to emergence can reduce the incidence of delirium in the recovery area.[49,53]

With treatment the patient improves. He is transferred to the floor and does well. He is discharged after 7 days.

DISCUSSION

EPIDEMIOLOGY AND PATHOGENESIS

Neuroblastoma is a relatively common cancer of childhood, affecting 650 children in the United States per year. Neuroblastomas are by far the most common cancer in infants with an incidence almost double that of leukemia. It accounts for 7.8% of all childhood cancers with an annual incidence of 9.5 per million children in the United States. The last epidemiological data representing the period 1975 to 1995 indicate that this incidence is stable. Neuroblastoma accounts for 15% of cancer-related deaths in children. There are no differences by sex or race for neuroblastoma.[54]

The etiology of neuroblastoma is unknown. However, the high incidence of infantile or even fetal cases begs an in utero explanation. Some maternal antepartum risk factors have been identified and include opiate, especially codeine, consumption[55]; folate deficiency[56]; and gestational diabetes.[57] In addition, there are some patient risk factors. Children diagnosed with neuroblastoma are more likely to have congenital abnormalities[57] or have been born at an extreme size (either large or small) for gestational age.[58] Syndromes associated with neuroblastoma include Kinsbourne, Aase-Smith,

Kunze-Riehm, Ondine, Rubinson-Taybi,[59] neurofibromatosis type I,[60] neurocristopathy,[61] and Weaver.[62] The vast majority of cases have no identifiable risk factor.

Neuroblastoma arises from primitive neural crest cells. They can arise anywhere along the sympathetic nervous system chain; 30% to 40% arise from the adrenal medulla, and the remainder from the parasympathetic ganglia, primarily in the abdomen. Neuroblastomas are biologically heterogenous with a wide range of clinical behavior. The primitive stage of the malignant transformation of the cells and the disparate pathways of their differentiation account for the heterogeneity of this disease. The genetics are complicated. There is no common genomic alteration, loss of heterozygocity, or genetic translocation specific to neuroblastoma, and there are few gene mutations that offer clues. *MYCN* oncogene amplification identifies an aggressive subset of tumors and is found in 20% of cases. *ALK* mutations are near-ubiquitous in familial neuroblastoma, which accounts for less than 1% of cases.[63]

CLINICAL MANIFESTATIONS

The clinical presentation of patients depends largely on where in the sympathetic chain the tumor arises and the extent of growth at presentation. The presentation is widely variable. Children often present with abdominal or pelvic masses that are either picked up on physical exam in the primary setting or during a workup for symptoms caused by mass effect, such as constipation or enuresis.[64] The vena cava is commonly involved due to its course close to the sympathetic chain. This can lead to congestion and edema of the upper or lower extremities.[65] Thoracic tumors can cause respiratory symptoms. These tumors can also extend into the mediastinum, causing tracheal deviation or compression. Cervical masses can cause Horner's syndrome.[66] Some children present with emergent spinal cord compression if the tumor moves centrally from the sympathetic chain.[67]

Some neuroblastomas are associated with paraneoplastic syndromes leading to symptoms that bring the child in for assessment. Neuroblastomas commonly secrete catecholamines and can cause hypertension, tachycardia, and, in rare and extreme cases, cardiomyopathy and heart failure.[68] Some tumors secrete VIP causing watery diarrhea, dehydration, and electrolyte disturbances.[69] Patients with opsoclonus-myoclonus syndrome present with rapid, multidirectional eye movements, ataxia, and behavioral changes. A full 50% of these kids have occult neuroblastoma. These symptoms are thought to be immune-mediated.[70]

DIFFERENTIAL

The differential diagnosis is wide and depends on where the tumor is located. Indeed, neuroblastoma must be distinguished from pretty much all other solid tumors, especially Wilm's, germ cell tumors, and Ewing's sarcoma. It can also mimic the presentation of lymphoma with a mediastinal mass and must be distinguished from leukemia if discovered on bone marrow aspirate.

DIAGNOSIS

Neuroblastoma must be proven by biopsy. Workup for the extent of disease and treatment planning includes imaging, usually computed tomography scan or magnetic resonance imaging, bone marrow aspirate to evaluate for metastatic disease, and laboratory work. This latter should include not only basics like blood count, electrolytes, liver panel, blood urea nitrogen, and creatinine but also the metabolites of catecholamines, urine vanillylmandelic acid, and homovanillic acid. VIP should be measured if the child has diarrhea. Metaiodobenzylguanidine scanning is helpful in measuring response to treatment.[71]

TREATMENT

Treatment depends on age of the patient, stage of disease, and histology of the tumor. In general, treatment algorithms include chemotherapy, surgery, and radiation.

Low-risk patients are often treated with surgery alone or are simply observed. The survival in this group is 97%. Intermediate-risk patients, similar to the patient presented in the case, are usually treated with low-dose chemotherapy to reduce the tumor burden and make it surgically resectable. Surgery is followed by ongoing chemotherapy. High-risk patients are treated aggressively adding radiation and myeloablative therapy with stem cell transplantation to chemotherapy and surgery. The chemotherapeutic regimens include some combination of etoposide, carboplatin, cyclophosphamide, vincristine, and doxorubicin.[72–74]

PROGNOSIS

The prognosis for patients with neuroblastoma varies based on multiple factors. Age, stage at diagnosis, histopathology of the tumor, and tumor genetics all play a role in patient prognosis.[75] Infants with neuroblastoma tend to have more favorable tumor characteristics and have a 5-year survival rate of 83%. Older children tend to get more aggressive tumors, and their survival is only 55% at 5 years. In general, children with resectable tumors have better cure rates and long-term outcomes than those with unresectable disease.[76] For those with unresectable disease, tumor cell and genetic factors play a larger role in prognosis and can be used to stratify risk.[77] In general, *MYCN* amplification confers a worse prognosis. However, a retrospective study of 118 patients showed that tumors expressing *MYCN* appeared to have a dichotomy in outcomes, either excellent or very poor, while those patients with tumors that did not express *MYCN* lacked this dichotomy.[78] Database studies have shown improved outcomes of patients with hyperdiploid tumors compared with diploid tumors.[79]

ANESTHETIC IMPLICATIONS

Children diagnosed with neuroblastoma, especially intermediate or high risk, spend a great deal of time in the hospital often in a tertiary care center far from home. They tend to need procedures, surgery, and imaging multiple times during their treatment course and are often well known to members of the anesthesia team. As "frequent flyers," these patients are extremely vulnerable emotionally, as are their caregivers. As such, it is critical that their experience be as pleasant and supportive as possible.

The children who require the most aggressive care are usually toddlers, as infants generally fare better and are often categorized as low risk. The tender age and specific developmental challenges of the higher risk patients present unique challenges to the anesthesia teams. Understanding their developmental stage and level of fatigue with their treatment is critical in taking good care of these patients.

Patients need sedation and anesthesia at every stage of their care, from their initial imaging scans, bone marrow aspirates, and major abdominal surgery all the way to daily radiation treatments and, hopefully, the removal of their central access when clear of disease. It is important to understand where they are in their treatment and the risks during each phase.

When the diagnosis is still unclear the greatest risk lies in the unknown. Imaging requires patients to lie flat and be sedated. Occult mediastinal masses must be considered. When chemotherapy begins, these children feel terrible and can have trouble maintaining nutrition due to vomiting and anorexia. Neutropenia puts them at risk of sepsis, and aseptic technique, especially with central lines, must be maintained.

The resection surgeries are often long cases as the tumors are poorly encapsulated and invasive to local structures. Their vascular nature and proximity to the vena cava can lead to heavy blood loss. Cases should be done with an arterial line, large bore access, and blood at the ready. Patients often spend a day or two in the acute setting sedated and intubated as they grapple with the fluid shifts related to their surgery and blood administration. An aggressive, multimodal approach to pain management in the first postoperative days is critical to early extubation, resolution of ileus, and mobility.

The road for these patients is long. It is fraught with complications of treatment. Each victory is hard-won, and each setback, devastating. Anesthesia teams play important roles at critical times in their treatment. Attention not only to the medically challenging aspects but also the emotional fragility of the families is critical to success in the treatment of this difficult and complicated disease.

CONCLUSIONS

- Neuroblastoma is a common childhood cancer. With surgery being an important treatment modality, anesthesiologists must be familiar with this disease.

- These children often come to the OR following neoadjuvant chemotherapy. The side effects of these medications must be factored into any anesthetic plan.

- Neuroblastoma tumors tend to be poorly encapsulated, making them harder to resect. These cases can be notable for large blood losses and fluid shifts.

- Risks of insufflation for laparoscopic surgery include collapse of smaller airways, reduced cardiac output, reduced renal blood flow, and hypercarbia.

- While laparoscopic resection of neuroblastoma is controversial, it does improve postoperative pain, ileus, time to extubation, and length of stay. Patient selection is key.

- Toddlers coming to the OR are at higher risk for emergence delirium. Limiting other risk factors, such as preoperative anxiety and postoperative pain can reduce the incidence.

- Postoperative pain management must be multimodal. Epidural catheter-delivered local anesthesia and PCA or nurse-delivered analgesia should be strongly considered.

REVIEW QUESTIONS

1. You are caring for a 27-month-old female undergoing laparoscopic excision of an adrenal neuroblastoma. The surgeon insufflates the belly, and your ventilator begins to alarm with high peak inspiratory pressures. You also note high plateau pressure. What is the **BEST** next step in management?

    A. Ask for reduction of insufflation.
    B. Increase respiratory rate.
    C. inhaled bronchodilator treatment
    D. needle decompression of chest

Answer: A
The increase in peak pressure in this patient is likely related to increased intra-abdominal pressure secondary to abdominal insufflation. Care must be taken to ensure insufflation pressures do not exceed 15 mmHg. Pneumothorax would be a less likely cause of this sudden increase in respiratory pressures, although it is in the differential. Bronchospasm causes increased peak pressures without changes in plateau pressures. Increasing the respiratory rate may further increase peak pressure.

2. You are caring for a 13-month-old patient undergoing laparoscopic resection of an adrenal mass. The surgeon is having difficulty with visualization of the mass and requests that the insufflation pressures be increased to 17 mmHg from 14 mmHg. The patient's blood pressure decreases to 65/32 mmHg. What is the next **BEST** step in management?

    A. Administer 1 L fluid bolus.
    B. Convert to open laparotomy.
    C. No intervention is necessary.
    D. Treat with norepinephrine.

Answer: B
The abdominal insufflation pressures required to facilitate surgical exposure are too high in this patient. For young children, insufflation pressure should not exceed 15 mmHg and should ideally be kept below 10 mmHg. Pressors may help temporarily; however, the best and quickest solution to this problem would be to reduce the intra-abdominal pressure and convert

to an open procedure. A fluid bolus of 1 liter is excessive and dangerous for a child of this age.

3. A 20-month-old male is induced uneventfully for open laparotomy for neuroblastoma resection. He is placed into lateral decubitus position for epidural catheter placement, which proceeds uneventfully. Test dose is administered, and no tachycardia is noted. Local anesthetic infusion is started, and shortly after administration he becomes profoundly hypotensive and bradycardic. What is the next **BEST** step in management?

    A. Administer glycopyrrolate.
    B. Increase epidural infusion rate.
    C. Remove the catheter and check for a pulse.
    D. Stop IV fluid administration.

Answer: C
The catheter is likely intrathecal, causing a high spinal block. Treatment is supportive and includes initiation of pediatric advanced life support, IV fluids, ephedrine, and slight Trendelenburg position. Increasing the rate of local anesthetic administration would worsen this problem. While glycopyrrolate will likely help the bradycardia, atropine is in the pediatric advanced life support algorithm.

4. A 27-month-old male presents for resection of adrenal neuroblastoma. He has been receiving cisplatin, cyclophosphamide, etoposide, and doxorubicin for tumor size reduction. What preoperative testing would be **MOST** helpful to evaluate this patient?

    A. C-reactive protein
    B. electrocardiogram
    C. pulmonary function testing
    D. renal ultrasound

Answer: B
Doxorubicin may cause myocardial damage, leading to conduction defects and cardiomyopathy. It has not been shown to cause pulmonary or renal abnormalities. C-reactive protein is nonspecific and will likely not alter management for this patient. Cisplatin does have renal toxicity, but an ultrasound would not rule this out or offer management guidance.

5. Which of the following is the **MOST** likely benefit of laparoscopic technique over open technique for abdominal surgery in children?

    A. better surgical visualization
    B. less hemodynamic instability
    C. shorter operative time
    D. shorter time to first meal

Answer: D
A laparoscopic approach may potentially lead to greater hemodynamic instability due to the effects of abdominal insufflation on cardiac output and ventilation/perfusion mismatch. Laparoscopic cases tend to take longer, and visualization may be more difficult. However, multiple studies have shown a shorter time to first meal in patients undergoing laparoscopic versus open abdominal surgery.

6. A 23-month-old female arrives for resection of neuroblastoma. She has received neoadjuvant chemotherapy, is anemic, and is extremely anxious. Which of the following will **MOST** likely increases the risk for difficulty with intubation?

    A. age over 1 year
    B. chemotherapy-induced vomiting
    C. cisplatin toxicity
    D. mediastinal tumor

Answer: D
Cisplatin is associated with renal toxicity but has not been associated with difficulty in airway management or changes in airway anatomy. The incidence of a difficult airway is higher in neonates and infants than in toddlers. Vomiting increases the chance of aspiration but not a difficult airway. Tumor encasement of the trachea can distort airway anatomy and may contribute to difficulty with intubation.

7. After an uneventful anesthetic, your 3-year old patient is screaming after extubation. He is disoriented and pulling at his lines. What is the **BEST** next step in management of his emergence delirium?

    A. Decrease anxiety with IV lorazepam.
    B. Reinduce with mask and sevoflurane.
    C. Sedate with IV dexmedetomidine.
    D. Treat disorientation IV haloperidol.

Answer: B
Propofol, dexmedetomidine, and opioids have all been successfully used to treat or prevent emergence delirium. Volatile anesthetics increase the risk of emergence delirium. Benzodiazepines are controversial as they can exacerbate emergence delirium. Haloperidol is not recommended to treat emergence delirium in children.

8. You are discussing the risks and benefits of an epidural catheter with the parents of a 3 year-old who presents for an abdominal neuroblastoma resection. Which of the following is the **MOST** common complication?

    A. block failure
    B. epidural hematoma
    C. Horner's syndrome
    D. postdural puncture headache

Answer: A
The most common complications of regional anesthesia in pediatric anesthesia are superficial infection (11%), failed block (2%), vascular puncture (2%), dural puncture (0.9%) with or without a postdural puncture headache, short-term neurologic sequelae such as Horner's (0.6%) or paresthesiae (1%), and respiratory complications (0.2%). Epidural hematoma and abscess are quite rare, but it is important to keep them in mind and to include them in conversations about risk with the parents.

9. You are waking up a 2-year-old patient from a general anesthetic with sevoflurane maintenance. Which of the following is the **GREATEST** risk factor for emergence delirium?

    A. abdominal surgery

B. catheter in the hand

C. glycopyrrolate use

D. preoperative anxiety

Answer: D

Preoperative anxiety, postoperative pain, the presence of a urinary catheter, and the administration of atropine have all been associated with emergence delirium or agitation. Otolaryngology surgeries such as tonsillectomy, adenoidectomy, or myringotomy tubes and ophthalmologic procedures such as strabismus surgery have been associated with emergence delirium. Abdominal surgeries do not carry additional risk. Glycopyrrolate does not cross the blood–brain barrier and is not associated with postoperative delirium in children. Children with emergence delirium will often pull out IVs placed in the hand, but they do not increase the risk.

10. Which of the following statements is the **MOST** accurate regarding blood transfusion in a child?

A. Acute hemolytic reactions are the leading cause of transfusion related death in children.

B. GVHD risk can be lowered by transfusing irradiated blood.

C. Transfusion-associated circulatory overload (TACO) is more common in children.

D. Transfusion-associated lung injury (TRALI) can occur up to 2 days after transfusion.

Answer: B

While TACO can occur in children, it is much more common in adults. TRALI, heralded by dyspnea, pulmonary edema, hypotension, and fever, occurs within 6 hours of completion of a transfusion. TRALI, not hemolytic reaction, is the leading cause of transfusion-related mortality. GVHD risk can be curtailed by administering irradiated blood.

QUESTIONS AND ANSWERS

This chapter has accompanying questions and answers which are available to subscribers as part of the Oxford eLearning platform. To access the questions, go to ✅ http://oxfordmedicine. com/pediatricanesthesiaPBL

REFERENCES

1. Matthay KK, Perez C, Seeger RC, et al. Successful treatment of stage III neuroblastoma based on prospective biologic staging: a Children's Cancer Group study. *J Clin Oncol.* 1998;16(4):1256–1264.

2. *Lexicomp.* http://online.lexi.com/lco/action/home. Accessed February 2017.

3. Chou R, Gordon DB, de Leon-Casasola OA, et al. Management of postoperative pain: a clinical practice guideline from the American Pain Society, the American Society of Regional Anesthesia and Pain Medicine, and the American Society of Anesthesiologists' Committee on Regional Anesthesia, Executive Committee, and Administrative Council. *J Pain.* 2016;17(2):131–157.

4. Goeller JK, Bhalla T, Tobias JD. Combined use of neuraxial and general anesthesia during major abdominal procedures in neonates and infants. *Paediatr Anaesth.* 2014;24(6):553–560.

5. McNeely JK, et al. Epidural analgesia improves outcome following pediatric fundoplication: a retrospective analysis. *Reg Anesth.* 1997;22(1):16–23.

6. Raghavan M, Montgomerie J. Anesthetic management of gastrochisis—a review of our practice over the past 5 years. *Paediatr Anaesth.* 2008;18(11):1055–1059.

7. Michelet D, et al. Factors affecting recovery of postoperative bowel function after pediatric laparoscopic surgery. *J Anaesthesiol Clin Pharmacol.* 2016;32(3):369–375.

8. Taenzer AH, et al. Asleep versus awake: does it matter? Pediatric regional block complications by patient state: a report from the Pediatric Regional Anesthesia Network. *Reg Anesth Pain Med.* 2014;39(4):279–283.

9. Polaner DM, et al. Pediatric Regional Anesthesia Network (PRAN): a multi-institutional study of the use and incidence of complications of pediatric regional anesthesia. *Anesth Analg.* 2012;115(6):1353–1364.

10. Wong GK, et al. Major complications related to epidural analgesia in children: a 15-year audit of 3,152 epidurals. *Can J Anaesth.* 2013;60(4):355–363.

11. Long E, Chung DH. Neuroblastoma. In: Ziegler MM, von Allmen D, Weber TR, eds. *Operative Pediatric Surgery.* 2nd ed. New York: McGraw Hill Education; 2014:1187–1197.

12. Faerber J, et al. Comparative safety of morphine delivered via intravenous route vs. patient-controlled analgesia device for pediatric inpatients. *J Pain Symptom Manage.* 2017;53(5):842–850.

13. Howard RF, et al. Nurse-controlled analgesia (NCA) following major surgery in 10,000 patients in a children's hospital. *Paediatr Anaesth.* 2010;20(2):126–134.

14. Walia H, et al. Safety and efficacy of nurse-controlled analgesia in patients less than 1 year of age. *J Pain Res.* 2016;9:385–390.

15. Mattei P. Minimally invasive surgery in the diagnosis and treatment of abdominal pain in children. *Curr Opin Pediatr.* 2007;19(3):338–343.

16. Blinman T, Ponsky T. Pediatric minimally invasive surgery: laparoscopy and thoracoscopy in infants and children. *Pediatrics.* 2012;130(3):539–549.

17. Peters CA. Complications in pediatric urological laparoscopy: results of a survey. *J Urol.* 1996;155(3):1070–1073.

18. Wedgewood J, Doyle E. Anaesthesia and laparoscopic surgery in children. *Paediatr Anaesth.* 2001;11(4):391–399.

19. De Waal EE, Kalkman CJ. Haemodynamic changes during low-pressure carbon dioxide pneumoperitoneum in young children. *Paediatr Anaesth.* 2003;13(1):18–25.

20. Gueugniaud PY, et al. The hemodynamic effects of pneumoperitoneum during laparoscopic surgery in healthy infants: assessment by continuous esophageal aortic blood flow echo-Doppler. *Anesth Analg.* 1998;86(2):290–293.

21. Sanders JC, Gerstein N. Arterial to endtidal carbon dioxide gradient during pediatric laparoscopic fundoplication. *Paediatr Anaesth.* 2008;18(11):1096–1101.

22. Liu SY, et al. Prospective analysis of cardiopulmonary responses to laparoscopic cholecystectomy. *J Laparoendosc Surg.* 1991;1(5):241–246.

23. McHoney M, et al. Carbon dioxide elimination during laparoscopy in children is age dependent. *J Pediatr Surg.* 2003;38(1):105–110.

24. Ott DE. Laparoscopic hypothermia. *J Laparoendosc Surg.* 1991;1(3):127–131.

25. Sodha S, et al. Effect of pneumoperitoneum on renal function and physiology in patients undergoing robotic renal surgery. *Curr Urol.* 2016;9(1):1–4.

26. Clinical Outcomes of Surgical Therapy Study Group, et al. A comparison of laparoscopically assisted and open colectomy for colon cancer. *N Engl J Med.* 2004;350(20):2050–2059.

27. Guillou PJ, et al. Short-term endpoints of conventional versus laparoscopic-assisted surgery in patients with colorectal cancer (MRC CLASICC trial): multicentre, randomised controlled trial. *Lancet.* 2005;365(9472):1718–1726.

28. Cai J, et al. A prospective randomized study comparing open versus laparoscopy-assisted D2 radical gastrectomy in advanced gastric cancer. *Dig Surg.* 2011;28(5–6):331–337.

29. Croome KP, et al. Total laparoscopic pancreaticoduodenectomy for pancreatic ductal adenocarcinoma: oncologic advantages over open approaches? *Ann Surg.* 2014;260(4):633–638; discussion 638–640.

30. de Lijster MS, et al. Minimally invasive surgery versus open surgery for the treatment of solid abdominal and thoracic neoplasms in children. *Cochrane Database Syst Rev.* 2010;3:CD008403.

31. Duarte RJ, et al. Laparoscopic nephrectomy for Wilms' tumor. *Expert Rev Anticancer Ther.* 2009;9(6):753–761.

32. Miller KA, et al. Experience with laparoscopic adrenalectomy in pediatric patients. *J Pediatr Surg.* 2002;37(7):979–982.

33. Monclair T, et al. The International Neuroblastoma Risk Group (INRG) staging system: an INRG Task Force report. *J Clin Oncol.* 2009;27(2):298–303.

34. Shirota C, et al. Laparoscopic resection of neuroblastomas in low- to high-risk patients without image-defined risk factors is safe and feasible. *BMC Pediatr.* 2017;17(1):71.

35. Yendt ER. Citrate intoxication. *Can Med Assoc J.* 1957;76(2):141–144.

36. Brown KA, et al. Hyperkalaemia during massive blood transfusion in paediatric craniofacial surgery. *Can J Anaesth.* 1990;37(4 Pt 1):401–408.

37. Li K, Xu Y. Citrate metabolism in blood transfusions and its relationship due to metabolic alkalosis and respiratory acidosis. *Int J Clin Exp Med.* 2015;8(4):6578–6584.

38. Roseff SD, Luban NL, Manno CS. Guidelines for assessing appropriateness of pediatric transfusion. *Transfusion.* 2002;42(11):1398–1413.

39. Pelszynski MM, et al. Effect of gamma irradiation of red blood cell units on T-cell inactivation as assessed by limiting dilution analysis: implications for preventing transfusion-associated graft-versus-host disease. *Blood.* 1994;83(6):1683–1689.

40. Bordet F, et al. Risk factors for airway complications during general anaesthesia in paediatric patients. *Paediatr Anaesth.* 2002;12(9):762–769.

41. Tiret L, et al. Complications related to anaesthesia in infants and children. A prospective survey of 40240 anaesthetics. *Br J Anaesth.* 1988;61(3):263–269.

42. Olsson GL. Bronchospasm during anaesthesia. A computer-aided incidence study of 136,929 patients. *Acta Anaesthesiol Scand.* 1987;31(3):244–252.

43. Cohen MM, Cameron CB. Should you cancel the operation when a child has an upper respiratory tract infection? *Anesth Analg.* 1991;72(3):282–288.

44. Difficult Airway Society Extubation Guidelines Group, et al. Difficult Airway Society Guidelines for the management of tracheal extubation. *Anaesthesia.* 2012;67(3):318–340.

45. Malarbi S, et al. Characterizing the behavior of children emerging with delirium from general anesthesia. *Paediatr Anaesth.* 2011;21(9):942–950.

46. Dahmani S, Delivet H, Hilly J. Emergence delirium in children: an update. *Curr Opin Anaesthesiol.* 2014;27(3):309–315.

47. Voepel-Lewis T, Malviya S, Tait AR. A prospective cohort study of emergence agitation in the pediatric postanesthesia care unit. *Anesth Analg.* 2003;96(6):1625–1630.

48. Hauber JA, et al. Dexmedetomidine as a rapid bolus for treatment and prophylactic prevention of emergence agitation in anesthetized children. *Anesth Analg.* 2015;121(5):1308–1315.

49. Makkar JK, et al. A comparison of single dose dexmedetomidine with propofol for the prevention of emergence delirium after desflurane anaesthesia in children. *Anaesthesia.* 2016;71(1):50–57.

50. van Hoff SL, et al. Does a prophylactic dose of propofol reduce emergence agitation in children receiving anesthesia? A systematic review and meta-analysis. *Paediatr Anaesth.* 2015;25(7):668–676.

51. Costi D, et al. Transition to propofol after sevoflurane anesthesia to prevent emergence agitation: a randomized controlled trial. *Paediatr Anaesth.* 2015;25(5):517–523.

52. Lee JR, et al. Comparison of propofol and fentanyl for preventing emergence agitation in children. *Br J Anaesth.* 2013;111(1):121–122.

53. Dahmani S, et al. Pharmacological prevention of sevoflurane- and desflurane-related emergence agitation in children: a meta-analysis of published studies. *Br J Anaesth.* 2010;104(2):216–223.

54. Goodman MT, Gurney, JG, Smith MA, Olshan AF. Sympathetic nervous system tumors. In: Ries L, Smith, MA, Gurney, JG, et al., eds. *Cancer Incidence and Survival among Children and Adolescents: United States SEER Program, 1975–1995.* Bethesda, MD: National Cancer Institute; 1999:65–72.

55. Cook MN, et al. Maternal medication use and neuroblastoma in offspring. *Am J Epidemiol.* 2004;159(8):721–731.

56. Olshan AF, et al. Maternal vitamin use and reduced risk of neuroblastoma. *Epidemiology.* 2002;13(5):575–580.

57. Chow EJ, Friedman DL, Mueller BA. Maternal and perinatal characteristics in relation to neuroblastoma. *Cancer.* 2007;109(5):983–992.

58. Rios P, et al. Risk of neuroblastoma, birth-related characteristics, congenital malformations and perinatal exposures: a pooled analysis of the ESCALE and ESTELLE French studies (SFCE). *Int J Cancer.* 2016;139(9):1936–1948.

59. Bissonnette B, Luginbuehl I, Marciniak B, Dalens BJ, eds. *Syndromes: Rapid Recognition and Perioperative Implications.* New York: McGraw-Hill Education, 2006.

60. Varan A, et al. Neurofibromatosis type 1 and malignancy in childhood. *Clin Genet.* 2016;89(3):341–345.

61. Nemecek ER, Sawin RW, Park J. Treatment of neuroblastoma in patients with neurocristopathy syndromes. *J Pediatr Hematol Oncol.* 2003;25(2):159–162.

62. Coulter D, Powell CM, Gold S. Weaver syndrome and neuroblastoma. *J Pediatr Hematol Oncol.* 2008;30(10):758–760.

63. Louis CU, Shohet JM. Neuroblastoma: molecular pathogenesis and therapy. *Annu Rev Med.* 2015;66:49–63.

64. Golden CB, Feusner JH. Malignant abdominal masses in children: quick guide to evaluation and diagnosis. *Pediatr Clin North Am.* 2002;49(6):1369–1392.

65. Ingram L, Rivera GK, Shapiro DN. Superior vena cava syndrome associated with childhood malignancy: analysis of 24 cases. *Med Pediatr Oncol.* 1990;18(6):476–481.

66. Pollard ZF, et al. Atypical acquired pediatric Horner syndrome. *Arch Ophthalmol.* 2010;128(7):937–940.

67. Trahair T, Sorrentino S, Russell SJ, et al. Spinal canal involvement in neuroblastoma. *J Pediatr.* 2017;188:294–298.

68. Carlson P, et al. Refractory dilated cardiomyopathy associated with metastatic neuroblastoma. *Pediatr Blood Cancer.* 2010;55(4):736–738.

69. Funato M, et al. Rapid changes of serum vasoactive intestinal peptide after removal of ganglioneuroblastoma with watery-diarrhea-hypokalemia-achlorhydria syndrome in a child. *J Pediatr Gastroenterol Nutr.* 1982;1(1):131–135.

70. Brunklaus A, et al. Investigating neuroblastoma in childhood opsoclonus-myoclonus syndrome. *Arch Dis Child.* 2012;97(5):461–463.

71. Brodeur GM, et al. Revisions of the international criteria for neuroblastoma diagnosis, staging, and response to treatment. *J Clin Oncol.* 1993;11(8):1466–1477.

72. *Neuroblastoma Treatment (PDQ(R)): Health Professional Version.* PDQ Cancer Information Summaries. Bethesda, MD: National Cancer Institute; 2002.

73. Strother DR, et al. Outcome after surgery alone or with restricted use of chemotherapy for patients with low-risk neuroblastoma: results of Children's Oncology Group Study P9641. *J Clin Oncol.* 2012;30(15):1842–1848.

74. Evans AE, et al. Successful management of low-stage neuroblastoma without adjuvant therapies: a comparison of two decades, 1972 through 1981 and 1982 through 1992, in a single institution. *J Clin Oncol.* 1996;14(9):2504–2510.

75. Bagatell R, et al. Outcomes of children with intermediate-risk neuroblastoma after treatment stratified by MYCN status and tumor cell ploidy. *J Clin Oncol.* 2005;23(34):8819–8827.

76. Owens C, Irwin M. Neuroblastoma: the impact of biology and cooperation leading to personalized treatments. *Crit Rev Clin Lab Sci.* 2012;49(3):85–115.

77. Sridhar S, et al. New insights into the genetics of neuroblastoma. *Mol Diagn Ther*. 2013;17(2):63–69.

78. Kushner BH, et al. Striking dichotomy in outcome of MYCN-amplified neuroblastoma in the contemporary era. *Cancer*. 2014;120(13):2050–2059.

79. Bagatell R, et al. Significance of MYCN amplification in international neuroblastoma staging system stage 1 and 2 neuroblastoma: a report from the International Neuroblastoma Risk Group database. *J Clin Oncol*. 2009;27(3):365–370.

34.

MYOTONIC DYSTROPHY

Andrea Johnson

STEM CASE AND KEY QUESTIONS

Jase is a 10-year-old boy referred for preoperative evaluation by an anesthesiologist for a muscle biopsy recommended by his pediatrician. His adoptive parents have brought him in today and have limited medical information regarding his biologic parents, but they do note that Jase's biologic mother had some "muscular" problems.

WHAT ARE THE MEDICAL REASONS TO GET A MUSCULAR BIOPSY?

Jase's past medical history is significant for attention deficit/ hyperactive disorder, anxiety, and mild intellectual and behavioral impairment. He was previously an active boy but has had to curtail his activity due to recent episodes of near syncope during sporting events. He also endorses pain in both legs and "stiffness" in his hands with cold weather or stress. Recent blood tests show an elevated serum creatinine kinase and given his family history of "muscular disease," his pediatrician is recommending a muscle biopsy and genetic workup.

WHAT PREOPERATIVE TESTING OR WORKUP SHOULD ONE CONSIDER ORDERING IN AN INDIVIDUAL WITH POSSIBLE NEUROMUSCULAR DISEASE (NMD)?

Based on Jase's recent history of near syncope, a complete blood count, basic metabolic panel, chest X-ray, and an electrocardiogram (EKG) are ordered. His chest X-ray and lab findings are with in normal limits, but his EKG shows a second degree atrioventricular block. He is scheduled to undergo muscle biopsy next week under general anesthesia.

WHAT ARE THE ANESTHETIC CONSIDERATIONS FOR AN INDIVIDUAL UNDERGOING A MUSCLE BIOPSY? WHAT ARE THE AMERICAN COLLEGE OF CARDIOLOGY/ AMERICAN HEART ASSOCIATION GUIDELINES FOR INDIVIDUALS WITH NMD AND ATRIOVENTRICULAR NODAL CONDUCTION ABNORMALITIES?

On the day of his surgery Jase underwent a smooth IV induction with 3mg/kg of propofol and 0.005 mg/kg of hydromorphone. Although the plan was to keep Jase spontaneously breathing on a 200 mcg/kg/min propofol infusion throughout the procedure, mechanical ventilation was required after hydromorphone was given. Postoperatively, Jase had frequent and substantial desaturation episodes. Upon further questioning of his family members, it was noted that Jase frequently has daytime somnolence and that his mother has witnessed "irregular breathing" at night with frequent apneic episodes.

WHAT ARE THE PERIOPERATIVE RECOMMENDATIONS FOR INDIVIDUALS WITH NMD AND CENTRAL SLEEP APNEA? WHAT DIAGNOSTIC TESTING SHOULD BE OFFERED TO THIS PATIENT AND FAMILY IN REGARDS TO HIS POTENTIAL SLEEP DISORDERED BREATHING?

Results from his muscle biopsy and genetic studies suggest that he has a rare form of muscular dystrophy type 1 that presents in childhood.

WHAT IS THE EXPECTED PROGRESSION OF DISEASE IN INDIVIDUALS WITH MYOTONIC DYSTROPHY (DM)? WHAT OTHER ORGAN SYSTEMS CAN BE AFFECTED?

DISCUSSION

DM (TYPE 1, TYPE 2)

DM is a multisystemic autosomal dominant disorder, and the most common DM among white individuals of European ancestry.[1-3] Individuals may present with symptoms at any age; however, pediatric patients typically will present before 10 years of age. The clinical features of DM differ depending on the type of dystrophy and the size of the trinucleotide repeat affecting the dystrophia myotonica protein kinase (DMPK) gene. Aberrant splicing and abnormal function of this gene leads to abnormal skeletal muscle chloride channel function and abnormal expression of insulin receptors and cardiac transcription factors. This leads to muscular dysfunction, insulin resistance, and cardiac conduction abnormalities. Affected individuals also commonly suffer from cataracts.

DM type 1 (DM1) is usually associated with earlier onset and the pediatric population. DM type 2 (DM2) is typically associated with young adults and adults, with symptoms usually presenting in the second or third decades of life. This chapter will discuss the differences between DM2 and DM1 as well as the 4 phenotypic subtypes of DM1: congenital, childhood, classic, and mild.

CLINICAL PRESENTATION

Congenital DM1

Congenital DM1 can present anytime during the fetal and the infantile period. Severity and onset of clinical presentation is related to the length of trinucleotide repeats on the DMPK gene. Clinical presentation in the fetal period is associated with trinucleotide repeats of greater than 1,000. Pregnant mothers often endorse reduced fetal movement and may suffer from prolonged labor (presumably due to subclinical disease of the uterine muscle).[4,5] Due to disturbances in fetal swallowing, ultrasound imagining may reveal polyhydramnios. Another common finding on ultrasound is a fetus with clubfoot. Congenital DM1 has almost exclusively a maternal inheritance pattern. In fact, affected mothers are often diagnosed with subclinical DM after giving birth to an affected neonate.[6–8] It is important to remember that these mothers and other individuals with subclinical DM are still at increased risk for cardiac conduction abnormalities and cardiomyopathy.

Most cases of congenital DM1 present after birth and within the first year of life. The clinical picture of facial paralysis (diplegia), poor feeding, and subsequent diagnosis of failure to thrive are typical. A characteristic V shape of the upper lip may be noted in infants with facial diplegia. Poor feeding associated with DM1 is thought to be due to dysphagia and hypotonic gastrointestinal motility. The profound hypotonia seen in congenital DM1 usually presents after the first year of life. At that time, myotonia and congenital joint contractures may become more prevalent as well. Respiratory involvement is common, and subsequent respiratory failure is the leading cause of death in the neonatal period with mortality rates approaching 20% during this stage of life.[9] In severely affected infants with congenital DM, morality rates approach 40%, likely due to the associated cardiomyopathy. These infants require intensive support to survive the first year of life.[9]

If the affected infant survives the first year of life, gradual improvement of motor function may occur in early childhood. In fact, the severity of congenital DM1 at birth has not demonstrated to be predictive of complications of disease in teen years. As children with DM1 age, their symptoms mimic those seen in classic, adult-onset DM1. Muscle weakness, myotonia, and EKG abnormalities become more prevalent. At 3 to 5 years of age, 50% to 60% of children will have associated learning or behavioral abnormalities.[10] By the second decade of life children with congenital DM1 should expect to have serious cardiac rhythm disturbances and a significant increase in rate of cardiorespiratory morbidity and mortality.[11]

Childhood (juvenile) DM1

Childhood DM1 typically presents before 10 years of age. Clinical features include cognitive and behavioral issues, low IQ, attention deficit disorders, executive dysfunction, anxiety, and other mood disorders. Muscle weakness and physical disability progress in a similar fashion to adult-onset classic DM1. It is important to note that cardiac rhythm disturbances will present even in asymptomatic adolescents or in those individuals with only mild signs of DM. One should not assume a patient with exercise tolerance is not at risk for cardiac disease. In addition, participation in sports and exercise will often precipitate arrhythmias. These patients also have a higher risk of congestive heart failure and structural cardiac abnormalities. Abnormal EKG findings such as QRS >120 ms and P–R interval >200 ms are predictive of finding regional wall motion abnormalities and left atrial enlargement on cardiac imaging.[12] Sleep disorders are also significant in this patient population and may be under recognized. Genetic studies suggest that patients with childhood DM1 tend to have trinucleotide repeats of about 800.[13]

Classic DM1

Patients with the classic form of DM1 typically become symptomatic in the second through fourth decades of life. Patients commonly present with skeletal and respiratory muscle weakness, myotonia, cataracts, cardiac arrhythmias, and excessive daytime somnolence. Genetic studies have shown that the classic form of DM1 generally have trinucleotide repeats of around 50–1,000.[14]

Mild DM1

Patients with mild DM1 will present with symptoms at 20–70 years of age, with a peak onset at 40 years of age. Mild DM1 is characterized by mild weakness, myotonia, and cataracts. Life expectancy in these individuals is normal. Genetic studies show trinucleotide repeats in the range of 50–150. Individuals who fall into this category may be diagnosed later in life, after giving birth to children with more severe forms of DM.

DM2

Patients with DM2 typically present between the second and fourth decades of life. Their symptoms tend to be less severe than classic DM1. DM2 is characterized by weakness of the proximal muscles especially the pelvic girdle and hip muscles. Patients may also suffer from myotonia, weakness, and cataracts. In contrast to DM1, there appears to be no correlation between trinucleotide repeat length on the DMPK gene and the severity of disease or age of onset.

Skeletal muscle

Skeletal muscle involvement varies depending on the type of DM. DM1 affects the facial muscles, sternocleidomastoid, distal muscles of the forearm, intrinsic muscles of the hand, and ankle dorsiflexors. In addition, the respiratory, palatal, pharyngeal, tongue, and extraocular muscles are also often affected. The characteristic facies associated with DM (long, narrow, high-arched palate; hollowed cheeks; and sagging jaw) is thought to be attributed to chronic facial muscle weakness. Clinicians should expect the muscle weakness in their patients with DM1 to decline by about 1% per year for proximal muscles and about 2% to 3% per year for distal muscles.[15]

In individuals with DM2, the most common presenting feature is weakness of the hip girdle. Patients presenting with symptoms in early stage DM2 may complain of weakness of the neck and finger flexors. Later symptoms include the impaired ability to rise from a chair or squatting position and difficulty climbing stairs due to weakness of thigh, hip flexor, and extensor muscles.

Myotonia

Myotonia is a slowed relaxation of a muscle following a normal muscle contraction. This inability to quickly relax a muscle is usually referred to as "muscle stiffness" by patients. Myotonia usually presents early during the natural progression of DM and is aggravated by cold and stress. The most common area patients experience myotonia is in facial, jaw, and hand muscles. Myotonia is a defining feature of DM1 while about 75% of patients have myotonia in DM2.[16] As the severity of DM progresses, skeletal muscle weakness becomes so severe that patients will eventually lose their myotonic symptoms.

Cardiovascular

DM1 and DM2 have significantly increased risk of cardiomyopathy, heart failure, conduction disorders, and arrhythmias.[17] One study found that risk of cardiac conduction disorders were 60 times more likely in patients with DM than the general population.[18] In DM1, arrhythmias or heart block may even be present before major neuromuscular symptoms have become clinically apparent. In DM1, structural cardiac abnormalities are also common and include abnormalities such as left ventricular hypertrophy, left ventricular dilation, left ventricular dysfunction, mitral valve prolapse, regional wall motion abnormalities, and left atrial dilation. One study correlated increasing age and trinucleotide repeat size to the relative risk of left ventricular systolic dysfunction. In DM1, the relative risk for left ventricular systolic dysfunction increases 1.9 for every decade of age and 2.8 for each 500 trinucleotide sequence repeats.[12] Thus, those patients with longer trinucleotide sequences, as they age, will have increasingly higher risk of left ventricular systolic dysfunction.

Respiratory

While respiratory muscle weakness is rare in DM2, it is often a defining characteristic of congenital and classic DM1. Respiratory complications stem from weaknesses in the pharyngeal muscles, weakness or myotonia of respiratory muscles, and possible alteration of the central respiratory drive.[19] Disease progression will lead to decreased vital capacity and alveolar hypoventilation. Respiratory failure is a constant threat to DM1 patients and, in fact, can be precipitated by general anesthesia because of heightened sensitivity to sedatives, inhalational anesthetics, and neuromuscular blocking agents.[20]

Sleep disturbance

DM 1 patients may have hypersomnia and excessive daytime sleepiness. The most likely cause is a central disorder of sleep regulation, though concurrent sleep disordered breathing is not improbable.[21]

Endocrine

Insulin hypersecretion is a common finding in patients with DM. The proposed mechanism is thought to be a compensatory beta cell response to tissue insulin resistance due to transcription of an insulin-resistant receptor. Prevalence of frank diabetes in DM1 is uncommon and more typically associated with DM2.[22]

Gastrointestinal

Disease involvement of the gastrointestinal tract can present in either DM1 or DM2 but tends to be associated with classic DM1. In these patients, dysphagia and weak pharyngeal muscles can lead to aspiration pneumonia, and increased morbidity and mortality. Severity of gastrointestinal symptoms correlates positively with the duration of skeletal muscle disease and poorly with the severity of muscle involvement.[23] Smooth muscle involvement is more likely in DM1 patients and often manifests as colic, constipation, diarrhea, and pseudo-obstruction. Patients may complain of irritable bowel-like symptoms.[24]

Gallstones are also more likely to occur in DM1 due to increased gallbladder sphincter tone.

Neurologic

Congenital DM1 patients will develop generalized cortical atrophy and abnormalities in frontal and anterior temporal lobes, leading to cognitive impairment consistent with mental retardation.[25] In general, lower IQ scores correlate with earlier age of disease onset and longer trinucleotide repeat expansions. There may be subtle cognitive impairment in individuals with classic DM1 and DM2. Cognitive impairment in these individuals is more likely to occur in the areas of the brain responsible for executive function and visual-spatial awareness.[25,26]

Due to underlying glucose intolerance, there may also be an increased incidence of axonal sensorimotor polyneuropathy in patients with DM.

Chronic pain

Lower extremity muscle pain is a common symptom of both DM1 and DM2. The muscles of the proximal legs are usually the source of pain and tend to be induced by exercise, palpation, or temperature change.

Pregnancy

Complications of pregnancy include an increased preterm labor rate, prolonged labor, increase in cesarean delivery rate, and increased risk of hemorrhage due to uterine atony.[27,28]

Workup/diagnostic testing

High clinical suspicion of DM usually prompts further workup such as muscle biopsy and genetic testing.

Muscle biopsy results of both DM1 and DM2 will typically display marked increase of internalized nuclei, severely atrophic muscle fibers with pyknotic nuclear clumps, muscle fiber necrosis, and regeneration of isolated muscle fibers. There may also be preferential atrophy of type 1 fibers.

Muscle biopsy findings suspicious for DM warrants genetic testing of the DMPK gene, which is considered the gold standard for definitive diagnosis of DM1. Children of individuals with expanded trinucleotide repeats in this gene are at an increased risk of inheriting a larger trinucleotide sequence and thus can have worse symptoms than their parentage.[8]

PREOPERATIVE ASSESSMENT OF NMD

Patients with suspected NMD often have multisystemic disease and are considered high risk for general anesthesia. Prior evaluations by a neurologist, cardiologist, and pulmonologist should be reviewed. Baseline EKG, echocardiogram, and pulmonary function tests should be investigated. American College of Cardiology/American Heart Association guidelines recommend EKG prior to every general anesthetic. Guidelines also suggest that individuals with DM and conduction delays may require pacemakers prior to undergoing general anesthesia for other elective procedures.[29]

Consultation with a metabolic specialist or neurologist regarding the suspected type of NMD and type of biopsy should be done. Understand the reasons for muscle biopsy, type of biopsy needed, and the anesthetic implications (Table 34.1).

ANESTHETIC CONSIDERATIONS FOR DM

The risks of anesthesia stem from the multisystemic features of DM. Each individual presenting to the perioperative arena should have a cardiac and pulmonary follow-up completed within the last year.

Table 34.1 TYPES OF MUSCLE BIOPSIES AND THEIR SUGGESTED ANESTHETICS

TYPE OF TESTING	SUGGESTED ANESTHETIC	SUSPECTED DISEASE
Malignant hyperthermia testing	Nontriggering anesthetic is essential.	Central core disease Multiminicore disease Nemaline rod myopathy King-Denborough syndrome Evans myopathy
Standard anatomical muscle biopsy	Nontriggering anesthetic	Muscular dystophy
Muscle mitochondrial enzyme analysis	Propofol and midazolam can lead to uncoupling of oxidative phosphorylation, thus should be avoided as they can affect enzyme assays.	Mitochondrial disorders
Standard anatomical nerve biopsy	No specific anesthetic requirements.	

Airway

The congenital and childhood forms DM1 have increased risk of a difficult airway. This is thought to be attributed to the long facies, high-arched palates, and limited temporomandibular joint motion common in these forms of DM.[30,31]

Muscle

Muscular weakness associated with DM can range from minimal to severe and can significantly increase risk of perioperative adverse events. To assess a patient's perioperative risk, a simple and reliable tool called the Muscular Impairment Rating Scale has been used by the Royal Children's Hospital of Melbourne, Australia to assess children with DM1. This tool has proven to be useful in planning the perioperative and postoperative care for patients with DM1.[32] Risk increases with general anesthesia, procedures lasting longer than 1 hour, and use of muscle relaxation without reversal (Table 34.2).

Myotonia triggers include medications (succinylcholine, reversal agents for neuromuscular blockers), potassium, hypothermia, shivering, and any mechanical or electrical stimulus. Intraoperatively patients should be kept warm as shivering has been known to trigger myotonia.

Medications

Although the diagnosis of DM does not increase the risk of true malignant hyperthermia, unpredictable responses to succinylcholine have been noted in the literature. Providers

Table 34.2 MUSCULAR IMPAIRMENT RATING SCALE

RATING	SYMPTOMS	RISK OF ADVERSE EVENT
1	No clinical muscle impairment	No increased risk
2	Myotonia, jaw and temporal wasting, facial or neck flexor weakness, ptosis, velopharyngeal insufficiency, nasal speech. No distal muscle weakness (except isolated digit flexor weakness).	Low risk
3	Distal muscle weakness. No other proximal muscle weakness (except isolated elbow extensor weakness).	Moderate risk
4	Mild to moderate proximal muscle weakness.	High moderate risk
5	Severe proximal weakness	High risk

should know that responses such as a rigid jaw or prolonged laryngospasm could result; thus, it is considered prudent to avoid of succinylcholine when possible.

Cardiac

Due to increased risks of cardiac rhythm conduction defects and potential progression of known conduction delays, all DM patients should have an EKG prior to any general anesthetic. Patients should be followed by a cardiologist to determine need for echocardiogram. Patients may also present with internal cardiac rhythm devices, and such devices should be interrogated prior to any anesthetic. Anesthetic providers should consider precautionary defibrillator pads during general anesthesia as risk for rhythm disturbances or progression of conduction delays increases with anesthesia.

Respiratory

The effects of DM on the respiratory system predispose patients to restrictive lung disease, dyspnea, and ineffective cough reflexes. In addition, diminished ventilatory responses to hypoxia and hypercapnia predispose these patients to increased sensitivity to volatile anesthetics and opiate derivatives. All of these factors result in an increased risk for pneumonia, aspiration, and other perioperative pulmonary complications. Vigilant monitoring of these patients is necessary as ventilatory failure and poor airway protection are often imminent. The perioperative team should prepare for prolonged mechanical ventilation or at the very least have plans to extubate to bi-level positive airway pressure or other home ventilation device. Postoperatively patients should undergo aggressive pulmonary toilet and use a mechanical cough-assistance device if necessary.

Central nervous system

The effects of DM on the central nervous system can further complicate care for these individuals. Behavioral and cognitive impairment can be significant and can complicate preoperative evaluation and induction of anesthesia. When considering premedication with sedatives, anxiolytics, or analgesics, remember hypersomnia in the DM population is common, as well as sleep disordered breathing and obstructive sleep apnea. Premedication of any kind should be administered with caution and in a stepwise fashion. Postoperative casualties have been noted and are often due to aspiration or hypoxia. During this period providers should be wary of increased agitation or confusion, as encephalopathy has been known to precede such events. Thus, patients should be transferred to a monitored floor postoperatively and discharged only after they have demonstrated a return to their cardiopulmonary and cognitive baselines. When considering discharge, management of postoperative pain without narcotics is ideal if not imperative.

Gastrointestinal

As DM affects gastrointestinal smooth muscle as well as skeletal muscle, providers should assume that all DM patients have prolonged gastric emptying time and gastrointestinal dysmotility. Dysphagia, diminished cough reflex, and small bowel pseudo-obstruction are also common findings. On induction of anesthesia, providers should anticipate aspiration but avoid the use of succinylcholine.

Extubation

Due to the multisystemic effects of DM, adherence to strict extubation criteria must be maintained. Patients and family should be mentally prepared for prolonged mechanical ventilation following anesthesia, as many patients will require mechanical ventilation well after consciousness has been regained.

Pregnancy

The anesthetic provider caring for a pregnant individual with DM has many things to consider in the perioperative arena. Preoperative evaluation of those organ systems affected by DM should be done by an anesthesiologist. Collaboration on a perioperative plan should be undertaken with an anesthesiologist, obstetrician, cardiologist, and pulmonologist present.

Regional versus general anesthesia

As general anesthesia presents a significant increase in perioperative risk for morbidity and mortality, regional or neuraxial anesthesia should be used whenever possible.

REVIEW QUESTIONS

1. DM is **MOST** closely associated with which of the following conditions?

A. cognitive dysfunction
B. congenital cardiac disease
C. malignant hyperthermia
D. osteogenic imperfecta

Answer: A

2. Myotonic reactions are **MOST** commonly triggered by which of following possible stimuli?

A. exercising
B. hyperthermia
C. shivering
D. metoclopramide

Answer: C

3. The inheritance of DM1 is **MOSTLY** attributed to which of the following mechanism?

A. autosomal dominant
B. autosomal recessive
C. sporadic genetic mutations
D. X-linked recessive inheritance

Answer: A

4. The **MOST** common cardiac finding associated with DM is which of following finding?

A. atrial fibrillation
B. coronary artery stenosis
C. restrictive cardiomyopathy
D. semilunar valve disease

Answer: A

5. If a patient with DM received a non-depolarizing neuromuscular blocking, the **BEST** option upon completion of surgery is which of the following treatments?

A. dantrolene
B. edrophonium
C. neostigmine
D. sugammadex

Answer: D

6. A pregnant mother presents for preoperative evaluation for her upcoming scheduled cesarean section. She has a history of classic DM1, currently uses a continuous positive airway pressure at night for central sleep apnea and has no history of cardiac arrhythmias. The **BEST** choice of anesthetic for this patient is which of the following options?

A. rapid sequence intubation using succinylcholine
B. epidural anesthesia using interval doses of chloroprocaine
C. modified rapid sequence intubation using rocuronium
D. spinal anesthesia using high-volumes of bupivacaine and morphine

Answer: B

7. According to the Muscular Impairment Rating Scale used by the Royal Children's Hospital of Melbourne, which DM patient would have the **LOWEST** risk of a perioperative adverse event?

A. 10-year-old with proximal muscle weakness undergoing general anesthesia for posterior spinal fusion
B. 15-year-old with distal muscle weakness undergoing regional anesthesia for muscle biopsy
C. 15-year-old with velopharyngeal insufficiency, myotonia and ptosis undergoing general anesthesia for strabismus surgery
D. 18-year-old with distal muscle weakness undergoing general anesthesia for laparoscopic gastrostomy tube placement

Answer: B

QUESTIONS AND ANSWERS

This chapter has accompanying questions and answers which are available to subscribers as part of the Oxford eLearning platform. To access the questions, go to ✓ http://oxfordmedicine. com/pediatricanesthesiaPBL

REFERENCES

1. Magee A, Nevin NC. The epidemiology of myotonic dystrophy in Northern Ireland. *Community Genet.* 1999;2:179–183.
2. Siciliano G, Manca M, Gennarelli M, et al. Epidemiology of myotonic dystrophy in Italy: re-appraisal after genetic diagnosis. *Clin Genet.* 2001;59:344.
3. Norwood FL, Harling C, Chinnery PF, et al. Prevalence of genetic muscle disease in Northern England: in-depth analysis of a muscle clinic population. *Brain.* 2009;132:3175.
4. Shore RN, MacLachlan TB. Pregnancy with myotonic dystrophy: course, complications and management. *Obstet Gynecol.* 1971;38:448.
5. Sarnat HB, O'Connor T, Byrne PA. Clinical effects of myotonic dystrophy on pregnancy and the neonate. *Arch Neurol.* 1976;33:459.
6. Thornton CA. Myotonic dystrophy. *Neurol Clin.* 2014;32:705.
7. Tsilfidis C, MacKenzie AE, Mettler G, et al. Correlation between CTG trinucleotide repeat length and frequency of severe congenital myotonic dystrophy. *Nat Genet.* 1992;1:192.
8. De Temmerman N, Sermon K, Seneca S, et al. Intergenerational instability of the expanded CTG repeat in the DMPK gene: studies in human gametes and preimplantation embryos. *Am J Hum Genet.* 2004;75:325.
9. Campbell C, Levin S, Siu VM, et al. Congenital myotonic dystrophy: Canadian population-based surveillance study. *J Pediatr.* 2013;163:120.
10. Roig M, Balliu PR, Navarro C, et al. Presentation, clinical course, and outcome of the congenital form of myotonic dystrophy. *Pediatr Neurol.* 1994;11:208.
11. Bassez G, Lazarus A, Desguerre I, et al. Severe cardiac arrhythmias in young patients with myotonic dystrophy type 1. *Neurology.* 2004;63:1939.
12. Bhakta D, Lowe MR, Groh WJ. Prevalence of structural cardiac abnormalities in patients with myotonic dystrophy type I. *Am Heart J.* 2004;147:224.
13. Ho G, Cardamone M, Farrar M. Congenital and childhood myotonic dystrophy: current aspects of disease and future directions. *World J Clin Pediatr.* 2015;4:66.
14. Turner C, Hilton-Jones D. Myotonic dystrophy: diagnosis, management and new therapies. *Curr Opin Neurol.* 2014;27:599.
15. Mathieu J, Boivin H, Richards CL. Quantitative motor assessment in myotonic dystrophy. *Can J Neurol Sci.* 2003;30:129.

16. Heatwole C, Johnson N, Bode R, et al. Patient-Reported Impact of Symptoms in Myotonic Dystrophy Type 2 (PRISM-2). *Neurology*. 2015;85:2136.

17. Fragola PV, Luzi M, Calò L, et al. Cardiac involvement in myotonic dystrophy. *Am J Cardiol*. 1994;74:1070.

18. Johnson NE, Abbott D, Cannon-Albright LA. Relative risks for comorbidities associated with myotonic dystrophy: a population-based analysis. *Muscle Nerve*. 2015;52:659.

19. Bogaard JM, van der Meché FG, Hendriks I, Ververs C. Pulmonary function and resting breathing pattern in myotonic dystrophy. *Lung*. 1992;170:143.

20. Klompe L, Lancé M, van der Woerd D, et al. Anaesthesiological and ventilatory precautions during cardiac surgery in Steinert's disease. *J Card Surg*. 2007;22:74.

21. Laberge L, Gagnon C, Dauvilliers Y. Daytime sleepiness and myotonic dystrophy. *Curr Neurol Neurosci Rep*. 2013;13:340.

22. Machuca-Tzili L, Brook D, Hilton-Jones D. Clinical and molecular aspects of the myotonic dystrophies: a review. *Muscle Nerve*. 2005;32:1.

23. Rönnblom A, Forsberg H, Danielsson A. Gastrointestinal symptoms in myotonic dystrophy. *Scand J Gastroenterol*. 1996;31:654.

24. Bellini M, Biagi S, Stasi C, et al. Gastrointestinal manifestations in myotonic muscular dystrophy. *World J Gastroenterol*. 2006;12:1821.

25. Modoni A, Silvestri G, Pomponi MG, et al. Characterization of the pattern of cognitive impairment in myotonic dystrophy type 1. *Arch Neurol*. 2004;61:1943.

26. Gaul C, Schmidt T, Windisch G, et al. Subtle cognitive dysfunction in adult onset myotonic dystrophy type 1 (DM1) and type 2 (DM2). *Neurology*. 2006;67:350.

27. Rudnik-Schöneborn S, Zerres K. Outcome in pregnancies complicated by myotonic dystrophy: a study of 31 patients and review of the literature. *Eur J Obstet Gynecol Reprod Biol*. 2004;114:44.

28. Rudnik-Schöneborn S, Schneider-Gold C, Raabe U, et al. Outcome and effect of pregnancy in myotonic dystrophy type 2. *Neurology*. 2006;66:579.

29. Epstein AE, DiMarco JP, Ellenbogen KA, et al. American College of Cardiology/American Heart Association Task Force on Practice Guidelines (Writing Committee to Revise the ACC/AHA/NASPE 2002 Guideline Update for Implantation of Cardiac Pacemakers and Antiarrhythmia Devices), American Association for Thoracic Surgery, Society of Thoracic Surgeons. *Circulation*. 2008;117(21):e350.

30. Moxley RT, Ciafaloni E, Guntrum D. Myotonic dystrophy. In: Darras BT, Jones R, Ryan MM, De Vivo DC, eds. *Neuromuscular Disorders of Infancy, Childhood, and Adolescence: A Clinician's Approach*. London: Elsevier; 2015:697–718.

31. Harper PS. *Myotonic Dystrophy*. 2nd ed. London: WB Saunders; 1989.

32. Sinclair JL, Reed PW. Risk factors for perioperative adverse events in children with myotonic dystrophy. *Ped Anesth*. 2009;19:740–747.

35.

DUCHENNE'S MUSCULAR DYSTROPHY

Tori N. Sutherland and Kirk Lalwani

STEM CASE AND KEY QUESTIONS

A 4-year old boy was assessed by his pediatrician. John's parents were concerned because he did not seem to be developing at the same pace as his older brother, Sam. John was becoming easily fatigued during playtime and would often crawl instead of walking up stairs. His vocabulary was limited to 2-word combinations and his speech was often not understandable. John's preschool teacher was also concerned because she noticed that he had started to use his hands to push himself up instead of sitting up like her other students. Because John had been adopted as an infant, his family history was unknown. His parents had been living abroad for a year and had not seen a pediatrician for almost 2 years. Upon returning, his pediatrician was alarmed and scheduled a follow-up appointment in 2 weeks to initiate a full workup.

DISCUSS THE DIFFERENTIAL DIAGNOSIS OF DELAYED MILESTONES AND MUSCLE WEAKNESS IN A CHILD THIS AGE.

Later that week, John's mother was worried when he complained of stomach pain and refused to eat dinner. He had a low-grade temperature of 100.5°F and vomited several times overnight. When he failed to improve the following morning, she took him to the local community hospital as his pediatrician's office was closed for the weekend. To the surprise of his mother, he tolerated the intravenous line placement for fluids and labs.

LIST THE COMMON CAUSES OF AN ACUTE ABDOMEN IN NEONATES, INFANTS, AND PRESCHOOL CHILDREN.

John was diagnosed with appendicitis and taken to the holding area for urgent laparoscopic appendectomy. The on-call anesthesiologist, who was responsible for adults and the rare pediatric case, made the decision to proceed with a rapid sequence induction because John continued to have episodes of emesis.

DISCUSS THE ADVANTAGES AND DISADVANTAGES OF PARENTAL PRESENCE AT INDUCTION (PPI) OF ANESTHESIA. WHAT INFORMATION WOULD YOU GIVE PARENTS TO PREPARE THEM FOR PPI AND ENSURE SAFETY OF THE CHILD DURING INDUCTION?

John's mother accompanied him to the operating room. He moaned as he was carried over to the operating table. She sung his favorite lullaby as he was preoxygenated, and monitors were applied. As he drifted off to sleep, she gave him a kiss and was escorted back to the waiting room. Five minutes later, she heard "Code blue—operating room" announced on the overhead intercoms. One hour later, her worst fears were confirmed when a tearful group of clinicians filtered into the room and the surgeon choked out, "I'm so terribly sorry, but we've lost your son."

LIST THE POTENTIAL CAUSES OF SUDDEN DEATH DURING ANESTHETIC INDUCTION IN A CHILD.

When John's parents asked "Why?," they were told that that he had experienced a cardiac arrest after induction. On preliminary laboratory analysis, his serum Potassium level was 8.5 mEq.

DISCUSSION

OVERVIEW

Duchenne's muscular dystrophy (DMD) is a progressive X-linked recessive disorder that affects boys and female carriers. It is the most common dystrophy with onset in childhood; the prevalence in the United States is nearly 2 per 10,000 males.[1] DMD is associated with severe, progressive proximal muscle weakening due to absence of dystrophin, which is found in skeletal and cardiac muscles. The classical presentation involves a young boy, around 4 years of age, with rapid onset of muscle weakness that begins in the pelvis and thighs and progresses to the shoulders and upper arms.[2] The affected patient first has difficulty running and standing up, followed by difficulty climbing stairs, and then loses the ability to ambulate by age 13.[3] Young boys with proximal lower extremity weakness will classically exhibit Gower's sign, meaning they must use their hands and arms to stand up from a sitting position by "walking up" their own body.

DMD is also associated with mild cognitive delay, involvement of the upper proximal muscles, cardiac fibrosis and dilated cardiomyopathy, and respiratory failure. Female carriers may develop cardiomyopathy. The most common causes of death are related to respiratory insufficiency, followed by cardiac complications. The development of new therapies, improved perioperative care, and expectant management of cardiac and pulmonary complications have resulted in improved quality of life and lifespan for DMD patients.[4]

When evaluating a preschool child with delayed milestones, a variety of conditions should be considered, including environmental toxin exposure, autism spectrum disorders, exposure to toxins in utero, cerebral palsy, genetic disorders such as Down's syndrome and Rett's syndrome in girls, and myopathies.[5] The combination of new-onset lower extremity weakness and delayed cognitive milestones in a boy between ages 2 and 5 should prompt a formal evaluation for muscular dystrophies.[6]

Related dystrophies include a variant of DMD, Becker muscular dystrophy, that generally has a later onset and more mild clinical course.[3] Other early-onset muscular dystrophies with a proximal to distal weakness progression pattern include the limb girdle dystrophies that are associated with a range of cardiomyopathies and spinal rigidity.[3]

With regard to common causes of an acute abdomen, the child's age should prompt the provider to consider distinct diagnoses. Abdominal pain is difficult to assess in young children and infants due to communication barriers. In neonates, the provider should rule out conditions such as Hirschsprung's disease, colitis, incarcerated hernia, intussusception, and volvulus.[7] Other causes of abdominal pain in patients younger than 2 years include urinary tract infection, constipation, and gastroenteritis. Among preschool aged children, a provider must also consider appendicitis and trauma and in rare circumstances, a sickle cell crisis, Henoch-Schonlein purpura, and mesenteric adenitis.[7]

ETIOLOGY AND PATHOGENESIS

DMD is an X-linked recessive condition caused by mutations in the dystrophin gene. The dystrophin gene is largest gene in the human body. It occupies 2.3 megabases on chromosome Xp21.2

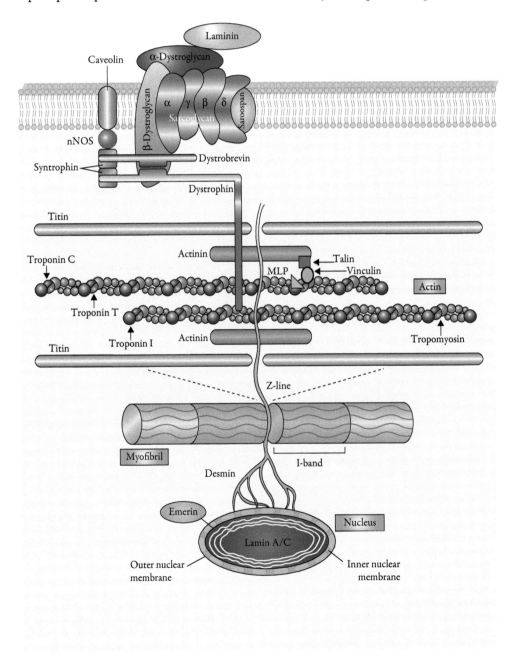

Fig. 35.1 Dystrophin and skeletal muscle.

and codes a 427 kilodalton protein.[8] Dystrophin is primarily expressed in skeletal and cardiac muscles, with smaller amounts located in the brain.[2] It is located on the intracellular sarcolemma membrane and is designed to stabilize muscle fibers during contraction.[2] The loss of dystrophin in the sarcomere membrane leads to instability, muscle fiber necrosis, and subsequent muscle replacement with fibrotic adipose tissue.[2] One third of DMD cases are caused by spontaneous mutations, while the other two thirds are inherited from a female carrier. 65% of mutations are large scale deletions, 25% are point mutations, and approximately 5% are attributable to duplications[2] (Figure 35.1).

CLINICAL PRESENTATION

1. **Cognitive**: DMD patients may be afflicted with mild, nonprogressive developmental delay; this is hypothesized to be secondary to decreased cerebral dystrophin levels.[2,6]

2. **Neuromuscular**: DMD's clinical course is well-documented and can only be delayed with steroid regimens and multidisciplinary interventions.[6] Males classically present as toddlers with mild delay of motor milestones and weakness during running and jumping.[6] They then develop weakness with standing and utilize their upper bodies and arms for assistance (i.e., Gower's maneuver).[6] By early adolescence, boys are wheelchair-bound, and the average age of death is 19 years.[6]

As DMD is a primary neuromuscular disease, progression is now divided into 5 stages: presymptomatic, early ambulatory, late ambulatory, early nonambulatory, and late nonambulatory.[6] Stage 2 is defined by Gower's sign, waddling gait, and toe walking.[6] Stage 3 is notable for inability to climb stairs and rise from sitting, while stage 4 is characterized by the decreased ability to maintain posture and the possibility of scoliosis development.[6] By stage 5 (late nonambulatory), patients lose function of the upper limbs and ability to maintain posture; nearly all patients develop scoliosis in this stage.[6]

Cardiac involvement

The natural history of cardiac involvement begins with electrocardiogram (EKG) changes and diastolic dysfunction (Figure 35.2). The disease then causes myocardial fibrosis that is detectable on magnetic resonance imaging and ventricular dilation. Patients develop systolic dysfunction and end-stage heart failure.[9] Individuals also have right ventricular failure that is often secondary to pulmonary hypertension.[10] Traditionally, conduction abnormalities involve the atrioventricular node, with significant fibrosis of the posterobasal left ventricular wall; EKG changes include tall right precordial R waves and deep waves in the lateral leads.[9,10]

Female mutation carriers have been reported to have high prevalence of cardiomyopathy. The highest estimates range from 54% in carriers less than 16 years of age and >90% in carriers over the age of 16.[11] This study did involve individuals ($n = 45$) who carried the less severe Becker's muscular dystrophy variant. Myocardial biopsy in carriers is notable for dystrophin anomalies at the endomyocardial layer.[11] A more recent study noted that 65% of DMD female carriers exhibited evidence of cardiomyopathy on imaging, including decreased ejection fraction and pathologic remodeling of the left ventricular free wall.[12]

Pulmonary involvement

Respiratory insufficiency is the most common cause of serious morbidity and mortality in DMD.[13] All patients develop loss of primary and accessory respiratory muscle strength over time; this leads to a functional restrictive disease pattern. Inspiratory function is preserved through the first decade of life; however, the expiratory muscles weaken earlier in the disease course.[14] Decreased muscle strength is associated with a weak cough and decreased or restrictive ventilation volumes.[13] Patients develop pneumonia and respiratory insufficiency requiring noninvasive ventilation.[13] Spirometry values correlate directly with disease prognosis and mortality risk[3,13] (Figure 35.3).

DIAGNOSIS

Early in the disease course prior to symptom onset, creatinine kinase (CK) levels are elevated (normal 75–230 IU/L).[15] Guidelines state that a DMD workup should be conducted for 3 reasons, without regard for a positive family history.[6] These include abnormal muscle function in a male, and detection of a high CK value, or increased transaminases.[6] The diagnosis is confirmed with genetic sequencing to detect a deletion or mutation in the dystrophin gene and with a muscle biopsy to demonstrate that the dystrophin protein is absent.[6]

MANAGEMENT

Daily corticosteroids for DMD patients are now considered to be the standard of care to improve motor, pulmonary, and cardiac outcomes. The recommended dose of prednisone is 0.75 mg/kg/day; deflazacort (Emflaza) has also recently received approval for use in the United States.[16] Lower steroid doses are associated with less systemic side effects but are also considered to be less effective.[17] However, dose modification should be considered in the presence of severe systemic side effects. Several biologic agents are in various phases are testing; they include a histone deacetylase inhibitor, cell-based replacement of dystrophin, and splicing therapy.[2]

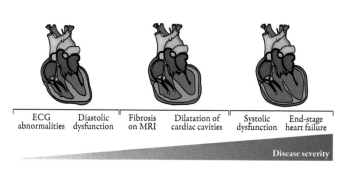

ECG abnormalities | Diastolic dysfunction | Fibrosis on MRI | Dilatation of cardiac cavities | Systolic dysfunction | End-stage heart failure

Disease severity

Fig. 35.2 Progression of cardiac disease in DMD.

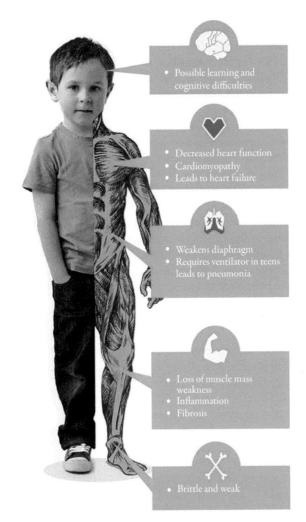

Fig. 35.3 Overview of systems affected by DMD.

- Possible learning and cognitive difficulties

- Decreased heart function
- Cardiomyopathy
- Leads to heart failure

- Weakens diaphragm
- Requires ventilator in teens leads to pneumonia

- Loss of muscle mass weakness
- Inflammation
- Fibrosis

- Brittle and weak

Early treatment of cardiac disease is important to reduce future morbidity and mortality. Prior to development of symptoms, clinical disease can be delayed with a combination of therapies, including angiotensin-converting-enzyme inhibitors, angiotensin-II-receptor blockers, beta-blockers, and mineralocorticoid-receptor antagonists.[9] When patients develop symptomatic disease, medical management includes use of agents such as digoxin, milrinone, and ivabradine, which inhibits the sodium–potassium (Na+/K+) channel at the sinoatrial node.[9] Nonpharmacologic interventions include pacemaker implantation, resynchronization therapy, and use of a ventricular assist device as a bridge to cardiac transplant for end-stage disease.[9] Other interventions that can moderate symptoms include surgery for scoliosis, noninvasive ventilation, and chronic pain management.[9]

With regard to management of respiratory involvement, patients treated with long-term steroids have improved prognostic indicators, including higher peak cough flow and respiratory muscle strength.[18] Therapies, including volume recruitment (indicated for forced vital capacity [FVC] <40% predicted), manual and assisted cough techniques, nocturnal ventilation, followed by daytime ventilation, and finally

tracheostomy, are introduced for management of worsening respiratory insufficiency.[4] During biannual assessments when vital capacity falls below 80% predicted or by age 12, patients should undergo spirometry and pulse oximetry and be evaluated for evidence of reflux, aspiration, asthma, and obstructive sleep apnea.[13]

SPECIAL ANESTHETIC CONSIDERATIONS

Broadly, conditions in children associated with sudden death include unrepaired cardiac lesions, specifically those that are cyanotic or ductus-dependent, and children with severe pulmonary hypertension or aortic stenosis.[19] Other causes of sudden cardiovascular collapse include lack of resuscitation in the presence of hypovolemic shock, anaphylaxis, inability to secure the airway with subsequent hypoxia, conduction disorders, and electrolyte abnormalities that may lead to cardiac arrest. Malignant hyperthermia is associated with high mortality risk but may not present immediately on induction. Patients with DMD are at risk of sudden death during anesthetic induction, secondary to severe hyperkalemia and intrinsic cardiac dysfunction.

Overview of anesthetic management

Apart from emergencies, DMD patients require evaluation for anesthesia for procedures to correct contractures and scoliosis.

Rhabdomyolysis and life-threatening hyperkalemia with succinylcholine and volatile agents. Patients are at high risk of rhabdomyolysis and subsequent hyperkalemic cardiac arrest linked to both succinylcholine and inhaled agent use.[20,21] Of note, patients are not at higher risk of developing malignant hyperthermia compared to the general population.[20] It is thought that in preadolescents atrophic muscle fibers continue to attempt to regenerate; these fibers carry higher risk of rhabdomyolysis after exposure to inhaled anesthetics.[21,22] High baseline intracellular calcium (Ca2+) levels continue to rise after exposure to inhaled agents or succinylcholine and promote extravasation of intracellular contents, such as potassium ions and CK.[21] A hypermetabolic response is then hypothesized to occur to re-establish membrane stability.[23]

Similar to patients with a malignant hyperthermia diagnosis, patients with DMD should receive a "trigger-free" total intravenous anesthetic with a machine that has been properly flushed.[4] Depolarizing paralytics should be avoided. If cardiac arrest or arrhythmia secondary to hyperkalemia develops, the anesthesiologist should first administer intravenous calcium chloride, even with knowledge of variable effects on this population, and then focus on interventions to shift potassium into the intracellular space.[24]

Primary intraoperative cardiac failure. It is well-established that patients with DMD develop dilation and fibrosis of the left ventricle over time that is often followed by pulmonary hypertension and right-heart involvement. Even if a patient does not demonstrate signs of cardiac remodeling, it is important to remember that the myocardium is affected at the cellular level. These patients are at risk of acute intraoperative hypotension, bradycardia, and tachyarrhythmias.[25] While the majority of intraoperative cardiac events are attributable to volatile agents and succinylcholine use, case reports document that young patients with stable cardiac baselines have acutely decompensated after unprovoked development of arrhythmias, hypotension, and left-sided systolic failure.[25] If a major surgery is planned, it is suggested that providers consider obtaining a stress echocardiogram.[25]

Preoperative evaluation

All patients undergoing general anesthesia should have a pulmonary evaluation, an echocardiogram, and EKG. For patients receiving moderate sedation or a regional anesthetic, these should be repeated if the prior studies were performed more than 1 year ago or if the patient had an abnormal echocardiogram between 7 and 12 months of age.[4] If the patient is receiving local anesthesia, a repeat echocardiogram is prudent if a prior abnormal result has been documented.[4]

Parental presence at induction

Parents of DMD patients should be well-educated if PPI is considered to be in the child's best interest. Evidence suggests than children older than 4 years, children with calm parents, and shy, inhibited children do experience decreased anxiety with parental presence.[26] If the anesthesiologist feels this is appropriate, the parent should receive standard education with regard to patient distress, physiologic responses to anesthesia, the possibility of decompensation on induction, and that they will be accompanied to a waiting room by a staff member. If a patient acutely decompensates on induction, the parent should be instructed to leave the room with the designated team member and that providers will give updates after the patient is stabilized.

Airway and positioning

Lordoscoliosis and tracheobronchomalacia have been reported to contribute to iatrogenic airway obstruction in the prone position for scoliosis repair; if this occurs, semilateral positioning may become necessary.[27] Contractures may also require modification for standard positioning. All patients should be evaluated for the possibility of a difficult airway. One retrospective review documented 8 difficult laryngoscopies among 91 DMD patients who underwent 232 general anesthetics.[28]

Concern for high blood loss

Compared to patients with idiopathic scoliosis, DMD patients lose up to 3 times the blood volume in spine procedures; this is attributed to decreased coagulation factors and need to fuse additional levels.[29] It is recommended that the anesthetic provider utilize invasive hemodynamic monitoring and take additional steps to minimize blood loss in the perioperative period such as the use of permissive hypotension and a cell-saver.[4] With regard to medical management, the use of an antifibrinolytic such as tranexamic acid is recommended for operations associated with significant blood loss.[30] It is suggested that compression boots or stockings be used in place of heparin to minimize deep-vein thrombosis risk.[4]

Neuromuscular blockade

DMD is associated with heightened sensitivity to non-depolarizing muscular blockade. One analysis found that onset time of low-dose rocuronium (0.3 mg/kg) is delayed over 100 seconds in DMD.[31] Recovery was delayed an average of 30 minutes compared to control patients.[31]

Respiratory concerns and extubation

Respiratory complications, such as postoperative reintubation and pneumonia, are common. Guidelines suggest that patients should be trained preoperatively in assisted cough techniques and use of noninvasive ventilation.[4] This is highly recommended for patients with FVC <50% of predicted and is considered essential if the FVC is <30% of predicted.[32] Incentive spirometry is not recommended given the weak musculature.[4]

Prior to an extubation attempt, the patient must have full reversal of paralysis with train-of-four confirmation. The patient must also demonstrate appropriate spontaneous tidal volumes (on a mL/kg basis) prior to any attempt at extubation. Patients with respiratory muscle involvement who do not effectively accept noninvasive ventilation and assisted cough techniques are at the highest risk of respiratory insufficiency.[33,34] Tracheostomy is indicated if a patient has failed 3 extubation attempts.[4]

CONCLUSIONS

- DMD is a progressive X-linked disorder that is characterized by proximal muscle wasting, mental impairment, dilated cardiomyopathy, and respiratory impairment.

- Pulmonary complications are related to progressive weakness of the diaphragm and respiratory muscles; 5-year survival falls to 8% when FVC <1 liter.[35]

- Patients with DMD are susceptible to the need for postoperative ventilation, intraoperative heart failure, hyperkalemia associated with succinylcholine use, and rhabdomyolysis induced by both succinylcholine and inhaled agents.

- The most common causes of death are pneumonia followed by cardiomyopathy and heart failure.

- Improvements in medical and airway management, standardized corticosteroid regimens, and promising biologic agents in development are leading to an improved quality of life and prolonging the lifespan for individuals with DMD.

REVIEW QUESTIONS

A 14-year-old boy has arrived for preoperative evaluation prior to undergoing surgery for scoliosis repair. He is wheelchair bound and reports good compliance with therapies ordered by his cardiologist and pulmonologist.

1. On standard cardiac work-up, what type of cardiomyopathy is **MOST** likely to be diagnosed in this patient?

   A. dilated cardiomyopathy
   B. hypertrophic cardiomyopathy
   C. ischemic cardiomyopathy
   D. restrictive cardiomyopathy

Answer: A
Dilated cardiomyopathy develops after early diastolic dysfunction and focal fibrosis.

2. Consider the scenario detailed in question 1. Because the patient has asymptomatic mild cardiac involvement without EKG changes, what intervention is **MOST** likely to be used to delay progression to symptomatic cardiac disease?

   A. beta-blockers
   B. calcium-channel blockers
   C. hyperpolarization-activated cyclic nucleotide-gated channel blocker
   D. phosphodiesterase-3 inhibitor

Answer: A
Prior to development of symptoms, clinical disease can be delayed with a combination of therapies, including angiotensin-converting-enzyme inhibitors, angiotensin-II-receptor blockers, beta-blockers, and mineralocorticoid-receptor antagonists.

3. Consider the scenario detailed in question 1. After undergoing an uncomplicated scoliosis repair, which of the following therapies, according to evidence-based medicine, is **LEAST** likely to reduce this patient's risk of postoperative reintubation?

   A. assisted cough techniques
   B. blow-by humidified oxygen
   C. mechanical insufflation-exsufflation
   D. noninvasive positive pressure ventilation

Answer: B
Respiratory complications, such as postoperative reintubation and pneumonia, are common. Guidelines suggest that patients should be trained preoperatively in assisted cough techniques and use of noninvasive ventilation. Postoperatively, oxygen therapies should be used with caution. Supplemental oxygen may improve saturation but not the underlying cause. It may also depress respiratory drive.

4. When reviewing a muscle biopsy for a patient with a genetic DMD diagnosis, what protein is **MOST** likely to be defective or missing?

   A. caveolin
   B. dysferlin
   C. dystroglycan
   D. dystrophin

Answer: D

5. The cardiac transplant group is evaluating a 15-year-old male with severe cardiac involvement and ejection fraction <10% for transplant. His disease progression has otherwise been well-controlled with evidence-based therapies. What cardiac alteration would you **MOST** likely see first in a patient with DMD?

   A. chamber dilation
   B. electrocardiogram changes
   C. pulmonary hypertension
   D. systolic dysfunction

Answer: B
The natural history of cardiac involvement begins with EKG changes and diastolic dysfunction. The disease then causes myocardial fibrosis that is detectable on magnetic resonance imaging, and ventricular dilation. Patients develop systolic dysfunction and end-stage heart failure.[9] Individuals also have right ventricular failure that is often secondary to pulmonary hypertension.[10]

6. You are evaluating a decade of records for a teenager with DMD who was recently transferred to your practice when his primary provider retired. Select the clinical finding that would be **LEAST** likely to be present in this patient.

   A. EKG with deep Q waves in I, aVL, and V5-6
   B. elevated CK levels prior to muscular weakness
   C. restrictive lung disease secondary to pulmonary fibrosis
   D. Holter record with supraventricular and ventricular arrhythmias

Answer: C

7. You are developing an anesthetic plan for a patient with DMD who will require an urgent exploratory laparotomy for pseudo-obstruction. Which anesthetic complication are you **MOST** concerned about with this patient?

   A. hyperkalemia from rhabdomyolysis.
   B. malignant hyperthermia from sevoflurane.
   C. postural headache from neuraxial anesthesia.
   D. urinary retention with benzodiazepines.

Answer: A

QUESTIONS AND ANSWERS

This chapter has accompanying questions and answers which are available to subscribers as part of the Oxford eLearning platform. To access the questions, go to ✓ http:// oxfordmedicine. com/pediatricanesthesiaPBL

REFERENCES

1. Romitti PA, Zhu Y, Puzhankara S, et al. Prevalence of Duchenne and Becker muscular dystrophies in the United States. *Pediatrics.* 2015;135:513–521.
2. Falzarano MS, Scotton C, Passarelli C, Ferlini A. Duchenne muscular dystrophy: from diagnosis to therapy. *Molecules.* 2015;20:18168–18184.
3. Mercuri E, Muntoni F. Muscular dystrophies. *Lancet.* 2013;381:845–860.
4. Bushby K, Finkel R, Birnkrant DJ, et al. Diagnosis and management of Duchenne muscular dystrophy, part 2: implementation of multidisciplinary care. *Lancet Neurol.* 2010;9:177–189.
5. Shevell M, Ashwal S, Donley D, et al. Practice parameter: evaluation of the child with global developmental delay: report of the Quality Standards Subcommittee of the American Academy of Neurology and the Practice Committee of the Child Neurology Society. *Neurology.* 2003;60:367–380.
6. Bushby K, Finkel R, Birnkrant DJ, et al. Diagnosis and management of Duchenne muscular dystrophy, part 1: diagnosis, and pharmacological and psychosocial management. *Lancet Neurol.* 2010;9:77–93.
7. Yang WC, Chen CY, Wu HP. Etiology of non-traumatic acute abdomen in pediatric emergency departments. *World J Clin Cases.* 2013;1:276–284.
8. Hoffman EP, Brown RH, Jr., Kunkel LM. Dystrophin: the protein product of the Duchenne muscular dystrophy locus. *Cell.* 1987;51:919–928.
9. Finsterer J, Cripe L. Treatment of dystrophin cardiomyopathies. *Nat Rev Cardiol.* 2014;11:168–179.
10. Finsterer J, Stollberger C. The heart in human dystrophinopathies. *Cardiology.* 2003;99:1–19.
11. Politano L, Nigro V, Nigro G, et al. Development of cardiomyopathy in female carriers of Duchenne and Becker muscular dystrophies. *JAMA.* 1996;275:1335–1338.
12. Florian A, Rosch S, Bietenbeck M, et al. Cardiac involvement in female Duchenne and Becker muscular dystrophy carriers in comparison to their first-degree male relatives: a comparative cardiovascular magnetic resonance study. *Eur Heart J Cardiovasc Imaging.* 2016;17:326–333.
13. Finder JD, Birnkrant D, Carl J, et al. Respiratory care of the patient with Duchenne muscular dystrophy: ATS consensus statement. *Am J Respir Crit Care Med.* 2004;170:456–465.
14. Ames WA, Hayes JA, Crawford MW. The role of corticosteroids in Duchenne muscular dystrophy: a review for the anesthetist. *Paediatr Anaesth.* 2005;15:3–8.
15. Zatz M, Rapaport D, Vainzof M, et al. Serum creatine-kinase (CK) and pyruvate-kinase (PK) activities in Duchenne (DMD) as compared with Becker (BMD) muscular dystrophy. *J Neurol Sci.* 1991;102:190–196.
16. Gloss D, Moxley RT 3rd, Ashwal S, Oskoui M. Practice guideline update summary: corticosteroid treatment of Duchenne muscular dystrophy: report of the Guideline Development Subcommittee of the American Academy of Neurology. *Neurology.* 2016;86:465–472.
17. Griggs RC, Moxley RT 3rd, Mendell JR, et al. Prednisone in Duchenne dystrophy. a randomized, controlled trial defining the time course and dose response. Clinical Investigation of Duchenne Dystrophy Group. *Arch Neurol.* 1991;48:383–388.
18. Daftary AS, Crisanti M, Kalra M, Wong B, Amin R. Effect of long-term steroids on cough efficiency and respiratory muscle strength in patients with Duchenne muscular dystrophy. *Pediatrics.* 2007;119:e320–e324.
19. Burch TM, McGowan FX, Jr., Kussman BD, Powell AJ, DiNardo JA. Congenital supravalvular aortic stenosis and sudden death associated with anesthesia: what's the mystery? *Anesth Analg.* 2008;107:1848–1854.
20. Gurnaney H, Brown A, Litman RS. Malignant hyperthermia and muscular dystrophies. *Anesth Analg.* 2009;109:1043–1048.
21. Hayes J, Veyckemans F, Bissonnette B. Duchenne muscular dystrophy: an old anesthesia problem revisited. *Paediatr Anaesth.* 2008;18:100–106.
22. Yemen TA, McClain C. Muscular dystrophy, anesthesia and the safety of inhalational agents revisited; again. *Paediatr Anaesth.* 2006;16:105–108.
23. Gronert GA, Fowler W, Cardinet GH 3rd, Grix A Jr., Ellis WG, Schwartz MZ. Absence of malignant hyperthermia contractures in Becker-Duchenne dystrophy at age 2. *Muscle Nerve.* 1992;15:52–56.
24. ECC Committee, Subcommittees and Task Forces of the American Heart Association. 2005 American Heart Association guidelines for cardiopulmonary resuscitation and emergency cardiovascular care. *Circulation.* 2005;112:IV1–203.
25. Schmidt GN, Burmeister MA, Lilje C, Wappler F, Bischoff P. Acute heart failure during spinal surgery in a boy with Duchenne muscular dystrophy. *Br J Anaesth.* 2003;90:800–804.
26. Kain ZN, Mayes LC, Caramico LA, et al. Parental presence during induction of anesthesia. A randomized controlled trial. *Anesthesiology.* 1996;84:1060–1067.
27. Yang JH, Bhandarkar AW, Lim BG, Modi HN, Suh SW. Intraoperative airway obstruction in a Duchenne muscular dystrophy patient. *Eur Spine J.* 2013;22(Suppl 3):S491–S496.
28. Muenster T, Mueller C, Forst J, Huber H, Schmitt HJ. Anaesthetic management in patients with Duchenne muscular dystrophy undergoing orthopaedic surgery: a review of 232 cases. *Eur J Anaesthesiol.* 2012;29:489–494.
29. Shapiro F, Sethna N. Blood loss in pediatric spine surgery. *Eur Spine J.* 2004;13(Suppl 1):S6–S17.
30. Shapiro F, Zurakowski D, Sethna NF. Tranexamic acid diminishes intraoperative blood loss and transfusion in spinal fusions for duchenne muscular dystrophy scoliosis. *Spine.* 2007;32:2278–2283.
31. Muenster T, Schmidt J, Wick S, Forst J, Schmitt HJ. Rocuronium 0.3 mg x kg-1 (ED95) induces a normal peak effect but an altered time course of neuromuscular block in patients with Duchenne's muscular dystrophy. *Paediatr Anaesth.* 2006;16:840–845.
32. Birnkrant DJ, Panitch HB, Benditt JO, et al. American College of Chest Physicians consensus statement on the respiratory and related management of patients with Duchenne muscular dystrophy undergoing anesthesia or sedation. *Chest.* 2007;132:1977–1986.
33. Lumbierres M, Prats E, Farrero E, et al. Noninvasive positive pressure ventilation prevents postoperative pulmonary complications in chronic ventilators users. *Respir Med.* 2007;101:62–68.
34. Bach JR, Sabharwal S. High pulmonary risk scoliosis surgery: role of noninvasive ventilation and related techniques. *J Spinal Disord Tech,* 2005;18:527–530.
35. Phillips MF, Quinlivan RC, Edwards RH, Calverley PM. Changes in spirometry over time as a prognostic marker in patients with Duchenne muscular dystrophy. *Am J Respir Crit Care Med.* 2001;164:2191–2194.

36.

ANESTHETIC MANAGEMENT FOR PATIENTS WITH CEREBRAL PALSY

J. Koh and I. Aliason

STEM CASE AND KEY QUESTIONS

JS is a 15-year-old young man with cerebral palsy (CP) scheduled for replacement of his baclofen pump. The patient's mother is unsure if the pump is currently functioning, since she has noticed that JS has had some increased spasticity in the past few weeks. In addition to CP, JS has a history of seizures, gastroesophageal reflux (GER), and developmental delay. His seizures are reasonably well controlled on his current medication. He has had multiple previous surgeries for contractures and ventriculoperitoneal shunt placement and revisions.

HOW IS CP MOST COMMONLY CLASSIFIED?

Mother states that JS has some spasticity in all 4 extremities, but his legs are more severely affected than his arms. He has been able to ambulate intermittently with braces and crutches. His baclofen pump has helped improve his ability to ambulate, and it has decreased his spasticity-associated discomfort. Mother states he does go to regular high school but attends special education classes.

IS COGNITIVE IMPAIRMENT COMMON IN PATIENTS WITH CP? HOW CAN YOU DETERMINE THE PATIENT'S COGNITIVE FUNCTION?

Mother states that JS functions at about a fourth-grade level but has some higher functioning in certain academic areas such as math. Mom feels he is able to understand almost all verbal communications reasonably well.

WHAT ARE OTHER KEY QUESTIONS YOU SHOULD ASK IN THE PERIOPERATIVE PERIOD?

JS uses a computer interface to communicate due to speech difficulty, and he has brought his communication kit with him to surgery. Mother states his seizures are variable in presentation including tonic-clonic and partial seizures. His seizures are well controlled on his current medications, but he will have increased seizure activity if he misses a medication dose. He can only take his seizure medication with applesauce or pudding. His GER seems well controlled, and he has no history of aspiration pneumonia. JS has never had any anesthetic complications, but he does have some preoperative anxiety due to previous traumatic hospital experiences.

SHOULD HE TAKE HIS REGULAR DOSE OF SEIZURE MEDICATION THE MORNING OF SURGERY?

Mom states that his seizure medication is usually given at 7 PM and 7 AM, and his surgery is planned for 8 AM. After discussion with the preoperative nurse, Mom agrees to give his evening dose the night prior to surgery. On the morning of surgery, she will give his seizure medication 2 hours early with a tablespoon of applesauce. Postoperatively she will adjust his dosing regimen back to his normal schedule.

WOULD YOU INSIST PLACE AN INTRAVENOUS (IV) LINE PREOPERATIVELY? IS PREMEDICATION APPROPRIATE?

When asked directly, JS states he is very nervous and would like something to help calm him. When asked about having an IV placed, he becomes very anxious. Mother states that they have had difficulty placing IVs with him awake due to his spasticity and contractures. Mother and JS agree with the plan for oral premedication with midazolam and inhalational induction.

WHAT ARE THE INTRAOPERATIVE CONCERNS RELATED TO THE PATIENT'S CONTRACTURES?

You note preoperatively that JS cannot extend his legs completely and has some flexion contractures of his elbows and wrists. He prefers to keep his neck flexed to the left side. On discussion with mom, she states he prefers to sleep in a flexed position but does seem to relax some with sleeping. There has been no difficulty with airway management reported in the past. Mother states that at times IV access has been difficult even when asleep.

SHOULD THE INTRAOPERATIVE ANESTHETIC PLAN DIFFER FROM A PATIENT WITHOUT CP?

JS has an uneventful inhalational induction. IV placement is successful after 3 attempts, and the patient is intubated using rocuronium without difficulty. Maintenance is planned with fentanyl, sevoflurane, and muscle relaxant. During the case, the patient does not seem to require much anesthetic but then will move during especially stimulating parts of the procedure despite regular dosing of rocuronium.

WHAT ANESTHETIC COMPLICATIONS CAN BE SEEN IN PATIENTS WITH CP?

His blood pressure is on the low side compared to preoperative values throughout the case. A fluid bolus is given with some improvement, and occasional low-dose ephedrine is required to allow a reasonable amount of anesthetic to be administered. You also note after the drapes are placed that the patient's temp is 33.2°C axillary. After changing the temperature probe and placing it in the esophagus, the temperature is 34.0°C. The surgeon comments that the surgical field is a little more bloody than usual; she requests that no ketorolac be given. A lower body forced air blanket is placed, and you cover the head and accessible upper body with a warm blanket.

HOW CAN POSTOPERATIVE PAIN BE ASSESSED IN THIS PATIENT?

JS arrives at in the postanesthesia care unit (PACU) in stable condition. He received 0.5 mcg/kg of fentanyl intraoperatively. He is initially quite sleepy but responsive. As he continues to recover, he becomes increasingly agitated. The recovery nurse is having difficulty communicating with JS to assess his pain level and is reluctant to give opioids. JS eventually is able to communicate that he wishes to see his mother. Once she arrives, she is able to interpret his behavior as being painful. Mother also has his communication kit, which allows JS to self-report his pain as being 8/10 at the surgical site.

ARE THERE ANY SPECIAL CONSIDERATIONS WHEN TREATING POSTOPERATIVE PAIN?

The recovery room nurse administers morphine in 0.03 mg/kg increments. Despite a total morphine dose of 0.1 mg/kg, JS still describes his pain as being 6/10. A dose of IV acetaminophen is administered, along with an additional dose of morphine. JS states that his incisional pain is much better, but he is having muscle spasms in his legs that are now the main source of his pain. A dose of IV diazepam is given, which relieves the muscle spasms. The patient is transferred to the floor after he states that his pain is well controlled.

WHAT ARE THE COMPLICATIONS THAT CAN BE SEEN WITH INTRATHECAL BACLOFEN ADMINISTRATION?

The baclofen pump is started in the PACU and appears to be functioning well. He has an uneventful night on the floor, and the plan is for him to be discharged home the next day. On morning rounds, the nurse notes that he is extremely sleepy and difficult to arouse. His oxygen saturation on room air is normal, but his respiratory rate is slow. He has not received

any opioids since leaving the PACU. Neurosurgery is immediately consulted, and the baclofen pump is interrogated, revealing a programming error resulting in an overdose. The pump is stopped immediately, and the patient is transferred to the pediatric intensive care unit for observation. He gradually wakes up over the next 24 hours and returns to his baseline mental status the next day. The baclofen pump is restarted at the proper rate. After additional observation, patient is transferred home without further incident.

DISCUSSION

Cerebral palsy encompasses a range of neurologic symptoms that can vary vastly from patient to patient. The main characteristics include abnormality of muscle tone, with or without movement disorder. The prevalence is reported to be in the range of 1 in 500 to 1,000 births.[1,2]

For many years, perinatal asphyxia was held as the primary cause of CP, resulting in a large number of litigations brought against obstetricians. We now understand that there are many perinatal etiologies that result in the picture of CP. Examples include antenatal infection, periventricular hemorrhage associated with prematurity, perinatal ischemic stroke, congenital anomaly, postnatal meningitis/encephalitis, or trauma. In most cases, the etiology is likely multifactorial rather than a singular event.[1] Of note, premature births account for about 50% of all cases of CP.[2] The neurologic insult is static in nature, as compared to other progressive degenerative neurological disorders. However, secondary manifestations such as muscle spasticity or GER may improve, worsen, or remain stable over time.

CLASSIFICATION

Classification of CP is most commonly centered on the characteristics of the motor symptoms that the patient presents with. Characteristics of muscle tone, distribution of extremity involvement, and movement disorders are usually included. One example is presented in Table 36.1.

Spastic CP is the most common type, with 70% of cases falling into this category.[2] Spastic CP can present as spastic quadriplegia, spastic diplegia, or spastic hemiplegia. Patients with spastic hemiplegia and spastic diplegia usually have the most potential for functional movement.

COGNITIVE ABILITY/COMMUNICATION

Patients with CP present with a wide variety of cognitive ability. It is important to understand that communication challenges do not necessarily correlate with intellectual ability.

Approximately two thirds of patients with CP have some degree of intellectual disability. Patients with spastic hemiplegia are most likely to be of normal intelligence whereas less than 30% of those with spastic quadriplegia will have normal intelligence. Learning disabilities are not uncommon, and patients can suffer from depression, attention deficit/

Table 36.1 CLASSIFICATION OF CEREBRAL PALSY

TYPE AND CAUSE	MOTOR DEFICITS	DISTRIBUTION	COMPLICATIONS
Hypotonic Syndromic Dysgenesis Insult: hypoxic-ischemia	Low axial tone Variable limb tone Deep tendon reflexes usually increased	Diffuse	Learning disability Contractures Epilepsy Feeding dysfunction Hearing or vision impaired Respiratory infections
Spastic Insult: hypoxia-ischemia; vascular	Increased tone: pyramidal type Increased deep tendon reflexes	Monoparesis Diparesis Hemiparesis Triparesis Tetraparesis	

Choreoathetoid
Insult: hypoxia-ischemia; neonatal
  hyperbilirubinemia; metabolic
	Involuntary movement; often
	  a mixture of choreaathetosis
	  dystonia
		May be diffuse (tetraparesis) or
		  confined to one or more limbs
		Often coexists with spasticity
			Hearing impairment
			Contractures
			Intellect often maintained

Ataxic
Cerebral dysgenesis
	Usually generalized truncal and
	  limb ataxia
	May coexist with spasticity
		May be diffuse but often
		  associated with diparesis
			Few, may be mild

Source. Reproduced from Crean P, Peake D. Essentials of Neurology and Neuromuscular Disorders. In Cote CJ, Lerman J, Anderson BJ. *A Practice of Anesthesia in Infants and Children.* 5th ed. Philadelphia, PA: Elsevier Saunders; 2013:476-477. Used with permission.

hyperactivity disorder, and emotional lability especially in adolescents.[1]

Communication abilities for patients with CP are influenced not only by their cognitive level of functioning but also by central nervous system or motor function disabilities that affect their ability to speak effectively and/or understand spoken information. Patients may use communication assist devices such as computers or communication boards to help them "speak." Sometimes simple communication strategies are developed such as looking right for "yes" and left for "no." Parents can provide critical information to care providers about their child's level of understanding, as well as usual methods for communicating. They will often know their child's approximate developmental age and if there are any specific areas of delay. Formal evaluation by a developmental pediatrician or a neuropsychologist may be documented in the patient's medical record as well.

PRESENTING SYMPTOMS/COMORBIDITIES

Spasticity is the most obvious presenting symptom for many patients and is the focus of much of the management of CP. Positioning restrictions often require custom-made seats and wheelchairs. Positioning for surgical procedures is often challenging and may require creative use of padding and positioning devices.

Some patients have significant discomfort associated with their spasticity as well. A variety of pharmacologic interventions can be used, including systemic muscle relaxants such as baclofen. If spasticity is preventing ambulation or causing significant discomfort or positioning challenges, a trial of intrathecal baclofen may be helpful. If clinical improvement is seen, a baclofen pump is often placed to allow for continuous administration of intrathecal baclofen.[3] There

are reports of baclofen withdrawal in circumstances of pump failure or inadvertent cessation of systemic baclofen. Overdose is unusual, with misprogramming of the pump being the most common cause. Intramuscular injections of botulinum toxin have also been found to be useful in certain cases, and orthopedic surgery for tendon release may be considered.[3]

Seizure disorders are common in children with CP, occurring in approximately 30% of patients. The most common seizure types are generalized tonic-clonic and complex partial. Seizures are most common in the spastic hemiplegia form of CP.[4] Patients are often on antiepileptic medications, and these should be continued throughout their perioperative course if possible. Seizure history should be obtained from parents including seizure frequency, duration, appearance of typical seizures, when the last seizure occurred, if/when abortive medications have needed to be given, and if seizures every result in physiologic compromise.

Although variable in severity, GER is also a prevalent comorbidity in this population. Gastric fundoplication may be required in patients with severe GER and history of aspiration pneumonias. However, based on a recent review, the overall risk of perioperative aspiration in patients with CP does not seem to be significantly higher than the general population.[3] Swallowing function may also be affected in patients with CP, which can also increase the risk for aspiration. In addition, some patients may not be able to take adequate oral nutrition due to swallowing difficulties and require feeding through a gastrostomy tube.

CONSIDERATIONS IN ANESTHETIC MANAGEMENT

Most patients with CP undergo a surgical procedure at some point in their lives, and they often undergo multiple procedures. The most common type of surgery is orthopedic, followed by dental restorations and general surgery procedures.[1]

As previously noted, it is important to complete a thorough history and physical to note patient factors such as comorbidities, medications, positioning restrictions, cognitive ability, communication methods, and parental concerns. In most cases, the patient should take all current home medications preoperatively, especially antiepileptic medications. In some circumstances, patients with swallowing difficulties may only be able to take their medication with some sort of soft food. The anesthesiologist will need to make a risk versus benefit decision about the relative need for the medication, timing of the administration, and risk of aspiration. One additional question is whether the patient would benefit from a premedication. The best person to answer this question is the patient if able, but the parents can also provide valuable input.

Induction of anesthesia can usually be either IV or inhalational, depending on the patient's condition and preferences. As noted, GER is common in this population, but aspiration pneumonia is relatively rare so rapid sequence induction for an elective procedure is not usually required.[3] In some circumstances, a pseudorapid sequence induction may be required with inhalational induction, cricoid pressure, and expeditious IV placement as the patient is being induced. The induction can then be completed rapidly with IV medication and the airway secured. However, it is important to remember that there is the potential for difficult IV placement due to contractures or movement disorders.

Maintenance of anesthesia can be performed using IV and/or inhalational agents. There is some suggestion in the literature that the maximum acceptable concentration for inhalation agents is lowered for patients with CP.[5,6] It is widely known that all patients on antiepileptic medications may be resistant to nondepolarizing muscle relaxants, this includes patients with CP.[7] However, if patients are receiving baclofen or dantrolene for muscle spasticity, they may be more sensitive to muscle relaxants. It is unknown if patients with CP inherently respond to nondepolarizing muscle relaxants differently, but it is likely clinically insignificant. Despite some degree of proliferation of extrajunctional acetylcholine receptors, patients with CP can safely receive succinylcholine without a hyperkalemic response.[4]

Patients with CP are often anemic and can be mildly coagulopathic at baseline due to poor nutrition and chronic disease. In addition, antiepileptic medications can also cause mild thrombocytopenia. Thus, they are at increased risk of bleeding and needing intraoperative blood transfusion. Antifibrinolytics are often used for surgeries with large expected blood loss (i.e., posterior spinal fusion for scoliosis.) If coagulation studies are normal, there is no contraindication to regional anesthesia in this patient population.[8]

There are no data to suggest this population responds differently to opioid administration, although there is some evidence that anesthesiologists tend to administer lower doses of opioid intraoperatively.[9,10] This did not correlate to increased pain postoperatively. This may indirectly suggest that opioid

requirements in this population are somewhat lower than the general population, but there is no clear evidence to support a difference.

ANESTHETIC COMPLICATIONS

Patients with CP are at increased risk for anesthetic complications. A recent review found that the incidence of perioperative adverse events was 63.1%.[3] By far, the most common events were hypothermia and hypotension, and when these were removed from analysis, the rate of adverse events was 13.1% (Figure 36.1). Delayed emergence is the next most common adverse event. Factors associated with higher risk in this population included American Society of Anesthesiologists score higher than 2, seizure disorder, upper airway hypotonia, general surgery procedures, and older age. Patients receiving baclofen or dantrolene for spasticity are at risk for respiratory insufficiency upon emergence from anesthesia as these medications contribute to weakness.

POSTOPERATIVE PAIN ASSESSMENT AND TREATMENT

Given the frequency of surgical procedures that patients with CP often undergo, adequate assessment and treatment of postoperative pain is essential.

It has become the standard to use self-report for healthy children over 5 years using a FACES scale, and for children older than 8 years, a 0 to 10 scale similar to that used in adults. As previously outlined, there is significant variability in the cognitive level and communication ability in patients with CP. The preoperative visit should include a discussion about how to best assess the patients pain. Fanurik et al.[11] showed that the majority of patients with mild to moderate cognitive impairment can use some form of self-report; this includes patients with CP. Parents can also provide very helpful interpretation of communications and/or behavior from patients that may be pain related. Considerable effort has been made to develop observational pain assessment tools specific for children with cognitive impairment. Collignon et al.[12] developed and validated a 10-item scale for patients with CP. Interestingly, many of the behaviors are similar to those found in tools developed for the general pediatric population, and, in fact, one group has shown that the FLACC (face, legs, activity, cry, consolability) scale can be an effective tool in patients with CP[13] (Table 36.2). As with all patients, the most effective method for assessing pain is to gather as much information as possible, including self-report, parent report, and nurse report, in addition to using behavioral assessment tools.

The management of postoperative pain does not differ from that of patients without CP. Multimodal therapy should be used as indicated, individualized to the patient and the surgical procedure. Similarly to intraoperative opioid use, there is no evidence that these patients as a population are more sensitive to opioids. However, some feel that some patients with CP may either be relatively insensitive to pain and therefore need less analgesia or be more sensitive to the effects of analgesics.

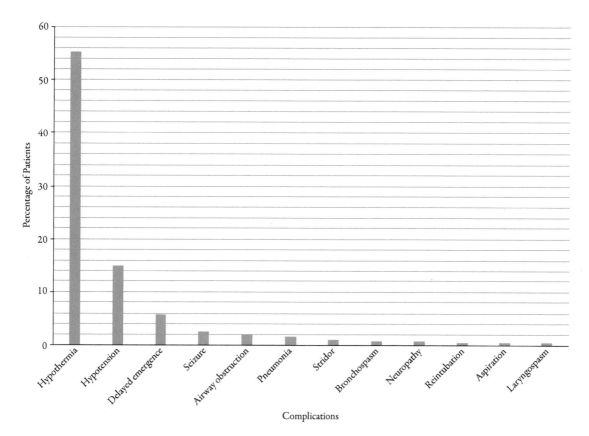

Fig. 36.1 Perioperative complications in patients with cerebral palsy. Reproduced with permission from Wass CT, Warner ME, Worrell GA, et al. Effect of general anesthesia in patients with cerebral palsy at the turn of the new millennium: a population based study evaluating perioperative outcome and brief overview of anesthetic implications of this coexisting disease. *J Child Neurol.* 2012;27(7):859–866.

Table 36.2 COMPARISON OF TWO BEHAVIORAL PAIN SCALES

PAIN EVALUATION SCALE ITEMS (COLLINGNON AND GIUSIAN)	FLACC SCALE ITEMS (VOEPEL-LEWIS ET AL.)
Crying	Face
Coordinated defensive reaction on exam of supposed painful area	Legs
Painful expression	Activity
Protection of painful areas	Cry
Moaning or inaudible cries	Consolability
Spontaneous interest in surroundings	
Aggravation of tonic troubles	
Ability to communicate with the nurse	
Increase in spontaneous movement	
Spontaneous antalgesic position	

Source. Adapted from Collignon P, Giusian B. Validation of pain evaluation scale for patients with cerebral palsy. *Eur J Pain.* 2001;5:433–442 and Voepel-Lewis T, Merkel S, Tait A, Trzcinka A, Malviya S. The reliability and validity of the face, legs, activity, cry, consolability observational tool as a measure of pain in children with cognitive impairment. *Anesth Analg.* 2002;95:1224–1229.

As with all patients, careful titration of opioids in the PACU is the best strategy for safely optimizing postoperative analgesia.

REVIEW QUESTIONS

1. What is the **MOST** common etiology of CP?

    A. chromosomal anomaly
    B. intrauterine drug exposure
    C. perinatal asphyxia
    D. prematurity/low birth weight

Answer: D

Prematurity/low birth weight accounts for approximately 50% of all cases of CP. There are many perinatal etiologies that result in the picture of CP. Examples include antenatal infection, periventricular hemorrhage associated with prematurity, perinatal ischemic stroke, congenital anomaly, postnatal meningitis/encephalitis, or trauma. In most cases, the etiology is likely multifactorial rather than a singular event.[1,2,4]

2. A 6-year-old boy with CP, spastic quadriplegia, and developmental delay is in the recovery room after a lower extremity contracture release. What is the **BEST** method to assess his pain?

    A. number of demands made on patient-controlled analgesia
    B. nurse report of patient behavior

C. parent report of patient behavior
D. patient use of FACES pain scale

Answer: C

It has become the standard to use self-report for healthy children over 5 years using a FACES scale, and for children older than 8 years, a 0 to 10 scale similar to that used in adults. As previously outlined, there is significant variability in the cognitive level and communication ability in patients with CP. In this case, the patient has developmental delay and use of pain scales may not be appropriate. Parents can provide very helpful interpretation of communications and/or behavior from patients that may be pain related, especially in nonverbal children. Children generally need to be at least 7 years old to use patient-controlled analgesia appropriately. As with all patients, the most effective method for assessing pain is to gather as much information as possible, including self-report, parent report, and nurse report in addition to using behavioral assessment tools.[11,14]

3. Of the following anesthetic complications, which are patients with CP at the **LOWEST** risk?

A. aspiration pneumonia
B. delayed emergence
C. difficult IV access
D. hypothermia

Answer: A

GER is a common comorbidity in patients with CP, but aspiration pneumonia is relatively rare so rapid sequence induction for an elective procedure is not usually required. Patients with CP are at increased risk for anesthetic complications.[3] A recent review found that the incidence of perioperative adverse events was 63.1%. By far, the most common events were hypothermia and hypotension. Delayed emergence is the next most common adverse event. There is the potential for difficult IV placement due to contractures or movement disorders.[3]

4. Cognitive disability **MOST** commonly correlates with which of the following findings?

A. brain magnetic resonance imaging abnormalities
B. bilateral inguinal hernias
C. degree of motor disability
D. past history of meningitis

Answer: C

The general observation is that the greater the degree of motor disability the higher the likelihood of cognitive impairment. Approximately two thirds of patients with CP have some degree of intellectual disability. Patients with spastic hemiplegia are most likely to be of normal intelligence, whereas less than 30% of those with spastic quadriplegia will have normal intelligence.[1]

5. Of the following common perioperative complications, which is the **LEAST** seen in patients with CP?

A. delayed emergence
B. hypothermia
C. hypotension
D. seizures

Answer: D

Patients with CP are at increased risk for anesthetic complications. A recent review found that the incidence of perioperative adverse events was 63.1%. By far, the most common events were hypothermia and hypotension. Delayed emergence is the next most common adverse event. Patients receiving baclofen or dantrolene for spasticity are at risk for respiratory insufficiency upon emergence from anesthesia as these medications contribute to weakness. A history of seizures increases the risk that a patient will have a perioperative complication; however, seizure itself is not a common complication. Factors associated with higher risk in this population included American Society of Anesthesiologists score higher than 2, seizure disorder, upper airway hypotonia, general surgery procedures, and older age.[3]

6. Of the following medications, which is **LEAST** likely to help relieve muscle spasticity in patients with CP?

A. baclofen
B. botulinum toxin
C. diazepam
D. levetiracetam

Answer: D

Levetiracetam is an antiepileptic medication used to treat seizures. Baclofen is a muscle relaxant and can be administered orally, intrathecally, or transdermally. Diazepam is a benzodiazepine, which can be administered orally, rectally, intramuscular, or intravenously. It is most commonly used to treat anxiety, alcohol withdrawal, muscle spasms, and seizure. Botulinum toxin is injected intramuscularly; it acts at the neuromuscular junction and inhibits the release of acetylcholine thereby blocking neuromuscular transmission in the particular muscle group where it was injected.[15]

7. Of the following symptoms, which is **LEAST** likely to be seen with baclofen overdose?

A. delirium
B. hypertension
C. hyperthermia
D. seizures

Answer: C

Baclofen overdose causes symptoms such as seizures, delirium/altered mental status, and nausea/vomiting. Severe toxicity can cause bradycardia, hypotension or hypertension, respiratory failure, hypothermia, coma, and death. Treatment consists of supportive care. Activated charcoal can be used in the event of acute oral ingestions. Hemodialysis can be used to increase the clearance of baclofen even in patients with normal renal function.[16]

QUESTIONS AND ANSWERS

This chapter has accompanying questions and answers which are available to subscribers as part of the Oxford eLearning platform. To access the questions, go to ✓ http:// oxfordmedicine. com/pediatricanesthesiaPBL

REFERENCES

1. Nolan J, Chalkiadis GA, Low J, Olesch CA, Brown TCK. Anaesthesia and pain management in cerebral palsy. *Anaesthesia*. 2000;55:32.

2. Lerman J. Perioperative management of the paediatric patient with coexisting neuromuscular disease. *Br J Anaesth*. 2011;107(Suppl 1):i79–i89.

3. Wass CT, Warner ME, Worrell GA, et al. Effect of general anesthesia in patients with cerebral palsy at the turn of the new millennium: a population based study evaluating perioperative outcome and brief overview of anesthetic implications of this coexisting disease. *J Child Neurol*. 2012;27(7);859–866.

4. Crean P, Peake D. Essentials of neurology and neuromuscular disorders. In: Cote C, Lerman J, Anderson B, eds. *A Practice of Anesthesia for Infants and Children*. 5th ed. Philadelphia, PA: Elsevier Saunders; 2013:476–477.

5. Yilbas AA, Ayhan B, Akinci SB, Saricaoglu F, Aypar U. The effect of different end-tidal desflurane concentrations on bispectral index values in normal children and children with cerebral palsy. *Turk J Aneasthesiol Reanim*. 2013:41(6)200–205.

6. Frei FJ, Haemmerle MH, Brunner R, Kern C. Minimum alveolar concentration for halothane in children with cerebral palsy and severe mental retardation. *Anaesthesia*. 1997;52:11056–11060.

7. Hepaguslar H, Ozzeybek D, Elar Z. The effect of cerebral palsy on the action of vecuronium with and without anticonvulsants. *Anaesthesia*. 1999;54:582–598.

8. Theroux M, Akins R. Surgery and anesthesia for children who have cerebral palsy. *Anesthesiol Clin North America*. 2005;23(4):733–743.

9. Long LS, Ved S, Koh J. Intraoperative opioid dosing in children with and without cerebral palsy. *Pediatr Anesth*. 2009;19:513–520.

10. Koh J, Fanurik D, Harrison R, Schmitz M, Norvell D. Analgesia following surgery in children with and without cognitive impairment. *Pain*. 2004;111(3):239–244.

11. Fanurik D, Koh J, Harrison R, Conrad T, Tomerlin C. Pain assessment in children with cognitive impairment. an exploration of self report skills. *Clin Nurs Res*. 1998;7(2):103–119; discussion 120–124.

12. Collignon P, Giusian B. Validation of pain evaluation scale for patients with cerebral palsy. *Eur J Pain*. 2001;5:433–442.

13. Voepel-Lewis T, Merkel S, Tait A, Trzcinka A, Malviya S. The reliability and validity of the face, legs, activity, cry, consolability observational tool as a measure of pain in children with cognitive impairment. *Anesth Analg*. 2002;95:1224–1229.

14. Fanurik D, Koh J, Schmitz M, Harrison R, Conrad T. Children with cognitive impairment: parent report of pain and coping. *J Dev Behav Pediatr*. 1999;20(4):228–234.

15. Davis E, Barnes M. Botulinum toxin and spasticity. *J Neurol Neurosurg Psychiatry*. 2000;69:143–149.

16. Jung M. Baclofen overdoses. Maryland Poison Center, University of Maryland School of Pharmacy. www.mdpoison.com. Accessed June 13, 2017.

ADDITIONAL READING

Sherwell S, Reid S, Reddihough D, Wrennall J, Ong B, Stargatt R. measuring intellectual ability in children with cerebral palsy: Can we do better? *Res Dev Disabil*. 2014;35(10):2558–2567.

Fanurik D, Koh J, Schmitz M, Harrison R, Roberson P, Killebrew P. Pain assessment and treatment in children with cognitive impairment: a survey of nurses' and physicians' beliefs. *Clin J Pain*. 1999;15(4):304–312.

SECTION 6

GASTROINTESTINAL SYSTEM

37.

HIRSCHSPRUNG DISEASE

Erica Sivak, Marcus Malek, and Denise Hall-Burton

STEM CASE AND KEY QUESTIONS

A 5 year-old boy, weighing 19 kilograms, presented to the gastroenterology clinic with a long history of constipation. He was diagnosed with Hirschsprung disease (HD) after a suction rectal biopsy revealed the absence of ganglion cells. Contrast enema identified a transition zone in the rectosigmoid. He was scheduled for a laparoscopic-assisted Soave primary pull-through procedure with intraoperative intestinal biopsies.

HOW DOES HD TYPICALLY PRESENT? WHAT IS THE DIFFERENTIAL DIAGNOSIS OF CHRONIC CONSTIPATION IN A CHILD? WHAT DIAGNOSTIC TESTS MAY BE USEFUL TO ESTABLISH DIAGNOSIS OF HD? WHAT ARE THE TREATMENT OPTIONS FOR HD?

On the day of surgery he was 19.3 kg and his blood pressure, heart rate, temperature, respiratory rate, and oxygen saturation were all within normal limits. He was born at 39 weeks gestation via vaginal delivery without complication. Preoperative evaluation revealed a remote history of reactive airway disease, but he had not required albuterol for 3 years. His physical exam was unremarkable with the exception of mild eczema on his legs and arms. He completed a bowel prep and was nil per os appropriate. He had never had an anesthetic, and there was no family history of problems with anesthesia. Although he had a runny nose and mild cough about 2 months ago, he has been well since. His parents report no known medication or food allergies. Routine preoperative blood work was unremarkable with electrolytes all within normal limits, a platelet count of 243,000 per mcL, hemoglobin of 14.2 g/dL, and hematocrit of 43 g/dL. Preoperative coagulation studies were within normal limits as well.

WHAT IS AN APPROPRIATE ANESTHETIC PLAN FOR THE LAPAROSCOPIC IDENTIFICATION OF THE TRANSITION ZONE AND PULL-THROUGH OPERATION?

After placing standard American Society of Anesthesiology monitors and an uneventful inhalation induction of general anesthesia with Sevoflurane, a 20 G angiocatheter was placed in the right saphenous vein and a 22 G angiocatheter was placed in the left hand. Propofol 2 mg/kg, fentanyl 12 mcg/kg, and rocuronium 0.6 mg/kg were given prior to direct laryngoscopy and placement of a 5.0 endotracheal tube. Endotracheal tube placement was confirmed using end-tidal carbon dioxide and bilateral pulmonary auscultation.

While placing an oral-gastric tube hives were noted on his chest and arms. His heart rate rose to 150 beats per minute and his end-tidal carbon dioxide tracing developed an obstructive pattern. Hypotension was also noted. Ventilation was switched from pressure control ventilation to bag-valve-mask. Auscultation revealed wheezing throughout all lung fields and high peak airway pressures were needed to effectively ventilate the patient. Intravenous (IV) fluid lines were opened wide and inhaled albuterol was given without significant hemodynamic or pulmonary improvement.

WHAT ARE THE MOST COMMON CAUSES OF ANAPHYLAXIS UNDER ANESTHESIA? HOW DO YOU DIFFERENTIATE BETWEEN THE TWO? WHAT IS THE TREATMENT FOR ANAPHYLAXIS?

His airway pressures, capnograph tracing, and wheezing rapidly improved with 1 mcg/kg IV epinephrine. Repeated doses of epinephrine were required and an intramuscular (IM) injection of epinephrine 10 mcg/kg was given into the quadriceps. Diphenhydramine 1 mg/kg and hydrocortisone 5 mg/kg were also administered.

IS THERE A WAY TO CONFIRM DIAGNOSIS OF ANAPHYLAXIS?

After resolution of his bronchospasm and hypotension, he was placed in a left lateral position and a single injection caudal block was performed with 10 mL of 0.2% ropivacaine injected. He was then again placed supine and prepped for the surgical procedure. Anesthesia was maintained with 1.0 vol% Isoflurane, 1.5 L/min oxygen, and 1.5 L/min air. Ventilator pressure and respiratory rate were adjusted to maintain a volume of 6 mL/kg and an end-expiratory carbon dioxide tension of 35 to 40 mmHg. His mean arterial pressures (MAP) were low normal and his heart rate was slightly tachycardic. Both his MAP and tachycardia improved with 10 mL/kg lactated ringers solution.

When inserting the Veress needle at the umbilicus, the surgeon reported needing increased force when initially inserting the needle followed by a sudden drastic release of that force. Upon trochar insertion the patient was again mildly tachycardic with MAPs in the low normal range. After establishment of pneumoperiteneum and insertion of the laparoscopic camera, there was no evidence of vascular trauma. Throughout the laparoscopic portion of the case, his mild tachycardia and hypotension continued to improve with intermittent fluid administration.

HOW COMMON IS VASCULAR INJURY DURING LAPAROSCOPY? HOW WOULD YOU RESPOND TO SUDDEN MASSIVE BLOOD LOSS IN YOUR PATIENT?

The contrast enema identified the transition zone in the rectosigmoid colon, and this was confirmed on initial inspection with the laparoscope. A seromuscular intestinal biopsy was taken just proximal to the presumed transition zone, which on frozen section analysis confirmed ganglion cells and the absence of hypertrophic nerves. After ligating and dividing the mesentery of the aganglionated segment, the healthy colon was mobilized so that it could reach the perineum for his pull-through anastomosis. At this point, the pneumoperitoneum was released and the surgeons moved down to the perineum to begin the pull-through portion of the operation.

Upon release of the pneumoperitoneum, however, the patient became tachycardic and hypotensive with only mild improvement with volume resuscitation. Hemoglobin and hematocrit (H/H) was assessed and found to be critically low at 6.2 g/dL and 18.7 g/dL. A repeat H/H and type and cross were sent while packed red blood cells, platelets, and fresh frozen plasma were requested from the blood bank. Uncross matched blood was immediately brought into the room. An 18 G angiocath was placed in the left arm and a 22 G angiocath was placed in the right radial artery. Due to the critical H/H and continued hypotension and tachycardia, uncrossed, universal donor blood was administered.

Upon re-insufflation and assessment of the abdominal cavity, a central retroperitoneal hematoma was visualized which was not present during the initial laparoscopy. The surgeon voiced concern for an iatrogenic vascular injury. A vascular surgeon was called and a large midline abdominal incision made. A defect was found in the patient's mesentery. An aortic injury was suspected so proximal and distal control of the aorta was obtained by the vascular surgeon and a 3 mm aortic laceration was identified. The aortic defect was quickly repaired. H/H, arterial blood gas (ABG) and thromboelastogram (TEG) were quickly sent. Although the ABG was unremarkable and his H/H had improved to 10.3 g/dL and 31 g/dL, the TEG revealed a maximum amplitude (MA) of 42 mm. Due to the decreased MA, platelets were administered. The patient's tachycardia and hypotension resolved. Due to the severity of the vascular injury the surgeon left a rectal stump after excising the aganglionated bowel segment and brought up the end of the healthy colon as a colostomy. It was decided that the patient should return in a few months for the pull-through portion of the procedure.

Coagulation studies were sent and found to be normal with an international normalized ratio of 1.3 and platelet count of 173,000 per mcL. After discussion with the surgeon, consent for an epidural nerve block catheter was obtained for postoperative analgesia. Upon completion of the surgical procedure, the patient was placed in left lateral position and prepared for the sterile placement of an epidural catheter between the eighth and ninth thoracic intervertebral space. The epidural space was found at 2.5 cm with an 18 G Touhy needle and a 20 G catheter was placed and secured at 7 cm without complication. After negative aspiration and a negative test dose with lidocaine and epinephrine, the epidural was bolused with 5 mL of 0.2% ropivacaine. After epidural placement the patient was successfully extubated and taken to the postanesthesia care unit (PACU).

WHAT ARE THE COMPLICATIONS OF CONTINUOUS EPIDURAL ANALGESIA IN PEDIATRIC PATIENTS? HOW WOULD YOU MANAGE A ONE-SIDED BLOCK?

In the PACU, repeat H/H and ABG were unremarkable and an epidural infusion of 0.2% ropivacaine at 8 mL/hr was started. Despite the epidural infusion, the patient consistently complained of pain on the left side of his abdomen that was only partially alleviated with Dilaudid. On exam, he had decreased sensation to pinprick along the right but not the left side of his abdomen from approximately the seventh to eleventh thoracic dermatomes. In the PACU his epidural dressing was taken down while maintaining sterility, the epidural catheter pulled back to 5.5 cm, and sterilely redressed. The epidural catheter infusion resumed and, within 45 minutes, adequate analgesia was obtained on both sides of his abdomen. He was transferred to the postsurgical ward with stable vital signs and minimal pain.

HOW DOES HD TYPICALLY PRESENT?

Most commonly HD is diagnosed during early infancy (80% of cases) after the patient is unable to pass stool, poor feeding, and abdominal distention. Some patients will present with life-threating enterocolitis and megacolon.[1] Patients may present outside of infancy with a complaint of chronic constipation.

WHAT IS THE DIFFERENTIAL DIAGNOSIS OF CHRONIC CONSTIPATION IN A CHILD?

Chronic constipation is a common pediatric complaint with a long list of etiologies. Causes include functional constipation, anatomic malformations, spinal cord abnormalities, metabolic causes, neuropathic disorders, including HD, drug use, and other systemic disorders.[2] A careful history and physical examination are the first steps in determining the cause of chronic constipation.

WHAT DIAGNOSTIC TESTS MAY BE USEFUL TO ESTABLISH DIAGNOSIS OF HD?

The absence of ganglion cells in the colon leads to an inability of the intestine to relax and allow the passage of stool. A variable segment of bowel may be affected and leads to dilation of the normal intestine proximal to the affected area. Although not definitive, this bowel dilation may be apparent on abdominal x-ray or contrasted enema (Fig. 37.1). Anorectal manometry measures the pressure in the anal sphincter and may be able to demonstrate incomplete relaxation in the affected area. Rectal biopsy may definitively diagnose HD but can be limited if a deep enough biopsy is not obtained. Multiple biopsies are frequently taken to increase sensitivity. Suction rectal biopsy does not require sedation or anesthesia. If a diagnosis cannot be established, a full thickness rectal biopsy may be required. Full thickness rectal biopsy does, however, require sedation or anesthesia.

WHAT ARE THE TREATMENT OPTIONS FOR HD?

HD can only be cured by complete surgical resection of the aganglionic bowel segment. The three most common operations include Swenson, Duhamel, and Soave (Fig. 37.2) each of which is a "pull-through" operation. The Swenson and Soave procedures involve the complete resection of the aganglionic bowel segment and the anastomosis of healthy bowel to the distal rectum, just above the dentate line. The Duhamel procedure involves anastomosis of the normal bowel in an end-to-side fashion to a rectal pouch that is aganglionated but left behind to function as a rectal reservoir. In order to define where the "transition zone or affected region of intestine extends; intraoperative intestinal biopsies with frozen section

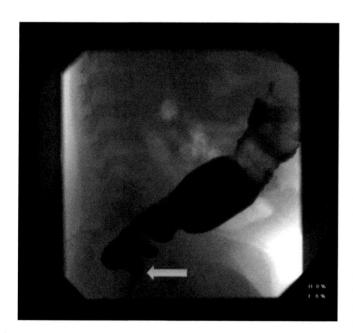

Fig. 37.1 Radiograph courtesy Marcus Malek, MD.

evaluation may be required. Occasionally a staged procedure must be performed for life threatening obstruction or enterocolitis and a colostomy created. After a recovery period the colostomy is then reversed and a pull-through procedure performed.

WHAT IS AN APPROPRIATE ANESTHETIC PLAN FOR THE LAPAROSCOPIC IDENTIFICATION OF THE TRANSITION ZONE AND PULL-THROUGH OPERATION?

General anesthesia with endotracheal intubation with or without muscle relaxation is appropriate for this procedure. Muscle relaxation may be helpful during abdominal insufflation. As blood loss is usually minimal for these procedures, only one to two peripheral IV catheters are usually required. Analgesia may be supplemented with regional anesthesia. A caudal block will provide excellent analgesia for the perineal portion, which is usually the most painful.

HOW DO YOU MAKE THE DIAGNOSIS OF ANAPHYLAXIS UNDER ANESTHESIA?

Anaphylaxis is a type I hypersensitivity reaction that may be caused by immunoglobin E (IgE) or non IgE (formerly called anaphylactoid reaction) activation of mast cells. This activation releases histamine, tryptase, and other chemokines and cytokines, causing an inflammatory reaction. The inflammatory reaction may result in cutaneous signs like erythema and urticaria, respiratory manifestations such as bronchospasm, or circulatory disturbances including tachycardia and hypotension. Reactions can be severe resulting in cardiac arrest. Diagnosis under anesthesia may be difficult—hypotension and tachycardia may be related to hypovolemia, bronchospasm could be secondary to mainstem intubation or light anesthesia, and surgical drapes may obscure cutaneous manifestations. Correct diagnosis must include the prompt exclusion of other possibilities and treatment must be immediate.

WHAT ARE THE MOST COMMON CAUSES OF ANAPHYLAXIS UNDER ANESTHESIA?

Neuromuscular blocking agents with a quaternary ammonium structure are responsible for 60% to 70% of immediate hypersensitivity reactions under anesthesia. Some populations have a higher incidence of anaphylaxis without prior exposure, raising concern that chemicals common to some populations may be the sensitizing agent.[3] Latex is another common cause of anaphylaxis. Patients with a history of atopy, allergy to some fruits (banana, mango, kiwi, and avocado), a history of exposure to latex products—specifically a history of myelomeningocele requiring urinary catheters—should raise concern. Penicillin is the most common antibiotic to cause anaphylaxis, but the cross rate of anaphylaxis from cephalosporins is small and they

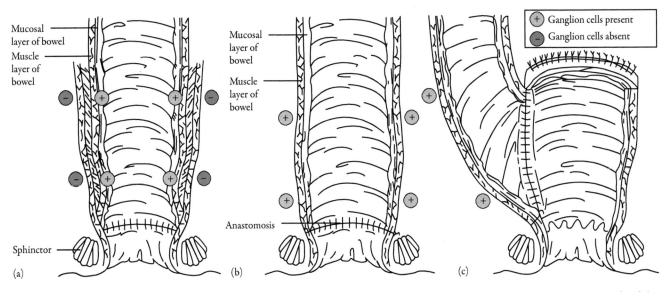

Fig. 37.2 The three most commonly preformed operations for Hirschsprung disease. (a) Swenson procedure: full thickness of rectum is removed and the normally innervated bowel is anastomosed just above the anal sphincter. (b) Soave procedure: the mucosa is stripped from the underlying muscle and the normally innervated bowel is brought through the rectal muscular "cuff" and anastomosed just above the anal sphincter. (c) Duhamel procedure: place behind the rectum is developed and the normally innervated bowel is brought down and anastomosed to the back of the native aganglion rectum just avoce the anal sphincter so that the result is a tube that has aganglionic rectum anteriorly and normally innervated bowel posteriorly. + ganglionic bowel, − aganglionic bowel. Adapted from Langer, Jacob C. Hirschsprung Disease. *Curr Opin Pediatr.* 2013:25(3):368–374.

may often be given safely. There are no case reports of anaphylaxis to any of the inhaled anesthetic agents. Colloid solutions, including albumin and dextrans, may also cause anaphylaxis. Skin preparatory solutions like iodine and chlorhexidine are potential offenders.[4]

WHAT IS THE TREATMENT FOR ANAPHYLAXIS?

Once the diagnosis is made the first step is to immediately halt administration or remove the offending agent if possible. Epinephrine is the next most important step—dose requirements depend on the clinical situation at time of administration. If true circulatory collapse with loss of pulse then pediatric advanced life support should be initiated and epinephrine 10 mcg/kg IV given as part of the pulseless electrical activity algorithm.[5] In the setting of hypotension and bronchospasm without circulatory collapse initiation of treatment with IM epinephrine 0.01 mg/kg to the thigh. An epinephrine infusion may be required with a dose of 0.1 to 1 mcg/kg/min to support blood pressure.[6] Histamine blockers diphenhydramine and ranitidine may also be useful but should not be given in place of epinephrine. Hydrocortisone or another corticosteroid may also be useful as anti-inflammatory agent and mast cell stabilizer, but its administration should not delay epinephrine.

IS THERE A WAY TO CONFIRM DIAGNOSIS OF ANAPHYLAXIS?

Frequently because of the number of medications administered simultaneously it is difficult to determine which medication caused anaphylaxis. It is also clinically impossible to determine if it was IgE or non-IgE mediated anaphylaxis during the event. It may be helpful to send the patient to an allergist for formal skin testing. Providing the allergist with a list of all medications administered will help to guide testing and evaluation.

HOW COMMON IS VASCULAR INJURY DURING LAPAROSCOPY?

Pediatric laparoscopy, when compared to open surgical procedures, leads to an earlier return to activities, reduced hospital stay, decreased hospital expense, and improved cosmetic results.[7,8] Laparoscopy, however, is not without risk. Iatrogenic visceral and vascular injury during laparoscopy is a rare but serious complication that can result in significant morbidity and mortality. As in our case, injury is most likely to occur during insertion of the Veress needle or trocars. Although pediatric specific data is not available, one adult study found an overall incidence of intra-abdominal trocar and Veress needle complications at 0.182% with vascular injury occurring in 0.049% and visceral injuries in 0.133% of cases.[9] Hemodynamic instability and unexpected hematoma formation should raise concern for vascular injury.

WHAT ARE THE COMPLICATIONS OF CONTINUOUS EPIDURAL ANALGESIA IN PEDIATRIC PATIENTS?

There are a variety of intraoperative and postoperative adverse events related to continuous neuraxial nerve block placement in pediatric patients. Intraoperative adverse events include dural puncture, vascular puncture, failed block, respiratory and cardiovascular compromise, neurologic injury, positive test dose, infection, local anesthetic toxicity (LAST), and inability to place the block. Postoperative epidural complications include unintentional unilateral blockade, prolonged blockade, excessive motor blockade, catheter complications, adverse drug reactions including LAST, respiratory and cardiovascular compromise, neurologic problems, hematoma, infection, and adverse reaction to materials used to secure the catheter. Multiple large multicenter studies have found that neurologic (lasting longer than 3 months), cardiovascular, respiratory, bleeding, and infection complications are rare.[10–13] One large multicenter study found that neuraxial adverse events occur more often when catheters are placed (vs. single injections) and that those events are most commonly catheter related—such as catheter dislodgement or kinking.[10] When compared to lumbar or caudal epidurals, thoracic epidurals have more catheter-related complications.[10] The pediatric regional anesthesia network also found that unilateral blockade, as in our patient, was more common in thoracic epidurals as well (2.2%).[10]

CONCLUSIONS

- HD results when ganglion cells do not migrate to the colon properly during development. The aganglionic bowel then fails to function properly resulting in constipation or obstruction and megacolon.

- The only cure for HD is complete excision of the aganglionic portion of the bowel. This can be accomplished through a variety of surgical techniques.

- Anaphylaxis under general anesthesia can be difficult to diagnose. The signs and symptoms of anaphylaxis can be difficult to assess and attribute to anaphylaxis. Anesthesiologists should remain vigilant and anaphylaxis should be included in many differential diagnoses in the operating room. The prompt diagnosis and treatment of anaphylaxis is crucial to minimizing morbidity and mortality.

- While neuromuscular blocking agents with quaternary ammonium structures, like rocuronium in the case here, are the most common cause of immediate hypersensitivity reactions under anesthesia, they are not always the offending drug. Determining which drug or substance is causing the reaction can be less clear.

- Laparoscopic surgery, although preferable to an open incision, is not without risk. Although, uncommon, vascular and visceral injuries can occur. Timely identification of the injury is essential to minimize significant morbidity and mortality from these events.

- Regional anesthesia is important both intraoperatively and postoperatively. Although generally safe, epidurals are not without risk or complication. Complications are more

likely when catheters are placed and most commonly involve the catheter itself.

REVIEW QUESTIONS

1. A stable 3-day-old full-term neonate presents with failure to pass meconium. On exam his abdomen is distended. After digital rectal exam, the passage of gas and meconium was noted. Contrast enema shows severely dilated colon suddenly tapering to a very narrow string-like section of contrast. What is the next **MOST** appropriate diagnostic test?

    A. chloride sweat test
    B. colonoscopy with biopsies
    C. exploratory laparotomy
    D. suction rectal biopsy

Answer: D

A is not correct. Although patients with cystic fibrosis will frequently present in the neonatal period with meconium ileus, bowel obstruction in these children is generally located in the small bowel. The patient's imaging shows dilated colon, making meconium ileus less likely. Answer B is not correct. Although there is increasing use of colonoscopy either with or without surgical intervention for the management of bowel obstruction, it is less common in pediatric patients. There is a significant suspicion of HD in this neonate and a tissue sample is required, rectal suction biopsy is the least invasive method to obtain a tissue sample. Answer C is not correct. Although the definitive cure for HD is surgical excision, the patient has not been definitively diagnosed with HD. In a stable patient, obtaining a tissue biopsy in the least invasive manner is prudent. The surgical approach for resection of aganglionic colon is also most commonly laparoscopic. Answer D is correct. HD most commonly presents in infants as an inability to pass stool, feeding difficulties, and abdominal distention. Although bowel dilation may be apparent on abdominal x-ray or contrast enema, these tests do not provide a definitive diagnosis. In a stable patient, suction rectal biopsy may provide evidence of aganglionic bowel and a definitive diagnosis without requiring general anesthesia.

2. An otherwise healthy 13-year-old female had an uncomplicated laparoscopic cholecystectomy for cholelithiasis and right upper quadrant pain 2 days ago. She was discharged on the day of surgery without complication. She now presents with abdominal pain and distention, fever, diarrhea, nausea and vomiting, and lethargy. What is the next **MOST** appropriate diagnostic step?

    A. Clostridium difficile stool samples
    B. flat and upright abdominal x-rays
    C. IV hydration and antiemetics
    D. urgent exploratory laparotomy

Answer: B

A is not correct. While patients with Clostridium difficile can present with abdominal pain, diarrhea, fever, nausea, and vomiting, it is an infrequent complication after abdominal surgery. In addition, Clostridium difficile stool testing can take hours to days to complete. Even in the setting of Clostridium difficile induced bowl perforation or toxic megacolon, abdominal imaging should not be delayed for stool testing. Answer B is correct. This patient's symptoms are consistent with peritonitis in the setting of recent laparoscopic surgery. It is possible that she is now presenting with a bowel perforation secondary to her recent laparoscopic cholecystectomy. Although uncommon, vascular and visceral injury are a known complication of laparoscopic surgery. Many times, bowel injuries are not recognized intraoperatively. Abdominal flat and upright x-rays looking for subdiaphragmatic free air, a visible falciform ligament, or an air-fluid level are quick, are noninvasive, have minimal radiation exposure, and can be diagnostic. Answer C is not correct. Although most patient presenting with abdominal pain, fever, vomiting, and diarrhea likely have a self-limiting viral infection, concern for more serious problems should be consider in a recent postoperative patient. Answer D is not correct. While this patient may require surgical intervention, proceeding with noninvasive imaging to better delineate the etiology of her acute abdominal pain is most appropriate.

3. A 15-year-old female presents for anterior cruciate ligament repair under general anesthesia. She has a history of rash with penicillin when she was a toddler. The surgeon is requesting perioperative antibiotics to be given. What is the **MOST** appropriate antibiotic given her history of reaction to penicillin?

A. ampicillin
B. cefazolin
C. clindamycin
D. vancomycin

Answer: B

A is not correct. Ampicillin is a beta-lactam antibiotic like penicillin. Ampicillin would not the first-choice antibiotic for this procedure and would not be indicated in a patient with history of reaction to penicillin. Answer B is correct. It is estimated that 1% of patients with true allergy to penicillin will also have a reaction to first-generation cephalosporins; thus, it is likely safe to give cefazolin in a patient without history of anaphylaxis.[14] Answers C and D are not correct. The first choice for antibiotic prophylaxis for this procedure is cefazolin. Vancomycin and clindamycin could be considered if patient had an allergy to cephalosporins.

4. After developing hives, wheezing, and hypotension following administration of neuromuscular blocking agent, what lab may be **MOST** helpful to confirm a diagnosis of anaphylaxis?

A. amylase level
B. eosinophil count
C. IgE level
D. tryptase level

Answer: D

Answer A is not correct. Amylase is produced by the pancreas and has no role in diagnosis or confirmation of anaphylaxis.

Answer B is not correct. Eosinophil count may be elevated following treatment of anaphylaxis secondary to steroid administration but is not specific or helpful to confirm anaphylaxis. Answer C is incorrect. IgE mediated anaphylaxis is caused by IgE antibodies activating mast cells to release tryptase and histamine. Obtaining levels of IgE is not helpful to make a diagnosis. Answer D is correct. Tryptase is elevated following anaphylaxis and may be helpful to allergist as part of further workup.

5. A 6-year-old patient presents for Soave pull-through procedure. Which of the following types of regional anesthesia would be **MOST** effective to cover perineal pain?

A. caudal block
B. ilioinguinal block
C. lumbar epidural
D. transverse abdominis plane blocks

Answer: A

Answer A is correct. Caudal block will cover perineal pain well for this type of procedure. Another alternative to consider would be pudendal block although this would require preforming bilateral blocks as opposed to one injection for a caudal. Answer B is not correct. Ilioinguinal block is useful to cover pain of inguinal region as well as anterior scrotum or labia. This block will not cover posterior perineal pain expected with a pull-through procedure. Answer C is not correct. A lumbar epidural may be effective but perineal coverage is not as reliable as with a caudal block. Answer D is not correct. Transverse abdominis plane blocks are peripheral nerve blocks which cover the anterior abdominal wall. This may be helpful for coverage of abdominal pain after laparoscopic surgery but will not cover perineal pain.

QUESTIONS AND ANSWERS

This chapter has accompanying questions and answers which are available to subscribers as part of the Oxford eLearning platform. To access the questions, go to ✔ http://oxfordmedicine. com/pediatricanesthesiaPBL

REFERENCES

1. Kessmann J. Hirschsprung's disease: diagnosis and management. *Am Fam Physician*. 2006;74(8):1319–1322.
2. Nurko S, Zimmerman LA. Evaluation and treatment of constipation in children and adolescents. *Am Fam Physician*. 2014;90(2):82–90.
3. Mertes PM, Aimone-Gastin I, Gueant-Rodriguez RM, et al. Hypersensitivity reactions to neuromuscular blocking agents. *Curr Pharmaceut Design*. 2008;14(27):2809–2825.
4. Mali S. Anaphylaxis during the perioperative period. *Anesth Essays Res*. 2012;6(2):124–133.
5. de Caen AR, Berg MD, Chameides L, et al. Part 12: pediatric advanced life support: 2015 American Heart Association guidelines update for cardiopulmonary resuscitation and emergency cardiovascular care. *Circulation*. 2015;132(18 Suppl 2):S526–S542.

6. Cheng A. Emergency treatment of anaphylaxis in infants and children. *Paediatr Child Health*. 2011;16(1):35–40.

7. Lugo-Vicente HL. Impact of minimally invasive surgery in children. *Bol Asoc Med P R*. 1997;89(1–3):25–30.

8. Luks FI LJ, Breuer CK, Kurkchubasche AG, Wesselhoeft CW Jr, Tracy TF Jr. Cost-effectiveness of laparoscopy in children. *Arch Pediatr Adolesc Med*. 1999;153(9):965–968.

9. Schäfer M, Lauper M, Krähenbühl L. Trocar and Veress needle injuries during laparoscopy. *Surg Endosc*. 2001;15(3):275–280.

10. Polaner DM TA, Walker BJ, Bosenberg A, Krane EJ, Suresh S, Wolf C, Martin LD. Pediatric Regional Anesthesia Network (PRAN): a multi-institutional study of the use and incidence of complications of pediatric regional anesthesia. *Anesth Analg*. 2012;115(6):1353–1364.

11. Ecoffey C, Lacroix F, Giaufré E, Orliaguet G, Courrèges P, Association des Anesthésistes Réanimateurs Pédiatriques d'Expression Française (ADARPEF). Epidemiology and morbidity of regional anesthesia in children: a follow-up one-year prospective survey of the French-Language Society of Paediatric Anaesthesiologists (ADARPEF). *Paediatr Anaesth*. 2010;20(12):1061–1069.

12. Giaufre E, Dalens B, Gombert A. Epidemiology and morbidity of regional anesthesia in children: a one-year prospective survey of the French-Language Society of Pediatric Anesthesiologists. *Anesth Analg*. 1996;83(5):904–912.

13. Llewellyn N, Moriarty, A. The national pediatric epidural audit. *Paediatr Anaesth*. 2007;17(6):520–533.

14. Campagna JD, Bond MC, Schabelman E, Hayes BD. The use of cephalosporins in penicillin-allergic patients: a literature review. *J Emerg Med*. 2012;42(5): 612–620.

38.

PEDIATRIC LIVER TRANSPLANTATION

Jonathon Nelson and Franklyn P. Cladis

STEM CASE AND KEY QUESTIONS

A full-term 6-month-old (7 kg) male is initially presented with progressive jaundice, light-colored stools, and dark urine. He was seen by his pediatrician 3 times and was reported to be fine. At 4 months of age he was seen by another pediatrician who performed blood work and a HIDA scan and cholangiogram.

WHAT ARE THE MOST COMMON CAUSES OF LIVER FAILURE IN THE PEDIATRIC POPULATION? WHAT BLOOD TESTS DO YOU THINK THE SECOND PEDIATRICIAN ORDERED AND WHY? WHAT IS A HIDA SCAN?

Your patient was found to have elevated liver enzymes including aspartate aminotransferase (AST), alanine aminotransferase (ALT), and gamma-glutamyl transpeptidase (GGT) and extrahepatic biliary atresia. His metabolic workup for alpha 1-antitrypsin as well as urine organic acids and plasma amino acids was negative. A liver biopsy confirmed the diagnosis of biliary atresia. He underwent a hepatoportoenterostomy (Kasai) at 4 months of age.

WHAT IS BILIARY ATRESIA? HOW DOES IT PRESENT AND HOW IS IT MANAGED? WHAT IS A KASAI PROCEDURE? WHEN DOES IT NEED TO BE PERFORMED? WHAT IS THE TYPICAL OUTCOME?

Unfortunately, your patient developed a coagulopathy and his liver enzymes continue to rise and he is listed for a liver transplant with a Pediatric End-Stage Liver Disease (PELD) score of 30. His family elects to have a living related liver transplant. On the day of surgery he is appropriately nil per os and he appears jaundice and lethargic. His parents noted a recent change in his behavior which they described as overly reactive to even the lightest touch.

HOW IS THE SEVERITY OF LIVER DISEASE CALCULATED IN PEDIATRIC PATIENTS? WHAT IS A PELD SCORE AND IS A SCORE OF 30 SIGNIFICANT? HOW WOULD YOU CLASSIFY HIS BEHAVIOR BASED ON THE WEST HAVEN ENCEPHALOPATHY CLASSIFICATION?

The surgeons ordered the following preoperative laboratory tests and exams:

Na = 130, K = 3.7, Cl = 99, HCO3 = 26, BUN = 9, Cr = 0.1, TBili = 23.9, ALT = 273 I units/ L, AST = 294 I units/L, GGT = 63 I units/L, Albumen = 2.5 g/dL

WBC; 14.4, HCT = 27.5, PLT = 67, PT = 22.7, INR = 1.9, PTT = 41

ECHO; Normal biventricular function, trivial tricuspid insufficiency, right ventricular systolic pressure estimate is normal

CXR: feeding tube at gastro-esophageal junction, right sided PICC line with tip at distal brachial cephalic junction, the lungs are clear, there is no cardiomegaly, there is no pleural effusion, and the bowel gas pattern is non-obstructive.

WHY DID THEY ORDER THESE TESTS? WHY DID THEY OBTAIN A CHEST X-RAY AND ECHOCARDIOGRAM? ARE YOU CONCERNED ABOUT ANY OF THE RESULTS? WILL THEY ALTER YOUR ANESTHETIC PLAN? HOW WOULD YOU INDUCE YOUR PATIENT? WHAT MONITORS ARE REQUIRED? WHERE WILL YOU PLACE THE CENTRAL LINE?

Induction of general anesthesia and endotracheal intubation were achieved without difficulties. Insertion of an internal

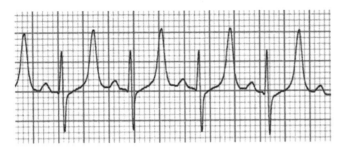

Fig. 38.1

jugular central line required several attempts but it transduced well and you were able to draw back a venous blood sample easily. Shortly after the start of surgery the end-tidal CO_2 ($ETCO_2$) decreased slightly. The peak airway pressures (PAP) increased to 40 cm/H2O.

IS THE CHANGE IN $ETCO_2$ SIGNIFICANT? WHY DID THE PAP INCREASE? WHAT IS YOUR DIFFERENTIAL DIAGNOSIS AND HOW WILL YOU MANAGE IT? WOULD YOUR MANAGEMENT BE DIFFERENT IF THE SYSTOLIC BLOOD PRESSURE DECREASED TO 50 MMHG?

Once the iatrogenic pneumothorax is addressed, surgery begins. During the dissection of the native liver, the patient experiences significant bleeding and requires 500 mL packed red blood cells, 500 mL fresh frozen plasma, and 3 units of platelets. The electrocardiogram (EKG) in Figure 38.1 is noted.

ARE YOU CONCERNED? WHAT IS YOUR DIFFERENTIAL DIAGNOSIS? WHAT TREATMENT MODALITIES ARE AVAILABLE TO YOU? IS THIS AN UNUSUAL COMPLICATION DURING LIVER TRANSPLANTATION? DESCRIBE THE SURGICAL STAGES OF THE LIVER TRANSPLANT AND THE ANESTHETIC CONCERNS FOR EACH.

Shortly after reperfusion of the liver, the thromboelastogram (TEG) is performed (see Fig. 38.2).

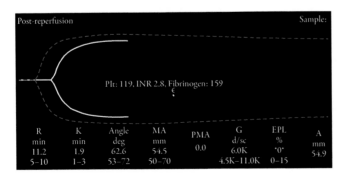

Post-reperfusion   Sample:

Plt: 119, INR 2.8, Fibrinogen: 159

R min	K min	Angle deg	MA mm	PMA	G d/sc	EPL %	A mm
11.2	1.9	62.6	54.5	0.0	6.0K	"0"	54.9
5–10	1–3	53–72	50–70		4.5K–11.0K	0–15	

Fig. 38.2

WHAT IS A THROMBOELASTOGRAM? WHAT DOES IT MEASURE? WHAT IS THE SIGNIFICANCE OF THE RESULT SHOWN? HOW WILL YOU MANAGE THIS? AT THE COMPLETION OF SURGERY, WILL YOU EXTUBATE IN THE OPERATING ROOM OR TAKE THE PATIENT TO THE INTENSIVE CARE UNIT INTUBATED? WHY WOULD YOUR PATIENT DEVELOP GRAFT FAILURE ON POSTOPERATIVE DAY 1? WHAT IS THE MOST LIKELY CAUSE?

We talk about hepatic artery thrombosis as a primary cause of graft failure in the text.

DISCUSSION

Cholestatic liver disease continues to be the most common pathology leading to hepatic failure and liver transplant in infants and children. Biliary atresia is the most common cholestatic disease and is the leading cause of hepatic failure in pediatric patients.[2] The data in Table 38.1 outlines the categories and incidence of liver pathology in patients from 0 to 18 years from the United Network of Organ Sharing (UNOS) database from 1988 to 2015.

BILIARY ATRESIA

Biliary atresia is a progressive disease of the intra- and extrahepatic biliary system in the infant that results in fibrosis and obstruction. It occurs in 1 in 8,000 to 1 in 18,000 infants and is characterized by persistent jaundice beyond the second week of life.[3] Patients present with jaundice, clay-colored stools, and dark urine. The evaluation includes blood work for total, direct, and indirect bilirubin, complete blood count, liver function tests, and electrolytes. Imaging studies include ultrasonography and biliary scintiscanning. Liver biopsy is the definitive test to confirm the diagnosis.[4] Alpa-1 antitrypsin deficiency and cystic fibrosis must also be ruled out since they are common causes of liver disease in infants.

The clinical stigmata of end-stage liver disease can be explained by liver failure and the development of portal hypertension. Liver failure from biliary atresia occurs secondary to the congenital obliteration of the extrahepatic biliary system. Bile is normally transported through the hepatic ducts to the gallbladder where it is stored and used to facilitate absorption of fat soluble vitamins (A, D, E, K). The ducts within the liver may be patent early on in life but become occluded quickly. The elevation of bile within the hepatic ducts results in destruction of hepatocytes and this leads to a reduction in synthetic function (vitamin K dependent clotting factors, albumin, and cholesterol). Metabolic toxins are also no longer removed by the liver and elevated levels of ammonia may result in hepatic encephalopathy.

The destruction of hepatocytes and the development of fibrosis results in reduced blood flow through the liver with subsequent development of portal hypertension. Portal hypertension results in esophageal varices, ascites, splenomegaly, and hemorrhoids. Esophageal varices are the source of bleeding and

Table 38.1 PRIMARY DIAGNOSIS OF LIVER DISEASE IN PEDIATRIC PATIENTS, 1988–2015

PRIMARY DIAGNOSIS	
Total	13,340
Cholestatic (total)	52%
Biliary atresia	
TPN-induced cholestasis	
Alagille syndrome	
Primary Sclerosing Cholangitis	
Secondary biliary cirrhosis	
Familiar cholestasis (Byler's, other)	
Biliary hypoplasia	
Primary biliary cirrhosis	
Neonatal cholestatic disease	
Other cholestasis	
Acute hepatic necrosis (total)	13.30%
Neonatal hepatitis	
Drug induced	
Hepatitis A	
Hepatitis B	
Hepatitis C	
Unknown	
Other	
Metabolic disorder (total)	12.90%
Alpha-1-antitrypsin	
Cystic fibrosis	
Wilson disease	
Tyrosinemia	
Oxalosis	
Glycogen storage disease	
Maple syrup urine disease	
Hemachromatosis	
Other	
Cirrhosis (total)	8%
Idiopathic	

Table 38.1 CONTINUED

PRIMARY DIAGNOSIS	
Autoimmune	
Hepatitis C	
Chronic active hepatitis	
Hepatitis B	
Drug/toxin	
Hepatitis A	
Combined exposure (alcohol, hepatitis A, B, C)	
Alcoholic	
Other	
Hepatic tumors (total)	4.80%
Hepatoblastoma	
Hepatocellular carcinoma	
Hemangioendothelioma	
Benign tumor	
Other	
Other (total)	8.40%
Congenital hepatic fibrosis	
Budd-Chiari syndrome	
Graft vs. host	
Trauma	
Other	

Note. TPN = total parenteral nutrition.

anemia. Ascites can cause restrictive lung pathology, decreased gastric emptying, and spontaneous bacterial peritonitis. Platelet sequestration and thrombocytopenia occur secondary to splenomegaly. Portal hypertension is also associated with pulmonary hypertension (portopulmonary hypertension) and abnormal pulmonary perfusion (hepatopulmonary syndrome).

Coagulopathy is often present as a result of thrombocytopenia and synthetic failure. Vitamin K dependent clotting factors will be reduced and result in an elevation in thromboplastin times and international normalized ratio (INR), although partial thromboplastin times (PTT) may also be elevated. Paradoxically, the coagulopathy may be balanced in patients with liver failure by a hypercoagulable state that develops from the synthetic reduction of Protein C and antithrombin III, and an elevation in factor VIII.[5,6] Anemia may be present from frequent blood draws and gastrointestinal loss. Hyponatremia is common and may result from diuretic

Table 38.2 GRADES OF ENCEPHALOPATHY (INFANTS AND TODDLERS)[7]

GRADE	CLINICAL FINDINGS	NEUROLOGIC EXAMINATION/ REFLEXES
I and II	Inconsolable crying, reversed sleep cycle	Normal or hyperreflexic
III	Somnolence, stupor, combativeness	Hyperreflexic
IV	Comatose, arouses with painful stimuli (IVa) or no response (IVb)	Absent, decerebrate, or decorticate posturing

use and syndrome of inappropriate antidiuretic hormone. Progressive hyponatremia may result in cerebral edema and death. Rapid correction may result in osmotic myelinolysis (central pontine myelinolysis).

HEPATIC ENCEPHALOPATHY

Hepatic encephalopathy is difficult to diagnose in infants and toddlers. Infants with liver failure may have altered mental status for a variety of reasons, and these require immediate evaluation (hypoglycemia, hyponatremia, cerebral edema, hepatic encephalopathy). The classification for hepatic encephalopathy is described by the West Haven Classification. It has been modified for infants and toddlers (Table 38.2) is separate from older children and adults (Table 38.3).[7,8] Based on the Infant and Toddler classification of encephalopathy, the infant's most appropriate grade would be 3. He is drowsy, lethargic, and arousable to voice.

KASAI PROCEDURE

A Kasai procedure is performed to bypass the blocked bile ducts in the liver as well as the gallbladder, ultimately replacing it with a segment of small intestine. The procedure is also known as a hepatoportojejunostomy or Roux-en-Y and is typically performed in infancy with the ultimate goal of allowing biliary drainage and preventing liver damage. Typical surgical outcomes include 33% of the patients requiring immediate liver transplant, 33% requiring a liver transplant during childhood, and 33% avoiding liver transplantation.[1] One future complication of a prior Kasai procedure includes adhesions

Table 38.3 WEST HAVEN CLASSIFICATION

GRADE	DESCRIPTION
0	Normal, needs neuropsychologic testing
1	Altered affect/sleep, altered orientation, short attention span
2	Drowsy, lethargic, slurred speech, asterixis
3	Somnolence, stuporous
4	Comatose

and an increased risk of intraoperative bleeding during future abdominal surgeries, including liver transplant.

PELD

The PELD scoring system is used for candidates under the age of 11 and utilizes the following components:

- Age
- Growth failure
- Serum albumin
- Bilirubin
- INR

This scoring system is utilized as a predictor of short-term mortality without a liver transplant and creates a priority order for the transplant allocation following all urgent Status 1 candidates. A PELD score of 30 is significant and increases the likelihood of a transplant.

LIVING RELATED LIVER TRANSPLANT

A living related transplant occurs when a living donor donates a portion of his or her liver, usually the left lobe. If the recipient is a pediatric patient, the donor's right lobe is used due to size restrictions. The donor is often a family member but not necessarily. This process has led to a reduced mortality in pediatric patients awaiting a liver transplant. There are several benefits including better graft quality, shorter ischemic times, and better immune compatibility.[5] Living donors are typically 18 to 60 years old and are ABO compatible with the pediatric

Table 38.4 PREOPERATIVE TESTING FOR PEDIATRIC LIVER TRANSPLANTATION

- Complete blood count -associated with anemia and platelet sequestration/thrombocytopenia

- Coagulation profile (PT, PTT, INR)
  o Increased PT, PTT, INR
  o Decreased fat-soluble vitamins (A, D, E, K)
  o Factor deficiency (II, VII, IX, X)

- Complete metabolic panel—associated with hypomagnesemia, hypocalcemia, hypo/hyperkalemia, hyponatremia, elevated blood urea nitrogen/Creatinine

- EKG—associated with prolonged QT, EKG changes associated with electrolyte abnormalities

- Echocardiogram—associated with congenital cardiac defects (Alagille), PPH
  o If concern for PPH, patient may benefit from cardiac catheterization to quantify pulmonary artery pressures and right ventricular dysfunction

Note. PT = prothrombin time; PTT = partial thromboplastin time; INR = international normalized ratio; EKG = electrocardiogram; PPH = portopulmonary hypertension.

recipient. There are several potential risks for the donor including exposure to blood products, peripheral nerve injuries, biliary leakage, abdominal wall defects, pleural effusions, pneumonia, pulmonary edema, and death.[5]

PREOPERATIVE ASSESSMENT

This patient will need to have blood work and diagnostic studies performed prior to transplantation. This includes blood work to assess his electrolyte and hematologic profile including coagulation studies. He will also require a preoperative echocardiogram to evaluate his right and left ventricular function as well as his pulmonary pressures. The presence of pulmonary hypertension increases his risk of morbidity and mortality.[9] A list of preoperative tests and associated anomalies is provided in Table 38.4.[10]

INTRAOPERATIVE MANAGEMENT

Infants and children with liver disease often suffer from the stigmata of portal hypertension. The ascites that develops may alter gastric motility and emptying. This may increase the risk of aspiration even when proper fasting guidelines are followed. A rapid sequence intravenous (IV) induction is most appropriate and indicated for this patient.

Infants and children with metabolic pathology like maple syrup urine disease do not develop portal hypertension because there is no destruction of the hepatocytes and subsequent fibrosis. These patients do not develop ascites and can be induced with a variety of techniques including inhalation with sevoflurane.

Liver transplant surgeries require adequate vascular access for resuscitation, as well as monitoring trends in blood pressure and volume status (central venous pressure) via a central venous catheter. Compared to liver transplants in adults, there are size limitations in most pediatric patients with regard to monitoring. Many pediatric institutions, in addition to standard American Society of Anesthesiologists monitors, will utilize at least 2 upper extremity IV catheters (upper extremity access is preferred because the inferior vena cava may be completely or partially cross clamped during the anhepatic phase), a central venous catheter, and noninvasive and invasive arterial blood pressure monitors. Transesophageal echocardiogram can aid in assessing cardiac function and volume status but is not routinely utilized in pediatric institutions. Furthermore, a pulmonary artery catheter (Swan-Ganz catheter) can assess pulmonary hypertension and portopulmonary hypertension intraoperatively and postoperatively in patients with these preoperative comorbidities, but patient size may limit their routine use. Point of care testing for blood gas analysis (iStat), electrolytes (iStat), glucose (glucometer), hemoglobin (Hemacue), lactate (iStat), and coagulation parameters (TEG or ROTEM) should be available in the operating room or in the immediate vicinity.

Central line placement location can be limited by scarring/thrombosis from prior line placements with previous surgeries, as well indwelling hemodialysis catheters. It is recommended to place the line under ultrasound guidance, and typically the internal jugular vein is accessed for central line placement. Placement of all invasive monitors in this patient population may be difficult and may require ultrasound guidance or surgical cut down. A preoperative ultrasound evaluation of common vascular sites may identify pre-existing thrombosis.

ANESTHETIC COMPLICATIONS

The decrease in ETCO$_2$ with the start of surgery may be due to an increase in ventilation secondary to a reduction in abdominal pressure from the drainage of ascites. However, with the increased peak airway pressures, it is important to consider the ventilator settings, ensure proper ventilator function, rule out circuit and endotracheal tube (ETT) kinking/obstruction/misplacement, as well as patient causes including bronchospasm, awakening/coughing, pneumothorax, and pulmonary edema. A quick pneumonic to diagnose the problem is DOPE (D = displaced ETT, O = obstruction, P = pulmonary pathology like pneumothorax, bronchospasm, pulmonary embolism, aspiration, atelectasis, etc., E = equipment failure). In order to manage and diagnose the cause, it is important to increase the fraction of inspired oxygen to 100% and switch to manual ventilation while auscultating for bilateral breath sounds and to assess for areas of consolidation/collapse. Next, the ETT may require repositioning and suctioning. Any obstruction (kink or foreign body) of the ETT and circuit should be identified. Increased peak airway pressure with unilateral breath sounds should increase the suspicion of a mainstem intubation or a pneumothorax. The surgeon may be able to examine chest movement and lung expansion and aid in the diagnosis of a pneumothorax. A portable chest x-ray can be performed to confirm the diagnosis of pneumothorax, pulmonary edema, pleural effusion, or aspiration.

If there is associated hypotension with the decrease in ETCO$_2$ and increase in PAP, especially with the recent placement of a central line, the leading diagnosis would be a tension pneumothorax. The surgeon should be immediately notified, and a needle thoracostomy decompression followed by placement of a chest tube should be performed. While these measures are taking place, the patient may require a fluid bolus and/or vasopressors to correct the hypotension and increase perfusion.

SURGICAL STAGES OF THE LIVER TRANSPLANT

There are four stages of the liver transplant, and each stage has several physiologic considerations which can each pose challenges for the anesthesia team.

The first stage is the hepatectomy/dissection/preanhepatic stage, and there may be substantial blood loss leading to hypovolemia and hypotension. This risk is typically larger in patients with prior abdominal surgeries (i.e., Kasai) from adhesions, as well as patients with coagulopathy. There can also be a large amount of third space losses, especially in patients with ascites. The combination of hypovolemia due to blood and third space losses often leads to the need for resuscitation with blood products, which can result in hypocalcemia, acidosis, hyperkalemia, and hypomagnesemia.[5] It is important to monitor for coagulopathy during this stage and to treat accordingly. At the start of the second stage of the liver transplant, clamping of the inferior vena cava can lead to a decrease in preload and cardiac output. The surgeon will often perform a test clamp to check the patient's response, and it may be required to fluid resuscitate further as well as start inotropic support (i.e. dopamine, epinephrine infusions) to achieve an adequate mean arterial pressure (MAP). The resuscitation strategy during the dissection phase is controversial. Some have advocated a restrictive fluid strategy with lower central venous pressure and hemoglobin to minimize dilution of clotting factors and exposure to blood products. There is an association with improved survival with reduced allogeneic blood exposure. Unfortunately, bleeding can be significant during this phase. This patient is at greater risk for significant bleeding because of his small size, previous abdominal surgery, and reduced graft size.[5] Prophylactic administration of fresh frozen plasma (FFP) is not recommended. Blood administration should be guided by point of care testing with TEG or ROTEM.

The second stage of the liver transplant is the anhepatic stage, which starts with cross clamping of the portal vein and hepatic veins and artery of the native liver and ends with the release of the cross clamp on the hepatic and portal veins of the graft. During this stage, it is important to maintain an adequate MAP through resuscitation and inotropic infusions and to correct any metabolic derangements from blood product administration (i.e., hypocalcemia, acidosis, hyperkalemia, and hypomagnesemia). One of the most important electrolyte levels to monitor during this stage is potassium in preparation for the third stage of the transplant, reperfusion. In order to decrease the potassium level prior to reperfusion, hyperventilation and/or sodium bicarbonate may be required. If the potassium continues to be elevated, the patient may require glucose and insulin, potassium-wasting diuretics (i.e., furosemide), and β_2 agonists (i.e., albuterol, salbutamol).

Unclamping and reperfusion of the graft marks the third stage and may result in an increase in right-sided heart filling pressures, potentially causing myocardial dysfunction, hyperkalemic associated arrhythmias, and cardiovascular collapse. Patients may require epinephrine boluses during this stage, as well calcium chloride for cardiac membrane stabilization due to hyperkalemia, as well as other treatments for hyperkalemia as discussed previously. There is a risk of bleeding and fibrinolysis during this stage. Due to a potential risk in pediatric patients for development of hepatic artery thrombosis or emboli, it is not recommended to normalize the PT, PTT, or hemoglobin. The goal hemoglobin in some centers is 8 to 9 g/dL.[5]

Biliary and hepatic artery reconstruction comprises the fourth and final stage of the liver transplant. During this time, the liver graft will start to function, potentially leading to a metabolic alkalosis and hypokalemia(11). It is crucial to maintain a normal CVP during this stage to decrease the risk of liver congestion and damage to the new graft. Depending on the institution, preventative treatment for hepatic artery thrombosis may be started with different anticoagulation medications including heparin infusions.

COMMON INTRAOPERATIVE COMPLICATIONS

The is EKG in Figure 38.3 demonstrates a sinus rhythm of approximately 100 beats per minute with peaked T-waves. The peaked T-waves are concerning for hyperkalemia. The potassium exposure from packed red blood cells vary based on age of the product and delivery technique. Pre-existing hyperkalemia and volume of packed red cells predicts hyperkalemia in pediatric patients and adult liver transplant patients.[12,13] Pediatric surgical patients typically receive fresh (less than 2 weeks old) blood and have a lower potassium exposure. This patient received a significant volume of blood (70 mL/kg). The EKG progression of hyperkalemia starts with peaked T-waves and then proceeds to a long PR interval, wide QRS complex, and then sinusoidal rhythm or ventricular fibrillation.[14,15] The treatment includes the following:

- Calcium gluconate 30 mg/kg or calcium carbonate 10 to 20 mg/kg (this stabilizes the cardiac membrane and raises the membrane threshold transiently)

- Dextrose 5% or 10%, administer 10 mL/kg with regular insulin 0.1 units/kg IV

- Albuterol 4 to 8 puffs (repeat until mild tachycardia)

- Sodium bicarbonate 1 to 3 mEq/kg

- Hyperventilation

- Furosemide 0.5 to 1 mg/kg

Extracellular potassium lowers the membrane potential and the membrane threshold making depolarization more likely. Calcium raises the membrane threshold of the cardiac cell and reduces early depolarization. Insulin with dextrose, albuterol, bicarbonate, and hyperventilation shifts the potassium from the extracellular space to the intracellular space. Furosemide removes potassium through renal excretion. Kayexalate should be used cautiously during the intraoperative period because it has been associated with bowel necrosis and perforations. Some of these complications have been described during the perioperative period.[16] A final but extreme step to remove potassium is intraoperative hemodialysis.

TEG

Patients with liver disease develop a coagulopathy related to decreased production of hepatically produced clotting

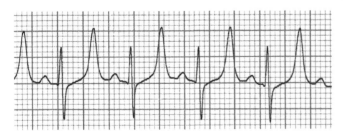

Fig. 38.3

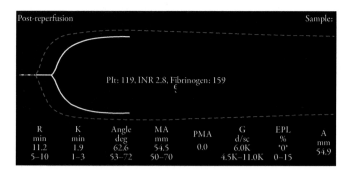

Fig. 38.4

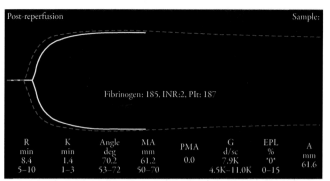

Fig. 38.5

factors (factors I [fibrinogen], II [prothrombin], V, VII, VIII, IX, X, XI, XIII, as well as protein C, protein S). These clotting factor deficiencies result in prolonged PT and INR. The severity of coagulopathy may predict severity of liver disease. In fact INR is used to calculate the PELD score and Child-Pugh score. Unfortunately, conventional clotting parameters like PT, PTT, and INR are poor markers for coagulopathy because they do not describe the dynamic clotting process (clot generation, stability, and degradation) and they fail to predict bleeding or hypercoagulability. Patients with liver disease are hypercoagulable secondary to a deficiency of protein C.

TEG provides dynamic clotting information that is more specific than conventional clotting parameters and it will identify hypercoagulable states. The r-time describes the time to fibrin formation. Abnormalities here relate to clotting factors and do not present until the factors are reduced to less than 20% to 30%. Administering FFP will correct this.[6] The TEG in Figure 38.4 demonstrates a prolonged r-time without other abnormalities (although the MA is low normal and improves with the administration of platelets). The administration of FFP (10–20 mL/kg) resulted in the TEG shown in Figure 38.4. Depletion of clotting factors can occur during the dissection phase with blood loss and dilution with the administration of crystalloid and colloid. Transplant protocols that adhere to fluid restriction have demonstrated reduced transfusion requirements.[17] The r-time may also be prolonged because of the release of endogenous heparinoid substances from the native liver and the graft after reperfusion. If the TEG is performed with heparinase, the r-time is corrected.[18] The other

TEG variables and management of specific abnormalities are outlined in Table 38.5.

POSTOPERATIVE MANAGEMENT

There is an association between postoperative intubation and reduced graft and recipient survival in the adult liver transplant literature.[19] This may be related to the postoperative respiratory complications associated with mechanical ventilation. Positive pressure ventilation may also alter venous flow, hepatic perfusion, and graft survival.[20] Retrospective data suggests that early extubation in the operating room is associated with reduced lengths of stay.[21] It is important to recognize that this is an association and the benefits seen after early extubation cannot yet be causally linked to this action. Patients that were selected for early extubation were likely healthier and received fewer blood products. Patients that failed to meet criteria for early extubation tended to have a higher Child-Pugh score, receive 6 or more units of blood, have acute liver failure, or undergo retransplantation.[22] Early extubation after pediatric liver transplantation is not well described. This patient is less than 1 year old and received a significant volume of blood products. Fast tracking this patient may not be clinically most appropriate. Respiratory failure with reintubation in the intensive care setting may result in other adverse events including hypoxia, excessive positive pressure ventilation, and hemodynamic instability.

Immediately after reperfusion, the liver graft should be functioning. Evidence of adequate graft function includes hemodynamic stability, normal neurologic examination, increasing factor V and VII levels, normalization of INR, reduction in lactate, correction of hypoglycemia, correction of aspartate aminotransferase/alanine aminotransferase/bilirubin, and patency of hepatic vessels with Doppler ultrasound.[23]

Graft failure occurs for several reasons. During the acute postoperative period, thrombosis is a significant concern and may occur in the hepatic artery, portal vein, or hepatic vein. The incidence of vascular thrombotic complications ranges from 1% to 10% and may be more common in patients weighing less than 10 kg.[23] The incidence of hepatic artery thrombosis in the pediatric population has been documented at 1% to 3%.[24] Other complications following pediatric liver transplantation include biliary leakage and stenosis, infection, and rejection. In fact, in the first 3 months after transplant, readmission is most likely related to sepsis and rejection.

Table 38.5

TEG VALUE	PHYSIOLOGY	MANAGEMENT
r-time	Initial fibrin formation	Fresh frozen plasma
k-value	Speed of clot strength	Fibrinogen
Angle (in degrees)	Rate of clot formation	Fibrinogen
MA (maximum amplitude)	Ultimate clot strength	Platelets (and/or fibrinogen)
LY 30 (lysis at 30 min)	Fibrinolysis	Antifibrinolytic (for primary only)

REVIEW QUESTIONS

1. A 5-year-old male presents to the operating room with end-stage liver disease for a liver transplant. Which neuromuscular blocking drug will **MOST** likely be prolonged and therefore should be utilized more cautiously intraoperatively?

    A. atracurium
    B. cisatracurium
    C. pancuronium
    D. vecuronium

Answer: D

Vecuronium is an intermediate-duration of action neuromuscular blocking medication and has 20% renal excretion (unchanged), 25% hepatic degradation, and 60% biliary excretion (unchanged). Due to this high percentage of both hepatic degradation and excretion, there is an increased risk for prolonged muscle relaxation. Therefore, utilization of vecuronium during a liver transplant should be utilized cautiously and monitored vigilantly with a nerve twitch monitor.

Answers A and B are incorrect due to both medications being hydrolyzed in the plasma via Hoffmann elimination. Due to this elimination, neither medication is significantly degraded or eliminated via the biliary system nor therefore will the duration of medication not be affected by liver failure.

Answer C is incorrect due to having 80% renal excretion (unchanged), 10% hepatic degradation, and 10% biliary excretion (unchanged). Although pancuronium is a long-duration neuromuscular medication, the duration of action is not changed significantly by liver failure.

It is also important to note that pseudocholinesterase levels can be decreased in advanced liver disease, leading to prolonged duration of action of ester-type local anesthetics (i.e., procaine), succinylcholine, and mivacurium.

2. A 6-year-old female with liver failure presents to the emergency room with confusion and increased drowsiness. Her labs show an increased ammonia level, leading to the diagnosis of hepatic encephalopathy. Which treatment would be the **LEAST** effective for this patient?

    A. flumazenil
    B. lactulose
    C. protein-rich diet
    D. neomycin

Answer: C

Ammonia production is increased in protein rich diets as well as amino acid-rich total parenteral nutrition and therefore will lead to further increase in ammonia levels and potentially progression of hepatic encephalopathy.

Answer A is incorrect because flumazenil will reverse hepatic encephalopathy symptoms for a short time. Answer B is incorrect due to lactulose decreasing the absorption of ammonia. Answer D is incorrect due to neomycin decreasing the production of ammonia.

3. Which coagulation factors are produced by the liver?

    A. antithrombin III
    B. factor III (tissue thromboplastin)
    C. factor IV (calcium)
    D. factor XII (Hageman factor)

Answer: A

The liver produces protein C, protein S, antithrombin III, as well as factor I, II, V, VII, IX, and X. Factor III, factor IV, and factor XII are not produced in the liver.

QUESTIONS AND ANSWERS

This chapter has accompanying questions and answers which are available to subscribers as part of the Oxford eLearning platform. To access the questions, go to ✓ http://oxfordmedicine. com/pediatricanesthesiaPBL

REFERENCES

1. Uejima T. Anesthetic management of the pediatric patient undergoing solid organ transplantation. *Anesthesiol Clin North America.* 2004;22:809–826.
2. https://optn.transplant.hrsa.gov/data/view-data-reports/national-data/
3. Sokol RJ, Shepherd RW, Superina R, Bezerra JA, Robuck P, Hoofnagle JH. Screening and outcomes in biliary atresia: summary of a National Institutes of Health workshop. *Hepatology.* 2007;46:566–581.
4. Bassett MD, Murray KF. Biliary atresia: recent progress. *J Clin Gastroenterol.* 2008;42:720–729.
5. Raffini L, Witmer C. Pediatric transplantation: managing bleeding. *J Thromb Haemost.* 2015;13(Suppl 1):S362–S369.
6. Mallett SV. Clinical utility of viscoelastic tests of coagulation (TEG/ROTEM) in patients with liver disease and during liver transplantation. *Semin Thromb Hemost.* 2015;41:527–537.
7. Newland CD. Acute liver failure. *Pediatr Ann.* 2016;45:e433–e438.
8. Squires RH Jr, Shneider BL, Bucuvalas J, et al. Acute liver failure in children: the first 348 patients in the pediatric acute liver failure study group. *J Pediatr.* 2006;148:652–658.
9. Condino AA, Ivy DD, O'Connor JA, et al. Portopulmonary hypertension in pediatric patients. *J Pediatr.* 2005;147:20–26.
10. Hammer GB, Krane EJ. Anaesthesia for liver transplantation in children. *Paediatr Anaesth.* 2001;11:3-18.
11. Xia VW, Du B, Tran A, et al. Intraoperative hypokalemia in pediatric liver transplantation: incidence and risk factors. *Anesth Analg.* 2006;103:587–593.
12. Juang SE, Huang CE, Chen CL, et al. Predictive risk factors in the development of intraoperative hyperkalemia in adult living donor liver transplantation. *Transplant Proc.* 2016;48:1022–1024.
13. Lee AC, Reduque LL, Luban NL, Ness PM, Anton B, Heitmiller ES. Transfusion-associated hyperkalemic cardiac arrest in pediatric patients receiving massive transfusion. *Transfusion.* 2014;54:244–254.
14. Parham WA, Mehdirad AA, Biermann KM, Fredman CS. Hyperkalemia revisited. *Tex Heart Inst J.* 2006;33:40–47.

15. Rossignol P, Legrand M, Kosiborod M, et al. Emergency management of severe hyperkalemia: guideline for best practice and opportunities for the future. *Pharmacol Res.* 2016;113:585–591.

16. Harel Z, Harel S, Shah PS, Wald R, Perl J, Bell CM. Gastrointestinal adverse events with sodium polystyrene sulfonate (Kayexalate) use: a systematic review. *Am J Med.* 2013;126: 264, e269–e224.

17. Massicotte L, Denault AY, Thibeault L, Hevesi Z, Nozza A, Roy A. Relationship between conventional coagulation tests and bleeding for 600 consecutive liver transplantations. *Transplantation.* 2014;98:e13–e15.

18. Kang Y. Coagulation and liver transplantation. *Transplant Proc.* 1993;25:2001–2005.

19. Yuan H, Tuttle-Newhall JE, Chawa V, et al. Prognostic impact of mechanical ventilation after liver transplantation: a national database study. *Am J Surg.* 2014;208:582–590.

20. Kaisers U, Langrehr JM, Haack M, Mohnhaupt A, Neuhaus P, Rossaint R. Hepatic venous catheterization in patients undergoing positive end-expiratory pressure ventilation after OLT: technique and clinical impact. *Clin Transplant.* 1995;9:301–306.

21. Taner CB, Willingham DL, Bulatao IG, et al. Is a mandatory intensive care unit stay needed after liver transplantation? Feasibility of fast-tracking to the surgical ward after liver transplantation. *Liver Transplant.* 2012;18:361–369.

22. Glanemann M, Langrehr J, Kaisers U, et al. Postoperative tracheal extubation after orthotopic liver transplantation. *Acta Anaesthesiol Scand.* 2001;45:333–339.

23. Rawal N, Yazigi N. Pediatric liver transplantation. *Pediatr Clin North America.* 2017;64:677–684.

24. Heffron TG, Welch D, Pillen T, et al. Low incidence of hepatic artery thrombosis after pediatric liver transplantation without the use of intraoperative microscope or parenteral anticoagulation. *Pediatr Transplant.* 2005;9:486–490.

IDIOPATHIC HYPERTROPHIC PYLORIC STENOSIS

Darlene Mashman and Carmen Mays

STEM CASE AND KEY QUESTIONS

A 6-week-old male infant is referred to the emergency department for evaluation of failure to thrive, nonbilious vomiting with feeds, and an abdominal mass. His weight is exactly the same as it was at 4 weeks of age. The patient's mother states that the baby "spits up" formula a lot and that she has been giving him smaller amounts of formula more frequently. Mom states that sometimes the emesis will "shoot across the room."

WHAT IS THE DIFFERENTIAL DIAGNOSIS FOR NONBILIOUS EMESIS IN THE INFANT?

The differential diagnosis includes gastroesophageal reflux disease (most common), inherited metabolic disease (e.g., urea cycle abnormality, adrenal insufficiency), esophagitis, gastritis, gastroenteritis, duodenal obstruction proximal to Ampulla of Vater and idiopathic hypertrophic pyloric stenosis (IHPS). The history of poor weight gain and worsening projectile vomiting over the course of several weeks without abdominal pain, diarrhea, or fever suggests IHPS.[1]

ARE THERE ANY INVESTIGATIVE MEANS TO IDENTIFY IHPS?

Abdominal ultrasound is used to confirm clinical suspicion and make the diagnosis. Upper gastrointestinal (GI) series are not done routinely for diagnosis due to increased aspiration risk with oral contrast.

On physical exam, the infant is quiet, with dry mucous membranes, sunken anterior fontanel, capillary refill >3 seconds, tenting with pinching his skin, and a dry diaper. Vital signs are: respiratory rate (RR) 22, blood pressure (BP) 68/30, heart rate (HR) 172, room air SPO$_2$ 95%. The infant's lab values show: Na+ 138, K+ 2.8, Cl–86, CO$_2$ –41, anion gap (AG) 10.8, glucose 78, blood urea nitrogen (BUN) 17, creatinine 0.3, Ca+ 10.2.

IS THIS PATIENT CLINICALLY DEHYDRATED?

Our patient is seriously dehydrated and in shock. He is tachycardic and hypotensive with altered mental status, dry mucous membranes, and poor skin turgor and capillary refill.[2,3] Physical exam findings can help determine the degree of dehydration (mild, moderate, or severe) and laboratory data help characterize the deficit.[2] Average normal infant vital signs are: HR 90–160 at rest, BP 72–104/37–59 (MAP 50–62), RR 30–53.[4]

WHAT IS YOUR ASSESSMENT OF THE PATIENT'S ELECTROLYTE AND ACID-BASE STATUS?

Some disease states result in specific types of dehydration and electrolyte losses. For example, diarrhea results in marked bicarbonate loss, metabolic acidosis, and progressive tachypnea whereas IHPS results in hypochloremic, metabolic alkalosis with progressive compensatory bradypnea.[2] Our patient's history, clinical presentation, and laboratory values are suggestive of IHPS.

DOES THE PYLOROMYOTOMY PROCEDURE NEED TO BE UNDERTAKEN EMERGENTLY?

IHPS is not a surgical emergency. The focus of preoperative preparation is to treat dehydration and electrolyte imbalance and minimize aspiration risk. The ultimate goal is to perform a sutureless myotomy of adequate length without compromising the pyloric mucosa.[5]

HOW SHOULD WE MANAGE INITIAL VOLUME RESUSCITATION IN OUR PATIENT?

Intravenous or intraosseous access must be established emergently in order to start isotonic parenteral rehydration and restore circulation. This is a medical (not surgical) emergency. We will give 20 mL/kg bolus of 0.9% normal saline (NS), and repeat 2 to 3 times, to restore organ perfusion as evidenced by improved capillary refill, skin color, and systolic blood pressure and decreased tachycardia. We may consider a volume expander (e.g. 10mL/kg of 5% albumin).[3] Serum glucose checks will rule out acute hypoglycemia, and laboratory analysis will guide correction of electrolyte imbalance. There are many regimens in the literature to guide subsequent hydration therapy for the patient with IHPS.[2,5–7] After restoration of circulation, we will begin infusing 5% dextrose solution 0.45% NS and add potassium chloride (KCl) to the solution when urine flow has been established.

Our patient has received the fluid infusions noted previously. His vital signs are now: RR 28, HR 148, BP 80/50, voided x1. Physical exam: Awake, Fontanel flat, capillary refill 1.5 seconds, mucous membranes dry.

HOW WOULD WE CONTINUE WITH THE FLUID MANAGEMENT OF THIS PATIENT?

We begin an infusion of 5% dextrose solution 0.45% NS with KCl 30 mEq/L at 1.5 × maintenance rate and recheck electrolytes, glucose, and acid base status 4 hours after initiating therapy, and again every 6 to 12 hours until normalized. If the patient has a nasogastric (NG) tube, we will replace the gastric output (1 mL: 1 mL) with 0.9% NS with 10 mEq/L of KCl.[2]

We will then adjust our final intravenous (IV) hydration therapy (e.g., 5% dextrose 0.45% NS solution with KCl 20 mEq/L at maintenance rate) to maintain our patient's normal nutritional state until he is able to return to oral feedings. Chloride (Cl−) deficiency has been found to be the best estimate of volume depletion in these patients.[6,8]

Follow-up laboratory values show: Na+ 138, K+ 4.8, Cl 110−, CO_2− 28, glucose 90, BUN 12, creatinine 0.1, calcium 10.2. On physical exam, the patient is awake, mucous membranes are pink and moist, capillary refill is <1.5 sec, HR 138, BP 95/48, RR 28, SPO_2 98% on room air and his diaper is wet.

WHAT ARE THE PREOPERATIVE HYDRATION GOALS IN PREPARING THE PATIENT FOR SURGERY?

There is limited evidence to suggest a safe level of alkalosis for general anesthesia.[7] Patients should be hydrated (evidenced by Cl ≥100 mEq/L) and alkalosis should be corrected (HCO3 ≤30 mmol/L) since this may contribute to postoperative apnea.[5] Our patient is adequately hydrated based on physical exam and repeat laboratory analysis results.

HOW WOULD YOU INDUCE ANESTHESIA FOR THIS PATIENT?

After confirmation of a working IV line and placement of a pulse oximeter, electrocardiogram and blood pressure cuff, we will pass an orogastric (OG) to decompress his stomach until no gastric fluid returns. We will suction the OG tube in the supine, right and left lateral positions. We will preoxygenate in preparation for a rapid sequence induction and intubation.[9]

WHAT SHOULD WE DO IN THE CASE OF PULMONARY ASPIRATION ON INDUCTION?

It is best to suction as much aspirate from the endotracheal tube as possible. Supportive care is provided to maximize oxygenation and ventilation. Preemptive steroids and antibiotics have not been shown to improve outcome.[10]

WHAT IS YOUR PLAN FOR MAINTENANCE OF ANESTHESIA?

Our goal during maintenance of anesthesia is to produce a stable operative field, appropriate plane of anesthesia, and airway protection for the patient. Air, oxygen, and sevoflurane plus a short acting non-depolarizing muscle relaxant (considering the procedure is usually short) may be needed. We will maintain oxygenation of the patient while avoiding hyperventilation. We will place rectal Tylenol suppository after the induction of anesthesia and request that our sugeon infiltrates the wounds with local anesthetic (laparoscopic procedure) or we will provide a regional block (open procedure) to achieve opioid-free analgesia. At the conclusion of the procedure, we will extubate the trachea with the infant awake.

DISCUSSION

IHPS, a condition considered to be easily corrected by surgery, presents with vomiting in the young infant. The pathologic cause for IHPS is unclear but there are strong familial tendencies, chromosomal implications, as well as numerous environmental associations.[11] The pyloromyotomy, first performed by Conrad Ramstedt in 1911, transformed the treatment of IHPS. Before the introduction of this minor and curative procedure, many infants would die from dehydration and malnutrition.[12] In the present day, the infant is usually ready for discharge from the hospital within 24 to 48 hours of surgery.[5]

EPIDEMIOLOGY

IHPS is the most prevalent condition necessitating surgery in the first few months of life. Among white individuals, the incidence is 1.5-3 per 1,000 live births.[13] In the United States, it appears to be less common in African American and Asian ethnicities. It is 4 to 5 times more likely to be seen in males.[12] The most consistently reported risk factors for IHPS are male sex, family history of pyloric stenosis, and being a first-born child. It appears to occur more frequently in infants with a maternal family history of IHPS.[13] Epidemiological studies suggest a genetic component, but it remains to be elucidated whether aggregation in families is mostly due to genes, maternal factors during pregnancy, or a common familial environment.

ETIOLOGY

The pathophysiology of IHPS at a molecular level is not known and a specific gene or sequence variant has not been identified to date. Nonsyndromic pyloric stenosis has been clearly shown to have a genetic predisposition. Nitric oxide plays a significant role in the relaxation of enteric smooth muscle. An abnormality with the synthesis of nitric oxide by nitrergic nerves of the enteric system is another possible cause of sustained contraction of pyloric smooth muscle. Five genetic loci have been discovered (IHPS 1−-5) that may be associated with IHPS. IHPS1 encodes the enzyme neuronal nitric oxide synthase. IHPS2 and IHPS3 may play a role in smooth muscle control and hypertrophy. Activity of NADPH diaphorase, a nitric oxide synthase, is usually present in an abundance of nerve fibers of the pyloric muscle. In patients with IHPS, the NADPH diaphorase activity is selectively absent in the circular musculature of the pylorus. The control and regulation of pyloric sphincter function is a complex system and heterogeneity at the molecular level seems likely because a defect in many different aspects of this system could cause IHPS.[12,14] IHPS is also associated with several genetic syndromes (e.g., Cornelia de Lange and Smith-Lemli-Opitz syndromes) and chromosomal abnormalities. Infants sleeping in the prone position (pooling of milk in antrum may lead to contractions in pylorus) and postnatal erythromycin (motilin receptor agonists can cause exaggerated pyloric motility) use are two environmental factors with biological explanations. Postnatal maternal smoking has also been investigated.[12,13]

CLINICAL PRESENTATION

The classic presentation of IHPS manifests within the 2nd and 12th week of life (peak incidence occurs in week 5) with nonbilious vomiting that occurs shortly after feeds, becoming progressively forceful over time as the pylorus hypertrophies. Patients are afebrile and do not usually have diarrhea but will occasionally (8%) present with bloody streaks in the emesis due to the development of gastritis or esophagitis.[15] Rarely (1.4%), patients present with bilious emesis.[16] Parents will often comment that the baby is very hungry soon after emesis. Patients with IHPS may also occasionally (5%) present with jaundice and indirect hyperbilirubinemia (ictopyloric syndrome) due to caloric deprivation and glucuronyl transferase deficiency that resolves after treatment.[1] Heightened physician awareness and a shift in practice to more widespread use of diagnostic ultrasound has led to a decrease in the frequency of severe dehydration and electrolyte abnormalities (hypokalemic, hypochloremic metabolic alkalosis), as patients are receiving earlier treatment.[11,17,18] That said, signs and symptoms of dehydration should be recognized and electrolyte abnormalities associated with IHPS must be treated appropriately. Some degree of metabolic alkalosis is expected in an infant with a history and clinical findings suggestive of severe dehydration and history consistent with IHPS. In their retrospective review of 100 infants that arrived to the emergency room with a history of vomiting, Oakley and Barnett found a positive predictive value of 88% for pyloric stenosis when the blood biochemical and acid/base values revealed a pH >7.45, Cl- <98 mmol/L, and base excess > +3.[19,20] Hydration status should be determined by inquiring about duration of illness, voiding patterns and estimated during the physical exam using normal vital signs as a standard of measure (HR 90–160 at rest, BP 72–104/37–59 [MAP 50–62], RR 30–53).[4] According to Nelson's Textbook of Pediatrics[2]:

Mild dehydration (4%–5% body weight loss; estimated 50 mL/kg fluid deficit) is present if the infant appears thirsty but alert with normal physical exam and vital signs. Pulse may be slightly increased and mucous membranes may be dry.

Moderate dehydration (6%–9% loss in body weight; estimated 90–100 mL/kg fluid deficit) is present if 2 or more of the following signs are present: irritability or drowsiness, rapid and possibly weak pulse, deep (sometimes rapid) respiratory rate, sunken anterior fontanel, low systolic blood pressure, poor skin turgor, capillary refill >1.5 seconds, sunken eyes, absent tears, dry mucous membranes or reduced, or dark urine output.

Severe dehydration (>10% loss in body weight; estimated fluid deficit 100–150 mL/kg) is present if 2 or more of the following signs are present: limpness/comatose, rapid, possibly impalpable pulse, very sunken fontanel, capillary refill >3 seconds, grossly sunken eyes, deep (sometimes rapid) respiratory rate, no tears, poor skin turgor, very dry mucous membranes, and oliguria.[2]

Laboratory data can characterize the electrolyte deficits. The metabolic alkalosis found in IHPS is multifactorial. It is due to (i) loss of H+ from stomach (primarily H+ and Cl- and to a lesser extent Na+ and K+), (ii) gastric cell release of HCO3- into the plasma, (iii) decreased pancreatic excretion of HCO3- into the serum due to small food volume in the small intestine, and (iv) renal response to electrolyte imbalance and dehydration. Early in the illness the urine is alkaline and normal serum pH is maintained by renal excretion of K+ in the urine in exchange for H+. The increased bicarbonate load overwhelms the absorptive capacity of the proximal and distal renal tubules, resulting in alkaline urine. Paradoxical aciduria ensues as gastric fluid loss continues and intravascular volume depletion worsens. The renal response shifts from maintenance of serum pH to maintenance of intravascular volume. Aldosterone secretion leads to Na+ absorption (in exchange for K+ excretion) and Cl- absorption in the distal tubules and collecting ducts to maintain (restore) intravascular volume at the expense of serum pH. The majority of the K+ deficit in patients with pyloric stenosis is due to this secondary hyperaldosteronism.[6] Severe hypokalemia is uncommon in infants and may be due to the reduced ability of the kidney to excrete potassium early in life. As serum Cl- diminishes with continued gastric losses, the kidney retains HCO_3^- to accompany the Na+ uptake,[20] exacerbating the metabolic alkalosis. Also, with decreased filtration of Cl-, the activity of the distal tubule Na+/Cl- symporter is reduced. Sodium uptake becomes dependent on the cation exchanger, which takes up Na+ in exchange for K+ (preferential in metabolic alkalosis) or H+. K+ is conserved at the expense of H+, leading to paradoxical aciduria, exacerbating alkalosis further.[21] Measuring urine chloride can aid in the assessment of dehydration status. In the IHPS patient with dehydration, a urine chloride concentration <20 mEq/L suggests maximal renal Cl- retention. Urine chloride concentration is >20 mEq/L when dehydration is treated.[2,8]

On physical exam, the hypertrophied pylorus can sometimes be palpated if the abdomen is relaxed. An OG or NG tube may be placed to decompress the stomach and improve success of this finding on exam. Occasionally, gastric peristaltic waves may be observed. Palpation of the hypertrophied pyloric muscle ("olive") has been reported to have a 99% positive predictive value in the infant with classical symptoms of pyloric stenosis.[22] In 2011, Glatstein et al. found only 13.6% of infants had a palpable olive in their retrospective review, compared to more than 50% of infants in older studies.[23] If the abdominal exam does not reveal an olive and ultrasound is negative then more extensive workup to evaluate suspected intestinal obstruction should be undertaken.[5]

IMAGING STUDIES

Abdominal ultrasound is often used for confirmation of diagnosis especially in the absence of physical or equivocal findings.[24] Early use of ultrasound to confirm the diagnosis is thought to play a major role in the earlier treatment of the illness.[18] Pyloric muscle thickness >3 mm and channel length greater than 15 mm (Fig. 39.1) is very sensitive and specific for IHPS.[5]

Upper GI series is not used routinely due to the increased aspiration risk with ingestion of contrast material. The classic elongated pyloric channel (string sign) often with bulging of pyloric muscle extending into the antrum of the stomach (shoulder signs) is diagnostic of poor gastric emptying in the presence of hypertrophied pyloric muscle. The presence of parallel streaks of barium in the narrowed pyloric channel sometimes produces a "double track sign" (Fig. 39.2).[1]

PREOPERATIVE PREPARATION

IHPS is not a surgical emergency. The focus of preoperative preparation is to minimize aspiration risk and treat dehydration and electrolyte imbalance. Infants are placed on gastric rest (nil per os) to minimize aspiration risk. OG tube placement may be used in cases of ongoing emesis to allow accurate measurement of output for replacement therapy (1 mL 0.9% NS with 10 mEq/L KCl for each mL of gastric output).[2] Some surgeons suggest placement of the OG tube should be

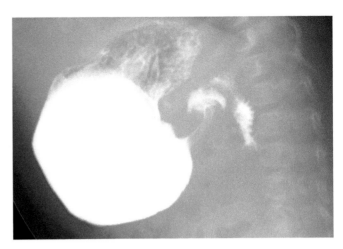

Fig. 39.2 Upper GI: String sign due to poor gastric emptying of contrast material through hypertrophied pyloric muscle into the (mushroom appearing) duodenum.

avoided (if possible) to minimize exacerbation of electrolyte losses.[25] An IV 0.9% NS bolus (20 mL/kg) is given to patients with signs of shock or moderate/severe dehydration to restore circulation.[3] This dose may be repeated if shock persists or adjusted for patients with cardiac disease.

Fluid replacement regimens vary after signs of shock are reversed and are modified based on electrolyte replacement needs. Potassium is usually withheld until the infant begins voiding. A maintenance fluid based on CL– deficiency has been found to be the best estimate of volume resuscitation in patients with IHPS.[2] For example, D5 ½ NS with 20 mEq KCl/L for serum chloride above 90 mEq/L, D5 ½ NS with 30 mEq KCl/L for serum chloride between 80 and 90 mEq/L and D5 ½ NS with 40 mEq KCl/L for chloride below 80 mEq/L. This fluid may be given at 1 to 1.5 × maintenance rate depending on the patient's hydration status. Another regimen recommends volume correction with 20 mL/kg 0.9% NS as above and then initial fluid therapy with 0.45% or 0.9% NS with D5 with 10 to 20 mEq/L of KCl at 150 mL/kg/day (1.5 × maintenance) which can be reduced to 100 mL/kg/day (maintenance) when serum bicarbonate is <25 mmol/L. Ongoing NG losses (if there is an NG tube in place) are replaced with mL for mL 0.9% NS with 10 mEq/L of KCl.[2]

Electrolytes, glucose and acid base status are checked every 4 to 6 hours after initiation of therapy and then every 6 to 12 hours until normalized. There is little evidence in the literature to suggest an acceptable level of metabolic alkalosis for an infant to safely undergo general anesthesia, but we do know that it is associated with apnea and extubation difficulty.[7] Patients should be hydrated (evidenced by Cl ≥100 mEq/L) and alkalosis should be corrected (HCO3 <30 mmol/L) since this may contribute to postoperative apnea.[5] Electrolyte and hydration status usually normalize within 12 to 48 hours of treatment initiation.

ANESTHETIC MANAGEMENT

The patient is scheduled for pyloromyotomy when hydration status and electrolytes are normalized. He should be placed on

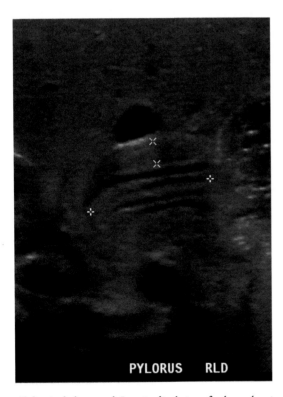

Fig. 39.1 Abdominal ultrasound: Longitudinal view of pylorus showing muscle thickness >3 mm (vertical markers) and channel length >15 mm (horizontal markers).

American Society of Anesthesiology standard monitors upon arrival to the operating room. A large bore OG suction should be used (whether the patient had a preoperative NG or not) to decompress the stomach (suctioning in the supine, right and left lateral position until no gastric fluid returns) prior to induction of general anesthesia. Using endoscopy, Cook-Sather et al. showed that infants with IHPS have substantial preoperative gastric fluid volumes that are not greatly decreased by preoperative NG tube suction and independent of the infant's fasting interval or having a barium study.[17,25] Furthermore, they can have more than 10 times the gastric fluid volume of the healthy fasted pediatric surgical patient; therefore, after preoxygenation, a rapid sequence induction (assuming there are no contraindications) is performed to secure the airway and decrease aspiration risk.[9,10,25] In their retrospective review of 269 cases, Scrimgeour et al. recommend considering inhaled induction of anesthesia (though they are careful to mention it is not more suitable than rapid sequence intubation [RSI]) and site the increased likelihood of hypoxemia along with increased difficulty of intubation when performing an RSI in the infant. It was noted that all patients in this series had an NG tube in situ and that their stomachs were suctioned. No additional details were given about how the infants' stomachs were suctioned or exactly what peak airway pressures were used during inhalation induction.[10,26] Of note, even with a peak airway pressure as low as 15 cm H2O during facemask ventilation, Bouvet et al. showed there is a 35% probability of having gastric insufflation using real-time ultrasonography. Real-time ultrasonography of the antrum led to the detection of gastric insufflation with high sensitivity.[27] After the airway is secure, a large-bore OG catheter attached to a 30 mL syringe using a stopcock is inserted into the stomach for injection of air. This is used to ensure integrity of the pyloric mucosa after the pyloromyotomy is performed.

Maintenance of anesthesia includes a short-acting muscle relaxant, a volatile anesthetic agent, as well as avoidance of opiates to prevent postoperative apnea. Hyperventilation could lead to a worsening alkalosis that can also depress respiratory drive. The infant is extubated awake at the conclusion of the procedure.

SURGICAL MANAGEMENT

There are 3 methods (open, circumumbilical, laparoscopic) of operative treatment of pyloric stenosis with the ultimate goal of performing sutureless extramucosal myotomy of adequate length which extends from the vein of Mayo on the duodenal side to the circular muscles of the stomach. When the myotomy is complete, the separated edges of the pyloric muscle move independently of each other[5] (Fig. 39.3). Instilling air into the indwelling OG catheter placed after induction of anesthesia confirms integrity of the mucosa as well as adequate passage of air into the duodenum.

Surgical management continues to evolve, but the fundamentals of pyloromyotomy have not changed for over 100 years.[1] The mortality rate of IHPS was 50% before Ramstedt developed the open pyloromyotomy (OP) in 1911 using a transverse incision in the right upper quadrant.[1,28]

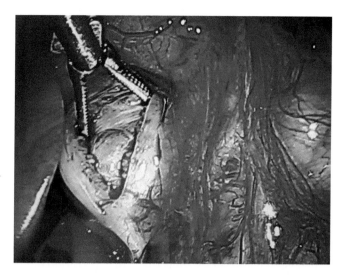

Fig. 39.3 Laparoscopic pyloromyotomy demonstrating spreading muscle layer of pylorus, exposing intact mucosa.

Even though the open approach leaves a scar, the mortality rate significantly improved and is now less than 0.5%.[1] Tan and Bianchi introduced a circumumbilical which improved the wound appearance.[29] The laparoscopic pyloromyotomy (LP) was introduced by Alain et al. in 1991.[30] Regardless of the approach, the procedure itself has remained unchanged and the potential postoperative complications include incomplete pyloromyotomy, mucosal perforation, and the need for reoperation.[8,31] Investigators have found benefits of laparoscopic technique include fewer doses of analgesic medication postoperatively, higher parental satisfaction with cosmetic appearance, and shorter time to the infant taking full feeds.[31,32] Adibe et al. found LP to be a safe and effective alternative to OP in a retrospective review of cases at their high-volume pediatric teaching hospital but commented that there appears to be an institutional learning curve when the technique is introduced, as reflected by the slightly higher rate of mucosal injury and incomplete pyloromyotomy.[33]

NONSURGICAL MANAGEMENT

Although surgical management is the mainstay of treatment for IHPS, there have been nonoperative approaches to treatment. Lukac et al. managed IHPS in 40 patients with oral atropine sulfate therapy. Ten of the patients did not respond to oral atropine therapy and received surgical management 5 to 7 days after the start of therapy. The remaining (75%) did not receive surgical management. When the vomiting ceased (between the 6th and 8th day of treatment), these to patients were discharged from the hospital and continued to take oral atropine medication for 4 to 6 weeks.[34] A 2013 meta-analysis review of the literature recommends that atropine therapy should be reserved only for treatment of extremely high-risk infants or for areas of the world with high mortality rates for neonatal surgery.[35] Interestingly, atropine therapy has been used successfully to treat incomplete pyloromyotomy in an infant presenting 14 days postoperatively.[36] Endoscopic balloon dilatation has also been used successfully in a patient with incomplete pyloromyotomy.[8]

POSTOPERATIVE CONCERNS AND MANAGEMENT

Postoperative respiratory depression, resolution of emesis postoperatively, and adequacy of analgesia are the primary concerns in the patient after pyloromyotomy. Postoperatively, patients are at increased risk for respiratory depression and oxygen desaturation can be significant.[37] This is thought to possibly be related to relative cerebrospinal fluid (CSF) alkalosis and hyperventilation[38] and possibly central residual effects of volatile agents.[39] Ph is one of the determinants of respiratory drive and CSF pH may remain increased for some time after correction of the serum electrolytes. Postoperative vomiting occurs in about half of the infants and is secondary to edema of the pylorus at the incision site. Current practice varies in regard to reintroduction of feeds. Debate continues regarding superiority of ad libitum versus incremental or protocol driven feeding.[40] A prospective, randomized trial of 150 infants compared ad libitum feeds (75 infants) with protocol feeds (75 infants) allowing oral electrolyte solution at 2 hours postoperative and progressed to full mild feeds in a standardized way. The ad libitum group reached goal feeds 7 hours faster than the protocol group, but there was no difference in length of hospital stay between the two groups, suggesting that other factors determine length of hospital stay.[41] Most infants will begin feeds within 12 to 24 hours and most are advanced within 36 to 48 hours. Persistent vomiting suggests incomplete pyloromyotomy, gastritis, gastroesophageal reflux disease, or other cause of obstruction. Rare occurrence of hypoglycemia has been reported postoperatively and was attributed to cessation of IV glucose infusion and depletion of liver glycogen stores while the patient's glycemic needs were not met by enteral progress.[15]

Rectal acetaminophen along with local infiltration of the wound can minimize the need for opioids in the postoperative period. Breschan et al. demonstrated that ultrasound-guided rectus sheath block is a simple and efficient adjuvant to general anesthesia, providing good intraoperative and postoperative analgesia for OP.[42]

The patient is discharged when he is afebrile, able to tolerate feeds, has acceptable pain tolerance, and is not experiencing apnea or bradycardia. He will follow up with the pediatrician in a few days and the surgeon within 1 month.[5]

REVIEW QUESTIONS

1. Which of the following abnormalities is **MOST** likely found in the 6-week-old infant experiencing nonbilious "spitting up"/vomiting with feeds?

    A. duodenal atresia
    B. esophageal atresia
    C. gastroesophageal reflux
    D. pyloric stenosis

Answer: C
The most common etiology of nonbilious "spitting up"/vomiting in infancy is gastroesophageal reflux.[43] IHPS is associated with nonbilious vomiting in the infant between 2 and 10 weeks of age and occurs in 1.5 to 3 per 1,000 live births.[13] Esophageal atresia is associated with nonbilious emesis and poor feeding tolerance in the neonatal period.[44] Duodenal atresia (incidence 1 in 10,000 live births) presents in the neonatal period shortly after birth and is associated with bilious vomiting.[13,43,44]

2. Which of the following is **MOST** consistently a risk factor for the patient with pyloric stenosis?

    A. bottle-feeding instead of breast-feeding
    B. family history of pyloric stenosis
    C. history of erythromycin use
    D. supine feeding position of infant

Answer: B
Of the choices listed, family history of IHPS is the only proven link to a person developing the condition.[13]

3. What clinical sign or symptom is **MOST** likely to be present in a patient diagnosed with pyloric stenosis in developed countries?

    A. hypochloremic metabolic alkalosis
    B. mild dehydration
    C. mild hypokalemia
    D. palpable "olive" or pyloric mass

Answer: B
Because IHPS is diagnosed earlier in the present-day secondary to high clinical acuity and increased use of ultrasound, the palpable "olive" as well as the traditional electrolyte and acid base changes are less likely to be seen.[1,17,18,45]

4. Normalization of which serum electrolyte is the **BEST** indicator of volume repletion in the infant with idiopathic hypertrophic pyloric stenosis requiring fluid resuscitation?

    A. chloride
    B. hemoglobin
    C. potassium
    D. sodium

Answer: A
Maintenance fluid based on chloride deficiency has been found to be the best estimate of volume resuscitation in these patients.[2] Miozzari et al. found a stronger correlation between chloride dose and change in circulating bicarbonate level than between potassium or water and changes in circulating bicarbonate. They emphasize the importance of chloride deficiency in these patients and use of this serum electrolyte in estimating fluid volume status for them. Patients should be rehydrated, and normalization of the chloride and bicarbonate levels should be assured prior to surgery.[2,6]

5. A 6-week-old term infant with a history of intolerance to feeds and worsening nonbilious, projectile vomiting has

physical exam findings significant for lethargy, weak pulses, and sunken fontanel. Which is the **BEST** initial fluid resuscitation plan?

    A. D_5 NS (0.9) IV infusion at 1.5 × maintenance
    B. fresh frozen plasma, 20 mL/kg IV or intraosseous bolus
    C. NS (0.9), 20 mL/kg IV or intraosseous bolus
    D. Pedialyte, ad libitum orally

Answer: C

The physical exam is consistent with severe dehydration. The initial fluid therapy goal is to restore circulating volume to treat shock. A 20 mL/kg bolus of isotonic fluid is recommended.[3] Repeat boluses may be necessary. Oral hydration is not reliable for the patient experiencing vomiting. An infusion of D_5 0.9 NS at 1.5 times maintenance is not adequate for resuscitation of the infant in shock due to dehydration. Fresh frozen plasma is not an appropriate intravascular volume expander.[3]

6. Which of the following findings are **MOST** closely associated with severe dehydration in an infant with IHPS?

    A. acidic urine
    B. hyperkalemia
    C. serum pH 7.0
    D. serum chloride 110 mEq/L

Answer: A

Prolonged vomiting in the infant with IHPS leads to depletion of sodium, potassium, chloride, and hydrogen ions in the gastric fluid loss. Prolonged illness due to IHPS is associated with hypochloremic, hypokalemic metabolic alkalosis. The urine is initially alkalotic because the kidney reabsorbs H+, excreting HCO_3^- to maintain serum pH. As the patient becomes progressively dehydrated, Na+ is absorbed and as Cl– availability diminishes, HCO_3^- is absorbed in its place. The Na+Cl– renal supporter activity is also replaced by a cation exchanger where Na+ is taken up and either K+ (preferentially in metabolic alkalosis) or H+ (if K+ is unavailable), thus worsening paradoxical aciduria in the face of metabolic alkalosis.[3,6,20,21]

7. Which of the following is the **MOST** commonly recommended method of anesthetic induction for a baby with pyloric stenosis *after* aspirating the stomach several times with a multiport OG tube?

    A. awake intubation
    B. inhaled induction/intubation
    C. inhaled induction with cricoid pressure
    D. rapid sequence IV induction

Answer: D

Although some anesthesiologists will perform awake intubation or inhaled inductions in the patient with IHPS, the recommended approach is to suction the patient's stomach several times with a multiport OG tube (until as much gastric contents can be removed as possible) and proceed with a rapid sequence induction.[15]

8. You are called to evaluate a lethargic infant on "heparin locked IV, ad libitum feeding protocol" 4 hours after undergoing an uneventful laparoscopic pyloromyotomy. His BP is 90/40, HR 148, SpO_2 100% RR 28, temperature 36.5. Which laboratory finding will **MOST** likely be abnormal?

    A. bicarbonate
    B. chloride
    C. glucose
    D. potassium

Answer: C

Edema of the pylorus is not uncommon after pyloromyotomy, and some vomiting during the early postoperative period is expected. Hypoglycemia should be considered in the patient scheduled for ad libitum feeds without dextrose-containing maintenance IV fluids infusing.[15]

9. What of the following signs would be **MOST** concerning after pyloromyotomy?

    A. fever
    B. irritability
    C. somnolence
    D. vomiting

Answer: A

It is important that the child is afebrile before being discharged in the event there is a wound infection. It is not uncommon for a patient to have some small, continued emesis after pyloromyotomy secondary to edema of the pylorus or irritability secondary to discomfort or hunger. It is also not unusual for the young infant to be somnolent after general anesthesia, as long as hypoglycemia has been ruled out.[5,15]

QUESTIONS AND ANSWERS

This chapter has accompanying questions and answers which are available to subscribers as part of the Oxford eLearning platform. To access the questions, go to ✔ http://oxfordmedicine. com/pediatricanesthesiaPBL

REFERENCES

1. Hunter AK, Liacourse CA. Hypertrophic pyloric stenosis. In Kliegman RM, ed. *Nelson's Textbook of Pediatrics.*19th ed. Philadelphia, PA: Elsevier Saunders; 2011: 1274–1275.
2. Greenbaum L. Maintenance and replacement therapy. In Kliegman RM, ed. *Nelson's Textbook of Pediatrics.*19th ed. Philadelphia, PA: Elsevier Saunders; 2011: 242–2245.
3. American Heart Association. Management of shock. In: Chameides L, Samson RA, Schexnayder SM, Hazinski MF, Ashcraft J, eds. *Pediatric Advanced Life Support Provider Manual.* Dallas, TX: American Heart Association; 2016: 197–233.
4. American Heart Association. Systematic approach to the seriously ill or injured child. In: Chameides L, Samson RA, Schexnayder SM, Hazinski MF, Ashcraft J, eds. *Pediatric Advanced Life Support Provider Manual.* Dallas, TX: American Heart Association; 2016: 29–67.stenosis. *Act Paediatr.* 2001;90:511–514.
5. Pandya S, Heiss K. Pyloric stenosis in pediatric surgery: an evidence-
6. Miozzari HH. Fluid resuscitation in infantile hypertrophic pyloric
7. Peters, Oomen MW, Kakx R, Benninga MA. Advances in infantile hypertrophic pyloric stenosis. *Expert Rev Gastroenterol Hepatol.* 2014;8:533–541.

8. Hall NJ, Eaton S, Seims A, et al. Risk of incomplete pyloromyotomy and mucosal perforation in open and laparoscopic pyloromyotomy. *J Pediatr Surg*. 2014;49:1083–1086.

9. Cook-Sather SD, Liacouras CA, Previte JP, Markakis DA, Schreiner MS. Gastric fluid measurement by blind aspiration in paediatric patients: a gastroscopic evaluation. *Can J Anaesth*. 1997;44(2):168–172.

10. Colombs JL. Aspiration Syndromes In Kliegman RM, ed. *Nelson's Textbook of Pediatrics*. 19th ed. Philadelphia, PA: Elsevier Saunders; 2011: 1469–1470.

11. Jobson M, Hall N. Contemporary management of pyloric stenosis. *Semin Pediatr Surg*. 2016;25: 219–224.

12. Georgoula C, Gardiner M. Pyloric stenosis 100 years after Ramstedt. *Arch Dis Child*. 2012; 97:741–745.

13. Krogh C, Fischer TK, Skotte L, et al. Familial aggregation and heritability of pyloric stenosis. *JAMA*. 2010;303(23):2393–2399.

14. Vanderwinden JM. Nitric oxide synthase in infantile hypertrophic pyloric stenosis. *N Engl J Med*. 1992; 327(8): 511–515.

15. Hammer G, Hall S and Davis P. Anesthesia for general abdominal, thoracic, urologic and bariatric surgery. In: Davis PJ, Cladis, FP, eds. *Smith's Anesthesia for Infants and Children*. 8th ed. Philadelphia, PA: Elsevier Mosby; 2011: 750–751.

16. Piroutek MJ, Brown L, Thorp AW. Bilious vomiting does not rule out infantile hypertrophic pyloric stenosis. *Clin Pediatr*. 2012;51(3):214–218.

17. Tutay GJ, Capraro G, Spirko B, Garb J, Smithline H. Electrolyte profile of pediatric patients with hypertrophic pyloric stenosis. *Pediatr Emerg Care*. 2013;29:465–468.

18. Hernanz-Schulman M. Pyloric stenosis: role of imaging. *Pediatr Radiol*. 2009;39:S134–S139.

19. Oakley EA, Barnett PLJ. Is acid base determination an accurate predictor of pyloric stenosis? *J Paediatr Child Health*. 2000;36:587–589.

20. Chen EA, Luks FI, Gilchrist DF, et al. Pyloric stenosis in the age of ultrasonography: fading skills, better patients? *J Pediatr Surg*. 1996;31(6):829–830.

21. Aspenlund G, Langer JC. Current management of hypertrophic pyloric stenosis. *Semin Pediatr Surg*. 2007;16:27–33.

22. de Laffolie J, Turial S, Heckmann M, Zimmer KP, Schier F. Decline in infantile hypertrophic pyloric stenosis in Germany in 2000–2008. *Pediatrics*. 2012;120:e901–e906.

23. Glatstein M, Carbell G, Boddu SK. The changing clinical presentation of hypertrophic pyloric stenosis: the experience of a large, tertiary care pediatric hospital. *Clin Pediatr*. 2011;50:192–195. based review. *Surg Clin N Am*. 2012:92:527–539.

24. Macdessi J, Oats RK. Clinical diagnosis of pyloric stenosis: a declining art. *BMJ*. 1993;306 (6877):553–555.

25. Cook-Sather, Tulloch H, Liacouras C, Schreiner MS. Gastric fluid volume in infants for pyloromyotomy. *Can J Anaesth*. 1997;440(3):278–283.

26. Scrimgeour G, Leather N, Perry R, et al. Gas induction for pyloromyotomy. *Pediatr Anesth*. 2015;25:677–680.

27. Bouvet L, Albert ML, Augris C, et al. Real-time detection of gastric insufflations related to facemask pressure-controlled ventilation using ultrasonography of the antrum and epigastric auscultation in nonparalyzed patients: a prospective randomized double blind study. *Anesthesiology*. 2014;120(2):326–334.

28. Ramstedt C. Zur operation der angeborenen pylorus-stenose. *Med Klin*. 1912;8:1702–1705.

29. Tan KC, Bianchi A. Circumumbilical incision for pyloromyotomy. *British J Surg*. 1986;78:399.

30. Alain J, Grousseau D, Terrier G. Extramucosal pyloromyotomy by laparoscopy. J Pediatr Surg. 1991;25:1191–1192.

31. Oomen MWN, Hoekstra LT, Bakx R, et al. Open versus laparoscopic pyloromyotomy for hypertrophic pyloric stenosis: a systematic review and meta-analysis focusing on major complications. *Surg Endosc*. 2012;26:2104–2110.

32. Vahdad MR, Nissen M, Semaan A, et al. Can a simplified algorithm prevent incomplete laparoscopic pyloromyotomy? *J Pediatr Surg*. 2015;50:1544–1548.

33. Adibe OO, Nichol PF, Flake AW, Matte P. Comparison of outcomes after laparoscopic and open pyloromyotomy at a high-volume pediatric teaching hospital. *J Pediatr Surg*. 2006;41:1676–1678.

34. Lukac M, Antunovic SS, Vujovic D, et al. Is abandonment of nonoperative management of pyloric stenosis warranted? *Eur J Pediatr Surg*. 2013;23:80–84.

35. Mercer AE, Phillips R. Question 2: can a conservative approach to the treatment of hypertrophic pyloric stenosis with atropine be considered a real alternative to surgical pyloromyotomy? *Arch Dis Child*. 2013;98:474–477.

36. Owen RP, Almond SI, Humphrey GM. Atropine sulfate: rescue therapy for pyloric stenosis. *Br Med J Case Rep*. 2012. doi:10.1136/bcr-2012-006489

37. Galinkin JL, Davis PJ, McGowan FX, et al. A randomized multicenter study of remifentanil compared with halothane in neonates and infants undergoing pyloromyotomy. II: perioperative breathing patterns in neonates and infants with pyloric stenosis. *Anesth Analg*. 2001;93:1387–1392.

38. Andropoulous DB, Heard MB, Johnson KL, Clarke JT, Rowe RW. Postanesthetic apnea in Full-term infants after pyloromyotomy. *Anesthesiology*. 1994;80:216–219.

39. Wolf AR, Lawson RA, Dryden CM, Davies FW. Recovery after desflurane anaesthesia in the infant: comparison with isoflurane. *Br J Anaesth*. 1996;76:362–364.

40. Graham KA, Laituri CA, Markel TA, Ladd AP. A review of postoperative feeding regimens in infantile hypertrophic pyloric stenosis. *J Pediatr Surg*. 2013;48(10):2175–2179.

41. Adibe OO, Iqbal CS, Sharp SW et al. Protocol versus ad libitum feeds after laparoscopic pyloromyotomy: a prospective randomized trial. *J Pediatr Surg*. 2014;49:129–132.

42. Breschan C, Jost R, Stettner H, et al. Ultrasound-guided rectus sheath block for pyloromyotomy in infants: a retrospective analysis of a case series. *Paedtr Anesth*. 2013;23:1199–1204.

43. Khan S, Orenstein S. Gastroesophageal reflux disease. In Kliegman RM, ed. *Nelson's Textbook of Pediatrics*. 19th ed. Philadelphia, PA: Elsevier Saunders; 2011: 1266–1269.

44. Brett C, Davis P. Anesthesia for general surgery in the neonate. In: Davis PJ, Cladis, FP, eds. *Smith's Anesthesia for Infants and Children*. 8th ed. Philadelphia, PA: Elsevier Mosby; 2011: 554–588.

45. Colletti J. Pyloric stenosis. *Can J Emerg Med*. 2004;6(6):444–445.

SECTION 7

RENAL AND URINARY SYSTEM

40.

BLADDER EXSTROPHY

Jason Bryant

STEM CASE AND KEY QUESTIONS

A 7-month-old male American Society of Anesthesiologists II presents to the operating theater for primary closure of bladder exstrophy. His surgical plan includes repair of his bladder and external genitalia with a pelvic osteotomy. He has a midline abdominal defect with mucosa externalized and bilateral hemipenis. He underwent an uncomplicated birth at 38 weeks with APGARs of 8 and 10, respectively. His condition was identified with a prenatal ultrasound and magnetic resonance imaging. His omphalocele was repaired on day 1 of life with placement of a colostomy, and he tolerated the procedure and anesthesia well.

THE PARENTS WANT TO KNOW ABOUT HOW MANY SURGERIES CHILDREN WITH BLADDER EXSTROPHY MUST UNDERGO. WHAT DO YOU TELL THEM?

The amount of surgeries is dependent on a variety of factors. Patients may need to undergo bladder neck reconstruction, which is dependent on whether he or she is able to have dry periods. There may be a few scar revisions and other cosmetic corrections as well. This question should be directed to the surgeon.

In our patient, hemocrit is 35% and his oxygen saturation is 100% on room air. His vital signs are appropriate for his age (temperature 37.5, heart rate 106, blood pressure 86/42, respiratory rate 20, SpO_2: 100% room air). His weight is 8 kg. He has no known drug allergies and is currently not on any medications. Focused physical exam reveals: HEENT: good oral opening, thyromental distance of 3 finger breaths, 2 teeth present (O,P), nonsyndromic appearing facies. Pulmonary: clear bilateral. Abdominal exam reveals a colostomy and a 3 cm midline mucosal cleft from below the umbilicus to just below the pubis with bilateral hemipenis.

WHAT IS BLADDER EXSTROPHY?

Bladder exstrophy is a rare congenital malformation in the pelvic floor and lower abdomen that results in a midline defect of the abdominal wall muscles, bladder, pelvis, and external genitalia. Incidence is reported between 1 in 200,000 births to 1 in 400,000.[1] Males are affected twice as much a

females.[2] This defect is believed to occur early in fetal development with the incomplete closure or rupture of the cloacal membrane during the fourth week of gestation.[3] This can affect the bladder and genitalia as well as associated structures including the pelvis, abdominal wall (omphalocele), spine, and bowel.[4,5]

WHAT ARE THE ANESTHETIC IMPLICATIONS OF BLADDER EXSTROPHY REPAIR?

The patient should be evaluated preoperatively for signs of dehydration, but these patients are usually well established, and with adequate teaching fluid balance can be maintained with an open bladder. With initial closure this may be more of a problem as the omphalocele will lead to greater loss of fluid through evaporation. The exposed bladder mucosa will still lose some fluid but is usually not clinically significant.

The major implication to anesthesia is related more to the pelvic osteotomies than the bladder repair. The pelvic osteotomies require prolonged immobilization postoperatively to maintain reapproximation and promote healing.[6] If these fail the abdominal suture will also be affected by increasing tension and may fail as well. To facilitate this prolonged immobilization, a tunneled lumbar epidural with a continuous infusion of local anesthetic is often used.

DURING YOUR INITIAL INTERVIEW WITH THE PARENTS, THEY RAISE CONCERNS ABOUT AN EPIDURAL, SPECIFICALLY THE RISK OF BACK PAIN OR PARESTHESIA LATER IN LIFE AND INFECTION. HOW WOULD YOU DISCUSS THE RISKS AND BENEFITS OF AN EPIDURAL IN THIS CASE?

Epidural analgesia has a safe and reliable record of use in infants and children.[7-9] To obtain informed consent from the parents, a detailed discussion of risks and benefits must be performed. The practitioner's choice of words should be easy to understand and limit the use of medical jargon. The risks that are usually discussed include neurologic damage, bleeding and hematomas, local anesthesia toxicity, and infection, including meningitis, respiratory, and cardiovascular changes including hypotension.

There is a large body of literature supporting the safe use of regional anesthesia in this age group. The pediatric regional anesthesia network has collected data from 2007 from multiple pediatric hospitals.[10] From 2007 to 2010, 2,946 neuraxial catheters were performed and analyzed. Catheter problems such as kinking, dislodgement, or malfunction were the most common complication occurring in one-third of the patients. Neurologic complications were very rare (0.1%), all of which resolved. There were no deep infections, abscess, or meningitis in this study (mean length of time was 2.2 days). There was a 0.2% incidence of respiratory complications and postoperative hypotension. There were no cases of local anesthetic toxicity or hematomas. This study and others can be quoted to the parents in a way to reassure them that the risk is low but that there are still inherent risks with any procedure. Having a dedicated pain service to follow up on these patients during their stay will also allow for careful observation.

The literature on tunneled epidural catheters and their prolonged use is not as extensive. One study included 25 pediatric patients where the catheter remained for a median of 11 days. [11] The range was from 4 to 240 days. Two of these were removed for possible infection. There was no signs of local anesthetic toxicity. Another study showed that tunneled catheters had a decreased incidence of colonization even in short-term use. There are, however, case reports of epidural catheters being used for weeks with a tunneled catheter without complications.

The benefit of using a tunneled lumbar epidural is that the outcomes of the surgery are improved secondary to the improved immobilization and healing of the pelvic osteotomies. Failure of this initial repair increases the risk of incontinence. Including pelvic osteotomies in the initial closure of the bladder can decrease the risk of bladder prolapse and dehiscence.

HOW WOULD YOU PREFORM THE TUNNELED EPIDURAL?

Most epidurals in pediatric anesthesia are performed under general anesthesia. This has been shown to be safe and effective.[12,13] The lumbar epidural can be placed in the lateral position usually L4-L5 under aseptic technique. An 18 gauge Touhy needle can be used to identify the space and a 20 gauge radiopaque catheter can be threaded using fluoroscopy to be placed L1-L2. To tunnel a second needle 22 gauge spinal needle can be used to create a tract starting at the first needle. A third 18 gauge epidural needle is slid over the 22 gauge spinal needle. The first 2 needles are removed leaving only the third needle and the catheter. The catheter then is threaded through the tip of the remaining 18 gauge epidural needle and then the needle is removed. Care must be taken to not pull the catheter out of the space during this maneuver. An alternative is to only use 2 epidural needles without the spinal needle as a guide. The distances can be recorded and used to determine if the catheter moves. A distance of 5 to 10 cm from the insertion site can be used depending on the size of the patient. The catheters should be secured with a sterile occlusive dressing. Detailed images provided in figures 40.1, 40.2, 40.3, and 40.4 shows the steps to tunnel epidural catheter.

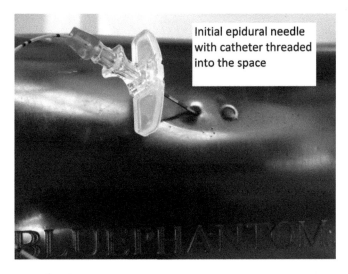

Fig. 40.1 Step 1

HOW CAN THE LEVEL OF THE EPIDURAL CATHETER TIP BE ASSESSED?

The use of flouroscopy and a radiopaque dye can be used to confirm the level of placement after insertion.[14,15] If the practitioner wishes to assess the level during insertion, electrical stimulation and ultrasound can be used. [14] Measuring the distance of the catheter does not guarantee the correct level, as it may not travel in a straight line or even in the correct direction.

WHAT ARE THE POSTOPERATIVE CONCERNS AFTER BLADDER EXTROPHY REPAIR WITH THE USE OF A TUNNELED EPIDURAL CATHETER?

Stabilization of the pelvic bones from decreased movement of the lower extremities and pain management are the main benefits from a tunneled epidural catheter. Intravenous

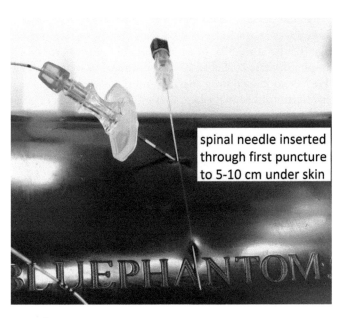

Fig. 40.2 Step 2

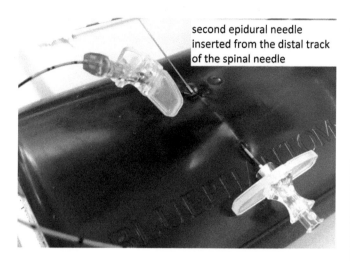

second epidural needle inserted from the distal track of the spinal needle

Fig. 40.3 Step 3

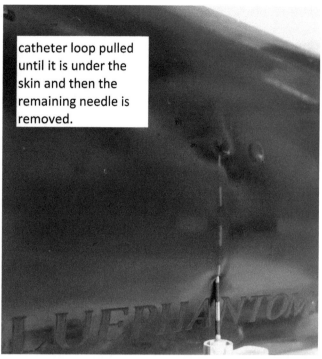

catheter loop pulled until it is under the skin and then the remaining needle is removed.

Fig. 40.5 Step 5

medications should also be used to reduce pain. Nonsteroidal and benzodiazepine medications can be used. The patient may be placed in traction or external fixation. This patient must be monitored for signs of infection, manipulation, respiratory depression and local anesthetic toxicity.

Epidural catheters have been shown to colonize with skin flora within 48 to 72 hours after placement. Infection is rare, however, when removed within 3 to 5 days.[8] Tunneling of the catheter decreases this rate for weeks. In one study none of the 23 catheters followed for weeks showed any signs of infection.[8]

Decreasing the manipulation of the catheter during the weeks of use can be difficult. Over one-third of epidurals in the Pediatric Regional Anesthesia Network database had complications from movement including kinking and unintentional removal, and these were all during shorter time

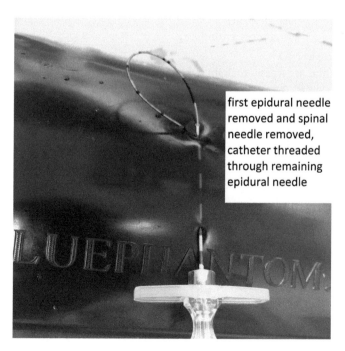

first epidural needle removed and spinal needle removed, catheter threaded through remaining epidural needle

Fig. 40.4 Step 4

periods.[10] Taping securely with loops to prevent direct traction can help. Careful nursing care and handling are key. Daily evaluation from a trained pain team can identify loose dressings or other issues before a catheter is unintentionally removed.

Local anesthetic toxicity risk is elevated in the neonate with lower serum protein levels and decreased metabolism. In patients older than 6 months this is less of a concern but must be considered. With lower serum proteins there is more "free" drug unbound leading to higher serum concentrations.[16] Local anesthetics that are metabolized by the liver such as bupivacaine, ropivicaine, and lidocaine can also build up, causing toxicity. Bupivacaine levels have been shown to rise especially after 48 hours in this age group and are highly cardiac toxic.[17,18] Lidocaine has been used in longer infusions to reduce the risk of accumulation. Lidocaine has the benefit of being shorter acting and easily measured in a blood test to obtain serum levels. The rate of infusion is also important in determining accumulation. Doses of a dilute lidocaine of 0.1% to 0.5% above 0.8 mh/kg/hr for more than 2 days are not recommended. Some institutions have started with a 0.1% bupivacaine infusion of 0.2 to 0.3 mg/kg/hr and switched to lidocaine on day 2 or 3. Levels of lidocaine should be measured regularly in the first few days can aid in reducing the risk of toxicity. 2-chloroprocaine is an ester anesthetic that is metabolized in the plasma by a cholinesterase and has a low toxicity level in the neonate as well. Even though plasma cholinesterases are lower in neonates, chloroprocaine is still rapidly metabolized in these patients. Rates of 0.5 mL/kg/hr of 1.5% chloroprocaine have been used safely in neonates. See local anesthesitic profile Table 40.1.

Table 40.1 LOCAL ANESTHESITIC PROFILES

BUPIVACAINE	LIDOCAINE	CHLOROPROCAINE
Rarely used in neonates	Used with lower infusions and careful monitoring in neonates	Used in neonates
Not usually easily measured in-house laboratory	Easily measured in-house laboratory	Not usually easily measured in-house laboratory but low risk of toxicity
Can accumulate in longer infusions	Lower risk to accumulate in longer infusions with a shorter half life	Metabolized in serum low risk for accumulation

Vigilance is important in the management of these patients postoperatively.

DISCUSSION

Bladder exstrophy is rare, with an incidence of 1:200,000 to 1:400,000. It can present as a mixed spectrum of abnormalities including the spine, pelvis, genitalia, and abdominal wall. An event in fetal development occurring as early as 6 weeks has been implicated. If the membrane in the early cloaca ruptures and there is a failure of separation of the gastrointestinal and urogenital structures, bladder exstrophy can occur. This occurs in a higher proportion of males to females. In males there are often 2 separate hemipenis that will need reconstructed during the bladder exstrophy surgery.

The timing of the surgery to correct the bladder exstrophy and pelvic instability usually is undertaken during the first year of life after there is enough tissue to ensure complete closure. If there is an associated omphalocele it must be repaired urgently as a neonate first. This is often performed with a diverting colostomy to separate the gastrointestinal tract and urogenital tract.

The goals of bladder reconstruction include continence, cosmetic, sexual function, and optimal quality of life. [19,20] Urinary continence is the primary outcome and is easy to measure as a long-term result. [21] The outcome of urinary continence has been tied to the success of the initial repair. Failure of the initial repair decreases the likelihood of long-term continence. [22] This is where the postoperative coarse and anesthetic plan can drastically improve the outcome. The closure the bladder and stabilize the pelvis with osteotomies, traction, and or external fixation are optimized with postoperative immobilization. Continuous epidural infusions have been used safely in this population to achieve this goal.

The use of a tunneled epidural catheter for weeks can help reduce the risk of failure and control postoperative pain. The tunneled catheter has a decreased risk of infection and colonization. Manipulation including inadvertent removal of the catheter is the highest risk complication. Signs of local anesthetic toxicity must be monitored, and careful management of the infusion and choice of drugs are important. A team approach to care of these complex patients will increase the vigilance of surveillance and care. Regional anesthesia use in the pediatric patient is safe and effective in the management of bladder exstrophy. Long-term outcome of these patients is improving and being followed as patients age and enter adulthood.

REVIEW QUESTIONS

1. Which of the following statement is **MOST** accurate regarding bladder exstrophy?

    A. Male to female ratio is 2:1
    B. Isolated finding in most cases
    C. Late developmental occurrence
    D. Incontinence risk is unalterable

Answer: A

Bladder exstrophy is rare with an incidence of 1:200,000 to 1:400,000. It can present as a mixed spectrum of abnormalities including the spine, pelvis, genitalia, and abdominal wall. This occurs twice as often in males than females. Postoperative management can improve the outcomes. An event in fetal development occurring as early as 6 weeks has been implicated. If the membrane in the early cloaca ruptures and there is a failure of separation of the gastrointestinal and urogenital structures, bladder exstrophy can occur not malrotation.

2. Which of the following compromised physiological functions is **MOST** responsible for the increased risk of local anesthetic toxicity in neonates?

    A. blood-brain-barrier permeability
    B. hepatic metabolism
    C. renal clearance
    D. serum protein binding

Answer: D

Local anesthetic toxicity risk is elevated in the neonate with lower serum protein levels and decreased metabolism. With lower serum proteins there is more "free" drug unbound leading to higher serum concentrations.

3. What is the **MOST** important benefit of using a tunneled epidural catheter for the postoperative management of bladder exstrophy?

    A. cervical analgesia
    B. immobilization
    C. family satisfaction
    D. early ambulation

Correct Answer: B

Bladder exstrophy repair requires prolonged immobilization post-operative to maintain reapproximation and promote healing. To facilitate this prolonged immobilization a tunneled lumbar epidural with a continuous infusion of local anesthetic is often used. There is an increased risk of local anesthetic toxicity in the neonate and prolonged infusions. Levels of analgesia should be maintained to cover only the lower abdomen not cervical.

4. Which of the following is **MOST** accurate about the use of epidural regional anesthesia in pediatric patients?

A. Anesthetic choice is unimportant.
B. Bacterial colonization is rare.
C. Catheter complications are common.
D. Efficacy has been demonstrated.

Correct Answer: C

There is a large body of literature supporting the safe use of regional anesthesia in this age group. The pediatric regional anesthesia network has collected data from 2007 from multiple pediatric hospitals. Epidural catheters have been shown to colonize with skin flora within 48 to 72 hours after placement. Catheter problems such as kinking, dislodgement, or malfunction are the most common complications occurring in one-third of the patients.

5. Which is the **MOST** accurate statement regarding serum levels with epidural lidocaine infusions?

A. high toxicity risk in neonates
B. longer lasting than bupivacaine
C. measured onsite by most hospitals
D. reduced by serum cholinesterase

Answer: C

Lidocaine has been used in longer infusions to reduce the risk of accumulation. Lidocaine has the benefit of being shorter acting and easily measured in a blood test in-house at most hospitals to obtain serum levels. Bupivacaine has been shown to accumulate significantly after the first 2 days. The rate of infusion is also important in determining accumulation. 2-chloroprocaine is an ester anesthetic that is metabolized in the plasma by a cholinesterase and has a low toxicity level in the neonate as well.

6, Which is the **MOST** accurate statement regarding bladder exstrophy repair?

A. Diverting colostomy timing is optional
B. Neonatal emergency considerations
C. Omphalocele repairs should be delayed
D. Tissue adequacy for closure paramount

Answer: D

The timing of the surgery to correct the bladder exstrophy and pelvic instability usually is undertaken during the first year of life after there is enough tissue to ensure complete closure. If there is an associated omphalocele, it must be repaired urgently as a neonate first. This is often performed with a diverting colostomy to separate the gastrointestinal tract and urogenital tract.

QUESTIONS AND ANSWERS

This chapter has accompanying questions and answers which are available to subscribers as part of the Oxford eLearning platform. To access the questions, go to ✓ http:// oxfordmedicine. com/pediatricanesthesiaPBL

REFERENCES

1. Nelson CP, Dunn RL, Wei JT. Contemporary epidemiology of bladder exstrophy in the United States. *J Urol.* 2005;173:1728–1731.
2. Muecke EC. The role of the cloacal membrane in exstrophy: the first successful experimental study. *J Urol.* 1964;92:659–667.
3. Vermeij-Keers C, Hartwig NG, Vanderwerff JF. Embryonic development of the ventral body wall and its congenital malformations. *Semin Pediatr Surg.* 1996;5(2):82–89.
4. Russell LJ, Weaver DD, Bull MJ. The axial mesodermal dysplasia spectrum. *Pediatrics.* 1981;67(2):176–182.
5. Diamond DA, Jeffs RD. Cloacal exstrophy: a 22 year experience. *J Urol.* 1985;133(5):779–782.
6. Hussman DA. Surgery insight: advantages and pitfalls of techniques for the correction of bladder exstrophy. *Nat Clin Pract Urol.* 2006;3:95–100.
7. Stratford MA, Wilder RT, Berde CB. The risk of infection from epidural analgesia in children: a review of 1620 cases. *Anesth Analg.* 195 80:234–238.
8. Kost-byerly S, Jackson E, Yaster M, Kolzowski L, Mathews R, Gearhart J. Perioperative anesthetic and analgesic management of newborn bladder exstrophy repair. *J Peadiatr Urol.* 2008;4:280–285.
9. Giaufre E, Dalens B, Gombert A. Epidemiology and morbidity of regional anesthesia in children: a one-year prospective survey of the French-Language Society of Pediatric Anesthesiologists. *Anesth Analg.* 1996;83:904–912.
10. Polaner DM, Taenzer AH, Walker BJ, et al. Pediatric Regional Anesthesia Network (PRAN): a multi-institutional study of the use and incidence of complications of pediatric regional anesthesia. *Anesth Analg.* 2012;115:1353–1364.
11. Aram L, Krane EJ, Kozloski LJ, Yaster M. Tunneled epidural catheters for prolonged analgesia in pediatric patients. *Anesth Analg.* 2001;99:1432–1438.
12. Massanyi EC, Gearhart JP, Kost-Byerly S. Perioperative management exstrophy. *Res Rep Urol.* 2013;5:67–75.
13. Burstal R, Wegener F, Hayes C, et al. Subcutaneous tunnelling of epidural catheters for post operative analgesia to prevent accidental dislodgement: a randomized controlled trial. *Anaesth Intensive Care.* 1998;26:147–151.
14. Tsui BC, Seal R, Koller J. Thoracic epidural catheter placement via the caudal approach in infants using electrographic guidance. *Anesth Analg.* 2001;93(5):1152–1155.
15. Valairucha S, Seefelder C, Houck CS. Thoracic epidural catheter placed by the caudal route in infants: the importance of radiographic confirmation. *Pediatr Anaesth.* 2002;1295:424–428.
16. Lerman J, strong HA, LeDez KM, et al. Effects of age on the serum concentration of alpha 1-acid glycoprotein and the binding of lidocaine in pediatric patients. *Clin Pharmacol Ther.* 1989;46:219–225.
17. Yaster M, Tobin JR, Kost-Byerly S. *Local Anesthetics: Pain in Infants, Children and Adolescents.* 2nd ed. Philadelphia, PA: Lippincott Williams and Wilkins; 2003.
18. Larsson BA, Lonnquist PA, Olsson GL. Plasma concentrations of bupivacaine in neonates after continuous epidural infusions. *Anesth Analg.* 1997;84(3):501–505.
19. Shnorhavorian M, Grady RW, Andersen A, Joyner BD, Mitchell ME. Long-term follow up of complete primary repair of exstrophy: the Seattle experience. *J Urol.* 2008;180:1615–1619.
20. Alpert SA, Cheng EY, Kaplan WE, Snodgrass WT, Wilcox DT, Kropp BP. Bladder neck fistula after the complete primary repair of bladder exstrophy: a multi-institutional experience. *J Urol.* 2005;174:1687–1689.
21. Ebert AK, Schott G, Bals-Pratsch M, Seifert B, Rosch WH. Long-term follow-up of male patients after reconstruction of the bladder-exstrophy epispadias complex: psychosocial status, continence, renal and genital function. *J Pediatr Urol.* 2010;691:6–10.
22. Palacios L, Salazar-Ramirez, KJ. Anaesthesia and analgesia for bladder exstrophy correction. *Case Rep Rev Colomb Anestesiol.* 2015;43(3):254–258.

41.

WILMS TUMOR

Graciela Argote-Romero

STEM CASE AND KEY QUESTIONS

A 4-year-old boy presents for a routine well-child visit with his primary care physician. Mom is a veterinarian. She states he has had issues with constipation for the last 3 to 4 months. The symptoms resolve intermittently with dietary changes. The patient continues to complain about mild persistent abdominal pain; he is otherwise healthy. Upon physical examination, the pediatrician discovers a firm abdominal mass on the right flank; it does not seem cross the midline, and it is not painful.

The mother reports feeling the mass while bathing the patient but thinking it was stool which correlated with the diagnosis of functional constipation.

The pediatrician decides to order a computed tomography (CT) of the abdomen and pelvis with and without contrast.

CT scan reveals a large unilateral renal mass. The patient is referred to the surgical oncologist for further evaluation. They request sedated magnetic resonance imaging (MRI).

WHAT PREOPERATIVE LABORATORY STUDIES WOULD YOU REQUEST AT THIS POINT? HOW OFTEN IS RENAL DYSFUNCTION PRESENT AT THE TIME OF DIAGNOSIS?

Complete blood count, liver function tests, coagulation studies and basic metabolic panel are normal, except for slightly elevated blood urea nitrogen.

THE PATIENT'S BLOOD PRESSURE (BP) IS ELEVATED, ABOVE 95% FOR AGE AND HEIGHT. WHAT IS THE PATHOPHYSIOLOGY BEHIND THIS FINDING? SHOULD THE CASE BE POSTPONED UNTIL BP IS WITHIN NORMAL RANGE?

During the preanesthesia evaluation, BP is retaken in 4 extremities, and it is consistently high. The preoperative echocardiogram reveals mild left ventricular hypertrophy with normal function. After premedicating with oral versed, BP is at 75th percentile and his mother is adamant the case should proceed as planned since staging is a crucial part of prognosis.

She requests to avoid general anesthesia and provide monitored anesthesia care instead for the case. After explaining the high risk of aspiration due to abdominal distention, she calls patient services and proceeds to describe in detail how

she felt her suggestions were dismissed by the medical team. A multispecialty emergency meeting is scheduled to explain in more detail the extent of the disease and the surgical plan, and to provide reassurance to the family. Mom cries inconsolably and asks for some time with her son before he is taken to MRI. While the mother is in the waiting room, a member of the medical team provides support; she discloses being emotionally overwhelmed by the diagnosis.

IS IT FEASIBLE TO ADDRESS PARENTAL ANXIETY IN THE IMMEDIATE PERIOPERATIVE ENVIRONMENT? SHOULD WE ALWAYS INCLUDE "DEATH" AS PART OF THE POSSIBLE COMPLICATIONS?

In general terms, the practice of anesthesia has evolved and is very safe. However, patients still face high levels of anxiety when facing the anesthesiologist for the first time, usually, moments before a surgical procedure.

CAN YOU DEFINE "EMPATHY" (EMOTIONAL, AFFECTIVE AND COGNITIVE COMPONENTS)?

Shortly after a rapid sequence induction the patient's BP drops about 40% from baseline. After a 20 mL/kg bolus, mean arterial pressure increases 5%. Pulse pressure variation indicates the patient is still fluid responsive; an additional bolus is given. Mean and systolic blood pressures increase by 20%. No other interventions are needed. Volume contraction due to preoperative hypertension could explain this intraoperative finding.

MRI shows the tumor extends into the inferior vena cava (Figs. 41.1 and 41.2). The plan is to proceed with transperitoneal radical nephrectomy with ipsilateral lymph node sampling. The plan is explained in detail to family members. They are willing to proceed but refuse an epidural; the mom had a low pressure headache after labor epidural, required 2 blood patches, and experienced low back pain for months after delivery.

WHAT OTHER ALTERNATIVES FOR INTRA- AND POSTOPERATIVE PAIN MANAGEMENT DO YOU RECOMMEND?

The acute pain team is consulted. They explain multiple ultrasound guided regional anesthesia techniques including

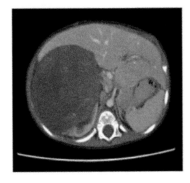

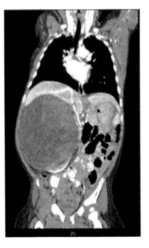

Fig. 41.1 Extensive Wilms tumor (Pictures courtesy of Dr Jennifer Aldrink, Surgery Department at Nationwide Childrens Hospital)

paravertebral blocks, transverse abdominis plane (TAP) blocks, and quadratus lumborum (QL) block. The family opts for the QL block. A patient controlled analgesia option is also discussed with the family.

ARE INVASIVE LINES NECESSARY FOR PERIOPERATIVE MANAGEMENT? IS THE LOCATION OF VASCULAR ACCESS IMPORTANT?

After premedication with intravenous (IV) versed, a rapid sequence induction with propofol, lidocaine, fentanyl, and rocuronium is well tolerated with stable vital signs. Two large bore IV lines are placed in the upper extremities; an arterial radial catheter is requested by the intensive care unit for frequent blood draws.

The patient has mild tachycardia during most of the procedure despite adequate opioid and fluid administration with low pulse pressure variation. An arterial blood gas (ABG) test shows normal electrolytes but partial pressure of oxygen (PO_2) is low relative to normal minute ventilation. The surgeon reports no ongoing blood loss. Right after renal vessels manipulation, $ETCO_2$ drops to 5 mmHg, and the patient becomes profoundly hypotensive. After ruling out acute hemorrhagic shock, arrhythmia, and monitor malfunction, the working diagnosis is pulmonary embolism. Epinephrine, atropine, and IV fluids are administered with rapid resolution of hypotension but $ETCO_2$ and saturation continues below normal levels. ABG confirms arterial hypoxemia and hypocapnia (pH:7.3, PCO_2 24mmHg, PO_2 75% on 100% fraction of inspired oxygen [FiO_2]). Intraoperative transesophageal echocardiography demonstrates mild right ventricular hypokinesis without right ventricular dilatation.

WHEN PULMONARY EMBOLISM IS SUSPECTED IN A PATIENT UNDER GENERAL ANESTHESIA, WHICH IS THE MOST SENSITIVE ABNORMALITY YOU WILL FIND IN AN ABG?

Surgery is completed without further complications and an ipsilateral QL catheter is placed for pain control.

The patient is transferred to the pediatric intensive care unit intubated and paralyzed. A spiral CT scan confirms segmental pulmonary embolism.

Eight hours after the surgery the patient is successfully extubated but continues to require supplemental oxygen via nasal cannula.

The family reports excellent pain for the first 18 hours. Intermittent morphine was added for breakthrough pain in addition to alternating IV acetaminophen and Toradol. The QT catheter is removed on the third postoperative day.

Pathology report shows favorable histology; the following day he is transferred to the oncology unit for chemotherapy.

DISCUSSION

Wilms tumor (WT), named after the German surgeon and pathologist Max Wilms,[1,2] has been widely studied since the early 1900s, leading to significant advancements in diagnosis, treatment, and impressive reduction in mortality. In general terms, survival rate in modern medicine is >90%, compared to 5% in the 1900, and 20% before the introduction of chemotherapy.[3]

Current multicenter collaborations focus on the continued reduction of mortality, toxicity from chemotherapy, and preservation of renal function.[4]

EPIDEMIOLOGY

WT is the most common primary malignant renal tumor and the second most frequent abdominal tumor in school-aged children. About 95% of all renal tumors in children younger than 15 years are WT.[5] The incidence in the United States is 8.1 per million children and is slightly higher in females. Median age at diagnosis is 3.5 years, with more than 80% of the total cases presenting in children <5 years of age. Males and bilateral tumors tend to be diagnosed at an earlier age.

ETIOLOGY

Most of the tumors arise from mutations of the tumor tissue, not from germline mutations.

WT1, the first gene mutation, was identified in 1990. WT is a tumor suppression gene, and the loss of both alleles leads to WT, but only one-fifth of patients have the mutation. These patients usually have a rapid progression of the disease. Congenital anomalies and syndromes are present in 10% of patients with WT. Anirida is caused by an abnormal *PAX6* gene, located adjacent to *WT1*. Up to 70% of patients with aniridia plus deletions of *WT1* will develop

WT. Denys–Drash syndrome (DDS; male pseudohermaphroditism, renal mesangial sclerosis, and WT) results from point mutation in *WT1*. Deletion of one WT allele results in WAGR syndrome (Wilms tumor, aniridia, genitourinary anomalies, and intellectual disability).

WTX, another tumor suppressor gene, has been associated with 30% of the cases.

Alterations at the chromosome 11p15 locus (*WT2*), known to host genes related with overgrowth syndromes such as Beckwith-Wiedemann, hemihypertrophy, Perlman and Soto syndromes, has been associated with a high risk of developing WT.

Other mutations have been linked to WT as well as environmental factors such as parental exposures, but nothing is conclusive to date.[4] Refer to Table 41.1 for syndromes associated.

PREOPERATIVE EVALUATION

Patients at high risk are screened with serial ultrasounds every 3 months despite the failure to demonstrate that early detection improves survival. There is wide variation of histologic patterns, but classic WT have favorable histology. The presence of anaplasia is associated with poor response to chemotherapy and grim prognosis.

WT are usually an incidental finding and is usually a large mass discovered by a family member or physician. Up to 20% of patients can have hematuria and hypertension at the time of diagnosis. Some cases can present with fever, failure to thrive, anorexia, and abdominal pain.

A preoperative laboratory evaluation should include a basic metabolic panel, calcium, complete blood count, liver profile, urinalysis, and coagulation studies. Most patients have normal renal function, and approximately 8% have von Willebrand disease (VWD). Children exposed to preoperative chemotherapy should have a cardiac evaluation prior to surgery.[11]

Outcomes depend on histopathology and tumor staging.

IMAGING

All patients need either a CT scan or MRI of the abdomen and pelvis with contrast to determine the extension of the tumor and possible involvement of vascular structures. A CT of the chest evaluates pulmonary metastasis, the most common site of metastasis.[6]

TREATMENT

A multimodal approach includes radical nephrectomy, chemotherapy, and possible radiotherapy.

Two large multicenter collaborations have different approaches to treatment, specifically timing of surgery. The Children's Oncology Group (COG) recommends pathologic staging after immediate nephrectomy. The European collaborative group International Society of Paediatric Oncology advocates for preoperative chemotherapy. Survival rates in both groups are similar.[8]

Preoperative chemotherapy is desired in some cases to reduce the size of the tumor or the presence of bilateral WT. The COG recommends 6 weeks of chemotherapy prior to radical nephrectomy. The main goal for these patients is tumor shrinkage and renal sparing surgery.[9] A smaller tumor also facilitates a laparoscopic approach.[7]

Relapse occurs in 15% of children with WT, long-term survival decreases to <30% after recurrence.[10] The most common relapse sites are the lungs followed by surgical field, abdomen, and liver.

Extension into the inferior vena cava occurs in 4% to 8% of the cases and half of the time is asymptomatic.

ANESTHETICS CONSIDERATIONS

The main preoperative concerns are delayed gastric emptying secondary to abdominal distension and possible hemorrhagic shock.

Significant abdominal distention would dictate the need for rapid sequence induction. Following induction of anesthesia, anticipating cross-clamping of the vena cava is reasonable; therefore, two large-bore IV lines should be placed preferably on the upper extremities or above the diaphragm. Arterial catheters are reserved for patients with large tumors or comorbidities at the discretion of the anesthesiologist.

One-fourth (25%) of the children presenting with WT have various degrees of hypertension at the time of diagnosis. Hypertension should be medically controlled before surgery.

Table 41.1 **SUMMARY OF SYNDROMES WITH ASSOCIATION TO WILMS TUMORS**

SYNDROME	GENETIC ABNORMALITY	ASSOCIATED ANOMALIES
WAGR syndrome	11p13 (*WT1*) deletion	Aniridia, Genitourinary anomalies, mental Retardation
Denys-Drash syndrome	*WT1* mutation	Nephropathy, intersex disorders
Beckwith-Wiedemann syndrome	11p15 (*WT2*) abnormalities	Macrosomia, macroglossia, visceromegaly, embryonal tumors, omphalocele, hypoglycaemia
Sporadic hemihypertrophy	Unknown	Enlargement of one side of the body or part of the body
Simpson-Golabi-Behmel syndrome	X-linked recessive	General overgrowth in height and weight with characteristic facial features

In most cases, hypertension is the result of increased renin levels, and most cases resolve after nephrectomy. Elevated levels of renin are not the only factors contributing to hypertension. Mean arterial pressure (MAP) is the product of cardiac output (CO) and systemic vascular resistance (SVR) (MAP = CO × SVR). If central venous pressure is significantly elevated, subtract it from MAP for accuracy. Factors increasing either CO or SVR should result in hypertension (HTN) unless a compensatory mechanism decreases proportionally.

The endothelium, proinflammatory mediators such as interleukin 1 beta and tumor necrosis factor, vasoconstrictor mediators, and the coagulation system (promoting platelet aggregation and a prothrombotic surface) have also been implicated in the pathogenesis of HTN.

Four to 10% of patients present with VWD, a coagulation defect presenting with mucosal bleeding, prolonged bleeding time, and decreased level of functional von Willebrand factor. Intranasal DDAVP in the preoperative period is one strategy to prevent intraoperative bleeding. WT-acquired VWD is usually infrequent, benign, and clinically insignificant. A complete bleeding history should be obtained to determine the severity of the disease. Not always, acquired VWD is benign. Baxter et al. presented a couple of cases that required intensive treatment, including plasmapheresis.[12]

The best strategy for pain control is multimodal. Regional techniques include thoracic epidural, paravertebral blocks, TAP block, or the most recent approach quadratus abdominis, described by Blanco in 2007.

REVIEW QUESTIONS

1. The risk of Wilms tumor is **LEAST** in which of the following syndromes?

    A. WAGR
    B. Denys-Drash
    C. Beckwith-Wiedemann
    D. Angelman

Answer: D

WT1, the first gene mutation, was identified in 1990. WT is a tumor suppression gene and the loss of both alleles leads to WT, but only one-fifth of patients have the mutation. These patients usually have a rapid progression of the disease. Congenital anomalies and syndromes are present in 10% of patients with WT. Aniridia is caused by an abnormal *PAX6* gene, located adjacent to *WT1*. Up to 70% of patients with aniridia plus deletions of *WT1* will develop WT. DDS (male pseudohermaphroditism, renal mesangial sclerosis and Wilms tumor) results from point mutation in WT1. Deletion of one WT allele results in WAGR syndrome (Wilms tumor, aniridia, genitourinary anomalies, and intellectual disability).

WTX, another tumor suppressor gene, has been associated with 30% of the cases.

Alterations at the chromosome 11p15 locus (*WT2*), known to host genes related with overgrowth syndromes such as Beckwith-Wiedemann, hemihypertrophy, and Perlman and Soto syndromes, has been associated with high risk of developing WT.

Other mutations have been linked to WT as well as environmental factors such as parental exposures, but nothing is conclusive to date.[4]

2. During a routine primary care visit, a 3-year-old girl is hypertensive and has a palpable abdominal mass. Which of the following laboratory studies are **MOST** diagnostic for WT?

    A. alpha-fetoprotein
    B. homovanillic acids
    C. lactic dehydrogenase
    D. none exist

Answer: D

Preoperative laboratory evaluation should include a basic metabolic panel, calcium, complete blood count, liver profile, urinalysis, and coagulation studies. Most patients have normal renal function, and approximately 8% have VWD. Children exposed to preoperative chemotherapy should have a cardiac evaluation prior to surgery.[11]

3. When placing an epidural for postoperative management of WT resection, what level would be **MOST** likely to providing optimal analgesia?

    A. L 2–3
    B. L 4–5
    C. T 5–6
    D. T 10–11

Answer: D

Ideally a low thoracic or high lumbar epidural will cover the area for adequate postoperative pain coverage. Caution should be taken regarding coagulation status prior to epidural placement or removal.

4. Which of the chemotherapy agents for the treatment of WT is **MORE** likely to cause heart failure?

    A. Cyclophosphamide
    B. Dactinomycin
    C. Doxorubicin
    D. Vincristine

Answer: C

Doxorubicin has been shown to be a cardiotoxic chemotherapeutic agent. If the patient has been known to have received chemotherapy with doxorubicin, cardiac function should be assessed.

QUESTIONS AND ANSWERS

This chapter has accompanying questions and answers which are available to subscribers as part of the Oxford eLearning platform. To access the questions, go to ✔ http://oxfordmedicine. com/pediatricanesthesiaPBL

REFERENCES

1. Zantinga AR, Coppes MJ. Max Wilms [1867–1918]: the man behind the eponym. *Med Pediatr Oncol.* 1992;20: 515–518.

2. Raffensperger J. Max Wilms and his tumor. *J Pediatr Surg.* 2015;50(2):356–359.

3. Ehrlich PF, Ritchey ML, Hamilton TE, et al. Quality assessment for Wilms' tumor: a report from the National Wilms' Tumor Study-5. *J Pediatr Surg.* 2005;40:208–212.

4. Grimsby G, Ritchey ML. Pediatric Urology Oncology: Renal and Adrenal. Section G, Ch 155;3567–3579.

5. Ali AN, Diaz R, Shu H-K, Paulino AC, Esiashvili N. A Surveillance, Epidemiology and End Results (SEER) program comparison of adult and pediatric Wilms' tumor. *Cancer.* 2012;118:2541–2551. doi:10.1002/cncr.26554

6. Meisel JA, Guthrie KA, Breslow N, et al. Significance and management of computed tomography detected pulmonary nodules: a report from the national Wilms Tumor Study Group. *Int J Rad Oncol.* 1999;44:579–585.

7. Duarte RJ, Denes FT, Cristofani LM, et al. Laparoscopic nephrectomy for Wilms' tumor. *Expert Rev Anticancer Ther.* 2009;9:753–761.

8. Kembhavi SA, Qureshi S, Vora T, et al. Understanding the principles in management of Wilms tumour: can imaging assist in patient selection? *Clin Radiol.* 2013;68:646–653.

9. Blute MI, Kelalis PP, Offord KP, et al. Bilateral Wilms' tumor. *J Urology.* 1987;138:968–973.

10. Grundy P, Breslow N, Green DM, Sharples K, Evans A, D'Angio GJ. Prognostic factors for children with recurrent Wilms tumor: results from the Second and Third National Wilms Tumor Study Group. *Pediatr Blood Cancer.* 2008;50;162–167.

11. Davis P, Cladis FP. Elsevier Mosby. Smith's Anesthesia for Infants and Children. 9th ed. Anesthesia for General Abdominal and Urologic Surgery. 2017;30:802–803

12. Baxter PA, Nuchtern JG, Guillerman RP, et al. Acquired von Willebrand syndrome and Wilms tumor: not always benign. *Pediatr Blood Cancer.* 2009;52(3):392–394.

42.

NEURONAL CEROID LIPOFUSCINOSES (BATTEN DISEASE)

Joshua C. Uffman

STEM CASE AND KEY QUESTIONS

A 5-year-old male with Batten disease with increasingly difficulty swallowing, feeding, and weight gain over last several months is scheduled for open gastrostomy tube insertion. Upon presentation to the preoperative holding area, he is found to have no allergies to medications, weight of 14.9 kg, and age-appropriate vitals (Temperature: 37.3°C, heart rate: 108, blood pressure: 95/53, respiratory rate: 28, blood oxygen saturation: 98% room air). His home medications include Levetiracetam, Famotidine, and Lorazepam (as needed), and he is reported to have a past medical history significant for Batten disease, developmental delay, progressing motor function loss (currently patient is able to sit only and roll side to side) seizures, chronic cough, and weight loss. He has had several prior anesthetics, including multiple magnetic resonance imaging (MRI) studies and vagal nerve stimulator implantation. His mother reports that he is slow to emerge after general anesthesia, and a review of the records for his prior anesthetics show no other significant issues. He has been managed via inhalational induction in the past with his airway successfully secured using both laryngeal mask airways and endotracheal tubes during prior anesthetics. Focused physical examination revealed: HEENT: Mallampati II, thyromental distance >3 finger breaths, limited oral exam secondary to patient cooperation but appears to have full range of motion. No loose teeth are reported or noted. Cardiac: regular rate and rhythm. Pulmonary: clear and unlabored. Neurological: global developmental delay, global hypotonia, but able to hold up head and uses wheelchair with head device for support.

WHAT IS BATTEN DISEASE AND HOW IS IT CATEGORIZED?

Neuronal ceroid lipofuscinoses (NCL) are a form of lysosomal storage disease and are the most common childhood neurodegenerative disorders characterized by accumulation of autoflourescent waxy lipopigments in the brain and other tissues. This group of disorders, resulting from the intracellular accumulation of lipopigment (ceroid lipofuscin) material, is autosomal recessive and leads to neuronal death.

There are 14 known phenotypes with 13 assigned genotypes[1] associated with NCL which are collectively referred to as Batten disease. Historically, patients were classified according to the age of symptom onset, which resulted in four variants of the disease: (i) infantile or Santavuori-Haltia, (ii) late infantile or Jansky-Bielschowsky, (iii) juvenile or Spielmeyer-Vogt, and (iv) adult or Kufs.[2] However, with improvements in genetic mutational analysis, diagnosis can be seen with childhood or adult onset phenotypes regardless of age of diagnosis and classification focuses on the genetic mutation.

WHAT ARE THE COMMON CLINICAL SYMPTOMS OF PATIENTS WITH BATTEN DISEASE?

Presenting symptoms of patients with Batten disease varies somewhat by the subtype, but the most common symptoms are language delay, seizures, blindness, and ataxia. As the disease progresses, patients will have loss of developmental milestones, loss of motor function often with muscle weakness, dementia, and premature death while neuroimaging will show cerebral and cerebellar atrophy.[3]

WHAT ARE THE ANESTHETIC IMPLICATIONS OF BATTEN DISEASE?

While it is easy to think of all children with Batten disease as one group since they share a similar phenotype, it is important to know which form of the disease they have along with elucidating specific symptoms and to what degree they are experiencing them from a thorough history and physical exam.

While difficult airway management has been reported,[4] absent typical predictors suggesting difficulty, providers have not routinely reported that patients with Batten disease are difficult to mask ventilate, nor present difficulty with supraglottic airway placement or endotracheal intubation. Ensuring adequate conditions for airway placement has successfully been reported with a myriad of techniques including intravenous administration of barbiturates (thiamylal),[5] propofol,[2] or etomidate[6] alone or in association with inhalational agents.[4,5,7] While there is reported concern for hyperkalemia after use of a depolarizing muscle relaxant such as succinylcholine,[5] because of the underlying neuromuscular disease, there are reports of use without clinical sequelae in the literature.[6,7] The response to non-depolarizing neuromuscular blocking agents may be unpredictable in the face of the neuromuscular disease;[8,9] however, they too have been used without apparent adverse events.[6,10,11]

While all Batten patients are at risk for autonomic dysfunction and perioperative hypothermia, children with neuronal ceroid lipofuscinosis (CLN1; infantile neuronal ceroid lipofuscinosis [INCL]) appear to experience perioperative hypothermia and bradycardia[12] to a greater degree than other forms of NCL. Regardless of disease subtype, special attention to maintenance of normothermia and preparation for treatment of autonomic dysfunction should be standard practice in the perioperative period.

While anesthesia-induced bradycardia may represent the most common cardiac anomaly seen while caring for patients with CLNs, other cardiac anomalies which may affect a safe anesthetic have been reported. Hofman et al.[13] reported that lipopigment accumulation in the cardiac musculature can result in cardiac conduction anomalies (including intraventricular conduction delays, supraventricular tachyarrhythmias, atrial and ventricular ectopic beats, and repolarization disturbances) fibrotic and degenerative changes, and ventricular hypertrophy.

Special attention should be paid to the patient's seizure status, including ensuring the child continues his or her anti-seizure medications on the normal schedule to reduce the likelihood of perioperative seizure activity. Careful evaluation of the degree of motor dysfunction including issues with gastroesophageal reflux and pulmonary aspiration are important in deciding the safest manner for airway support.

Patients on antiepileptic medications are known to have a reduced anesthetic requirement.[9,14] In addition to the reduction in intraoperative anesthesia requirements, delayed emergence in patients with NCLs has also been reported.[6] Tailoring an anesthetic plan to minimize the risk of delayed emergence, such as using short-acting inhalational agents, short-acting narcotics, non-narcotic analgesia, and regional anesthesia techniques, should be considered.

DURING YOUR PREANESTHETIC EVALUATION, THE MOTHER REPORTS THAT THE CHILD'S EMERGENCE FROM ANESTHESIA HAS BEEN DELAYED WHEN HE HAS RECEIVED PROPOFOL FOR PAST ANESTHETICS. SHE COMMUNICATES HER CONCERNS THAT ITS METABOLISM MAY WORSEN HIS DISEASE PROGRESSION AND ASKS THAT YOU NOT USE IT. IS THERE EVIDENCE TO SUPPORT THIS?

Propofol is a commonly used medication to provide sedation and general anesthesia for children and adults. Propofol infusion syndrome (PIS) is a rare but well-known potential adverse event, characterized by metabolic acidosis, rhabdomyolysis, renal failure, and death.[15] Prolonged administration of relatively high doses (>5 mg/kg/h for 48 hours) is thought to be a risk factor;[16,17] however, PIS has been reported after shorter exposures. While the mechanism has not been fully elucidated, it is thought to be the result of propofol's direct or metabolic byproduct disrupting normal mitochondrial activity.[18] While the use of propofol is typically minimized or avoided in patients with known mitochondrial deficiencies, there are numerous reports of minimal or no clinical effects of its use in patients with known mitochondrial disease,[19] leaving many questions unanswered.

NCLs are lysosomal storage defects and result in accumulation of autofluorescent lipopigment deposits in neuronal and extraneural tissue and are not thought to affect the mitochondria or electron transport chain. Use of propofol in Batten patients without significant adverse events has been well documented.[2,7,12] While children with Batten disease may be prone to delayed emergence, given the lack of mitochondrial effects of the disease and the relatively large number of successful patients treated with propofol, routine elimination of its use in the population does not appear warranted.

IS THERE A BENEFIT TO USING A REGIONAL ANESTHETIC FOR THIS PATIENT? IF SO, WHAT ARE THE BEST OPTIONS?

Given the degree of hypotonia and location of the proposed incision (left mid to upper quadrant), the child may be at higher risk for postoperative pulmonary complications. An anesthetic plan that includes a regional anesthetic to minimize the need for intra- and postoperative narcotics and minimizes postoperative pulmonary compromise from pain would be beneficial.

While there are several options, including epidural, transversus abdominis plane (TAP) and paravertebral block, the TAP block will likely meet the goals of minimizing narcotic requirements and maximizing postoperative pulmonary function with the lowest risks.

A TAP block is intended to provide analgesia for procedures on the abdominal wall and has been successfully used for patients undergoing appendectomy, cholecystectomy cesarean section, and other laparoscopic procedures.[20] The TAP block was originally described as an injection of local anesthetic between the internal oblique and transversus abdominis muscles via an injection in the lower abdomen at the triangle of Petit: located in the region bounded inferiorly by the iliac crest, posteriorly by the latissimus dorsi and anteriorly by the external oblique. Advances in the use of ultrasound guidance, however, have extended the use of the TAP block along the entire abdomen, including the subcostal region with local anesthesia reaching as far cephalad as T7 (Figs. 42.1 and 42.2).[21–23]

YOU PLAN FOR AN INHALATION INDUCTION, INSERTION OF PERIPHERAL INTRAVENOUS CATHETER, ENDOTRACHEAL INTUBATION WITHOUT MUSCLE RELAXATION, AND TAP BLOCK FOR INTRA- AND POSTOPERATIVE PAIN RELIEF. WHAT IS THE MAJOR LIMITATION OF USING A TAP BLOCK FOR THIS CASE?

Sensory innervation to the anterior abdominal wall comes from the anterior divisions of the T7-L1 nerves which innervate the skin and three muscle layers (external and internal obliques and transversus abdominis) and their fascial

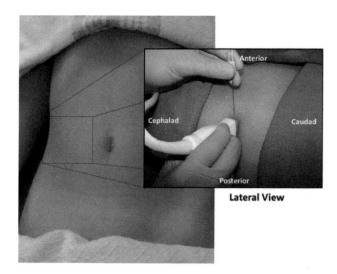

Fig. 42.1 Patient and probe positioning for ultrasound guided TAP block. (Photos courtesy of Tarun Bhalla, MD, MBA. Nationwide Children's Hospital, Columbus, OH).

sheaths.[24] Local anesthetic blockade of these segmental nerve fibers as they traverse the transversus abdominis muscle results in anesthesia of the parietal peritoneum, muscles, and skin.[20] Successful TAP blocks do not, however, provide anesthesia to deeper structures and will not likely provide comparable muscle relaxation to neuromuscular blockade with a paralytic agent.

While complications of TAP blocks are rarely reported to occur in children,[25] especially when done under ultrasound guidance, it is important to remember that peritoneal structures, including bowel, spleen, and liver, are a short distance from the intended target of the needle tip. Farooq[26] reported an unintentional puncture of the liver using a blind technique in an adult, and Long et al.[25] reported one peritoneal puncture and one vascular aspiration (out of 1,994 reported pediatric TAP blocks) from the Pediatric Regional Anesthesia Network database.

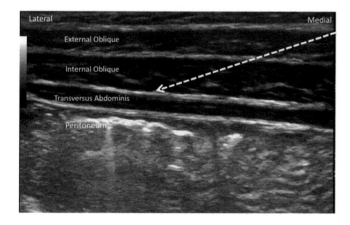

Fig. 42.2 Ultrasound images of TAP block. Dotted line represents needle trajectory with tip of arrow the intended location for local anesthetic. (Photo courtesy of Tarun Bhalla, MD, MBA. Nationwide Children's Hospital, Columbus, OH).

THIRTY MINUTES INTO THE PROCEDURE YOU NOTICE THE CHILD'S TEMPERATURE HAS INCREASED TO 38.2°C. ARE PATIENTS WITH BATTEN DISEASE AT INCREASED RISK FOR MALIGNANT HYPERTHERMIA? ARE THEY PRONE TO TEMPERATURE ABNORMALITIES? IF SO, WHAT IS THE MOST COMMON ISSUE WITH TEMPERATURE REGULATION?

Attention to maintenance of normothermia is an important part of an anesthetic plans. While hypothermia is most commonly seen during routine care of NCL patients due to environmental and physiological changes occurring during routine anesthesia care, hyperthermia can also be seen. When intraoperative hyperthermia occurs, malignant hyperthermia (MH) is often at the top of the differential because of the life-threatening nature of the disease even though it is extremely rare. MH is thought to affect 1:15000 children and results from a disorder in calcium homeostasis in the sarcoplasmic reticulum of skeletal muscle resulting in abnormal relaxation after a muscle contracture.[9] Over the years, there have been several neuromuscular diseases which have been linked to MH, only to be found not to have a direct association. Duchenne's muscular dystrophy and mitochondrial myopathies are two examples of diseases once thought to be linked to MH, only later to be disproven. Currently only central core disease (CCD) and King-Denborough syndrome have been positively linked to MH.[9,27] Patients with NCL are prone to autonomic dysfunction and have been shown to be at higher risk for hypothermia, which may be difficult to treat.[5,10,12]

WHAT ARE THE POSTOPERATIVE CONCERNS FACING A PATIENT WITH BATTEN DISEASE?

Depending on the degree of neurological deterioration, delay in emerging from anesthesia may be a significant concern,[6] which can be exacerbated by the choice of anesthetic and pain management plan. Consideration for nonopioid pain management techniques and short-acting opioids may be beneficial. Care to avoid postoperative pulmonary dysfunction should also be addressed in patients with significant preoperative pulmonary disease. Careful assessment to ensure adequate reversal of neuromuscular blockade will minimize normal postoperative pulmonary changes seen after general anesthesia. Lastly, for patients with significant preoperative pulmonary dysfunction, planned extubation to noninvasive respiratory support such as continuous positive airway pressure or bilevel positive airway pressure has been advocated.[2]

DISCUSSION

HISTORY AND PATHOGENESIS

NCLs are the most common neurodegenerative diseases of childhood and adolescence first thought to be described in 1826 by Otto Christian Stengel with characterization of variants by the age of symptom onset by Frederick Batten (1903), Jan

Jansky(1908), Max Bielschowsky (1913), Hugh Kufs (1925), and Haltia (1973). The result is four clinical classifications of NCLs: infantile (INCL), late-infantile (LINCL), juvenile (JNCL), and adult (ANCL), which are also referred to as Haltia-Santavuori, Jansky-Bielschowdy, Batten-Spielmeyer-Vogt, and Kufs diseases, respectively. Often, however, the term Batten disease is used to refer to the group as a whole in addition to specifically referring to the juvenile form.[3]

Fourteen gene mutations (CLN1–14) have been implicated in NCLs, each resulting in lysosomal accumulation of autofluorescent pigment in neural and extraneural cells.[3,28] While technically a lysosomal storage disease (LSD), the accumulated material is not specific to the disease subtype as is usually the case in LSDs. The incidence of the disease ranges from 0.6/100,000 to almost 14/100,000 livebirths depending on population and study (1.6–2.4/100,000 in the United States).[3,29,30] CLN3 followed closely by CLN2 and CLN1 are the three most common genetic defects with CLN7, CLN6, and CLN5 being a distant fourth, fifth, and sixth, respectively.[31] Like many other LSDs, NCLs are typically autosomal recessive with variable expression. For example, defects in the CLN1 gene result in INCL and JNCL forms of the disease 53% and 47% of the time, respectively, while defects in CLN6 result in INCL in virtually 100% of cases.[31] Because of this heterogeneity in the age of presentation and advances in diagnostic testing, there is a trend away from categorization based on age of onset toward the affected gene (CLN1–14).

CLINICAL FEATURES AND DIAGNOSTIC CRITERIA

Clinical presentation of patients with an NCL is variable in terms of symptoms and age of onset but tend to include some combination of seizures, blindness, ataxia and cerebellar atrophy, myoclonus, loss of developmental milestones (motor and cognitive) or dementia, and premature death.[3,31,32] The combination of low incidence and relatively nonspecific symptoms can make diagnosing NCL difficult. In addition, diagnosis is often delayed while other more common diagnoses are first entertained unless there is a pre-existing knowledge of the disease in the family.[28] Most patients will have had electroencephalogram, basic blood work, diagnostic imaging such as a MRI, as well as an ophthalmologic examination before a diagnosis is made. MRI typically shows cerebellar and cerebral atrophy as well as changes to both gray and white matter.[28] Attention to the possibility of an NCL is typically entertained when other more common diagnoses are excluded and the patient exhibits more than a single symptom.

Once the diagnosis of NCL is entertained based on clinical symptoms and exclusion of other diseases, attention shifts to diagnostic imaging and electron microscopic changes consistent with NCL. Finally, an NCL gene panel is obtained for confirmation of disease and clarification of the type. Electron microscopic findings consistent with NCL include granular osmiophilic deposits, curvilinear profiles, fingerprint profiles, and rectilinear complex. The gene panel looks for known genetic defects associated with NCLs, and specific protein activity can be assayed for many of the CLN subtypes (Table 42.1).

TREATMENT

Treatment focuses on symptom management in all forms of the disease, and, for a limited number of subtypes, there are ongoing experimental treatments for which a patient may qualify. While a complete review of the current experimental treatments is beyond the scope of this discussion, one area of promise which may affect the anesthesia team focuses on enzyme replacement therapy directed to the central nervous system (CNS), often requiring sedation or general anesthesia to administer.

Patients with the CLN2 form of the disease are deficient in the enzyme tripeptidyl peptidase I (TTP1). Injection of a viral vector containing a portion of a normal CLN2 gene into the cerebrospinal fluid of mice resulted in increased TTP1 enzyme activity in neural structures, reduced brain pathology, and increased survival.[33] Based on this favorable data, clinical trials are ongoing looking at the efficacy of enzyme replacement in humans.[34] Delivery of the vectors to the CNS thus far has included at least a portion delivered directly to the CNS via either an implanted CNS reservoir or via intrathecal injection via lumbar puncture. Disease progression is monitored both clinically and radiologically (MRI most commonly), which often requires sedation or general anesthesia to complete.

If viral directed gene therapy is proven effective for any of the diseases subtypes, the exposure of the anesthesia team to patients with CLN can be expected to increase because of increased therapeutic options requiring anesthesia services as well as increased duration of survival increasing the need for other surgical interventions.

CONCLUSION

NCLs, collectively referred to as Batten disease, are the most common neurodegenerative disorder of childhood and can present unique challenges to the anesthesia team responsible for providing a safe anesthetic. While there are multiple forms of NCL, most share a common set of symptoms that needs to be evaluated including seizures, motor dysfunction, loss of developmental milestones, and cognitive function. Early concerns for NCL patients having anesthesia have generally not held true; however, there are some key points to remember. First, there appears to be an increased risk for hypothermia, decreased anesthetic requirements, and prolonged emergence from anesthesia. Second, some forms of the disease may have higher risks for autonomic dysfunction than others. For instance, patients with CLN1 form of the disease may have increased risk for bradycardia while under anesthesia. Regardless of the genetic defect, based on the current published knowledge of caring for patients with Batten disease, the primary focus should be on recognition of an individual patient's current symptoms and their severity with the goal of providing an anesthetic while minimizing the risks associated with them.

Table 42.1 RELATIONSHIP BETWEEN GENOTYPE, PHENOTYPE, AND EFFECTED PROTEINS

GENOTYPE	PRIMARY CLINICAL PHENOTYPE	SECONDARY CLINICAL PHENOTYPE	EFFECTED PROTEIN
CLN 1	INCL	JNCL	Palmitoyl protein thioesterase 1
CLN 2	LINCL	JNCL	Tripeptidyl peptidase 1
CLN 3	JNCL	INCL	CLN 3
CLN 4	JNCL	NA	Dnaj homolog
CLN 5	LINCL	JNCL	CLN 5
CLN 6	LINCL	NA	CLN 6
CLN 7	INCL	JNCL	Major facilitator superfamily
CLN 8	LINCL	NA	CLN 8
CLN 9	JNCL	NA	Unknown
CLN 10	JNCL	ANCL	Cathepsin D
CLN 11	ANCL	NA	Granulins
CLN 12	JNCL	NA	Probable cation-transporting
CLN 13	ANCL	NA	Cathepsin F
CLN 14	NA	NA	BTB/POZ domain-containing

Note. INCL = infantile neuronal ceroid lipofuscinoses (NCL); LINCL = late-infantile NCL; JNCL = juvenile NCL; ANCL = adult NCL; NA = not applicable or unknown.

Source. Adapted from Nita DA, Mole SE, Minassian BA. Neuronal ceroid lipofuscinoses. *Epileptic Disord.* 2016;18(Suppl 2):S73–S88; Aungaroon G, Hallinan B, Jain P, Horn PS, Spaeth C, Arya R. Correlation among genotype, phenotype and histology in neuronal ceroid lipofuscinoses: an individual patient data meta-analysis. *Pediatr Neurol.* 2016;60:42–48.

REVIEW QUESTIONS

1. Which clinical problem has the **LEAST** association with Batten disease?

   A. language delay
   B. renal dysfunction
   C. seizure disorders
   D. vision loss

Answer: B
Language delay, seizures, blindness, and ataxia are the hallmark presenting symptoms of Batten disease. In addition, generalized weakness, blindness, myoclonus, cardiac arrhythmias, and premature death have been reported.[3,13] Renal dysfunction is not commonly associated with patients with CLNs.

2. Which of the following has the **LOWEST** risk of occurring when anesthetizing a patient with Batten disease?

   A. bradycardia
   B. delayed emergence
   C. hypothermia
   D. malignant hyperthermia

Answer: D
Hypothermia and delayed emergence are commonly seen across all CLN variants while bradycardia is more likely to occur with the CLN1 defect.[6,12] According to the Malignant Hyperthermia Association of the United States, the only two diseases linked to malignant hyperthermia are CCD and King-Denborough syndrome.[9,27]

3. When a TAP block is administered subcostally, what is the **HIGHEST** sensory level expected?

   A. T3
   B. T5
   C. T7
   D. T10

Answer: C
T7 is the cephalad most dermatome reached by a TAP block but is reported to occur in approximately 40% of the cases depending on how cephalad the local anesthetic is injected and the number of injections.[21,22,23] On the other hand, T9 appears to be consistently reached with >90% on injections.[22]

4. Of the following procedures, for which will a TAP block be the **LEAST** affective in providing analgesia?

   A. bilateral inguinal hernia repair
   B. laparoscopic cholecystectomy
   C. percutaneous nephrostomy tube
   D. renal transplantation

Answer: C

Sensory innervation to the anterior abdominal wall comes from the anterior divisions of the T7-L1 nerves which innervate the skin, muscle layers, and their fascial sheaths.[24] A TAP block is intended to provide analgesia for procedures on the abdominal wall and has been successfully used for patients undergoing appendectomy, cholecystectomy, cesarean section, and other laparoscopic procedures.[20] Percutaneous nephrostomy tubes are placed posteriorly and would not be covered by a TAP block.

5. What is the **MOST** accurate nomenclature style when referring to a patient with Batten disease?

    A. age of onset (e.g., INCL)
    B. Batten disease + primary symptom
    C. genetic defect (e.g., CLN1)
    D. name of person who originally described the form of disease (Jansky-Bielschowsky)

Answer: C

Early classifications of patients with these constellation of symptoms were referred to as Batten disease, and variants focused on age of onset of symptoms and the names of those who originally described them. Over time, there was recognition that these were NCLs, a form of LSD. With improvements in genetic mutational analysis, diagnosis can be seen with childhood or adult onset phenotypes regardless of age of diagnosis and classification now focuses on the genetic mutation (CLN1–14). However, this switch has been slow, and the multitude of naming regimens can prove challenging for many practitioners not well versed on the disease.

QUESTIONS AND ANSWERS

This chapter has accompanying questions and answers which are available to subscribers as part of the Oxford eLearning platform. To access the questions, go to ✓ http://oxfordmedicine.com/pediatricanesthesiaPBL

REFERENCES

1. Schulz A, Kohlschütter A, Mink J, Simonati A, Williams R. NCL diseases—clinical perspectives. *Biochim Biophys Acta*. 2013 Nov;1832(11):1801–1806.
2. Kako H, Martin DP, Tobias JD. Perioperative care of a patient with neuronal ceroid lipofuscinoses. *Saudi J Anaesth*. 2013 Jul;7(3):336–340.
3. Nita DA, Mole SE, Minassian BA. Neuronal ceroid lipofuscinoses. *Epileptic Disord*. 2016;18(Suppl 2):S73–S88.
4. Pereira D, Pereira M, Caldas F. Anesthesia management in neuronal ceroid lipofuscinoses. *Paediatr Anaesth*. 2006;16:352–358.
5. Yamada Y, Doi K, Sakura S, Saito Y. Anesthetic management for a patient with Jansky-Bielschowsky disease. *Can J Anaesth*. 2002;40:81–83.
6. Defalque RJ. Anesthesia for a patient with Kufs' disease. *Anesthesiology*. 1990;73:1041–1402.
7. Gopalakrishnan S, Sidduiqui S, Mayhew JF. Anesthesia in a child with Batten disease. *Paediatr Anaesth*. 2004;14:890–891.
8. Azar I. The responses of patients with neuromuscular disorders to the muscle relaxants: a review. *Anesthesiology*. 1984;61:173–187.
9. Lerman J. Perioperative management of the paediatric patient with coexisting neuromuscular disease. *Br J Anaesth*. 2011;107(Suppl 1):i79–i89.
10. Hiramori T, Goto S, Kuroiwa K, et al. Anesthetic management of patients with neuronal ceroid lipofuscinoses. *Masui*. 2011;60:1207–1210.
11. Nationwide Children's Hospital, Department of Anesthesiology. Internal data. Accessed July 25, 2017.
12. Miao N, Levin SW, Baker EH, et al. Children with infantile neuronal ceroid lipofuscinosis have an increased risk of hypothermia and bradycardia during anesthesia. *Anesth Analg*. 2009;109:372–378.
13. Hofman IL, van der Wal AC, Dingemans KP, Becker AE. Cardiac pathology in neuronal ceroid lipofuscinosis—a clinicopathologic correlation in three patients. *Eur J Paediatr Neurol*. 2001;5:213–217.
14. Ouchi K, Sugiyama K. Required propofol dose for anesthesia and time to emerge are affected by the use of antiepileptics: prospective cohort study. *BMC Anesthesiol*. 2015;15:34.
15. Rosenfeld-Yehoshua N, Klin B, Berkovitch M, Abu-Kishk I. Propofol use in Israeli PICUs. *Pediatr Crit Care Med*. 2016;16(17):e117–e120.
16. Cremer OL, Moons KGM, Bouman EAC, et al. Long term propofol infusion and cardiac failure in adult head-injured patients. *Lancet*. 2001;357:117–118.
17. Wolf AR, Potter F. Propofol infusion in children: when does an anesthetic tool become an intensive care liability? *Pediatr Anaesth*. 2004;14:435–438.
18. Kam PCS, Cardone D. Propofol infusion syndrome. *Anaesthesia*. 2007;62(7):690–701.
19. Finsterer J, Frank M. Propofol is mitochondrion-toxic and may unmask a mitochondrial disorder. *J Child Neurol*. 2016;31(13):1489–1494.
20. Bhalla T, Dewhirst E, Jagannathan N, Tobais JD. Ultrasound-guided trunk and core blocks in infants and children. *J Anesth*. 2013;27(1):109–123.
21. Barrington MJ, Ivanusic JJ, Rozen WM, Hebbard P. Spread of injectate after ultrasound-guided subcostal transversus abdominis plane block: a cadaveric study. *Anaesthesia*. 2009 Jul;64(7):745–750.
22. Hernandez MA, Vecchione T, Boretsky K. Dermatomal spread following posterior transversus abdominis plane block in pediatric patients: our initial experience. *Paediatr Anaesth*. 2017;27(3):300–304.
23. McDonnell JG, O'Donnell BD, Farrell T, et al. Transversus abdominis plane block: a cadaveric and radiological evaluation. *Reg Anesth Pain Med*. 2007;32(5):399–404.
24. McDonnell JG, O'Donnel B, Curley G, Heffernan A, Power C, Laffey JG. The analgesic efficacy of transversus abdominis plane block after abdominal surgery: a prospective randomized controlled trial. *Anesth Analg*. 2007;104:193–197.
25. Long JB, Birmingham PK, De Oliveira GS, et al. Transversus abdominis plane block in children: a multicenter safety analysis of 1994 cases from the PRAN (Pediatric Regional Anesthesia Network) database. *Anesth Analg*. 2014;119:395–399.
26. Farooq M, Carey M. A case of liver trauma with a blunt regional anesthesia needle while performing a transversus abdominis plane block. *Reg Anesth Pain Med*. 2008;33:274–275.
27. Associated conditions: how to be prepared. https://www.mhaus.org/healthcare-professionals/be-prepared/associated-conditions/. Accessed August 20, 2017.
28. Fietz M, Moeenaldeen A, Burke D, et al. Diagnosis of neuronal ceroid lipofuscinosis type 2 (CLN2 disease): expert recommendations for early detection and laboratory diagnosis. *Mol Genet Metab*. 2016;119:160–167.
29. Sleat DE, Gedvilaite E, Zhang Yeting, Lobel P, Xing J. Analysis of large-scale whole exome sequencing data to determine the prevalence of genetically distinct forms of neuronal ceroid lipofuscinosis. *Gene*. 2016;593:284–291.
30. Uvebrant P, Hagberg B. Neuronal ceroid lipofuscinoses in Scandinavia: epidemiology and clinical pictures. *Neuropediatrics*. 1997;28:6–8.
31. Aungaroon G, Hallinan B, Jain P, Horn PS, Spaeth C, Arya R. Correlation among genotype, phenotype and histology in neuronal ceroid lipofuscinoses: an individual patient data meta-analysis. *Pediatr Neurol*. 2016;60:42–48.
32. Simonati A, Williams RE, Nardocci N, et al. Phenotype and natural history of variant late infantile ceroid-lipofuscinosis 5. *Dev Med Child Neurol*. 2017;59(8):815–821.
33. Mink JW. Neuronal ceroid lipofuscinoses (Batten's disease). Paper presented at the American Academy of Neurology annual meeting, 2010.
34. Richa, F. Anaesthesia and orphan disease: a child with neuronal ceroid lipofuscinosis. *Eur J Anaesthesiol*. 2015;32:207–220.

43.

PEDIATRIC RENAL TRANSPLANTATION

Kristin Chenault

STEM CASE AND KEY QUESTIONS

A 12-year-old Caucasian male, with end-stage renal disease (ESRD), presents to the operating room for living-related donor (LRD) kidney transplantation from his adult sibling. His past medical history is significant for vesicoureteral reflux and anemia. The patient has never required dialysis.

DOES THE TIMING OF DIALYSIS MAKE A DIFFERENCE ON TIMING OF AN ELECTIVE CASE?

The patient has no known drug allergies. He is adequately fasted for solid foods and clear liquids. The patient's lab values are as follows: hemoglobin 10.4 g/dL, hematocrit 32%, platelet count 156 K/mm^3, Na 143 mmol/L, K 5.2 mmol/L, Cl 103 mmol/L, glucose 84. He is visibly anxious regarding his surgery.

WHAT IS THE ANESTHETIC INDUCTION PLAN FOR THIS PATIENT? HOW WOULD YOUR PLAN DIFFER IF THE PATIENT WAS PRESENTING FOR A CADAVERIC DONOR TRANSPLANT?

Considering that this patient has arrived from home for a scheduled procedure, either an inhalation or intravenous induction is acceptable. Potentially nephrotoxic agents should be avoided.

WHAT ARE COMMON NEPHROTOXIC DRUGS TO AVOID? WHAT DRUGS ARE SAFE IN ESRD PATIENTS?

Preoperative sedation with oral midazolam (0.3–0.5 mg/kg) can be helpful to create a cooperative patient for inhalation induction with sevoflurane (with or without nitrous oxide). If an intravenous (IV) line is in place preoperatively, IV midazolam (0.1 mg/kg) may be administered for anxiolysis and sedation. Propofol (2–4 mg/kg) may be used for IV induction. Ketamine (1–3 mg/kg) can also be used if hypovolemia is a significant concern, such as from recent dialysis.

Tracheal intubation is facilitated by the use of neuromuscular blocking agents. It is advisable to use agents that are not dependent on the kidneys for excretion, such as cisatracurium. Vecuronium and rocuronium may be used, but these agents undergo partial renal excretion and their duration of action may be prolonged. Succinylcholine is usually avoided, except in emergencies, mainly due to the increase in serum potassium after administration.[1,2]

After induction and tracheal intubation, anesthesia is maintained with isoflurane, desflurane, or sevoflurane.

If the patient were presenting for a cadaveric donor transplant, preoperative fasting status becomes a significant consideration. The pediatric patient may not be adequately fasted, thereby eliminating the possibility of an inhalational induction and requiring a rapid sequence induction. In this case, a preinduction IV line is necessary. Rapid sequence induction and intubation may be accomplished with any of the induction agents discussed earlier.

WHAT TYPE OF INTRAOPERATIVE MONITORING IS NEEDED FOR THIS CASE? WHAT ABOUT ARTERIAL LINE ACCESS? CENTRAL VENOUS ACCESS?

Intraoperative monitoring of pediatric patients for renal transplantation starts with standard monitors: electrocardiogram, pulse oximetry, noninvasive blood pressure, end-tidal CO_2 and gas analysis, and temperature. Advanced monitoring with central venous pressure (CVP) or arterial line may help guide hemodynamic management.

Arterial line monitoring can be useful in infants and small children undergoing renal transplant who require cross-clamping of the aorta to facilitate arterial anastomosis. Reperfusion under these circumstances can result in significant hypotension, and the immediate data provided by arterial line monitoring can minimize treatment delays. Of note, the arterial line must be placed in an upper extremity if cross-clamping is anticipated.[1]

Central venous pressure monitoring can also be useful in small children undergoing renal transplantation. A central line provides additional IV access (if peripheral access is difficult) and allows the administration of certain immunosuppressive medications that may only be given centrally, such as thymoglobulin and OKT3. The CVP can also be used to help guide fluid management intraoperatively and ensure adequate hydration prior to reperfusion.[1]

THIS PATIENT IS RECEIVING A KIDNEY FROM A SIBLING. DOES THE AGE OF SIBLING MATTER? DO LIVING RELATED DONOR TRANSPLANTS HAVE A HIGHER RATE OF SUCCESS THAN CADAVERIC DONOR TRANSPLANTS?

Yes, the age of the sibling does matter. In general, most transplant programs do not allow donors under the age of 18 years.[1] The stance of the American Academy of Pediatrics is that a minor may ethically serve as a living organ donor for a minor sibling but only in specific, limited circumstances.[3,4] The US Live Organ Donor Consensus Group specifies 4 conditions which must be met for a minor to ethically serve as an organ donor: both the potential donor and recipient are highly likely to benefit, the surgical risk for the donor is extremely low, all other opportunities for transplantation have been exhausted (no potential adult living donor is available and timely and/or effective transplantation from a cadaver donor is unlikely), and the minor freely agrees to donate without coercion.[4] The most common scenario where a minor sibling may be used as an organ donor is in the case of identical twins. Transplantation between identical twin siblings eliminates the need for immunosuppression in the recipient sibling.

Living-related renal transplantation is the most effective therapy for children with ESRD.[8] The use of LRD grafts minimizes cold ischemia time of the kidney as well as reducing allelic differences between donor and recipient.[5] LRD grafts have a higher degree of graft survival at one and three years posttransplant.[6] More recently, graft survival rates at one year for children over the age of 1 range from 94% to 96%.

WHAT IS THE PLAN FOR ANESTHETIC MAINTENANCE IN THIS PATIENT? IS SEVOFLURANE CONTRAINDICATED? ARE THERE ANY SPECIFIC MEDICATIONS TO AVOID IN THIS PATIENT?

Anesthetic maintenance is accomplished with isoflurane, sevoflurane, or desflurane. It is important to note that all potent inhalational agents can cause a dose-dependent decrease in renal blood flow and glomerular filtration rate.[2] The main concern with potent inhalation agents and renal function is the association between inorganic fluoride ions and high output renal failure. Serum fluoride levels as low as 20 micromol/l can cause a decrease in urine concentrating ability, and nephrotoxicity is seen at levels of 50 micromol/l and greater.

Studies have not shown an advantage of one inhalational agent over another. Isoflurane has traditionally been the agent of choice due to the minimal amount of fluoride produced from its metabolism.[2] Recently, studies have looked at the safety of sevoflurane and desflurane in patients with renal failure. Teixeira et al. compared sevoflurane and isoflurane for maintenance of anesthesia in adult renal transplants and found no significant differences in the immediate start of diuresis; need for postoperative dialysis; postoperative creatinine levels at 1, 3, or 6 months; or the incidence of rejection.[7] Sevoflurane has been shown to protect against ischemia-reperfusion injury

via an anti-inflammatory effect.[2] Desflurane is also a reasonable choice is this patient population.

Morphine should be avoided in patients with chronic renal failure due to an accumulation of morphine-6-glucuronide.[2,8] High or repeated doses of meperidine can lead to an accumulation of normeperidine, which can produce seizures.[2] Pain control can be safely achieved with fentanyl, sufentanil, or remifentanil.

WHAT IS THE EMERGENCE PLAN FOR THIS PATIENT? CAN HE BE EXTUBATED IN THE OPERATING ROOM AT THE CONCLUSION OF THE CASE? IS SUGAMMADEX A SAFE CHOICE FOR NEUROMUSCULAR REVERSAL IN THIS PATIENT?

At the completion of surgery, the vast majority of patients are able to have neuromuscular blockade reversed and extubate in the operating room. Sugammadex is a modified gamma-cyclodextrin used to reverse the effects of rocuronium and vecuronium. The dose of sugammadex administered is based on the degree of neuromuscular blockade present. Sugammadex and the complex formed when bound to rocuronium or vecuronium are both excreted mainly via the kidneys; it has been demonstrated that the sugammadex-rocuronium complex can be detected up to 7 days after administration in patients with severe renal impairment.[9] Previous studies in adults with severe renal impairment have shown that sugammadex-mediated reversal of neuromuscular blockade was slower when compared to patients with normal renal function.[9] Two case reports describe the use of sugammadex to reverse rocuronium-induced neuromuscular blockade in pediatric patients after renal transplantation.[10] Reversal of neuromuscular blockade was rapidly reversed with sugammadex, and the patients were extubated in the operating room. The authors hypothesize that the pathway for renal clearance of sugammadex is available within 24 hours of reperfusion of the transplanted kidney.[10] At this point, data to support the use of sugammadex in patients undergoing renal transplantation is limited, and further study is needed before its use can be recommended in this patient population.

WHAT IS THE POSTOPERATIVE PAIN MANAGEMENT PLAN FOR THIS PATIENT? IS EPIDURAL ANALGESIA A VIABLE OPTION FOR PAIN CONTROL POSTOPERATIVELY?

Postoperative pain can be managed in a multitude of ways. Patient-controlled analgesia (or caregiver- or nurse-controlled analgesia, depending on the patient's age and presence or absence of developmental delays) with fentanyl, morphine, or hydromorphone is commonly utilized.[1] Acetaminophen is a useful adjunct to opioids. Nonsteroidal anti-inflammatory drugs (NSAIDs) may reduce renal glomerular perfusion pressure via prostaglandin inhibition and are therefore contraindicated. Epidural analgesia has also been used with success in this patient population. Some concerns about the use of epidural analgesia in this population include risk of epidural hematoma/abscess formation and vascular instability resulting in decreased graft perfusion. It has been demonstrated that the use of epidural analgesia in pediatric renal transplantation can result in increased intraoperative hemodynamic stability;[11] no difference in the quality of pain control postoperatively was demonstrated.

YOU GO TO SEE THE PATIENT ON POSTOPERATIVE DAY 1 AND THE PATIENT STATES THAT HE REMEMBERS HEARING THE SURGEON TALK DURING THE SURGERY AND FEELING THINGS IN HIS ABDOMEN BUT WAS UNABLE TO LET ANYONE KNOW HE WAS AWAKE. DID THIS PATIENT EXPERIENCE INTRAOPERATIVE AWARENESS? WHAT IS THE INCIDENCE OF INTRAOPERATIVE AWARENESS IN THE PEDIATRIC POPULATION? WHAT SHOULD YOUR NEXT COURSE OF ACTION BE FOR THIS PATIENT?

It is possible that this patient did experience intraoperative awareness under general anesthesia. The incidence of awareness under general anesthesia is roughly 1 to 2 per 1,000 patients (0.2%) during general surgery.[12] The incidence of recall or awareness in pediatrics is higher, with 2 recent studies reporting an incidence of 0.6% and 0.8%. [13,14] Auditory and tactile sensations are most frequently reported, as opposed to pain, paralysis, or anxiety. It is important to note that children may not spontaneously report recall experiences. Data from children who do experience recall reveals that they are unlikely to suffer any long-term psychological consequences from their experience.[14]

There are several well-defined risk factors in the adult population for intraoperative recall including cesarean delivery, cardiopulmonary bypass, trauma surgery, higher American Society of Anesthesiologists (ASA) physical status, use of neuromuscular blocking agents, and small doses of anesthetic.[14] Possible risk factors for intraoperative recall in pediatric patients are the use of neuromuscular blocking agents, multiple intubation attempts, and endoscopic procedures.[13–15]

The next course of action in assessing this patient should include a structured interview to assess exactly what the patient experienced. A referral for psychological therapy should be offered.

DISCUSSION

There are roughly 700 renal transplants performed in the United States on a yearly basis. Approximately one-third of these transplants are from living-related donors, with the rest being cadaveric donors. Renal transplantation is the treatment of choice in pediatric patients with ESRD. This is because transplantation is associated with improved patient survival, better growth, and lower cost than chronic dialysis.[16]

Chronic kidney disease (CKD) and ESRD carry with it many complications, including growth failure, poor nutrition, renal osteodystrophy, cardiovascular disease, anemia,

and even neurocognitive effects. CKD can lead to significant stunting of height and growth failure; these effects are even more pronounced if renal failure develops early in life. Height discrepancies can begin in the first several months of life. Onset of puberty is often delayed by approximately 2 years and results in a reduced height velocity and duration. Additionally, a rapid decline in renal function often coincides with puberty. Use of growth hormone can allow for catch-up growth and increase final adult height. It is important to note that renal transplant will not fully correct the growth disturbance and catch-up growth posttransplant is limited.[17]

Cardiovascular disease is the leading cause of death in children with CKD. The risk of death is 1,000 times higher in pediatric patients with ESRD when compared to age-matched non-CKD patients. Nearly half of children with CKD have dyslipidemia (44%), 21% demonstrate abnormal glucose metabolism, and 15% are obese (BMI >95th percentile). Hypertension is also prevalent in this population with an incidence of 54%. Nearly half of children with CKD are anemic; anemia has been linked to poor outcomes and neurocognitive ability in CKD patients.[17]

ESRD is less common in children than in adults, with an overall incidence of approximately 14 per million in children ages 0 to 19 years. This is in contrast to the incidence in the adult population, which is approximately 120 per million in adults ages 20 to 24 years. In addition to differing in incidence, the causes of renal failure differ in children versus adults (Table 43.1). Congenital lesions, such as hypoplastic or dysplastic kidneys or obstructive nephropathy, and glomerulonephritis, such as focal segmental glomerulosclerosis, are the most common causes of ESRD in pediatrics, accounting for 60% of cases.[6] In patients less than 5 years of age, nearly 50% have a congenital lesion as the cause of renal failure compared to older children (ages 13–17 years), where various forms of glomerulonephritis are the most frequent causes of renal failure.[6] Approximately 30% of pediatrics patients are dialysis naïve at transplant, a distinct difference compared to the adult population. Of pediatric patients who have received dialysis

Table 43.1 PRIMARY DIAGNOSES IN PEDIATRIC VERSUS ADULT KIDNEY TRANSPLANT RECIPIENTS

Pediatric Diagnose	Adult Diagnoses
Aplastic/hypoplastic/dysplastic kidney	Diabetes mellitus
Obstructive nephropathy	Glomerulonephritis
Focal segmental glomerulosclerosis	Secondary glomerulonephritis/vasculitis
Reflux nephropathy	Interstitial nephritis/pyelonephritis
Chronic glomerulonephritis	Hypertension
Polycystic disease	Cystic/congenital/hereditary disease
Medullary cystic disease	Neoplasms/tumors

prior to transplant, half have undergone peritoneal dialysis and the other half hemodialysis.[1]

The following indications for pediatric renal transplant were published in 1998 by the Pediatric Committee of the American Society of Transplantation: patients with ESRD unresponsive to medical management, patients with developmental delays, patients with growth failure despite maximal nutritional management, patients with progressive renal osteodystrophy despite optimal medical management, and patients with failure to thrive.

Timing of patients who are on dialysis and coming to the operating room is also a concern due to possible postoperative hypotension.[18] This may be of more concern when there is an organ to be transplanted. Deng et al. showed that patients who came to the operating room within 7 hours of their dialysis were more prone to having hypotension. Previous studies also have shown hypotension and arrhythmias are associated postoperatively with dialysis patients.[19–22] After dialysis, patients are relatively hypovolemic with lower oncotic pressures. Preoperatively, this can be mitigated with increased sodium consumption. However, this can lead to thirst and increased fluid intake. Unless an emergency, the best possible course is to avoid elective surgery soon after dialysis.

There are some distinct differences in surgical technique for kidney transplantation depending on the age and size of the donor as well as the recipient. When the donor kidney is from a child less than 5 years of age or weighing less than 21 kg, the kidneys are usually transplanted en block to avoid small vessel anastomoses. En block transplantation is more commonly performed in adult patients. This technique is associated with an increased risk of technical complications, thrombosis, and early graft failure.[23] Transplantation of very small donor kidneys to very small recipients occurs rarely. Regardless, graft survival of very small pediatric donor kidneys is significantly lower when compared to ideal adult donor kidneys.[23]

In children weighing more than 20 kg, a lower flank incision with a retroperitoneal approach is used and the kidney is placed in the pelvis, similar to an adult kidney transplant. The renal artery is sutured to the common iliac or hypogastric artery and the renal vein to the common iliac or external iliac vein. The ureter is then attached to the bladder. When transplanting an adult kidney into a child weighing less than 20 kg, the renal artery is anastomosed directly to the aorta and the renal vein to the inferior vena cava (IVC). A retroperitoneal or peritoneal approach may be used to access the aorta and vena cava. When transplanting an adult-sized kidney into a small child, the aorta and vena cava are cross-clamped to accomplish the anastomoses; therefore, systemic heparinization (50–100 mg/kg) is often utilized.[1] When cross-clamping of the aorta is anticipated, placement of an arterial catheter can be beneficial.

After induction of general anesthesia and tracheal intubation, preparations for reperfusion of the new kidney can begin. Hemoglobin, hematocrit, and electrolytes should be checked. In older children, blood transfusion is usually not needed unless the hemoglobin falls below 8 gm/dL. Sodium bicarbonate may be necessary if the pH is less than 7.25 despite mild hyperventilation or if there is a largely negative base excess. If a CVP monitor is in place, fluids should be administered to maintain a CVP between 12 and 14 mmHg. Mannitol (0.5 g/kg) and furosemide (1 mg/kg) are given to aid diuresis in the new kidney. The systolic blood pressure is maintained around 100 to 120 mmHg; this higher blood pressure helps to prevent hypotension after clamp release and reperfusion. If the patient becomes hypotensive (systolic blood pressure [SBP] < 90 mmHg) after reperfusion, administration of a vasopressor may be necessary if the blood pressure does not respond to fluid therapy.[1] One study has identified dopamine use as an independent risk factor for delayed graft function in deceased donor grafts.

It is still important to avoid nephrotoxic drugs during renal transplantation since new kidneys may not be functional immediately. Table 43.2 shows a list of common drugs to avoid and their reasons. Table 43.3 also summarizes which common drugs are renal independent/dependent.

Table 43.2 MEDICATIONS TO AVOID IN PATIENTS WITH RENAL FAILURE

CLASS	DRUG	AVOID IF	REASON
Analgesic	Pethidine	GFR <60	Convulsions
Antibiotic	Cefepime	GFR <30	Central nervous system toxicity
Pyschotropic	Lithium	GFR <60	Nephro/neurotoxicity
Diabetic	Glibenclamide, gimepiride Metformin	GFR <60	Hypoglycemia Lactic acidosis
Diuretic	Spironolactone, eplerenone	GFR <30	Hyperkalemia
Immune suppressant	Methotrexate	GFR <60	Myelotoxicity
Contrast media	Gadolinium	GFR <30	Nephrogenic systemic fibrosis
LMW-heparin	Enoxaparin	GFR <60	Hemorrhage

Source. Adapted from Hartman B, Czock D, Keller R. Drug therapy in patients with chronic renal failure. Dtsch Arzteb Int. 2010;107(37):649–650

Table 43.3 MEDICATIONS THAT DO AND DO NOT DEPEND ON RENAL FUNCTION

CLASS	DEPENDENT ON RENAL FUNCTION	INDEPENDENT OF RENAL FUNCTION
Analgesic(s)	Morphine, pethidine	Fentanyl
Antibiotic	Ciprofloxacin, levofloxacin	Moxifloxacin
Diabetic	Glibenclamide, glimepride	Gliquidone, gliclacide
	Nateglinide	Pioglitazone
	Sitagliptine	
Antirrthymic drug(s)	Sotalol	Amidarone
Anticonvulsants	Gabapentin, pregabalin, lamotrigine, levetiracetam	Carbamazepine, phenytoin, valproate
Antihypertensives	Atenolol	Carvedilol, metoprolol, propranolol
Cholesterol-lowering drugs	Bezafibrate, fenofibrate	Simvastatin, niacin
Rheumatological drugs	Methotrexate	Colchicine, hydroxychloroquine, leflunomide
Cardiovascular drugs	Digoxin	Digitoxin
Pyschoactive drugs	Lithium	Amitriptyline, citalopram (metabolites?), haloperidol, risperidone
Antiviral drugs	Acyclovir	Brivudine
Cytostatic drugs	Actinomycin D, bleomycin, capecitabine, carboplatin, cisplatin, cyclophosphamide, doxorubicin, epirubicin, etoposide, gemcitabine (dFdU), ifosfamide, irinotecan, melphalan, methotrexate, oxaliplatin, topotecan	Anastrozole, docetaxel, doxorubicin-peg-liposomal, erlotinib, fluorouracil, gefitinib, leuprorelin, megestrol, paclitaxel, tamoxifen, terozol, vincristine, trastuzumab

Source. Adapted from Hartman B, Czock D, Keller R. Drug therapy in patients with chronic renal failure. *Dtsch Arzteb Int.* 2010;107(37):649–650.

Reperfusion of an adult-sized kidney in an infant or very small child is more challenging to manage. The aorta and IVC are cross-clamped for anastomosis of the renal artery and vein. During cross-clamp, the lower extremities are not perfused. With release of the cross-clamps, ischemic by-products from the kidney, as well as those accumulated in the lower extremities, are released to the central circulation, leading to vasodilation and hypotension. The new kidney will also sequester a significant amount of circulating blood volume, up to 300 mL. A large influx of potassium from the preservative solution in the new kidney can lead to arrhythmias. The new kidney is also cold; the release of the cold preservative solution can lead to hypothermia, which can depress cardiac function and affect coagulation and platelet function. Prior to reperfusion when transplanting an adult-sized kidney into an infant or very small child, it is recommended to raise the CVP to 18 mmHg and to raise the SBP to 20% higher than preoperative values in order to minimize hemodynamic changes with cross-clamp release. This can be accomplished with fluids, blood transfusion, decreasing anesthetic gas concentration, and/or vasopressors.[1] Often atropine and calcium chloride are administered just before cross-clamp release. Atropine (20mcg/kg) helps prevent vagally mediated bradycardia resulting from a sudden decrease in systemic vascular resistence from cross-clamp release. Calcium chloride (10 mg/kg) helps to stabilize the myocardium during the sudden influx of potassium from the newly perfused organ. Sodium bicarbonate (1mmol/kg) may be necessary to help neutralize the lactate accumulated during cross-clamping.[1]

At the conclusion of the procedure, most children are extubated in the operating room, recover in the postanesthesia care unit, and then are transferred to the intensive care unit for overnight monitoring. Urine output is carefully monitored and replaced milliliter per milliliter with half-normal saline for 2 days postoperatively. Electrolytes are monitored frequently.[1]

Graft thrombosis is the primary cause of graft loss in the first year after pediatric renal transplantation.[1] Children under the age of 5 have a higher incidence of early graft loss, mainly due to graft thrombosis, primary graft nonfunction, acute rejection, or technical or immunologic factors. While young children have a decrease in early graft survival, adolescents experience overall lower graft survival long term, most secondary to chronic rejection. While medication noncompliance is a significant concern for graft loss in the teenage population, the data does not support this hypothesis. It has also been demonstrated that race is a predictor of graft survival in patients receiving a LRD transplant. Overall, LRD graft survival among African American patients was 11% less than among Caucasians and 14% less than Hispanics at 7 years posttransplant. The reasons for these disparities are not well understood.[5]

REVIEW QUESTIONS

1. Which of the following muscle relaxants exhibits the **GREATEST** prolongation of duration of action in patients with renal failure?

    A. cisatracurium
    B. pancuronium
    C. rocuronium
    D. succinylcholine

Answer: B
Cisatracurium is eliminated via Hoffman elimination and therefore not affected by renal function. Rocuronium undergoes partial renal elimination (10%–25%). The duration of action of succinylcholine is not affected by renal function. The main mode of elimination for pancuronium is the kidney (85%).

2. In an infant undergoing renal transplantation, calcium chloride is often administered prior to removal of cross-clamps and reperfusion of the new organ in order to prevent which **MOST** likely complication?

    A. arrhythmias
    B. coagulopathy
    C. hypotension
    D. seizures

Answer: A
Calcium chloride is often administered prior to reperfusion of the transplanted kidney in infants receiving an adult donor kidney. There can be a large influx of potassium from the organ preservative solution, and the administration of calcium chloride can help to stabilize the myocardium and prevent arrhythmias related to hyperkalemia.

3. Of the following risk factors for intraoperative recall, which is the **LEAST** cited as a cause?

    A. cardiopulmonary bypass
    B. higher ASA physical status
    C. intraoperative narcotics
    D. neuromuscular blockade

Answer: C
All of the following are risk factors for intraoperative recall: cesarean delivery, cardiopulmonary bypass, trauma surgery, higher ASA physical status, use of neuromuscular blocking agents, and small doses of anesthetic. Possible risk factors for intraoperative recall in pediatric patients are the use of neuromuscular blocking agents, multiple intubation attempts, and endoscopic procedures.

4. At which age do children with chronic renal disease **MOST** often experience a significant decrease in renal function?

    A. early adulthood
    B. preschool years
    C. puberty
    D. school age

Answer: C
A rapid decline in renal function is often seen during puberty.

5. Which of the following medications would be **MOST** appropriate for postoperative pain control in a pediatric patient after renal transplantation?

    A. fentanyl
    B. ketorolac
    C. meperidine
    D. morphine

Answer: A
Ketorolac, along with all NSAIDs, are contraindicated after renal transplant due to prostaglandin inhibition resulting in reduced renal glomerular perfusion pressure. In the early postoperative period after renal transplant, medications that undergo renal metabolism or clearing should be avoided until the graft is functioning well. Meperidine is a poor choice in this population because of the accumulation of normeperidine which can lead to seizures. Morphine should be avoided due to an accumulation of morphine-6-glucuronide.

7. Of the following conditions, which is the **LEAST** likely after reperfusion during kidney transplantation?

    A. arrhythmias
    B. hyperkalemia
    C. hyperthermia
    D. hypotension

Answer: C
Hyperkalemia, cardiac arrhythmias (resulting from hyperkalemia), and hypotension can be seen after reperfusion in children undergoing renal transplant. Hypothermia can also occur due to the influx of cold preservative solution and new blood flow through the cold donor organ. Hyperthermia is extremely unlikely.

8. Which of the following inhaled anesthetics is **MOST** associated with Compound A formation?

    A. desflurane
    B. isoflurane
    C. nitrous oxide
    D. sevoflurane

Answer: D
Compound A is formed by the interaction of sevoflurane with carbon dioxide absorbents in the anesthesia machine. The patient inhales compound A. Compound A has been shown to produce transient renal injury in rats. The US Food and Drug Administration recommends the use of sevoflurane with fresh gas flow rates at least 1 L/min for exposures up to 1 hour and at least 2 L/min for exposures greater than 1 hour.

QUESTIONS AND ANSWERS

This chapter has accompanying questions and answers which are available to subscribers as part of the Oxford eLearning platform. To access the questions, go to ✓ http:// oxfordmedicine. com/pediatricanesthesiaPBL

REFERENCES

1. Scott II VL, Wahl KM, Soltys K, Belani KG, Beebe DS, Davis PJ. Anesthesia for organ transplantation. In: Davis PJ, Cladis FP, Motoyama E, eds. *Smith's Anesthesia for Infants and Children.* 8th ed. Philadelphia, PA: Elsevier; 2011:931–938.
2. SarinKapoor H, Kaur R, Kaur H. Anaesthesia for renal transplant surgery. *Acta Anaesthesiol Scand.* 2007;51:1354–1367.
3. Joseph JW, Thistlethwaite JR Jr, Josephson MA, Ross LR. An empirical investigation of physicians' attitudes toward intrasibling kidney donation by minor twins. *Transplantation.* 2008;85:1235–1239.
4. Ross LF, Thistlethwaite JR Jr, Committee on Bioethics. Minors as living solid-organ donors. *Pediatrics.* 2008;122:454–461.
5. Ishitani M, Isaacs R, Norwood V, Nock S, Lovo P. Predictors of graft survival in pediatric living-related kidney transplant recipients. *Transplantation.* 2000;70:288–292.
6. McEnery PT, Stablein DM, Arbus G, Tejani A. Renal transplantation in children. *N Engl J Med.* 1992;326:1727–1732.
7. Teixeira S, Costa G, Costa F, da Silva Viana J, Mota A. Sevoflurane versus isoflurane: does it matter in renal transplantation. *Transplant Proc.* 2007;39:2486–2488.
8. Schmid S, Jungwirth B. Anaesthesia for renal transplant surgery: an update. *Eur J Anaesthesiol.* 2012;29:552–558.
9. Panhuizen IF, Gold SJA, Buerkle C, et al. Efficacy, safety and pharmacokinetics of sugammadex 4mg/kg for reversal of deep neuromuscular blockade in patients with severe renal impairment. *Br J Anaesth.* 2015;114:777–784.
10. Carlos RV, Torres ML, de Boer HD. The use of rocuronium and sugammadex in paediatric renal transplantation: two case reports. *Eur J Anaesthesiol.* 2015;32:1–4.
11. Coupe N, O'Brien M, Gibson P, DeLima J. Anesthesia for pediatric renal transplantation with and without epidural analgesia—a review of 7 years experience. *Paediatr Anaesth.* 2005;15:220–228.
12. Kent CD, Posner KL, Mashour GA, et al. Patient perspectives on intraoperative awareness with explicit recall: report from a North American anaesthesia awareness registry. *Br J Anaesth.* 2015;i114–i121.
13. Blusse van Oud-Alblas HJ, van Dijk M, Liu C, Tibboel D, Klein J, Weber F. Intraoperative awareness during paediatric anaesthesia. *Br J Anaesth.* 2009;102:104–110.
14. Malviya S, Galinkin JL, Bannister CF, et al. The incidence of intraoperative awareness in children: childhood awareness and recall evaluation. *Anesth Analg.* 2009;109:1421–1427.
15. Lopez J, Habre W, Laurencon M, Haller G, Van der Linden M, Iselin-Chaves IA. Intra-operative awareness in children: the value of an interview adapted to their cognitive abilities. *Anaesthesia.* 2007;62:778–789.
16. Furth SK, Pushkal PG, Neu A, Hwang W, Fivush BA, Powe NR. Racial differences in access to the kidney transplant waiting list for children and adolescents with end-stage renal disease. *Pediatrics.* 2000;106:756–761.
17. Kaspar CDW, Bholah R, Bunchman TE. A review of pediatric chronic kidney disease. *Blood Purif.* 2016;41:211–217.
18. Deng J, Lenart J, Applegate RK. General anesthesia soon after dialysis may increase postoperative hypotension: a pilot study. *Heart, Lung, Vesel.* 2014;6(1):52–59.
19. Della Rocca G, Costa MG, Bruno K, et al. Pediatric renal transplantation: anesthesia and perioperative complications. *Pediatr Surg Int.* 2001;17:175–179.
20. Kabutan K, Mishima M, Takehisa S, Morimoto N, Ta-niquchi M. Postoperative pancreatitis after total hip replacement under general anesthesia with sevoflurane in a patient with chronic renal failure on hemodialysis. *Masui.* 2000;49:309–311.
21. Maruyama K, Agata H, Ono K, Hiroki K, Fujihara T. Slow induction with sevoflurane was associated with complete atrioventricular block in a child with hypertension, renal dysfunction, and impaired cardiac conduction. *Paediatr Anesth.* 1998;8:73–78.
22. Figueroa W, Alankar S, Pai N, Dave M. Subxiphoid peri-cardial window for pericardial effusion in end-stage renal disease. *Am J Kidney Dis.* 1996;27:664–667.
23. Ardissino G, Dacco V, Testa S, et al. Epidemiology of chronic renal failure in children: data from the ItalKid Project. *Pediatrics.* 2003;111:e382–e387.

SECTION 8

ENDOCRINE AND METABOLIC SYSTEM

44.

PHEOCHROMOCYTOMA

Ralph J. Beltran

STEM CASE AND KEY QUESTIONS

A 14-year-old male high-school student presents to his pediatrician's office accompanied by his parents for evaluation of intermittent headache, sweating episodes, and associated palpitations. The patient had been seen recently in the local emergency department for moderate to severe headache. He was not experiencing visual changes or nausea at the time.

WHEN SHOULD ONE GET A COMPUTER TOMOGRAPHY (CT) SCAN?

He was advised to take acetaminophen and ibuprofen for pain relief and to follow up with his primary care physician if symptoms recurred. Incidentally, his parents were told he had a remarkably elevated blood pressure (BP) reading during his visit. The patient was not currently on any medications and had had no prior medical or psychological history. His vital signs were as follows: temperature 36.8°C, heart rate 120 bpm, BP 178/88 mmHg, oxygen saturation 98% on room air. On examination the patient appeared restless, noted diaphoretic, and complained of moderate headache but did not appear to be in acute distress. His neurological exam was within normal limits, his lungs were clear and devoid of crackles, he was tachycardic but with a regular rhythm, and his neurological examination was within normal limits.

WHAT DIAGNOSTIC STUDIES ARE APPROPRIATE FOR INITIAL SCREENING?

As this young patient's blood pressure remained consistently elevated during outpatient consultation with this physician, the patient was admitted to the local children's hospital for observation. A 24-hour fractionated urinary metanephrine and catecholamine measurement was ordered as part of a comprehensive workup. Obtained results were abnormal with noted significantly elevated metanephrine levels. Subsequently magnetic resonance imaging (MRI) of the abdomen and pelvis was obtained which demonstrated the presence of a right intraadrenal mass.

HOW IS PHEOCHROMOCYTOMA OR PRESUMED PARAGANGLIOMA INITIALLY TREATED? HOW LONG DO YOU NEED TO WAIT AFTER TREATMENT? WHAT IS THE TARGET BLOOD PRESSURE?

Following confirmation of adrenal tumor presence by biochemical assay and radiological imaging, the patient was initiated on phenoxybenzamine with a starting dose of 0.25 mg/kg per day. This dose was adjusted based on continuous monitoring of symptoms and blood pressure. After several days of steady BP and headache pain improvement, a beta-blocker was added to his regimen. An inpatient surgical consultation was also requested, and the patient was deemed a candidate for surgical tumor excision. The patient was subsequently discharged to home with close follow-up with his pediatrician for continued BP management.

WHAT IS THE TIMING OF SURGERY?

Two weeks after diagnosis, the patient underwent laparoscopic surgical adrenalectomy, and the specimen was sent for pathological analysis. During resection and tumor isolation, significant swings in BP were noted. These acute changes were adequately controlled with vasodilating therapy during episodes of moderate to severe hypertension. Following tumor excision, moderate hypotension was noted, and this was treated with fluid administration and discrete doses of norepinephrine when necessary. Subsequently, the patient achieved hemodynamic stability and underwent uneventful emergence from anesthesia and successful extubation.

WHAT STEPS ARE GENERALLY FOLLOWED AFTER TUMOR EXCISION?

Postoperatively, the patient was admitted to the intensive care unit for continued monitoring after successful tumor removal and emergence of anesthesia. Once there, he had an uneventful postoperative course with noted BP return to normal range within a few days. This event was followed by termination of previous medications, and he was at that point discharged to home. During follow-up with his pediatric surgeon, tissue pathology results confirmed the presence of pheochromocytoma without signs of local or regional invasion. After discussion with patient and family it was determined that similar problems had occurred with other family members in the distant past.

WHAT IS MULTIPLE ENDOCRINE NEOPLASIA TYPE 2 (MEN 2 SYNDROME)?

A geneticist consultation was requested by the surgical team. During the discovery interview and assessment, similarities of symptoms and presentation became evident in other close family members. At this point, the patient was screened for commonly associated gene mutations and shown to be positive for the RET gene mutation. Additional workup included screening for medullary thyroid carcinoma and primary hyperparathyroidism.

DISCUSSION

Pheochromocytoma is a rare neoplasm in children.[1] Pheochromocytoma is a tumor of neural crest cell origin and is confined to the adrenal medulla. Tumors found in extraadrenal locations are termed paragangliomas. The cause for the symptoms associated with pheochromocytomas centers around the production of catecholamines including norepinephrine, epinephrine, and dopamine. In one study, determination between benign tumors and malignant ones could not be made on the basis of tissue analysis but could only be made on a clinical basis. Tumors were defined as malignant when distant metastases were present, when regional tissue invasion of nearby structures was found, or if the tumor recurred following surgical resection.[2]

CLINICAL FEATURES

The most typically linked signs to pheochromocytoma are headache, sweating, tachycardia, and hypertension in adults. Few adults may present with all the initial signs at the same time.[3] In children, hypertension is usually continuous rather than intermittent in nature.[4] Pheochromocytoma is associated with several familial conditions including von Hippel-Lindau disease or as a feature of MEN syndrome types 2A or 2B.[5-7]

DIAGNOSIS

Sympathetic activity may be increased in a number of conditions affecting children, and differentiating between them becomes critical in the treatment of conditions such as pheochromocytoma. Conditions resembling pheochromocytoma's presentation may include other sympathomimethic tumors of neural origin such as neuroblastoma or ganglioneuroma, which may similarly secrete catecholamines. Additional conditions to include in a differential diagnosis are essential hypertension, Cushing syndrome, hyperthyroidism, adrenal cortical tumors, cerebral disorders, diabetes mellitus or insipidus, ingestion of sympathomimethic drugs, and panic disorder.[5,8] Panic disorder by virtue of leading to a surge in endogenous sympathomimetic activity can resemble the hypertension seen with pheochromocytoma. This phenomenon may need special consideration particularly in adolescent children who are treated with tricyclic antidepressants.[9] Separately, ingestion or consumption of substances such as cocaine, or products containing phenylephrine, epinephrine, and amphetamine, among others, may lead to symptoms resembling pheochromocytoma due to their effect, and their presence may need to be ruled out as part of the differential diagnosis.

The best initial screening test recommended for children in suspected pheochromocytoma may be up for debate but is reduced to two options. The first is measurement of fractionated metanephrine and catecholamines using a 24-hour urine collection.[10] The other primary screening test is obtaining plasma free metanephrines, which has high sensitivity and specificity.[5] The later test may be particularly amenable for use in young children, but age-specific values need be used when interpreting results.[11] Following laboratory data acquisition, radiologic tumor localization and characterization is necessary. To this end, CT and MRI of the abdomen and pelvis are typically the two most commonly used modalities.[4,5] MRI may be helpful in differentiating between pheochromocytoma versus other kinds of adrenal tumors. Additional tests may be necessary as well such as metaiodobenzylguanidine, metaiodobenzylguanidine (MIBG), and positron emission tomography (PET), for aid in tumor localization and to determine the presence of multicentric disease given that up to 40% of children diagnosed with a paraganglioma may have multiple different concomitant tumor sites.[12]

PREOPERATIVE ASSESSMENT AND PREPARATION

Evaluation of renal and cardiac function is important in preparation for surgery. Obtaining electrolytes, glucose sampling, electrocardiogram, and echocardiography can assist in defining the impact of pheochromocytoma on homeostasis. In addition, determining whether other coexisting endocrinopathies are present, as may occur in multiple endocrine neoplasia, may also be necessary.

The basis for preoperative treatment of hypertension is alpha-adrenergic blockade. This can be accomplished successfully with phenoxybenzamine, but other alpha-1 selective inhibitors have also been used such as doxazosin. Phenoxybenzamine may be initiated at once daily dosing and titrated to a maximum total dose of 10mg per day. The effectiveness of phenoxybenzamine revolves around its mechanism of action, specifically its noncompetitive antagonism of the alpha-receptor, thus yielding effective blockade despite potentially high levels of plasma catecholamine.[1,13] Treatment with phenoxybenzamine may require time for optimization up to a few weeks as it is gradually adjusted. The advantage of phenoxybenzamine resides in its longer lasting effect. Beta-blockade may only be used after initiation of alpha-blockade and should not be used as initial therapy as this may lead to exacerbation of vasoconstriction and hypertension, progressing to potential cardiac failure with resulting pulmonary edema.[5] A beta-blockade's principal use is to assist difficult-to-control hypertension, tachycardia, or dysrhythmia. Newer approaches in adults involves using other antihypertensive categories such as calcium channel blockers and metyrosine.[14] Metyrosine works by virtue of blocking production of catecholamines via inhibition of the enzyme tyrosine hydroxylase; however, this is not considered first-line treatment, and it is generally reserved for patients who cannot tolerate the side effects of alpha- and beta-blockade combinations.

Regarding premedication and anxiolysis, oral and intravenous midazolam, as well as oral clonidine, have all been used successfully. Opioid agent administration may be used as an adjunct.

INTRAOPERATIVE MANAGEMENT

Many different anesthetics agents have been used to provide adequate surgical conditions with good results. Regarding intravenous agents, propofol and etomidate have been used successfully for induction, and propofol has been reported as a central agent in total intravenous anesthesia techniques for these cases. However, specific anesthetics leading to significant sympathomimetic activity or histamine release are typically avoided. For these reasons ketamine is generally contraindicated. Inhalational induction of anesthesia with sevoflurane has been used successfully, and both sevoflurane and isoflurane are well tolerated for maintenance of anesthesia. Desflurane has also been reported as inhalational agent for these cases, but its potential for tachycardia and hypertension during rapid titration offer a word of caution when considering it for maintenance of anesthesia.[13] Neuromuscular blockers like rocuronium and vecuronium are also well tolerated.[1,13] Placement of an arterial catheter is mandatory for monitoring of blood pressure and blood sampling during the course of surgery but may be placed after induction of anesthesia if necessary.[13] In preparation for the possible hemodynamic changes that may occur during laryngoscopy and intubation, several agents have proven useful. Intravenous lidocaine, high dose opioid fentanyl or remifentanil, magnesium, and esmolol administration have all been used during this perilous period.[1,15,16] Other periods of potential hemodynamic instability include skin incision, insufflation for laparoscopic cases, and abdominal exploration.[17]

During the intraoperative course, three different problems may be anticipated: hypertension, dysrhythmias, and hypotension. As described, hypertension may be experienced during the period of induction of anesthesia, laryngoscopy, and intubation but also at other times such as during tumor handling and excision. Several vasodilating agents have been used successfully in pediatrics. Sodium nitroprusside has a long track record, as well as nitroglycerin, but other infusion agents such as nicardipine, clevidipine, magnesium sulfate, and esmolol have also proven useful and effective. When using magnesium infusions, one must be aware of its potential effect in prolongation of neuromuscular blockade and possible need for postoperative ventilation.[13,15,16]

Dysrhythmia may appear at any time during the course of anesthesia, but the period of underlying tumor excision may be of highest risk. Treatment of dysrhythmia will depend upon its presentation and etiology. Hypotension may manifest itself after excision and removal of the tumor. Episodes of hypotension may be managed initially by ceasing use of vasodilating infusions and by providing fluid and blood product administration as necessary. Patients may benefit from fluid administration during the initial stages of the anesthetic as the chronically elevated plasma concentration of catecholamines would frequently lead to intravascular volume contraction. If hypotension proves refractory to these measures, vasoconstrictive agents may be used including norepinephrine and epinephrine for hemodynamic stabilization and to improve circulation. Vasopressin has also been used in this instance as reported by Deutsch and Tobias.[5,18] The use of vasopressin may be important intraoperatively and postoperatively in the presence of refractory hypotension, as this may be the result of catecholamine-resistant vasoplegia. Since vasopressin does not rely on adrenergic receptors to exert its vasoconstrictive effect by working independently via the V1 receptor, this may be an important option during instances of refractory shock.[17] Intraoperative monitoring of glucose is of particular importance as its levels may fluctuate depending on acute changes in plasma catecholamine concentration. These changing conditions may give way to either hyperglycemia or hypoglycemia requiring treatment. The effects of elevated levels of epinephrine in particular can lead to hyperglycemia and insulin suppression. Conversely, removal of the secretory tumor with subsequent precipitous decrease in plasma levels of epinephrine may lead to hyperinsulinism and significant hypoglycemia. It is also worth acknowledging that patients receiving preoperative or intraoperative beta-blockade may not exhibit signs and symptoms consistent with hypoglycemia, therefore bringing into focus the importance of consistent glucose level monitoring. In addition, epidural continuous infusion of local anesthetic alone, or in combination with fentanyl, can be used for pain management of open procedures, but it can also be helpful in adding to the management of hypertension.[5,13] For postoperative pain management following laparoscopic procedures, patient-, nurse-, or parent-controlled analgesia may be used with opioid-based therapy. Spinal anesthesia has been used successfully in adults; however, the level of hypotension as a result of sympathectomy maybe profound.[17]

POSTOPERATIVE CARE

Following emergence and extubation as determined by patient monitoring and decision by the anesthesia team, close postoperative observation may proceed in a pediatric intensive care unit. Resolution of hypertension is expected after removal of the tumor and return to the normotensive range expected within a few days. The presence of hypertension beyond 1 week removed from surgery may be a concerning sign and may signal residual disease necessitating investigation.[4,5,18]

Complications in the postoperative arena are related to significant or profound hypotension, hypertension, or hypoglycemia. Hypotension may be persistent or refractory as described earlier, and different agents may be used including vasopressin.[19] Persistent hypotension may occur in up to 50% of patients. Hypertension may be amenable to the intraoperative medications discussed previously, but other agents deserve consideration such as magnesium and calcium channel blockers like nicardipine and clevidipine. Clevidipine is a very short-acting medication metabolized by plasma esterases and can be used effectively to achieve adequate hemodynamic control.[17] Regarding blood sugar monitoring, hypoglycemia will remain a concern secondary to possible rebound hyperinsulinism and require at least 48 hours of continuous postoperative monitoring.[20] Patients who may have undergone bilateral adrenalectomy are likely to require steroid replacement therapy, and consultation with an endocrinology team is necessary. Single adrenalectomy patients need steroid replacement in rare cases.[21]

Patient follow-up after resection is necessary to monitor for tumor recurrence or incomplete resection. Plasma metanephrine levels may be obtained a few weeks postresection. If the screening test is positive, imaging may be obtained. Under normal follow-up conditions, the patient may be seen yearly and for a period of up to 10 years. If the patient has a known familial or genetic predisposition, or had young age at presentation, life-long follow up may be necessary.[17]

GENETICS

In most instances pheochromocytoma may present as isolated disease in adults, but in the pediatric population its incidence has a stronger correlation with familial disease. Several conditions may be associated with the presence of pheochromocytomas, and those include MEN; MEN, types 2A and 2B; von Hippel-Lindau syndrome; and neurofibromatosis type 1 (NF-1). Since these conditions have a genetic basis as their common denominator, pheochromocytoma is directly linked to several gene mutations including RET protooncogene, von Hippel-Lindau syndrome (VHL), and succinate dehydrogenase complex subunits B, C, and D.[2]

MEN syndromes are a complex group of entities classified in several subcategories and encompassing a wide variety of diseases. MEN 1, also known as Wermer syndrome, involves the development of neuroendocrine tumors arising from the adrenal cortex, the anterior pituitary, and the parathyroid glands. It does not include pheochromocytoma as part of its spectrum.

MEN 2 is also known as Sipple syndrome, considered an autosomal dominant disorder, and is further subdivided into three groups: MEN 2A, MEN 2B, and familial medullary thyroid carcinoma. For reference, MEN 2B is also known as MEN 3.[22] Pheochromocytoma is a feature of both MEN 2A and 2B and may occur in up to half of patients diagnosed with MEN 2. Pheochromocytoma does not typically constitute part of the initial presentation for either syndrome, but it may be discovered during screening for medullary thyroid carcinoma (MTC). MTC is a staple of these two subclassifications of MEN syndrome. Patients with MEN 2A may exhibit primary hyperparathyroidism in association with primary parathyroid hyperplasia. A subgroup within the MEN 2A patients may also experience Hirschsprung's disease, affecting them via the absence of ganglion cells in the colon thus leading to chronic constipation, possible megacolon, and obstruction.

Patients in the MEN 2B group may exhibit both MTC and pheochromocytoma, but primary hyperparathyroidism is absent.[22] When both disorders are present, the initial treatment recommended is resection of the pheochromocytoma.

The clinical suspicion of MEN 2 syndrome is linked to the presence of RET mutations, and when these mutations are detected they are associated with an earlier presentation of both MTC and pheochromocytoma.[23] Furthermore, the presence of pheochromocytoma may affect up to half of all patients diagnosed with MEN 2.

Recently a new entity was defined as MEN 4 and includes parathyroid and anterior pituitary tumors. Other types of tumors may be present in this condition as well, including gastrinomas and bronchial and gastric carcinoids, but pheochromocytoma is not part of this clinical picture. Patients with MEN 4 may exhibit a mutation in the *CDKN1B* tumor suppressor gene (see Table 44.1).

Other conditions associated with pheochromocytoma include von Hippel-Lindau syndrome and NF-1. The incidence of pheochromocytoma for patients with VHL resides between 10% and 20%. The incidence of pheochromocytoma for NF-1 is estimated between 1% and 5%.[7] Additional conditions include Sturge-Weber syndrome, ataxia-telangiectasia, and tuberous sclerosis (see Table 44.2).

CONCLUSION

- Pheochromocytoma is a rare disease in children, and its diagnosis is more closely related to familial and genetic conditions relative to adults.

Table 44.1 **SYNDROMES AND DISEASE ASSOCIATIONS**

SYNDROMES	DISEASE ASSOCIATION	COMMON MUTATIONS
MEN 1, Wermer syndrome	Neuroendocrine tumors • Pancreas • Anterior pituitary • Parathyroid • Adrenal cortex	Germline mutations MEN1 gene chromosome 11q13
MEN 2A, Sipple syndrome	• MTC • Pheochromocytoma • Parathyroid tumors	RET oncogene chromosome 10q11.21[a]
MEN 2B, formerly MEN 3	• MTC • Pheochromocytoma	RET oncogene chromosome 10q11.21[a]
MEN 4	• Parathyroid tumors • Anterior pituitary tumors	CDKN1B[b]

Note. MEN = multiple endocrine neoplasia; MTC = medullary thyroid carcinoma.

[a] Multiple exons identified. [b] Tumor suppressor gene.

Sources. Walls GV. Multiple endocrine neoplasia (MEN) syndromes. *Semin Pediatr Surg.* 2014;23:96–101; Wells S, Asa S, Dralle H, et al. Revised American Thyroid Association guidelines for the management of medullary thyroid carcinoma. *Thyroid.* 2015;25:567–610.

Table 44.2 PHEOCHROMOCYTOMA AND ASSOCIATED SYNDROMES

TUMOR	FAMILIAL SYNDROME, CONDITION
	MEN 2A
	MEN 2B
	VHL
Pheochromocytoma	NF-1
	Sturge-Weber syndrome
	Tuberous sclerosis
	Ataxia-Telangiectasia

Note. MEN = multiple endocrine neoplasia; VHL = von Hippel-Lindau syndrome; NF-1 = neurofibromatosis type 1.

Sources. Walther M, Reiter R, Keiser H, et al. Clinical and genetic characterization of pheochromocytoma in von Hippel-Lindau families: comparison with sporadic pheochromocytoma gives insight into natural history of pheochromocytoma. *J Urol.* 1999;162:659–664; Walls GV. Multiple endocrine neoplasia (MEN) syndromes. *Semin Pediatr Surg.* 2014;23:96–101.

- Pheochromocytoma is a neurondocrine type-tumor confined to the adrenal gland. Similar tumors found outside the adrenals are termed paragangliomas.

- Benign versus malignant pheochromocytomas cannot be distinguished on the basis of function or histopathology.

- Diagnosis of pheochromocytoma in children may be associated with syndromes such as MEN 2, VHL, and NF-1, among other conditions.

- Preoperative preparation for surgical resection of pheochromocytoma may require medications to control blood pressure and heart rate.

- Common intraoperative complications with pheochromocytoma include hypertension, hypotension, dysrhythmia, and glycemic derangements.

- After resection of pheochromocytoma at an early age, life-long follow-up to include biomarkers and imaging may be necessary.

REVIEW QUESTIONS

1. A 2-year-old male, with history of elevated blood pressure readings and intermittent tachycardia, is suspected of having a possible pheochromocytoma. What would be the **BEST** test to substantiate your diagnosis?

    A. 24-hour urine collection for metanephrines
    B. CT scan of the abdomen and pelvis
    C. free plasma levels for metanephrines
    D. MRI of the abdomen and pelvis

Answer: C

It would be difficult to reliably obtain a 24-hour urine collection in such a young patient, so obtaining free plasma metanephrines would be the first option. MRI and CT scans would also be indicated if the patient proved to have elevated metanephrines on initial screen.[5,9,11]

2. A 14-year-old male presents to the emergency department with symptoms of diaphoresis, tachycardia, and hypertension. He recently was preparing arduously for his SAT exam. He was recently prescribed amitriptyline by his pediatrician to help with previous "episodes." The parents are concerned that these events are occurring more frequently. There is no family history of MEN, VHL, or any other known heritable condition. What is the **MOST** likely diagnosis?

    A. medullary thyroid carcinoma
    B. panic disorder
    C. pheochromocytoma
    D. primary hyperthyroidism

Answer: B

Panic disorders may mimic signs and symptoms resembling pheochromocytoma due to the elevation of sympathomimetic activity it may lead to. Panic disorder is prevalent in the pediatric teenage population. Primary hyperparathyroidism may lead to similar symptoms, and it is associated with MEN syndrome; however, this patient does not have a history of familial disorders which would include MEN syndrome. Patients with MEN 2A or 2B are at increased risk of MTC.[9]

3. A 4-year-old girl presents with hypertension, tachycardia, and diaphoresis. Her laboratory workup and imaging is consistent with high suspicion of pheochromocytoma. You are consulted to begin medical treatment for her hypertension. What initial medication is **MOST** commonly suggested for blood pressure control?

    A. doxazosin
    B. metoprolol
    C. metyrosine
    D. phenoxybenzamine

Answer: D

4. Of the following conditions and syndromes, which is **LEAST** associated with pheochromocytoma?

    A. MEN 1 syndrome
    B. MEN 2A syndrome
    C. neurofibromatosis
    D. VHL

Answer: A

Pheochromocytoma is strongly associated with MEN 2A and 2B syndromes. Both conditions follow autosomal dominant transmission. VHL and neurofibromatosis are also linked to pheochromocytoma. Pheochromocytoma is not associated with MEN 1 syndrome.[22,23]

5. Which of the following medications is **BEST** described as an ultra-short acting calcium channel blocker metabolized by plasma esterases which may be used intraoperatively for blood pressure control during hypertensive episodes?

    A. clevidipine
    B. isradipine

C. nicardipine

D. nifedipine

Answer: A

All of these medications are calcium channel blockers, but only clevidipine is an ultra-short acting agent metabolized by plasma esterases.[17]

6. Which of the following medications is **BEST** described as preoperative anti-hypertensive medication which has as its mechanism of action the decrease of catecholamine production?

A. doxazosin

B. metoprolol

C. metyrosine

D. phenoxybenzamine

Answer: C

Metyrosine binds to the enzyme tyrosine hydroxylase and affects the production of catecholamines. Phenoxybenzamine is the preoperative anti-hypertensive medication of choice because it has a long-half life and binds noncompetitively to the alpha-adrenergic receptor. Phenoxybenzamine does not affect the production of catecholamines. Doxazosin is a short-acting alpha-1 receptor blocker, and metoprolol is a beta-blocker. Doxazosin and metoprolol do not affect catecholamine production.

7. Which of the modes of genetic transmission is **MOST** closely associated with the presence of pheochromocytoma as part of MEN 2 syndrome?

A. autosomal dominant

B. autosomal recessive

C. homozygote dominant

D. heterozygote recessive

Answer: A

MEN 2 syndromes are characterized by autosomal dominant transmission with variant penetrance. When one autosomal chromosome with abnormality is inherited, this may in turn be enough to lead to expression of the disease.

8. A 12-year-old boy presents to the emergency department with extreme hypertension, diaphoresis, and headache. After comprehensive testing he is positive for grossly elevated urine metanephrines. His comprehensive metabolic panel shows an elevated glucose level with normal calcium levels. An MRI of the abdomen and pelvis confirms he has an area within the adrenal gland suspicious for pheochromocytoma. The boy's father shares with you that the patient's younger brother passed away after a battle with "throat cancer" recently. A genetics consult was recommended at the time, but they were unable to attend due to recent problems in the family farm. What syndrome is this young patient **MOST** at risk for?

A. MEN 1

B. MEN 2A

C. MEN 2B

D. MEN 4

Answer: B

Pheochromocytoma is part of the clinical presentation for MEN 2 syndrome. Medullary thyroid carcinoma is also part of MEN 2 syndrome. Patients with MEN 2B may present with a form of MTC that appears at a young age and in a more aggressive form. MEN 2B does not feature primary hyperparathyroidism. MEN 1 and MEN 4 syndromes do not include pheochromocytoma.

9. While investigating scenario in question 8, you are able to discuss the case with your institution's geneticist. After you update her with all the background information, she convinces you to order a test to confirm your suspicions. Which mutation is **MOST** likely present?

A. CDKN1B

B. MEN1 germline

C. NF-1

D. RET oncogene

Answer: D

MEN 2 syndromes are strongly linked to RET oncogene chromosome mutations. Several mutations have been identified and directly linked to the presentation of pheochromocytoma. MEN 1 germline mutation is not linked to pheochromocytoma. CDKN1B is linked to MEN 4 and not related to pheochromocytoma.[22]

10. A 14-year-old boy is taken to the operating room for right laparoscopic adrenalectomy after he being diagnosed with pheochromocytoma. Preoperatively he receives phenoxybenzamine and metoprolol. In the preoperative area his vital signs do not show elevated blood pressure or significant tachycardia. After uneventful intravenous induction and intubation, the surgical team is able to isolate the tumor and successfully remove the right adrenal gland. During routine intraoperative monitoring of blood sampling, your arterial blood gas shows a blood sugar level of 30 mg/dL. You begin to treat the patient immediately. What is the most likely diagnosis?

A. hyperinsulinism due to elevated catecholamine concentration

B. hyperinsulinism due to low catecholamine concentration

C. hypoinsulinism due to elevated catecholamine concentration

D. hypoinsulinism due to low catecholamine concentration

Answer: B

Changes in plasma glucose concentration can be observed intraoperatively and postoperatively. These levels may fluctuate depending upon catecholamine plasma concentration. After removal of the pheochromocytoma, plasma concentrations of epinephrine can decrease dramatically, thus leading to rebound hyperinsulinism with resulting hypoglycemia. Continuous monitoring intraoperatively and postoperatively is necessary to ensure the patient remains euglycemic during and after surgery. Preoperative beta-blockade may mask the signs and symptoms of hypoglycemia.[20]

QUESTIONS AND ANSWERS

This chapter has accompanying questions and answers which are available to subscribers as part of the Oxford eLearning platform. To access the questions, go to ✔ http://oxfordmedicine.com/pediatricanesthesiaPBL

REFERENCES

1. Ein S, Pullerits J, Creighton R. Pediatric pheochromocytoma. A 36-year review. *Pediatr Surg Int.* 1997;12:595–598.
2. Pham T, Moir C, Thompson G, et al. Pheochromocytoma and paraganglioma in children: a review of medical and surgical management at a tertiary care center. *Pediatrics.* 2006;118:1109–1117.
3. Baguet J, Hammer L, Mazzuco T, Chabre O, Mallion J, Sturm N, Chaffanjon P. Circumstances of discovery of phaeochromocytoma: a retrospective study of 41 consecutive patients. *Eur J Endocrinol.* 2004;150:681–686.
4. Caty M, Coran A, Geagen M, Thompson N. Current diagnosis and treatment of pheochromocytoma in children: experience with 22 consecutive tumors in 14 patients. *Arch Surg.* 1990;125:978–981.
5. Maxwell L, Goodwin S, Mancuso T, et al. Systemic disorders. In: Davis PJ, Cladis FP, Motoyama E, eds. *Smith's Anesthesia for Infants and Children.* 8th ed. Philadelphia, PA. Elsevier;2011:1110–1111.
6. Pomares F, Canas R, Rodriguez J, Hernandez A, Parrilla P, Tebar F. Differences between sporadic and multiple endocrine neoplasia type 2a phaeochromocytoma. *Clin Endocrinol.* 1998;48:195–200.
7. Walther M, Reiter R, Keiser H, et al. Clinical and genetic characterization of pheochromocytoma in von Hippel-Lindau families: comparison with sporadic pheochromocytoma gives insight into natural history of pheochromocytoma. *J Urol.* 1999;162:659–664.
8. Stein P, Black H. A simplified diagnostic approach to pheochromocytoma: a review of the literature and report of one institution's experience. *Medicine.* 1991;70:46–66.
9. Louie A, Louie E, Lannon R. Systemic hypertension associated with tricyclic antidepressant treatment in patients with panic disorder. *Am J Cardiol.* 1992;70:1306–1309.
10. Gardet V, Gatta B, Simonnet G, Tabarin A, Chene G, Ducassou D, Corcouff JB. Lessons from an unpleasant surprise: a biochemical strategy for the diagnosis of pheochromocytoma. *J Hypertens.* 2001;19:1029–1035.
11. Weise M, Merke D, Pacak K, Walther M, Eisenhofer G. Utility of plasma free metanephrines for detecting childhood pheochromocytoma. *J Clin Endocrinol Metab.* 2002;87(5):1955–1960.
12. Whalen R, Althausen A, Daniels G. Extra-adrenal pheochromocytoma. *J Urol.* 1992;147:1–10.
13. Hack HA. The perioperative management of children with phaeochromocytoma. *Pediatr Anaesth.* 2000;10:463–476.
14. Lebuffe G, Dosseh E, Tek G, et al. The effect of calcium channel blockers on outcome following the surgical treatment of phaeochromocytomas and paragangliomas. *Anaesthesia.* 2005;60:439–444.
15. Zakowski M, Kaufman B, Berguson P, Tissot M, Yarmush L, Turndorf H. Esmolol use during resection of a pheochromocytoma. *Anesthesiology.* 1989;70(5):875–877.
16. James MF. The use of magnesium sulfate in the anesthetic management of pheochromocytoma. *Anesthesiology.* 1985;62:188–190.
17. Naranjo J, Dodd S, Martin Y. Perioperative management of pheochromocytoma. *J Cardiothorac Vasc Anesth.* 2017;31:1427–1439.
18. Perel Y, Schlumberger M, Marguerite G, et al. Pheochromocytoma and paraganglioma in children: a report of 24 cases of the French Society of Pediatric Oncology. *Pediatr Hematol Oncol.* 1997;14:413–422.
19. Deutsch E, Tobias J. Vasopressin to treat hypotension after pheochromocytoma resection in an eleven-year-old boy. *J Cardiothorac Vasc Anesth.* 2006;20:394–396.
20. Lenders J, Duh Q, Eisenhofer G, et al. Pheochromocytoma and paraganglioma: an endocrine society clinical practice guideline. *J Clin Endocrinol Metab.* 2014;99:1915–1922.
21. Shen W, Lee J, Kebebew E, Clark O, Duh Q. Selective use of steroid replacement after adrenalectomy: lessons from 331 consecutive cases. *Arch Surg.* 2006;141:771–774.
22. Walls GV. Multiple endocrine neoplasia (MEN) syndromes. *Semin Pediatr Surg.* 2014;23:96–101.
23. Wells S, Asa S, Dralle H, et al. Revised American Thyroid Association guidelines for the management of medullary thyroid carcinoma. *Thyroid.* 2015;25:567–610.

45.

ANESTHETIC MANAGEMENT OF PEDIATRIC CRANIOPHARYNGIOMA

Adele King and Christopher McKee

STEM CASE AND KEY QUESTIONS

A 12-year-old female presents to the ophthalmology outpatient with a 12-month history of increasing visual loss and a 6-month history of worsening headaches and vomiting. Initial ophthalmic examination found severe compromise of visual acuity in the right eye, with right-sided optic atrophy. Left-sided visual acuity and fundal findings were normal. The pupils were noted to be unequal and the direct light response was absent in the right eye. Magnetic resonance imaging (MRI) of the brain was obtained and showed a solid sellar mass and cystic suprasellar mass causing compression of the optic chiasma. The radiological findings were suggestive of a craniopharyngioma (CP).

THE CLINICAL PRESENTATION OF CP IS DEPENDENT ON THE SITE OF INVOLVEMENT AS WELL AS THE PRESENCE OF COMPRESSION OF VITAL STRUCTURES. WHAT ARE OTHER COMMON PRESENTING SYMPTOMS?

On further questioning the family reported a history of lethargy and increased thirst but denied any changes in appetite or growth problems. On examination the girl was prepubertal, her height was + 0.8 SD and weight + 1.3 SD.

HYPOTHALAMIC DAMAGE AND ENDOCRINE DISTURBANCES ARE COMMON IN CHILDREN WITH CP. WHAT LABORATORY WORKUP IS REQUIRED PREOPERATIVELY?

Initial laboratory investigations showed a normal prolactin with undetectable alpha-feto protein and beta-human chorionic gonadotrophin levels. Thyroid function tests were indicative of central hypothyroidism (thyroid stimulating hormone [TSH] was 0.2 mL/UL, free T4 0.6 ng/dL, and free T3 2.75 pg/mL). Morning cortisol levels, as well as adrenocorticotrophic hormone, follicle stimulation hormone, luteinizing hormone, prolactin, and growth hormone were low normal. Serum and urine osmolality were within normal limits, as was serum sodium level. Thyroxine and oral hydrocortisone therapy were commenced 2 weeks prior to surgery.

WHAT ARE THE TREATMENT OPTIONS AVAILABLE FOR CP?

The patient underwent a right pterional (fronto-temporo-spenoidal) osteoplastic craniotomy, and trans-sylvian subtotal tumor removal was carried out. Histological examination confirmed the diagnosis of CP. Postoperative computed tomography of the head revealed some remaining solid tumor in the sella with left-sided residual capsule. The patient was discharged with regular follow-up.

WHAT ARE THE INTRAOPERATIVE CONCERNS WHEN ANESTHETIZING A PATIENT WITH A CP, AND HOW DO YOU APPROACH THEM?

On the morning of surgery the patient received her usual doses of both hydrocortisone and thyroxine. Prior to induction, routine American Society of Anesthesiologists monitoring was instituted.

DO YOU NEED ADDITIONAL MONITORS? ARTERIAL LINE? CENTRAL LINE? WHY OR WHY NOT?

A balanced intravenous (IV) induction was performed with fentanyl, propofol, and rocuronium. The airway was then secured with a size 6.5 cuffed endotracheal tube. Partial pressure of arterial carbon dioxide was maintained between 30 and 35 mmHg. Following intubation, an arterial cannula was placed. Two large-bore IV cannulas were then inserted and, following this, 1 mg/kg of hydrocortisone was administered and subsequently repeated 6 hourly as stress dosing. A Foley catheter was placed to allow assessment of urine output and for temperature measurement.

WHAT IS YOUR CEREBRAL PERFUSION PRESSURE GOAL?

Balanced anesthesia was achieved with sevoflurane in 50% air/oxygen mix, rocuronium boluses guided by nerve stimulation, and a remifentanil infusion, maintaining cerebral perfusion pressure and avoiding increases in intracranial pressure.

WHAT ARE THE POTENTIAL INTRAOPERATIVE COMPLICATIONS THAT CAN OCCUR DURING SURGERY FOR CP?

Two hours into the surgery, the patient began passing large quantities of urine and continued to do so over the subsequent 2 hours. Measured urine output was >4 mL/kg/hr during this time with rising sodium on serial blood gases (142–148-154 mmol/l). Of note, blood sugar levels were normal and no osmotic therapies had been administered. Initial treatment consisted of replacement of fluid deficits and blood loss using central venous pressure monitoring as a guide. Serum and urine osmolality levels were 442 and 224, respectively, and formal serum sodium levels were 156. A diagnosis of intraoperative central diabetes insipidus (CDI) was made. A vasopressin infusion was commenced and adjusted to achieve urine output <2 mL/kg/hr. Fluids were maintained at two-thirds maintenance with 0.9% normal saline with hourly monitoring of serum sodium.

WHAT ARE THE COMMON POSTOPERATIVE COMPLICATIONS FOLLOWING SURGERY FOR CP?

The patient responded appropriately to verbal commands and had no neurological sequelae following extubation. She was subsequently transferred to the intensive care unit (ICU) where she continued to have CDI requiring treatment with vasopressin.

Ophthalmic review showed no improvement in visual acuity from the preoperative testing.

Postoperative investigations revealed a decreased TSH level. She was prescribed thyroxine and dexamethasone and was discharged on day 10 with surgical follow-up.

DIABETES INSIPIDUS (DI) IS A COMMON POSTOPERATIVE COMPLICATION OF CP. HOW DO YOU DIFFERENTIATE IT BETWEEN SYNDROME OF INAPPROPRIATE ANTIDIURETIC HORMONE (SIADH) AND CEREBRAL SALT WASTING (CSW)?

DI initially occurred intraoperatively requiring treatment with a vasopressin infusion. This was later transitioned to oral desmopressin (DP) when diet resumed.

DISCUSSION

CP are rare and histologically benign neuroepithelial tumors that arise from the anterior margin of the sella turcica and predominantly involve the sella and suprasellar space.[1] They were first identified by Zenker in 1857, but it was not until 1899 that the histological origin of these tumors from the hypophyseal duct of Rathke's pouch was first postulated by Mott and Barrett.[2] Cushing was the first to coin the term craniopharyngioma in 1932.[2] Despite their benign microscopic appearance, they often aggressively infiltrate into critical parasellar structures and have high recurrence rates, leading to significant morbidity and mortality.[3]

The incidence of CP is 0.13 to 2 cases per 100,000 persons per year with 30% to 50% of cases presenting in childhood and adolescence.[4] CP account for 1% to 3% of all brain tumors and 5% to 10% of brain tumors in children.[5] Distribution by age is bimodal, with peak incidence in children at aged 5 to 14 years and in adults at age 50 to 75 years.[6] No sex or genetic predilection exists.[7]

ETIOLOGY AND PATHOGENESIS

The World Health Organization classifies CP into two types, adamantinomatous and papillary.[8] The adamantinomatous type arises from epithelial remnants of the Rathke pouch or the craniopharyngeal duct and is the most frequently occurring type in childhood.[8] According to the location of the tumor, they may be further classified as sellar, suprasellar, parasellar, retrosellar and infrasellar, or multicompartmental.

PRESENTATION

The clinical presentation of CP may vary depending on the proximity to and the subsequent pressure effects of the tumor on vital structures of the brain, visual tracts, brain parenchyma, ventricular system, major blood vessels, and hypothalamo-pituitary system.[9] Severity of the symptoms is dependent upon on the location, the size, and the growth potential of the tumor.[10] Initial diagnosis is usually delayed form the initial onset of symptoms by 1 to 2 years due to the slow-growing nature of the tumor.[2]

1. **Raised intracranial pressure:** In children the initial presentation is often dominated by manifestations of raised intracranial pressure (headaches and nausea and vomiting), either due to mass effect or due to cerebrospinal fluid (CSF) flow obstruction at the level of the third ventricle, foramen of Monro, and the sylvian aqueduct.[11]

2. **Visual defects:** Visual impairment is present in 62% to 84% of cases[12] and is due to compression of the adjacent optical nerve tract. Bitemporal hemianopia is the most common visual manifestation (49%); other manifestations include homonymous anopsia, scotoma, and optic atrophy with papilloedema.[13]

3. **Endocrine deficits:** Endocrine deficits are present in 52% to 87% of cases and are commonly caused by disturbance of the hypothalamic-pituitary axes that effect growth hormone secretion (75%), gonadotrophins (40%), TSH (25%), and adrenocorticotropic hormone (25%). Short stature, obesity, and lethargy are common in children.[13] Forty to 87% of patients have at least one hormonal deficit present at diagnosis. In the perioperative period, other endocrine symptoms such as CDI are present in 17% to 27% of all patients.[12]

4. Miscellaneous: Other presenting symptoms include neck stiffness and seizures due to rupture of the cyst contents and decreased functional activity and behavioral changes due to local invasion of the hypothalamus. In children hypothalamic involvement and endocrine disturbances are more common and occur before the onset of visual symptoms. Those patients with involvement of the thalamus and frontal lobe may present with hyperphagia, psychomotor retardation, short-term memory deficits, emotional immaturity, apathy, and incontinence.[14]

Clinical presentation may be distinct in various age groups. In young children symptoms of raised intracranial pressure are most commonly reported; in adolescents sexual immaturity is most common; and visual deficits and symptoms of hypopituitarism occur most often in young and middle-aged adults.[15]

DIAGNOSIS AND WORKUP

A suspicion of CP is based on clinical and radiological findings. Diagnosis is confirmed by histology.

1. Endocrine evaluation: An endocrine evaluation should include the assessment of anterior and posterior pituitary functions and should include:
- Adrenocorticotropic hormone (or corticotropin)
- Growth hormone and insulin growth factor 1
- Cortisol
- Prolactin
- Luteinizing hormone
- Follicle-stimulating hormone
- Testosterone (males)/estradiol (females)
- TSH
- Triiodothyronine
- Thyroxine
- Serum electrolytes and osmolality
- Urine osmolality

Any abnormalities should be corrected and treated preoperatively.

2. Neuroimaging: Cranial computer tomography (CT) and/or magnetic resonance imaging (MRI) with and without contrast enhancement, are part of the neuroradiological evaluation of CP. Calcifications and bony structures are best evaluated on CT, while MRI is best at assessing the delineation of tumor size and the involvement of neighboring structures.[16]

Tumor location (e.g., sellar or chiasmatic) and appearance (dystrophic calcification, cystic component, contrast-enhancing solid component) are suggestive of CP.

MRI: MRI with and without contrast is the preferred imaging approach.[17] On T1–weighted images, the cystic component is often hyperintense and the solid component is iso dense, with enhancement of the tumor nodule. On T2–weighted images, both the cystic and solid components are hyperintense.[17]

CT: On CT, 90% of tumors are at least partially cystic, 90% have calcifications, and 90% have rim or nodular enhancement.

3. Ophthalmology testing: In order to delineate any defect including papilledema, ophthalmological evaluation should include visual acuity testing, visual field perimetry, and optic disk evaluation (visual evoked potentials).

TREATMENT

The current treatment of CP includes a multimodal approach in which the aim is disease control and improved preservation of quality of life. Management should involve the multidisciplinary team (neurosurgery, endocrinology, ophthalmology, psychology, oncology, and radiation oncology) and be individualized for each patient.

The type of surgical approach depends the location, the consistency, the degree of calcification, the shape and size of the tumor, as well as the surgeon's preference and experience.[18] Surgical treatment options range from gross total resection (GTR) to more conservative surgery (subtotal resection [STR] or biopsy only) followed by postoperative radiotherapy (RT). Other less invasive procedures include endoscopic cyst fenestration or placement of an Ommaya reservoir into the tumor cyst for delivery of antineoplastic agents, namely bleomycin or interferon alpha.[8] Over previous years the management of CP has taken a more conservative path in an attempt to balance tumor control with quality of life. Historically, open cranial surgery with the goal of achieving GTR has been the treatment of choice, but the tendency of theses tumors to invade nearby critical neurovascular structures often leads to significant morbidity.[19] Mortality rates post-GTR have been reported as high as 20% with 80% to 86% of patients requiring permanent hormone replacement and 10% to 33% having worsening vision.[20] These results would support the conclusion that GTR is very often associated with a high surgical morbidity and has shaped clinical practice toward a more conservative surgical approach, including STR +/– postoperative RT. No significant difference in progression-free survival at 5 years between GTR and STR + RT exists; however, STR without RT has significantly increased recurrence rates.[18]

For small tumors restricted to the sella without significant extension laterally into the suprasellar space or without encasement of vessels, a transsphenoidal approach has been shown to provide higher rates for GTR (66%–69% vs. 48%), with lower reoccurrence (18% vs. 28%), lower rates of permanent DI (27%–32% vs. 48%), and less visual deterioration (1.7% vs. 11%) when compared to open surgery.[21]

Medical management includes hormonal replacement therapy for any identified endocrine abnormalities. Systemic chemotherapy with interferon alpha 2b has been trialed in children with recurrent disease. Table 45.1 criteria associated with a favorable prognosis in CP.

PREOPERATIVE SPECIAL CONSIDERATIONS

1. **Endocrine**—All patients with identified endocrine deficiency should be assessed and managed by an endocrinologist.

    a. **Cortisol**—Optimization of cortisol levels is required for those children with identified low cortisol levels before elective surgery. In the paediatric population, hydrocortisone is given in an oral dose of 10 to 15 mg/m2/day either in 2 or 3 divided doses.[2] It is the responsibility of the anesthesiologist to ensure that all patients have appropriate steroid replacement during the preoperative evaluation.

    b. **Salt/water imbalance**—CDI typically presents with polyuria and polydipsia, but symptoms may not be obvious in milder forms of the disorder or may be masked by secondary hypocortisolism. Adequate assessment of volume status, maintenance of intravascular volume, and monitoring and correction of electrolyte imbalances is paramount to management. DI treatment is a combination of fluid management and vasopressin or DP. DP can be used safely in an oral dose of 0.05 mg twice daily in children.[23]

    c. **Thyroid**—TSH levels are used to guide thyroid hormone replacement in the preoperative period. Oral thyroxine is administered in a dose of 4 to 5 micrograms/kg/day and adjusted as TSH levels dictate.[2]

RISK STRATIFICATION

3. **Surgical grading**—A preoperative grading system is proposed in children in an attempt to balance the advantages of aggressive surgical resection against the risk of significant morbidity. The system considers the extent of hypothalamic invasion by the tumor.[24]

Table 45.1 CONDITIONAL CRITERIA REQUIRED FOR FAVORABLE CRANIOPHARYNGIOMA PROGNOSIS

Age	More than 5 years
Tumour size	Less than 4 cm
Endocrine involvement	Absence of severe endocrine dysfunction
Surgery	Complete surgical removal

Modified from Moningi S. Anaesthetic management of children with craniopharyngioma. *J Neuroanaesthesiol Crit Care.* 2017;4(Suppl S1):30–37.

- Type 0—The tumor represents no hypothalamic involvement
- Type 1—The tumor distorts or elevates the hypothalamus but the latter is still visible
- Type 2—The hypothalamus is no longer visible

Subsequently it was proposed that a GTR be attempted for type 0 and type 1 tumors and a STR be attempted for a type 2 tumor, leaving the hypothalamic component remaining.

INTRAOPERATIVE SPECIAL CONSIDERATIONS

Position. Surgical positioning is dependent on the surgical approach. Transsphenoidal pituitary surgery generally requires a degree of head-up positioning making venous air embolism a risk.

Tumor location and surgical approach. Due to the close proximity to the internal carotid artery (ICA) and other vessels of the circle of Willis, intraoperative hemorrhage is a major concern. In the case of inadvertent ICA damage, deliberate hypotension can be employed in an attempt to minimize blood loss.[25] Typically, transsphenoidal surgery is associated with minimal blood loss, with moderate venous oozing from cavernous sinuses occurring more commonly than damage to the ICA.[25] Large-bore IV access and invasive arterial blood pressure monitoring is required as well as calculation of maximal permissible blood loss to guide effective blood transfusion and volume replacement.

Craniotomy for CP usually requires elevation of the optic chiasma and manipulation of the optic nerve with the potential for deterioration in vision postoperatively. However, there is no strong evidence to suggest the use of routine visual evoked potential monitoring, due to its sensitivity to anesthetic agents.[26] The conventional craniotomy also involves frontal lobe retraction and manipulation, thus increasing the potential for seizures postoperatively. Intraoperative seizure prophylaxis should be considered in these cases.

Disturbances to the hypothalamus may result in the loss of temperature homeostasis and cardiovascular changes (ST–T alterations) due to stimulation of the anteromedial hypothalamus.

In cases of widespread invasion that requires radical tumor excision, injury to the mammillothalamic tract, thalamus, and basal forebrain may result. Brain stem injury is rare but will result in a comatose state postoperatively.[2]

Endocrine. For children undergoing major surgery or those with a deficit preoperatively, steroid replacement is essential. Hydrocortisone 0.5 mg to 1 mg/kg is required every 6 hours for at least 72 hours.

DI is the most common intraoperative complication and is due to injury to the pituitary stalk or hypothalamus, resulting in decreased antidiuretic secretion and inability to concentrate urine. Treatment consists of volume replacement with continuous monitoring of acid-base, osmolality, electrolyte changes, and glucose.

Other. In the transsphenoidal approach following resection of the tumor, a Valsalva maneuver may be required to test for a CSF leak.

POSTOPERATIVE SPECIAL CONSIDERATIONS

Salt/water imbalance is an issue. Surgery for CP involving the hypothalamic-pituitary area is often accompanied by abnormalities in fluids, electrolytes, and osmoregulation due to handling and/or vascular compromise of the neurohypophysis.[27] Abnormalities in blood osmolality and sodium levels can be life-threating if not managed properly. Patients observed to have fluid and electrolyte imbalances postoperatively have been reported to have a longer hospital stay and higher mortality when compared to patients with normal sodium levels.[28] Postoperative management should involve accurate recording of fluid intake and output 6–8 hourly. A Foley catheter is required for accurate urine output. Other losses such as stool or CSF should be recorded and accounted for. Paired plasma and urine osmolality and electrolytes should be measured initially postoperatively and repeated every 8 hours, but changes in plasma sodium >5 mmol require more frequent testing (4–6 hours).[29]

CDI is the most common postoperative complication, occurring in 83% of patients with intrasellar and parasellar tumors. It usually becomes evident 24 to 48 hours postoperatively.[28] With the advent of improved surgical techniques, the incidence has decreased to 50% to 55% in recent years. The risk factors for development of CDI are younger age, male gender, CSF leak, and extent of surgery.[28] When considering a diagnosis of CDI, it is important to rule out other causes of polyuria and polydipsia, namely diabetes mellitus and administration of osmotic therapies (furosemide, mannitol).

The course of postoperative CDI can be transient, permanent, or triphasic. In the triphasic pattern, the initial phase of CDI is followed 3 to 5 days later by a second oliguric phase of SIADH, and then 7 to 10 days later permanent CDI occurs. The initial phase of triphasic CDI or transient DI is thought to be due to transient dysfunction of antidiuretic hormone (ADH)-producing neurones due to oedema or from alternations in the blood supply. Transient CDI resolves when the neurones regain function. The second oliguric phase of SIADH is due to uncontrolled release of ADH from the degenerating posterior pituitary or from the remaining magnocellular neurons whose axons have been damaged. Severe and long lasting SIADH can be a predictor for the occurrence of permanent CDI. The final phase of CDI results from the degeneration of hypothalamic ADH-secreting neurons.

In addition, some patients may develop CSW syndrome, which can develop as a primary neuronal insult or as a secondary response to SIADH. In CSW there is a defect in renal conservation of sodium leading to extracellular fluid volume depletion and hyponatraemia.

CP located within the hypothalamic region may cause patients to develop thirst abnormalities such as adipsia or hypodipsia, leading to hypernatremia and wide fluctuations in osmolality. Thirst abnormalities can often coexist with CDI.[30]

CDI

The diagnosis of CDI is made on the basis of clinical and biochemical findings. Typical findings include

- Polyuria (urine output >2.5 mL/kg) and polydipsia, usually within 24 to 48 hours postoperatively
- Plasma osmolality >300 mosm/l
- Urine osmolality <200 mosm/l
- Hypernatraemia
- Urine/plasma osmolality ratio <1

Assessment of the thirst mechanism is paramount postoperatively as those patients with an intact thirst mechanism and access to oral fluids may not develop hypernatremia and hyperosmolality. As long as fluids are replaced, CDI is not life-threatening. Those patients who are adipsic or those unable to drink enough to maintain normal biochemistry should be encouraged to increase their oral fluid intake. If required, IV fluid supplementation with 0.9% normal saline can be introduced at two-thirds maintenance with replacement volume for volume for other fluid losses.[31] Fluids can be replaced by water given orally or via a nasogastric tube or by 0.45% saline intravenously in eunatraemic patients. DP can be administered alongside fluid replacement to reduce the total daily fluid intake/output and need for IV fluid replacement. An "on demand policy" of DP administration is adopted in order to minimize the risk of water intoxication and hypernatremia in resolving transient CDI. In a pediatric intensive care setting, low-dose DP (0.1–0.2 μg s.c./i.m) or dilute arginine ADH (0.25–3 mU/kg/h) by a continuous IV infusion is often used in the first 24 to 48 hours postoperatively.[29] Doses should be titrated according to the daily urine output.

SIADH

SIADH can be transient in the postoperative period or occur after the initial phase of CDI. It is clinically characterized by a significant reduction in urine output in the presence of euvolaemia and hypervolemia, and patients often report increased thirst.[29] Biochemical classification of SIADH includes[32]

- Low plasma osmolality (<270 mosm/kg)
- Inappropriately high urine osmolality (>100 mosm/kg)
- Hyponatraemia
- Urine sodium loss >20 mmol/L
- Decreased plasma renin activity
- Low hematocrit
- Low plasma urea and uric acid

Fluid restriction is the mainstay of treatment for SIADH. In severe cases, only insensible losses (300 mL/body surface area in m2) should be replaced. Sodium replacement may only be required in prolonged cases resulting in total body sodium depletion. Symptomatic, severe hyponatraemia with a clinical picture of cerebral oedema requires treatment with a 3% hypertonic saline infusion at a rate of 0.5 to 1 mmol/kg/hr for 2 to 3 hours followed by conservative adjustments.[32] This is a temporary measure only to increase sodium levels to a safer level. Overcorrection should be avoided by limiting the rate of correction to <10 to 12 mmol/l during the initial 24 hours. Rapid correction of hypernatremia can result in permanent neurological damage secondary to cerebral pontine myelinolysis and death.

CSW

CSW is characterized by polyuria and natriuresis. It is caused by a defect in the tubular absorption of sodium leading to extracellular volume depletion. The pathophysiology of CSW is unclear, but it is postulated that it is due to the release of natriuretic peptides (NP), namely atrial NP and brain NP, from the injured brain and the loss of sympathetic stimulation to the kidney.[33] Release of atrial and/or brain NP causes natriuresis, diuresis, vasodilation, and suppression of the renin angiotensin system. Sympathetic stimulation normally causes tubular reabsorption of sodium, therefore any depression of sympathetic stimulation leads to reduced sodium absorption in the proximal tubule and an increase in sodium to the distal tubule. This in turn leads to a reduction in effective arterial blood volume that triggers the baroreceptor response to release ADH in order to maintain intravascular volume. A reduction in renin and aldosterone also occur as a result of decreased sympathetic stimulation, further inhibiting sodium retention.[29] The differences between SIADH and CSW are outlined in Table 45.2.

Patients with CSW and SIADH both can present with hyponatraemia following CP surgery. Distinguishing between these two entities is vital as the management for each condition differs. The primary treatment for CSW is water and salt replacement whereas fluid restriction is the principal treatment for SIADH.[29]

Treatment of CSW is comprised of appropriate fluid therapy and sodium supplementation. Depending on the severity and clinical symptoms of hyponatremia, isotonic or hypertonic fluids should be given to correct volume depletion. Severe cases may require intensive care admission to allow aggressive fluid replacement and central venous pressure monitoring.[29]

ANTERIOR/POSTERIOR PITUITARY DYSFUNCTION

Pituitary function will return to normal in 27% of patients with a preoperative deficit. After 24 to 48 hours of supraphysiological doses of steroids the dose is then tapered down, depending on morning cortisol levels. Those with cortisol levels <10 mcg/dL will require ongoing steroid replacement.[2] The majority of patients with normal pituitary function preoperatively will retain this postoperatively; however, all patients should be screened for hypopituitism.[33]

Table 45.2 **THE MAIN DIFFERENCES BETWEEN CSW AND SIADH**

	SIADH	CSW
Body weight	Increased	Same or decreased
Plasma volume	High	Low
Evidence of volume depletion	No	Yes
Plasma sodium	Low	Low
Urine sodium	High	High
Net sodium loss	Normal	High
Urine output	Usually low	Very high
Plasma osmolality	Low	Low
Urine osmolality	High	High
Urine/plasma osmolality ratio	>1	>1
Plasma urea	Low	Normal/high
Serum uric acid	Low	Normal
Haematocrit	Low	Normal/high
Plasma renin	Suppressed	Normal/high/suppressed
Plasma aldosterone	Normal/high	Suppressed
Plasma ADH	High	Suppressed
Plasma NP	High	High

Note. CSW = cerebral salt wasting; SIADH = syndrome of inappropriate antidiuretic hormone; ADH = antidiuretic hormone; NP = natriuretic peptides.

Modified from Edate S, Albanese A. Management of electrolyte and fluid disorders after brain surgery for pituitary/suprasellar tumours. *Horm Res Paediatr.* 2015;83:293–330.

VISUAL AND NEUROLOGICAL

Risk factors for visual impairment include prechiasmatic tumor location and severe presurgical deficits. Forty to 48% of patients with a preoperative visual impairment will gain some improvement postsurgery. Outcomes are improved with transsphenoidal surgery.[34]

Most neurological sequelae are transient and include epilepsy, hemiparesis, and cranial nerve deficits. The chances of long-term sequelae increases from 8% to 36% for larger size tumors.[33]

HYPOTHALAMIC DYSFUNCTION

Thirty-five percent of patients with CP will have symptoms related to hypothalamic dysfunction at diagnosis, namely obesity, behavioral changes, somnolence and imbalances in regulation of temperature, heart rate, thirst, and or blood pressure. Postoperatively, the rate of hypothalamic dysregulation increases up to 80%.[34]

1. A 15-year-old previously healthy female presents with a history of progressive visual loss and amenorrhea. Physical examination shows poorly developed secondary sexual characteristics and left-sided optic atrophy. An MRI brain scan is suspicious for CP. Which of the following radiological findings are **MOST** suspicious for CP?

    A. infrasellar solid mass without evidence of cystic elements (brain MRI)

    B. partially cystic mass without calcification or rim enhancement (brain CT)

    C. sellar and suprasellar mass with solid and cystic elements (brain MRI)

    D. sellar destruction and suprasellar flocculonodular calcification (skull x-ray)

Answer: C

Answer A is not correct as 75% of CP are suprasellar and CP are typically cystic in nature. Answer B is not correct as 90% of CP have calcifications and 90% have rim enhancement on CT scan. Answer D is not correct as MRI is the preferred diagnostic screening modality for CP.

2. Clinical presentation of CP may vary depending on the age of the child. Which of the following clinical presentations is the **LEAST** likely?

    A. 6-year-old male complaining of headaches and vomiting

    B. 7-year-old female complaining of decreasing vision

    C. 16-year-old female with amenorrhea and lack of pubic hair

    D. 19-year-old female with weight gain and cold intolerance

Answer: B

On presentation younger children present with symptoms of raised intracranial pressure (headaches, nausea, and vomiting) and rarely complain of changes in vision.

3. A 12-year-old girl with a high suspicion of CP on MRI brain scans undergoes preoperative endocrine evaluation which reveals a TSH level of 0.1 mU/L (normal 0.27 to 4.2 mU/L), a free thyroxine level of 13 pmol/L (normal 10 to 24 pmol/L), a free triiodothyronine level of 3.8 pmol/L (normal 3 to 6.5 pmol/L), and a low morning cortisol level (95 nmol/L). Which is the **MOST** appropriate course of action?

    A. transsphenoidal surgery

    B. hydrocortisone 5–10 mg/m2/day TID

    C. hydrocortisone 10–15 mg/m2/day TID and oral thyroxine 8–10 mcg/kg/day

    D. oral thyroxine 4–5 mcg/kg/day

Answer: D

Answer A is wrong as children should not proceed to elective surgery until correction of cortisol and TSH levels. The appropriate dosing regime is hydrocortisone 10 to 15 mg/m2/day in 2 to 3 divided doses and oral thyroxine 4 to 5 mcg/kg/day.

4. A 10-year-old underwent transsphenoidal resection of a CP. Surgery was complicated by injury to ICA resulting in bleeding and localized oedema. While in the ICU, the patient developed central diabetes insipidus lasting for 4 days, which then converted to SIADH. When is urine output **MOST** likely to normalize on its own?

    A. never

    B. 24 hours

    C. 48 hours

    D. 3 to 6 months

Answer: A

Answer B, C, and D are wrong as CDI followed by SIADH is suggestive of the triphasic pattern of CDI in which permanent CDI ensues and hence urine output does not normalize without treatment.

5. A 6-year-old female is recovering from craniopharyngioma resection in the ICU. Due to tumor extension toward the hypothalamus and third ventricle, a transcranial approach was employed to increase the likelihood of complete resection. On postoperative day 3, she is noted to have decreased skin turgor, sunken eyes, and dry oral mucosa. Laboratory testing reveals a low serum sodium, low plasma osmolarity, and high urine osmolarity. What is the **MOST** likely diagnosis?

    A. CDI

    B. CSW

    C. hypocortisolemia

    D. SIADH

Answer: B

In the SIADH the child would have a high plasma volume with no signs of volume depletion. In CDI the patient would be hypernatraemic with a high plasma osmolality and low urine osmolality.

6. Which of the following findings are **MOST** likely seen in a patient with SIADH?

    A. decreased serum sodium, normal urine sodium, increased urine osmolality

    B. decreased serum sodium, increased urine sodium, increased urine osmolality

    C. increased serum sodium, decreased urine sodium, decreased urine osmolality

    D. normal serum sodium, decreased urine sodium, decreased urine osmolality

Answer: B

In SIADH, ADH release leads to absorption of water in the collecting ducts causing hyponatraemia, inappropriately high urine osmolality, and urine sodium loss >20 mmol/L. CWS also causes hyponataraemia with high urine sodium loss and high urine osmolality but, in the case of CSW, patients are volume depleted. Answer C refers to CDI.

7. A 4-year-old child presents to the emergency department with a 3-day history of increased urine output and sudden onset of mental status changes. Parents report that he had recently been having a hard time seeing television screen and an ophthalmology appointment was scheduled for next week.

Prior to coming to emergency department, he was difficult to arouse from afternoon nap and remains somnolent in the emergency department. A CT brain scan reveals large CP. Serum chemistry is notable for serum sodium of 157 mmol/L. What is the **MOST** appropriately fluid therapy for this child?

A. 0.2% NaCl in 5% dextrose in infused at maintenance rate
B. 0.45% NaCl infused at a half maintenance rate plus urine replacement
C. 0.9% NaCl infused at a 2x maintenance rate plus urine replacement
D. 0.9% NaCl infused at two-thirds maintenance rate plus urine replacement

Answer: D

This patient is suffering from CDI and, due to his somnolence, may not be able to maintain adequate fluid intake. In this scenario 0.9% NACL is recommended at a two-thirds maintenance rate with replacement volume for volume for fluid losses; 0.45% NaCl is recommended for fluid replacement in eunatraemic patients; 5% dextrose solutions can lead to hyponatraemia, hyperglycemia, and seizures and hence are not recommended.

QUESTIONS AND ANSWERS

This chapter has accompanying questions and answers which are available to subscribers as part of the Oxford eLearning platform. To access the questions, go to ✓ http://oxfordmedicine. com/pediatricanesthesiaPBL

REFERENCES

1. Stamm AC, Vellutini E, Balsalobre L. Craniopharyngioma. *Otolaryngol Clin North Am.* 2011;44:937–952, viii.
2. Moningi S. Anaesthetic management of children with craniopharyngioma. *J Neuroanaesthesiol Crit Care.* 2017;4(Suppl S1):30–37.
3. Gleeson H, Rakesh A, Maghnie M. "Do no harm" management of craniopharyngioma. *Eur J Endocrinol.* 2008;159:S95–S99.
4. Stiller CA, Nectoux J. International incidence of childhood brain and spinal tumours. *Int J Epidemiol.* 1994;23(3):458–464.
5. Garre ML, Cama A. Craniopharyngioma: modern concepts in pathogenesis and treatment. *Curr Opin Pediatr.* 2007;19(4):471–479.
6. Bunin GR, Surawicz TS, Witman PA, Preston-Martin S, Davis F, Bruner JM. The descriptive epidemiology of craniopharyngioma. *Neurosurg Focus.* 1997;3(6):e1.
7. Sanford RA, Muhlbauer MS. Craniopharyngioma in children. *Neurol Clin.* 1991;9(2):453–465.
8. Crotty TB, Scheithauer BW, Young WF, et al. Papillary craniopharyngioma: a clinicopathological study of 48 cases. *J Neurosurg.* 1995;83(2):206–214.
9. Weiner HL, Wisoff JH, Rosenberg ME, et al. Craniopharyngiomas: a clinicopathological analysis of factors predictive of recurrence and functional outcome. *Neurosurgery.* 1994;35:1001–1010.
10. Petito CK, De Girolami U, Earle K. Craniopharyngiomas: a clinical and pathological review. *Cancer.* 1976;37:1944–1952.
11. Muller HL, Heinrich M, Bueb K, et al. Perioperative dexamethasone treatment in childhood craniopharyngioma—influence on short-term and long-term weight gain. *Exp Clin Endocrinol Diabetes.* 2003;111(6):330–334.
12. Müller, H.L. Risk adapted, long term management in childhood-onset craniopharyngioma. *Pituitary.* 2017;20:267.
13. Parisi JE, Mena H. Nonglial tumors. In: Nelson JS, Parisi JE, SchochetJr SS, eds. *Principles and Practice of Neuropathology.*1st ed. St. Louis, MO: Mosby; 1993:203–266.
14. Kuratsu J, Ushio Y. Epidemiological study of primary intracranial tumours in childhood: a population-based survey in Kumamoto Prefecture, Japan. *Pediatr Neurosurg.* 1996;25:240–246.
15. Lustig RH. Hypothalamic obesity after craniopharyngioma: mechanisms, diagnosis, and treatment. *Front Endocrinol.* 2011;2:60.
16. Garnett M. R., Puget S., Grill J., Sainte-Rose C. Craniopharyngioma. *Orphanet J Rare Dis.* 2007;2:18. doi:10.1186/1750-1172-2-18
17. Jagannathan J, Dumont AS, Jane JA Jr, Laws ER Jr. Pediatric sellar tumors: diagnostic procedures and management. *Neurosurg Focus.* 2005;18(6A):E6.
18. Habrand JL, Ganry O, Couanet D, et al. The role of radiation therapy in the management of craniopharyngioma: a 25-year experience and review of the literature. *Int J Radiat Oncol Biol Phys.* 1999;44:255–263.
19. Clark AJ, Cage TA, Aranda D, et al. A systematic review of the results of surgery and radiotherapy on tumour control for pediatric craniopharyngioma. *Childs Nerv Syst.* 2013;29:231–238.
20. Cohen M, Bartels U, Branson H, Kulkarni AV, Hamilton J. Trends in treatment and outcomes of pediatric craniopharyngioma, 1975–2011. *Neuro Oncol.* 2013;15:767–774.
21. Komotar RJ, Starke RM, Raper DM, Anand VK, Schwartz TH. Endoscopic endonasal compared with microscopic transsphenoidal and open transcranial resection of craniopharyngiomas. *World Neurosurg.* 2012;77:329–341.
22. Reddy GD, Hansen D, Patel A, et al. Treatment options for pediatric craniopharyngioma. *Surg Neurol Int.* 2016;7:85.
23. Mishra G, Chandrashekhar SR. Management of diabetes insipidus in children. *Indian J Endocrinol Metab.* 2011;15(Suppl 3):S180–S187.
24. Puget S, Garnett M, Wray A, et al. Pediatric craniopharyngiomas: classification and treatment according to the degree of hypothalamic involvement. *J Neurosurg.* 2007;106(1 Suppl):3–12.
25. Fukushima T, Maroon JC. Repair of carotid artery perforations during transsphenoidal surgery. *Surg Neurol.* 1998;50:174–177.
26. Nemergut EC, Dumont SA, Barry TU, Laws ER. Perioperative management of patients undergoing transsphenoidal pituitary surgery. *Anesth Analg.* 2005;101:1170–1181.
27. Müller HL. Craniopharyngioma. *Endocr Rev.* 2014;35:513–543.
28. Sherlock M, O'Sullivan E, Agha A, et al. Incidence and pathophysiology of severe hyponatraemia in neurosurgical patients. *Postgrad Med J.* 2009;85:171–175.
29. Edate S, Albanese A. Management of electrolyte and fluid disorders after brain surgery for pituitary/suprasellar tumours. *Horm Res Paediatr.* 2015;83:293–330.
30. Dabadghao P. Craniopharyngiomas: postoperative assessment of fluid and electrolyte imbalances. *Neurol India.* 2015;63:663–664.
31. Spoudeas HA, ed. Paediatric endocrine tumours. In: *A Multidisciplinary Consensus Statement of Best Practice from a Working Group Convened under the Auspices of the British Society for Paediatric Endocrinology and Diabetes (BSPED) and the United Kingdom Children's Cancer Study Group (UKCCSG).* Crawley: Novo Nordisk; 2005:16–46.
32. Liamis G, Milionis HJ, Elisaf M. Endocrine disorders: causes of hyponatremia not to neglect. *Ann Med.* 2010;43:1–9.
33. Liamis G, Milionis HJ, Elisaf M. Endocrine disorders: causes of hyponatremia not to neglect. *Ann Med.* 2010;43:1–9.
34. Momi J, Tang CM, Abcar AC, Kujubu DA, Sim JJ. Hyponatremia—what is cerebral salt wasting? *Perm J.* 2010;14:62–65.

46.

PERIOPERATIVE MANAGEMENT OF DIABETES MELLITUS TYPE 1 AND 2

Vidya T. Raman

STEM CASE AND KEY QUESTIONS

A 15-year-old with diabetes mellitus type 2 is scheduled for an endoscopy.

DOES IT MATTER WHAT TIME OF THE DAY HIS CASE IS SCHEDULED?

Generally, diabetic patients are scheduled as first cases due to challenges of glycemic control especially when eating and drinking is restricted. The patient is on monotherapy of metformin.

WHEN SHOULD HE STOP HIS METFORMIN PRIOR TO HIS OPERATION AND WHY?

His past medical history was significant for an episode of hyperosmolar nonketosis (HONK).

WHAT IS HONK AND HOW IS IT DIFFERENT FROM DIABETIC KETOACIDOSIS (DKA)?

His glycolated hemoglobin or HbA1C test is 8.

IS THAT HBA1C OKAY TO PROCEED?

His body mass index is over 99%; his vital signs are: blood pressure 140/78; respiratory rate 12; heart rate 87; oxygen saturation is 98% in room air.

His family history is significant for diabetes. He has severe needle phobia, and last time he had a blood draw he fainted. He stated he last ate a muffin about 5.5 hours ago because he forgot and was so hungry.

IS HE AT INCREASED RISK OF ASPIRATION VERSUS A NON-DIABETIC?

After discussing it with the gastroenterologist, the team decides to delay the case another 2.5 hours. Mom is not happy but wants to get this endoscopy done today.

SHOULD HE HAVE ANOTHER SUGAR CHECKED? SHOULD WE GET ANOTHER GLUCOSE WHILE WAITING? SHOULD WE PLACE AN INTRAVENOUS LINE WHILE WAITING?

His sugar during this time is checked and comes back at 375 g/dL.

WHAT ARE PREOPERATIVE GLUCOSE VALUES THAT CAUSE CONCERN? IS THERE ANY EVIDENCE-BASED GUIDELINES OF GLUCOSE LEVELS TO CANCEL?

You also obtain a urine sample for ketones.

IF HE IS NEGATIVE FOR KETONES, DOES THAT MEAN HE IS SAFE? WHAT IS YOUR INDUCTION PLAN? INTRAOPERATIVE PLAN FOR GLUCOSE MONITORING? YOU ELECT TO DO THIS SHORT CASE WITH GENERAL ANESTHESIA WITH AN ENDOTRACHEAL PLACEMENT. AFTER INTUBATION, YOU PLACE A SUCTION INTO HIS STOMACH AND OBTAIN ABOUT 100 CC OF A THICK BROWN PARTICULATE MATTER. IS THIS UNUSUAL?

The rest of the case proceeds without incident. Your patient's trachea was extubated safely and he goes to the postoperative care unit.

WHAT IS HIS POSTOPERATIVE PLAN FOR HIS DIABETES?

In the postoperative unit, his glucose is checked and is 200 g/dl. His room air oxygen saturations are 97%. He is discharged home when PACU criteria are met.

DISCUSSION

OVERVIEW

Diabetes management offers unique challenges in children and adolescents versus adults especially in the perioperative environment. The obvious challenges of monitoring dietary intake plus possible communication barriers with increased risk of DKA and hypoglycemia. Almost 30% of children will present with DKA as their first presenting sign.[1] Data from diabetes mellitus type 2 is just becoming available. Almost 50% of these children are not able to maintained on oral monotherapy.[2]

Consideration of each child's specific glycemic control and planned surgery makes it imperative to have a perioperative plan. There are standardized guidelines which have been shown to improve care and possibly lower cost. [3]

CLASSIFICATION AND EPIDEMIOLOGY IN CHILDREN

See Table 46.1 for most common types of diabetes encountered. We do not expand on other classifications (genetics, endocrinopathies, drug induced, etc.), which are beyond the scope of this chapter. Also, we touch briefly on screening and diagnosis of diabetes. However, if there are clinical suspicions of a diagnosis in the perioperative environment, it would be best to consult a pediatric endocrinologist to ensure not only proper management but teaching for the family and underscore the importance of the diagnosis.

The SEARCH trials in United States since 2000 have established prevalence and incidence of diabetes in those under 20 years old. Type I is the most common form of diabetes with the greatest number (2 per 1,000) found among non-Hispanic Caucasians.[4,5]

SCREENING/DIAGNOSIS

See Tables 46.2 and 46.3.

GENERAL MANAGEMENT PRINCIPLES

Type 1 diabetes always requires a treatment of insulin. Types and delivery of insulin are numerous. Generally, treatment includes a long- or medium-acting insulin to provide basal coverage and a short-acting insulin to cover meals. (See Table 46.4 for types and pharmokinetic profiles.)

Many children are managed with an insulin pump that delivers rapid-acting insulin subcutaneously. This basal rate is supplemented with more insulin with meals and snacks. Younger and smaller children may need diluted insulin to achieve appropriate levels.

Type 2 diabetes patients are mostly managed with either metformin alone or in combination with insulin. Metformin

Table 46.1 **CHARACTERISTICS AND PREVALENCE OF DIFFERENT TYPES OF DIABETES**

	TYPE IA	TYPE 2	MODY	ATYPICAL DIABETES MELLITUS
Prevalence	Common	Increasing	< 5% in Caucasians	>10% in African Americans
Age of presentation	Throughout childhood	Pubertal	Pubertal	
Onset	Acute severe	Insidious to severe	Gradual	Acute severe
Ketosis at onset	Common	>33%	Rare	Common
Affected relative	5%–10%	75%–90%	100%	>75%
Female: male	1:1	2:1	1:1	Variable
Inheritance	Polygenic	Polygenic	Autosomal dominant	Autosomal dominant
Ethnicity	All, Caucasian	All	Caucasian	African American/Asian
Insulin secretion	Decreased/absent	Variable	Variable decreased	Decreased
Insulin sensitivity	Normal when controlled	Decreased	Normal	Normal
Insulin dependence	Permanent	Episodic	Infrequent	Variable
Obesity	No	>90%	Uncommon	Varies with population
Acanthosis Nigerians	No	Common	No	No
Pancreatic autoantibodies	Yes	No	No	No

Note. MODY = maturity onset diabetes of the young.

Adapted from Botero D, Wolfsdorf JI. Diabetes mellitus in children and adolescents. *Arch Med Res.* 2005;36:281–290.

Table 46.2 SCREENING CRITERIA FOR DIABETES
MELLITUS TYPE 2 IN CHILDREN

Consider for children who are overweight plus 2 of the following:

- Family history of diabetes in first- or second-degree relative
- Native American, African American, Latino, Asian American, or Pacific Islander
- Signs of insulin resistance or conditions associated with insulin resistance
- Maternal history of gestational diabetes during the child's gestation

Adapted from American Diabetes Association. Standards of medical care in diabetes. *Diabetes Care.* 2016;39(Suppl 1):S1–S106.

is the oral hypoglycemic approved for use in children (see Table 46.5). There are many types available, but not all may be appropriately used in children.

HYPERGLYCEMIC HYPEROSMOLAR SYNDROME (HHS) AND DKA

DKA occurs more commonly in pediatric patients. However, the clinical presentation differs mainly in the presence of ketones and the degree of hyperosmolality. Insulin, which is the cornerstone of DKA treatment, is not warranted upfront with HHS and may be detrimental. Instead, vigorous fluid resuscitation is enough to treat the intravascular depletion which in turn dilutes the glucose. Also particular to HHS is the incidence of thrombosis and malignant hyperthermia. Dantrolene is the advocated treatment for children who manifest fever along with increasing creatinine kinase.[6]

Children are thought to be infrequently susceptible to HHS. HHS occurs when there is hyperglycemia and hyperosmolality without ketosis; this is also known as HONK. Sometimes patients can present with a mixed picture. (See Table 46.6.)

GLYCEMIC TARGETS FOR SURGERY

The optimal target for glycemic control among children during the perioperative period is debated. Surgical stress causes a hyperglycemic, catabolic state. Insulin actually may need to be increased to counter the neuroendocrine stress. Infection is unfortunately associated with hyperglycemia.[7] The general glycemic target is to maintain glucose 90 to 180

Table 46.3 SCREENING FOR DIABETES MELLITUS
TYPE 2 USING A1C

Test every 3 years using A1C at age 10 or onset of puberty

- Body mass index >85th percentile for age and sex; or weight >120% of ideal body weight
- Acanthosis nigrans, hypertension, hyperlipidemia, polycystic ovarian syndrome, small for gestational age, birth weight

Adapted from American Diabetes Association. Standards of medical care in diabetes. *Diabetes Care.* 2016;39(Suppl 1):S1–S106.

Table 46.4 INSULIN PREPARATIONS AND
PHARMOKINETIC PROFILES

	ONSET (HOURS)	PEAK (HOURS)	DURATION (HOURS)
Insulin Lispro (Humalog)	<0.25	0.5–2.5	<5
Insulin aspart (Novolog)	<0.25	1–3	3–5
Insulin Glulisine (Apidra)	<0.25	0.5–1.5	3–5
Regular (soluble)	0.5–1	2–4	5–8
NPH (isophane)	1–2	2–8	14–24
Insulin Glargine (Lantus)	2–4	No peak	20–24
Insulin Detemir (Levemir)	1–2	3–9	Up to 24

Adapted from Rhodes ET, Ferrari LR, Wolfsdorf JI. Perioperative management of the pediatric surgical patient with diabetes mellitus. *Anesth Analg.* 2005;101:986–999.

mg/dL intraoperatively.[8] However, most of the pediatric trials have shown unacceptable rates (up to 25%) of hypoglycemia associated with tighter glycemic controls even if infection, inflammatory responses, and mortality improved.[9,10]

PREOPERATIVE ASSESSMENT OF CHILDREN WITH DIABETES

Children with diabetes should have an assessment of electrolytes, glycemic control, and ketones (urine or blood) a few days prior to surgery. Delay of surgery is ideal if there is poor glycemic control. Admission may be necessary to achieve optimal control.

Also important prior to the day of the surgery is to establish whether this is a major surgery or minor surgery. Minor surgery generally takes less than 2 hours, which should not cause glucose fluctuations. Some examples are adenotonsillectomies and endoscopies. The child is expected to go home after a brief monitoring period.

Table 46.5 CHARACTERISTICS OF METFORMIN
USED TO TREAT CHILDREN AND ADOLESCENTS
WITH DIABETES MELLITUS TYPE 2

ORAL HYPOGLYCEMIC	MECHANISM OF ACTION
Metformin	<ul><li>First-line therapy</li><li>Improves insulin responsiveness by increasing insulin-mediated glucose uptake</li><li>Decreases hepatic insulin production</li><li>Weight loss</li></ul>

Adapted from Coté CJ, Lerman J, Todres ID. *A Practice of Anesthesia for Infants and Children.* Philadelphia, PA: Elsevier Health Sciences; 2012.

Table 46.6 **CHARACTERISTICS OF HYPERGLYCEMIC HYPEROSMOLAR SYNDROME**

- Serum glucose concentration >600 g/dL
- Serum osmolality >330 mOsm/kg
- Absence of ketosis and acidosis (serum bicarbonate concentration >15 mEq/L, urine ketones concentration (15 mg/dL or trace on urine dipstick)

Adapted from Zeitler P, Haqq A, Rosenbloom A, Glaser N. Hyperglycemic hyperosmolar syndrome in children: pathophysiological considerations and suggested guidelines for treatment. *J Pediatrics.* 2011;158(1):9–14.

Major surgeries are defined as more than 2 hours and the patient is expected to be admitted after. Preoperative glycemic control is very important. Elective surgeries should be delayed if that cannot be achieve preoperatively.[8] (See Table 46.7.)

PREOPERATIVE CARE RECOMMENDATIONS

On the morning of surgery it is recommended that no rapid-acting or short-acting insulin be given unless glucose is over 250 mg/dL. A target glucose range of 150 mg/dL is desired. The child's established sliding scale or "correction factor" can be used. This can be calculated by 1,500 divided by the total daily dose of the child's insulin. That will give the amount of glucose that will be decreased by 1 unit. If the child is on a split-mixed insulin regimen between a long-acting insulin such as NPH and a short-acting insulin. Generally, anywhere from half to the full dose of the long-acting dose given on day of surgery. The short-acting insulin is held while the child is fasting.[3]

Insulin pumps should be kept at the basal rate for minor <2 hour surgeries with the exception being sedation for magnetic resonance imaging (MRI). Generally these pumps are not compatible with MRI machines and the patient should be switched to a continuous intravenous infusion. If there is concern about hypoglycemia, a glucose infusion should be started.[11]

For patients on oral hypoglycemics, metformin should be held at least 24 to 48 hours prior to surgery.[3] More complex diabetes management requires an endocrinologist to work closely with the anesthesiologist to help manage glycemic control in the perioperative environment.

Table 46.7 **TARGET GLYCOLATED HEMOGLOBIN IN PREOPERATIVE ASSESSMENT**

AGE (YEARS)	HBA1C TARGET
<6	<8.5%
6–12	<8%
13<	<7.5%

Adapted from Coté CJ, Lerman J, Todres ID. *A Practice of Anesthesia for Infants and Children.* Philadelphia, PA: Elsevier Health Sciences; 2012.

There are no strict evidence-based guidelines on when to cancel for increased glucose. Certain institutions such as Yale New Haven Hospital uses 400 g/dL as a cut-off.

INTRAOPERATIVE MANAGEMENT

The administration of insulin and dextrose containing intravenous fluids in the intraoperative period is dependent mainly on duration of the procedure. Procedures longer than 2 hours should definitely have insensible losses replaced. Generally an isotonic fluid is preferred such as lactated ringers or normal saline. Glucose should be frequently used in procedures longer than 2 hours. Temperature can affect subcutaneous glucose levels, so consider intravenous blood measurements in hypothermic patients.[12] If glucose levels exceed >250 g/dL, it is advised to check for ketones either via blood or urine to make sure the patient is not in DKA. The Glucose-Insulin-Potassium (GIK) technique can be utilized. GIK has been shown to be an effective inotropic, metabolic therapy in disease states.[13] However, using this technique to provide myocardial stability may not allow a more finely tuned glycemic control.[14]

POSTOPERATIVE MANAGEMENT

It is imperative for the perioperative team to work in conjunction with the endocrinologist in the postoperative period. Catabolic stresses during surgery may cause huge derangements in glucose management. Also, dietary restrictions can make glycemic control more challenging. Close monitoring of glucose plus ketones may be warranted. Generally, metformin should not be restarted for 48 hours.[3]

REVIEW QUESTIONS

1. Which is the **MOST** accurate statement regarding HHS?

   A. Insulin is the primary treatment.
   B. Ketosis is frequently present.
   C. It is often misdiagnosed as DKA.
   D. It is more common in children than DKA.

Answer: C

DKA occurs more commonly in pediatric patients. However, the clinical presentation differs mainly in the presence of ketones and the degree of hyperosmolality. Insulin, which is the cornerstone of DKA treatment, is not warranted upfront with HHS and may be detrimental. Instead, vigorous fluid resuscitation is enough to treat the intravascular depletion which in turn dilutes the glucose. Also particular to HHS is the incidence of thrombosis and malignant hyperthermia. Dantrolene is the advocated treatment for children who manifest fever along with increasing creatinine kinase.[6]

Children were thought to be infrequently susceptible to HHS. HHS occurs when hyperglycemia and hyperosmolality is present without ketosis; this is also known as HONK. Sometimes patients can present with a mixed picture.

2. Which of the following statements is the **LEAST** accurate?

 A. Glucose monitoring is not needed for surgeries less than 2 hours.
 B. Diabetic patients should be scheduled as the first case of the day.
 C. Metformin is the only Food and Drug Administration (FDA)-approved oral hypoglycemic in children.
 D. Metformin should be taken, as scheduled, until the day of surgery.

Answer: D

Metformin should be held 24 to 48 hours before surgery due to possible lactic acidosis. The rest of the statements are true. Glucose monitoring intraoperatively is dependent on duration and type of surgery performed. Being the first case of the day helps diabetic patients control their glucose better. Metformin is the only FDA-approved oral hypoglycemic.

3. A 4-year-old insulin-dependent diabetic is scheduled to go to surgery in a week. He is extremely compliant. His HbA1C is most likely which of the following values?

 A. 8.5%
 B. 9%
 C. 10%
 D. 10.9%

Answer: A

4. Which of the following statements regarding prevalence and characteristics of diabetes mellitus type 2 is **MOST** accurate?

 A. Boys are more likely to be affected.
 B. Ketosis is rarely present at onset.
 C. Insulin sensitivity is often decreased.
 D. Inheritance is autosomally dominant.

Answer: C

5. Which of the following characteristics is **MOST** likely found in HHS?

 A. bicarbonate <15 mEQ/L
 B. glucose >300 g/dL
 C. glucose >600 g/dL
 D. serum osmolality <220 mosm/kg

Correct Answer: C

QUESTIONS AND ANSWERS

This chapter has accompanying questions and answers which are available to subscribers as part of the Oxford eLearning platform. To access the questions, go to ✓ http://oxfordmedicine.com/pediatricanesthesiaPBL

REFERENCES

1. Rewers A, Klingensmith G, Davis C, et al. Presence of diabetic ketoacidosis at diagnosis of diabetes mellitus in youth: the Search for Diabetes in Youth Study. *Pediatrics.* 2008;121(5):e1258–e1266. doi:10.1542/peds.2007-1105
2. TODAY Study Group, Zeitler P, Hirst K, et al. A clinical trial to maintain glycemic control in youth with type 2 diabetes. *N Engl J Med.* 2012;366(24):2247–2256. doi:10.1056/NEJMoa1109333
3. Coté CJ, Lerman J, Todres ID. *A Practice of Anesthesia for Infants and Children.* Philadelphia, PA: Elsevier Health Sciences; 2012.
4. Mayer-Davis EJ, Lawrence JM, Dabelea D, et al. Incidence trends of type 1 and type 2 diabetes among youths, 2002–2012. *N Engl J Med.* 2017;376(15):1419–1429. doi:10.1056/NEJMoa1610187
5. Hamman RF, Bell RA, Dabelea D, et al. The SEARCH for Diabetes in Youth study: rationale, findings, and future directions. *Diabetes Care.* 2014;37(12):3336–3344. doi:10.2337/dc14-0574
6. Wolfsdorf J, Glaser N, Sperling MA. American Diabetes Association. Diabetic ketoacidosis in infants, children, and adolescents: a consensus statement from the American Diabetes Association. *Diabetes Care.* 2006;29(5):1150–1159. doi:10.2337/diacare.2951150
7. Kaufman FR, Devgan S, Roe TF, Costin G. Perioperative management with prolonged intravenous insulin infusion versus subcutaneous insulin in children with type I diabetes mellitus. *J Diabetes Complicat.* 1996;10(1):6–11.
8. Rhodes ET, Gong C, Edge JA, Wolfsdorf JI, Hanas R. International Society for Pediatric and Adolescent Diabetes. ISPAD clinical practice consensus guidelines 2014: management of children and adolescents with diabetes requiring surgery. *Pediatr Diabetes.* 2014;15(Suppl 20):224–231. doi:10.1111/pedi.12172
9. Macrae D, Grieve R, Allen E, et al. A randomized trial of hyperglycemic control in pediatric intensive care. *N Engl J Med.* 2014;370(2):107–118. doi:10.1056/NEJMoa1302564
10. Srinivasan V, Agus MSD. Tight glucose control in critically ill children—a systematic review and meta-analysis. *Pediatr Diabetes.* 2014;15(2):75–83.
11. Boyle ME, Seifert KM, Beer KA, et al. Guidelines for application of continuous subcutaneous insulin infusion (insulin pump) therapy in the perioperative period. *J Diabetes Sci Technol.* 2012;6(1):184–190. doi:10.1177/193229681200600123
12. Sudhakaran S, Surani SR. Guidelines for perioperative management of the diabetic patient. *Surg Res Pract.* 2015;2015(5):284063–284068. doi:10.1155/2015/284063
13. Puskarich MA, Runyon MS, Trzeciak S, Kline JA, Jones AE. Effect of glucose-insulin-potassium infusion on mortality in critical care settings: a systematic review and meta-analysis. *J Clin Pharmacol.* 2009;49(7):758–767. doi:10.1177/0091270009334375
14. Fath-Ordoubadi F, Beatt KJ. Glucose-insulin-potassium therapy for treatment of acute myocardial infarction: an overview of randomized placebo-controlled trials. *Circulation.* 1997;96(4):1152–1156.

47.

MITOCHONDRIAL DISEASE

Ajay D'Mello

STEM CASE AND KEY QUESTIONS

A 4-year-old male with developmental delay, hypotonia, and seizures has been referred by neurology for a muscle biopsy due to concerns of mitochondrial disease (MD). The child presents with his mother, who states that the child recently had an magnetic resonance imaging (MRI) of his brain under a general anesthetic at another hospital. Vitals obtained are in the normal range for his age. He was given Pedialyte until 2 hours ago and is adequately nil per os. His mother states that he had to be admitted following his last anesthetic as he was slow to wake up and that he only received an intravenous (IV) anesthetic.

ROUTINE PREOPERATIVE LABS REVEAL NORMAL COMPLETE BLOOD COUNTS AND ELECTROLYTES WITH AN ELEVATED LACTATE. WHAT IS THE SIGNIFICANCE OF THE ELEVATED LACTATE? IS PREOPERATIVE CARDIAC TESTING NECESSARY BEFORE PROCEEDING WITH SURGERY?

MD with a dysfunction of the electron transport chain results in decreased production of adenosine triphosphate (ATP). Low levels of ATP result in the upregulation of glycolysis, which results in an overproduction of pyruvate that is either transaminated to alanine or reduced to form lactate.[1]

In a study by Munich et al., elevated venous lactate was found in only 30% of patients with mitochondrial disorders. It should be noted that <10% of mitochondrial disorders in children are due to mitochondrial DNA mutations[2] and lactic acidosis is found more commonly in patients with mitochondrial DNA mutations.[3] Hence, the presence of lactic acidosis is not specific to mitochondrial disorders, and other causes for an elevated lactate that include hypoxia, hypoperfusion, sepsis, hepatic and renal dysfunction, and seizures should be considered.

Patients with MD are at higher risk for conduction abnormalities, pre-excitation syndromes, cardiomyopathy, and sudden death.[3] Ideally, all patients with neuromuscular disease (NMD) will have a screening electrocardiogram (EKG). Abnormal EKGs should prompt a cardiology consult. Syndromes of mitochondrial dysfunction that are known to be associated with cardiac involvement include Kearns-Sayre, ocular myopathy, myoclonic

epilepsy with ragged-red fibers (MERRF), and mitochondrial encephalomyopathy with lactic acidosis and stroke-like episodes (MELAS). An echocardiogram performed within the past year is recommended prior to anesthesia for patients with known cardiac disease.

YOU BECOME AWARE THAT THE PATIENT IN ON A KETOGENIC DIET. HOW WILL THIS INFORMATION CHANGE YOUR MANAGEMENT OF THE PATIENT?

Ketogenic diets are composed of high-fat, moderate protein, and low-carbohydrate components. Some patients with MD are placed on a ketogenic diet for control of seizures.[4] This group of patients should not have glucose added to their maintenance IV fluids as they may become hyperglycemic. Perioperative serum glucose monitoring is recommended.

ARE PATIENTS WITH MD SUSCEPTIBLE TO MALIGNANT HYPERTHERMIA (MH)?

A true association with MH is known to exist only with King Denborough syndrome and central core disease.[5,6] However, succinylcholine should not be administered in patients with myopathy (most patients with MD) due to concern for upregulation of skeletal muscle nicotinic acetylcholine receptors leading to rhabdomyolysis and hyperkalemic cardiac arrest.

WHAT IS YOUR ANESTHETIC PLAN FOR THIS PATIENT?

Since patients with MD have a variety of presentations, the anesthetic plan should be tailored to the patient. The anesthetic goals include maintaining normoglycemia while preventing further metabolic stress and complications that worsen lactic acidosis.

One of the steps to achieve these goals is minimizing preoperative fasting time to avoid hypovolemia. Prolonged fasting in patients with MD results in metabolic stress, limiting ATP production. Patients are also prone to hypoglycemia due to an inability to maintain energy requirements from fatty acid oxidation during periods of fasting and surgical stress. It would be prudent to allow patients to take clear liquids until 2 hours prior to anesthesia or have IV fluids started on arrival to the preoperative area. Admission for IV hydration the night before surgery may need to be considered. Due to the possibility of deranged lactate metabolism in this group of patients, IV fluids that contain lactate should be avoided and the administration of glucose-containing fluids is considered essential in all but the shortest of procedures due to the tendency toward hypoglycemia. Perioperative monitoring of glucose and electrolytes is warranted, especially in patients with prior episodes of hypoglycemia. Ideally the case should be scheduled as the first case of the day.

Premedication for anxiolysis and sedation should be used cautiously due to the risk of respiratory depression, undiagnosed sleep apnea, and impaired response to hypoxia and hypercarbia. Patients with MD may also have impaired upper airway and lower esophageal sphincter tone with a predisposition to reflux and aspiration.

A variety of anesthetic techniques have been used safely, including inhalational anesthetic agents and propofol. However, case reports suggest susceptibility to propofol infusion syndrome in patients with MD, especially with prolonged exposure. Since propofol has been shown to affect mitochondrial function, it is likely that some patients with MD are more susceptible to adverse reactions due to propofol. Based on the current literature, propofol, especially prolonged infusions, may not be the anesthetic of choice in patients with MD. Titrated administration of a single bolus of propofol is acceptable and appears to be well tolerated.[7,8]

Other interventions aimed at decreasing metabolic stress and complications during the surgical procedure include careful titration of inhalational and parenteral anesthetics to minimize hemodynamic changes, cautious use of muscle relaxants in patients with pre-existing myopathy, maintaining normothermia, and measures to decrease incidence of postoperative nausea and vomiting (opioid-sparing techniques with the use of nonsteroidal analgesics and regional techniques if appropriate).[8]

THE CHILD IS EXTUBATED
AT THE END OF THE PROCEDURE AND
IS TRANSFERRED TO THE POSTANESTHESIA
CARE UNIT, WHERE HE APPEARS
UNCOMFORTABLE. WHAT ARE YOUR
POSTOPERATIVE CONCERNS?

The anesthetic plan for MD should include an aggressive plan for pain management to blunt the effects of surgical stress. Opioid-sparing techniques with the use of nonsteroidal anti-inflammatory drugs (NSAIDs) and local and regional anesthesia should be considered as patients with MD manifesting with hypotonia and myopathy are at higher risk for airway obstruction, hypoventilation, hypercarbia, and consequent acidosis.

Patients with MD may have an increased sensitivity to toxicity from bupivacaine, which has been shown to inhibit carnitine-acylcarnitine translocase. Lidocaine and ropivacaine have less inhibitory effects on mitochondrial function when compared to bupivacaine and would be preferred agents.[9]

NSAIDs have been used safely. However, repeated doses of acetaminophen should be used with caution due oxidative stress on the liver.[10]

DISCUSSION

Mitochondria are cellular organelles often referred to the as "powerhouses" of the cell due their generation of ATP, which is the principal molecule for storing and transferring energy in cells by the oxidization of glucose and fatty acids. Apart from the principle role of ATP production and energy hemostasis, mitochondria are also involved in the synthesis of heme and phospholipids, calcium hemostasis, apoptosis, and cell death.[11] As a result of its multiple roles, the study of mitochondrial dysfunction has expanded beyond the respiratory chain, and defects in mitochondrial functions have been linked to metabolic disorders, cancers, and neurogenerative disorders like Parkinson's disease.[12]

MD or cytopathies are a heterogeneous group of disorders that occur due to a structural or functional abnormality of mitochondria causing dysfunction of the mitochondrial respiratory chain. MDs are the result of DNA mutations of either nuclear or mitochondrial DNA.[13] The mitochondrial respiratory chain is the final common pathway for aerobic metabolism. Hence, organs that are highly dependent on aerobic metabolism are most likely to be affected. The presence of mitochondria in every cell of the body (except red blood cells) results in their dysfunction, manifesting with a wide range of neurological, cardiac, musculoskeletal, gastrointestinal, and endocrine disorders.

The diagnosis of MD is challenging and is based on clinical, histological, biochemical, molecular, neuroimaging, and enzymatic findings, along with several diagnostic criteria.[14] Of note, some of the laboratory evidence for diagnosis involves a presentation for a general anesthetic: invasive muscle biopsy for histology, electron microscopy, and enzymatic assays.[15]

The classification of MD is difficult and continues to evolve. MD can present at any age and usually presents as a multisystem disease although single-organ manifestations may occur (e.g., Leber hereditary optic neuropathy). When compared to adults who present with recognizable mitochondrial syndromes, presentations in children appear to be more nonspecific.[1]

SYSTEMIC MANIFESTATIONS OF MD

SYSTEMS	MANIFESTATION
Head, ears, eyes, nose, and throat	Ptosis, ophthalmoplegia, optic atrophy, hearing loss
Central nervous system	Developmental delay, hypotonia, seizures, ataxia, stroke

SYSTEMS	MANIFESTATION
Respiratory	Obstructive/central sleep apnea, recurrent respiratory infections
Cardiovascular	Conduction defects, predisposition to arrhythmias (Wolff-Parkinson-White), cardiomyopathy (dilated or hypertrophic)
Gastrointestinal	Swallowing difficulties, gastroesophageal reflux disease, aspiration risk, deranged hepatic function
Hematologic	Anemia (most frequent), leukopenia, thrombocytopenia, or thrombocytosis
Endocrine	Diabetes mellitus, hypoparathyroidism, hypothyroidism, growth hormone deficiency
Musculoskeletal	Exercise intolerance, muscle weakness, and atrophy

Patients with MD may display clinical features that fall into discrete clinical syndromes. However, there is clinical variability in presentation. Examples of syndromes of mitochondrial dysfunction include: Kearns-Sayre syndrome, chronic progressive external ophthalmoplegia, MELAS, MERRF, and Leigh syndrome.[13]

The anesthetic management of a child with hypotonia of uncertain etiology raises a dilemma for an anesthesiologist when faced with a patient who could have either a muscular dystrophy or a mitochondrial disorder. An understanding of the differences in the management of the two families of disorders is important for the formulation of an appropriate anesthetic plan. The main concern is the risk of MH or rhabdomyolysis due to the underlying condition and the effect on perioperative morbidity based on the chosen anesthetic technique.[16] Flick et al. have estimated the risk of a patient with NMD to have MH or rhabdomyolysis from exposure to a volatile anesthetic at less than or equal to 1.09%, while the estimated risk of an MH-susceptible child developing an episode of MH after a no-triggering anesthetic is lower at 0.46%.[17]

It has been suggested that children with hypotonia and suspicion of a NMD be anesthetized with nontriggering agents including omitting inhalant agents in the anesthetic plan to avoid the issue of MH and or rhabdomyolysis.[18,19] Total intravenous anesthesia (TIVA) with propofol was considered the preferred technique for patients susceptible to MH. It is now known that only central core disease and King-Denborough syndrome have been linked to MH and the association between mitochondrial myopathies and MH have mostly been dismissed.[6]

Propofol is now known to depress mitochondrial function at the level of complex I, complex IV, cytochrome C, and acylcarnitine transferase, as well as uncoupling oxidative phosphorylation.[20] Hence, it seems likely that some patients with mitochondrial dysfunction may develop adverse reactions to propofol. While propofol has been used in this patient population, the choice of a TIVA with propofol may no longer be considered the anesthetic of choice in this group of patients. Also, there exists the concern of propofol infusion syndrome with a short duration of high-dose propofol in a child with impaired fatty acid utilization.[21,22] Other agents such as dexmedetomidine, ketamine, or etomidate should be considered when deciding between the risks and benefits associated with the planned technique.

Volatile agents have been found to depress oxidative phosphorylation, with complex I being most sensitive.[23,24] The currently used volatile anesthetics are minimally metabolized when compared to IV anesthetics. The increased sensitivity that patients with MD may exhibit are well tolerated provided there is careful monitoring and titration of anesthetic dose and depth.[8,25] It would appear that the choice for TIVA for a patient with muscular dystrophy and the use of an inhaled agent for a child with mitochondrial myopathy would be appropriate. However, for those who consider the risk of around 1% for MH or rhabdomyolysis from exposure to a volatile anesthetic, when presented with a child with an undiagnosed myopathy, a TIVA technique with propofol can be considered provided dosing is moderate and the duration is short.[16]

At this time, it does not appear that any particular anesthetic technique is safer than another. Several case reports have documented that patients with MD may face a higher risk during the perioperative period.[26–28] There are also reports of patients with profound respiratory depression and central nervous system white matter degeneration in patients who had an uneventful anesthetic course and who appeared to be only mildly affected preoperatively.[29–31] It is fortunate that most anesthetics for patients with MD are uneventful.

Mitochondrial disorders are a heterogeneous group of disorders representing a variety of molecular defects and diseases. It is likely that some of these defects are more sensitive to anesthetic inhibition and hence are more prone to adverse effects. It is hence imperative for the anesthesiologist to thoroughly review the patient's history while formulating an anesthetic plan to minimize the risk of perioperative adverse events.

REVIEW QUESTIONS

1. A 12-year-old female with idiopathic scoliosis and MD presents for posterior spine decompression and fusion. The **PRINCIPAL** defect in MD is

A. ATP production dysfunction
B. carnitine deficiency
C. hexose monophosphate (HMP) shunt defect
D. ryanodine receptor defect

Answer: A

MD occurs due to a structural or functional abnormality of mitochondria, which causes dysfunction of the mitochondrial respiratory chain that leads to inadequate ATP production resulting in a variety of clinical manifestations. Option B is incorrect. Carnitine deficiency, which results from inadequate intake of, or inability to, metabolize the amino acid carnitine, is important in lipid metabolism. Option C is incorrect as the HMP shunt is a cytoplasmic process. Erythrocytes lack mitochondria and are not able to generate energy from the Krebs cycle. The HMP shunt is one of the pathways that provides for the metabolic needs of the erythrocyte and is critical to erythrocyte survival. Option D is incorrect as ryanodine receptor defects are associated with MH.

2. A 5-year-old male with developmental delay, hypotonia, and seizures attributed to MD presents for a upper gastrointestinal endoscopy. Regarding management of this patient, which statement is **MOST** accurate?

    A. Inhalational anesthetic agents are contraindicated.
    B. Dystrophin protein defects mandate avoidance of succinylcholine.
    C. Lactate-containing IV fluids should be avoided.
    D. Malignant hyperthermia risk is higher than in the general population.

Answer: C
Option C is correct because patients with MD are prone to lactic acidosis. Hence, IV fluids that contain lactate should be avoided and the administration of glucose-containing fluids is considered essential in all but the shortest of procedures due to the tendency toward hypoglycemia. Option A is incorrect because a variety of anesthetic techniques have been used safely including inhalational anesthetic agents and propofol. Option B is incorrect because dystrophin protein defects are associated with muscular dystrophies and not mitochondrial disorders. Option D is incorrect as a true association with MH is known to exist with only King Denborough syndrome and central core disease.

3. A 4-year-old male with MD who underwent bilateral hernia repair and orchidopexy is not waking up after an uneventful general anesthetic with sevoflurane. A caudal was placed after securing the airway with an appropriate dose of 0.2% ropivacaine. A 0.05 mg/kg dose of morphine was administered for analgesia. The child had an 8-hour fast for both solids and liquids and received normal saline during the procedure. Which is the **MOST** appropriate next step in the treatment for this patient?

    A. CT brain scan
    B. $D_{25}W$ bolus
    C. intralipid bolus
    D. naloxone push

Answer: B
It is prudent to limit prolonged fasting in patients with MD, as these patients are prone to hypoglycemia due to an inability to maintain energy requirements from fatty acid oxidation during periods of fasting and surgical stress. This patient had a prolonged fast and did not receive intraoperative dextrose. Option B is correct as a dextrose bolus will correct hypoglycemia. Option A is incorrect as the more common causes of prolonged awakening have not been excluded. Option B is incorrect as it appears that the anesthetic was otherwise uneventful with no hemodynamic instability. Option D is incorrect as the dose of morphine would be considered appropriate for the procedure, and it would be more appropriate to first rule out hypoglycemia.

4. Which of the following agents **LEAST** depresses mitochondrial function?

    A. bupivacaine
    B. desflurane
    C. dexmedetomidine
    D. propofol

Answer: C
The mitochondrial effects of dexmedetomidine on humans are unknown, with no adverse mitochondrial effects reported as yet. Dexmedetomidine is generally considered safe in patients with a mitochondrial disorder. However, it should be used with caution in patients with arrhythmia or heart block because bradycardia is a known risk and asystole can occur. Option A is incorrect as patients with MD may have an increased sensitivity to toxicity from bupivacaine, which has been shown to inhibit carnitine-acylcarnitine translocase. Option B is incorrect as volatile agents have been found to depress oxidative phosphorylation, with complex I being most sensitive. Option D is incorrect as propofol is now known to depress mitochondrial function at the level of complex I, complex IV, cytochrome C, and acylcarnitine transferase, as well as uncoupling oxidative phosphorylation.

5. A 4-year-old male with muscle weakness and concern for MD presents for muscle biopsy. Which of the following drugs is **BEST** to avoid?

    A. dexmedetomidine
    B. etomidate
    C. ketamine
    D. succinylcholine

Correct Answer: D
While there is no known accepted association between MD and MH, it would be best to avoid succinylcholine in patients with myopathy (which is most patients with MD) due to the risk of rhabdomyolysis and hyperkalemic cardiac arrest. Option A is incorrect as no adverse mitochondrial effects have been reported with dexmedetomidine, and it is generally considered safe in patients with MD. Options B and C are incorrect as the IV agents etomidate and ketamine have been used safely in patients with MD despite their inhibition of mitochondrial function at concentrations within the clinical range.

QUESTIONS AND ANSWERS

This chapter has accompanying questions and answers which are available to subscribers as part of the Oxford eLearning platform. To access the questions, go to ✓ http://oxfordmedicine.com/pediatricanesthesiaPBL

REFERENCES

1. Koenig MK. Presentation and diagnosis of mitochondrial disorders in children. *Pediatr Neurol.* 2008;38(5):305–313. doi:10.1016/j.pediatrneurol.2007.12.001
2. Lamont PJ, Surtees R, Woodward CE, Leonard JV, Wood NW, Harding AE. Clinical and laboratory findings in referrals for mitochondrial DNA analysis. *Arch Dis Child.* 1998;79:22–27.
3. Munnich A, Chretien RD, Cormier V, et al. Clinical presentation of mitochondrial disorders in childhood. *J Inherited Metab Dis.* 1996;19:521–527.
4. Steriade C, Andrade DM, Faghfoury H, Tarnopolsky MA, Tai P. Mitochondrial encephalopathy with lactic acidosis and stroke-like episodes (MELAS) may respond to adjunctive ketogenic diet. *Pediatr Neurol.* 2014;50(5):498–502.
5. Lerman J. Perioperative management of the paediatric patient with coexisting neuromuscular disease. *Br J Anaesth.* 2011;107(Suppl 1):i79–i89.
6. Associated conditions: how to be prepared. https://www.mhaus.org/healthcare-professionals/be-prepared/associated-conditions/
7. Driessen J, Willems S, Dercksen S, Giele J, van der Staak F, Smeitink J. Anesthesia-related morbidity and mortality after surgery for muscle biopsy in children with mitochondrial defects. *Paediatr Anaesth.* 2007;17(1):16–21.
8. Niezgoda J, Morgan PG. Anesthetic considerations in patients with mitochondrial defects. *Paediatr Anaesth.* 2013;23(9):785–793.
9. Weinberg GL, et al. Bupivacaine inhibits acylcarnitine exchange in cardiac mitochondria. *Anesthesiology.* 2000; 92(2):523–528.
10. Hsieh VC, et al. Mitochondrial disease and anesthesia. *J Inborn Errors Metab Screen.* 2017;5:1–5. doi:10.1177/2326409817707770
11. Susin SA, Lorenzo HK, Zamzami N, et al. Molecular characterization of mitochondrial apoptosis-inducing factor. *Nature.* 1999;397:441–446.
12. Nunnari J, Suomalainen A. Mitochondria: in sickness and in health. *Cell.* 2012;148:1145–1159.
13. Chinnery PF. Mitochondrial disorders overview. In: Pagon RA, Adam MP, Ardinger HH, et al., eds. *GeneReviews®.* Seattle: University of Washington; 2014. https://www.ncbi.nlm.nih.gov/books/NBK1224/
14. Frye RE, Rossignol DA. Mitochondrial dysfunction can connect the diverse medical symptoms associated with autism spectrum disorders. *Pediatr Res.* 2011;69(5 Pt 2):41R–47R. doi:10.1203/PDR.0b013e318212f16b
15. Morava E, van den Heuvel L, Hol F, et al. Mitochondrial disease criteria: diagnostic applications in children. *Neurology.* 2006;67:1823–1826.
16. Kinder Ross A. Muscular dystrophy versus mitochondrial myopathy: the dilemma of the undiagnosed hypotonic child. *Pediatr Anesth.* 2007;17:1–6.
17. Carr AS, Lerman J, Cunliffe M, et al. Incidence of malignant hyperthermia reactions in 2,214 patients undergoing muscle biopsy. *Can J Anaesth.* 1992;42:281–286.
18. Yemen TA, McClain C. Muscular dystrophy, anesthesia and the safety of inhalational agents revisited; again. *Pediatr Anesth.* 2006;16:105–108.
19. Goresky GV, Cox RG. Inhalational anesthetics and Duchenne muscular dystrophy. *Can J Anaesth.* 1999;46:525–528.
20. Chidambaran V, Costandi A, D'Mello A. Propofol: a review of its role in pediatric anesthesia and sedation. *CNS Drugs.* 2015;29(7):543–563. doi:10.1007/s40263-015-0259-6
21. Liolios A, Guerit JM, Scholtes JL, et al. Propofol infusion syndrome associated with short-term large dose infusion during surgical anesthesia in an adult. *Anesth Analg.* 2005;100:1804–1806.
22. Vasile B, Rasulo F, Candiani A, et al. The pathophysiology of propofol infusion syndrome: a simple name for a complex syndrome. *Intensive Care Med.* 2003;29:1417–1425.
23. Cohen PJ. Effect of anesthetics on mitochondrial function. *Anesthesiology.* 1973;39(2):153–164.
24. Kayser EB, Suthammarak W, Morgan PG, Sedensky MM. Isoflurane selectively inhibits distal mitochondrial complex I in *Caenorhabditis elegans. Anesth Analg.* 2011;112(6):1321–1329.
25. Morgan P, Hoppel CL, Sedensky MM. Mitochondrial defects and anesthetic sensitivity. *Anesthesiology.* 2002;96:1268–1270.
26. Bolton P, Peutrell J, Zuberi S, Robinson P. Anaesthesia for an adolescent with mitochondrial encephalomyopathy-lactic acidosis-stroke-like episodes syndrome. *Paediatr Anaesth.* 2003;13(5):453–456.
27. Shipton EA, Prosser DO. Mitochondrial myopathies and anaesthesia. *Eur J Anaesthesiol.* 2004;21(3):173–178.
28. Thompson VA, Wahr JA. Anesthetic considerations in patients presenting with mitochondrial myopathy, encephalopathy, lactic acidosis, and stroke-like episodes (MELAS) syndrome. *Anesth Analg.* 1997;85(6):1404–1406.
29. Casta A, Quackenbush EJ, Houck CS, Korson MS. Perioperative white matter degeneration and death in a patient with a defect in mitochondrial oxidative phosphorylation. *Anesthesiology.* 1997;87(2):420–425.
30. Cooper MA, Fox R. Anesthesia for corrective spinal surgery in a patient with Leigh's disease. *Anesth Analg.* 2003;97(5):1539–1541.
31. Grattan-Smith PJ, Shield LK, Hopkins IJ, et al. Acute respiratory failure precipitated by general anesthesia in Leigh's syndrome. *J Child Neurol.* 1990;5(2):137–141.

48.

GLYCOGEN STORAGE DISEASES

Tammy Wang, Jocelyn Wong, and Anita Honkanen

STEM CASE AND KEY QUESTIONS

An 18-month-old male infant presents to your preoperative clinic 1 week prior to a complex hypospadias repair and gastrostomy tube placement. His initial surgery was scheduled at 6 months of age but was postponed when he was hospitalized for seizures due to severe hypoglycemia and subsequently diagnosed with glycogen storage disease (GSD) type 1 (von Gierke's).

WHAT IS VON GIERKE DISEASE? WHAT IS THE USUAL AGE OF PRESENTATION? HOW DO PATIENTS TYPICALLY PRESENT?

GSDs are due to deficiencies in enzymes or transport proteins in the glycogen metabolism pathway. Type 1, or von Gierke's, is an autosomal recessive disorder that is due to a deficiency in glucose-6-phosphatase (type 1a) or the enzyme's transport protein (type 1b). These defects result in insufficient hepatic conversion of glucose-6-phosphate to glucose.

Patients typically present as infants with hepatomegaly and seizures due to hypoglycemia. Symptoms often begin at age 3 to 6 months when periods between feedings are extended and they begin to sleep through the night. Classically, these children have "doll-like" faces with chubby cheeks, thin extremities, and a protuberant abdomen.

WHAT LABS AND STUDIES WOULD YOU OBTAIN?

Laboratory evaluation should include a complete metabolic panel in addition to lactic acid, uric acid, and triglycerides. Patients may demonstrate hypoglycemia, lactic acidosis, hyperuricemia, and hyperlipidemia. If the plasma triglycerides are significantly elevated, the blood may have a milky appearance. Liver transaminases are often normal or nearly normal despite hepatomegaly.

ARE THESE PATIENTS AT AN INCREASED RISK OF BLEEDING? IF SO, WHY?

While the synthetic function of the liver is normally not affected, platelet function can be abnormal. If patients describe easy bruising and/or epistaxis, a complete blood count should be ordered to evaluate hemoglobin and platelets, and platelet function assays should be considered. Even with normal platelet numbers, aggregation and adhesion may be abnormal and the bleeding time prolonged.

Careful glucose control for 24 to 48 hours prior to surgery can correct abnormal bleeding times. DDAVP can also reduce bleeding complications.

WHAT SPECIFIC PREOPERATIVE INSTRUCTIONS WOULD YOU GIVE THE FAMILY REGARDING PREOPERATIVE FASTING?

Maintenance of normal blood glucose levels is the goal. This is commonly achieved via either a nasogastric or gastrostomy tube for continuous enteral feeds or oral administration of uncooked cornstarch. Children younger than 2 years of age typically need cornstarch administered at least every 4 hours which is not compliant with current American Society of Anesthesiologists fasting guidelines.

It is important to note that fructose and galactose cannot be converted directly to glucose in GSD patients, so sucrose, fructose, lactose, and sorbitol should be avoided. A soy-based or elemental enteral formula may be used.

Consideration should be made for patients to be admitted the day prior to surgery and started on dextrose-containing intravenous (IV) fluids to maintain euglycemia during the preoperative fasting period, while prolonged fasting times should be avoided.

After an uneventful anesthetic induction, intubation, and caudal placement, the urologist begins. A propofol infusion is used for maintenance of anesthesia and D10 ½ normal saline is running. Early in the case you infused 30 mL/kg of lactated ringers to maintain the patient's blood pressure at 80s/40s.

WHAT IS DIFFERENTIAL DIAGNOSIS FOR THE PATIENT'S HYPOTENSION? WHAT ARE YOUR NEXT STEPS?

You suspect continued hypotension is due to the vasodilation from the caudal you placed. While re-draping for the gastrotomy tube placement portion of the case, you attempt to obtain a venous sample to run a blood sugar and venous blood gas (VBG) from your peripheral IV. Unfortunately, it appears to have infiltrated. A new IV is placed and the result of your VBG is

pH 7.19

pCO_2 35

pO2 161

BE –8.2

HCO3 16.4

Glucose 42

WHAT DERANGEMENT DOES THIS VBG SHOW? WHAT COULD BE THE CAUSE?

This VBG shows hypoglycemia and a metabolic acidosis. The hypoglycemia is likely from failure to deliver dextrose due to IV infiltration. The metabolic acidosis is likely related to the lactate in the lactated ringer's solution given earlier.

The recommendation by the American College of Medical Genetics and Genomics is to start D10 ½ normal saline at 1.25 to 1.5 times the maintenance rate and to maintain blood glucose levels >70 mg/dL.

Lactic acid levels are recommended to be monitored during long procedures.

On POD #2, during your postoperative check, the patient's mother reports repeated episodes of abdominal pain and emesis since oral feeds have been reinitiated. The pain requires narcotics for treatment and the surgeons feel it is out of proportion to normal postoperative pain. The following labs are obtained:

Amylase 402

Lipase 2341

AST 45

ALT 63

Total bilirubin 0.9

WHAT IS THE LIKELY DIAGNOSIS? DO ANY COMMON ANESTHETICS PREDISPOSE PATIENTS TO THIS DISEASE STATE?

Abdominal pain and emesis with ingestion, accompanied by elevated amylase and lipase, are signs of acute pancreatitis. Pancreatitis in adults is typically caused by gallstones or alcohol abuse. In pediatrics, the causes are diverse and the etiology is often unknown. More common causes include abdominal trauma, pancreaticobiliary anomalies, multisystem disease, drugs and toxins, and viral illness.

In von Gierke's, elevated triglycerides and cholesterol cause the lipid abnormality that predisposes patients to pancreatitis. Propofol-induced pancreatitis has been described in the literature when propofol was used as one of the induction agents, although the causal relationship is unclear. A suggested mechanism is that propofol increases serum triglycerides in patients where this is already elevated. Given that a single dose of propofol may cause pancreatitis, an infusion may place the patient at even higher risk.

DISCUSSION

GSD: OVERVIEW

GSDs are a set of disorders caused by malfunctions of various enzymes involved in the metabolism of glycogen, the large branched molecular complex that acts as a storage reservoir for glucose. Abnormal deposition of glycogen and/or fat is responsible for the primary organ effects and dysfunction seen in many of the disorders. Difficulty in producing glucose at a steady rate during fasting causes hypoglycemic symptoms and growth retardation in several of the types. Manifestations may vary depending on the degree of enzyme function maintained, and some of the disorders will manifest marked phenotypic changes over time as patients age (Fig. 48.1). As each of the disorders has a somewhat varied presentation and anesthetic considerations, a brief overview for the long-recognized forms follows. Details in organ systems affected, highlights of clinical presentations, and primary long-term management considerations are summarized in Table 48.1. Key considerations in anesthetic management are summarized in Table 48.2. Additional related disorders are being identified regularly. See Figures 48.1 and 48.2.

GSD TYPE 0: GLYCOGEN SYNTHASE DEFICIENCY 1

Clinical presentation and systems affected

Patients present with fasting hypoglycemia, hypoalaninemia, ketosis, and postprandial hyperglycemia and lactic acidemia. Ketotic hypoglycemia responds to ingestion of protein-containing foods. If untreated, growth retardation/short stature and osteopenia may result.

Basic treatment

Administer frequent protein-rich meals, avoid fasting, and provide un-cooked cornstarch prior to sleep.

Confirming diagnosis

Liver biopsy, or analysis of the GYS2 gene in leukocyte DNA; glycogen synthase activity is low to un-measurable in liver with low glycogen content, and normal enzyme activity in fibroblasts.

Anesthetic considerations

Avoid prolonged fasts due to dysregulation of plasma glucose, monitor intraoperatively.

GSD TYPES 1A (VON GIERKE DISEASE) AND 1B: GLUCOSE-6-PHOSPHATASE AND GLU-6-PHOSPHATASE TRANSLOCATE DEFICIENCIES

Clinical presentation and systems affected

GSD type 1a and 1b are clinically indistinguishable and children usually present early in life, at about age 3 to 4 months.[2]

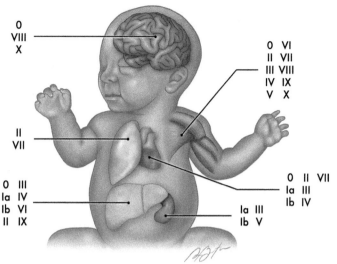

Fig. 48.1 Illustration of infant highlighting the primary organ systems affected by the various types of Glycogen Storage Disease. (By Ryan Charles Leung Brewster)

Prevalence is 1:100,000. Both renal and hepatic enlargement occur due to deposition of glycogen and fat. While neonates can present with severe hypoglycemia, it is more common for unrecognized and untreated infants to develop some combination of lactic acidosis, hyperuricemia, hyperlipidemia, hypertriglyceridemia, and hypoglycemic seizures.[3] Physical manifestations include "doll-like" facies with fat cheeks, thin extremities, short stature, and protuberant abdomen. Platelet and neutrophil functions can be affected with resultant tendency to infection (oral and mucosal ulcers) and bleeding (epistaxis). Antifibrinolytics and/or DDAVP may be used cautiously to treat this Von Willebrand-like manifestation of bleeding related to platelet dysfunction. Treated children do well, with normal growth and puberty. However, if untreated, several severe long-term consequences result: growth retardation, osteoporosis, delayed puberty, gout, pulmonary hypertension, polycystic ovaries, pancreatitis, and brain function changes. In particular, kidney effects can lead to end-stage renal disease, eventually necessitating transplant. Liver adenomas have malignant transformation potential; thus these patients may present for interventions for adenoma ablation.

Basic treatment

Diet regulation to maintain normal blood glucose levels is key. Note that even a short fast of 2 to 4 hours can produce hypoglycemia and lactic acidosis. Patients will often be on a cornstarch supplement and/or nighttime nasogastric infusions of glucose to help maintain a stable glucose concentration in the blood. Other treatments include diet restrictions for fructose,

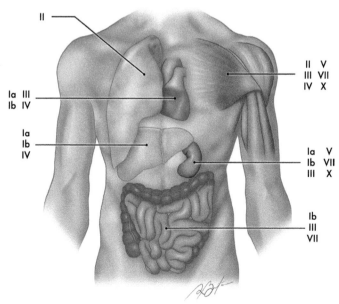

Fig. 48.2 Illustration of adolescent/adult highlighting the primary organ systems affected by the various types of Glycogen Storage Disease. (By Ryan Charles Leung Brewster)

Table 48.1 GLYCOGEN STORAGE DISEASE TYPES SUMMARIZING KEY ORGAN SYSTEMS AFFECTED, PATHOLOGY AND CONSIDERATIONS FOR TREATMENT. FOR REFERENCES, SEE TEXT

GLYCOGEN STORAGE DISEASES

TYPE 0		ORGAN SYSTEMS INVOLVED		CLINICAL PRESENTATION		LONG-TERM MANAGEMENT CONSIDERATIONS
Common Name	Glycogen synthase deficiency	Neuro		Fasting ketotic hypoglycemia	Cardiomyopathy	Frequent feedings to prevent hypoglycemia and seizures
Genetic Defect	GYS2 gene	Cardiac		Postprandial hyperglyccmia	Seizures, developmental delay	Address cardiomyopathy if present
Enzyme Defect	Glycogen synthase	Hepatic		Hyperlactatemia	Growth failure	
Inheritance Pattern	Autosomal recessive			Hepatic steatosis	Muscle cramping	

TYPE IA		ORGAN SYSTEMS INVOLVED		CLINICAL PRESENTATION		LONG-TERM MANAGEMENT CONSIDERATIONS
Common Name	von Gierke	Cardiac	Heme	Doll-like facies and fat cheeks	Renal enlargement, calcifications; hyperuricemia with uric acid stones and gout	Maintain low-sucrose, low-fructose diet; limit galactose and lactose intake; consider corn starch PO to maintain blood glucose levels (1.6 g/kg)
Genetic Defect	G6PC gene	Hepatic	GI	Short stature with protuberant belly and thin extremities	Systemic hypertension; atherosclerotic disease; possible pulmonary hypertension	Liver ultrasound every 1–2 years until 16 years old, then CT or MRI with contrast every 6–12 months for hepatic adenomas
Enzyme Defect	Glucose-6-phosphatase	Renal	GU	Hepatomegaly, with benign hepatic adenomatous nodules. Possible malignant transformation of nodules	Platelet dysfunction with easy bruising and bleeding; anemia; neutropenia or impaired neutrophil function	Echocardiography every 3 years after 10 years old to screen for pulmonary hypertension
Inheritance Pattern	Autosomal recessive			Hypoglycemia (often with illness); pancreatitis	Vit D deficiency; osteoporosis and osteopenia	Platelet function can be improved with DDAVP or intensive glucose therapy; treatment with human granulocyte colony-stimulating factor for recurrent infections

TYPE IB		ORGAN SYSTEMS INVOLVED		CLINICAL PRESENTATION		LONG-TERM MANAGEMENT CONSIDERATIONS
Common Name	None	Cardiac	Heme	Same as for Type 1A along with:	Oral lesions, i.e. hyperplastic gingiva	Same as for Type 1A
Genetic Defect	SLC37A4 gene	Hepatic	GI		Crohn's disease, chronic IBD	
Enzyme Defect	Glucose-6-phosphate translocase	Renal	GU		Perianal abscesses	
Inheritance Pattern	Autosomal recessive					

TYPE II		ORGAN SYSTEMS INVOLVED		CLINICAL PRESENTATION		LONG-TERM MANAGEMENT CONSIDERATIONS
Common Name	Pompe infantile	Neuro	Pulmonary	Cardiomyopathy by 2–3 months of age; ventricular hypertrophy	Hepatomegaly	Often fatal in 1st year of life from respiratory failure or cardiomyopathy

GLYCOGEN STORAGE DISEASES						
Genetic Defect	Acid-alpha glucosidase gene	Cardiac	GI	EKG findings: LVH, wide QRS, shortened PR, T-wave inversion	Feeding difficulties due to macroglossia, tongue weakness, poor oromotor skills	EKG to assess for LVH or biventricular hypertrophy; Holter monitor if concerned for arrhythmias
Enzyme Defect	Lysosomal acid-maltase	Hepatic	Musculoskeletal	Outflow obstruction from LV septal hypertrophy	Hypotonia, respiratory insufficiency	Chest X-ray to evaluate for cardiomegaly. ECHO to assess for hypertrophic cardio-myopathy +/− left ventricular outflow tract obstruction and dilated cardiomyopathy
Inheritance Pattern	Autosomal recessive					Begin recombinant α-glucosidase as soon as diagnosed to decrease cardiac manifestations
TYPE II		**ORGAN SYSTEMS INVOLVED**		**CLINICAL PRESENTATION**		**LONG-TERM MANAGEMENT CONSIDERATIONS**
Common Name	Pompe late onset, juvenile and adult	Pulmonary		Compared to infantile onset: greater skeletal involvement, minimal cardiac involvement	Scoliosis and/or hyperlordosis	Monitor for arteriopathy (Ectasias of basilar and carotid arteries, dilation of ascending thoracic aorta, etc.)
		Musculoskeletal		More proximal muscle weakness and respiratory insufficiency	Gower sign	
TYPE III		**ORGAN SYSTEMS INVOLVED**		**CLINICAL PRESENTATION**		**LONG-TERM MANAGEMENT CONSIDERATIONS**
Common Name	Debrancher deficiency	Cardiac	GI	Doll-like facies	Hypertrophic cardiomyopathy	Can present similar to type I but marked clinical variability; often improves after puberty
Genetic Defect	AGL gene	Hepatic	GU	Hypoglycemia, storage of short-branch polysaccharide in all tissues	Hepatomegaly, fibrosis leading to cirrhosis and hepatocellular carcinoma	Monitor blood glucose between 2–4 AM or urine ketones upon awakening
Enzyme Defect	Glycogen debrancher enzyme		Musculoskeletal	Macroglossia	Renal tubular acidosis: very rare	Consider high-protein diet (3 g/kg) or cornstarch (1 g/kg) after 1 year old to maintain euglycemia
Inheritance Pattern	Autosomal recessive			Muscular weakness and wasting, with truncal obesity	Osteoporosis and osteopenia	Progressive liver failure common in Japanese patients. Consider liver transplantation
TYPE IV		**ORGAN SYSTEMS INVOLVED**		**CLINICAL PRESENTATION**		**LONG-TERM MANAGEMENT CONSIDERATIONS**
Common Name	Andersen	Cardiac		Hypotonia	Abnormally branched glycogen accumulates in muscle and liver, altered glucose release	Routine LFTs, coagulation profile, liver ultrasound, EKG, and ECHO
Genetic Defect	GBE1 gene	Hepatic		Muscle atrophy	Hepatic failure with cirrhosis and associated symptoms/signs	Prevent nutritional deficiencies
Enzyme Defect	Glycogen branching enzyme	Renal		Delayed milestones	CHF rare but can occur with amylopectin storage in heart	Neurological and neurodevelopmental assessment

Table 48.1 CONTINUED

(Continued)

GLYCOGEN STORAGE DISEASES

Inheritance Pattern	Autosomal recessive	Musculoskeletal		Growth retardation	5 different subtypes, with varying degrees of severity	Often requires liver transplant to improve cirrhosis and decrease amylopectin storage in heart

TYPE V		ORGAN SYSTEMS INVOLVED		CLINICAL PRESENTATION		LONG-TERM MANAGEMENT CONSIDERATIONS
Common Name	McArdle syndrome	Renal		Infantile and late-onset form	Myoglobinuria after intense exercise can cause renal impairment	Moderate-intensity aerobic training to increase fitness and muscle oxidative capacity
Genetic Defect	PYGM gene	Musculoskeletal		Accumulation of glycogen in muscle, causing myopathy	Creatinine kinase levels elevated at rest	Simple carbohydrates prior to exercise to prevent exercise-induced rhabdomyolysis
Enzyme Defect	Muscle phosphorylase			Stiffness, pain, cramps with moderate exertion; improves with rest	Possible conduction block	Low-dose creatinine supplementation to improve ischemic exercise
Inheritance Pattern	Autosomal recessive			Easy fatigability, with muscle wasting in upper extremities	Often diagnosed as adolescents due to asymptomatic childhood. Boys > Girls	Avoid heavy static contractions or activities that induce severe myalgia

TYPE VI		ORGAN SYSTEMS INVOLVED		CLINICAL PRESENTATION		LONG-TERM MANAGEMENT CONSIDERATIONS
Common Name	Hers disease	Hepatic		Mild to moderate hypoglycemia	Muscle hypotonia and fatigue with exercise	Prevention of hepatomegaly and hypoglycemia by administration of uncooked cornstarch 1–3 times/day; avoid simple sugars, glucagon, and growth hormone
Genetic Defect	PGYL gene	GU		Prominent hepatomegaly with possible hepatic adenomas or malignancy	Growth retardation	Normal response to glucagon
Enzyme Defect	Glycogen phosphorylase	GI		Potential for cirrhosis	Delayed puberty	Monitor blood glucose and blood ketones when physically active, ill, or pregnant
Inheritance Pattern	Autosomal recessive			Mild ketosis	Osteoporosis and osteopenia	Routinely monitor blood glucose between 2–4 AM or urine ketones upon awakening

TYPE VII		ORGAN SYSTEMS INVOLVED		CLINICAL PRESENTATION		LONG-TERM MANAGEMENT CONSIDERATIONS
Common Name	Tarui disease, (infantile form)	Cardiac	Heme	Death secondary to respiratory complications	Severe infantile form: CNS and cardiac muscle abnormalities, severe myopathy and arthrogryposis	Note: exercise intolerance worsens after meals rich in carbohydrates due to glucose-inhibiting lipolysis
Genetic Defect	PFKM gene	Pulmonary	GI	Cardiomyopathy		Avoidance of strenuous exercise, carbohydrate meals, glucose infusions, and statins

Table 48.1 CONTINUED

Table 48.1 CONTINUED

GLYCOGEN STORAGE DISEASES						
Enzyme Defect	Phosphofructo-kinase M-subunit	Musculoskeletal	GU	Arthrogryposis		Avoid hyperthermia while undergoing anesthesia
Inheritance Pattern	Autosomal recessive			See VII(late-onset form) for other clinical features		
TYPE VII		**ORGAN SYSTEMS INVOLVED**		**CLINICAL PRESENTATION**		**LONG-TERM MANAGEMENT CONSIDERATIONS**
Common Name	Tarui disease, (late-onset form)	Musculoskeletal	GU	Exercise intolerance, with myoglobinuria with exertion	Hyperuricemia	See infantile form
		GI	Heme	Mild hemolytic anemia, erythrocytosis	Gallstones	
TYPE VIII		**ORGAN SYSTEMS INVOLVED**		**CLINICAL PRESENTATION**		**LONG-TERM MANAGEMENT CONSIDERATIONS**
Common Name	Muscle phosphorylase b kinase deficiency	Neuro		Mild cognitive impairment		Similar to type V but milder
Genetic Defect	PJKalpha, PHKbeta	Hepatic		Exercise intolerance with cramping and weakness		Consider simple carbohydrates prior to exercise
Enzyme Defect	Phosphorylase b kinase	Musculoskeletal		Myoglobinuria		Consider low-dose creatinine supplementation
Inheritance Pattern	X-linked recessive			Male predominance		
TYPE IX		**ORGAN SYSTEMS INVOLVED**		**CLINICAL PRESENTATION**		**LONG-TERM MANAGEMENT CONSIDERATIONS**
Common Name	Fanconi-Bickel	Cardiac (rare)		Possible hypotonia or muscle weakness; mild motor delay	Rare form with cardiac specific enzyme: death in infancy due to massive cardiac glycogen deposition	Prevention of hypoglycemia with frequent daytime feedings of complex carbohydrates and protein
Genetic Defect	PHKA1 or PHKA2	Hepatic		Hypoglycemia in infancy with fasting ketosis	Growth retardation	Monitor blood glucose and blood ketones when initially diagnosed, and when physically active, ill, or pregnant
Enzyme Defect	Phosphorylase kinase	Musculoskeletal		Liver fibrosis, rarely leading to cirrhosis; elevated liver transaminases	Delayed puberty	Routine LFTs, BMP, coagulation profile, lipid panel, and serum CK
Inheritance Pattern	75%: X-linked recessive, 25%, autosomal recessive			Hypercholesterolemia and hypertriglyceridemia	Improvement in disease with age	If <18 years old, perform liver ultrasound every 12–24 months; if >18 years old consider CT or MRI with IV contrast
TYPE X		**ORGAN SYSTEMS INVOLVED**		**CLINICAL PRESENTATION**		**LONG-TERM MANAGEMENT CONSIDERATIONS**
Common Name	Phosphoglycerate mutase 2 deficiency	Hepatic		Hemolytic anemia		Similar to type V but milder

(Continued)

Table 48.1 **CONTINUED**

GLYCOGEN STORAGE DISEASES						
Genetic Defect	PGAM-M	Musculoskeletal		Neurologic features possible: Parkinsonism +/– learning difficulties		Consider simple carbohydrates prior to exercise
Enzyme Defect	Phosphoglycerate mutase			Myopathy with exertion		Consider low-dose creatinine supplementation
Inheritance Pattern	Autosomal recessive			Myoglobinuria and rhabdomyolysis with exercise		

Note. GI = gastrointestinal; GU = genitourinary; CT = computed tomography; MRI = magnetic resonance imaging; IBD = irritable bowel disease; EKG = electrocardiogram; LVH = left ventricle hypertrophy; LV = left ventricle; ECHO = echocardiogram; LFT = liver function test; CHF = congestive heart failure; CNS = central nervous system; BMP = basic metabolic panel; CK = creatine kinase; IV = intravenous.

sucrose, galactose, and lactose; medications to help control lipid levels and uric acid concentration; citrate supplements for urinary calculi prevention; and angiotensin-converting enzyme inhibitors to decrease micro-albuminuria.

Confirming diagnosis

Various genomic tests provide the definitive diagnosis; alternatively, an enzyme assay from liver biopsy will confirm levels of activity, usually less than 10% of normal. If the diagnosis is in question, a Glucagon or Epinephrine challenge test may clarify the patient's status, with little to no increase in glucose with administration of these drugs, in contrast to large increases in serum lactate.

Anesthetic considerations

Prolonged fasting must be avoided to ensure maintenance of adequate glucose concentrations. Patients may need admission the night prior to surgery for administration of glucose containing IV fluids. If unable to admit the patient, nothing-by-mouth instructions should be modified to take this into account, with no more than 2 hours of fasting after clear glucose-containing fluids. It is often best for patients to be scheduled as the first case in the morning to avoid prolonged or variable fasting periods.

GSD TYPE II (POMPE'S DISEASE): ACID-ALPHA-GLUOSIDASE DEFICIENCY (GAA)

Clinical presentation and systems affected

GSD type II presents in one of 2 forms, related to age of onset, organs involved, rate of progression, and severity of manifestations.[3,4] The infantile form is life-threatening, usually presenting in the first 2 months of life. Muscle is primarily involved, thus signs include hypotonia and generalized muscle weakness, cardiomegaly with hypertrophic

cardiomyopathy, feeding difficulty related to swallowing problems resulting in failure to thrive, and respiratory distress. Cardiac enlargement can compress lungs and bronchi, and glycogen deposition causes conduction defects with shortened PR interval seen on electrocardiogram. Hearing loss occurs as well. The non-classic form of infantile-onset Pompe alternatively is marked by severe respiratory muscle involvement, presenting over the first year of life with motor delays and ultimately resulting in death in early childhood (cardiac involvement is usually not seen). Creatinine kinase is uniformly elevated in the infantile forms but may be normal in the late onset, adult form, which is marked by proximal muscle weakness and respiratory insufficiency with minimal cardiac involvement.

Basic treatment

The only treatment is enzyme replacement therapy, without which, in the classic form, death is the normal outcome in the first year related to left ventricular outflow tract obstruction. These patients may have unusual responses to cardiac medications and should receive individualized approaches.

Confirming diagnosis

Diagnosis is confirmed with GAA enzyme activity level, with levels of less than 1% normal activity associated with infantile forms and levels between 2% and 40% associated with non-classic infantile and late onset forms.

Anesthetic considerations

Digoxin, inotropes, diuretics, and afterload-reducing agents may worsen left ventricular outflow obstruction and should be avoided, as should hypotension and volume depletion. Anesthesia in general should be carefully titrated due to respiratory and cardiac concerns, with surgery or procedures requiring anesthesia avoided unless critically needed.

Table 48.2 KEY ANESTHETIC CONSIDERATIONS FOR GLYCOGEN STORAGE DISEASES. NOTE THAT NEW UNDERSTANDINGS ARE BEING DISCOVERED AT A RAPID PACE IN THIS AREA AND RECOMMENDATIONS FOR ANESTHETIC MANAGEMENT MAY CHANGE

ANESTHETIC CONSIDERATION AND PREPARATION	TYPE OF GLYCOGEN STORAGE DISEASE													
	0	IA	IB	II-I	II-L	III	IV	V	VI	VII-I	VII-L	VIII	IX	X
Organ System Checks and Preparation														
Avoid prolonged preop fasting without glucose	✔	✔✔	✔			✔	✔	✔	✔				✔	
Assess renal function		✔	✔											
Check for platelet dysfunction		✔	✔											
Check for anemia		✔	✔							✔	✔			
Assess liver function						✔	✔		✔				✔	
Assess cardiac function				✔	✔	✔	✔			✔				
Check for GI lesions			✔											
Management Considerations														
Not appropriate for outpatient surgery	✔			✔										
Increased risk of aspiration due to poor clearance				✔	✔									
Large tongue can cause airway obstruction				✔	✔	✔								
Cardiomegaly can compress bronchi				✔										
Consider regional or neuraxial anesthesia if no cardiac disease				✔	✔			✔						
Avoid myocardial depressant effects				✔										
Advanced myopathy may require post op ventilation					✔									
Avoid prolonged use of tourniquets					✔			✔				✔		✔
Maintenance														
Avoid lactate in maintenance IVFs (chronic lactic acidosis)		✔	✔											
Monitor glucose and IVFs with glucose added	✔	✔✔	✔			✔	✔	✔	✔				✔	
Medication Considerations														
Propofol may increase urinary uric acid excretion		✔	✔								✔			
Propofol may induce acute postoperative pancreatitis		✔	✔											
Caution with succinylcholine if muscle weakness (risk of hyperkalemia)				✔	✔	✔	✔	✔				✔		✔
Reports of cardiac arrest with sevoflurane induction				✔	✔									
Reports of Torsade de pointes with ketamine induction				✔	✔									
May be sensitive to nondepolarizing muscle relaxants								✔						

Note. GI = gastrointestinal; IVF = intravenous fluid

GSD TYPE III (CORI DISEASE OR DEBRANCHER DEFICIENCY): DEBRANCHING ENZYME DEFICIENCY

Clinical presentation and systems affected

GSD type III involves varying degrees of liver, cardiac muscle, and skeletal muscle affects.[5] The IIIa subtype affects 85% of this subset of patients and includes cardiac muscle and liver involvement, while the IIIb subtype is limited to involvement of the liver. Liver manifestations present as ketotic hypoglycemia and hyperlipidemia, with hepatomegaly and elevated transaminases. This will be present in infants and young children. In type IIIa, cardiac hypertrophy and myopathy develops in early childhood, with a broad range of presentation, from asymptomatic to severe dysfunction, congestive heart failure, and, in the rare individual, sudden death. In contrast, skeletal muscle weakness in type IIIb is usually not evident until later adolescence, with progression to prominent weakness in adulthood. In adolescence, the liver manifestations are less prominent, with hepatic fibrosis. However, for that small percentage who develop cirrhosis with severe dysfunction and/or hepatocellular carcinoma, liver transplant may be necessary.

Basic treatment

A high-protein diet with short feeding intervals helps avoid hypoglycemia in infants. Fructose and galactose are acceptable, and cornstarch can be used as well.

Confirming diagnosis

Diagnosis is supported by a constellation of signs and lab results including hepatomegaly, ketotic hypoglycemia with fasting, and elevated transaminases and creatinine kinase. Fasting glucose levels should increase with glucagon administration after a short fast of less than 2 hours but will not after a prolonged fast.

Anesthetic considerations

Hypoglycemic concerns are highest in infants and young children. This improves with age. Anesthetic regimens should take into consideration possible cardiomyopathy for type IIIa patients.

GSD TYPE IV: DEBRANCHER DEFICIENCY

Clinical presentation and systems affected

GSD type IV represented only 3% of GSDs, with an incidence of 1:600,000 to 1:800,000.[6] It presents with a range of phenotypes at varying ages: (i) fatal perinatal neuromuscular in which fetal hydrops and polyhydramnios are present and death usually occurs in the neonatal period due cardiopulmonary compromise; (ii) congenital neuromuscular in which hypotonia causing respiratory distress and dilated cardiomyopathy present in the neonatal period with death in infancy; (iii) classic progressive hepatic with normal appearance at birth, followed by failure to thrive, liver dysfunction and cirrhosis, hypotonia and cardiomyopathy, with the need for liver transplant prior to age 5; (iv) nonprogressive hepatic in which hepatomegaly, myopathy, and hypotonia occur but cardiac, skeletal muscle, and neurologic involvement are absent; and (v) rare childhood variant presents in the second decade with mild disease and/or progresses to cause death in the third decade.

Basic treatment

Treatment includes liver transplantation if liver failure develops, monitoring by a cardiologist for signs of cardiomyopathy and subsequent supportive care, possible cardiac transplantation, prevention of nutritional deficiencies (in particular fat-soluble vitamins), and physical therapy for motor developmental delay.

Confirming diagnosis

Muscle or liver biopsy reveals abnormally branched glycogen accumulation, and glycogen branching enzyme deficiency is demonstrated in liver, muscle, or skin fibroblasts. May also identify biallelic pathogenic variants in GBE1.

Anesthetic considerations

These patients will have liver involvement, so a review of liver function tests is important to evaluate for coagulopathy. Fresh-frozen plasma administration may be required preoperatively. Cardiomyopathy is likely to develop. Echocardiograms should be reviewed every 3 months in infants, followed by every 6 months in childhood years, and annually from adolescence and thereafter.

GSD TYPE V: MUSCLE GLYCOGEN PHOSPHORYLASE DEFICIENCY, MCARDLE DISEASE

Clinical presentation and systems affected

Prevalence is 1:100,000 to 1:170,000.[7,8] Metabolic myopathy causes exercise intolerance with rapid fatigue and cramping in exercising muscles and an improvement after a brief period of rest. Onset in the first decade is common with up to 25% of affected individuals developing fixed muscle weakness, particularly of proximal muscle groups. Acute renal failure related to recurrent episodes of myoglobinuria may develop in up to 50% of affected patients.

Basic treatment

Treatment includes a consistent exercise program to increase cardiorespiratory fitness and muscle oxidative capacity. Ingestion of simple carbohydrates, such as in sports drinks, prior to exercise can improve tolerance and protect against rhabdomyolysis.

Confirming diagnosis

Lab findings of elevated resting serum creatinine kinase activity is suggestive; gene testing for variants of PYGM (encoding glycogen phosphorylase, muscle form) is definitive, but assay of myophosphorylase enzyme activity can confirm the diagnosis if genetic tests are unclear.

Anesthetic considerations

General anesthesia may cause acute muscle damage, related to use of muscle relaxants and inhaled anesthetics. This is a rare occurrence in practice but practitioners should try to prevent muscle ischemia.

GSD TYPE VI: HERS DISEASE, HEPATIC GLYCOGEN PHOSPHORYLASE DEFICIENCY

Clinical presentation and systems affected

Types VI and IX are phenotypically indistinguishable, and together they account for 25% to 30% of all GSDs. Prevalence is estimated at 1:100,000 for both together, with type IX being more common.[9] If untreated, it presents in childhood with hepatomegaly and ketotic hypoglycemia after overnight fasting, or mild hypoglycemia with prolonged fasting as in illness. The disease is usually mild, with diagnosis in infancy or childhood, but it can demonstrate severe and recurrent hypoglycemia with severe hepatomegaly.

Signs and symptoms resolve with age, with most adults being completely asymptomatic.

Basic treatment

Small frequent meals and uncooked cornstarch 1 to 3 times/day can help normalize blood glucose and prevent ketosis. Pre-bedtime cornstarch administration can improve overall energy in patients with subclinical glucose swings. Excessive simple sugars should be avoided, and glucagon administration is an effective rescue therapy for hypoglycemia.

Confirming diagnosis

Molecular genetic testing for the PYGL gene (the only gene with pathogenic variants related to GSD VI) is preferred due to false negatives when glycogen phosphorylase enzyme activity is tested in erythrocytes/leukocytes or liver cells.

Anesthetic considerations

During surgical procedures, the patient's blood glucose needs monitoring especially during prolonged fasts/anesthetics. Exogenous glucose may need to be given.

GSD TYPE VII: TARUI DISEASE, PHOSPHOFRUCTOKINASE DEFICIENCY

Clinical presentation and systems affected

There are rare reports of type VII, which is more prevalent in the Ashkenazi Jewish population.[10,11] The classic form presents with exercise intolerance, muscle cramps and pain. After intense physical exercise, patients may experience nausea and vomiting, as well as jaundice with elevated creatinine kinase, hyperuricemia, reticulocytosis, and increased serum bilirubin. The late-onset form presents with cramps and myalgias in later life with mild muscle weakness in the 5th decade, progressing to severe disability. The infantile form is associated with hypotonia ("floppy babies"), and patients die in their first year of life, with arthrogryposis and mental retardation. The hemolytic form presents with hereditary non-spherocytic hemolytic anemia without muscle symptoms.

Basic treatment

Patients should avoid meals rich in carbohydrates prior to exercise (tolerance is worsened related to glucose inhibiting lipolysis) and avoid strenuous exercise; glucose infusions will not be effective at improving exercise tolerance, and may induce exertional fatigue. Patients should also avoid statins, due to concern for statin induced myositis.

Confirming diagnosis

Genetic testing and enzyme tests for PFK activity is required to confirm diagnosis, which is absent in muscle biopsies.

Anesthetic considerations

Patients may be anemic with increased hemolysis, particularly in the hemolytic form.

GSD TYPE VIII: PHOSPHORYLASE B KINASE DEFICIENCY

Clinical presentation and systems affected

There are rare reports of Type VIII in the literature.[12–14] Older literature cites primarily central nervous system involvement and mental retardation while more recent literature states the most common presentation in childhood or adolescence is exercise intolerance and cramps and weakness of exercising muscles. There is one recent case report of mild cognitive impairment as the only clinical feature.

Basic treatment

No specific treatments are noted in the literature but the usual recommendations for maintenance of euglycemia should be considered.

Confirming diagnosis

Classically, diagnosis comes from detection of giant glycogen particles in axon cylinders and synaptic vesicles in biopsy specimens. Genetic testing with mutation in the PHKA1 gene can be performed.

Anesthetic considerations

No specific considerations are noted in the literature but the usual recommendations for surveillance and prevention of hypoglycemia and caution with neuromuscular blockade should be considered.

GSD TYPE IX: PHOSPHOPHORYLASE KINASE DEFICIENCY

Clinical presentation and systems affected

Prevalence is 1:100,000.[14–17] This form has several subtypes (depending on the subunit affected by a mutation) that are inherited either as autosomal recessive or X-linked recessive. The range of clinical symptoms is variable with hepatomegaly and fasting hypoglycemia. The most seriously affected patients may have delayed motor and mental development, but the majority of patients are normal. Short stature may be present in some individuals.

Basic treatment

Uncooked cornstarch with a high-protein supplement may be helpful in some patients. Treat hypoglycemia or ketosis with oral fruit juice or IV glucose. Symptoms usually improve with age.

Confirming diagnosis

Diagnosis can come from enzyme testing with a deficiency but not an absence of phosphorylase kinase. Liver biopsy can be helpful. Molecular genetic testing for specific genes is advocated.

Anesthetic considerations

No specific recommendations are noted in the literature but practitioners should consider the usual concerns for surveillance and prevention of hypoglycemia.

GSD TYPES X, XI, XII, XIII: PHOSPHOGLYCERATE MUTASE DEFICIENCY (GSD X), LACTATE DEHYDROGENASE DEFICIENCY (GSD XI), ALDOLASE A DEFICIENCY (GSD XII), B-ENOLASE DEFICIENCY (GSD XIII)

Clinical presentation and systems affected

Prevalence is unknown.[11] Presentation includes some combination of myalgias, exercise intolerance, myoglobinuria, increased creatinine kinase values, and rhabdomyolysis that occurs after strenuous exercise.

Basic treatment

See type V recommendations.

Confirming diagnosis

Diagnosis is confirmed through genetic testing. Enzyme activities will be very low (2%–11%).

Anesthetic considerations

No specific considerations are noted in the literature but practitioners should use caution with neuromuscular blockade and engage in careful monitoring of renal function.

REVIEW QUESTIONS

1. You are evaluating a child in a preoperative clinic who was recently diagnosed with a GSD. His mother cannot remember which type. However, she does confirm frequent nosebleeds and has been referred by genetics to the hematology clinic. Which of the following GSD does the child **MOST** likely have?[2,18,19]

    A. type I
    B. type II
    C. type III
    D. type IV

Answer: A

Frequent nosebleeds are often an indicator of bleeding disorders. GSD type I is associated with impaired platelet function and/or acquired Von Willebrand-like disease. Type I can present with frequent nosebleeds, easy bruising, menorrhagia, and increased surgical bleeding. Consequently, patients may also be anemic.

The degree of platelet function impairment correlates with the degree of dyslipidemia. Platelet count and platelet function should be assessed prior to surgery. Platelet function can be improved with DDAVP or intensive glucose therapy. Neuraxial anesthesia can be considered, as there have been successful case reports of epidural and spinal anesthesia performed without complications.

Of note, there are two types of GSD type 1: type 1a and type 1b. Severe anemia is associated with hepatic adenomas in patients with GSD type 1a, while GSD type 1b patients with severe anemia often have enterocolitis.

Type II, III, and IV are not associated with bleeding diathesis.

2. Which of the following GSD is **LEAST** likely to be associated with cardiomyopathy?[2,3,5,6]

    A. type I
    B. type II
    C. type III
    D. type IV

Answer: A

Cardiomyopathy is associated with GSD type II, III, IV, and VII (infantile) but not type I.

Type I typically presents during infancy with hepatomegaly, lactic acidosis, hyperuricemia, hypercholesterolemia, and hypoglycemic seizures. Due to the enzymatic defect in either glucose-6-phosphatase or glucose-6-phosphate translocase, glycogen and fat accumulation results in hepatomegaly and renomegaly but not cardiomegaly. However, atherosclerotic disease and pulmonary arterial hypertension may be present in GSD type I. Close metabolic control may reduce the risk of atherosclerotic disease. Periodic screening echocardiography should be performed to assess for pulmonary artery hypertension.

GSD type II has two variants, classic infantile-onset Pompe disease and late-onset juvenile and adult Pompe disease. GSD type II infantile Pompe disease often presents with cardiomegaly, cardiomyopathy, left ventricular hypertrophy, and hypotonia. Cardiomyopathy, due to left ventricular septal hypertrophy, often presents by 2 to 3 months of age. If left untreated, left ventricular septal hypertrophy can cause outflow obstruction and result in death within the first year of life. GSD type II late-onset juvenile and adult Pompe disease typically exhibit minimal cardiac involvement. Type II late-onset juvenile and adult Pompe disease are associated with greater skeletal involvement.

GSD type III can present with hypertrophic cardiomyopathy, beginning in childhood. Other forms of cardiac dysfunction include congestive heart failure and sudden cardiac death. Periodic electrocardiogram and echocardiogram should be performed. Both skeletal and cardiac myopathies can improve with a high-protein, low-carbohydrate diet.

GSD type IV, also known as Andersen disease, is further subdivided into five subtypes. Three subtypes, the congenital neuromuscular, the classic hepatic, and the childhood neuromuscular subtype, can present with cardiomyopathy. Routine echocardiograms are required.

3. Which of the following GSD is **MOST** likely to affect males more than females?[15,16]

    A. type I
    B. type IV
    C. type VI
    D. type IX

Answer: D

The following lists the genetic inheritance of the GSD types:

Type I: Autosomal recessive

Type IV: Autosomal recessive

Type VI: Autosomal recessive

Type IX: 75% X-linked recessive, 25% autosomal recessive

4. Which type of GSD is **MOST** likely to be associated with decreased fetal movement and arthrogryposis?[2,5,20]

    A. type I
    B. type III
    C. type VII
    D. type IX

Answer: C

GSD type VII, also known as Tarui disease, has two subtypes: the infantile form and the late-onset form. The infantile form can present with severe cardiomyopathy, arthrogryposis, and severe myopathy.[5]

Type III and type IX can present with hypotonia and muscle weakness but are not associated with arthrogryposis. Type I is not associated with hypotonia, muscle weakness, or arthrogryposis.

5. Your patient was diagnosed with GSD after he developed dark red urine following a high school track meet. What type of GSD does he **MOST** likely have?[5,6,8,9]

    A. type III
    B. type IV
    C. type V
    D. type VI

Answer: C

Dark red urine in this situation is due to myoglobinuria. GSD type V, also known as McArdle syndrome, results in an accumulation of glycogen in muscle (skeletal and cardiac), resulting in myopathy. Intense exercise can cause stiffness, pain, muscle cramping, and elevated creatinine kinase levels due to myopathy. Simple carbohydrates prior to intense exercise have been shown to reduce the risk of exercise-induced rhabdomyopathy.

Type III can present with muscle weakness and muscle wasting, but it is not associated with myoglobinuria.

Type IV can result in an accumulation of abnormally branched glycogen in muscle. Muscle atrophy is often present, but myoglobinuria from muscle breakdown is not present during moments of intense exercise.

Type VI, also known as Hers disease, can present with muscle hypotonia and fatigue with exercise but will not result in myoglobinuria.

6. Which of the following cardiac findings is **LEAST** likely in a patient with GSD type II?[2,3]

    A. cardiomyopathy in infancy
    B. pulmonary hypertension
    C. septal hypertrophy with left ventricle (LV) outflow obstruction
    D. T-wave inversions, wide QRS and short PR interval

Answer: B
GSD type II is associated with cardiomyopathy causing septal hypertrophy. Electrocardiogram findings are consistent with LV hypertrophy. Periodic echocardiograms are required to assess for possible LV outflow obstruction.

Pulmonary hypertension is not related to GSD type II. Pulmonary hypertension can be seen with GSD type I.

7. Which of the following GSD is clinically **MOST** similar to von Gierke's but shows significant symptoms improvement after adolescence?[5,6,8,20]

    A. type III
    B. type IV
    C. type VI
    D. type VII

Answer: A
Von Gierke's GSD, also known as type Ia, is characterized by hepatomegaly and renomegaly due to glycogen and fat accumulation in the liver and kidneys. Type Ia also presents with doll-like facies, short stature, hypoglycemia, platelet dysfunction, and anemia.

GSD type III can present like type I but with marked clinical variability. Often, clinical presentation will improve after puberty.

8. An anesthesiologist can be the **LEAST** concerned about perioperative glucose monitoring in which of the following type of GSD?[20]

    A. type 0
    B. type Ia
    C. type II
    D. type IV

Answer: C
Types 0, 1a, and IV can present with hypoglycemia secondary to enzymatic defects in accessing glycogen stores.

9. In which of the following GSDs should succinylcholine be used with the **MOST** caution?[20]

    A. type 0
    B. type Ia
    C. type III
    D. type VII

Answer: C
GSD types II, III, IV, and V are associated with hypotonia, muscle weakness, and muscle atrophy. Succinylcholine should be used with caution in these patients due to concerns for acetylcholine receptor upregulation and resultant life-threatening hyperkalemia after succinylcholine exposure.[20]

GSD types 0, Ia, and VII are not associated with muscle wasting.

10. Of the following GSDs, which has the **STRONGEST** contraindication against the use of propofol?[19,21]

    A. type 0
    B. type Ib
    C. type III
    D. type V

Answer: B
There have been case reports of patients developing postoperative pancreatitis when propofol was used. Given the degree of hyperlipidemia, it has been postulated that propofol's lipid emulsion can cause propofol-induced hypertriglyceridemia and precipitate acute pancreatitis in GSD type I patients. Propofol should be used with caution in patients with GSD type I. Propofol may also alter uric acid metabolism and may increase urinary acid excretion in GSD type Ia and type Ib.

QUESTIONS AND ANSWERS

This chapter has accompanying questions and answers which are available to subscribers as part of the Oxford eLearning platform. To access the questions, go to ✔ http://oxfordmedicine.com/pediatricanesthesiaPBL

REFERENCES

1. Craigen WJ, Firth HV, Deputy D, TePas E. Liver glycogen synthase deficiency (glycogen storage disease 0), Wolters Kluwer, UpToDate, www.uptodate.com, last updated Mar 14, 2017.
2. Bali DS, Chen YT, Austin S, Goldstein JL. Glycogen storage disease type I. In: Pagon RA, Adam MP, Ardinger HH, et al., eds. *GeneReviews(R)*. Seattle: University of Washington; 1993.
3. Lesli N, Tinkle BT. Glycogen Storage Disease type II (Pompe Disease) 2007 Aug 31 [Updated 2013 May 9] In: Pagon R, Adam M, Bird T, et al., eds. *GeneReviews®[internet]*. Seattle: University of Washington; 2013.
4. Al Atassi A, Al Zughaibi N, Naeim A, Al Basha A, Dimitriou V. Anesthesia management in an infant with glycogen storage disease type II (Pompe disease). *Middle East J Anaesthesiol*. 2015;23(3):343–346.
5. Dagli A, Sentner CP, Weinstein DA. Glycogen storage disease type III. In: Pagon RA, Adam MP, Ardinger HH, et al., eds. *GeneReviews(R)*. Seattle: University of Washington; 1993.
6. Magoulas PL, El-Hattab AW. Glycogen storage disease type IV. In: Pagon RA, Adam MP, Ardinger HH, et al., eds. *GeneReviews(R)*. Seattle: University of Washington; 1993.
7. Bollig G. McArdle's disease (glycogen storage disease type V) and anesthesia—a case report and review of the literature. *Pediatr Anesth*. 2013;23(9):817–823.

8. Martin MA, Lucia A, Arenas J, Andreu AL. Glycogen storage disease type V. In: Pagon RA, Adam MP, Ardinger HH, et al., eds. *GeneReviews(R)*. Seattle: University of Washington; 1993.

9. Dagli AI, Weinstein DA. Glycogen storage disease type VI. In: Pagon RA, Adam MP, Ardinger HH, et al., eds. *GeneReviews(R)*. Seattle: University of Washington; 1993.

10. Nakajima H, Raben N, Hamaguchi T, Yamasaki T. Phosphofructokinase deficiency; past, present and future. *Curr Mol Med*. 2002;2(2):197–212.

11. Toscano A, Musumeci O. Tarui disease and distal glycogenoses: clinical and genetic update. *Acta Myologica*. 2007;26(2):105–107.

12. Echaniz-Laguna A, Akman HO, Mohr M, et al. Muscle phosphorylase b kinase deficiency revisited. *Neuromusc Dis*. 20(2):125–127.

13. Kornfeld M, LeBaron M. Glycogenosis type VIII. *J Neuropathol Exp Neurol*. 1984;43(6):568–579.

14. Mahler RF. Disorders of glycogen metabolism. *Clin Endocrinol Metab*. 1976;5(3):579–598.

15. Godfrey R, Quinlivan R. Skeletal muscle disorders of glycogenolysis and glycolysis. *Nat Rev Neurol*. 2016;12(7):393–402.

16. Goldstein J, Austin S, Kishnani P, Bali D. Phosphorylase kinase deficiency. In: Pagon RA, Adam MP, Ardinger HH, et al., eds. *GeneReviews(R)*. Seattle: University of Washington; 1993.

17. Roscher A, Patel J, Hewson S, et al. The natural history of glycogen storage disease types VI and IX: long-term outcome from the largest metabolic center in Canada. *Mol Genet Metab*. 2014;113(3):171–176.

18. Christian Erker MM. Anaesthesia recommendations for patients suffering from glycogen storage disease type I. Orphananesthesia; 2015. http://www.orphananesthesia.eu/en/rare-diseases/published-guidelines/doc_view/229-glycogen-storage-disease-type-i.html. Accessed May 27, 2017.

19. Kishnani PS, Austin SL, Abdenur JE, et al. Diagnosis and management of glycogen storage disease type I: a practice guideline of the American College of Medical Genetics and Genomics. *Genet Med*. 2014;16(11):e1.

20. Kliegman R, Stanton B, St. Geme JW, Schor NF, Behrman RE, Nelson WE. *Nelson Textbook of Pediatrics*. Philadelphia, PA: Saunders; 2016.

21. Bustamante SE, Appachi E. Acute pancreatitis after anesthesia with propofol in a child with glycogen storage disease type IA. *Paediatr Anaesth*. 2006;16(6):680–683.

49.

MUCOPOLYSACCHARIDOSES

Ashley Smith

STEM CASE AND KEY QUESTIONS

A 25-kg, 6-year-old male, with classic features of Hurler syndrome, presents for bilateral proximal femoral osteotomies.

WHAT ARE KEY COMPONENTS OF A PREOPERATIVE ASSESSMENT FOR A PATIENT WITH MUCOPOLYSACCHARIDOSIS (MPS) I?

Preoperative assessment for patients with Hurler syndrome involves review of recent patient testing and physical exam. Patients are frequently followed by a multidisciplinary team. Figure 49.1 shows the recommended testing schedule for patients with Hurler syndrome.

The patient has a history of snoring, and a previous sleep study showed mild obstructive sleep apnea (OSA), now status post-tonsillectomy and adenoidectomy (T&A) at age 5.

IS OSA VERY COMMON IN HURLER PATIENTS? HOW ABOUT POST-ADENOTONSILLECTOMY? WHAT IS THE WORKUP FOR OSA?

The pediatrician has suggested another sleep study since there has been clinical signs of sleep-disordered breathing (i.e., snoring). Parents have not yet returned to the sleep lab. They also do not know if patient would comply with continuous positive airway pressure (CPAP).

The anesthetic chart from previous T&A noted a grade 3 airway with direct laryngoscopy with a Miller 2 blade.

On physical exam, the patient shows moderate developmental delay and shortened height. The patient will not fully comply with a Mallampati exam but does have an enlarged tongue, limited mouth opening, thick neck, and moderate kyphosis.

IS AN ECHOCARDIOGRAM NECESSARY TO PROCEED WITH GENERAL ANESTHESIA?

Cardiac examination shows regular rhythm and rate, with Grade III holosystolic murmur. An echocardiogram from 6 months ago shows normal ejection fraction, left ventricle hypertrophy, and thickened mitral valve with regurgitation. On auscultation of chest, patient has decreased chest sound in bilateral bases and noisy transmitted upper airway sounds.

He is currently on enzyme replacement therapy medication, laronidase.

A discussion was held with the orthopedic surgeon on whether to consider placement of an epidural for postoperative pain management.

WOULD NEURAXIAL ANESTHESIA BE A GOOD OPTION FOR THIS PATIENT OR ONE WITH ANY TYPE OF MPS?

There have been case reports of paralysis after combined general and neuraxial anesthesia in a patient with Hurler syndrome as well as several documented cases of spinal cord infarction after combined technique in patients with Morquio syndrome.[1-3] All three case episodes occurred with an orthopedic lower extremity surgery. It is postulated that areas of kyphoscoliosis and cord narrowing mixed with blood loss and low mean arterial pressures result in cord ischemia.[4] Neuraxial anesthesia led to significant delay in discovering the weakness postoperatively. These cases were reported to WakeUp Safe, which then made the recommendation to avoid epidurals or neuraxial blocks in patients with MPS. It is also recommended to obtain an x-ray or magnetic resonance imaging in all patients with kyphosis, as well as to consider intraoperative neuromonitoring for patients with long non-spine procedures. Careful positioning of kyphotic patients and special attention to blood loss and maintaining spinal cord perfusion is paramount to avoid such complications.[5] Finally, there has been a case report of a failed epidural in one patient with Hurler syndrome, postulated to be secondary to glycosaminoglycan (GAG) deposition around the epidural space preventing local anesthetic effect.[6] Both of these considerations should be taken into account before deciding to proceed with neuraxial analgesia.

The patient proceeded with uneventful mask induction. Visualization with direct laryngoscopy revealed an airway of grade 4.

CAN THE AIRWAY EXAM CHANGE WITH TIME IN HURLER PATIENTS?

Placement of a laryngeal mask airway (LMA) is done atraumatically and a fiberoptic is called into the room. The airway is then secured.

	Every 6 month	Every year	Every other year
General physical exam	x		
Neurologic			
CT or MRI Brain			x
MRI spine			x
Median nerve EMG			x
Cognitive testing		x	
Audiometry		x	
Retinal/corneal exam		x	
Head circumference	x		
Respiratory			
Spirometry	x		
Sleep study		x	
Cardiac			
Echo			x
EKG			x
Skeletal Survey			x
Gastrointestinal			
Spleen/liver volume			x
Urinary Glycosaminoglycan level (in those on ERT)	x		

Fig. 49.1 Recommended assessment of patients with MPS I. From Scott HS, Bunge S, Gal A, Clarke LA, Morris CP, Hopwood JJ. Molecular genetics of mucopolysaccharidosis type I: diagnostic, clinical, and biological implications. *Hum Mutat*.1995;6(4):288–302.

HOW COMMON IS A DIFFICULT AIRWAY IN A PATIENT WITH MPS I? CAN THE DIFFICULT AIRWAY ALGORITHM BE APPLIED TO HURLER PATIENTS?

Despite the advances in treatment for MPS I, anesthetic and airway management can still be difficult. In the age of hematopoietic stem cell transplantation (HSCT) and enzyme replacement therapy (ERT), the incidence of difficult airway is still being studied. Before these treatments were available, incidence of difficult airway was as high 25% in children in all forms of MPS, with overall failed intubation rate at 8%, a difficult airway rate of 54%, and a failed intubation rate of 23% in MPS I.[7] A more recent study after initiation of HSCT and ERT has shown a decrease in numbers of patients with difficult airway for Hurler syndrome (12%) but maintained higher numbers for Hunter syndrome patients (35%)[7]. Recent anesthetic records of successful direct laryngoscopy can be of some use, but caution should be used as changes to airway structure can be dramatic in short time frames. Pediatric mask fit can be challenging because of abnormal facies. Increased oral secretions may warrant anticholinergic premedication. Cervical spine precautions should be observed secondary to prevalence of atlantoaxial instability. Direct laryngoscopy increases in difficulty with age. Oral airways can increase airway obstruction by moving the epiglottis downward into the larynx. Nasal airways may be useful; however, they may not be successfully passed secondary to dense tissue. All of these components can make a "cannot intubate" situation even worse if it evolves into a "cannot mask ventilate" emergency. Children with MPS I also have distorted anatomy and thickened tissues, making rescue cricothyroidotomy, retrograde intubation, or emergency tracheostomy for an airway emergency very difficult[8,9,10]. Furthermore, in many MPS I patients it is not feasible to perform an awake fiberoptic intubation secondary to age and developmental delay. Laryngeal mask airways, videolaryngoscopes, and fiberoptic techniques have been utilized for intubation.[8,11,12] Fiberoptic intubation *through* a supraglottic device can be attempted, and occasionally LMA alone can be used for the entirety of a case if seated well and appropriate for the type of case.

The difficult airway algorithm can and should be used, with the knowledge that awake intubation pathway is not always feasible and that surgical airway access pathway will not be timely in an airway emergency.

The case completes. The surgeon asks you if this patient needs the intensive care unit (ICU).

DOES THIS PATIENT NEED AN ICU FOR POSTOPERATIVE MONITORING?

Since the degree of sleep-disordered breathing or OSA is unknown, it may be advisable to place the patient in the ICU, especially for postoperative pain management.

DISCUSSION

MPS I can occur across all ethnicities, and the incidence is 1 in 100,000 live births.[13] Of those diagnosed with MPS I, an estimated 50% to 80% have the severe phenotype.[14] This severity of disease may reflect an ascertainment bias, as the severe phenotype is typically diagnosed earlier than milder forms. Diagnostic delay frequently occurs for MPS I patients because of the heterogeneity of symptoms that occurs. Severe MPS I initial symptoms include dysmorphic facies, progressive skeletal deformities, frequent respiratory infections, and enlarged head circumference. Hurler syndrome can be diagnosed with urinary GAG levels, which is sensitive but not specific for MPS I. Definitive diagnosis can be done by identifying deficient a-L-iduronidase activity on serum assay.

Treatments for different types of MPS are based on the enzyme that is deficient in each type (Table 49.1). Hurler and Hunter syndromes can be treated with palliative care, ERT, or HSCT from cord blood or bone marrow. ERT for Hurler syndrome replaces the enzyme alpha-L-Iduronidase, known as laronidase, and Hunter ERT treatment involves idursulfase to replace iduronate sulfatase. ERT is given as infusions for the entirety of a patient's life. Neither of these ERTs crosses the blood brain barrier, and so cognitive changes can continue.

HSCT works by replacing enzyme-deficient macrophages with donor macrophages that have working enzymes. Working macrophages then travel to distance sites with GAG buildup. Timing is very important in the consideration of HSCT. Treatment before cognitive delay starts results in the best clinical outcome.[15] A developmental quotient of greater than 70 and age less than 2 results in the best outcomes with HSCT for patients with Hurler syndrome.[14] HSCT has improved with time, and in one large retrospective analysis the mortality rate was 15% and survival with intact engraftment was 56%.[16] While HSCT for Hurler syndrome is not curative, it does attenuate cardiac disease, decreases airway obstruction, and increases life expectancy.[15] Neurologic outcomes are variable. Importantly, heart failure and tachycardia has been shown to improve 1 year after successful HSCT, and improvement in myocardia function and coronary artery patency has been shown for 14 years after engraftment.[15] HSCT for Hunter syndrome is more controversial and studies are ongoing, as it does not appear to attenuate neurodegeneration at all. As improvements are continuously made to HSCT, these treatments are being attempted more frequently for other types of MPS.

Therapy with ERT while preparing for HSCT can be utilized and has been shown to improve mortality and engraftment rates. ERT is used as bridge to HSCT and is typically discontinued afterward if full engraftment takes place. ERT can be continued if there is unsuccessful HSCT.

The difficulty of intubation and mask ventilation that occurs in patients with MPS I was described before treatment with either HSCT or ERT was developed. With improvement in detecting patients with MPS I, earlier initiation of HSCT and ERT, as well as improvement in HSCT as a treatment, it has been postulated that patients with Hurler syndrome should not have as high an anesthetic airway risk as in the past. Advanced airway tools have also improved outcome for difficult airway management in the same time frame as these treatments. Several studies have subsequently looked at anesthetic complications in patients who had undergone treatment.[9,12,13] Frawley et al. found a decrease in airway difficulty in patients with MPS I who had undergone HSCT at an early age. Kirkpatrick et al. found that patients treated with HSCT had a much lower incidence of airway complications, at 14%, with no episodes of failed intubations. This study found that failed intubations occurred in patients who only received ERT, and these were in other types of MPS, not MPS I. Kirkpatrick et al.'s study also found that their practice included an inhalation induction, spontaneous respiration during induction, use of a planned fiberoptic intubation, and possible use of LMA. This planning and use of difficult airway equipment could also contribute to the change in complication rate compared to studies conducted in the 1990s. Anesthetic risk can be increased in all types of MPS, secondary to difficult airway or cardiac disease, and is summarized in Table 49.1.

In HSCT, the largest component of morbidity is failure to achieve complete engraftment as well as the development of graft versus host disease. Patients can also be susceptible to pulmonary hemorrhage after treatment.[15] Patients receiving ERT require frequent intravenous (IV) dosing of the medication, typically every 1 to 2 weeks for life. The most common side effects of ERT include IgG-mediated hypersensitivity reactions characterized by flushing, headache, fever, and urticaria. Symptoms are concurrent with infusion and can be ameliorated by slowing the infusion rate or pretreating the patient with antihistamines and prednisone. More serious IgE anaphylaxis reaction can occur with any of the ERT treatments,[17] and, because treatment is essential, patients may undergo desensitization protocols to continue treatment despite their reactions.[18] IgE anaphylaxis can be devastating to MPS patients who may already have a compromised airway;

rapid lip and mucosal swelling combined with narrowed larynx, baseline obstructed airway, and restrictive airway disease results in very rapid respiratory failure. Treatment of anaphylaxis includes rapid recognition and treatment with epinephrine, securing a difficult airway, and continuing treatment with prednisone and H1 and H2 blocker. In phase 3 of the clinical trial of laronidase, one patient developed anaphylaxis that required tracheostomy.[14] IgG antibodies occur in up to 90% of patients treated with laronidase in the first several months of treatment.[19] It is postulated these antibodies can decrease the efficacy of GAG clearing from effected tissues; however, further research is ongoing as to the clinical impact of this change.[18]

MPS share several features; however, some characteristics are more common in one syndrome than another. The following is a summary of shared and unique characteristics based on organ system.

RESPIRATORY COMPLICATIONS

Patients with MPS may have coarse facial features, gingival hyperplasia, and dental changes. They may also have large swollen tongues and enlarged tonsils, adenoids, and floppy long epiglottises. All of these changes in the upper airways may lead to difficult mask ventilation or airway obstruction with even mild sedation.

Patients can be particularly susceptible to recurrent pneumonias. This combined with kyphoscoliosis can over time cause restrictive lung disease. They can also have obstructive and central sleep apnea. Patients may present with tracheobronchomalacia, otitis media, laryngitis, and tonsillitis.

CARDIAC COMPLICATIONS

Cardiac disease can include valvulopathy, more commonly mitral and aortic, ventricular hypertrophy, systolic and/or diastolic dysfunction, conduction abnormalities, and coronary artery disease.[20,21] Hurler, Hunter, and Morquio patients are prone to develop valvulopathy. Conduction abnormalities and arrhythmias can develop in Hunter, Hurler, and Maroteaux-Lamy patients. Cardiac complications occur earlier and are more severe in MPS I, II, and VI and appear to be linked to those syndromes that involve metabolism of dermatan sulfate. Chronic pulmonary disease can lead to right ventricular dysfunction and heart failure in all types of MPS.

Cardiac complications can develop silently, usually at young ages, and can contribute to significant mortality. Because patients with MPS I cannot endorse typical features of exercise intolerance, such as chest pain with stair climbing, it can be difficult to assess a decrease in cardiac capacity that warrants angiography. An echocardiogram and electrocardiogram are recommended every other year even in asymptomatic children;[14] however, there is no consensus for the optimal technique to assess coronary artery involvement.[21] Coronary artery disease occurs most frequently in MPS I and II and is caused by deposition of GAGs within the intima of large epicardial arteries. MPS I and II patients

Table 49.1 CHARACTERISTICS OF MPS TYPES

TYPE	SYNDROME NAME	GAGS INCREASED	ENZYME DEFICIENCY	INHERITANCE	KEY CLINICAL FEATURES	ENT/AIRWAY MANIFESTATIONS	TREATMENT	ANESTHETIC RISK[3,9]
MPS I H	Hurler	HS +DS	alpha-L iduronidase	AR	Course facial features, severe developmental delay, corneal clouding, heart valve disease, atlantoaxial instability	Sleep apnea, recurrent URI, otitis media, adenotonsillar hypertrophy, sensorineural hearing loss, difficult airway that increases over time	ERT with Laronidase, HSCT for severe disease	Very high
MPS I H/S	Hurler Scheie				Intermediate phenotype			High
MPS I S (used to be MPS V)	Scheie				Least severe, can be diagnosed in adulthood, normal intelligence			Mildly high
MPS II	Hunter	HS +DS	Iduronate sulfatase	X-linked recessive	Severe course, similar to MPS I; milder course, later manifestation; mild phenotype, survival to adulthood without developmental delay	Otitis media, adenotonsillar hypertrophy, sensorineural hearing loss, difficult airway that increases over time	ERT with Idursulfase Possible HSCT	High
MPS III A	Sanfilippo A	HS	Heparan-N-sulfatase	AR	Clinically indistinguishable from one another, severe neurodegeneration, behavior problems, aggression	Otitis media, adenotonsillar hypertrophy, can have difficult airway with age but low risk	Possible intrathecal enzyme therapy in future	Generally, not increased
MPS III B	Sanfilippo B		a-N-acetylglucosaminidase					
MPS III C	Sanfilippo C		AcetylCoA a-glucosamine acetyltransferase					
MPS III D	Sanfilippo D		N-acetylglucosamine 6-sulfatase					
MPS IV A	Morquio A	KS	Galactosamine 6-sulfate sulfatase	AR	Skeletal dysplasia, joint laxity, spondyloepiphyseal dysplasia, short stature final height <125 cm, heart valve disease, atlantoaxial instability, normal intelligence	Otitis media, adenotonsillar hypertrophy	ERT with Elosulfase alfa	Very high
MPS IV B	Morquio B		B-galactosidase		Same as MPS IV A, final height >125 cm		NA	
MPS VI	Maroteaux-Lamy	DS	N-acetylgalactamine 4-sulfatase	AR	Hurler facies, corneal clouding, Normal intelligence	Otitis media, adenotonsillar hypertrophy, progressive diffuse airway narrowing	ERT with Galsulfase Possible HSCT	High
MPS VII	Sly	HS+DS	B-glucuronidase	AR	Similar variability in severity as Hurler, cardiac valve disease, short stature, unstable cervical spine	Otitis media, adenotonsillar hypertrophy	NA	High
MPS IX	Natowicz	Hyaluronan	Hyaluronidase 1	AR	Short stature, normal intelligence, painful joint swelling	NA	NA	Generally, not increased

Note. MPS = mucopolysaccharidosis; GAGs = glycosaminoglycans; ENT = ear, nose, throat; URI upper respiratory tract infection; HS = heparan sulfate; DS = dermatan sulfate; KS = keratin sulfate; AR = autosomal recessive; HSCT = hematopoietic stem cell transplantation; ERT = enzyme replacement therapy

may also have narrowing of the aorta, and systemic hypertension is common. Besides treatment with HSCT and ERT, many patients are treated for the underlying cardiac disease with common medications for heart failure and hypertension. They can undergo valve replacements, coronary artery bypass, and other surgical interventions to treat their heart disease. Anesthetic techniques must be tailored on a case-by-case basis.

ORTHOPEDIC COMPLICATIONS

Patients with MPS commonly have short stiff necks, with minimal ability to flex or extend. They may have full body joint stiffness, including the temporomandibular joint. The only MPS that instead presents with ligamentous laxity is Morquio A and B. There are many problems that can arise in the spine, including odontoid instability, atlantoaxial instability, kyphoscoliosis, and possible spinal cord compression. They can develop hip dysplasia and valgus/varus knees.

NEUROLOGIC COMPLICATIONS

Developmental delay occurs in most types of MPS. Mental retardation can be progressive in Hurler, the severe variant of Hunter syndrome, and Sly syndromes. Sanfilippo A syndrome patients can have aggressive behavior and sleep disorders as well as developmental delay. Sanfilippo B patients display progressive dementia. Notably, Morquio A and Maroteaux-Lamy syndrome patients are cognitively intact. All types can frequently have sensorineural hearing loss and blindness from corneal opacities or glaucoma. Patients may develop communicating hydrocephalus, particularly in Hurler, Hunter, and Sanfilippo A syndromes. Hunter and Hurler patients may also develop seizure disorders.

GASTROINTESTINAL COMPLICATIONS

Patients can have hepatosplenomegaly. Hurler and Hunter syndrome patients are particularly susceptible to umbilical and inguinal hernias.

SUMMARY

Children with MPS have significant airway and other organ system challenges that require careful preoperative assessment and intraoperative planning. Not all MPS patients represent the same anesthetic risk, and so knowing if a patient has received proper treatment as well as norms for the specific disease can aid in making anesthetic choices.

REVIEW QUESTIONS

1. A 3-year-old male with Hurler syndrome is scheduled for tonsillectomy under general anesthesia. Which of the following feature, of this syndrome, will **MOST** likely cause postoperative complication?

    A. joint hyperflexibility
    B. large glottic opening
    C. lower airway infections
    D. obstructive lung disease

Answer: C
Hurler's syndrome patients are at risk of obstructive sleep apnea,[2,3] postoperative complications due to underlying OSA, persistent upper and lower airway infections, and restrictive lung disease. They may present with a small glottis opening

due to increase in tissue from GAG deposition. They typically have immobile stiff joints instead of joint flexibility. Patients with Morquio syndrome present with joint laxity.[3]

2. A 16-month-old male presents with coarse facial features, progressive hydrocephalus, severe mixed sleep apnea, and recurring respiratory infections. He is found to have severe MPS II. Which of the following treatments will this patient **LEAST** likely receive?

    A. HSCT
    B. idursulfase, ERT
    C. laronidase, ERT
    D. quality of life improvement interventions

Answer: C
Hunter syndrome patients can be treated with palliative care, the enzyme replacement therapy Idursulfase, and possibly with HSCT. Laronidase is the ERT used to treat patients with MPS I or Hurler syndrome.

3. What is the **MOST** appropriate sleep study schedule for patients with severe MPS I, 2 years of age or older?

    A. every 6 months
    B. once symptomatic
    C. one time per year
    D. stop after T&A

Answer: C
Patients with MPS 1 should be monitored closely by a pulmonologist. Sleep studies are recommended to take place yearly in patients with severe MPS I after the age of 2 to 3.[2]

4. A 20 kg 4-year-old male presents to his in-hospital multidisciplinary clinic to receive his Laronidase infusion for MPS I. This is his third month of weekly infusions. He has not had any adverse effects in the past. Today, after 5 minutes of infusion he develops facial edema and stridor. A quick check shows a blood pressure of 80/45. Which of the following intravenous intervention is the **BEST** treatment for this patient?

    A. diphenhydramine 100 mg
    B. epinephrine 200 mcg
    C. famotidine 10 mg
    D. methylprednisone 100 mg

Answer: B
The first-line treatment of acute anaphylaxis is epinephrine as it acts to prevent mast cell degranulation and increases blood pressure. IV epinephrine can be given and titrated to effect, or intramuscular epinephrine (such as an EpiPen) can be used. IV methylprednisone should be dosed at 1 mg/kg for treatment of anaphylaxis to stop the histamine reaction. H1 and H2 blockers such as famotidine and diphenhydramine are also an appropriate adjunct to anaphylaxis, but they are not first-line drugs. Attempts to quickly secure the patient's airway if respiratory failure is impending is also essential.

5. A 10-year-old child with Morquio A syndrome has severe aortic regurgitation and pulmonary hypertension. Recent cardiac catheterization shows elevated pulmonary artery pressure that is two-thirds of systemic pressures. If this patient needed an anesthetic, which of the following conditions would

MOST likely lead to acute right ventricular failure, if not adequately managed intraoperatively?

A. alkalemia
B. awareness
C. hyperthermia
D. hypocarbia

Answer: B
Hypoxia, hypercapnia, acidosis/acidemia, hypothermia, atelectasis, and light anesthesia can lead to an acute pulmonary hypertensive crisis in patients with underlying pulmonary hypertension.

6. Which of the following cardiac abnormality is seen **MOST** often in mucopolysaccharidoses?

A. aortic insufficiency
B. ejection fraction reduction
C. left ventricular dilation
D. mitral regurgitation

Answer: D
In echocardiographic evaluations in patients aged 2 to 14 in with all types of MPS, left ventricular dilation and mitral stenosis was the least prevalent finding. Left valvular lesions, including mitral regurgitation, aortic valve thickening, and aortic regurgitation, as well pulmonary hypertension and obstructive sleep apnea, were the most common.[20]

7. Which of the following is the **MOST** appropriate treatment for a 7 y-year-old male 40-kg patient with Hunter syndrome with a history of snoring and an apnea hypopnea index (AHI) of 35 during polysomnography?

A. adenotonsillectomy
B. nighttime CPAP
C. tracheostomy
D. weight reduction

Answer: B
The AHI measures the number of episodes of apnea and hypopnea in 1 hour on polysomnography. Mild OSA has an AHI of 5 to 15 episodes an hour, Moderate OSA has an AHI of 15 to 30 per hour, and severe OSA has an AHI of >30 episodes per hour. Weight loss is unlikely to improve this patient's sleep apnea, as increased pharyngeal tissue from GAG deposits is the likely contributing issue. While T&A may help with some of the airway obstruction, CPAP at night is the definitive treatment for severe OSA and should be started immediately.

8. A 6-year-old female with Hurler Sheie syndrome presents for hiatal hernia repair. She requires CPAP at night for severe OSA. She has been diagnosed with significant gastroesophageal reflux disease (GERD), currently treated with omeprazole. Her most recent anesthetic was for an esophagogastroduodenoscopy and was completed using an LMA. Which of the following plans for induction of anesthesia would be the **LEAST** appropriate for this patient?

A. intubating LMA with fiberoptic scope
B. intubation without muscle relaxants
C. rapid sequence intubation
D. video-assisted laryngoscopy

Answer: C
Anticipation of a difficult airway is very important when taking care of any child with MPS. Spontaneous ventilation until there is assurance of an easy mask ventilation is vital to prevent a "cannot intubate" situation becoming a "cannot ventilate" emergency in patients known to be a difficult intubation. Despite the patient's underlying GERD and hiatal hernia, it would be safest to continue the patient's home omeprazole the day of surgery and avoid a rapid sequence intubation. Having advanced airway equipment, such as a video-assisted laryngoscopy or fiberoptic scope and intubating LMA, are important for a pediatric difficult airway, as awake fiberoptic intubations is not typically feasible.

9. Which MPS syndrome is the **SAFEST** to anesthetize?

A. Maroteaux-Lamy syndrome (MPS VI)
B. Morquio syndrome (MPS IV)
C. Sanfilippo syndrome (MPS III)
D. Sly syndrome (MPS VII)

Answer: C
Compared to other MPS syndromes, Sanfilippo syndrome has less systemic organ system involvement and more central nervous system impairment. Cognitive decline and behavior issues are a key clinical component, but difficult airway, neck instability, and other cardiac disease are uncommon. Patients with Sly syndrome have significant cervical spine and cardiac disease, placing them at greater anesthetic risk. Morquio and Maroteaux-Lamy syndrome patients can present with difficult airways as they age.

10. An 8-year-old male with a history of Hurler syndrome treated with ERT is scheduled for tympanoplasty. He is intubated after an inhalation induction and elective fiberoptic intubation through an intubating LMA. No direct laryngoscopy was attempted due to previous difficulty with this technique T&A at age 4. Although all reasonable, which of following preventative measures is **LEAST** advisable in a patient with Hurler syndrome?

A. decreasing endotracheal tube size to avoid postintubation croup
B. deep endotracheal extubation to prevent bucking and coughing
C. heightened vigilance for postobstructive pulmonary edema
D. ICU admission for postoperative monitoring

Answer: B
Patients with Hunter syndrome may need postoperative care in the ICU, especially if they have underlying OSA or restrictive lung disease. Initial downsizing of an endotracheal tube from the age-appropriate size is important to avoid airway edema postoperatively in these patients. A smaller tube may also be required secondary to a narrowed airway from GAG deposits. Postoperative pulmonary edema can occur after extubation due to underlying obstructive disease in these patients. Breathing forcefully against a closed glottis can lead to pulmonary edema. While it is important to avoid coughing and straining after

tympanoplasty, a patient with a difficult airway should not be extubated deep.

QUESTIONS AND ANSWERS

This chapter has accompanying questions and answers which are available to subscribers as part of the Oxford eLearning platform. To access the questions, go to ✓ http://oxfordmedicine. com/pediatricanesthesiaPBL

REFERENCES

1. Pruszczynski B, Mackenzie WG, Rogers K, White KK. Spinal cord injury after extremity surgery in children with thoracic kyphosis. *Clin Orthop Relat Res.* 2015;473(10):3315–3320.
2. Drummond JC, Krane EJ, Tomatsu S, Theroux MC, Lee RR. Paraplegia after epidural-general anesthesia in a Morquio patient with moderate thoracic spinal stenosis. *Can J Anaesth.* 2015;62(1):45–49.
3. Tong CK, Chen JC, Cochrane DD. Spinal cord infarction remote from maximal compression in a patient with Morquio syndrome. *J Neurosurg Pediatr.* 2012;9(6):608–612.
4. Farley CW, Curt BA, Pettigrew DB, Holtz JR, Dollin N, Kuntz C 4th. Spinal cord intramedullary pressure in thoracic kyphotic deformity: a cadaveric study. *Spine.* 2012;37(4):E224–E230.
5. Spinello CM, Novello LM, Pitino S, et al. Anesthetic management in mucopolysaccharidoses. *ISRN Anesthesiol.* 2013:791983. doi:10.1155/2013/791983
6. Vas L, Naregal F. Failed epidural anaesthesia in a patient with Hurler's disease. *Paediatr Anaesth.* 2000;10:95–98.
7. Walker RW, Darowski M, Morris P, et al. Anaesthesia and mucopolysaccharidoses: a review of airway problems in children. *Anaesthesia.* 1994;49:1078–1084.
8. Frawley G, Fuenzalida D, Donath S, et al. A retrospective audit of anesthetic techniques and complications in children with muccopolysaccharodoses. *Paediatr Anaesth.* 2012;22:737–744.
9. Seyedhejazi M, Sheikzadeh D, Sharabiani B. Cardiac arrest in a case of mucopolysaccharidosis after tracheostomy. *J Cardiovasc Thorac Res.* 2010;2:51–53.
10. Diaz JH, Belani KG. Perioperative management of children with Mucopolysaccharidosis. *Anesth Analg.* 1993;77:1261–1270.
11. Osthaus WA, Harendza T, Witt LH, et al. Pediatric airway management in mucopolysaccharidoses I: a retrospective case review. *Eur J Anesthesiol.* 2012;29:204–207.
12. Kirkpatrick K, Ellwood J, Walker RWM. Mucopolysaccharidosis type I (Hurler syndrome) and anesthesia: the impact of bone marrow transplantation, enzyme replacement therapy, and fiberoptic intubation on airway management. *Paediatr Anaesth.* 2012;22:745–751.
13. Scott HS, Bunge S, Gal A, Clarke LA, Morris CP, Hopwood JJ. Molecular genetics of mucopolysaccharidosis type I: diagnostic, clinical, and biological implications. *Hum Mutat.* 1995;6(4):288–302.
14. Muenzer J, Wraith J, Clarke L. Mucopolysaccharidosis I: management and treatment guidelines. *Pediatrics.* 2009;123(1):19–29. doi:10.1542/peds.2008-0416
15. Peters C, Steward CG. Hematopoietic cell transplantation for inherited metabolic diseases: an overview of outcomes and practice guidelines. *Bone Marrow Transplant.* 2003;31(4):229–239.
16. Boelens JJ, Wynn RF, O'Meara A, et al. Outcomes of hematopoietic stem cell transplantation for Hurler's syndrome in Europe: a risk factor analysis for graft failure. *Bone Marrow Transplant.* 2007;40(3):225–233.
17. Kim J, Park MR, Kim DS, et al. IgE-mediated anaphylaxis and allergic reactions to idursulfase in patients with Hunter syndrome. *Allergy.* 2013;68:796–802.
18. Giugliani R, Vieira TA, Carvalho CG, et al. Immune tolerance induction for laronidase treatment in muccopolysaccharidosis I. *Mol Genet Metab.* 2017;10:61–66.
19. Xuea Y, Richards SM, Mahmood A, Cox GF. Effect of anti-laronidase antibodies on efficacy and safety of laronidase enzyme replacement therapy for MPS I: A comprehensive meta-analysis of pooled data from multiple studies. *Mol Genet Metab.* 2016;117(4):419–426.
20. Leal GN, Paula AC, Leone C, Kim CA. Echocardiographic study of paediatric patients with mucopolysaccharidosis. *Cardiol Young.* 2010;20:254–261. doi:10.1017/S104795110999062X
21. Braunlin EA, Harmatz PR, Scarpa M, et al. Cardiac disease in patients with mucopolysaccardosis: presentation, diagnosis and management. *J inherit Metab Dis.* 2011;34:1183–1197.

SECTION 9

HEMATOLOGIC SYSTEM

50.

HEMOPHILIAS

Nicole M. Elsey

STEM CASE AND KEY QUESTIONS

A 17-year-old, 70.4-kg male with a history of severe hemophilia A presents to an outside hospital with severe abdominal pain for 24 hours associated with nausea, vomiting, and diarrhea. Physical exam demonstrated tenderness to palpation in the right lower abdominal quadrant with associated guarding; no masses were noted and there was no rebound or other concerning peritoneal signs noted. Labs obtained in the emergency department included the following: Na+ 139 mmol/L, K+ 4.1 mmol/L, Cl– 100 mmol/L, bicarb 27 mmol/L, BUN 7 mg/dL, Cr 0.83 mg/dL, U/A specific gravity 1.03 with negative leukocyte esterase and nitrites. A complete blood count showed a white blood count 11.2 K/mm³ (no bands, 72% segs), hemoglobin 14.9 g/dL, plt 276 K/mm³. Coagulation studies revealed a prothrombin time (PT) 13.7, international normalized ratio 1.02, activated partial thromboplastin time (aPTT) 63, and a fibrinogen level of 250.

WHAT ARE THE DIFFERENT TYPES OF HEMOPHILIA AND HOW ARE THEY DIAGNOSED?

A computed tomography scan of the abdomen demonstrated an enlarged appendix with adjacent inflammation, consistent with appendicitis without abscess or rupture. The patient was subsequently transferred to a pediatric institution for surgical and hematologic management.

WHAT ARE THE COMMON CLINICAL MANIFESTATIONS SEEN PRIOR TO A DIAGNOSIS OF HEMOPHILIA?

The patient was diagnosed with hemophilia A at 2 weeks of age after severe bleeding occurred during/after a circumcision. Since that time, he has had multiple bleeding episodes involving the hip, hands, shoulder, knee, ankle, and foot.

WHAT ARE THE DIFFERENT TREATMENT MODALITIES AVAILABLE FOR PATIENTS WITH HEMOPHILIA?

The patient's factor VIII levels are consistently less than 1%, with no identified inhibitors up to this point. Due to the severity of disease, the patient receives infusions at home of factor VIII (Advate, Baxalta US Inc, Westlake Village, CA, USA), 40 IU/kg on Monday, Wednesday, and Friday via a peripherally inserted central catheter. He had been doing well with his prophylaxis and has been self-administering his factor VIII at home. Prior to his arrival to the hospital, the patient denies any bruising or bleeding symptoms or blood in his urine or stool. After obtaining lab work and having a peripheral intravenous (IV) line started in the emergency department, the patient does note that they are unable to obtain hemostasis at the site of IV placement. Furthermore, the patient reported that he did not receive his usually scheduled factor VIII infusion on the day of presentation to the hospital.

HOW ARE PATIENTS WITH HEMOPHILIA MANAGED IN THE PREOPERATIVE SETTING?

Upon the patient's arrival to the emergency department, a hematology consult was obtained. Given the need for surgical management of acute appendicitis, the hematologist recommended a bolus dose of factor VIII (Advate), 50 IU/kg, to be given over 3 to 5 minutes, followed by the initiation of a continuous infusion of Advate at 5 IU/kg/hr. Immediately after initiating the continuous infusion, a factor VIII assay was to be obtained, with a goal factor VIII level of 80% to 100%.

HOW ARE PATIENTS WITH HEMOPHILIA MANAGED IN THE POSTOPERATIVE SETTING?

Factor VIII assay levels obtained immediately after the patient received a bolus dose were 102%. The patient was then cleared by hematology to proceed to the operating room to undergo a laparoscopic appendectomy. The surgical procedure and anesthetic proceeded without any complications. Postoperatively, the patient was managed by the hematology service. The Advate was maintained throughout postoperative day (POD) 1 at 5 IU/kg/hr. A repeat factor VIII assay level was obtained on the morning of POD 2 and was found to be 214% of normal. Based on this result, the continuous Advate infusion was decreased to 4 IU/kg/hr. Factor VIII assay levels on POD 3 and 4 were 92% and 83% of normal, respectively. On POD 4 the patient was given a bolus dose of Advate, 25 IU/kg, prior to discontinuing the continuous infusion. The bolus dosing was administered every 12 hours for 3 days, then changed to 50 IU/kg every day for 1 week before resuming his home prophylactic regimen of 40 IU/kg every Monday, Wednesday, and Friday.

DISCUSSION

The group of bleeding disorders classified as hemophilia, including hemophilias A, B, C, and acquired hemophilia A, are considered rare bleeding disorders. Hemophilia A (factor VIII) and B (factor IX) are sex-linked recessive disorders that almost exclusively affect males, although they can occur in homozygous females, with a reported prevalence of 1 in 5,000 and 1 in 30,000 live male births, respectively.[1,2] Hemophilia C (factor XI) is an inherited autosomal recessive disorder that primarily affects the Ashkenazi Jewish population, at an estimated frequency of 1 in 450 for the severe form of the disease and 1 in 11 for the heterozygous type.[2,3] Acquired hemophilia A occurs as a result of autoantibodies that develop against factor VIII and has an estimated incidence of 1.3 to 1.5 per million.[1] Hemophilia A is by far the most common form of the disorder, accounting for nearly 85% of the individuals diagnosed with a hemophilia, while hemophilias B and C represent 14% and 1% of the hemophiliac population, respectively.[4] Known family history of the disorder is a clinical indication for testing; however, nearly 30% of hemophiliac patients have no known family history of the disease.[4]

CLINICAL CHARACTERISTICS OF HEMOPHILIA

Individuals with hemophilia A present with varying degrees of bleeding episodes depending on the severity of the disease and level of factor VIII clotting activity. Any individual who presents with hemarthrosis, deep-muscle hematomas, intracranial hemorrhage (in a neonate or in the absence of significant head trauma), or prolonged bleeding/oozing from minor injury or surgeries should be suspected of and tested for a bleeding disorder. Patients with hemophilia A are classified as having a severe, moderate, or mild form of the disease. Table 50.1 provides a summary of the clinical characteristics of hemophilia A based on the disease severity.[5] The clinical

characteristics of hemophilia B are quite similar to those of hemophilia A. Hemophilia C, on the other hand, lacks the presence of soft tissue hematomas or hemarthrosis.

DIAGNOSIS OF HEMOPHILIA

Figure 50.1 provides an overview of the clotting cascade, including the intrinsic, extrinsic and common pathways. Clinical signs and symptoms concerning for a bleeding disorder or a known family history of a bleeding disorder would be an indication for workup and laboratory testing, especially in the surgical or perioperative setting. In assessing for hemophilia, the presence of a prolonged aPTT with a normal PT and normal bleeding time (BT) is suspicious for either hemophilia A or B. Further testing for specific factor assays would then demonstrate a deficiency of factor VIII coagulant activity in patients with hemophilia A or a deficiency of factory IX coagulant activity and factor concentration in the setting of hemophilia B.[2,4] A diagnosis of hemophilia C would occur with a prolonged aPTT, normal PT, normal BT, and a factor assay demonstrating a deficiency in factor XI levels.[2,4]

Activation of the clotting cascade occurs when tissue factor, a membrane-bound protein on the surface of fibroblasts found primarily in the extravascular tissue, is exposed to the vascular endothelium. Tissue factor then initiates a series of factor activations, beginning with factor VII. Each factor circulates as an inactive proenzyme, which becomes active by cleavage of a portion of the molecule. In each step of the coagulation pathway, the active form of the clotting factor will then interact with the next factor to initiate activation until the formation of thrombin (factor IIa) has occurred. Thrombin serves to amplify the coagulation process by way of 4 main functions including activation of adjacent platelets, activation of factor V, cleavage of the von Willebrand factor (vWF)–factor VIII complex to activate factor VIII, and activation of factor XIII.

Although the clotting cascade plays a substantial role in the successful development of hemostasis, it is important to remember that there are several cellular components that are also vital to the process. In the cellular model of coagulation, 3 stages (activation, amplification, and propagation) are

Table 50.1 **DISEASE SEVERITY CLASSIFICATION OF HEMOPHILIA A**

DISEASE SEVERITY	AGE OF DIAGNOSIS	CLINICAL SIGNS/SYMPTOMS	FACTOR VIII COAGULANT ACTIVITY LEVELS
Severe	Before age 2	Intracerebral hemorrhage, hemarthrosis, soft tissue hematomas, spontaneous hemorrhage, prolonged/excessive bleeding from MINOR injuries or procedures	<1%
Moderate	Before age 5–6	-Prolonged bleeding/oozing from MINOR trauma or surgery -RARELY experience spontaneous bleeding	1%–5%
Mild	Adolescent to adulthood	-Prolonged bleeding/oozing from MAJOR trauma or surgery -No spontaneous bleeding	6%–30%

Source. Konkle BA, Hutson H, Nakaya Fletcher S. Hemophilia A. In: Pagon, RA, Adam MP, Ardinger HH, et al., eds. *GeneReview*®. Seattle: University of Washington; 1993–2017. https://www.ncbi.nlm.nih.gov/books/NBK1404/

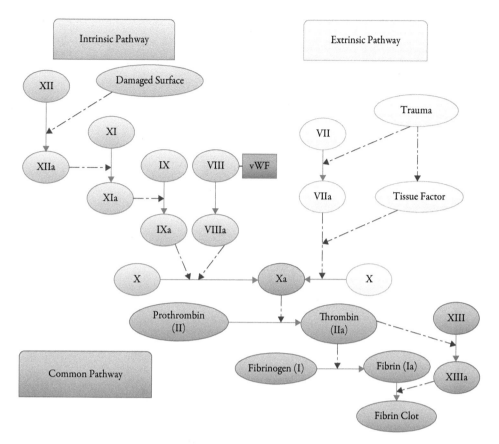

Fig. 50.1 Review of the clotting cascade.

combined to ultimately form a stable fibrin clot and achieve hemostasis. In this specific model, the activation phase focuses on the clotting cascade and the production of thrombin, which is the crucial component needed for amplification of the cascade and activation of platelet components needed for aggregation and adhesion.[2,4]

The formation of a clot and activation of the coagulation process are crucial to maintaining hemostasis in the event that an injury occurs with a resultant breach in the endothelial lining. However, there also has to be a mechanism in place that serves as a checks-and-balance system to prevent the extension of the clot beyond the site of injury. The vascular endothelium serves as the primary defense mechanism to prevent rampant extension of a clot through the synthesis of several products to inhibit coagulation and to control platelet aggregation and fibrinolysis. In addition to the regulatory properties provided by the vascular endothelium, there are several other coagulation-inhibition systems that serve to limit and localize clot formation. The 4 main antithrombotic mechanisms are depicted in Figure 50.2.

LABORATORY EVALUATION OF HEMOSTASIS

Laboratory testing mechanisms of hemostasis can be divided into 2 categories: those testing for primary hemostasis and those evaluating coagulation. Table 50.2 provides a brief overview of the different laboratory tests available to evaluate these two pathways.

Thromboelastrography (TEG) is a testing method to evaluate the efficiency of blood clotting by measuring the elastic properties of blood as clot formation is occurring in relation to time. The primary advantage of TEG is that it provides a real-time analysis of all elements involved in the hemostatic process including platelet aggregation, coagulation, and fibrinolysis.[2,6] TEG is commonly used intraoperatively to assess hemostasis during liver transplants, severe trauma, obstetric surgeries, and cardiac procedures. In these settings, abnormalities in the TEG pattern can help guide the administration of blood and blood component products during periods of resuscitation and bleeding. Figure 50.3 depicts the appearance of a normal TEG with the variables measured.

When evaluating a TEG, the reaction time (R) demonstrates the amount of time until clot formation begins, a process that requires the formation of thrombin. Abnormalities in the R value can be indicative of deficiencies in factors of the intrinsic pathway of the clotting cascade. Prolonged R values indicate the need for fresh frozen plasma (FFP), cryoprecipitate, or additional protamine (in the setting of prior heparinization). Like R, K is a measure of clot formation time until the clot achieves a fixed strength; prolongation of K can be indicative of intrinsic pathway factor deficiencies. The maximum amplitude (MA), which typically occurs between 30 and 60 minutes, is a reflection of platelet count and function, as it measures the strength of the fully formed clot. A decrease in MA would indicate a need for platelet administration. Fibrinolysis begins from MA to the

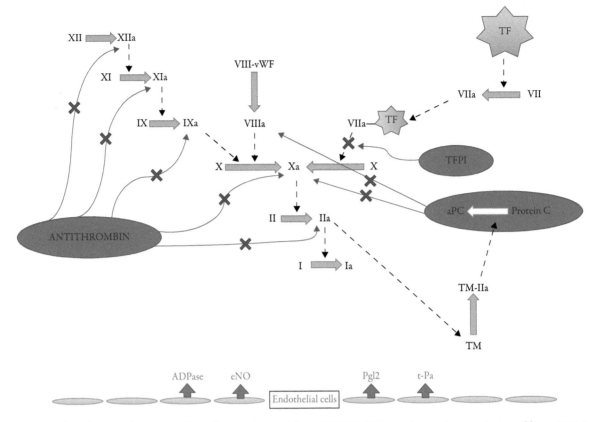

Fig. 50.2 Intrinsic antithrombotic mechanisms: 1. Tissue factor pathway inhibitor (TFPI) inhibits extrinsic pathway activation of factor X; 2. Activated protein C (aPC) inhibits activated factor VIII (VIIIa) and activated factor X-V complex (Xa-Va); 3. Intact vascular endothelium releases adenosine diphosphatase (ADPase), nitric oxide (eNO), prostacyclin (PGI₂), and tissue plasminogen (t-Pa), all of which have platelet-inhibiting and clot-lysing effects; 4. Antithrombin III binds to and inhibits activated factors XII (XIIa), XI (XIa), IX (IXa), X (Xa), and II (IIa).

time in which the clot has resolved and is reflected by LY-30 or LY-60. Shortened LY-30 or LY-60 values can prompt the administration of antifibrinolytics.

MANAGEMENT OF HEMOPHILIA

The World Federation of Hemophilia (WFH) currently recommends the use of prophylactic factor replacement therapy for the management of both hemophilia A and B. These recommendations come after several studies demonstrated that individuals with moderate hemophilia (i.e., factor levels greater than 1 IU/dL) rarely experienced spontaneous bleeding events and maintained better joint function.[7] Prophylaxis can be administered episodically, continuously, or intermittently, as defined in Table 50.3.

The WFH currently recognizes 2 prophylaxis protocols, the Malmo and the Utrecht, which are outlined in Table 50.4, for the management of both hemophilia A and B. It is important to note that factor replacement prophylaxis has not been shown to reverse joint damage that has occurred from prior hemathroses; however, it can help reduce the frequency of large joint bleeds, which can lead to a slower progression of joint disease and an improved functional status with increased quality of life.[7] Ideally, once prophylaxis therapy has been initiated and long-term vascular access has been established, hemophilia patients can be transitioned to home therapy.

A thorough evaluation should be performed at least every 12 months to assess venous access, issues related to hemostasis, functional status of large joints, the response to factor replacement, the development of factor inhibitors, and the overall psychosocial status of the patient.

The management of hemophilia patients within the surgical setting can require additional planning and extensive health care resources. For hemophilia patients requiring surgery, preoperative laboratory assessment should include complete blood count, liver and renal function tests, coagulation profile (PT, aPTT, fibrinogen), factor inhibitor screening and assay, blood type and crossmatch, and, for those with known inhibitors, a quantification of the titer to determine if the patient is a high or low responder.[6,7] Consultation with a hematologist is also recommended to determine appropriate factor replacement dosing pre-, intra-, and postoperatively. The target factor level for a surgical procedure varies depending on the type of procedure involved; regardless of the type of surgery, it is imperative to determine the patient's factor level immediately after preoperative replacement to ascertain that the response to therapy is appropriate. Several studies have indicated that use of a continuous infusion for factor replacement, following a bolus dose, provides improved hemostatic management to repeated, intermittent bolus dosing while reducing the overall total of factor required for replacement and better maintaining desired target factor level.[7–9] The

Table 50.2 LABORATORY TESTS FOR PRIMARY HEMOSTASIS AND COAGULATION

LABORATORY TEST	METHOD	NORMAL VALUES
Primary Hemostasis		
Platelet Count	Manual count performed from peripheral blood smear or automated by impedance counters	150,000 to 440,000/mm³
Bleeding Time	Directly assess platelet function by measuring the amount of time needed for a clot to form after a 1 mm deep by 10 mm long is placed on the volar surface of the forearm and blotted every 30 seconds	2 to 9 minutes
Platelet Aggregometry	An in vitro measurement of platelet activation and platelet-to-platelet aggregation when exposed to various agonists (adenosine diphosphate, epinephrine, collagen, arachidonic acid, thrombin, and ristocetin)	Reported as percentage (%) maximal aggregation; results vary depending on the agonist being utilized
Coagulation Pathway		
Prothrombin Time	Used to evaluate the classic extrinsic coagulation pathway, specifically tissue factor, fibrinogen, and factors II, V, VII, and X. Measures the time to fibrin clot formation when calcium and thromboplastin are added to a blood sample.	10 to 12 seconds
Activated Partial Thromboplastin Time	Used to evaluate the intrinsic and final common pathway of the coagulation cascade by adding calcium, a contact activator and partial thromboplastin to a blood sample. Tests for deficiencies/abnormalities of high-molecular-weight kininogen, prekallikrein, and factors I, II, V, VIII, IX, X, XI, XII.	25 to 35 seconds
Activated Clotting Time	Used to evaluate the intrinsic coagulation pathway with the addition of factor XII activators to whole blood. Coagulation requires adequate intrinsic amounts of platelet phospholipids. Most commonly used to monitor heparin therapy or the degree of heparin reversal following protamine administration.	90 to 120 seconds
Thrombin Time	Measures thrombin's ability to convert fibrinogen to fibrin when exogenous thrombin is added to citrated plasma.	10 to 15 seconds
Fibrinogen Levels	Automated electromagnetic detection of fibrinogen present in plasma.	160 to 350 mg/dL

Source. Carabini LM, Ramsey G. Hemostasis and transfusion medicine. In: Barash PG, Cullen BF, Stoelting RK, et al, eds. *Clinical Anesthesia.* 8th ed. Philadelphia, PA: Wolters Kluwer Health; 2017

WFH has published guidelines for desired factor levels in the perioperative setting; these guidelines are outlined in Table 50.5.[7,10]

In mild to moderate hemophilia A patients, desmopressin (1-deamino-8-D-arginine vasopressin, also known as DDAVP [Ferring Pharmaceuticals Inc, Parsippany, NJ, USA]) can be used to raise factor VIII to appropriate therapeutic levels. A single dose of DDAVP has been shown to raise circulating levels of factor VIII and vWF between three- and sixfold, with a peak response seen approximately 60 minutes after the dose has been administered.[7] A patient's response to DDAVP can be variable, closely spaced administrations of the medication can result in tachyphylaxis, and water retention with associated hyponatremia can occur as a result of DDAVP use. It is important to note that DDAVP has no effect on factor IX levels and therefore is not indicated for the management of hemophilia B.

In patients with severe hemophilia, the WFH strongly recommends factor replacement through the use of viral-inactivated plasma-derived products or recombinant concentrates over the use of FFP or cryoprecipitate.[7,10] Dosing guidelines for treatment in the surgical setting are listed in Table 50.4.[3,6,7,12] Plasma-derived factor VIII is commercially available as MonoclateP (CSL Behring LLC, Kankakee, IL, USA) and Hemofil-M (Baxalta US Inc, Westlake Village, CA, USA). Recombinant factor VIII is marketed as Recombinate (Baxter Healthcare Corporation, Westlake Village, CA, USA), Kogenate FS (Bayer HealthCare LLC, Whippany, NJ, USA), Helixate FS (Bayer HealthCare LLC, Whippany, NJ, USA), Advate (Baxalta US Inc, Westlake Village, CA, USA), and Xyntha (Wyeth Pharmaceuticals Inc, Philadelphia, PA, USA). Humate P (CSL Behring GmbH, Marburg, Germany) and Wilate (Octapharma USA, Inc, Hoboken, NJ, USA) are two products that are a plasma derived factor VIII–vWF combination. For the management of hemophilia B, plasma derived factor IX is available as Alphanine SD (Grifols Biologicals Inc, Los Angeles, CA, USA) and Mononine (CSL Behring LLC, Kankakee, IL, USA), while recombinant factor IX products

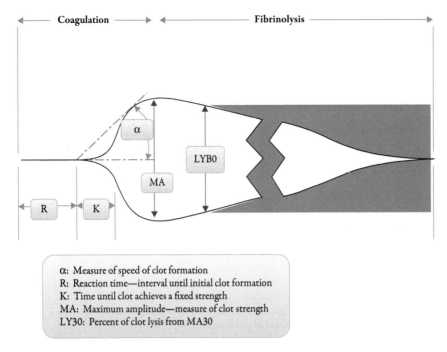

α: Measure of speed of clot formation
R: Reaction time—interval until initial clot formation
K: Time until clot achieves a fixed strength
MA: Maximum amplitude—measure of clot strength
LY30: Percent of clot lysis from MA30

Fig. 50.3 Thromboelastogram.

are BeneFIX (Wyeth Pharmaceuticals Inc, Philadelphia, PA, USA) and Rixubis (Baxter Healthcare Corporation, Westlake Village CA, USA). In the absence of inhibitors, each unit of

Table 50.3 FACTOR REPLACEMENT PROTOCOL DEFINITIONS PER WORLD FEDERATION OF HEMOPHILIA

PROTOCOL	DEFINITION
Episodic (on-demand)	Factor administration given at the time of bleeding event
Continuous Prophylaxis	Factor replacement intended for 52 weeks of the year, with a minimum administration of at least 45 weeks a year Treatment initiated based on the following criteria: – absence of osteochondral joint disease determined by physical exam or imaging – started before the second major bleeding event into a large joint* – started before the age of 3 years
Secondary Prophylaxis	Treatment initiated based on the following criteria: – started after the second large joint bleeding event – absence of osteochondral joint disease determined by physical exam or imaging
Tertiary Prophylaxis	Treatment initiated after the onset of osteochondral joint disease
Intermittent Prophylaxis	Intended factor replacement administered to prevent bleeding events for less than 45 weeks per year

*large joint includes ankles, knees, hips, elbows and shoulders.

Source. Srivastava A, Brewer AK, Mauser-Bunschoten P, et al. Guidelines for the management of hemophilia. *Haemophilia*. 2013;19:e1–e47.

factor VIII and IX infused per kilogram of body weight will raise the plasma factor level by 2 IU/dL and 1 IU/dL, respectively.[3,7] In the event that commercially produced factor products are not available, cryoprecipitate is preferred over FFP for the replacement of factor VIII. Cryoprecipitate contains 3 to 5 IU/mL of factor VIII, along with vWF, fibrinogen and factor XIII; however, cryoprecipitate contains no factor IX so is not indicated for the treatment of hemophilia B.[3,7] Lastly, if FFP is the only available factor component available for replacement, it can be used for both hemophilia A and B; however, 1 mL of FFP contains only 1 unit of active factor. Therefore, large volumes of FFP are often required, and, even still, it is difficult to achieve factor VIII and IX levels above 30 IU/dL and 25 IU/dL, respectively.[3,7]

The development of factor inhibitors (IgG antibodies that interfere with clotting factors) can further complicate the perioperative management of both hemophilia A and B patients, with the highest risk in patients suffering from a severe form of the disease. It is estimated that 20% to 30% of severe hemophilia A patients and 1% to 6% of severe hemophilia B patients will develop inhibitory antibodies during their lifetime.[6,7,11] The development of inhibitory antibodies is, quite possibly, the most severe complication of factor replacement therapy in hemophilia, as inhibitors render factor replacement ineffective. Patients with inhibitors are classified as either low responders or high responders based on the level of antibodies, measured in Bethesda Units, following exposure to replacement factor. Low responder inhibitors can be managed with high-dose factor replacement to overwhelm the antibody inhibitor; however, high responder inhibitors require agents that bypass the need for factors VIII or IX to establish hemostasis. The management of hemophilia patients with inhibitors is outlined in Tables 50.4 and 50.6.

Table 50.4 PROPHYLACTIC AND TREATMENT OPTIONS FOR HEMOPHILIA A AND B

MILD TO MODERATE HEMOPHILIA A

Desmopressin (DDAVP)	Intravenous: 0.3 μg/kg Intranasal: Adult: 150 μg in each nare Pediatric: 150 μg in one nare

Severe Hemophilia A

Recombinant Factor VIII	Prophylaxis: Malmo protocol: 25–40 IU/kg 3×/week Utrecht protocol: 15–30 IU/kg 3×/week Treatment: Pt weight (kg) × 50 IU/kg to reach 100% factor VIII level, q8-12h
Fresh Frozen Plasma	Not recommended for factor VIII replacement If required, starting dose 15–20 mL/kg
Cryoprecipitate	Preferred over FFP 70–80 units FVIII per 30–40 mL of cryoprecipitate

Hemophilia A with High Responding Inhibitors (See Table 50.6)

Hemophilia A with Low Responding Inhibitors

Recombinant Factor VIII	Loading dose: 10,000 to 15,000 U Maintenance dose: 1000 U/h
Porcine Factor VIII	50–100 U/kg q8h

Hemophilia B

Recombinant Factor IX	Prophylaxis: Malmo protocol: 25–40 IU/kg 2×/week Utrecht protocol: 15–30 IU/kg 2×/week Treatment: Adult: Pt weight (kg) × desired factor level (IU/dL) × 0.8 Pediatric: Pt weight (kg) × desired factor level (IU/dL) × 0.7
Pure Factor IX	Treatment: Pt weight (kg) × desired factor level (IU/dL)
Fresh Frozen Plasma	Not recommended for factor IX replacement If required, starting dose 15–20mL/kg
Cryoprecipitate	Not indicated for factor IX replacement

Hemophilia B with Inhibitors (See Table 50.6)

Sources. Lee J. von Willibrand disease, hemophilia A and B, and other factor deficiencies. *Int Anesthesiol Clin.* 2004;42:59–76; Kulkarni R. Comprehensive care of the patient with haemophilia and inhibitors undergoing surgery: practical aspects. Haemophilia. 2013;19:2–10; Srivastava A, Brewer AK, Mauser-Bunschoten P, et al. Guidelines for the management of hemophilia. *Haemophilia.* 2013;19:e1–e47; Rodriquez-Merchan EC, Rocino A, Ewenstein B, et al. Consensus perspectives on surgery in haemophilia patients with inhibitors: summary statement. *Haemophilia.* 2004;10(Suppl 2):50–52.

Advancements in modern medicine, in the form of gene therapy, may someday render factor replacements unnecessary. Current gene therapy studies are using viral vectors, such as

Table 50.5 DESIRED FACTOR LEVELS IN THE PERIOPERATIVE PERIOD

	HEMOPHILIA A	HEMOPHILIA B
	DESIRED LEVEL (IU/DL) **DURATION (DAYS)**	**DESIRED LEVEL (IU/DL)** **DURATION (DAYS)**
Major Surgery	80–100	60–80
Preoperative	60–80 (1–3)	40–60 (1–3)
Postoperative	40–60 (4–6)	30–50 (4–6)
	30–50 (7–14)	20–40 (7–14)
Minor Surgery	50–80	50–80
Preoperative	30–80 (1–5, depending on procedure)	30–80 (1–5, depending on procedure)
Postoperative		

Note. Major surgery = intra-abdominal, intracranial, orthopedic; minor surgery = skin excisions, arthroscopy

Source. Srivastava A, Brewer AK, Mauser-Bunschoten P, et al. Guidelines for the management of hemophilia. *Haemophilia.* 2013;19:e1–e47.

retrovirus, adenovirus, and adeno-associated virus, to incorporate intact gene copies into selected somatic cells that are administered via intramuscular injection.[3] Greater success has been seen in the treatment of hemophilia B, with gene defect correction lasting up to 17 months in dogs; human clinical trials of this model are now underway as well.

COMMON COMORBIDITIES IN PATIENTS WITH HEMOPHILIA

As a result of the use of prophylactic factor replacement and the improved medical management of hemophilia, patients with hemophilia are now living longer. While increasing the lifespan of patients in this population is a positive outcome, it has resulted in an increase in comorbidities among hemophiliacs that are commonly seen in the general population such as chronic pain, obesity, and psychosocial issues. The impact of obesity on patients with hemophilia is of significant concern, given the increased prevalence of osteoarthritis and joint disease in the obese population.[13] Furthermore, limited data suggests that obese patients with hemophilia are at elevated risk for hemophilic joint disease.[13–15] Recurrent intra-articular bleeding, either spontaneous or trauma-related, is a common complication of severe hemophilia A and B. Repeated hemarthroses is associated with acute pain during the bleeding episode and chronic pain over time due to irreversible joint damage and the development of hemophilic arthropathy. The European Hemophilia Therapy Standardization Board has defined chronic pain in hemophilia patients as pain that is continuous or intermittent, occurs more than 1 time per week, and persists for 3 or more months.[16] Chronic pain in the hemophiliac population is a well-documented comorbidity, with 50% of respondents in the Hemophilia Experiences, Results and Opportunities (HERO) study reporting constant pain, irrespective of the severity of their hemophilia.[13,16–18]

Table 50.6 HEMOSTATIC DOSING FOR HEMOPHILIA PATIENTS WITH INHIBITORS UNDERGOING SURGERY

	PREOPERATIVE DOSING	POSTOPERATIVE DOSING	
		DAYS 1–5	DAYS 6–14
rFVIIa			
Minor Surgery	Adult: 90–120 μg/kg q2h Pediatric: 120–150 μg/kg q2h	90–120 μg/kg q2h up to 4 times then q3–6h for 24h	
Intermediate/Major Surgery	Adult: 120 μg/kg q2h Pediatric: 150 μg/kg q2h	Day 1: 90–120 μg/kg q2h Day 2: 90–120 μg/kg q3h Day 3–5: 90–120 μg/kg q4h	90–120 μg/kg q6h
Continuous Infusion	15–50 μg/kg/h	15–50 μg/kg/h	15–50 μg/kg/h
aPCC			
Minor Surgery	50–75 U/kg	50–75 U/kg q12–24h 1 or 2 times	
Intermediate/Major Surgery	75–100 U/kg	75–100 U/kg q8–12h	75–100 U/kg q12h

Note. rFVIIa = recombinant-activated factor VII; aPCC = activated prothrombin complex concentrate.

Sources. Kulkarni R. Comprehensive care of the patient with haemophilia and inhibitors undergoing surgery: practical aspects. *Haemophilia*. 2013;19:2–10; Rodriquez-Merchan EC, Rocino A, Ewenstein B, et al. Consensus perspectives on surgery in haemophilia patients with inhibitors: summary statement. *Haemophilia*. 2004;10(Suppl 2):50–52.

The management of both acute and chronic hemophilic joint pain can be challenging, and the lack of evidence-based pain management practice guidelines to aid health care providers can make effective treatment of patients with bleeding disorders that much more difficult. Currently, the only available recommendations for the management of pain in hemophilia patients are provided by the WFH. Acetaminophen, nonsteroidal anti-inflammatory drugs (NSAIDs), selective cyclo-oxygenase 2 (COX-2) inhibitors, and opioids are the primary medications used for the treatment of hemophilic arthropathy. However, each of these medications are not without their own limitations. Acetaminophen is recommended for the treatment of mild to moderate joint pain since it has no effect on platelet function or BTs; however, there are concerns that it is less effective than NSAIDs or COX-2 inhibitors for the reduction of inflammatory pain.[19] Furthermore, achieving therapeutic doses of acetaminophen over a prolonged period can be problematic due its potential to elevate liver enzymes.[19] Both NSAIDs and COX-2 inhibitors are recommended for the management of chronic joint pain as a result of their anti-inflammatory qualities, but they should be strictly avoided during times of acute intra-articular bleeding due to their interference with platelet function. Long-term use of either of these medications can also be of concern given the increased risk of gastrointestinal bleeding and cardiovascular thrombo-occlusive events.[16,19] When acetaminophen, NSAIDs, or COX-2 inhibitors become ineffective at managing pain, opioids should be initiated.[16,20] For acute pain events, short-acting, immediate-release opioids in combination with acetaminophen or an NSAID are preferred, with an attempt to discontinue use as soon as possible. The use of long-acting opioids in combination with a short-acting opioid available as needed for breakthrough pain is recommended when managing chronic pain.[16,19]

Alternative pharmacological options to acetaminophen, NSAIDs, and opioids for the management of chronic pain have been reported and include tramadol, anticonvulsants (pregabalin or gabapentin), and antidepressants known to improve neuropathic pain.[16] Nonpharmacological methods to manage pain, including behavioral strategies, physiotherapy, complementary therapies, and invasive interventions, have all been reported to be beneficial in hemophiliacs.[16,19] Behavioral techniques to improve pain include distraction, reinterpreting pain, self-hypnosis, biofeedback, and cognitive behavioral therapy.[19,21,22] Although behavioral strategies have been proposed as methods to reduce hemophilia-related pain, no studies currently exist on this topic. Table 50.7 demonstrates other nonpharmacological methods used for pain management in the hemophilia population with associated references demonstrating benefit, either in the form of case report or small studies.

The psychosocial impact of hemophilia on patients is also important. Eighty-nine percent of all patients who responded in the HERO study indicated that pain interfered with their daily activities and caused functional impairment.[17,18] Furthermore, when the young adult population (age 18–30 years) was evaluated in the HERO study, over one-third of the respondents indicated that they had experienced and/or been treated for anxiety and depression.[17] In addition, 37% of the young adult respondents indicated that hemophilia had a negative impact on their ability to develop and maintain a close relationship with a partner.[17] Last, 76% of young adult patients with hemophilia reported that the disease

Table 50.7 NONPHARMACOLOGIC HEMOPHILIA-RELATED PAIN MANAGEMENT TECHNIQUES

PHSYIOTHERAPY[16,21,23–26]	COMPLEMENTARY[16,27,28]	INVASIVE INTERVENTIONS[19,29]	SURGICAL INTERVENTIONS[16,19,30]
Protection, rest, ice, compression, elevation	Acupuncture	Viscosupplementation (intra-articular hyaluronic acid injection)	Synovectomy
Stretching and strengthening	Music therapy		Total joint replacement
Splinting	Meditative breathing	Intra-articular steroid injections	
Orthotics			
Transcutaneous electrical neurostimulation			
Hydrotherapy			
Therapeutic ultrasound			

had negatively impacted their employment, either in terms of choice of career, ability to adequately communicate with employers, or their capacity to fulfill work responsibilities.[17,18] Given these findings from the HERO study, ongoing psychosocial assessments should be a routine component of the medical management of hemophilia patients.

REVIEW QUESTIONS

1. When treating a patient with hemophilia B, all of the following are indicated **EXCEPT**

A. recombinant factor IX
B. FFP
C. cryoprecipitate
D. activated prothrombin complex concentrate

Answer: C
In hemophilia B, factor IX is deficient. Cryoprecipitate does not contain factor IX and therefore is not indicated for the treatment of hemophilia B. All of the other options contain factor IX for replacement.

2. A full-term male newborn presents to an urgent care center with excessive bleeding and oozing at his circumcision site 24 hours after having an uncomplicated circumcision. There is no known family medical history of bleeding disorders. Coagulation studies obtained at the urgent care center reveal a platelet count of $153,000/mm^3$, a PT of 12 seconds, an aPTT of 67 seconds, and a fibrinogen level of 183 mg/dL. Which of the following is the most appropriate next step?

A. administer vitamin K
B. obtain specific factor assays
C. obtain a thrombin time
D. perform a bone marrow aspiration and biopsy

Answer: B
A prolonged aPTT in the setting of a normal platelet count, normal PT, and a normal fibrinogen level is indicative of a factor deficiency, specifically factors VIII, IX, or XI. In a patient with vitamin K deficiency, the PT would be prolonged as an indication of factor VII depletion. In the setting of a normal fibrinogen level, an abnormal thrombin time would be unlikely as an elevated thrombin time is indicative of inadequate fibrinogen levels. A bone marrow aspiration and biopsy should be considered when thrombocytopenia is noted on coagulation studies.

3. Which of the following does **NOT** contribute to clot formation?

A. tissue factor
B. calcium
C. phospholipids
D. protein C

Answer: D
Protein C, when activated, is part of the intrinsic antithrombotic pathway to prevent overextension of clot formation, by inhibiting factor VIII and factor X–V complex.

4. All of the following cause prolongation of the aPTT that is unresponsive to the administration of FFP **EXCEPT**

A. factor IX inhibitor
B. factor VIII inhibitor
C. heparin
D. factor VII inhibitor

Answer: D
The aPTT tests for factors of the intrinsic pathway of coagulation; prolongation of the aPTT would be indicative of a deficiency in intrinsic pathway factors (i.e., factors VIII, IX, XI, XII). The use of FFP to repleat the deficient factors should result in correction of the aPTT. When FFP administration fails to normalize the aPTT, it is indicative of the presence of factor inhibitors or the presence of heparin in the testing sample. Factor VII is a component of the extrinsic coagulation pathway, which is reflected in the PT, not the aPTT.

5. Which of the following statements is **FALSE**?

A. Congenital factor IX deficiency is inherited as a sex-linked recessive disorder.
B. Hemophilia C is an inherited autosomal recessive disorder primarily affecting the Ashkenazi Jewish population.
C. Factor VIII has a half-life of 24 hours.
D. Long-term complications of severe hemophilia A can include chronic pain, joint arthropathy, and acquisition of transfusion-related infections (i.e., hepatitis B, hepatitis C, HIV).

Answer: C
Factor VIII has a half-life of 8 to 12 hours.

6. A 31-year-old male with hemophilia A presents to the emergency department with gross hematuria in the absence of any recent trauma or history of genitourinary pathology. Physical

examination is unremarkable, and initial laboratory findings demonstrate a hemoglobin of 8.2 g/dL. All of the following can used in the treatment of hemophilia A **EXCEPT**

A. DDAVP
B. plasmapheresis
C. FFP
D. cryoprecipitate

Answer: B
The goal of treatment for hemophilia A is to replace or increase factor VIII levels. FFP and cryoprecipitate both contain factor VIII. DDAVP can be used in the management of mild hemophilia; it functions to increase the release of numerous clotting factors and vWF from the liver to aid in hemostasis. Plasmapheresis does not increase production of factor VIII or function as a form of replacement of factor VIII; therefore, it plays no role in the treatment of hemophilia A.

7. Which one of the following statements about hemophilia A is **TRUE**?

A. Hemophilia B is more common than hemophilia A.
B. Rebleeding 5 days after an injury is common.
C. A patient with a factor VIII coagulant activity level of 4% would be classified as severe hemophilia A.
D. Hemophilia A is inherited as an autosomal recessive disease.

Answer: B
Rebleeding after surgery or an injury is very common with hemophilia A and is one of the hallmarks of the disease due to weakness of the initial clot that forms. The other statements are false. Hemophilia A is the most common form of the diseases classified as hemophilia, accounting for nearly 85% of the individuals diagnosed with hemophilia. A factor VIII coagulant activity level of 4% would classify as moderate disease. Hemophilia A is inherited in a sex-linked recessive pattern.

8. Which one of the following is the **MOST** common inherited bleeding disorder?

A. von Willebrand disease
b. hemophilia B
C. hemophilia A
D. Bernard Soulier disease

Answer: A
Of the inherited bleeding disorders, von Willebrand disease is the most common, affecting approximately 1% to 3% of the population, although many of those individuals are undiagnosed.

9. All of the following are crucial components of the intrinsic antithrombotic mechanism **EXCEPT**

A. intact vascular endothelium releases adenosine diphosphatase, nitric oxide, prostacyclin, and tissue plasminogen
B. activated protein C
C. tissue factor pathway inhibitor
D. activated factor X

Answer: D
Activated factor X is the common pathway between the intrinsic and extrinsic pathways of the clotting cascade. The formation of activated factor X results in the activation of thrombin and fibrinogen to achieve a stable fibrin clot.

10. When evaluating a TEG, which one of the following associations is **INCORRECT**?

A. prolonged LY-30: administer antifibrinolytic
B. decreased MA: administer platelets
C. prolonged R value: administer protamine or FFP
D. low α-angle: administer FFP or cryoprecipitate

Answer: A
Explanation: LY-30 is a measure of fibrinolysis. A shortened LY-30 or LY-60 indicates that clot breakdown is occurring faster than normal; in this scenario, administration of an antifibrinolytic is indicated.

QUESTIONS AND ANSWERS

This chapter has accompanying questions and answers which are available to subscribers as part of the Oxford eLearning platform. To access the questions, go to ✔ http://oxfordmedicine. com/pediatricanesthesiaPBL

REFERENCES

1. Livnat T, Barg AA, Levy-Mendelovich S, Kenet G. Rare bleeding disorders—old diseases in the era of novel options for therapy. *Blood Cells Mol Dis.* 2017;67:63–68. http://dx.doi.org/10.1016/j.bcmd.2017.02.003
2. Carabini LM, Ramsey G. Hemostasis and transfusion medicine. In: Barash PG, Cullen BF, Stoelting RK, et al., eds. *Clinical Anesthesia.* 8th ed. Philadelphia, PA: Wolters Kluwer Health; 2017:419–458.
3. Lee J. von Willibrand disease, hemophilia A and B, and other factor deficiencies. *Int Anesthesiol Clin.* 2004;42:59–76.
4. Graetz TJ, Despotis GJ. Hemophilia and coagulation disorders. In: Yao F, Malhotra V, Fong J, Skubas N, eds. *Yao and Artusio's Anesthesiology: Problem-Oriented Patient Management.* 8th ed. Philadelphia, PA: Wolters Kluwer Health; 2016:675–694.
5. Konkle BA, Hutson H, Nakaya Fletcher S. Hemophilia A. In: Pagon, RA, Adam MP, Ardinger HH, et al., eds. *GeneReview*®. Seattle: University of Washington; 1993–2017. https://www.ncbi.nlm.nih.gov/books/NBK1404/
6. Kulkarni R. Comprehensive care of the patient with haemophilia and inhibitors undergoing surgery: practical aspects. *Haemophilia.* 2013;19:2–10.
7. Srivastava A, Brewer AK, Mauser-Bunschoten P, et al. Guidelines for the management of hemophilia. *Haemophilia.* 2013;19:e1–e47.
8. Batorova A, Holme P, Gringeri A, et al. Continuous infusion in haemophilia: current practice in Europe. *Haemophilia.* 2012;18:753–759.
9. Batorova A, Martinowitz U. Intermittent injections vs continuous infusion of Factor VIII in haemophilia patients undergoing major surgery. *Br J Haematol.* 2000;110:715–720.
10. Rickard KA. Guidelines for therapy and optimal dosages of coagulation factors for treatment of bleeding and surgery in haemophilia. *Haemophilia.* 1995;1(Suppl 1):8–13.

11. Escobar M, Maahs J, Hellman E, et al. Multidisciplinary management of patients with haemophilia with inhibitors undergoing surgery in the United States: perspectives and best practices derived from experienced treatment centres. *Haemophilia*. 2012;18:971–981.

12. Rodriquez-Merchan EC, Rocino A, Ewenstein B, et al. Consensus perspectives on surgery in haemophilia patients with inhibitors: summary statement. *Haemophilia*. 2004;10(Suppl 2):50–52.

13. Witkop ML, Peerlinck K, Luxon BA. Medical co-morbidities of patients with hemophilia: pain, obesity and hepatitis C. *Haemophilia*. 2016;22(Suppl 5):47–53.

14. Wong TE, Majumdar S, Adams E, et al. Overweight and obesity in hemophilia A: systematic review of the literature. *Am J Prev Med*. 2011;6(Suppl 4):s369–s375.

15. Majumdar S, Ahmad N, Karlson C, et al. Does weight reduction in haemophilia lead to a decrease in joint bleeds? *Haemophilia*. 2011;18:e82–e84.

16. Young G, Tachdjian R, Baumann K, Panopoulos G. Comprehensive management of chronic pain in haemophilia. *Haemophilia*. 2014;20:e113–e120.

17. Witkop M, Guelcher C, Forsyth A, et al. Treatment outcomes, quality of life, and impact of hemophilia on young adults (age 18–30 years) with hemophilia. *Am J Hematol*. 2015;90:S3–S10.

18. Forsyth AL, Gregory M, Nugent D, et al. Haemophilia Experiences, Results and Opportunities (HERO) Study: survey methodology and population demographics. *Haemophilia*. 2014;20:44–51.

19. Humphries TJ, Kessler CM. Managing chronic pain in adults with haemophilia: current status and call to action. *Haemophilia*. 2015;21:41–51.

20. World Health Organization's pain ladder. http://www.who.int/cancer/palliative/painladder/en/. Accessed July 28, 2017.

21. Riley RR, Witkop M, Hellman E, Akins S. Assessment and management of pain in haemophilia patients. *Haemophilia*. 2011;17:839–845.

22. Santavirta N, Bjorvell H, Solovieva S, et al. Coping strategies, pain and disability in patients with hemophilia and related disorders. *Arthritis Care Res*. 2001;45:48–55.

23. Witkop M, Lambing A, Divine G, et al. A national study of pain in the bleeding disorders community: a description of haemophilia pain. *Haemophilia*. 2012;18:e115–e119.

24. Witkop M, Lambing A, Kachalsky E, et al. Assessment of acute and persistent pain management in patients with haemophilia. *Haeomphilia*. 2011;17:612–619.

25. Heijnen L, de Kleijn P. Physiotherapy for the treatment of articular contractures in haemophilia. *Haemophilia*. 1999;5:16–19.

26. Raffini L, Manno C. Modern management of haemophilic arthropathy. *Br J Haematol*. 2007;136:777–787.

27. Lambing A, Kohn-Converse B, Hanagavadi S, et al. Use of acupuncture in the management of chronic haemophilia pain. *Haemophilia*. 2012;18:613–617.

28. Wallny TA, Brackmann HH, Gunia G, et al. Successful pain treatment in arthropathic lower extremities by acupuncture in haemophilia patients. *Haemophilia*. 2006;12:500–502.

29. Carulli C, Civinini R, Martini C, et al. Viscosupplementation in haemophilic arthropathy: a long-term follow-up study. *Haemophilia*. 2012;18:e210–e214.

30. Wang K, Street A, Dowrick A, et al. Clinical outcomes and patient satisfaction following total joint replacement in haemophilia—23 year experience in knees, hips, and elbows. *Haemophilia*. 2012;18:86–93.

51.

SICKLE CELL DISEASE

Lynne R. Ferrari

STEM CASE AND KEY QUESTIONS

A 16-year-old African American male presents to the emergency department with right upper quadrant pain. He has a history of sickle cell disease and has been admitted to the hospital on many prior occasions for treatment of vaso-oclusive crisis. He has been vomiting and appears to be mildly dehydrated on physical examination. Abdominal ultrasound reveals chronic cholelithiasis and, after consultation with the general surgeon on call, cholecystectomy is recommended.

WHAT ARE THE ADVANTAGES OF LAPAROSCOPIC CHOLECYSTECTOMY VERSUS AN OPEN PROCEDURE?

The surgeon tells the family he will be using the laparoscopic approach. He tells them this results in less postoperative pain and an improved ability to breathe comfortably. The decreased postoperative pain will promote better respiratory excursion, prevent respiratory compromise, allow the patient to take deep breaths, improve and maintain adequate functional residual capacity, and decrease the risk of atelectasis, hypoxia, and ventilation/perfusion mismatch. In most circumstances, the surgical time for the laparoscopic approach is shorter, thus decreasing the risk of postoperative complications and painful crisis.

SHOULD THE PATIENT BE TRANSFUSED PREOPERATIVELY?

The patient's lab work shows his hemoglobin is 8.4 mg/dL. A decision is made to call a hematology consult prior to proceeding to the operating room and also to help postoperative management. You begin hydration at 1.5 times maintenance.

WHAT OTHER SUBSPECIALISTS SHOULD YOU CONSULT PRIOR TO PLANNING HIS ANESTHETIC MANAGEMENT?

In light of his previous vaso-occlusive episodes, the acute pain service has been also consulted. Since a laparoscopic procedure is planned, an epidural was considered but the family declined.

WHAT ARE THE INTRAOPERATIVE RISKS?

The surgery proceeds without incident and the patient goes to the postanesthesia care unit with a temperature of 35.4°C despite aggressive warming in the operating room. The patient complains of pain 4/10. The pain team is called to assist with postoperative pain management.

WHAT IS THE BEST PAIN MANAGEMENT PLAN?

The family wants to know what the best pain management plan is for this patient after the procedure.

Pain in patients with sickle cell disease is often chronic due to the relapsing nature of the disease. Management usually begins with oral medication, including acetaminophen, nonsteroidal anti-inflammatory agents, and occasionally opioids.[1,2] When oral medication is ineffective, admission to the hospital for multimodal pain management is warranted. Hydration and oxygenation should be optimized to aid in pain management. Intravenous administration of ketorolac in conjunction with opioids including morphine, fentanyl, and hydromorphone may be effective. Regional anesthesia with an indwelling catheter would be a good choice for management of postoperative pain in this patient.

DISCUSSION

Sickle cell disease is a congenital hemaglobinopathy. Sickle hemoglobin differs from normal adult hemoglobin by one amino acid substitution, glutamic acid for valine, at position 6 on the beta chain.[3-5] Affected homozygous HbSS individuals have severe hemolytic anemia as a result of poorly deformed and unstable sickled cells (Fig. 51.1).

Pharmacologic therapy with the amino acid L-glutamine to reduce the complications associated with sickle cell disease has been approved for children over age 5 years with sickle cell disease. Individuals with sickle cell trait who are heterozygous for HbAS have no signs or symptoms of sickle cell disease and are resistant to falciparum malaria. Occasionally, these patients have painless hematuria. The red blood cells in individuals with sickle cell trait contain 30% to 40% of HbS and as a result sickling does not occur under normal circumstances.

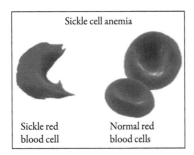

Fig. 51.1 Red blood cell morphology.

Painful vaso-occlusive episodes are a result of microvascular occlusions secondary to hemolysis. Intravascular hemolysis resulting in a decreased production of nitric oxide and endothelia dysfunction contributes to pathologic findings and the development of multiorgan dysfunction. The pathophysiology in sickle cell disease is mediated by inflammation, vascular endothelial abnormalities, platelet aggregation, and the activation of the coagulation cascade. These changes contribute to the development of vaso-occlusive crisis. The most common sites include the phalanges, long bones, ribs, sternum spine, and pelvis. Micro-occlusion in the mesenteric vessels may cause pain that mimics an acute surgical abdomen. Other common clinical manifestations of sickle cell disease include cerebrovascular accidents, acute chest syndrome, gallbladder disease, hematuria, renal concentrating defect, cardiomyopathy, and recurrent infections. Additional sequelae of microvascular occlusion include stroke, lung infarction and myocardial infarction, priapism, pulmonary hypertension, and skin breakdown. Additional risk for vaso-occlusive crisis may occur in conditions such as hypotension, shock, high altitude, or extreme exercise. Severe pain accompanies many of these conditions. As a result or chronic pain and recurring episodes of sickle cell crisis, patients may exhibit a variety of psychological problems including depression and school failure.

Vaso-occlusive episodes are managed with hydration, environmental warming, and pain management with antiinflammatory agents and opioids. A calm, stress-free environment will also aid in pain reduction. Oral hydroxyurea therapy in children has some effectiveness in reducing the number of vaso-occlusive episodes.

Preoperative considerations include an assessment of hematocrit and the need for red blood cell or exchanged transfusion. Patients should be encouraged to liberally drink fluids preoperatively to avoid dehydration and intravascular volume depletion. If this is not possible or if dehydration is already present, admission to the hospital for intravenous fluid therapy is warranted. Preoperative antibiotics should be administered to those patients with fever, elevated white count, or other evidence of infection.

Transfusion is considered for perioperative symptomatic anemia. Prophylactic transfusion is not warranted, especially if a laparoscopic approach is chosen. In patients who have a hematocrit less than 30%, red blood cell transfusion may be considered for procedures with the potential of significant blood loss or long duration defined as greater than 45 minutes. If the HbS level is below 30%, red blood cell transfusion is not indicated. For those patients who have a HbS level greater than 30%, transfusion may be beneficial.

Adequate hydration should be provided intraoperatively with careful consideration of renal function. Oxygenation should be optimized to prevent hypoxia and the subsequent associated morbidity. Hypothermia and acidosis should be avoided to maintain red cell integrity. The operating room should be warm; fluids should be administered through a warming device and forced air warmers utilized to maintain optimal core body temperature. Regional anesthesia is an important consideration and should be considered as the primary anesthetic when feasible or an adjunct to general anesthesia for postoperative pain management.

The goal of intraoperative management is to avoid sickle cell crisis.[6] This is best accomplished by avoiding hypotension, hypothermia, hypovolemia, acidosis, and hypoxia. Careful attention must be given to positioning to reduce venous stasis and mechanical vascular occlusion. The use of a tourniquet, although not needed for this procedure, should be avoided.

Acute exacerbations of the disease, especially acute chest syndrome and pain crisis, frequently occur during the perioperative period. Adequate control of postoperative pain is essential as is effective pulmonary toilet in the immediate postoperative period. Fever and infection as well as transfusion-related events occur in 5% to 10% of patients.

Early mobilization is important to encourage during the postoperative period. Aggressive pain management, rigorous pulmonary toilet, oxygen therapy, bronchodilators, red blood cell transfusion to optimize hematocrit, and a supportive, calm environment will contribute to a successful postoperative outcome.

PREOPERATIVE WORKUP

The status of specific organ function is an essential component of the preoperative preparation. Perioperative morbidity is directly related to exacerbations of specific organ damage.

Hematology. A discussion regarding the need for a standard red blood cell transfusion versus exchange transfusion should be part of the preoperative plan. A history of functional asplenia should be sought, as well as history of hemolytic episodes. Bone marrow function should be determined, especially if a history of bone marrow depression is present. Preoperative antibiotics should be administered to patients who have compromised splenic or bone marrow function.[7,8]

Pulmonary. Acute chest syndrome is defined by pulmonary hyperreactivity, new pulmonary infiltrates, fibrosis, and restrictive lung disease. Patient current status, history of prior pulmonary events, and prevention strategy should be discussed.

Neurologic. A history of previous stroke or central nervous system infarction should be sought. The vasculature may be weakened as a result of chronic damage as well as occluded due to progressive hyperplasia of arterial intima and accumulation of red cells.

Renal. Renal function should be assessed since papillary necrosis and glomerular disease may result in chronic renal insufficiency with loss of concentrating ability due to renal medulla infarction.

Gastrointestinal. Laboratory evaluation of liver function and electrolytes should be obtained prior to anesthesia. Adequate preoperative oral fluid intake is essential in preventing perioperative dehydration, hypotension, and intravascular hyperviscosity, all of which may lead to sickle cell crisis.

MISCELLANEOUS SYMPTOMS

The acute chest syndrome may occur as a complication of postoperative atelectasis and is the leading cause of death in children over 10 years of age.[9,10] Initially, the patient may not appear severely ill, but the condition can progress rapidly (Fig. 51.2). The illness clinically and radiographically resembles bacterial pneumonia, with fever, leukocytosis, pleuritic chest pain, pleural effusion, and cough (Fig. 51.3). In contrast to bacterial pneumonia, multiple lobe involvement and recurrent infiltrates are common, and the duration of clinical illness and radiologic clearing of infiltrates are prolonged to 10 to 12 days. The syndrome includes hypoxemia, infiltration on chest radiograph, and pulmonary infection. Acute chest syndrome is a frequent cause of hospitalization for patients with sickle cell disease, second only to painful crisis, and recurrent episodes may cause debilitating chronic pulmonary disease accounting for 25% of deaths in patients with sickle cell disease. Early detection of pulmonary compromise in any patient with sickle cell disease followed by vigorous treatment with chest physical therapy and incentive spirometry are essential in preventing the high rate of mortality in patients with this condition.

Orthopedic symptoms and complications of sickle cell disease include osteonecrosis and osteomyelitis. Distal vascular compromise may result in leg ulcers and skin breakdown due to

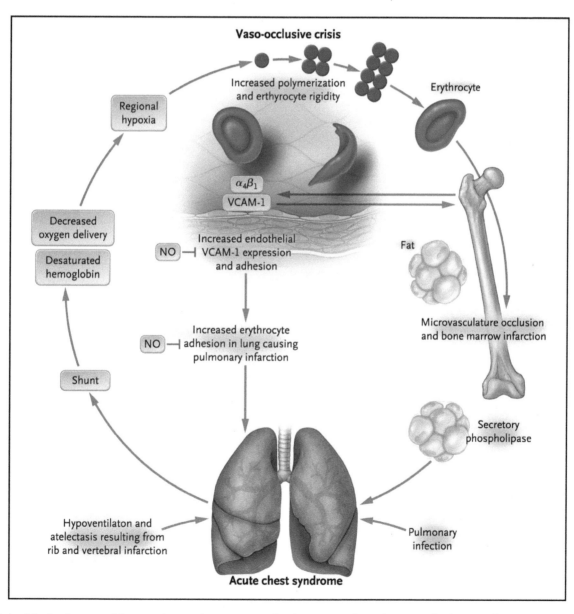

Fig. 51.2 Cycle of the development of the acute chest syndrome. Reprinted with permission from *The New England Journal of Medicine*.

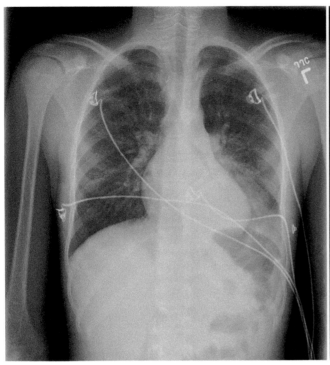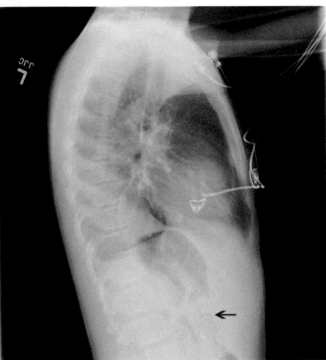

Fig. 51.3 13-year-old with sickle cell disease presenting with cough and fever. Note the abdominal clip from a previous cholecystectomy. (Courtesy of Ilse Castro-Aragon MD, Boston Medical Center.)

microvascular occlusion. The immune system is compromised and may lead to autoimmunization and hemolytic transfusion reactions. Hemolytic anemia, aplastic anemia, bone marrow failure, and splenic infarction and fibrosis are common findings.

DIAGNOSTIC MODALITIES

Neonatal screening was instituted in 1975, and the diagnosis of sickle cell trait is made with hemoglobin electrophoresis. Chronic hemolytic anemia is a hallmark of the disease, and most patients have a hemoglobin level of 5 to 9 g/dL. Specific preoperative laboratory values of hemoglobin and hemoglobin S should be measured. Hemoglobin electrophoresis should be performed to determine the hemoglobin subtype and a complete blood count obtained to determine white cell count and bone marrow function. An electrocardiogram and chest radiograph should be obtained as well as a measure of pulmonary function. Measurement of serum electrolytes and a urine dipstick should be completed to assess renal function.

TREATMENTS

Pain crisis is best treated with adequate analgesia, consisting of acetaminophen, nonsteroidal anti-inflammatory agents, NMDA agonists, and intravenous opiates. A calm environment and psychological support are also important components of treatment. Steroids may be beneficial in certain cases.

Acute chest syndrome is avoided by early postoperative ambulation, vigorous chest physical therapy, and incentive spirometry. Treatment includes oxygen therapy, bronchodilators,

antibiotics, and adequate analgesia. Red cell transfusion to treat hypoxia in the setting of relative anemia may be considered. Steroids or nitric oxide as well as mechanical ventilation may be useful in severe cases.

CONCLUSIONS

The hallmark of sickle cell disease is a disruption of intravascular function resulting in clinical crisis of multiple etiologies. Painful crises of bones, abdomen, chest, and other organs caused by sickling red cells leading to ischemia are a result of vaso-occlusive episodes in small arterial vessels. Aplastic crisis due to bone marrow failure may also be present and result in non-hemolytic anemia and neutropenia. Sequestration crisis may result in serious infarction in multiple organs including central nervous system, kidney, and spleen. Hemolytic crisis, growth retardation, osteonecrosis, osteomyelitis especially with salmonella, renal papillary necrosis, priapism, splenomegaly, cholelithiasis, acute chest syndrome, retinopathy, and cerebral vascular accidents are clinical features that must be considered throughout the perioperative episode of care.

REVIEW QUESTIONS

1. The **MOST** dangerous aspect of pneumococcal infections in children with sickle cell disease is which of following?

   A. It was the leading cause of death in children over 30 years ago.

B. Penicillin prophylaxis dramatically drops the infection rate.
C. Pneumococcal vaccine is not effective in young children.
D. Reaction to penicillin occurs in 1% to 10% of the population.

Answer: C
The polyvalent pneumococcal vaccines that are currently available have poor immunogenic activity in children under the age of 5 years. Prophylactic penicillin is effective in preventing serious pneumococcal infection in younger children. Full up-to-date immunization status is therefore especially important in children with sickle cell disease.

2. The **LEAST** important treatment for vaso-occlusive crisis is which of the following therapies?

A. analgesia
B. antibiotics
C. hydration
D. oxygenation

Answer: B
Children with chronic painful conditions are frequently difficult to assess. They may present with a flat affect, which makes determining the degree of pain and discomfort unreliable, and observers may underestimate the need for therapy. Analgesics should be offered early and in adequate doses. The goal of treatment is to prevent complications and sequelae such as acute chest syndrome. Infection such as pneumonia or osteomyelitis should be treated with appropriate antibiotics. Adequate hydration, nutrition, oxygen (if indicated) and comfort are essential for recovery.

3. The **MOST** important postoperative advantage of a laparoscopic surgery in a patient with sickle cell disease is which of following?

A. Infection risk is reduced.
B. Respiratory function is improved.
C. Sickling risk is decreased.
D. Surgical duration is shorter.

Answer: B
Abdominal surgery in patients with sickle cell disease is not uncommon. One of the most frequently performed procedures is cholecystectomy, via either an open or laparoscopic approach. The laparoscopic approach results in less postoperative pain and improved ability to breathe comfortably. Compared to a right upper quadrant incision required when the open approach is performed, laparoscopy will result in a minimal incision and less discomfort. Less pain will allow for better respiratory excursion, prevent respiratory compromise, allow the patient to take deep breaths, improve and maintain adequate functional residual capacity, and decrease the risk of atelectasis, hypoxia, and ventilation/perfusion mismatch. A laparoscope approach may be associated with a shorter intraoperative duration but is institution and surgeon specific.

4. Of the following therapies, which is the one that will decrease risk in the perioperative setting the **LEAST**?

A. fluid administration
B. environmental warming
C. oxygenation optimization
D. patient-controlled analgesia (PCA)

Answer: D
Adequate hydration should be provided intraoperatively with careful consideration of renal function. Oxygenation should be optimized to prevent hypoxia and the subsequent associated morbidity. Hypothermia and acidosis should be avoided to maintain red cell integrity. The operating should be warm; fluids should be administered through a warming device and forced air warmers utilized to maintain optimal core body temperature.

Most important are the avoidance of hypoxemia, hypocarbia, and hypothermia. In a hypoxic environment, hemoglobin S will polymerize and cause erythrocytes to become rigid. These distorted red blood cells cause structural damage in the cell membrane, which alters the rheologic properties of the cell, impairs blood flow through the microvasculature, and leads to hemolysis and vaso-occlusive crisis. Organ regions such as renal medulla and tissue such as bone will suffer repeat damage in the setting of sickling and poor perfusion. Pain control is essential in children with vaso-occlusive crises, but PCA is not the only method to deliver analgesics.

5. What clinical manifestation of sickle cell anemia is seen **MOSTLY** in very young children?

A. acute chest syndrome
B. aplastic anemia
C. hand-foot syndrome
D. splenic sequestration

Answer: C
Clinical manifestations are rarely seen before 6 months of age, with the hand-foot syndrome most often seen in children ages 1 to 2 years. Sickle cell disease is a chronic hemolytic anemia with associated crises such as splenic sequestration, aplastic crisis, and vaso-occlusive crisis. Pain crisis is the most common type of vaso-occlusive crisis.

6. The **MOST** accurate statistic about the prevalence of and mortality related to sickle cell disease is which of the following?

A. 8% of African Americans
B. 60 years life expectancy
C. 100,000 Americans
D. 10 million worldwide

Answer: C
There are an estimated 100,000 people living with sickle cell anemia in the United States. Sickle cell trait is found in approximately 8% of African American populations and approximately 3% of the Hispanic population in North America. It is also found in less than 1% of other racial groups. The estimated number of people with sickle trait, worldwide, is 10 million. The average life expectancy of an American with sickle cell anemia is less than 50 years of age—on average 42 years for men and 48 years for women.

7. The **MOST** likely cause of sickle cell anemia related death in children, after the age of 10 years, is which of following?

    A. acute chest syndrome
    B. cerebral vascular accident
    C. end-stage renal disease
    D. haemophilus influenzae sepsis

Answer: A

Acute chest syndrome is only seen in children with sickle cell disease and is the leading cause of death in children over the age of 10 years and adults. It is a constellation of hypoxemia, infiltrates on chest radiograph, and pulmonary infection. It is best treated with nebulized bronchodilators and vigorous hydration.

8. The **BEST** indicator for preoperative red blood cell transfusion in patients with sickle cell disease is which of the following?

    A. frequent vaso-occlusive crises
    B. hemoglobin <10 mg/dL
    C. hemoglobin S >50%
    D. red blood cell antibodies documented

Answer: B

Empiric prophylactic transfusion is not warranted. In patients who have hemoglobin measurement less than 10 mg/dL, red blood cell transfusion may be considered for procedures with the potential of significant blood loss or long duration.

QUESTIONS AND ANSWERS

This chapter has accompanying questions and answers which are available to subscribers as part of the Oxford eLearning platform. To access the questions, go to ✔ http://oxfordmedicine. com/pediatricanesthesiaPBL

REFERENCES

1. Brandow AM, Weisman SJ, Panepinto JA. The impact of a multidisciplinary pain management model on sickle cell disease pain hospitalizations. *Pediatr Blood Cancer*. 2011;56(5):789–793.
2. Krishnamurti L, Smith-Packard B, Gupta A, Campbell M, Gunawardena S, Saladino R. Impact of individualized pain plan on the emergency management of children with sickle cell disease. *Pediatr Blood Cancer*. 2014;61(10):1747–1753.
3. Firth PG. Anaesthesia for peculiar cells—a century of sickle cell disease. *Br J Anaesth*. 2005;95(3):287–299.
4. Firth PG. Anesthesia and hemoglobinopathies. *Anesthesiol Clin*. 2009;27(2):321–336.
5. Firth PG, Head CA. Sickle cell disease and anesthesia. *Anesthesiology*. 2004;101(3):766–785.
6. Firth PG, McMillan KN, Haberkern CM, Yaster M, Bender MA, Goodwin SR. A survey of perioperative management of sickle cell disease in North America. *Paediatr Anaesth*. 2011;21(1):43–49.
7. Abboud MR, Yim E, Musallam KM, Adams RJ, STOP II Study Investigators. Discontinuing prophylactic transfusions increases the risk of silent brain infarction in children with sickle cell disease: data from STOP II. *Blood*. 2011;118(4):894–898.
8. Fu T, Corrigan NJ, Quinn CT, Rogers ZR, Buchanan GR. Minor elective surgical procedures using general anesthesia in children with sickle cell anemia without pre-operative blood transfusion. *Pediatr Blood Cancer*. 2005;45(1):43–47.
9. Gladwin MT, Vichinsky E. Pulmonary complications of sickle cell disease. *N Engl J Med*. 2008;359(21):2254–2265.
10. Platt OS, Brambilla DJ, Rosse WF, et al. Mortality in sickle cell disease: life expectancy and risk factors for early death. *N Engl J Med*. 1994;330(23):1639–1644.

52.

ANESTHETIC MANAGEMENT OF ANTERIOR MEDIASTINAL MASSES IN CHILDREN

Mehdi Trifa and Candice Burrier

STEM CASE AND KEY QUESTIONS

A previous healthy 2-year-old male, weighing 10 kg, presented to the emergency department because of a 1-month history of cough, stridor, and progressively increasing shortness of breath, worsening with the supine positioning. The child presented for a chest computed tomography (CT) scan.

WHAT IS THE SIGNIFICANCE OF THE SYMPTOMS THAT THE CHILD PRESENTS?

On examination, the patient could not tolerate the supine position. He was tachypneic and had a SpO2 of 93% on room air. The heart rate (HR) was 115 bpm and the blood pressure (BP) was normal. There was decreased air entry to the left lung on pulmonary auscultation. The cardiac auscultation was normal. There was no head or neck edema.

WHAT IS THE MAIN RISK ASSOCIATED WITH ANESTHESIA IN THIS PATIENT? WOULD YOU PROCEED?

Consultations were made to anesthesiology, interventional radiology, oncology, and pediatric surgery. Anesthesia was avoided for the CT scan. The CT was obtained with the assistance of parental presence and child life distraction techniques.

WHAT ADDITIONAL INFORMATION DO YOU NEED TO OPTIMIZE YOUR PREOPERATIVE ASSESSMENT?

The chest CT scan revealed a large mass in the anterior mediastinum extending to left hemithorax narrowing 50% of trachea and left main bronchial lumen. The echocardiography showed mild compression of the right ventricular outflow tract with normal right and left ventricular function. There was no pericardial effusion. The patient was scheduled for a minimally invasive extrathoracic tissue biopsy of the mass the next day by interventional radiology under local anesthesia.

WHAT WOULD BE YOUR ANESTHETIC TECHNIQUE FOR THE BIOPSY? WHAT ARE YOUR CONCERNS?

ENT and cardiac surgery were consulted. The child had an awake intravenous (IV) line placement. The biopsy was obtained utilizing gentle titrated sedation with dexmedetomidine and ketamine along with local anesthesia by the interventional radiologist. The child was kept breathing spontaneously. ENT was on standby for rescue rigid bronchoscopy.

The examination of a tissue biopsy of the mass showed that the tumor had a poor sensitivity to chemotherapy and radiation. The decision of the multidisciplinary meeting was to proceed with a surgical resection of the tumor via a thoracoscopy following a course of chemotherapy and radiation to shrink the tumor burdon in the anterior mediastinum.

WHAT IS THE MAIN RISK ASSOCIATED WITH GENERAL ANESTHESIA IN THIS PATIENT? WHAT WOULD BE YOUR MONITORING FOR THIS CASE? WHO WOULD YOU WANT TO BE PRESENT ON THE INDUCTION OF ANESTHESIA? WHAT WOULD BE YOUR ANESTHETIC TECHNIQUE (DRUGS FOR INDUCTION, AIRWAY MANAGEMENT, MAINTENANCE OF ANESTHESIA)? WHAT ARE THE MAIN INTRAOPERATIVE COMPLICATIONS THAT YOU WOULD BE CONCERNED ABOUT?

The resection of the tumor proceeded under general anesthesia and was without complications.

DISCUSSION

INTRODUCTION

The anterior mediastinum is bordered by the sternum anteriorly, the heart and great vessels posteriorly, the thoracic inlet superiorly, and the diaphragm inferiorly. Anterior mediastinal masses (AMMs) are a heterogeneous collection of primary or secondary, benign or malignant tumors. However, primary lesions are uncommon in children.[1] Pediatric AMMs differ from adults in the histology and symptomatology.[2] The most common tumor types in children are lymphoblastic lymphoma and Hodgkin's disease.[3] There is also an increased incidence of neurogenic tumors in pediatrics.[4]

The management of children with an AMM presents an anesthetic challenge since these tumors can precipitate severe and life-threatening complications related to airway obstruction and/or cardiovascular compression.[5–13] The incidence of perioperative complications in children with AMM undergoing general anesthesia varies from 9% to 20%.[5,14,15] These complications can vary from a brief decrease in BP or a minor airway obstruction to a severe cardiopulmonary collapse leading to cardiac arrest and even death.[9] The risk of anesthesia with an AMM is even higher in children than adults, as the majority of deaths have occurred in children.[16]

PATHOPHYSIOLOGY OF AMM SYMPTOMS

Children with an AMM can experience symptoms by extrinsic compression of vital structures within or bordering the anterior mediastinum including the tracheobronchial tree, the superior vena cava (SVC), the right cardiac chambers, and the pulmonary arteries or veins. Symptoms are due to the competition for mediastinal space with cardiovascular and respiratory structures. Patients presenting with AMM can experience respiratory and/or cardiovascular symptoms including cough, stridor, orthopnea, shortness of breath, cyanosis, jugular vein distension, or SVC syndrome.[17,18]

Infants and young children are at a higher risk of respiratory compromise for several reasons. First, their airways tend to be more compressible than older children or adults. Furthermore, minor diminutions in airway diameter are more likely to lead to a clinically significant decrease in the diameter of the tracheal and bronchial lumens.[19] Children may experience more symptoms than adults because of their smaller intrathoracic volume, the more frequent central position of the AMM, and the higher potential for malignancy and infiltration of tumors in childhood.[17] However, the absence of significant symptoms does not eliminate the possibility of developing cardiorespiratory collapse during the induction of general anesthesia.[20]

Children with AMM are also at risk for cardiovascular compression and cardiac symptoms. Compression of the cardiac structures typically involves compression of the right cardiac structures, the SVC, or the pulmonary veins. The obstruction of the right atria and the main pulmonary artery are uncommon since these structures are protected by the aorta. The compression of any of these cardiovascular structures can result in decreased left ventricular preload and therefore decreased cardiac output.[21,22] Right ventricular outflow obstruction can lead to right ventricular failure from increased strain on the right heart. The compression of the

SVC leads to clinical symptoms together known as SVC syndrome. SVC compression can lead to venous distention of the upper body with edema of the head and neck. The venous distention of SVC syndrome can result in respiratory signs because of venous engorgement of the airway and alteration in consciousness due to cerebral venous engorgement. Lastly, compression of pulmonary veins could be responsible for pulmonary edema.

PATHOPHYSIOLOGY OF AAM AND ANESTHESIA

Anesthesia can precipitate life-threatening cardiorespiratory events in children with AMM.[23] This effect depends on patient position, depth of anesthesia, mechanical versus spontaneous ventilation, and use of muscle relaxants. We discuss the pathophysiology of each of these variables.

Patient positioning can be critically important when caring for a child with a mediastinal mass. Anesthesia is typically provided in the supine position. However, the supine position, due to the effects of gravity on the mass, can cause compression of the more posterior structures of the heart and airways. An alternative position must be considered to offload the effects of gravity. Alternative positions include head of bed elevated, the prone position, and the right lateral decubitus position. In the case of cardiorespiratory collapse under anesthesia, one rescue maneuver should be to change the patient position.

Depth of anesthesia can contribute to respiratory collapse. As the depth of anesthesia increases, there is progressive relaxation of the airway smooth musculature, a decrease in the transpleural pressure gradient, and a decrease in airway diameter thereby increasing the risk of airway collapse under the pressure of the mass.[24,25] This effect is more likely to happen in younger patients in whom airway tissue is more collapsible. Furthermore, as the depth of anesthesia increases, you may see the negative inotropic effects of anesthetic agents contributing to cardiovascular collapse. Under general anesthesia as compared to sedation, you will see a loss of functional residual capacity contributing to small airway collapse and impaired oxygenation, potentiating the effects of AMM on oxygenation.

In children with AMM, spontaneous ventilation preserves the negative intrathoracic pressure to counterbalance the gravity effects of the tumor, preventing airway collapse.[26] The application of positive pressure ventilation leads to the loss of the normal negative thoracic pressure, which shifts the balance of pressures in favor of gravity, increasing the risk of the compression of the airway, the heart, and great vessels by the tumor.[18] Furthermore, positive pressure ventilation can cause diminution of the venous return due to a change from negative to positive intrathoracic pressure.[27]

Lastly, the administration of neuromuscular blockade agents could aggravate the degree of airway collapse due to the induced muscular relaxation of the chest wall, neck, and supraglottic structures.[17]

PERIOPERATIVE MANAGEMENT OF AMM

PREOPERATIVE EVALUATION

The aim of the preoperative evaluation of children with AMM is to identify those with higher risk of perioperative complications before initiating any procedure under anesthesia. The patient's history and physical examination should focus on the compressive cardiorespiratory symptoms and their possible exacerbation by exercise and positioning. Specific signs and symptoms of cardiopulmonary compression should be elicited. Signs and symptoms of airway compression may include stridor, tachypnea, hemoptysis, dyspnea, cough, or cyanosis. Signs and symptoms of SVC syndrome may include head, neck, and upper extremity swelling; swelling of the nasal passages and larynx causing stridor; cough, hoarseness, or dyspnea; and signs of cerebral edema including altered mental status. Cardiovascular compression can cause signs and symptoms of chest pain, hypotension, orthopnea, dyspnea, dizziness, syncope, or fatigue. Exacerbating and remitting factors should be elicited. It is recommended to determine a potential "rescue position" causing less symptomatic compression for the patient. This position should be considered as part of the anesthetic plan if the child develops a worsening of his or her cardiopulmonary symptoms under anesthesia. The preoperative assessment must also consider previous chemotherapy or radiation and potential anesthetic implications.

The clinical assessment should be followed with laboratory and imagining investigations. Basic laboratory tests including a complete blood count and basic metabolic panel should be obtained.[28] A chest CT scan with IV contrast provides the bulk of information about the anatomic location of the mass, its static assessments, and its extension and effects on surrounding cardiorespiratory structures.[29] The CT scan will inform about the level and degree of tracheal, bronchial, and/or cardiac compression and the existence of a pleural or pericardial effusion.

The role of pulmonary function testing (PFT) is limited in the workup for children with AMM, since it does not provide further information in addition to history, physical examination, and chest CT scanning.[17,18,27,30] Also, cooperation and age is an important barrier in obtaining accurate PFT in children. However, an adult study has demonstrated that the risk of postoperative respiratory complications increases with mixed obstructive and restrictive findings on PFT.[14]

The echocardiography of the heart and the mediastinal structures is essential for the preoperative assessment of patients with AMM, especially if the chest CT scan shows compression of cardiovascular structures. It provides information about the myocardial function, the degree of compression of the heart and great vessels, the pericardial extension of the mass, and the presence of a pericardial effusion.[26]

Once the assessment has been completed, a multidisciplinary consultation between the specialists involved, including surgeons, oncologists, anesthesiologists, pediatric intensivists, interventional radiologists, and radiation oncologists, should precede anesthesia in order to obtain a definitive diagnosis in a safe fashion.

To obtain a definitive diagnosis, the lowest risk techniques (pleural fluid cytology, bone marrow aspiration, and biopsy) should be attempted first, especially in patients with obstructive symptoms. Backup plans to manage cardiorespiratory complications during anesthesia should be discussed with the operating room team, since the absence of preoperative cardiorespiratory dysfunction does not exclude the risk of cardiorespiratory collapse under general anesthesia.[26]

In severely compromised patients, the choice between a risky anesthetic to obtain tissue biopsy and a presumptive treatment with steroids, empiric chemotherapy, and/or radiotherapy prior to surgery in order to reduce symptoms before attempting anesthesia for tissue biopsy is controversial. This presumptive treatment could cause shrinkage of the tumor, reduce cardiorespiratory compression, improve the patient's condition, and hopefully reduce the risk of anesthesia.[17] However, pretreatment may affect the accuracy of the histological diagnosis of some tumors, such as T-cell lymphomas, once the biopsy is secondarily taken, which could compromise the ultimate therapeutic success.[5,8,16,24,26] The limitation of steroid treatment's duration to 5 days could be an acceptable balance between reducing the general anesthesia risks and obtaining an accurate histological diagnosis of the tumor.[5]

When considering the available evidence, there is a controversy regarding the predictive clinical or radiological signs of intraoperative complications in children with AMM undergoing general anesthesia.[5] Ng et al. demonstrated in a series of 63 children that patients presenting with respiratory symptoms, signs of tracheal and vascular compression, or chest infection had a higher risk of developing perioperative complications.[31] Lam et al. reported that airway narrowing or displacement on imaging, histologic diagnosis of lymphoma, and evidence of SVC obstruction, pericardial or pleural effusion increased the anesthesia-related complications in children with AMM.[32] Stridor was the only symptom predicting an anesthetic complication in the Hack et al. series, in which the authors also concluded that the risk of intraoperative airway collapse was higher if the tracheal cross-sectional area was either less than 30% or less than 70% with associated bronchial compression.[5] Anghelescu et al. found in a large series of 117 children with malignant mediastinal masses that orthopnea, upper body edema, and great vessel compression increased the risk of general anesthesia.[15] These anesthesia-related complications in children with AMM were also identified in the Freud et al. series.[33] However, the absence of significant clinical or radiological symptoms of airway or cardiovascular compression does not exclude the possibility of a perioperative cardiorespiratory collapse, especially in the supine position, with the loss of spontaneous ventilation and the institution of positive pressure ventilation.[12,23,26]

Even though there is limited evidence of correlation between preoperative findings and the risk of perioperative

Table 52.1 CLINICAL SIGNS AND SPECIAL INVESTIGATIONS' FINDINGS THAT MAY BE ASSOCIATED WITH HIGHER RISK OF PERIOPERATIVE COMPLICATIONS

CLINICAL SYMPTOMS	SPECIAL INVESTIGATIONS' FINDINGS
– Orthopnea – Stridor – Cyanosis – SVC obstruction – Collapse/dizziness	– Tracheal compression >70% – Tracheal cross-sectional area <70% with bronchial compression – Great vessel compression, SVC obstruction – Pericardial effusion, tamponade – Pulmonary artery outflow obstruction – Ventricular dysfunction – Supine peak expiratory flow rate ≤50% predicted

Note. SVC = superior vena cava.

complications, some authors have published guidelines to stratify children with AMM into categories based on their clinical signs and the results of the investigations they underwent (Table 52.1).[5,17,18,20]

INDUCTION AND MAINTENANCE OF ANESTHESIA

Anesthesia for children with AMM may be indicated for chest CT scan, biopsy of the tumor, central line placement, or resection of the mass. Cardiac arrests, severe airway obstructions, and even deaths have been reported during general anesthesia in children with AMM.[9] Thus, general anesthesia should be avoided, if possible, in high-risk patients undergoing imaging and diagnostic tissue biopsy procedures. One consideration as an alternative to anesthesia for tissue diagnosis is biopsy of an extra mediastinal site performed under local anesthesia.[20,34–36] However, in some circumstances local anesthesia may not be feasible due to an uncooperative child or challenging tumor location.

If anesthesia is mandatory, a careful and specific perioperative care plan must be formulated. Sedation should be initiated with caution, as even light sedation can cause relaxation of resting muscle tone and further collapse and compression of tissue underlying the AMM. Sedation should proceed with the same precautions as general anesthesia.

In a high-risk patient proceeding with general anesthesia, a rescue plan for cardiorespiratory collapse needs to be in place prior to the start of the procedure. That plan may include rapid change to rescue position, rigid bronchoscopy to stent open collapsed airways, and either extracorporeal membrane oxygenation (ECMO) or cardiopulmonary bypass (CPB). Appropriate consultations to otolaryngology, general surgery, or cardiac surgery should be placed. If airway compression is a concern and rigid bronchoscopy may be needed, the equipment should be set up and the otolaryngologist on immediate standby. If cardiovascular collapse is a concern, a perfusionist, a primed ECMO circuit, or a CPB circuit and a cardiac surgeon must be on immediate standby. Some authors have advocated for preinduction initiation of ECMO as the time needed for the initiation of ECMO may result in significant neurologic ischemia.[18]

Additional airway equipment should be available prior to the start of anesthesia. A fiberoptic bronchoscope should be available to confirm correct placement of the endotracheal tube (ETT). A reinforced ETT may help combat tracheal compression. If distal tracheal or bronchial compression is an issue, a long ETT may be necessary to stent open the airway.

Careful consideration should be given to patient position. Supine position may not be tolerated by the child, and the anesthesiologist should consider the position associated with best cardiorespiratory function for the induction of anesthesia. Keeping the head of the bed elevated or the patient in lateral decubitus position could help to prevent airway collapse and reduce cardiovascular compression.[34]

Preinduction monitoring must include pulse oximetry, continuous electrocardiography, and noninvasive BP. The placement of an arterial line prior to induction, if feasible, is very helpful to detect hemodynamic variations during the induction of anesthesia. The monitoring of the end-tidal CO_2 is mandatory in these patients, as the capnography graph could alert to bronchial obstruction or a sudden drop in cardiac output before the occurrence of a cardiac arrest.[26]

Age-appropriate large-bore IV access must be secured. Upper extremity IVs may need to be avoided in patients with a right-sided mediastinal tumor or a preoperative evidence of SVC syndrome, in whom venous return from upper extremities could be compromised. Some authors recommend the insertion of an IV catheter before induction of anesthesia.[26] For surgical resection, bleeding is a potential complication, especially with a large AMM, an AMM encasing major vasculature, or in the case of SVC obstruction with venous engorgement and the development of venous collaterals. The patient should have a type and screen, and, after consultation with the surgeon, blood may need to be available.

Premedication should be avoided in patients with compromised cardiorespiratory function. For induction of anesthesia, either inhalational and IV inductions have been described and various anesthetic agents have been used (ketamine, propofol, dexmedetomidine, inhalational agents) in children with AMM. No agent seems to be superior to others as long as spontaneous ventilation is maintained and muscular relaxation and positive pressure ventilation are avoided.[17,18,24,26] However, dexmedetomidine and ketamine may have advantages due to their minimal effect on respiratory function.[18] If muscle relaxation is absolutely necessary for the procedure, the anesthesiologist should start by assessing if the child will safely tolerate positive-pressure ventilation and if so administrating a short-acting muscle relaxant, such as succinylcholine, before giving a longer-acting paralytic agent.[17] Some authors have reported the safe use of muscle relaxants and positive-pressure ventilation in children with AMM.[5,37]

The interventions for rescue from airway or cardiovascular collapse during anesthesia include[18,20,29,38]:

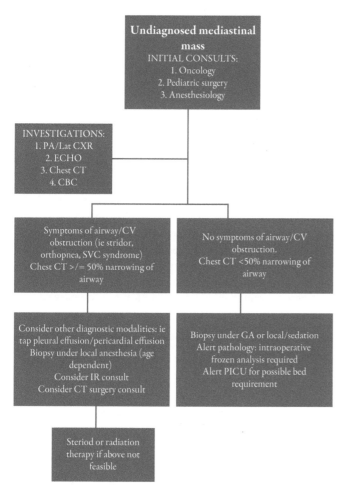

Undiagnosed mediastinal mass
INITIAL CONSULTS:
1. Oncology
2. Pediatric surgery
3. Anesthesiology

INVESTIGATIONS:
1. PA/Lat CXR
2. ECHO
3. Chest CT
4. CBC

Symptoms of airway/CV obstruction (ie stridor, orthopnea, SVC syndrome) Chest CT >/= 50% narrowing of airway

No symptoms of airway/CV obstruction. Chest CT <50% narrowing of airway

Consider other diagnostic modalities: ie tap pleural effusion/pericardial effusion Biopsy under local anesthesia (age dependent) Consider IR consult Consider CT surgery consult

Biopsy under GA or local/sedation Alert pathology: intraoperative frozen analysis required Alert PICU for possible bed requirement

Steriod or radiation therapy if above not feasible

Fig. 52.1 Mediastinal mass management algorithm. PA/Lat CXR: posterior anterior/lateral chest x-ray, CV: cardiovascular, CT: computed tomography, CBC: complete blood count, SVC: superior vena cava, GA: general anesthesia, IR: interventional radiology, PICU: pediatric intensive care unit. From Tobias JD, Cambier G, Balla T. Mediastinal mass management algorithm. In: *Intraoperative management guidelines.* Columbus, OH: Department of Anesthesiology and Pain Medicine, Nationwide Children's Hospital.

- Awakening the patient.

- Repositioning the child to a preplanned "rescue" position (semi-sitting, lateral decubitus, or prone) to displace the mass and to take its weight off the airway or the cardiovascular structures.

- Utilizing rigid bronchoscopy to mechanically open the obstructed airway and restore effective ventilation and oxygenation distal to the obstruction.

- Performing an immediate sternotomy and a surgical elevation of the mass off of the cardiovascular structures in case of compression of the great vessels.

- Instituting cardiopulmonary bypass or extra corporeal membrane oxygenation in unresponsive cases.

Many authors and institutions have established guidelines for the management of children AMM.[5,20,23,39,40] We suggest the algorithm in Figure 52.1 based on the most recent evidence.[40]

CONCLUSION

Acute cardiorespiratory collapse could be precipitated by the induction of anesthesia in children with AMM. The initial management of these patients should involve a multidisciplinary team discussion in regard to the type of procedure, the benefit/risk of prebiopsy treatment, the appropriate timing, and the associated risks of surgery and anesthesia. Institutions should have algorithms for the management of children with AMM, identifying high-risk patients and recommending an appropriate strategy depending on the case presentation.

1. Which of the following statements regarding AMM in children is **MOST** accurate?

  A. Masses tend to be less centrally located.
  B. Symptoms are less common on presentation.
  C. Thymomas are very common neoplasms.
  D. Tumors have a higher risk for malignancy.

Answer: D

Anesthesia can precipitate life-threatening cardiorespiratory events in children with AMM.[23] This effect depends on patient position, depth of anesthesia, mechanical versus spontaneous ventilation, and use of muscle relaxants. The most common tumor types in children are lymphoblastic lymphoma and Hodgkin's disease.[3]

Infants and young children are at a higher risk of respiratory compromise for several reasons. First, their airways tend to be more compressible than older children or adults. Furthermore, minor diminutions in airway diameter are more likely to lead to a clinically significant decrease in the diameter of the tracheal and bronchial lumens.[19] Children may experience more symptoms than adults because of their smaller intrathoracic volume, the more frequent central position of the AMM, and the higher potential for malignancy and infiltration of tumors in childhood.[1]

2. A previously healthy 4-year-old boy presents with orthopnea, tachypnea, and SpO2 of 90%. Symptoms have become progressively worse over the past couple of days. A chest x-ray reveals a large AMM. You are called to provide anesthesia to obtain a CT scan. The patient is sitting quietly with his parents but when the team tries to move him to the CT scanner he is uncooperative. He had breakfast a few hours ago. The **BEST** next step would be

  A. Consult with hematology, otolaryngology, pediatric surgery, and pediatric intensive care unit.
  B. Sedate with dexmedetomidine, maintaining responsiveness to light touch.
  C. Postpone the procedure until this young child is appropriately nil per os.
  D. Induce anesthesia with sevoflurane, maintaining spontaneous respiration.

Answer: A

If an AMM is suspected, it is best to have a multidisciplinary approach. A multidisciplinary consultation between the specialists involved, including surgeons, oncologists, anesthesiologists, pediatric intensivists, interventional radiologists, and radiation oncologists, should precede anesthesia in order to obtain a definitive diagnosis in a safe fashion. At times, sedation/general anesthesia may be needed to get through even the initial assessment (CT, echocardiogram, etc.) and the safest manner to proceed.

Some institutions even have formalized clinical pathways developed as how to proceed.

3. A CT scan is obtained in the previous patient that demonstrates a large mediastinal mass with 70% luminal narrowing of the carina and 50% narrowing of the left mainstem bronchus. The echocardiogram is normal. Labs are unremarkable: Vitals are as follows: HR 115, BP 94/45, respiratory rate (RR) 45, SpO2 95%. The patient is on 2L NC. The team would like to proceed with tissue biopsy. The next **BEST** step is

    A. Biopsy a supraclavicular lymph node using local anesthesia.
    B. Discuss all options at a multidisciplinary conference.
    C. Induce endotracheal general anesthesia for a tissue biopsy.
    D. Shrink the tumor with radiation prior to the biopsy.

Correct Answer: B
The management of children with an AMM presents an anesthetic challenge since these tumors can precipitate severe and life-threatening complications related to airway obstruction and/or cardiovascular compression.[5-13] The incidence of perioperative complications in children with AMM undergoing general anesthesia varies from 9% to 20%.[5,14,15] These complications can vary from a brief decrease in BP or a minor airway obstruction to a severe cardiopulmonary collapse leading to cardiac arrest and even death.[9] The risk of anesthesia with an AMM is even higher in children than adults, as the majority of deaths have occurred in children.[16]

4. Of the following respiratory measurements that differ in children as compared to adults, which contributes the **LEAST** to their increased risk for respiratory compromise with AMMs?

    A. lower closing volume
    B. more compressible airways
    C. smaller intrathoracic volume
    D. smaller tracheal diameter

Answer: A
Infants and young children are at a higher risk of respiratory compromise for several reasons. First, their airways tend to be more compressible than older children or adults. Furthermore, minor diminutions in airway diameter are more likely to lead to a clinically significant decrease in the diameter of the tracheal and bronchial lumens.[19] Children may experience more symptoms than adults because of their smaller intrathoracic volume, the more frequent central position of the AMM, and the higher potential for malignancy and infiltration of tumors in childhood.[17] However, the absence of significant symptoms does not eliminate the possibility of developing cardiorespiratory collapse during the induction of general anesthesia.[20] Infants and younger children have higher closing volumes than adults.

Children with AMM are also at risk for cardiovascular compression and cardiac symptoms. Compression of the cardiac structures typically involves compression of the right cardiac structures, the SVC, or the pulmonary veins. The obstruction of the right atria and the main pulmonary artery are uncommon since these structures are protected by the aorta. The compression of any of these cardiovascular structures can result in decreased left ventricular preload and therefore decreased cardiac output.[21,22] Right ventricular outflow obstruction can lead to right ventricular failure from increased strain on the right heart. The compression of the SVC leads to clinical symptoms together known as SVC syndrome. SVC compression can lead to venous distention of the upper body with edema of the head and neck. The venous distention of SVC syndrome can result in respiratory signs because of venous engorgement of the airway and alteration in consciousness due to cerebral venous engorgement. Lastly, compression of pulmonary veins could be responsible for pulmonary edema

5. Of the following symptoms, which one is **LEAST** likely due to compression of SVC by an AMM?

    A. altered mental status
    B. hoarseness and coughing
    C. pulmonary edema
    D. upper extremity swelling

Answer: C
Signs and symptoms of SVC syndrome may include head, neck, and upper extremity swelling; swelling of the nasal passages and larynx causing stridor; cough, hoarseness, or dyspnea; and signs of cerebral edema including altered mental status.

6. Anesthesia can precipitate life-threatening events in the presence of AMM. Which of following physiological change, seen with inhaled anesthetics, is the **MOST** dangerous in children with AMM?

    A. skeletal muscle relaxation
    B. decreased transpleural pressure
    C. decreased cardiac contractility
    D. loss of functional residual capacity

Answer: B
Depth of anesthesia can contribute to respiratory collapse. As the depth of anesthesia increases, there is progressive relaxation of the airway smooth musculature, a decrease in the transpleural pressure gradient, and a decrease in airway diameter thereby increasing the risk of airway collapse under the pressure of the mass.[24,25] This effect is more likely to happen in younger patients in whom airway tissue is more collapsible. Furthermore, as the depth of anesthesia increases, you may see the negative inotropic effects of anesthetic agents contributing to cardiovascular collapse. Under general anesthesia as compared to sedation, you will see a loss of functional residual capacity contributing to small airway collapse and impaired oxygenation, potentiating the effects of AMM on oxygenation.

In children with AMM, spontaneous ventilation preserves the negative intrathoracic pressure to counterbalance the gravity effects of the tumor, preventing airway collapse.[26] The application of positive pressure ventilation leads to the loss of the normal negative thoracic pressure, which shifts the balance of pressures in favor of gravity, increasing the risk of the compression of the airway, the heart, and great vessels by the tumor.[18] Furthermore, positive pressure ventilation can cause diminution of the venous return due to a change from negative to positive intrathoracic pressure.[27]

Lastly, the administration of neuromuscular blockade agents could aggravate the degree of airway collapse due to the induced muscular relaxation of the chest wall, neck, and supraglottic structures.[17] Sevoflurane, at clinically relevant dose, has no effect on skeletal muscle strength or contractility.

7. The **MOST** important aspect of the preoperative evaluation of children with AMM is which of following?

 A. electrocardiogram
 B. history and physical exam
 C. pulmonary function tests
 D. pulse oximetry values

Answer: B
The role of PFT is limited in the workup for children with AMM, since it does not provide further information in addition to history, physical examination, and chest CT scanning.[17,18,27,30] Also cooperation and age is an important barrier in obtaining accurate PFT in children. Pulse oximetry and electrocardiogram results may possibly make some contribution to a preoperative evaluation, but the history and physical exam are essential in assessing the degree of compromise a patient with an AMM is experiencing.

8. A 14-year-old girl presents with progressive weakness and fatigue over the past several weeks. She presented to the emergency room after feeling dizzy and briefly collapsing. She complains of dyspnea, chest pain, and fatigue. On exam, her extremities are cold and clammy. Heart sounds are muted. Lungs are clear to auscultation. Her HR is 140, BP is 80/65, RR is 30, SpO2 is 96%. She exhibits pulsus paradoxus. Chest x-ray reveals a large AMM. There is low QRS voltage on the electrocardiogram. The patient **MOST** likely has which of the following complications of an AMM?

 A. pericardial tamponade
 B. pulmonary artery outflow obstruction
 C. SVC syndrome
 D. ventricular dysfunction

Answer: A
The three signs of cardiac tamponade are muffled heart sounds, increased jugular vein distention, and hypotension. This is also known as Beck's Triad. Patients can also present with SVC syndrome, pulmonary artery outflow obstruction, and ventricular dysfunction.

9. A 2-year-old boy presents with a 1-month history of cough, stridor, and progressively increasing shortness of breath worsening in the supine position. On exam he is tachypneic and SpO2 is 93% on room air. HR is 115 and BP is 85/62. There is decreased air entry to the left lung

on pulmonary auscultation. The cardiac exam is normal. A chest CT reveals a large AMM extending to the left hemithorax narrowing 50% of the trachea and left main bronchial lumen. The echocardiography showed mild compression of the right ventricular outflow tract with normal right and left ventricular function. Tissue biopsy obtained under local reveals that the tumor has poor sensitivity to chemotherapy and radiation and the decision of a multidisciplinary meeting is to proceed with thoracoscopy under general anesthesia. Who would you **LEAST** need to be immediately available?

 A. cardiac surgeon
 B. otolaryngologist
 C. pediatric intensivist
 D. perfusionist

Answer: C
In a high-risk patient proceeding with general anesthesia, a rescue plan for cardiorespiratory collapse needs to be in place prior to the start of the procedure. That plan may include rapid change to rescue position, rigid bronchoscopy to stent open collapsed airways, and either ECMO or CPB. Appropriate consultations to otolaryngology, general surgery, or cardiac surgery should be placed. If airway compression is a concern and rigid bronchoscopy may be needed, the equipment should be set up and the otolaryngologist on immediate standby. If cardiovascular collapse is a concern, a perfusionist, a primed ECMO circuit or CPB circuit, and a cardiac surgeon must be on immediate standby. Some authors have advocated for preinduction initiation of ECMO as the time needed for the initiation of ECMO may result in significant neurologic ischemia.[18]

Additional airway equipment should be available prior to the start of anesthesia. A fiberoptic bronchoscope should be available to confirm correct placement of the ETT. A reinforced ETT may help combat tracheal compression. If distal tracheal or bronchial compression is an issue, a long ETT may be necessary to stent open the airway.

10. The **MOST** important consideration of an anesthetic plan, for a patient with a mediastinal mass, is to maintain which of the following?

 A. baseline oxygenation
 B. optimal surgical exposure
 C. spontaneous ventilation
 D. surgical plane of anesthesia

Answer: C
In children with AMM, spontaneous ventilation preserves the negative intrathoracic pressure to counterbalance the gravity effects of the tumor, preventing airway collapse.[26] The application of positive pressure ventilation leads to the loss of the normal negative thoracic pressure, which shifts the balance of pressures in favor of gravity, increasing the risk of the compression of the airway, the heart, and great vessels by the tumor.[18] Furthermore, positive pressure ventilation can cause diminution of the venous return due to a change from negative to positive intrathoracic pressure.[27]

QUESTIONS AND ANSWERS

This chapter has accompanying questions and answers which are available to subscribers as part of the Oxford eLearning platform. To access the questions, go to ✔ http://oxfordmedicine. com/pediatricanesthesiaPBL

REFERENCES

1. Franken EA Jr, Smith JA, Smith WL. Tumors of the chest wall in infants and children. *Pediatr Radiol.* 1977;6:13–18.
2. Takeda S, Miyoshi S, Akashi A, et al. Clinical spectrum of primary mediastinal tumors: a comparison of adult and pediatric populations at a single Japanese institution. *J Surg Oncol.* 2003;83:24–30.
3. King RM, Telander RL, Smithson WA, et al. Primary mediastinal tumors in children. *J Pediatr Surg.* 1982;17:512–520.
4. Azarow KS, Pearl RH, Zurcher R, et al. Primary mediastinal masses: a comparison of adult and pediatric populations. *J Thorac Cardiovasc Surg.* 1993;106:67–72.
5. Hack HA, Wright NB, Wynn RF. The anaesthetic management of children with anterior mediastinal masses. *Anaesthesia.* 2008;63:837–846.
6. Azizkhan RG, Dudgeon DL, Buck JR, et al. Life-threatening airway obstruction as a complication to the management of mediastinal masses in children. *J Pediatr Surg.* 1985;20:816–822.
7. Bray RJ, Fernandes FJ. Mediastinal tumour causing airway obstruction in anaesthetised children. *Anaesthesia.* 1982;37:571–575.
8. Ferrari LR, Bedford RF. General anesthesia prior to treatment of anterior mediastinal masses in pediatric cancer patients. *Anesthesiology.* 1990;72:991–995.
9. Keon TP. Death on induction of anesthesia for cervical node biopsy. *Anesthesiology.* 1981;55:471–472.
10. Levin H, Bursztein S, Heifetz M. Cardiac arrest in a child with an anterior mediastinal mass. *Anesth Analg.* 1985;64:1129–1130.
11. Prakash UB, Abel MD, Hubmayr RD. Mediastinal mass and tracheal obstruction during general anesthesia. *Mayo Clin Proc.* 1988;63:1004–1011.
12. Viswanathan S, Campbell CE, Cork RC. Asymptomatic undetected mediastinal mass: a death during ambulatory anesthesia. *J Clin Anesth.* 1995;7:151–155.
13. Todres ID, Reppert SM, Walker PF, Grillo HC. Management of critical airway obstruction in a child with a mediastinal tumor. *Anesthesiology.* 1976;45:100–102.
14. Bechard P, Letourneau L, Lacasse Y, Cote D, Bussieres JS. Perioperative cardiorespiratory complications in adults with mediastinal mass: incidence and risk factors. *Anesthesiology.* 2004;100:826–834; discussion 5A.
15. Anghelescu DL, Burgoyne LL, Liu T, et al. Clinical and diagnostic imaging findings predict anesthetic complications in children presenting with malignant mediastinal masses. *Paediatr Anaesth.* 2007;17:1090–1098.
16. Victory RA, Casey W, Doherty P, et al. Cardiac and respiratory complications of mediastinal lymphomas. *Anaesth Intensive Care.* 1993;21:366–369.
17. Pearson JK, Tan GM. Pediatric anterior mediastinal mass: a review article. *Semin Cardiothorac Vasc Anesth.* 2015;19:248–254.
18. Blank RS, de Souza DG. Anesthetic management of patients with an anterior mediastinal mass: continuing professional development. *Can J Anaesth.* 2011;58:853–867.

19. Vas L, Naregal F, Naik V. Anaesthetic management of an infant with anterior mediastinal mass. *Paediatr Anaesth.* 1999;9:439–443.
20. Hammer GB. Anaesthetic management for the child with a mediastinal mass. *Paediatr Anaesth.* 2004;14:95–97.
21. Abdelmalak B, Marcanthony N, Abdelmalak J, Machuzak MS, Gildea TR, Doyle DJ. Dexmedetomidine for anesthetic management of anterior mediastinal mass. *J Anesth.* 2010;24:607–610.
22. Redford DT, Kim AS, Barber BJ, Copeland JG. Transesophageal echocardiography for the intraoperative evaluation of a large anterior mediastinal mass. *Anesth Analg.* 2006;103:578–579.
23. Garey CL, Laituri CA, Valusek PA, St Peter SD, Snyder CL. Management of anterior mediastinal masses in children. *Eur J Pediatr Surg.* 2011;21:310–313.
24. Neuman GG, Weingarten AE, Abramowitz RM et al. The anesthetic management of the patient with a mediastinal mass. *Anesthesiology.* 1984;60:144–147.
25. Johnson D, Hurst T, Cujec B, Mayers I. Cardiopulmonary effects of an anterior mediastinal mass in dogs anesthetized with halothane. *Anesthesiology.* 1991;74:725–736.
26. Lerman J. Anterior mediastinal masses in children. *Semin Anesth.* 2007;26:133–140.
27. Narang S, Harte BH, Body SC. Anesthesia for patients with a mediastinal mass. *Anesthesiol Clin North America.* 2001;19:559–579.
28. Gothard JW. Anesthetic considerations for patients with anterior mediastinal masses. *Anesthesiol Clin.* 2008;26:305–314.
29. Slinger P, Karsli C. Management of the patient with a large anterior mediastinal mass: recurring myths. *Curr Opin Anaesthesiol.* 2007;20:1–3.
30. Rath L, Gullahorn G, Connolly N, Pratt T, Boswell G, Cornelissen C. Anterior mediastinal mass biopsy and resection: anesthetic techniques and perioperative concerns. *Semin Cardiothorac Vasc Anesth.* 2012;16:235–242.
31. Ng A, Bennett J, Bromley P, Davies P, Morland B. Anesthetic outcome and predictive risk factors in children with mediastinal tumors. *Pediatr Blood Cancer.* 2007;48:160–164.
32. Lam JC, Chui CH, Jacobsen AS, Tan AM, Joseph VT. When is a mediastinal mass critical in a child? An analysis of 29 patients. *Pediatr Surg Int.* 2004;20:180–184.
33. Freud E, Ben-Ari J, Schonfeld T, Blumenfeld A, Steinberg R, Dlugy E, Yaniv I, Katz J, Schwartz M, Zer M. Mediastinal tumors in children: a single institution experience. *Clin Pediatr.* 2002;41:219–223.
34. Pullerits J, Holzman R. Anaesthesia for patients with mediastinal masses. *Can J Anaesth.* 1989;36:681–688.
35. Perger L, Lee E, Shamberger R. Management of children and adolescents with a critical airway due to compression by an anterior mediastinal mass. *J Pediatr Surg.* 2008;43:1990–1997.
36. Ricketts RR. Clinical management of anterior mediastinal tumors in children. *Semin Pediatr Surg.* 2001;10:161–168.
37. Stricker PA, Gurnaney HG, Litman RS. Anesthetic management of children with an anterior mediastinal mass. *J Clin Anesth.* 2010;22:159–163.
38. Shamberger RC. Preanesthetic evaluation of children with anterior mediastinal masses. *Sem Pediatr Surg.* 1999;8:61–68.
39. Cheung S, Lerman J. Mediastinal masses and anesthesia in children. *Anesthesiol Clinics North America.* 1998;16:893–910.
40. Tobias JD, Cambier G, Balla T. Mediastinal mass management algorithm. In: *Intraoperative management guidelines.* Columbus, OH: Department of Anesthesiology and Pain Medicine, Nationwide Children's Hospital.

SECTION 10

PEDIATRIC PAIN

53.

MULTIMODAL APPROACH TO ACUTE PAIN MANAGEMENT AFTER NUSS BAR PLACEMENT AND OTHER PAIN SCENARIOS

Christina D. Diaz and Steven J. Weisman

STEM CASE AND KEY QUESTIONS

Your patient is a 16-year-old 65-kg young man who presents for a thoracoscopic Nuss bar placement during his summer break. He runs track and reports some chest discomfort when running and would like to have his pectus excavatum repaired. In the preoperative area, he and his mother appear very anxious and his mother answers all the preoperative questions for the patient. When you discuss the postoperative pain management options, you suggest an epidural be placed but also offer patient-controlled analgesia (PCA) with morphine. The father informs you that the surgeon had suggested the epidural and he states that is what they want.

WHAT ARE THE BENEFITS OF AN EPIDURAL BLOCK FOR NUSS BAR PLACEMENT? WHAT ARE THE ASSOCIATED RISKS WITH PLACEMENT OF AN EPIDURAL CATHETER? CAN ANYTHING BE DONE TO MINIMIZE THE RISKS OF THE EPIDURAL PLACEMENT? WOULD YOUR PLAN FOR PLACING AN EPIDURAL CHANGE IF THIS WERE A 2-YEAR-OLD PATIENT OR A 16-YEAR-OLD WITH SEVERE DEVELOPMENTAL DELAY?

The epidural is placed with the patient awake and sitting on the operating room bed. He is cooperative with instructions after the administration of midazolam and fentanyl. The epidural is placed at the T8 level, and there is a negative test dose with 3 mL of 1.5% lidocaine with 1:200,000 epinephrine. The patient is then placed under a general anesthetic and intubated, and the surgeon places the Nuss bar uneventfully. A pharmacist delivers the epidural infusion containing ropivacaine 0.1% and morphine 10 mcg/mL, and it is run throughout the 1-hour case at 10 mL/hour. The patient is extubated and taken to the recovery room. In the recovery area, he is tachycardic, hypertensive, and screaming "it really hurts." He rates his pain as 15 out of 10 on the verbal numeric pain scale.

WHAT APPROACHES CAN THE ANESTHESIOLOGIST USE TO DETERMINE IF THE EPIDURAL IS WORKING? ARE THERE ANY IMAGING TECHNIQUES THAT MAY BE HELPFUL? IF THE LEVEL OF ANALGESIA IS INAPPROPRIATE, WHAT OPTIONS ARE AVAILABLE TO AID THIS PATIENT USING THE EPIDURAL?

Using an icepack, the patient reports that he has a narrow band of "numbness" below his nipple line and is begging you to help him with his pain. Since the block is present and bilateral, you give a loading dose of 10 mL ropivacaine and morphine from his epidural infusion pump. Approximately 20 minutes later, the patient looks calmer and describes a block from T6-T12. The patient continues to report his pain as 8 out of 10.

WHAT ADDITIONAL PAIN ADJUNCTS CAN YOU PROVIDE THIS PATIENT?

After a discussion with the surgeon, the patient is given scheduled intravenous (IV) acetaminophen (15 mg/kg every 6 hours; 1000 mg maximum), to be followed by oral acetaminophen (15 mg/kg every 6 hours; 1000 mg maximum) when he is tolerating clear liquids. He also is given scheduled IV ketorolac (15 mg every 6 hours) to be followed by oral ibuprofen (10 mg/kg every 6 hours). His epidural infusion rate is increased to 12 mL/hour to maintain the larger block spread. Forty-five minutes later, the patient's blood pressure and heart rate have returned to his preoperative baseline, and he appears sleepy. His mother joins him at the bedside, and he reports to her that he is in "incredible pain" and "can't breathe." This upsets his mother, which also seems to worsen the patient's state of anxiety and pain. A bedside chest radiograph is performed in the recovery room, and it does not show any significant pathology. The anesthesiologist reassures the mother and patient that his oxygen saturation is appropriate.

WHAT ADDITIONAL STEPS MAY BE OF BENEFIT TO THIS PATIENT?

This patient and his mother were already very anxious prior to the procedure. While his epidural is now providing him an appropriate block, the change in his chest wall dynamics may be causing significant anxiety. Although his oxygen saturation remains normal, his chest wall constriction from the costal Nuss bar attachments may be inducing a sense of air hunger. The patient is given low-dose IV diazepam (0.05 mg/kg), as a muscle relaxant/anxiolytic, with improved pain/anxiety control.

The following morning, the pain service is notified that the patient reports leg weakness, and he is reluctant to get out of bed because he is very sleepy. When you review the chart, you learn that the previous evening the call physician was summoned emergently because the patient woke up at 2 AM "writhing and screaming" in pain. The call physician responded by redosing the epidural catheter with 12 mL of the infusate followed by a rate increase to 14 mL/hour. When you inform the patient and his family that you would like to decrease the infusion rate to allow the patient to regain function of his legs, they worry about having pain similar to the previous evening.

WHAT OPTIONS CAN YOU OFFER THE FAMILY AS A COMPROMISE TO SIMPLY LOWERING THE EPIDURAL INFUSION RATE?

The morphine is removed from the epidural infusion and the infusion rate is lowered back to the previous setting (12 mL/hour.). The block shrinks back to between T7-T12 after several hours. As part of the compromise with the family, a morphine PCA without a basal infusion rate (set at 20 mcg/kg/dose every 8 min; 1 mg/kg/hour maximum) is initiated to allow the patient more control over his own pain management regimen. He is continued on his scheduled acetaminophen and ibuprofen, and the diazepam is available as needed.

Three days later the epidural is removed and the patient continues to report a significant amount of pain. His morphine use has increased since removing the epidural, and he reports burning pain around the left chest wall incision site. The patient is tolerating a regular diet.

WHAT OPTIONS ARE THERE TO TREAT THE PATIENT'S INCREASING PAIN? WHAT TYPES OF MEDICATIONS CAN THE PATIENT USE TO GO HOME?

The patient is started on oral oxycodone (0.1 mg/kg/dose every 4 hours, as needed). In addition, he is started on oral gabapentin 300 mg/dose 3 times a day (approximately 5 mg/kg/dose). He is discharged later that day, on postoperative day 4, with oxycodone and gabapentin and is instructed to continue his scheduled acetaminophen and ibuprofen.

DISCUSSION

EPIDURAL

Pectus excavatum is one of the most common congenital chest deformities, affecting males greater than females at a ratio of 4:1.[1] The Nuss procedure, which is one technique used to correct pectus excavatum, can result in significant pain and discomfort as it changes the structure of the chest. During the procedure a U-shaped bar is placed under the sternum via blunt dissection at the point of greatest concavity, and the bar is flipped into place, elevating the chest depression. The bar is fixed to the ribs on both sides of the chest. Multiple approaches for pain management have been advocated with regard to this procedure, including the thoracic epidural regional block, PCA with an opioid, incisional infusion catheters, and paravertebral nerve blocks/catheters.[1] The two most frequently reported approaches are epidural block catheter placement and PCA analgesia with the addition of multimodal analgesia to either approach. Both approaches appear to be efficacious,[2–4] with some studies reporting better pain scores in the epidural group immediately postoperatively.[2,4]

The thoracic epidural block management involves placement of a catheter into the epidural space ideally at the level of innervation of the surgical site and Nuss bar placement. Local anesthetic, and possibly low-dose opioid, is then infused into the epidural space. The risks of placing this catheter include bleeding and infection at the site of insertion; spinal headache/dural puncture; unilateral block; block failure; reaction to the medication including high spinal, seizure, and cardiac arrest; and nerve and spinal cord injury.[5,6] However, when placed successfully, the epidural catheter can reduce pain at the sites of incisions and bar placement.[1,2,4] With successful placement of the epidural block, the patient may have less splinting due to pain and, therefore, easier respiratory mechanics.[7] The patient may also have a faster return of bowel function by limiting the overall opioid exposure.[7]

The anesthesiologist must choose the local anesthetic (commonly ropivacaine or bupivacaine) and may elect to add an opioid such as fentanyl, sufentanil, morphine, or hydromorphone, with or without clonidine, as pain adjuncts. Epidural clonidine has been shown to lengthen the duration of analgesia and thereby decrease the need for rescue medication.[8] Side effects commonly experienced by the patient from these local anesthetics include urinary retention and lower extremity motor weakness.[7] Pruritus, nausea, vomiting, urinary retention, and sedation are common side effects caused by the addition of opioid to the infusion. Urinary retention, postoperative nausea, and vomiting have been particularly associated with higher doses of morphine.[1] The use of an opioid in the epidural catheter can improve the patient's overall pain control and may limit the total amount of systemic opioid needed.[7] If the patient experiences ringing in the ears, a metallic taste, respiratory depression, arm weakness, seizures, loss of consciousness, or significant bradycardia, the epidural infusion must be stopped and the patient reassessed and possibly treated for local anesthetic toxicity or the presence of a high spinal.

Placement of the epidural catheter in a cooperative awake adult patient is a common practice. This practice may decrease the risk of nerve injury and may allow earlier detection of a malpositioned catheter. An awake patient can report to the provider if there are any shooting or sharp pains and can report pain as the needle advances into bone or other inappropriate structures. Also, with the administration of local anesthetics, an awake patient can report symptoms immediately in the event of an intravascular injection. The Nuss bar is commonly placed in patients during their teen or early adult years. This cohort of patients is likely to cooperate with their anesthesiologist during epidural placement while awake or lightly sedated. Younger children and developmentally delayed patients, who are not able to understand the consequences of moving during the epidural catheter placement or in whom reliable report of symptoms is unlikely, are inappropriate candidates for an awake placement and it is safer to place the epidural while under anesthesia. While this practice has raised concern in the past, Taenzer et al. demonstrated, after reviewing more than 50,000 regional blocks from the Pediatric Regional Anesthesia Network database, that placement of the block in pediatric patients under general anesthesia is as safe as placing the block in an awake or sedated child. They further suggest that placing the block in an anesthetized child remains the standard of care.[9]

Epidural placement should target the level that centers on the dermatomes involved in the bar placement. Therefore, it is imperative that the anesthesiology team discuss the level of sternal and costal bar placement with the surgeon. Once this location is determined, patients will need epidural coverage at least 3 dermatomes above and below this central location. In most Nuss bar procedures, the epidural catheter should be placed at the T5-T7 level.

Because Nuss bar procedures are frequently performed in teenage patients with restrictions in movement after surgery, the surgeon may wish to start the patient on an antithrombotic medication. Guidelines have been established by the American Society of Regional Anesthesia[10,11] and should be reviewed when initiating antithrombotic therapy in conjunction with an epidural catheter block. Generally, unfractionated heparin (5,000 IU BID or TID) and prophylactic enoxaparin are felt to have a lower risk of epidural bleed as long as the medication, per the guideline, is held the appropriate length of time prior to placing and removing the catheter.[10,11]

The catheter placement can be examined via radiographic imaging. If the catheter is one of the flexible wire-reinforced varieties, a simple anterior/posterior chest X-ray can identify the insertion site and the tip location of the catheter. The stiffer nylon or polyvinyl chloride catheters often are hard to visualize without dye. The anesthesiologist can shoot an epidurogram by injecting 0.5 to 2 mL of water soluble contrast dye into the catheter to see the distribution of the dye in the epidural space. Common clinical approaches for determining the level of the analgesic block are to use cold sensation (ice packs or alcohol wipes) and sharp sensation (such

Table 53.1 **EPIDURAL DOSING**

	BOLUS DOSE	INFUSION RATE
Thoracic	0.25–0.5 mL/kg	0.1–0.15 mL/kg/hr
Lumbar	0.5 mL/kg	0.2 mL/kg/hr
Caudal	0.75 mL/kg	0.3 mL/kg/hr

as scratching the patient lightly with a sharp object, broken tongue depressor, or a needle).

There really are no standardized formulas for administration of epidural medications in children. Although infusions can consist of local anesthetic alone, most contain a mixture of opioids and local anesthetic. Guidelines exist for the rate of epidural infusions and loading bolus doses (Table 53.1). Studies of bupivacaine and ropivacaine levels suggest that doses be limited to 0.4 mg/kg/hour to avoid neurotoxicity. Infusions should be preceded by a bolus load of local and opioid. In the case of Nuss bar placement, some clinicians advocate for a denser block administered at a lower rate (0.2% ropivacaine at 0.05–0.1 mL/kg/hour). In addition, in order to avoid neuraxial opioid toxicity, some clinicians advocate running a local anesthetic-only epidural, which is then combined with intravenous PCA opioid. There are no studies defining superiority of any of these techniques.

MULTIMODAL ANALGESIA

Multimodal analgesia has been advocated for the past 20 years, due to its potential additive analgesic properties and the limitation of negative opioid side effects. The concept has come to the forefront as enhanced recovery after surgery pathways push for increased quality and efficiency of patient care, with decreased cost, and also because the United States is currently facing an opioid addiction epidemic. The multimodal analgesic approach attempts to use analgesics from different medication classes as well as regional blocks, muscle relaxants, acupuncture, and biophysical feedback to attenuate a patient's pain. Classes of analgesic medications include nonsteroidal anti-inflammatory drugs (NSAIDs), acetaminophen, gabapentanoids, local anesthetics, tramadol, and N-methyl-D-aspartate (NMDA) receptor antagonists.[7] NSAIDs and acetaminophen should be scheduled, instead of given on an as-needed basis, for best efficacy.[7] NSAIDS have not been shown to increase surgical site bleeding, which is often a concern for the surgeon.[12,13] Of note, the US Food and Drug Administration recently issued a black box warning regarding the use of tramadol and codeine in children. This states that tramadol is contraindicated in children less than 12 years old when used to treat pain after surgery and also in children 12 to 18 years old after airway surgery.[14]

A multimodal approach to a patient's pain control has been shown to be superior to a single modality approach.[15] The early initiation of multimodal analgesia has also been linked to a reduced likelihood of an opioid-related adverse event,

Table 53.2 **EPIDURAL SOLUTIONS**

	THORACIC	LUMBAR	CAUDAL
Bupivacaine	0.1%–0.2%	0.0625%–0.1%	0.1%
Ropivacaine	0.1%–0.2%	0.1%	0.1%
Fentanyl	2 mcg/mL	2–5 mcg/mL	2–5 mcg/mL
Morphine	10–20 mcg/mL	10–20 mcg/mL	10–20 mcg/mL
Hydromorphone	2–4 mcg/mL	2–4 mcg/mL	2–4 mcg/mL
Clonidine	1–2 mcg/mL	1–2 mcg/mL	1–2 mcg/mL

including respiratory depression, other life-threatening events, the use of naloxone, or an intensive care unit admission.[16] It should be noted that children that require supplemental oxygen at the time of discharge from the postanesthesia care unit are at increased risk for these opioid-associated adverse events.[16] In the patient with a working epidural, the addition of scheduled intravenous acetaminophen has the benefit of improving pain control via a different mechanism of action, and acetaminophen is tolerated well if the patient is nauseated. Assuming there is no contraindication, an NSAID, such IV ketorolac or oral ibuprofen also tends to be opioid-sparing.[7] Intravenous ketorolac has been shown to be a good rescue medication in conjunction with the epidural for breakthrough pain and provides an additional analgesic mechanism via the inhibition of cyclooxygenase and prostaglandin synthesis.[2]

Anxiety, stress, and sleep deprivation can contribute to making a patient's perception of pain worse. In addition, the development of postoperative constipation can significantly contribute to overall discomfort. Muscle spasms and bladder spasms also may contribute to a patient's pain and can be addressed pharmacologically or with nonpharmacological approaches, such as heat packs, massage, or acupuncture. Mood and depression affect a patient's processing of pain and may need to be addressed to allow the patient to improve. The patient described above had signs of an adequate epidural block and received several analgesic adjuvants, but he continued to report significant pain. His complaints, however, were more focused on a sense of respiratory impingement, and he was surrounded by anxious, overbearing parents. The addition of diazepam, which has the dual benefit of being an anxiolytic and a muscle relaxant, most likely contributed to the beneficial effects described.

PCA

PCA provides the patient with an on-demand medication bolus with the press of a button connected to a programmable pump. This provides the patient with a significant amount of control over his or her own pain regimen and has been shown to lead to greater satisfaction in both adult and pediatric pain patients.[17] Patients do not need to wait for a nurse or physician to provide their medication, and they can administer their own small dose of medication preemptively, if they expect to have an increase in pain, such as in anticipation of physical therapy or ambulation. The PCA button can be used with an epidural, the administration of an opioid, or even the NMDA receptor antagonist ketamine. The PCA program settings provide a timed (hourly or four hourly) maximum of medication the patient may administer and also sets a lockout time between doses. This allows patients to safely administer their own medication and minimizes the risk of excessive use. The PCA can also be used with a continuous infusion (the basal rate) that is administered without the participation of the patient. If a basal rate is present, then the timed maximum

Table 53.3 **PATIENT-CONTROLLED ANALGESIA DOSING**

	BOLUS DOSE MCG/KG)	LOCK OUT (MIN)	BASAL RATE (MCG/KG/HR)	1 HOUR MAXIMUM (MCG/KG)
Fentanyl	0.5	6–10	0.5–2	2–5
Morphine	10–20	6–10	10–20	60–120
Hydromorphone	2–4	6–10	2–4	12–24

medication delivered includes the basal rate. (See Table 53.3 for dosing.)

Proxy PCA has been advocated at many institutions.[18,19] This can be set up so that the nurse alone administers all doses or so that other caretakers, such as parents, also have the authority to dose the patient. This approach is appropriate for patients under the age of 7 to 8 years, who may not yet understand how the PCA works. It can also be employed in patients with significant developmental delay and some clinicians even advocate PCA use in very young infants.[20]

In the adult literature, the presence of the basal rate has been linked to an increase in opioid-related side effects, such as nausea, pruritus, sedation, and respiratory depression, without an improvement in efficacy.[21] The American Society of Anesthesiologists 2012 practice guideline no longer recommended the use of a basal infusion with PCA use because there is no evidence of increased efficacy in pain management. Because the pediatric patient may not control the initiation of the bolus (parent/nurse controlled), and there is a concern about inadequate analgesia when the patient or caregiver is asleep or unavailable, Hayes et al. performed a meta-analysis reviewing studies that compared pediatric PCA with a basal rate versus PCA without a basal rate. Their meta-analysis did not find a significant difference in efficacy with the addition of basal opioid to the PCA bolus function. The analysis also did not demonstrate an increased risk of opioid-induced adverse events, such as nausea, emesis, or sedation, when a basal infusion was present. The analysis regarding respiratory depression was inconclusive.[22]

When a patient describes neuropathic pain, such as burning, pins and needles, or shooting pain, the addition of a gabapentinoid (gabapentin or pregabalin) or a low-dose tricyclic antidepressant (amitriptyline or nortriptyline) might be beneficial for the patient.[17] The most common side effect of adding these medications is drowsiness and constipation. This improves with time, and these medications are generally well tolerated. The gabapentinoids do not interact with most other commonly used analgesics. In the very unlikely event that severe continued pain seems to warrant use of long-term opioids, methadone may be an ideal choice, since it is both a mu-receptor agonist as well as an NMDA receptor antagonist, which may offer beneficial effects for neuropathic type pain.[17]

ADDITIONAL CASE SCENARIO

A 6-month-old boy with a history of apnea of prematurity, that has since resolved, presents for hypospadias repair. His family is very concerned about the anesthetic and the potential for postoperative apnea in their young child and would like to know if there are any options other than opioids to help control his pain after the surgery. You discuss the choice of a caudal epidural block, penile nerve block (PNB), or morphine. Together, you elect to perform a caudal epidural block.

WHAT ARE THE RISKS AND BENEFITS OF A CAUDAL EPIDURAL BLOCK? HOW IS CAUDAL PLACEMENT DIFFERENT THAN AN EPIDURAL CATHETER PLACEMENT? HOW IS A PENILE BLOCK PLACED? WOULD A SPINAL ANESTHETIC HAVE BEEN AN OPTION? IS MORPHINE CONTRAINDICATED IN A 6-MONTH-OLD INFANT?

Neuraxial anesthesia has been successfully used in children for many years.[23] The caudal epidural anesthetic has been the gold standard in pediatric regional anesthesia for lower abdominal and extremity surgery.[8] The single-shot caudal block can provide analgesia below the umbilicus for 6 to 9 hours, depending on the local anesthetic utilized.[24] The anesthesia provider may choose to place only local anesthetic or, when appropriate, administer another adjunvant into the epidural/caudal space, such as morphine or clonidine. A caudal block is most commonly placed in pediatric patients using anatomic surface landmarks, although ultrasound guidance and fluoroscopy have also been described. The placement by surface landmarks or "blind technique" in pediatric patients has a success rate of 96%.[25] In the landmark technique, the caudal epidural block is initiated by placing the patient in a lateral position and identifying the sacral cornua, which straddle the sacral hiatus. Covering the sacral hiatus is the sacrococcygeal ligament (SCL). After appropriately cleaning the overlying skin, a needle is inserted into the sacral hiatus between the cornua, and a "loss" or change in resistance is generally noted when the needle passes through the SCL, into the sacral canal/epidural space.[26] The local anesthetic is deposited into the space, and the needle is removed. An epidural catheter can be placed into the epidural space through the sacral canal and then threaded higher into the epidural space. Recent studies have demonstrated that the local anesthetic volume, as compared to the speed of injection or the concentration of the local anesthetic, correlates in a positive way with the cranial spread of the medication and the increased length of time until adjunct analgesia is needed.[8,24] The risks of caudal epidural block placement are similar to placement of an epidural catheter. The most common complication for a caudal block includes block failure, usually due to subcutaneous injection, vascular

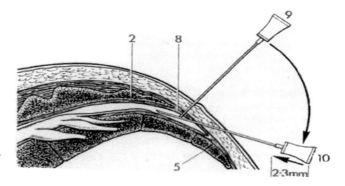

Fig. 53.1 Diagram of caudal block placement.

puncture with a positive test dose, and dural puncture.[27] Major complications such as seizure (0.02% incidence), cardiac arrest (0.02% incidence), and spinal cord injury[6] are rare events and should not limit the pediatric anesthesiologist from offering a caudal block to patients.[27]

Placing local anesthetic around the two dorsal penile nerves, which are the terminal endings of the pudendal nerves, results in a PNB. Dalens and Vanneuville describe the PNB as follows: The patient is placed supine, and the penis is pushed downward.[28] The needle is inserted 0.5 to 1 cm lateral to the pubic symphysis and inferior to the pelvic rami and directed posteriorly, slightly medially, and caudally at a 70 to 80 degree angle. The practitioner will feel two changes in resistance as the needle passes through the superficial fascia of the abdomen and Scarpa's fascia. After negative aspiration, the local anesthetic (0.5–2 mL) is deposited into the subpubic space, and the procedure is repeated on the contralateral side. More recently, greater block efficacy during the first hour and greater length of time until the patient requires adjuvant analgesia has been reported when using ultrasound guidance for placing a PNB.[29]

Spinal anesthesia has been used successfully in infants and children worldwide. The benefits of a spinal anesthetic are the avoidance of a general anesthetic and rapid anesthesia recovery when compared to a general anesthetic. The "spinal" provides cardiopulmonary stability and less apnea and respiratory complications.[8] Recent evidence from the GAS study supports that spinals can be used safely in infants and children and shows that spinal anesthesia was the only technique noted to decrease postoperative apnea in pediatric patients.[30] However, all spinal anesthetics have a limited duration depending on the choice of local anesthetic. Because hypospadias surgery can involve an intricate and possibly lengthy repair, the spinal anesthetic may not be the best anesthetic choice for this patient, even if it has the benefit of decreased apnea. While opioids are one of the more common causes of apnea, they are not contraindicated in 6-month-old infants or even neonates and can be dosed appropriately based on weight and tolerance to opioids, taking care to use doses about ½ of those recommended in older infants and children.

ADDITIONAL CASE SCENARIO: "MY HEAD IS KILLING ME!"

A 15-year-old young woman presents to the emergency department with "the worst headache of her life." She reports that it started with her eyes bothering her. It has not gone away for the last 12 hours and she had to go home early from school. Acetaminophen and ibuprofen did not relieve the pain, and her mother brought her to the emergency room. The computer tomography scan does not show any sinusitis, intracranial bleed, tumor, or hydrocephalus. She is admitted to the floor for pain control, and a pain consult is placed. When the pain service arrives, they find the patient irritable and crying in a darkened room. The patient's mother reports her daughter routinely has headaches, and she has been stressed because of final exams. However, they have never experienced anything like this before. The patient reports nausea without emesis, light sensitivity, sound sensitivity, and a "horrible pulsing pain" at her temples. Mom denies any previous history of severe headaches and also adds that her daughter is adopted.

WHAT SHOULD BE INCLUDED IN THE DIFFERENTIAL DIAGNOSIS? ASSUMING THE HEADACHE IS CONSISTENT WITH A MIGRAINE, WHAT TREATMENT OPTIONS ARE AVAILABLE FOR THIS PATIENT? IF THE PATIENT'S MIGRAINE DOES NOT RESOLVE AFTER 3 DAYS OF TREATMENT, WHAT TREATMENTS ARE AVAILABLE FOR STATUS MIGRAINOSUS IN A PEDIATRIC PATIENT?

The following sections discuss different classifications of migraine headaches.[31]

MIGRAINE WITHOUT AURA

Previously used terms

Common migraine; hemicrania simplex.

Description

Recurrent headache disorder manifesting in attacks lasting 4 to 72 hours. Typical characteristics of the headache are unilateral location, pulsating quality, moderate or severe intensity, aggravation by routine physical activity, and association with nausea and/or photophobia and phonophobia.

Diagnostic criteria

A. At least five attacks[1] fulfilling criteria B–D

B. Headache attacks lasting 4-72 hours (untreated or unsuccessfully treated)[2,3]

C. Headache has at least two of the following four characteristics:
   1. unilateral location
   2. pulsating quality
   3. moderate or severe pain intensity
   4. aggravation by or causing avoidance of routine physical activity (e.g., walking or climbing stairs)

D. During headache at least one of the following:

   1. nausea and/or vomiting
   2. photophobia and phonophobia

E. Not better accounted for by another ICHD-3 diagnosis.

Notes

1. One or a few migraine attacks may be difficult to distinguish from symptomatic migraine-like attacks. Furthermore, the nature of a single or a few attacks may be difficult to understand. Therefore, at least 5 attacks are required. Individuals who otherwise meet criteria for 1.1 *Migraine without aura* but have had fewer than 5 attacks should be coded 1.5.1 *Probable migraine without aura*.

2. When the patient falls asleep during a migraine attack and wakes up without it, duration of the attack is reckoned until the time of awakening.

3. In children and adolescents (aged under 18 years), attacks may last 2 to 72 hours (the evidence for untreated durations of less than 2 hours in children has not been substantiated).

MIGRAINE WITH AURA

Previously used terms

Classic or classical migraine; ophthalmic, hemiparaesthetic, hemiplegic, or aphasic migraine; migraine accompagnée; complicated migraine.

Description

Recurrent attacks, lasting minutes, of unilateral fully reversible visual, sensory, or other central nervous system symptoms that usually develop gradually and are usually followed by headache and associated migraine symptoms.

Diagnostic criteria

A. At least two attacks fulfilling criteria B and C

B. One or more of the following fully reversible aura symptoms:
   1. visual
   2. sensory
   3. speech and/or language
   4. motor
   5. brainstem
   6. retinal

C. At least two of the following four characteristics:
   1. at least one aura symptom spreads gradually over ≥5 minutes, and/or two or more symptoms occur in succession
   2. each individual aura symptom lasts 5–60 minutes[1]
   3. at least one aura symptom is unilateral[2]
   4. the aura is accompanied, or followed within 60 minutes, by headache

D. Not better accounted for by another ICHD-3 diagnosis, and transient ischemic attack has been excluded.

Notes

1. When, for example, three symptoms occur during an aura, the acceptable maximal duration is 3 × 60 minutes. Motor symptoms may last up to 72 hours.

2. Aphasia is always regarded as a unilateral symptom; dysarthria may or may not be.

OVERVIEW

Migraine headache commonly presents in childhood or the teenage years and is inherited in 60% to 90% of cases.[32,33] The prevalence of migraines is higher in female patients than in their male counterparts. While the presentation can vary, migraine headaches tend to present with light and sound sensitivity, nausea, and emesis. Patients may also describe abdominal pain, lightheadedness, fatigue, and an inability to think well. While not always consistent, the headache is often described as a severe, throbbing head pain and may be unilateral or over bilateral temples and forehead.[32] The diagnosis of migraine is a clinical determination through a physical exam and a thorough history, often after other secondary causes of head pain, such as intracranial bleed, tumor, or stroke, have been excluded from the differential diagnosis. The majority of childhood headaches are primary headaches, consisting of migraines or tension headaches, and their incidence has increased over the past 30 years.[33] Tension headaches are also seen in the pediatric population and are described as bilateral, mild to moderate pain anywhere in the cranium or occiput. The pain is not aggravated by physical activity, while migraine symptoms may be worsened by activity. Tension headaches may be exacerbated by stress and anxiety. Migraine sufferers may also have an increased tendency toward anxiety and depression; however, the link does not appear to be statistically significant.[33]

Outpatient treatment of migraine headache in pediatric patients usually consists of acetaminophen, an NSAID including ibuprofen or naproxen, and, commonly, a "triptan," such as sumatriptan or rizatriptan.[32,34] Patients with recurrent migraine that impacts their ability to function at school or work should be started on a preventative medication. The drugs commonly used include a beta-blocker, like propranolol (contraindicated in asthmatic patients); a tricyclic antidepressant, such as amitriptyline; an antihistamine, like cyproheptadine; or an antiepileptic, such as topiramate or divalproex.[32] Other successful long-term treatments include cognitive behavioral therapy to restructure coping mechanisms and pain perception[35,36] and repeated acupuncture treatments, which lead to decreased pain intensity and frequency.[37,38]

When the patient presents to the emergency department after not being able to break the migraine at home, common treatments include intravenous hydration with a 20 mL/kg fluid bolus, an antiemetic (such as prochlorperazine, metoclopramide, or ondansetron), intravenous ketorolac (NSAID), and, the empiric addition of diphenhydramine. The patient is likely to fall asleep and have an improvement in the headache, particularly if a sedating antiemetic is employed. Of note, repeated doses of neuroleptic drugs may cause extrapyramidal symptoms or prolongation of the QT interval. The patient should be closely monitored for this known side effect. Other treatments include antiepileptic drugs, such as valproic acid, magnesium sulfate, or steroids.[32,34,35,39] If the migraine does not improve, the patient is frequently admitted for pain control and to manage nausea and hydration.

Status migrainosus is characterized by an intense migraine that has not resolved after 72 hours and may warrant an admission to the hospital for treatment.[35,39] Kabbouche et al. described the successful use of dihydroergotamine (DHE) in children and adolescents with 74.4% of the patients reporting they were headache-free at the time of discharge. Their approach included aggressive intravenous hydration (20 mL/kg load of D_5 normal saline) and premedication half an hour before administration of the DHE with an antiemetic, such as prochlorperazine, metoclopramide, or ondansetron, to combat nausea. Administration of 1 mg DHE every 8 hours was given to the patient until the symptoms resolve or a maximum of 20 doses was reached. For children less than 9 years old or weighing less than 25 kg, the dose was decreased to 0.5 mg. It should be noted that anxiety, severe nausea, increased blood pressure, and, occasionally, worsening of the headache have been reported before there is any noted improvement in the headache.[34] Kabbouche et al. recommends administering 5 doses prior to determining if there is a response to treatment.

REVIEW QUESTIONS

1. A 3-month-old infant, born at 24 weeks postconceptual age, is brought to the operating room for inguinal hernia repair prior to discharge home. His parents agree to a caudal block for postoperative analgesia. Of the following, which is the **LEAST** common complication from placing a caudal block?

    A. block failure
    B. dural puncture
    C. Horner's syndrome
    D. intravascular injection

Answer: C
Inadvertent dural puncture is a potential complication of a caudal block, due to the proximity of the dural sac to the needle tip within the caudal epidural space. Because of the blood vessels that are present in the spinal column, there is also a risk of unintentional intravascular injection of local anesthetic. Block failure is one of the more common complications of the caudal block if the medication is placed into the wrong space. With novice trainees, local anesthetic is commonly placed subcutaneously instead of into the caudal space.

Horner's syndrome affects the sympathetic nervous system and is more likely to been seen with an interscalene or stellate ganglion block. Horner's syndrome is highly unlikely with a caudal block because the medication is placed at the most distal part of the spine.

2. Of the following reactions to local anesthetic, which is **LEAST** likely to be a sign of toxicity?

    A. apnea
    B. cardiac arrest
    C. seizures
    D. urticaria

Answer: D
Signs of local anesthetic toxicity include tinnitus, blurred vision, circumoral numbness, metallic taste, and dizziness and can progress to seizures, apnea, arrhythmias, and cardiovascular collapse. Urticaria is more commonly an indication of an allergic reaction.

3. While rounding on the pain service, you are called about a patient who arrived to his hospital room after a large abdominal surgery. While transferring beds, his epidural catheter got caught, and the nurse is concerned about the integrity of the epidural catheter. On inspection, the dressing is intact, but the catheter has been pulled out by 2 cm. Of the following confirmatory approaches, which is **LEAST** likely to be helpful in the evaluation epidural catheter placement?

    A. AP and lateral chest x-rays
    B. epidurogram
    C. patient's ability to walk
    D. medication test dosing

Answer: C
When determining the depth of the remaining catheter, it is helpful to know where the loss of resistance was and thereby the presumed depth of the epidural space with that particular pass of the needle. Then, by looking at the markings on the epidural catheter, one can calculate the approximate length of the catheter within the epidural space. Without this information, one may use a chest x-ray to determine the placement of the catheter if the catheter is radiopaque or inject contrast into the catheter (epidurogram) to determine the location of the tip of the catheter. Using a test dose of local anesthetic medication and then examining the patient for a change in his block may also help determine if the catheter remains in place. Evaluating the patient's ability to walk is not an indicator of appropriate epidural placement. Depending on the location of the epidural and the concentration of the medication, the patient may be able to walk with a fully functional epidural. Also, if the catheter was just removed, the duration of the local anesthetic may last hours before one can see a change in the patient's block.

4. The patient's epidural block appears to be covering the dermatomes affected by surgery. However, the patient still reports pain levels of 6/10. Which is the **BEST** description of multimodal analgesia to treat his pain?

    A. adding nonanalgesics to sedate recalcitrant patients
    B. reserving nonpharmacologic treatments for later

C. prescribing multiple medications but only as needed

D. targeting different analgesic receptors and pathways

Answer: D

Multimodal therapy includes opioids, scheduled NSAIDs (e.g., acetaminophen, ibuprofen), muscle relaxants, possible neuropathic pain medications when indicated, heating pads, ice packs, acupuncture, and stress and behavioral management. By using multiple modalities, pain is treated through different receptors and pathways, with the goal of increasing efficacy and decreasing side effects of the medications by limiting the quantity of each medication. Multimodal therapy has been shown to be more efficacious than any single approach to pain management and, in an era of opioid abuse, has been shown to be opioid-sparing. In the past, there was a concern that NSAID use postoperatively would result in an increased risk of bleeding. With certain exceptions, such as patients with bleeding disorders, NSAIDs are now commonly and successfully used for postoperative pain management, including for tonsillectomies.

5. During a patient's 2-month follow-up visit with his surgeon after thoracotomy, he reports burning and tingling over the right T7 dermatome. The surgeon wishes to employ a prescription medication. His pain will be **LEAST** effectively treated with the following medications?

    A. amitriptyline

    B. diazepam

    C. gabapentin

    D. pregabalin

Answer: B

What the patient appears to be describing is neuropathic pain, most likely due to a nerve injury associated with the surgery. Gabapentin, pregabalin, and amitriptyline all treat neuropathic pain and would be a better choice than diazepam. Diazepam is more commonly used as an antianxiety medication and muscle relaxant, which does not directly treat this patient's problem.

6. Of the following, which is the **LEAST** accurate statement regarding PCA use in pediatric patients?

    A. Basal rates are not needed in all patients.

    B. Explanation of PCA use and function is unnecessary.

    C. Individual control of analgesia improves satisfaction.

    D. Medication doses are weight based.

Answer: B

PCA and parent/nurse-administered analgesia have been successfully used in children of all ages, including in neonates. They have been shown to increase satisfaction scores among nurses, patients, and family members because the patient can immediately receive medication instead of having to wait for the nurse to administer it. This provides the patient with a certain amount of control over his or her care. With guidance from their nurse and parents, children can successfully self-administer the PCA. Because pediatric patients vary so much in size, the dose is calculated by weight. While some physicians may wish to run a basal infusion rate on the PCA so that the child continues to get some

medication while asleep, possibly providing a more restful night, studies have shown that a basal rate is not necessary to achieve good pain control.

8. A 12-year-old girl presents to the emergency department with her dad because of headache for the past week. Dad reports she has missed school for the last 2 weeks, the first week because they had to attend a funeral for his mother and the second week because of this headache. Of the following factors, which one is **LEAST** likely a contributing factor to the child's head pain?

    A. family history of migraines

    B. grandmother's death

    C. multiple food allergies.

    D. stress from missing school

Answer: C

The cause of headaches is often multifactorial and can be associated with mood, stress, and a family history of migraines or headaches. Food allergies are not a common trigger for headaches.

9. Of the following therapies, which is the **LEAST** appropriate as a first-line treatment for headaches?

    A. acetaminophen

    B. hydration

    C. ketorolac

    D. methadone

Answer: D

For a new headache, NSAIDs, hydration, rest, and time for the symptoms to abate are the most appropriate first steps. Opioids are not considered first-line therapy for headaches, and a long-acting medication such as methadone is inappropriate as a first choice.

QUESTIONS AND ANSWERS

This chapter has accompanying questions and answers which are available to subscribers as part of the Oxford eLearning platform. To access the questions, go to ✔ http:// oxfordmedicine. com/pediatricanesthesiaPBL

REFERENCES

1. Frawley G, Frawley J, Crameri J. A review of anesthetic techniques and outcomes following minimally invasive repair of pectus excavatum (Nuss procedure). *Paediatr Anaesth*. 2016;26(11):1082–1090.

2. Densmore JC, Peterson DB, Stahovic LL, et al. Initial surgical and pain management outcomes after Nuss procedure. *J Pediatr Surg*. 2010;45(9):1767–1771.

3. Gasior AC, Knott E, Weesner KA, Poola A, St. Peter SD. Long term patient perception of pain control experience after participating in a trial between patient-controlled analgesia and epidural after pectus excavatum repair with bar placement. *J Surg Research*. 2013;179(2):343.

4. Stroud, AM, Tulanont DD, Coates TE, Goodney PP, Croitoru DP. Epidural analgesia versus intravenous patient-controlled analgesia following minimally invasive pectus excavatum repair: a systematic review and meta-analysis. *J Pediatr Surg*. 2014;49(5):798–806.

5. Llewellyn N, Moriarty A. The National Pediatric Epidural Audit. *Pediatr Anesth*. 2007;17(6):520–533.

6. Meyer MJ, Krane EJ, Goldschneider KR, Klein NJ. Neurological complications associated with epidural analgesia in children. *Anesth Analg*. 2012;115(6):1365–1370.

7. Wick EC, Grant MC, Wu CL. Postoperative multimodal analgesia pain management with nonopioid analgesics and techniques. *JAMA Surg*. 2017;152(7):691–697.

8. Stein ALS, Baumgard D, Del Rio I, Tutiven JL. Updates in pediatric regional anesthesia and its role in the treatment of acute pain in the ambulatory setting. *Curr Pain Headache Rep*. 2017;21(2):11.

9. Taenzer AH, Walker BJ, Bosenberg AT, et al. Asleep versus awake: does it matter? Pediatric regional block complications by patient state: a report from the Pediatric Regional Anesthesia Network. *Reg Anes Pain Med*. 2014;39(4):279–283.

10. Horlocker, TT, Wedel DJ, Rowlingson JC, et al. Regional anesthesia in the patient receiving antithrombotic or thrombolytic therapy. *Reg Anes Pain Med*. 2010;35(1):64–101.

11. Narouze S, Benzon HT, Provenzano DA, et al. Interventional spine and pain procedures in patients on antiplatelet and anticoagulant medications: guidelines from the American Society of Regional Anesthesia and Pain Medicine, the European Society of Regional Anaesthesia and Pain Therapy, the American Academy of Pain Medicine, the International Neuromodulation Society, the North American Neuromodulation Society, and the World Institute of Pain. *Reg Anes Pain Med*. 2015;40(3):182–212.

12. Gobble RM, Hoang HLT, Kachniarz B, Orgill DP. Ketorolac does not increase perioperative bleeding. *Plastic Recon Surg*. 2014;133(3):741–755.

13. Riggin L, Ramakrishna J, Sommer DD, Koren G. A 2013 updated systematic review and meta-analysis of 36 randomized controlled trials; no apparent effects of non steroidal anti-inflammatory agents on the risk of bleeding after tonsillectomy. *Clin Otolaryn*. 2013;38(2):115–129.

14. FDA Drug Safety Communication. FDA restricts use of prescription codeine pain and cough medicines and tramadol pain medicines in children; recommends against use in breastfeeding women. https://www.fda.gov/Drugs/DrugSafety/ucm549679.htm.Accessed April 20, 2017.

15. Chou R, Gordon DB, de Leon-Casasola OA, et al. Management of postoperative pain: a clinical practice guideline from the American Pain Society, the American Society of Regional Anesthesia and Pain Medicine, and the American Society of Anesthesiologists' Committee on Regional Anesthesia, Executive Committee, and Administrative Council. *J Pain*. 2016;17(2):131–157.

16. Voepel-Lewis T, Wagner D, Burke C, et al. Early adjuvant use of nonopioids associated with reduced odds of serious postoperative opioid adverse events and need for rescue in children. *Pediatr Anesth*. 2012;23(2):162–169.

17. Mathew E, Kim E, Zempsky W. Pharmacologic treatment of pain. *Sem Pediatr Neurol*. 2016;23(3):209–219.

18. Czarnecki ML, Salamon KS, Jastrowski Mano KE, Ferrise AS, Sharp M, Weisman SJ. A preliminary report of parent/nurse-controlled analgesia (PNCA) in infants and preschoolers. *Clin J Pain*. 2011;27(2):102–107.

19. Monitto CL, Greenberg RS, Kost-Byerly S, et al. The safety and efficacy of parent-/nurse-controlled analgesia in patients less than six years of age. *Anesth Analg*. 2000;91(3):573–579.

20. Czarnecki ML, Hainsworth K, Simpson PM, et al. Is there an alternative to continuous opioid infusion for neonatal pain control? A preliminary report of parent/nurse-controlled analgesia in the neonatal intensive care unit. *Pediatr Anesth*. 2014;24(4):377–385.

21. Looi-Lyons LC, Chung FF, Chan VW, McQuestion M. Respiratory depression: an adverse outcome during patient controlled analgesia therapy. *J Clin Anesth*. 1996;8(2):151–156.

22. Hayes J, Dowling JJ, Peliowski A, Crawford MW, Johnston B. Patient-controlled analgesia plus background opioid infusion for postoperative pain in children. *Anesth Analg*. 2016;123(4):991–1003.

23. Hannallah RS, Broadman LM, Belman AB, Abramowitz MD, Epstein BS. Comparison of caudal and ilioinguinal/iliohypogastric nerve blocks for control of post-orchiopexy pain in pediatric ambulatory surgery. *Anesthesiology*. 1987;66(6):832–833.

24. Hong, JY, Han SW, Kim WO, Cho JS, Kil HK. Comparison of high volume/low concentration and low volume/high concentration ropivacaine in caudal analgesia for pediatric orchiopexy. *Surv Anesth*. 2010;54(3):128–129.

25. Dalens B, Hasnaoui A. Caudal anesthesia in pediatric surgery: success rate and adverse effects in 750 consecutive patients. *Anesth Analg*. 1989;68(2):83–89.

26. Kao SC, Lin CS. Caudal epidural block: an updated review of anatomy and techniques. *BioMed Res Int*. 2017;2017:1–5.

27. Suresh S, Long J, Birmingham PK, De Oliveira GS. Are caudal blocks for pain control safe in children? An analysis of 18,650 caudal blocks from the Pediatric Regional Anesthesia Network (PRAN) database. *Anesth Analg*. 2015;120(1):151–156.

28. Dalens B, Vanneuville G, Dechelotte P. Penile block via the subpubic space in 100 children. *Anesth Analg*. 1989;69(1):41–45.

29. Faraoni D, Gilbeau A, Lingier P, Barvais L, Engelman E, Hennart D. Does ultrasound guidance improve the efficacy of dorsal penile nerve block in children? *Pediatr Anesth*. 2010;20(10):931–936.

30. Davidson AJ, Disma N, De Graaff JC, et al. Neurodevelopmental outcome at 2 years of age after general anaesthesia and awake-regional anaesthesia in infancy (GAS): an international multicentre, randomized controlled trial. *Lancet*. 2016;387(10015):239–250.

31. Headache Classification Committee of the International Headache Society. The International Classification of Headache Disorders, 3rd edition (beta version). *Cephalalgia*. 2013;33(9):629–808. doi:10.1177/0333102413485658

32. Teleanu RI, Vladacenco O, Teleanu DM, Epure DA. Treatment of pediatric migraine: a review. *Maedica*. 2016;11(6):136–143.

33. Özge A, Termine C, Antonaci F, Natriashvili S, Guidetti V, Wöber-Bingöl C. Overview of diagnosis and management of paediatric headache. Part I: diagnosis. *J Headache Pain*. 2011;12(1):13–23.

34. Marmura MJ, Wrobel Goldberg S. Inpatient management of migraine. *Curr Neurol Neurosci Rep*. 2015;15(4):13. doi:10.1007/s11910-015-0539-z

35. Powers SW, Kashikar-Zuck SM, Allen JR, et al. Cognitive behavioral therapy plus amitriptyline for chronic migraine in children and adolescents: a randomized clinical trial. *JAMA*. 2013;310(24):2622–2630.

36. Ng QX, Venkatanarayanan N, Kumar L. A systematic review and meta-analysis of the efficacy of cognitive behavioral therapy for the management of pediatric migraine. *Headache*. 2016;57(3):349–362.

37. Brittler M, Le Pertel N, Gold MA. Acupuncture in pediatrics. *Curr Problems Ped Adolesc Health Care*. 2016;46(6):179–183.

38. Pintov S, Lahat E, Alstein M, Vogel Z, Barg J. Acupuncture and the opioid system: implications in management of migraine. *Pediatr Neurol*. 1997;17(2):129–133.

39. Kabbouche MA, Powers SW, Segers A, et al. Inpatient treatment of status migraine with dihydroergotamine in children and adolescents. *Headache*. 2009;49(1):106–109.

54.

PEDIATRIC COMPLEX REGIONAL PAIN SYNDROME TYPE 1

A FUNCTIONAL AND WELLNESS RESTORATION THERAPY

Bobbie Riley and Navil Sethna

STEM CASE AND KEY QUESTIONS

A 13-year-old, otherwise healthy young girl twisted her left ankle 6 weeks earlier and presents with severe foot and leg pain that is described as constant burning and is exacerbated with normal contact with skin and any movement of the affected extremity. She is intolerant to wearing socks, washing the extremity, or bearing weight and walks with crutches. She holds the foot in plantar flexion and inversion. Pain persists despite conservative treatment. She cannot engage in outpatient physical and occupational therapies effectively due to excruciating pain and distress associated with light skin touch and movement of joints.

WHAT ARE THE DIFFERENTIAL DIAGNOSES, LABORATORY TESTS, AND CONSULTATIONS THAT MAY BE CONSIDERED?

Differential diagnoses include

- posttraumatic musculoskeletal disorders (stress fracture, ligament and/or muscle tear, tendonitis, joints hematoma) or posttraumatic neuralgia or neuropathy.

- infection (osteomyelitis).

- juvenile idiopathic arthritis, autoimmune diseases, erythromelalgia, or malignancy.

Laboratory tests could include a basic metabolic panel, complete blood count with differential, erythrocyte sedimentation rate, C-reactive protein, vitamin D3, rheumatoid factor, antinuclear antibody, plain x-ray, magnetic resonance imaging (MRI) right foot, and bone scan.

Consultations with orthopedic, rheumatology, and/or neurology should be requested to rule out a specific condition in the differential diagnosis.[1]

WHAT ARE THE CURRENT INTERNATIONAL ASSOCIATION OF STUDY OF PAIN (IASP) DIAGNOSTIC CRITERIA FOR COMPLEX REGIONAL PAIN SYNDROME (CRPS) AND WHAT ARE THE CHALLENGES?

According to the IASP, CRPS type 1 (CRPS-1) is a chronic pain condition likely due to dysfunction in the central and/or peripheral nervous systems while type 2 (CRPS-2) results from identifiable damage or disease of the nervous system.[2,3]

CRPS-1 is characterized by pain in combination with sensory, autonomic, trophic, and motor abnormalities. CRPS was originally diagnosed in children in the 1970s. CRPS-1 was previously called reflex neurovascular dystrophy or reflex sympathetic dystrophy, and CRPS-2 was previously termed causalgia. These syndromes were ultimately renamed CRPS-1 and CRPS-2 in an effort to de-emphasize the role of the sympathetic nervous syndrome as the primary pathophysiologic mechanism.[2,3]

The IASP endorsed the Orlando criteria in 1994 and, more recently, the revised Budapest criteria, which have a higher sensitivity of 0.99 and specificity of 0.68 and include motor features to be used for clinical and research diagnostic CRPS criteria in adults.[4] However, the validity of the Budapest criteria has not been confirmed in children. The Budapest criteria are as follows:

1. Continued pain, disproportionate to any inciting event.

2. Patient must report at least 1 symptom in 3 out of 4 of the following categories:
   a. Sensory report of hyperesthesia and/or allodynia.
   b. Vasomotor report of temperature asymmetry and/or skin color change and/or skin color asymmetry.
   c. Sudomotor/edema report of edema and/or sweating change and/or sweating asymmetry.

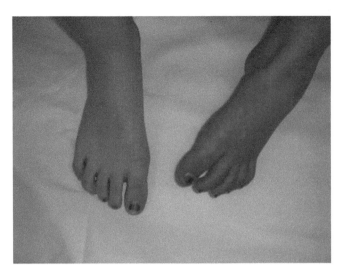

Fig. 54.1 CRPS-1 showing skin discoloration, swelling and inversion dystonia.

    d. Motor/trophic changes of decreased range of motion and/or motor dysfunction (weakness, tremor, dystonia) and/or trophic change in hair, nail, and skin.

3. Patient must display at least 1 sign at time of evaluation in 2 or more of the following categories (Fig. 54.1):

    a. Sensory: evidence of hyperesthesia to sharpness and/or allodynia to light touch and/or deep somatic pressure and/or joint movement.

    b. Vasomotor: evidence of temperature asymmetry and/or skin color changes and/or skin color asymmetry.

    c. Sudomotor/edema: evidence of edema and/or sweating changes and/or sweating asymmetry.

    d. Motor/trophic: evidence of decreased range of motion and/or motor dysfunction (weakness, tremor, dystonia) and/or trophic changes (hair, nail, skin).

4. No other diagnosis better explains the signs and symptoms.

ARE THERE LABORATORY OR IMAGING TESTS THAT CAN CONFIRM THE DIAGNOSIS OF CRPS?

CRPS-1 is a clinical diagnosis based on the patient's medical history, signs, and symptoms as outlined previously. No specific biochemical markers have been identified for its diagnosis. Laboratory and imaging tests are helpful for excluding other underlying causes or conditions that may mimic CRPS-1.[1]

CRPS-2 presents with similar clinical manifestations, but there is demonstrable damage or disease of a specific nerve or nerves by laboratory test, positive nerve conduction and electromyography studies, and imaging tests (e.g., focal or generalized neuropathy involving large myelinated fibers).

Bone scintigraphy/bone densitometry is not recommended for establishing the diagnosis of CRPS-1 because of low specificity, correlating more with the vasomotor changes or osteoporosis due to disuse atrophy, rather than presence or absence of CRPS-1.[5]

Quantitative sensory testing is helpful in diagnosing small fiber neuropathies and abnormal function of the various small fibers (unmyelinated C-fibers and myelinated A-delta) but does not confirm nor rule out the diagnosis of CRPS-1 because of considerable heterogeneity of mechanical and thermal sensory abnormalities among children with CRPS-1.

Skin biopsy may demonstrate defects in small fiber axons and nerve density that is not specific to CRPS.[6]

Diagnostic selective sympathetic nerve block is controversial because failure to respond does not exclude the diagnosis, and successful response may confirm sympathetically medicated pain, but not necessarily the presence of CRPS-1.

Laser Doppler flowmetry and sweat axon reflex tests can detect local sympathetic function changes, such as cutaneous reflex blood vessel vasoconstriction and local sweat responses, respectively, but do not confirm the presence of CRPS-1.

WHAT IS THE INCIDENCE AND PREVALENCE IN CHILDREN AND ADOLESCENTS?

The precise incidence of CRPS in the pediatric population is unknown. In a retrospective cohort study of 3,752 hospitalized children with chronic pain, CRPS constituted 26% of the chronic pain diagnoses. There are differences in children's responses to CRPS.[7] The duration of CRPS-1 is usually shorter in children compared to adults and so trophic changes are less frequent.[3] Also, certain recognized comparisons of childhood to adult CRPS include a predominance of

- Onset in preadolescent females 5–7:1 male.

- Lower extremity involvement 4–6:1 upper extremity.

- Less often preceded by major trauma or surgery. Nearly 10% of patients recall no specific injury or triggers.

- High stress in family and school environment and with peer interactions.

- Favorable response to physical and psychological therapies and complete recovery in most children, compared to adults, probably due to resilient developmental and nervous system plasticity as well as higher compliance with rehabilitative therapy.

WHAT IS NEUROPATHIC PAIN? WHAT IS THE DIFFERENCE BETWEEN CRPS-1 AND CRPS-2? WHAT IS THE PATHOPHYSIOLOGY OF CRPS? DO GENETICS PLAY A ROLE?

Neuropathic pain originates from a lesion or disease affecting the peripheral and/or central somatosensory system.

CRPS-1 usually occurs after noxious events or immobilization, such as a tight cast, and without demonstrable specific nerve injury. Symptoms and signs spread across multiple dermatomes. CRPS-2 results from direct injury to the central and/or peripheral nerve(s).

The exact mechanism and pathophysiology of CRPS-1 is unknown. Several mechanisms have been postulated, such as small fiber nociceptor or dorsal horn neuron dysfunction, sympathetic dysregulation, tissue hypoxia and reperfusion injury, inflammation, autoimmune antibodies, and central and cortical reorganization. With improved understanding of the pathophysiology over the past decades, 3 major pathways have been identified: aberrant inflammatory/immune mechanisms, vasomotor dysfunction, and maladaptive brain neuroplasticity. The psychological factors have a considerable role in contributing to the severity of pain perception and maintenance. Ultimately, the somatosensory, motor, and sympathetic nervous systems have all been implicated in CRPS-1 patients; no one mechanism fully explains CRPS-1.[1,8]

CRPS-1 sometimes occurs in several family members with siblings of CRPS-1 patients having increased risk for developing CRPS-1, consistent with a possible genetic association of different human leukocyte antigens and CRPS phenotypes, although this association is not yet confirmed.

Chronic pain is a complex experience and best understood as interactions between an individual child's psychological, social, and environmental (school, peers, family, and health care providers) factors. These factors play a strong role in perception of pain severity, belief system about the pain, and the extent of disability (i.e., pain is a biopsychosocial disorder). Thus, as with all chronic pain disorders, CRPS-1 is best understood with a biopsychosocial model and managed by an interdisciplinary team of physicians, psychologists, nurses, and physical and occupational therapists.[8–10]

HOW DO YOU MANAGE A CHILD WITH CRPS-1?

The primary goal of management of CRPS-1 is to reverse or diminish the negative impact of immobilization and psychological distress, to allow the child to regain the use of the affected limb, and to avoid long-term secondary musculoskeletal structural impairment. The impact of CRPS-1 is complicated by each individual child's specific and unique set of physical, psychological, and social characteristics. Therefore, treatment requires coordination of multiple medical, psychological, and physical medicine disciplines, in the context of a biopsychosocial approach, to maximize restoration of function to pre-pain onset levels. The pain relief is usually gradual, and pain level diminishes after return of active range of movement and physical functioning. Optimally, this goal is achieved by the efforts of a collaborative, interdisciplinary team, educating the patient and family about fear avoidance versus fear of activity-related harm, managing mood difficulties (e.g., anxiety, depression), and shifting the locus of control (active self-management and independent re-engagement in normal daily activities) to the patient for complete recovery and wellness.[8–10] This is best accomplished by the following.

1. Physical and occupational therapy modalities aid in mobilization of the affected limb through active self-management skills of active range of movement, strengthening, stretching, balance and coordination, dexterity training, gait education, passive and active textural desensitization of the nociceptors to normalize sensations, gradual exposure therapy, and stress loading activities.

2. Cognitive-behavioral therapy (CBT) aims to educate and teach patients cognitive, behavioral, and coping skills necessary to diminish the stress of participation in painful physical and occupational therapies. These strategies are accomplished best by lessening fear avoidance and catastrophic thoughts, tolerating the graded exposure to uncomfortable movements, conditioning of aerobic fitness, and regulating sleep. The ultimate goals are gradual normalization of daily activities, such as school attendance, socialization, and recreational activities. CBT also incorporates a school reintegration plan in collaboration with school educators to support the child's return to age-appropriate sports and academic success.

IS THERE EVIDENCE FOR THE EFFECTIVENESS OF ANALGESICS FOR MANAGING PAIN AND OTHER SYMPTOMS?

Medications, procedural interventions, and alternative therapies may offer limited benefit when incorporated in a functional restoration and rehabilitation plan.

No prospective randomized controlled trials have evaluated analgesics in treatment of children with CRPS-1. Treatment, when initiated, often includes anticonvulsant therapy (e.g., gabapentin, pregabalin, etc.), mood stabilizers (e.g., selective serotonin reuptake inhibitors [SSRIs], tricyclic antidepressant agents [TCAs], clonidine, etc.), nonsteroidal anti-inflammatory drugs (NSAIDs) to alleviate secondary muscle soreness, and sleep-promoting agents. The efficacy of anti-inflammatory, antioxidants, sodium-channel blockers, and NMDA-receptor blockers in the form of topical analgesics, dimethyl sulfoxide, N-acetylcysteine, and intravenous lidocaine and ketamine infusion await assessment in controlled trials in children. Vitamin C (antioxidant) has been demonstrated as most effective in preventing development of CRPS-1 after limb surgery in adults. Opioids provide little to no benefit and are not recommended due to lack of efficacy and potential for significant adverse effects. Other analgesic agents, such as calcium channel blockers, beta agents, clonidine, corticosteroids, muscle relaxants, hyperbaric oxygen, and immune modulators are controversial as they have neither been investigated in randomized controlled trials or demonstrated benefits in alleviating pain or restoring physical function. TCAs and sleep promoting medications are prescribed as sleep aids to improve insomnia. SSRIs and norepinephrine reuptake inhibitors as well as anxiolytics are prescribed to manage anxiety, depression, and mood difficulties that could be barriers to effective compliance in functional restoration therapy.[11] To date, there are no randomized controlled trials to demonstrate a role for analgesics in improving function.

HOW ARE ACUTE PAIN AND OTHER SYMPTOMS, SUCH AS DYSTONIA, MANAGED?

Focal dystonia is the most common movement disorder associated with CRPS-1. It is still rare, and the precise incidence is unknown. It is characterized by involuntary painful sustained muscle spasms that interfere with use of affected limb. The cause of dystonia in CRPS-1 is unknown, and it responds poorly to physical therapy and pharmacological agents (muscle relaxants, antispastic agents, anticholinergic medications, botulinum toxin injections). Persistent focal dystonia can lead to contractures, requiring surgical correction.[12]

DO SYMPATHETIC AND/OR SOMATIC NEURAL BLOCKADE PLAY A ROLE IN THE DIAGNOSIS AND/OR TREATMENT OF CRPS-1?

Interventional chronic pain management techniques can play a part in the multidisciplinary management of CRPS-1 and have a limited role when pain is unrelieved by conventional treatment modalities. Most existing data regarding the efficacy of interventional procedures are uncontrolled studies and have failed to examine the long-term benefit of these interventions in relieving pain and/or restoring function. A recent review of invasive treatments (sympathetic or epidural blocks with local anesthetics, peripheral and plexus nerve blocks, intravenous agents, surgical and chemical sympathectomy, implantable spinal cord simulator, and intrathecal opioid pumps) for pediatric CRPS found 36 publications involving 173 patients over 40 years. There were only 2 controlled trials in a small number of patients. The study concluded that the level of evidence for invasive interventional therapies is poor, consisting of only a few case reports and small retrospective reviews, lacking standardization and failing to report diagnostic criteria and outcome measures, missing long-term follow-up, and focusing on pain reduction as the outcome rather than improvement in function.[13–15]

Despite shortcomings in these invasive interventions, continuous peripheral, plexus, and epidural nerve block analgesia with indwelling catheters are offered as part of biopsychosocial treatment in selected patients to accelerate functional recovery or to transiently relieve pain.

WHAT IS THE INCIDENCE OF RELAPSE, AND WHAT IS THE LONG-TERM PROGNOSIS?

CRPS-1 is associated with transient relapses as a rule. The incidence of recurrence in children ranges from 20% to 30%. Flares may occur spontaneously, by induced physical and emotional stress, or following reinjury. The overall prognosis for children is favorable following interdisciplinary management. Recovery is usually complete, and chronicity is rare. Relapse is relatively common and treatable with aggressive implementation of learned self-management strategies, including desensitization, use of coping strategies to keep moving, and mobilization of the affected limb. Early institution of outpatient physical and occupational therapies may be necessary for severe relapse, and interventional therapy may be used as a rescue measure to facilitate the physical rehabilitation.[15]

In summary, in view of our limited understanding of CRPS-1 mechanisms, the treatment can be frustrating. CRPS-1 is a complex disorder, caused by various mechanisms in different individuals and based on diverse triggers, environmental factors, and genetic predisposition that lead to the unpredictable responses to treatment. As with other chronic pain disorders, treatment is challenging and most successful with a multidisciplinary rehabilitative approach.[16]

REVIEW QUESTIONS

1. Which of the following mechanisms is **MOST** consistent with the proposed pathophysiology of CRPS-1?

    A. Disinhibition of the descending modulating pathways.
    B. Inflammation and reperfusion injury.
    C. Sensitization of primary efferent neurons.
    D. Ventral horn neurons.

Answer: B
Review the key question discussion for "What is neuropathic pain? What is the difference between CRPS-1 and CRPS-2? What is the pathophysiology of CRPS? Do genetics play a role?" There have been multiple suggested mechanisms underlying the pathophysiology of CRPS: sympathetic dysregulation, inflammation and reperfusion injury, facilitation of nociceptive pathways, and/or disinhibition of descending modulating pathways. The mechanism of CRPS may be distinct in different patients based on the inciting event.

2. Which of the following is **NOT** a component of the Budapest criteria?

    A. Continued pain, disproportionate to an inciting event.
    B. At least 1 symptom in 3 out of 4 categories of sensory, vasomotor, sudomotor/edema, and motor/trophic changes.
    C. At least 1 sign at the time of examination in 3 out of 4 categories of sensory, vasomotor, sudomotor/edema, and motor/trophic changes.
    D. No other diagnosis better explains the signs and symptoms.

Answer: C
Review the key question discussion for "What are the current International Association of Study of Pain (IASP) diagnostic criteria for complex regional pain syndrome (CRPS) and what are the challenges?" The criteria include at least 1 sign in 2 or more of the categories listed.

3. An 11-year-old female sustains an open fracture of the left distal radius while bouncing with friends on a trampoline. Which of the following **MOST** predisposes her to developing CRPS?

    A. Athletic ability.

B. Female gender.
C. Source of injury.
D. Type of injury.

Answer: B

In children, CRPS is most commonly identified in preadolescent females and in the lower extremities. See the key question discussion for "What is the incidence and prevalence in children and adolescents?" to review the incidence and prevalence and predisposing factors.

4. A 10-year-old boy with a history of anxiety and left lower extremity CRPS-1 two years ago presents with spontaneous onset of severe pain, swelling of the left lower extremity, and difficulties with sleep due to excruciating pain from contact with bed sheets. CRPS flare-up is suspected. Which of the following tests **BEST** helps confirm the diagnosis?

    A. Elevation of blood inflammatory markers.
    B. None exist, CRPS is a clinical diagnosis.
    C. Qualitative sensory testing.
    D. Response to sympathetic nerve block.

Answer: B

CRPS-1 remains a clinical diagnosis. Imaging and blood tests may be helpful to rule out other underlying pathology that may mimic CRPS symptoms but will not help confirm or rule out the diagnosis of CRPS-1. Qualitative sensory testing is a test for diagnosis of small fiber neuropathy, and there are no distinct characteristics of this test to verify or exclude CRPS-1. Pain alleviation or lack thereof after selective sympathetic nerve blockade is no longer considered diagnostic. The sympathetic system is not primarily involved in the mechanism of CRPS-1, even when clinical presentation is suggestive of sympathetic system dysfunction. Review the key question discussion for "Are there laboratory or imaging tests that can confirm the diagnosis of CRPS?"

5. A 12-year-old girl presents for follow up of ongoing posttraumatic CRPS-1 pain and fixed inversion posture of the right foot. Previous MRI showed complete healing of the original injury and shortening of the anterior talo-fibular ligament and calcaneo-fibular ligament. Her pain has not improved at a 6-month follow-up visit despite participation in physical therapy, psychology/psychiatric counseling, and a trial of oral and repeated intramuscular Botox injections. What is the next **BEST** therapeutic action?

    A. Orthopedic consultation for fixed contracture.
    B. Repeat intramuscular Botox injections.
    C. Repeat lumbar sympathetic nerve blockade.
    D. Serial casting to correct ankle joint to neural position.

Answer: A

Focal dystonia is the most common movement disorder of CRPS. Because the underlying pathophysiology is poorly understood, when there is a persistently poor response to physical therapy, analgesics, Botox injections, psychological counseling, and psychopharmacological therapy, it is important to consult with an orthopedic surgeon for an evaluation of fixed contracture and the possible need for release of the contractures and restoration of normal joint position and function. Review the key question discussion for "How are acute pain and other symptoms, such as dystonia, managed?"

6. A 14-year-old female adolescent presents with posttraumatic significant pain and swelling in the right lower extremity. The distribution of pain and cutaneous hypersensitivity do not follow a specific nerve territory. A comprehensive evaluation has been negative for an anatomic etiology, nerve conduction and electromyography tests are normal, and she meets Budapest criteria for CRPS. She has been unable to ambulate and attend school due to pain. What is the **BEST** initial management for this patient?

    A. Elastic compression bandage wrap, icing, elevation and oral NSAID.
    B. Physical therapy including weight bearing, opioid and gabapentin for severe pain.
    C. Physical therapy for desensitization and mobilization CBT.
    D. Pneumatic walking boot, crutches for partial weight bearing and analgesics.

Answer: C

Review the key question discussion for "What is neuropathic pain? What is the difference between CRPS-1 and CRPS-2? What is the pathophysiology of CRPS? Do genetics play a role?" With the primary goal being to reverse the negative impact from immobilization and psychological distress, a biopsychosocial approach with psychotherapy and CBT is the most impactful at improving function and alleviating pain symptoms. Immobilization of the limb will reinforce pain avoidance, fear of movement, and the negative behavior, leading to worsening of the CRPS-1 signs and symptoms, pain-associated distress, and disability.

7. A 14-year-old adolescent with a lower extremity CRPS-1 returns to clinic and complains of worsening pain and a lack of progress after 4 weeks of physical therapy and psychological counseling. She reports distress related to pain-related insomnia and inability to wash the affected limb, move the ankle joint, or bear weight. Along with physical therapy and cognitive-behavioral support, what is the next **BEST** approach to managing this patient?

    A. Extended-release opioid and a short-acting opioid.
    B. Implantable spinal cord stimulator.
    C. Inpatient continuous peripheral nerve catheter block.
    D. Outpatient serial lumbar sympathetic nerve blocks.

Answer: C

See the review of key question "Do sympathetic and/or somatic neural blockade play a role in the diagnosis and/or treatment of CRPS-1?" While procedural interventions offer a limited and transient benefit, as a rescue intervention, it may reduce pain and enable mobilization of the ankle joint and a return to outpatient management. Two recent studies suggest that continuous somatic neural blockade may sufficiently alleviate pain and allay fear of movement to encourage patients to effectively participate in physical therapy.

8. A 15-year-old female presents with a history of painful left foot and a diagnosis of a tarsal coalition that required surgical correction. She has completed her postsurgical physical therapy; however, pain has persisted for several postsurgical weeks. Postsurgical imaging studies reveal no structural abnormalities, and the medial foot operative scar appears healthy. The constant pain gradually spread to the proximal region of the leg and is associated with skin hypersensitivity, intermittent discoloration, temperature changes, and swelling and limited range of motion of the ankle. Her findings are **MOST** consistent with

    A. CRPS-1.
    B. Non-union of the bones.
    C. Postsurgical neuroma.
    D. Saphenous neuropathy.

Answer: A
Refer to the description of the key question "What are the current International Association of Study of Pain (IASP) diagnostic criteria for complex regional pain syndrome (CRPS) and what are the challenges?" Postoperative pain normally resolves within a few days after uncomplicated surgery, and patients should be able to bear weight and engage in physical therapy. This patient meets the Budapest criteria for CRPS. The patient's presentation is not consistent with known complications after surgery. Postoperative imaging studies excluded infection, inflammation, bony non-union, or failed surgical procedure. Neuroma and saphenous neuropathy are possible, but these conditions should present with distinct manifestations. Neuroma pain is localized and visible on MRI. Saphenous neuropathy most likely presents with numbness along the saphenous nerve distribution or hypersensitivity (i.e., CRPS-2), but this is unlikely because the incision is remote from the saphenous nerve course.

QUESTIONS AND ANSWERS

This chapter has accompanying questions and answers which are available to subscribers as part of the Oxford eLearning platform. To access the questions, go to ✔ http://oxfordmedicine. com/pediatricanesthesiaPBL

REFERENCES

1. Marinus J, Moseley GL, Birklein F, et al. Clinical features and pathophysiology of complex regional pain syndrome. *Lancet.* 2011;10:637–648.
2. Wilder RT. Management of pediatric patients with complex regional pain syndrome. *The Clinical journal of pain.* 2006;22(5): 443–448.
3. Wilder RT, Berde CB, Wolohan M, et al. Reflex sympathetic dystrophy in children: clinical characteristics and follow-up of seventy patients. *J Bone Joint Surg Am.* 1992;74:910–919.
4. Harden RN, Bruehl S, Perez RSGM, et al. Validation of proposed diagnostic criteria (the "Budapest Criteria") for complex regional pain syndrome. *Pain.* 2010;150(2):268–274.
5. Ringer R, Wertli M, Bachmann LM, Buck FM, Brunner F. Concordance of qualitative bone scintigraphy results with presence of clinical complex regional pain syndrome 1: meta-analysis of test accuracy studies. *Eur J Pain.* 2012;16(10):1347–1356.
6. Sethna NF, Meier PM, Zurakowski D, Berde CB. Cutaneous sensory abnormalities in children and adolescents with complex regional pain syndromes. *Pain.* 2007;131(1–2):153–161.
7. Coffelt TA, Bauer BD, Carroll AE. Inpatient characteristics of the child admitted with chronic pain. *Pediatrics.* 2013;132(2):e422–e429.
8. Logan DE, Carpino EA, Chiang G, et al. A day-hospital approach to treatment of pediatric complex regional pain syndrome: initial functional outcomes. *The Clin J Pain.* 2012;28(9):766–774.
9. Lee BH, Scharff L, Sethna NF, et al. Physical therapy and cognitive-behavioral treatment for complex regional pain syndromes. *J Pediatr.* 2002;141:135–140.
10. Simons LE, Sieberg CB, Conroy C, et al. Children with chronic pain: response trajectories after intensive pain rehabilitation treatment. *J Pain.* 2018;19(2):207–218.
11. Williams G, Howard R. The pharmacological management of complex regional pain syndrome in pediatric patients. *Paediatr Drugs.* 2016;18(4):243–250.
12. Majumdar A, Lopez-Casas J, Poo P, et al. Syndrome of fixed dystonia in adolescents—short term outcome in 4 cases. *Eur J Paediatr Neurol.* 2009;13(5):466–472.
13. Cucchiaro G, Craig K, Marks K, Cooley K, Cox TKB, Schwartz J. Short- and long-term results of an inpatient programme to manage complex regional pain syndrome in children and adolescents. *Br J Pain.* 2017;11(2):87–96.
14. O'Connell NE, Wand BM, Gibson W, et al. Local anaesthetic sympathetic blockade for complex regional pain syndrome. *Cochrane Database Syst Rev.* 2016;28:CD004598.
15. Zernikow B, Wager J, Brehmer H, Hirschfeld G, Maier C. Invasive treatments for complex regional pain syndrome in children and adolescents: a scoping review. *Anesthesiology.* 2015; 122(3):699–707.
16. Donado C, Lobo K, Velarde-Alvarez MF, et al. Continuous regional anesthesia and inpatient rehabilitation for pediatric complex regional pain syndrome. *Reg Anesth Pain Med.* 2017;42(4):527–534.

55.

NEURAXIAL ANESTHESIA AND ANALGESIA FOR PEDIATRIC SURGERY

Heather Ballard, Ravi Shah, and Santhanam Suresh

STEM CASE AND KEY QUESTIONS

A 2-month-old ex-31-week male presents for bilateral inguinal hernia repair prior to discharge from the neonatal intensive care unit. His hospital course is significant for respiratory distress at birth, requiring intubation for 2 weeks, and multiple episodes of apnea and bradycardia. He is currently hemodynamically stable on room air, he weighs 2.6 kg, and his medications include caffeine.

The patient is brought to the operating room and monitors are placed. Using sucrose solution via pacifier to calm the infant, the arms and legs are held together in an upright fetal position, and the lower back is prepped with betadine solution. A 2.5 cm, 25G styletted spinal needle is used for dural puncture and, after noting cerebrospinal fluid (CSF), 0.2 mL/kg (total volume 0.5 mL) of preservative-free bupivacaine 0.5% is slowly injected. The block duration is sufficient for the 55-minute operation. The patient spends the next 24 hours under observation due to his age and history of apneic spells. The observation period is uneventful, and the patient is discharged home the following day with oral acetaminophen as needed for pain control.

WHAT ARE POTENTIAL ADVANTAGES TO PERFORMING SPINAL ANESTHESIA IN THE PEDIATRIC POPULATION?

Spinal anesthesia has shown to be safe and effective for patients undergoing lower abdomen, urological, and lower extremity surgeries.[1] This technique can be used as a sole anesthetic in pediatric surgery, primarily in infants. Advantages of using spinal anesthesia include avoiding general anesthesia and endotracheal intubation, minimizing opioid requirements, and reducing time to emergence.[2] The avoidance of sedatives is particularly important in premature infants, who are susceptible to postoperative apnea. A study has shown that spinal anesthesia reduced the incidence of early apnea in infants less than 60 weeks postconceptional age but not the incidence of apnea overall.[3]

WHAT ARE THE RELEVANT DIFFERENCES BETWEEN NEONATAL AND ADULT SPINAL ANATOMY?

Though spinal anesthesia can be successfully performed in both populations, there are important differences between the neonatal and adult spinal cord. The neonatal spinal cord terminates at the L3 vertebra, whereas the adult spinal cord terminates 2 levels higher at L1.[4] Due to this difference, there is a preference for accessing the L4/L5 vertebral interspace for neonatal spinal placement to avoid nerve injury. Locating an appropriate interspace is difficult using surface anatomy; ultrasound may improve accuracy by visualization of bony landmarks.

Infants are typically not cooperative patients; however, anatomical differences improve the likelihood of successful subarachnoid block. Infants have flexible spines that allow positioning to increase intervertebral space. There is also a shorter distance between the skin and arachnoid space, limiting the depth required for each needle pass.[5] The neonatal spinal canal has a 70% width compared to the adult canal; this larger width relative to body size allows adequate space for needle entry. When dural puncture is successful, the infant's flat spinal column permits even spread of intrathecal medications.[6]

WHAT IS THE TYPICAL HEMODYNAMIC RESPONSE IN NEONATES UNDERGOING SPINAL ANESTHESIA? HOW ARE SPINAL BLOCKS DOSED IN THE PEDIATRIC POPULATION?

Unlike adult patients, neonates tend to have minimal hemodynamic changes when undergoing spinal anesthesia. This is independent of whether a fluid bolus is given prior to initiation of nerve block.[7] The sympathectomy associated with spinal block has little effect on neonates because parasympathetic tone predominates.[8] Classically, the teaching is that the first sign of a high level during an infant spinal is apnea. In premature infants, there is little to no autonomic response to spinal anesthesia.

Infant spinals are dosed with much higher amounts of local anesthetic than would be predicted based upon body weight. The reason for this larger dose is the relatively larger spinal canal of the infant, leading to a larger volume of CSF per kilogram of body weight. A typical dose for an infant spinal is bupivacaine 0.5% 0.8 mg/kg (range 0.5–1 mg/kg.) The milligram per kilogram dosing decreases as patient size increases.[9,10]

STEM CASE AND KEY QUESTIONS

A 7-month-old female with a past medical history of cystic fibrosis presents for ileostomy stoma reversal after neonatal surgery for meconium ileus. Other significant past medical history includes prolonged postoperative intubation following ileostomy due to difficulties with ventilation and opioid tolerance from prolonged sedation. After uneventful induction of general anesthesia and timeout, the patient is placed in the lateral decubitus position and the back prepped with chlorhexidine antiseptic. A 5-cm 20-gauge Tuohy needle is inserted into the T10-T11 epidural space, and a 21-gauge epidural catheter is inserted under ultrasound guidance.

An initial test dose of 0.4 mL lidocaine 1% with epinephrine 1:200,000 is injected with negative aspiration of blood or CSF. No hemodynamic or electrocardiographic changes are observed. A bolus of 2.5 mL ropivacaine 0.25% is administered, followed by a continuous infusion of 1 mL/hr ropivacaine 0.1% during surgical closure. No opioids are given during surgery. The patient is extubated uneventfully at the end of the case. She remains comfortable in recovery and the epidural is removed 3 days later, at which point intravenous acetaminophen and ketolorac are administered for acute pain management.

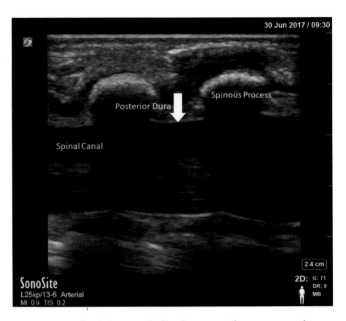

Fig. 55.1 Longitudinal ultrasound of lumbar region shows posterior dura located between two spinous processes. The paramedian longitudinal approach is often needed in older infants and children due to ossification of spinous processes. The spinal canal with cerebrospinal fluid is seen deep to the posterior dura.

HOW DOES EPIDURAL CATHETER PLACEMENT DIFFER IN PEDIATRIC PATIENTS WHEN COMPARED TO ADULTS?

Thoracic and lumbar epidural catheters can provide effective analgesia for thoracic, abdominal, and lower extremity surgery in both adults and children. However, practitioners must be aware of anatomical differences between these groups to avoid dural puncture. Pediatric patients have a shallower depth to the epidural space.[11] A rough rule of thumb is that this distance can be approximated by 0.1 centimeter per kilogram of body weight (i.e., 1.5 cm for a 15-kg child.) In addition, the loss of resistance (LOR) may not feel as obvious in young children because there is less ossification of the ligamentum flavum.

WHAT IS THE ROLE OF ULTRASOUND GUIDANCE IN LUMBAR AND THORACIC EPIDURAL CATHETER PLACEMENT?

Although the LOR technique is widely used to localize the epidural space, ultrasound is a good adjunct. This is especially true in infants and young children because the tactile feel of LOR may be subtle due to lack of ligamentous ossification. Figure 55.1 shows a longitudinal image of an infant lumbar spine including spinal processes and dura mater. The ultrasound can be utilized to measure the depth to the ligamentum flavum and dura. In obese patients where landmarks may be harder to palpate, ultrasound can be used to identify spinous processes and identify midline.[12]

Ultrasound beam penetration is particularly effective in infants and neonates because the posterior vertebral column is mostly cartilaginous. This visibility of spinal structures decreases with age because the vertebral column starts to ossify.

The epidural catheter may be difficult to visualize using ultrasound due to its lack of echogenicity; correct catheter placement is indirectly confirmed by viewing extradural spread of local anesthetic injected through the catheter.

CAN LUMBAR AND THORACIC EPIDURAL CATHETERS BE PLACED SAFELY IN ANESTHETIZED PEDIATRIC PATIENTS?

Yes; lumbar and thoracic epidural catheters can be placed in either the awake or asleep state. Though the awake state is preferable because the patient can give feedback regarding paresthesias and signs of local anesthetic toxicity, children may not be able to give this feedback or be cooperative. It may be safer to place the epidural in an asleep, motionless patient than to attempt placement in an awake, moving child.[13] Utilization of ultrasound may lead to reduced risk of neurological injury if nerve structures can be identified and correct catheter placement can be confirmed.

HOW IS AN EPIDURAL CATHETER BEST MANAGED AFTER PLACEMENT AND FOR POSTOPERATIVE PAIN CONTROL?

After placement, the epidural catheter should be aspirated for blood or CSF and injected with a test dose to ensure proper placement. An example of a test dose is 0.1 mL/kg of lidocaine 1% with 1:200,000 epinephrine.[14] With a negative test dose, the epidural catheter can be used during surgery to reduce general anesthetic or sedation requirements. The epidural catheter can also be used for postoperative analgesia—its use has been shown to provide superior analgesia compared to opioids alone and can be part of a multimodal postoperative

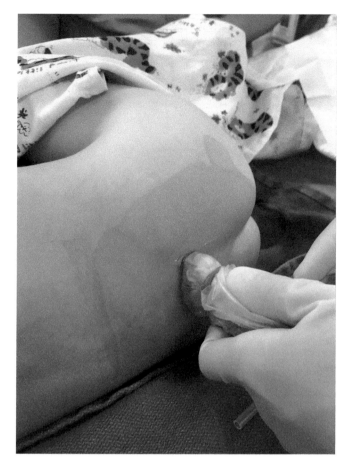

Fig. 55.2 The patient is positioned in the left lateral decubitus position with hips and knees flexed and skin prepped with chlorhexidine paint. An assistant is positioned on the other side of the bed to ensure safety. The ultrasound is placed in a transverse location relative to the patient's spine.

pain regimen. As with any invasive catheter, nursing staff should be educated to examine the site daily and monitor for any complications. An organized pain service is particularly effective, providing adjuncts for optimizing pain control and easing the transition to oral medications.[15]

STEM CASE AND KEY QUESTIONS

A 2-month-old female with a past medical history of bilateral clubfoot deformity presents for bilateral achilles tenotomy and casting. The anesthetic plan is to perform an awake caudal epidural block with 3% 2-chloroprocaine. After application of standard monitors, caudal epidural is performed with the patient in lateral position using a landmark-based technique with a 20-gauge angiocatheter. The test dose is negative, as is aspiration for blood or CSF. Chloroprocaine 3% is administered in 3 incremental doses of 2 mL for a total of 6 mL. Bilateral motor block developed over the next 2 to 3 minutes. The surgical procedure began, and patient was tolerating the procedure well. Eight minutes later, she began to exhibit bilateral eyelid twitching and upper extremity shaking, which was concerning for seizure activity.

Respirations were supported with positive pressure bag mask ventilation with 100% oxygen, and intravenous access

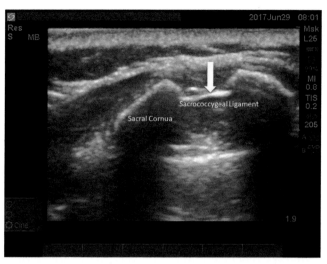

Fig. 55.3 The ultrasound image shows the sacrococcygeal ligament located between the sacral cornua. A transverse image is usually obtained initially to confirm midline positioning; this is especially helpful in patients with bony abnormalities or difficult-to-palpate landmarks.

was obtained. Within 30 seconds, the seizure self-resolved, vital signs remained stable, and the infant began to cry. After discussion with family, the decision was made to complete the operation as adequate sensory and motor block were

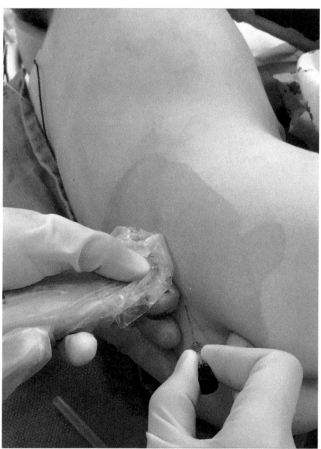

Fig. 55.4 The ultrasound probe is rotated 90 degrees to the longitudinal plane. This allows real-time guidance of needle advancement and local anesthetic injection.

already achieved. Postoperatively, the patient was admitted overnight for additional monitoring and consultation with a neurologist. Further workup, including an electroencephalogram, creatinine kinase, and pseudocholinesterase levels, were unremarkable.

WHAT ARE SOME COMMON INDICATIONS FOR CAUDAL BLOCKADE IN CHILDREN? WHAT IS THE SAFETY PROFILE OF CAUDAL ANESTHESIA IN PEDIATRICS?

Caudal anesthesia is a popular technique for surgical anesthesia and postoperative analgesia in the pediatric population. Single injections can be used for lower extremity, urological, and abdominal surgeries.[16] If a catheter is placed, the upper abdomen and thoracic surgical sites can also be covered.[17] When utilized in addition to general anesthesia, caudal anesthesia lowers sedative requirements potentially reducing the time to discharge.[18]

The decision to use a single dose of local anesthetic versus placing a caudal catheter depends on many factors—surgical location, duration, and anticipated postoperative pain control requirements. The use of caudal blockade is safe in pediatrics. This has been confirmed by the limited complications recorded in the 18,000 single-shot caudal blocks in the Pediatric Regional Anesthesia Network (PRAN) database.[19] Despite the safety profile, it is prudent to remain within the limits of local anesthetic toxicity for caudal anesthesia dosing.

WHAT IS THE RELEVANT ANATOMY FOR PERFORMING A CAUDAL BLOCK? HOW IS THE PATIENT POSITIONED, AND WHAT IS DONE TO IDENTIFY APPROPRIATE LANDMARKS?

The caudal epidural space is located deep to the sacrococcygeal membrane at the sacral hiatus. Needle entry into the caudal space is typically easier in infants and young children because the sacrococcygeal ligament is not completely ossified until 8 years of age. In addition, the sacral cornua are easier to palpate because the sacral fat pad is absent in children.[20]

In order to perform caudal anesthesia, the patient is positioned prone or lateral decubitus. Figure 55.2 demonstrates lateral decubitus position with adequate skin preparation using chlorhexidine. Flexion of the knee, leg, and neck has been shown to shift the dural sac cephalad; this may lead to a greater margin of safety due to the increased distance needed for dural puncture.[21] The relevant surface landmarks are the sacral cornua located midline rostral to the sacral hiatus. Alternatively, an equilateral triangle may be drawn between the 2 posterior superior iliac spines and the sacral hiatus at the apex. In clinical practice, a common error is needle entry that is too low on the sacrum.

DESCRIBE THE TECHNIQUE INVOLVED IN SAFELY DELIVERING CAUDAL ANESTHESIA.

Using surface landmarks, the needle is inserted at a 45-degree angle into the midline at the level of the sacral cornua. The skin is punctured, and the needle is advanced through the

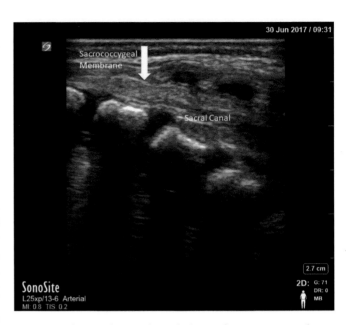

Fig. 55.5 This ultrasound image shows the hyperechoic sacrococcygeal ligament superficial to the sacral canal. The dural sac is seen as a hypoechoic structure on the right side of the sacral canal.

sacrococcygeal ligament with a "pop." Using a blunt tip needle may increase tactile sensation through the sacrococcygeal membrane in comparison to a steeper beveled cutting needle. Once this LOR is encountered, the needle angle is decreased and advanced slightly into the caudal space. The needle is aspirated to ensure there is no return of blood or CSF. In addition, a test dose should be given to further confirm there is no inadvertent injection into a blood vessel or dural sac.[22] Divided doses of local anesthetic are administered with electrocardiographic monitoring of changes indicative of intravascular injection.[14] High pressure during injection and swelling of subcutaneous tissue should alert the practitioner to misplacement of the needle.

CAN CAUDAL ANESTHESIA BE PERFORMED WITH ULTRASOUND GUIDANCE?

Ultrasound guidance for block placement can be a useful tool, especially in patients with difficult to palpate surface landmarks or bony abnormalities. Relevant structures such as the sacral cornua, hiatus, and sacrococcygeal membrane can be easily identified.[23,24] As seen in Figures 55.2–55.3, the linear high-frequency probe is first used in the transverse plane to find the midline prior to needle insertion. The probe is then rotated to the longitudinal direction for needle advancement—paramedian orientation is utilized for older children due to bony shadows from the ossified vertebral column. Figures 55.4–55.5 demonstrate the position of the ultrasound probe relative to the spine for a longitudinal view and the corresponding ultrasound image in a young infant. Imaging local anesthetic injection avoids inadvertent placement into the intrathecal space or subcutaneous tissue. Correct needle location is confirmed with ultrasound by the anterior displacement of the posterior dura.[25] In addition, viewing the injection of local anesthetic through the caudal catheter can help estimate whether the catheter is threaded to the appropriate level for optimal analgesia.

WHAT LOCAL ANESTHETICS AND CONCENTRATIONS ARE APPROPRIATE? CAN ADJUVANTS BE ADDED?

Several local anesthetics have been utilized in caudal anesthesia. For postoperative analgesia, 0.2% ropivacaine or 0.125% to 0.25% bupivacaine/levobupivacaine are acceptable options. Ropivacaine has gained favor in some institutions due to its potential greater margin of safety and reduced motor blockade.[26,27] As a sole anesthetic, higher concentrations, such as 0.5% ropivacaine, 0.5% bupivacaine (levobupivacaine,) or 3% 2-chloroprocaine, must be used to ensure a denser nerve block. 3% 2-chloroprocaine is often chosen for short cases as a sole anesthetic due to its safety profile, rapid onset, and relatively dense motor block; 1 mL/kg dosing of local anesthetic is recommended to ensure a T10 level. Several adjuncts have been added to the epidural space to prolong blockage time, but each drug may have unintended side effects. Epinephrine is often added to epidural solutions to act as a vascular marker, but its vasoconstriction can prolong the duration of certain local anesthetics. Epidural opioids may lead to respiratory depression, itching, nausea, and vomiting. Though clonidine has been shown to prolong neuraxial analgesia, sedation and hypotension have been attributed to its use. Ketamine has also been used as an adjunct to increase the duration and density of blockage, but usage has been decreased out of concerns for neurotoxicity.[28–30]

DESCRIBE THE APPROACH TO MANAGING LOCAL ANESTHETIC SYSTEMIC TOXICITY (LAST) IN PEDIATRIC PATIENTS.

Resuscitation measures must be initiated immediately after LAST. Neurotoxicity (seizures) can be treated with barbiturates and benzodiazepines in addition to supportive care. Recent evidence indicates that the most successful treatment for LAST-related cardiotoxicity is the administration of a lipid emulsion, which is now considered first-line therapy. Case reports have described rapid bolus injections of lipid emulsion reversing the toxic effects of local anesthetics in pediatric patients. Safe dosing limits for lipid resuscitation are important to establish in pediatrics because complications from lipid overload have been reported in neonates receiving intravenous nutritional support. The suggested dose of 20% Intralipid' for pediatric patients is 2 to 5 mL/kg. This dose is repeated (up to 10 mL/kg) if cardiac function does not return to baseline. Although the exact mechanism of lipid emulsion therapy is unknown, it can be a life-saving measure for treating LAST in pediatric patients, as has been reported to the LipidRescue registry (www.lipidrescue.org).

DISCUSSION

Neuraxial analgesia is a powerful tool in the anesthesiologist's armamentarium. Whether utilized as a sole anesthetic or in addition to a general anesthesia, spinals and epidurals can provide effective analgesia and reduce sedation requirements.

Decreasing sedatives may decrease the incidence of postoperative apnea and lower risks associated with anesthetic exposure to the developing brain.[31,32] There are a limited number of contraindications to performing neuraxial anesthesia—these are listed in Table 55.1. Caudal, thoracic, and lumbar epidurals are invaluable for opioid-sparing postoperative pain control, potentially limiting undesirable narcotic side effects, such as nausea/vomiting, respiratory depression, and pruritus.[33] Though neuraxial analgesia has a safe track record in anesthetic practice, the risks of these invasive procedures must be considered.

Due to the density of block, spinal anesthesia can be a sole anesthetic for many lower orthopedical, urological, and gastrointestinal surgeries. Time is a limiting factor because a single-shot spinal reliably only provides 60 to 90 minutes of motor blockade. The rate of spinal failure is low, but reports vary widely from 1% to 15%.[1,34,35] Differences in success rate may be attributed to provider and institutional experience. The use of ultrasound to identify landmarks may reduce the number of failures, especially in inexperienced hands.[36,37] Other complications of spinal placement include epidural hematoma, meningitis, subcutaneous infection, backache, postdural puncture headache, and total spinal. Postdural puncture headache is less common in infants and neonates, but its true incidence in this population remains unknown due to difficulties in assessment. In older children (2–15 years old), the incidence is reported to be similar to adults at around 5%.[38]

A high level of neuraxial blockade can be seen with spinal and epidural analgesia. Adults typically present with

Table 55.1 **ABSOLUTE AND RELATIVE CONTRAINDICATIONS TO NEURAXIAL ANESTHESIA**

Absolute
Patient or parent refusal
Coagulopathy
Sepsis
Hemodynamic instability
Infection of placement site
Allergy to local anesthetic
Relative
Congenital anomaly of spine
Neurologic disease
Increased intracranial pressure
Unknown duration of surgery
Distant infection
Valvular heart disease
Prior spine surgery

hemodynamic findings from sympathectomy (hypotension and bradycardia) before respiratory distress and loss of consciousness occur. In contrast, infants have stable hemodynamics with sympathetic blockade due to their dominant parasympathetic tone; apnea and loss of consciousness (if no sedation administered) may be the first sign of a high spinal or epidural. The differential diagnosis for apnea after neuraxial blockade also includes medication overdose or error, breathing circuit obstruction, laryngospasm, severe bronchospasm, cardiovascular collapse, and apnea of prematurity. Early recognition of a high spinal level is of utmost importance to avoid complications; treatment involves sedation, airway support, and hemodynamic monitoring.[39]

Despite the potential for adverse reactions, epidural anesthesia has demonstrated a low incidence of complications. The national pediatric epidural audit of over 10,000 catheters demonstrated only 1 patient with sequelae 12 months after epidural placement.[40] In the PRAN database, 2 cases out of 7,617 reported neuraxial catheters had complications.[13] One patient had symptoms of local anesthetic toxicity, and another patient had a seizure. The complications from epidural anesthesia can range from mild annoyances, such as delayed micturition, to the devastating complication of nerve damage.[41] Many centers choose to leave urinary catheters in patients with epidural catheters to avoid issues with urinary retention. Neurological injury from epidural catheter placement can occur from several mechanisms: epidural abscess, epidural hematoma, and direct nerve injury from needle. Luckily, the incidence of these serious complications is rare. A reported risk unique to caudal placement is that epidermoid tumors can develop if nonstyletted needles are utilized due to tracking of skin cells into the epidural space.[42]

Though the incidence of LAST is rare in children, these events can be severe and life-threatening. Local anesthetic toxicity can occur from either intravascular injection of local anesthetics or high levels of systemic absorption. Caudal blocks and epidurals have the highest rates of intravascular absorption after intercostal nerve blocks. Diagnosing LAST in children is particularly difficult because most neuraxial techniques are performed under general anesthesia. Test doses can be unreliable for detection, and seizure activity may be masked by sedatives and muscle relaxants. The differential diagnosis for seizure under anesthesia includes LAST, febrile seizure, underlying seizure disorder, drug effect, hypoxia, and electrolyte disorder. The first sign of local anesthetic toxicity may be dysrhythmias or even cardiac arrest. Children, especially infants under 4 months, are at greater risk for LAST due to decreased protein binding and clearance of amide local anesthetics. This risk is heightened with use of continuous local anesthetic infusions for postoperative pain control. Using divided doses of local anesthetics, paying attention to drug dosages, and administering a test dose can help to mitigate risk. Recommended maximum dosages for commonly used local anesthetics in neuraxial anesthesia are listed in Table 55.2. If the local anesthetic is lipophilic, LAST can be treated with lipid rescue therapy with improved outcomes.[43] Safe-dosing guidelines of local anesthetics has facilitated acceptance of pediatric regional anesthesia practice.

Table 55.2 **LOCAL ANESTHETIC MAXIMUM DOSAGE AND DURATION**

LOCAL ANESTHETIC	MAXIMUM DOSE IN MG/KG (WITH EPINEPHRINE)	LOCATION	DURATION IN HOURS
Lidocaine	5 (7)	Epidural	1–2
Tetracaine	1.5 (2.5)	Spinal	1–1.5
2-chloroprocaine	8 (10)	Epidural	0.5–1
Bupivacaine	2.5 (3)	Epidural	2–5
Bupivacaine	2.5 (3)	Spinal	1
Ropivacaine	3	Epidural	2–6

REVIEW QUESTIONS

1. The vertebral level that the spinal cord terminate in neonates and adults is **BEST** described as which of following?

    A. L2 and L1
    B. L2 and L3
    C. L3 and L1
    D. L3 and L2

Answer: C

The lower termination of spinal cord in neonates (L3 vs. L1 in adults) has important clinical implications. Spinal needle placement should be attempted at lower lumbar levels (L4-L5) in infants to avoid injury to the spinal cord. If a child has a history of spina bifida or any syndrome associated with spinal cord abnormalities, an ultrasound or magnetic resonance imaging study should be conducted prior to the performance of neuraxial anesthesia to rule out tethered cord or abnormally low spinal cord location.[4,44]

2. Which of the following feature of the infants, relative to adults, **MOST** often impedes successful placement of spinal blockade?

    A. greater flexibility
    B. reduced lordosis
    C. uncooperativeness
    D. wider spinal canal

Answer: C

Despite the lack of cooperation in infants, there are several features of infant anatomy that facilitate spinal placement. Infant spines demonstrate greater flexibility, which allows for better positioning to increase the space between vertebral bodies. The distance from skin to subarachnoid space is relatively short, and the infant spinal canal is wider than what would be expected for body size.[5] These factors decrease the distance and increase the target size for needle placement. In terms of drug delivery, the flattened spinal column promotes an even spread of medication.[6] These factors help to account for the low failure rate seen in infant spinal anesthesia of 1% to 15%.[1,35]

3. Which of the following caudal dosing volumes would **MOST** likely achieve blockade to the T10 level?

    A. 0.1 mL/kg
    B. 0.5 mL/kg
    C. 0.75 mL/kg
    D. 1.0 mL/kg

Answer: D

In comparison to adult neuraxial dosing, a much higher volume of local anesthetic is required to achieve a sufficient sensory level. The infant and child's larger volume of CSF per body weight may account for this difference, as local anesthetics are diffusing into a larger space of CSF.[10] The upper limit for adult epidural blousing is typically 20 to 30 mL (0.3–0.5 mL/kg) of local anesthetic. In order to maintain a consistent sensory level to T10, 1.0 mL/kg of local anesthetic is administered. Depending on the concentration utilized, this amount of local anesthetic borders on the recommended limits for safe dosing. Careful attention must be applied when administering local anesthetics for caudal anesthesia because there is a high rate of intravascular absorption.[16]

4. Which of the following findings is **MOST** consistent with a high spinal block in an infant?

    A. apnea
    B. bradycardia
    C. hypotension
    D. tachycardia

Answer: A

Unlike adults, infants maintain relatively stable hemodynamics with high spinal blockade. The bradycardia and hypotension that occurs in adults undergoing sympathectomy is largely absent. This phenomenon is due to the infant's possession of a predominantly parasympathetic tone.[8] Apnea may be the first sign of a high spinal, followed by loss of consciousness. It may be difficult to differentiate an infant's baseline apnea of prematurity from a high spinal block. The treatment for high spinal is to support the infant's airway and monitor hemodynamic parameters.[39]

5. Epidural catheter placement failure in pediatric patients as compared to adults is **MOST** likely due to which anatomical difference?

    A. greater ossification of ligamentum flavum
    B. higher volume of CSF
    C. narrower intravertebral spaces
    D. shallower depth of epidural space

Answer: D

Epidural catheter placement has been shown to have a low incidence of complications in both the national pediatric epidural audit and PRAN database.[13,40] However, anesthesiologists must recognize the differences between adult and pediatric anatomy to minimize risk of dural puncture. Pediatric patients have a shorter distance to the epidural space. A rough rule of thumb is the distance to LOR is around 0.1 centimeters per kilogram of body weight. The tactile feel of LOR may be less pronounced in children despite using the same type of needle because the ligamentum flavum is less ossified. The anesthesiologist may have to support the epidural needle throughout catheter placement because only a small percentage of the needle length is inside the patient. Despite these differences, epidural catheter placement can be successful even in neonates.[11]

6. Blood levels after local anesthetic injection are **HIGHEST** for which of the following?

    A. caudal epidural
    B. lumbar epidural
    C. subcutaneous infiltration
    D. thoracic epidural

Answer: A

Despite a long history of safety using single-shot caudal blocks in pediatric anesthesia, care must be given when administering any local anesthetic. Local anesthetic system toxicity can occur from direct intravascular injection or systemic absorption. Negative aspiration and the use of a test dose reduce the likelihood of injecting into a blood vessel.[14,22] The epidural space is known to have large amounts of veins, especially in the sacral plexus. This predisposes caudal epidurals to have the highest amounts of systemic vascular absorption, followed by thoracic and lumbar epidurals. Local anesthetic is absorbed from the epidural space into nearby veins; Starling forces determine this rate of transfer. In order to limit the amount of systemic absorption, injection of local anesthetic should be administered in divided doses with low amounts of driving pressure.

7. Which of the following factors render infants more susceptible than adults to neurological or cardiac toxicity related to excessive local anesthetic blood concentration?

    A. decreased volume of distribution
    B. greater receptor binding
    C. increased drug clearance
    D. lower protein binding

Answer: D

Infants have a double-edged sword with respect to local anesthetic toxicity—lower protein binding and decreased drug clearance. Lower protein binding to albumin and alpha 1-acid glycoprotein ensures that more of the active form of the drug is available to cause toxicity. In addition, infant's immature hepatic function decreases the amount of drug metabolized and cleared from the body. This combination increases the susceptibility to LAST, especially when continuous infusions are employed. If symptoms of LAST occur, administration of local anesthetic should be discontinued immediately and supportive therapy should be instituted. If the local anesthetic is lipophilic, such as bupivacaine or ropivacaine, a bolus of lipid emulsion 20% 1.5 mL/kg should be administered followed by an infusion of 0.25 mL/kg/min. Further guidelines for the treatment of LAST are available at www.lipidrescue.org.

QUESTIONS AND ANSWERS

This chapter has accompanying questions and answers which are available to subscribers as part of the Oxford eLearning platform. To access the questions, go to ✓ http:// oxfordmedicine. com/pediatricanesthesiaPBL

REFERENCES

1. Williams RK, Adams DC, Aladjern EV, et al. The safety and efficacy of spinal anesthesia for surgery in infants: the Vermont Infant Spinal Registry. *Anesth Analg.* 2006;102(1):67–71.

2. Cote CJ, Zaslavski A, Downes JJ, et al. Postoperative apnea in former preterm infants after inguinal herniorrhaphy: a combined analysis. *Anesthesiology.* 1995;82(4):809–822.

3. Davidson AJ, Morton NS, Arnup SJ, et al. Apnea after awake regional and general anesthesia in infants: The General Anesthesia Compared to Spinal Anesthesia Study—comparing apnea and neurodevelopmental outcomes, a randomized controlled trial. *Anesthesiology.* 2015;123:38–54.

4. Van Schoor AN, Bosman MC, Bosenberg AT. Descriptive study of the differences in the level of the conus medullaris in four different age groups. *Clin Anat.* 2015;28(5):638–644.

5. Bosenberg AT, Gouws E. Skin-epidural distance in children. *Anaesthesia.* 1995;50(10):895–897.

6. Hirabayashi Y, Shimizu R, Saitoh K, Fukuda H, et al. Spread of subarachnoid hyperbaric amethocaine in adolescents. *Br J Anaesth.* 1995;74(1):41–45.

7. Dohi S, Naito H, Takahashi T. Age-related changes in blood pressure and duration of motor block in spinal anesthesia. *Anesthesiology.* 1979;50(4):319–323.

8. Oberlander TF, Berde CB, Lam KH, Rappaport LA, Saul JP. Infants tolerate spinal anesthesia with minimal overall autonomic changes: analysis of heart rate variability in former premature infants undergoing hernia repair. *Anesth Analg.* 1995;80(1):20–27.

9. Gupta A, Saha U. Spinal anesthesia in children: a review. *J Anaesthesiol Clin Pharmacol.* 2014;30(1):10–18.

10. Kokki H. Spinal blocks. *Paediatr Anaesth.* 2012;22(1):56–64.

11. Rapp HJ, Folger A, Grau T. Ultrasound-guided epidural catheter insertion in children. *Anesth Analg.* 2005;101(2):333–339.

12. Tsui BC, Suresh S. Ultrasound imaging for regional anesthesia in infants, children, and adolescents: a review of current literature and its application in the practice of neuraxial blocks. *Anesthesiology.* 2010112(3):719–728.

13. Taenzer AH. Walker BJ, Bosenberg AT, et al. Asleep versus awake: does it matter? Pediatric regional block complications by patient state: a report from the Pediatric Regional Anesthesia Network. *Reg Anesth Pain Med.* 2014;39(4):279–283.

14. Varghese E, Deepak KM, Chowdary KV. Epinephrine test dose in children: is it interpretable on ECG monitor? *Paediatr Anaesth.* 2009;19(11):1090–1095.

15. Lonnqvist PA, Morton NS. Postoperative analgesia in infants and children. *Br J Anaesth.* 2005;95(1):59–68.

16. Johr M, Berger TM. Caudal blocks. *Paediatr Anaesth.* 2012;22(1):44–50.

17. Bosenberg AT, Bland BA, Schulte-Steinberg O, Downing JW. et al. Thoracic epidural anesthesia via caudal route in infants. *Anesthesiology.* 1988;69(2):265–269.

18. Peutrell JM, Hughes DG. Epidural anaesthesia through caudal catheters for inguinal herniotomies in awake ex-premature babies. *Anaesthesia.* 1993;48(2):128–131.

19. Suresh S, Long J, Birmingham PK, De Oliveira GS Jr. et al. Are caudal blocks for pain control safe in children? An analysis of 18,650 caudal blocks from the Pediatric Regional Anesthesia Network (PRAN) database. *Anesth Analg.* 2015;120(1):151–156.

20. Chen CP, Tang SF, Hsu TC, et al. Ultrasound guidance in caudal epidural needle placement. *Anesthesiology.* 2004;101(1):181–184.

21. Koo BN, Hong JY, Kim JE, Kil HK, et al. The effect of flexion on the level of termination of the dural sac in paediatric patients. *Anaesthesia,.*2009;64(10):1072–1076.

22. Tobias JD. Caudal epidural block: a review of test dosing and recognition of systemic injection in children. *Anesth Analg.* 2001;93(5):1156–1161.

23. Marhofer P, Bosenberg A, Sitzwohl C, et al. Pilot study of neuraxial imaging by ultrasound in infants and children. *Paediatr Anaesth.* 2005;15(8):671–676.

24. Kil HK, Cho JE, Kim WO, et al. Prepuncture ultrasound-measured distance: an accurate reflection of epidural depth in infants and small children. *Reg Anesth Pain Med.* 2007;32(2):102–106.

25. Schwartz D, Raghunathan K, Dunn S, Connelly NR, et al. Ultrasonography and pediatric caudals. *Anesth Analg.* 2008;106(1):97–99.

26. Chipde S, Banjare M, Arora K, Saraswat M, et al. Prospective randomized controlled comparison of caudal bupivacaine and ropivacaine in pediatric patients. *Ann Med Health Sci Res.* 2014;4(Suppl 2):S115–S118.

27. Khalil S, Campos C, Farag AM, et al. Caudal block in children: ropivacaine compared with bupivacaine. *Anesthesiology.* 1999;91(5):1279–1284.

28. Bosenberg A. Adjuvants in pediatric regional anesthesia. *Pain Manag.* 2012;2(5):479–486.

29. Vetter TR, Carvallo D, Johnson JL, et al. A comparison of single-dose caudal clonidine, morphine, or hydromorphone combined with ropivacaine in pediatric patients undergoing ureteral reimplantation. *Anesth Analg.* 2007;104(6):1356–1363.

30. Wheeler M, Patel A, Suresh S, et al. The addition of clonidine 2 microg.kg-1 does not enhance the postoperative analgesia of a caudal block using 0.125% bupivacaine and epinephrine 1:200,000 in children: a prospective, double-blind, randomized study. *Paediatr Anaesth.* 2005;15(6):476–483.

31. Davidson AJ, Morton NS, Arnup SJ, et al. Apnea after awake regional and general anesthesia in infants: the general anesthesia compared to spinal anesthesia study—comparing apnea and neurodevelopmental outcomes, a randomized controlled trial. *Anesthesiology.* 2015;123(1):38–54.

32. Rappaport BA, Suresh S, Hertz S, et al. Anesthetic neurotoxicity--clinical implications of animal models. *N Engl J Med.* 2015;372(9):796–797.

33. Walker SM, Yaksh TL. Neuraxial analgesia in neonates and infants: a review of clinical and preclinical strategies for the development of safety and efficacy data. *Anesth Analg.* 2012;115(3):638–662.

34. Kachko L, Simhi E, Tzeitlin E, et al. Spinal anesthesia in neonates and infants—a single-center experience of 505 cases. *Paediatr Anaesth.* 2007;17(7):647–653.

35. Puncuh F, Lampugnani E, Kokki H. Use of spinal anaesthesia in paediatric patients: a single centre experience with 1132 cases. *Paediatr Anaesth.* 2004;14(7):564–567.

36. Arthurs OJ, Simhi E, Tzeitlin E, et al. Ultrasonographic determination of neonatal spinal canal depth. *Arch Dis Child Fetal Neonatal Ed.* 2008;93(6):F451–F454.

37. Nomura JT, Leech SJ, Shenbagamurthi S, et al. A randomized controlled trial of ultrasound-assisted lumbar puncture. *J Ultrasound Med.* 2007;26(10):1341–1348.

38. Kokki H, Tuovinen K, Hendolin H. Spinal anaesthesia for paediatric day-case surgery: a double-blind, randomized, parallel group, prospective comparison of isobaric and hyperbaric bupivacaine. *Br J Anaesth.* 1998;81(4):502–506.

39. Suresh S, Hall SC. Spinal anesthesia in infants: is the impractical practical? *Anesth Analg.* 2006;102(1):65–66.

40. Llewellyn N, Moriarty A. The National Pediatric Epidural Audit. *Paediatr Anaesth.* 2007;17(6):520–533.

41. Aprodu GS, Munteanu V, Filciu G, Gotia DG, et al. [Caudal anesthesia in pediatric surgery]. *Rev Med Chir Soc Med Nat Iasi.* 2008;112(1):142–147.

42. Guldogus F, Baris YS, Baris S, et al. Comparing tissue coring potentials of hollow needles without stylet and caudal needles with stylet: an experimental study. *Eur J Anaesthesiol.* 2008;25(6):498–501.

43. Weinberg G, Ripper R, Feinstein DL, Hoffman W. Lipid emulsion infusion rescues dogs from bupivacaine-induced cardiac toxicity. *Reg Anesth Pain Med.* 2003;28(3):198–202.

44. Oulego-Erroz I, Mora-Matilla M, Alonso-Quintela P, et al. Ultrasound evaluation of lumbar spine anatomy in newborn infants: implications for optimal performance of lumbar puncture. *J Pediatr.* 2014;165(4): 862–865.

56.

PERIPHERAL NERVE BLOCKADE IN THE PEDIATRIC PATIENT

Joel Stockman and Lisa Lee

STEM CASE AND KEY QUESTIONS

An 8-year-old, 25-kg boy presents to the hospital emergency department (ED) after suffering an ankle fracture while skateboarding with his older brother. The boy's medical history is significant for a history of T-cell acute lympho-blastic leukemia. His disease is currently in remission fol-lowing extensive treatment including chemotherapy. He has undergone multiple anesthetics including port placement (and subsequent removal) as well as numerous lumbar punc-ture procedures with methotrexate administration. He is cur-rently in remission following 2 years of maintenance therapy. Approximately 2 months prior to this admission, the patient was found to have a platelet count in the $50s \times 10^9/L$. Further workup resulted in an isolated finding of thrombocytopenia, which was diagnosed as immune thrombocytopenic purpura. He has been undergoing treatment with oral prednisolone with improvement. His bloodwork during this admission is significant for a platelet count of $59 \times 10^9/L$. His radiographic studies show a displaced, unstable fibula fracture (Fig. 56.1).

The orthopedic surgeon places the patient in a splint in the ED but would like to proceed with an open reduction and internal fixation of the distal fibula. The patient's parents are concerned about recovery, as the boy has experienced intol-erance (e.g., nausea and vomiting) to multiple opioids in the past, and his parents request an opioid-free anesthetic, if pos-sible. Furthermore, the patient has had a delayed emergence in the past during general anesthesia. The patient has not had solid food or liquids in over 8 hours.

> WHAT ARE POTENTIAL CONSIDERATIONS
> FOR UNDERGOING ANESTHESIA IN THIS
> PATIENT? WHAT ARE THE BENEFITS
> OVER GENERAL ANESTHESIA WITH OPIOIDS?
> IS THE PATIENT'S PLATELET COUNT
> AN ABSOLUTE CONTRAINDICATION
> TO UNDERGOING A REGIONAL PROCEDURE?
> WHAT ARE OTHER CONTRAINDICATIONS
> TO DOING REGIONAL ANESTHESIA? IS
> THE BLOCK/CATHETER PLACEMENT SAFE
> TO PERFORM UNDER GENERAL ANESTHESIA?

The anesthesiologist reviews the options with the patient and family. They have significant concerns about postoperative management, specifically pain control. The orthopedic team, in discussion with the anesthesiologist and family, would like regional anesthesia. The surgeon will utilize a calf tourniquet during surgery. The plan includes premedication with intra-venous (IV) midazolam, followed by anesthesia induction with propofol. A laryngeal mask airway is placed to secure the airway for surgery and to provide general anesthesia with sevoflurane. Limited narcotics may be used to account for tourniquet pain. Positioning for the case will be supine.

> WHAT ARE THE KEY LANDMARKS IN THE
> POPLITEAL FOSSA ANATOMY? DISCUSS
> THE GENERAL PRINCIPLES OF ULTRASOUND
> AND NERVE STIMULATION FOR BLOCK
> ADMINISTRATION. WHAT LOCAL ANESTHETIC
> WILL YOU USE FOR THE PROCEDURE? WHAT
> ABOUT FOR INFUSION THROUGH THE
> CATHETER AFTER THE PROCEDURE? WILL
> YOU ADD ANY ADJUNCTS TO THE LOCAL
> ANESTHETIC? HOW WILL YOU GAUGE BLOCK
> EFFECTIVENESS? WHAT ARE YOUR CONCERNS
> REGARDING LOCAL ANESTHETIC TOXICITY?
> WHAT CAN YOU DO TO ACCOMMODATE
> A SURGEON THAT WISHES TO CHECK
> NEUROLOGIC FUNCTION IMMEDIATELY
> AFTER SURGERY?

All American Society of Anesthesiologists monitors were previously applied prior to induction. The anesthesiologist performs a timeout with all staff present. The patient's left leg is elevated with a stack of blankets. The posterior left lower extremity is cleaned with chlorhexidine gluconate from mid-thigh to posterior knee. Under ultrasound guidance, a catheter is placed near the sciatic nerve in the posterior mid-thigh location. Ropivacaine (0.25%) is injected incremen-tally (10 mL) through the catheter with frequent aspiration. Ultrasonography allows for monitoring the influx of local an-esthetic through the catheter and observation of the spread around the nerve sheath in real time. The catheter is secured with 2-octylcyanoacrylate glue (at the needle puncture site) and covered with clear, occlusive tape. An elastomeric pump containing 0.2% ropivacaine is attached to the catheter (with a fixed flow rate of 4 mL/hour), allowing continuous adminis-tration of local anesthetic.

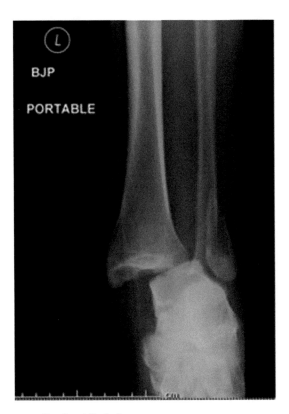

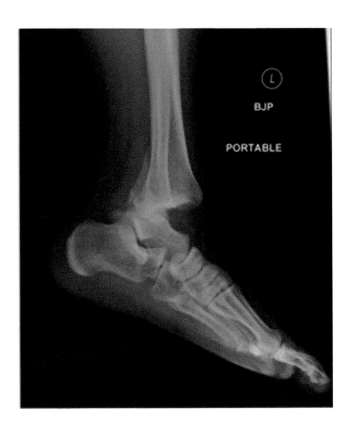

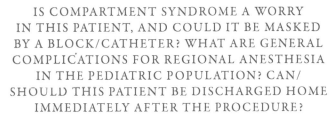

Fig. 56.1 Displaced fibula fracture.

IS COMPARTMENT SYNDROME A WORRY
IN THIS PATIENT, AND COULD IT BE MASKED
BY A BLOCK/CATHETER? WHAT ARE GENERAL
COMPLICATIONS FOR REGIONAL ANESTHESIA
IN THE PEDIATRIC POPULATION? CAN/
SHOULD THIS PATIENT BE DISCHARGED HOME
IMMEDIATELY AFTER THE PROCEDURE?

The patient is observed in the hospital overnight. The family is educated on the maintenance of the pain pump with further instructions regarding removal after 3 to 4 postoperative days. The acute pain service will follow up with the patient and family on a daily basis until the catheter is removed. The patient continues scheduled oral acetaminophen and is provided with a prescription for an opioid medication, if necessary, for breakthrough pain.

DISCUSSION

It is not uncommon for patients to experience an intolerance to opioid medications. Opioid medications, in normal doses, may cause respiratory depression, itching, nausea and vomiting, constipation, urinary retention, and confusion. However, orthopedic surgical procedures will often require pain relief with opioid medications during and, for at least a short period, following surgery. Regional anesthesia involving a local anesthetic is an alternative analgesic method, which can significantly reduce pain during the perioperative period. It can be combined with general anesthesia to potentially use less anesthetic and allow for a faster recovery. Regional

anesthesia, in the form of a perineural catheter, can substantially decrease, if not eliminate, the need for opioids for this patient in the immediate days after surgery. Patients often generally report dissatisfaction with their pain control following surgery.[1] Regional anesthesia, as a component of multimodal therapy, improves postoperative analgesia leading to greater patient satisfaction.

In this case, opioid-free anesthesia would likely be limited to a peripheral or central block/catheter. Peripheral nerve interventions can provide similar analgesia to neuraxial interventions without the hemodynamic consequences (less sympathetic effect) and with fewer complications.[2–4] However, unlike the brachial plexus, a single perineural infusion may not cover all surgical sites. Therefore, regional interventions may not provide optimal analgesia without supplementation of additional analgesics. Continuous perineural infusions have shown other benefits over epidural analgesia. After knee arthroplasty, regional intervention showed a decreased time to achieve flexion goals, improved analgesia, and lower analgesic requirements.[5] After foot and ankle surgery, utilization of a continuous peripheral nerve catheter has been shown to decrease hospital costs and length of stay, although savings are often limited.[6] Decreased opioid use leads to lower incidence of opioid-related side effects including nausea, vomiting, sedation, and pruritus. Patients also demonstrate improved sleep and are generally more satisfied when receiving regional interventions as compared to general anesthesia with systemic analgesia.[7]

Both relative and absolute contraindications must be considered prior to any regional procedure. Contraindications include patient/parent refusal, site infection, amide local anesthetic allergy, pre-existing neuropathy, and coagulopathy. Few reports exist of significant complications associated with peripheral nerve blocks secondary to hemorrhage. Therefore, the associated risk after peripheral techniques remains undefined.[8] However, the coagulopathy risk is significantly higher when considering a neuraxial technique. Most practitioners would consider neuraxial procedures as long as the platelet count is maintained at greater than $75 \times 10^9/L$, assuming no other risk factors. A popliteal fossa sciatic block is characterized as a superficial perivascular block and thus constitutes a moderate risk for patients with coagulopathies.[9] This patient's thrombocytopenia, like other coagulopathies, is considered a relative contraindication. Coagulation guidelines provided by the American Society of Regional Anesthesia and Pain Medicine (ASRA) and other organizations are meant to help ascertain risk. One must determine the individual patient's risk and formulate a plan for that circumstance. The patient and his family should be given all the information they need to make an informed decision.

Pediatric patients often undergo an inhalational induction prior to surgical procedures. There are few contraindications to this practice, and it allows for a painless anesthetic. A premedication, such as oral midazolam, may be administered at the discretion of the anesthesia provider. Furthermore, given this patient's young age, a nerve block or catheter would likely require deep sedation or even general anesthesia for completion. In the pediatric patient, general anesthesia is the accepted practice for placement of regional and neuraxial blocks, as supported by both the European Society of Regional Anaesthesia and Pain Therapy (ESRA) and the ASRA.[10] The idea is that such a procedure is safer when performed on an immobile target rather than one that may be distressed. Their guidelines are based primarily on a few large-scale, multicenter studies: (i) 1996 French-Language Society of Paediatric Anaesthesiologists (ADARPEF) study involving 24,409 anesthetics utilizing regional techniques (38% of these were regional blocks). The complication rate of regional anesthesia was 0.9 per 1,000, and all complications were deemed minor. All complications occurred after central blocks.[11] (ii) 2007 UK Prospective National Pediatric Epidural Audit involving 10,633 epidurals, with the vast majority placed under general anesthesia. Overall, there were 96 reported incidents, with 5 noted to be serious (1 per 2,000) and 9 noted to be major (1 per 1,100). One child had persistent symptoms (paresthesia) that lasted beyond the 12-month follow-up period. Four patients developed compartment syndrome, but the presence of an epidural did not appear to mask the condition.[12] (iii) 2010 ADARPEF study involving 29,870 anesthetics utilizing regional techniques (66% of these were regional blocks). Complications occurred in 40 patients with an overall incidence of 1.2 per 1,000 and were significantly higher for central (6 times) than for peripheral blocks.[13] (iv) 2014 Pediatric Regional Anesthesia Network study involving 56,564 children. Neurological complications occurred at a rate of 0.93 per 1,000 in children who underwent procedures under general anesthesia versus 6.82 per 1,000 in sedated and awake patients. One

incident of postoperative neurological symptoms was noted and lasted over 6 months.[14]

The sciatic nerve, at the level of the popliteal fossa, is bounded by the biceps femoris laterally, the semimembranosus and semitendinosus muscles superiorly, and the popliteal artery and vein inferiorly (Fig. 56.2). The sciatic nerve splits into the tibial nerve and common peroneal nerve several centimeters above the popliteal crease. The distance varies depending on the age of the patient. The block should be performed at or above the level of the bifurcation for adequate surgical anesthesia and analgesia. It is important to note that the popliteal block does not provide full analgesic coverage to the entire lower extremity below the knee. An adductor canal block would need to be performed in order to anesthetize the saphenous nerve that supplies the medial aspect of the lower leg and ankle.

The use of ultrasound in regional anesthesia began in the late 1980s and early 1990s.[15,16] Ultrasound technology has greatly improved since then. The use of the ultrasound can be helpful in localizing the target nerve, visualizing spread of local anesthetic around the nerves, and detecting intraneural or intravascular injection. The most recent ASRA assessment of literature in the pediatric population[17] suggests that the use of ultrasound in peripheral nerve blockade results in faster block onset, higher rate of success when compared to nerve stimulation alone, and lower volumes of local anesthetic. However, it also found that analgesia consumption was not different in patients who had peripheral nerve blocks done with nerve stimulation alone when compared to ultrasound alone. Nerve stimulation can be used in conjunction with ultrasound guidance. The person performing the block should be careful to observe for nerve swelling during injection, as no intraneural stimulation at 0.2 mA does not preclude intraneural needle placement.[18] If the block is performed under general anesthesia, the use of a long-acting muscle relaxant will also preclude the use of nerve stimulation.

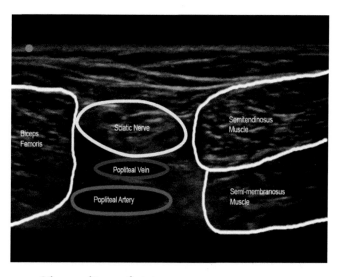

Fig. 56.2 Ultrasound image of sciatic nerve.

For the sciatic nerve block at the level of the popliteal fossa, patient positioning would depend on whether the block will be performed with the patient under general anesthesia or if the patient is able to tolerate having the block done under mild sedation. Generally, the performance of the block under general anesthesia would restrict positioning to the supine position. The operative leg should be raised with the knee bent at 90 degrees and a stack of towels or blankets supporting the foot and ankle for ease of access. The block can also be performed in the lateral or prone position if the block can be done awake. This position is technically easier for beginners, but the patient's ability to do this may be limited by pain or orthopedic hardware, such as an external fixator device.

Depending on the size of the patient, a 13-6 MHz, 6-cm probe or 10-5 MHz, 9-cm probe should be used for an optimal view of the sciatic nerve. Traditionally, the nerve is targeted above the level of the bifurcation of the sciatic nerve into the tibial and common peroneal nerve. Placement of the probe depends on the size and age of the patient. Based on a linear regression model of the magnetic resonance imaging studies of 59 patients,[19] the bifurcation of the sciatic nerve occurs around 27+4 (age, in years) mm above the popliteal crease.

Various kits are available commercially for perineural catheter insertion. A catheter with or without an electrically conductive connection to its tip can be placed by using the needle as a conduit for the catheter, or the block can be performed with the catheter over the needle (similar to IV insertion). Care should be taken to maintain aseptic technique during the performance of the block since the catheter will be an indwelling foreign body. There have been case reports of serious infectious complications of peripheral nerve blocks in immunocompromised patients.[20] The catheter can be tunneled beneath the skin to decrease the risk of accidental dislodgement and then secured with a transparent bio-occlusive dressing. Careful consideration should be taken in securing the catheter to avoid areas to be included in the sterile field during surgery and to avoid securing the catheter hub in a location where the patient will be likely to lie on top of it during the surgery or during sleep afterwards. The catheter should be clearly labeled as a peripheral nerve catheter.

Any local anesthetic can be used depending on the goals of onset and duration of the blockade needed. The characteristics of each individual local anesthetic are determined by its concentration, hydrophobicity, and degree of ionization. Generally speaking, local anesthetics with a faster onset also have a shorter duration of action while longer-acting local anesthetics have a longer duration of action (Table 56.1).

A local anesthetic with a faster onset of action may be preferred in a situation where the block is the primary surgical anesthetic, and it is less of a concern when general anesthesia will be used. 0.25% bupivacaine or 0.2% ropivacaine at a dose of 0.2 to 0.3 mL/kg for larger nerves and 0.1 to 0.2 mL/kg for sensory nerves are most commonly used for single-shot peripheral nerve blocks for the lower extremity.[21] Care should be taken to not to exceed the maximum local anesthetic dose (Table 56.2).

The toxicity profile of the local anesthetic should also be considered in the selection of an appropriate agent. Bupivacaine and ropivacaine bind more avidly to cardiac conduction channels than other lower potency local anesthetics, such as lidocaine, so cardiac toxicity symptoms are more likely with more potent local anesthetics.[22] Thus, with lidocaine, it is more common to observe central nervous system (CNS) toxicity symptoms before cardiotoxic symptoms when compared to bupivacaine. While levobupivacaine and ropivacaine are marketed as being less cardiotoxic than bupivacaine, it should be stressed that, despite the introduction of these two less cardiotoxic drugs in the late 1980s, cardiotoxicity continues to be a problem.[23] Any local anesthetic, when given at a high enough concentration or dose, has the potential to produce local anesthetic toxicity. Local anesthetic toxicity is discussed further in a later section.

For the purposes of postoperative pain relief, lower concentrations of longer-acting local anesthetics, such as 0.25% bupivacaine and 0.2% ropivacaine, would be a good choice for the patient in this case. However, a selection of

Table 56.1 **PROPERTIES OF LOCAL ANESTHETICS**

LOCAL ANESTHETIC	ONSET (MIN)	DURATION OF ANESTHESIA (HR)	DURATION OF ANALGESIA (HR)
3% 2-Chloroprocaine (with bicarbonate)	10–15	1	2
3% 2-Chloroprocaine (with bicarbonate + epinephrine)	10–15	1.5–2	2–3
2% Lidocaine (with bicarbonate + epinephrine)	10–20	2–5	3–8
0.5% Ropivacaine	15–30	4–8	5–12
0.5% Bupivacaine (with epinephrine)	15–30	5–15	6–30

Adapted from NYSORA website (http://www.nysora.com/regional-anesthesia/foundations-of-ra/3492-local-anesthetics-clinical-pharmacology-and-rational-selection.html).

Table 56.2 MAXIMUM DOSES FOR COMMONLY USED LOCAL ANESTHETICS

LOCAL ANESTHETIC	DOSE LIMIT (MG/KG)
Lidocaine without epinephrine	4
Lidocaine with epinephrine	7
Bupivacaine with/without epinephrine	2.5
Ropivacaine with/without epinephrine	3
2-Chloroprocaine	10

local anesthetics could be used, depending on goals for duration of block (Table 56.3).

If an amide type local anesthetic is chosen, the dose should be decreased by 50% in infants under the age of 6 months because they have limited liver enzymatic activity, decreased protein binding, and immature drug clearance.[24] If the infusion will continue for greater than 3 days, the rate should be reduced by an additional 30% after 48 hours. Because 2-chloroprocaine is an ester-type local anesthetic that is hydrolyzed by plasma cholinesterase, a decrease in dose for patients below the age of 6 months is not necessary.

Epinephrine has been commonly added to local anesthetic in order to increase the duration of the block. The proposed mechanism of action is that epinephrine acts as a vasoconstrictor to limit systemic absorption of the local anesthetic away from the injection site. Ropivacaine has some intrinsic vasoconstrictive properties that allow for a greater duration of blockade compared to other local anesthetics, which have vasodilatory properties or no effect, such as lidocaine and bupivacaine.[25] Therefore, the addition of epinephrine to ropivacaine may be of limited benefit. Epinephrine may be added for other reasons, including detecting intravascular injection.

The use of other adjuncts have been more controversial. There have been studies demonstrating that the use of dexamethasone with local anesthetic prolongs both motor and sensory block without any adverse effect.[26] However, other studies have demonstrated equivalence between perineural

Table 56.3 COMMON CONTINUOUS LOCAL ANESTHETIC INFUSION RATES

LOCAL ANESTHETIC (CONCENTRATION)	<6 MONTHS (MG/ KG/HR)	>6 MONTHS (MG/KG/HR)
Lidocaine (0.1%)	0.8	1.6
Bupivacaine (0.1%)	0.2	0.4
Ropivacaine (0.1%)	0.3	0.5
2-Chloroprocaine (1%)	10	10

Adapted from Berde CB. Convulsions associated with pediatric regional anesthesia. *Anesth Analg.* 1992;75164.

and IV administration,[27,28] suggesting that the increase in sensory block time may be a systemic effect.

A recent systematic qualitative review found that perineural buprenorphine, clonidine, dexamethasone, dexmedetomidine, and magnesium most consistently demonstrated prolongation of peripheral nerve blocks.[29] However, there have been animal studies demonstrating that clonidine, buprenorphine, dexamethasone, and midazolam can increase local anesthetic neurotoxicity when used with ropivacaine.[30] Additionally, currently none of these drugs has Food and Drug Administration approval for use as a perineural adjuvant, and further studies need to be conducted.

The ability to gauge block effectiveness will be determined by whether or not the block is performed while the patient is awake but sedated or under general anesthesia. If the block can be performed while the patient is awake and able to respond, sensory changes over the intended surgical site can be tested using ice or an alcohol swab. If general anesthesia is induced, the hemodynamic response of the patient to surgical stimuli would be assessed, and the appropriate analgesics should be given.

In order to avoid local anesthetic toxicity, steps need to be taken to reduce the risk and be vigilant for possible signs and symptoms of toxicity. Measures to decrease the risk of local anesthetic toxicity include using the lowest local anesthetic dose necessary. The use of ultrasound guidance may help achieve this goal. Aspiration should be performed prior to each injection, and the injection should be done incrementally (0.1–0.2 mL/kg) while observing for signs and symptoms of local anesthetic toxicity. The addition of 5 mcg/mL of epinephrine as a means to detect intravascular injection may also be helpful. According to the 2015 ESRA/ASRA Practice Advisory,[10] the use of a test dose is discretionary with a B3 to B4 level of evidence. It should be kept in mind that a negative test dose does not necessarily rule out an intravascular needle or catheter. Careful observation for electrocardiogram (EKG) changes (T wave changes), increases in heart rate above 10 beats per minute, and systolic blood pressure of greater than 10% above baseline should be done. Central nervous system toxicity and cardiac toxicity can be delayed for up to 30 minutes,[22] and local anesthetic toxicity should be considered in any patient with altered mental status, neurological symptoms, and/or hemodynamic instability after the administration of a local anesthetic.

Early symptoms of CNS toxicity include excitation, confusion, twitching, or seizures. The later signs of CNS toxicity are depressive in nature and can include drowsiness, obtundation, and coma. Nonspecific signs include reports of a metallic taste, perioral numbness, tinnitus, light-headedness, and diplopia. Depending on the dose, type of local anesthetic, or if the block was performed under general anesthesia, cardiovascular instability may be the only sign of local anesthetic toxicity. Initially, the cardiovascular response may be hyperdynamic with hypertension and tachycardia. Later, there may be progressive hypotension, conduction block, bradycardia, asystole, or other ventricular arrhythmias.[31]

Should signs of toxicity occur, 20% intralipid should be administered at a dose of 1.5 mL/kg followed by 0.25 mL/kg/

min infusion to be continued for at least 10 minutes after cardiac stability is achieved. A second bolus of 1.5 mL/kg may be repeated 1 to 2 times for persistent asystole. It is important to note that propofol is not a substitute for 20% intralipid. While Pediatric Advanced Life Support should be provided to support the patient, it is important to note that epinephrine can reduce lipid efficacy. Smaller doses of epinephrine (<1 mcg/kg) should be used for treating hypotension.

Depending on motor nerve involvement, long-duration local anesthetic administration will inhibit motor function for an extended time. Therefore, testing motor function after surgical intervention may not be possible. An alternative approach involves placing a nerve catheter under ultrasound and/or nerve stimulator guidance and administering local anesthetic only after the surgeon has evaluated the patient's motor function.[32]

Compartment syndrome occurs when a fascial compartment cannot adequately expand to accommodate a fluid load. The compartment subsequently is deprived of blood flow, leading to tissue anoxia. Unrecognized compartment syndrome can lead to neuronal cell death. Acute compartment syndrome could happen after any severe injury that compromises tissue perfusion. Common orthopedic causes include tibial and forearm fractures.[33] Compartment syndrome has rarely occurred after isolated ankle fracture.[34] The threshold for fascietomy is 30 mmHg in the adult literature.[35] However, this may not be accurate for small children, as they tend to have higher baseline compartment pressures than adults.[36] Symptoms of acute compartment syndrome include (i) severe pain out of proportion to the perceived injury, (ii) a burning sensation, and (iii) numbness and/or tingling (late sign). Diagnosis and treatment in infants and toddlers can be very difficult due to the variability of presentation and an inability to communicate.[37]

Dense nerve blocks are thought to mask the signs of acute compartment syndrome. However, there does not seem to be evidence to support this claim.[38] Furthermore, peripheral nerve catheters offer the benefit of sufficient pain control with titratable concentrations and volumes of local anesthetic. Breakthrough pain in a patient with a previously functional block warrants further investigation for acute compartment syndrome. Regardless of the type of analgesia, patients at risk deserve close observation. Ongoing assessment and timely measurement of compartment pressures are necessary for early diagnosis.[39]

A recent meta-analysis conducted by Walker et al.[40] in 2015 reinforced the safety associated with pediatric regional anesthesia. The overall complication rate was 12.1%, and the rate of serious complications was 0.04%. Catheter malfunctions (e.g., dislodgement and occlusion) and block failure were the most common complications. Site infection was uncommon and could be minimized by limiting catheter placement to 72 hours. Overall, these findings were similar to adult complication data.

Continuous peripheral nerve blocks deliver prolonged analgesia and offer an alternative to opioid-based pain therapy for procedures with all projected pain types—mild to severe.

When appropriate, patients can typically be discharged home on the day of surgery. Appropriate patient selection is vital, as not all patients will be capable of accepting the responsibility of the added catheter/pump system. Patients at risk for compartment syndrome require thorough education including return instructions, so that they may be evaluated in a timely manner if the need arises. This patient's health condition warrants a complete discussion with the surgery team regarding the need for overnight observation. Once the patient is discharged, he or she will need frequent follow-up by phone with an established regional anesthesia provider. This provider must be equipped to troubleshoot any catheter-related issues that may arise.

REVIEW QUESTIONS

1. Of the following doses of local anesthetic, which is the **LEAST** appropriate for use in the pediatric patient?

A. bupivacaine 0.25%—6 mL in a 5-month-old (6 kg)
B. bupivacaine 0.5%—10 mL in a 6-year-old (20 kg)
C. lidocaine 1%—7.5 mL in a 4-year-old (15 kg)
D. ropivacaine 0.2%—18 mL in a 3-year-old (13 kg)

Answer: A

2. Which of the following risks is the **LEAST** likely to be an advantage of peripheral nerve blocks over neuraxial anesthesia?

A. apnea in former preterm infants
B. local anesthetic toxicity
C. urinary retention in supine boy
D. weakness of treated extremities.

Answer: C

3. A 3-year-old presents for clubfoot repair. Peripheral nerve blocks are requested for postoperative pain relief. Which one of the following block(s) would provide the **MOST** complete analgesia?

A. ankle block
B. femoral nerve block and sural nerve block
C. popliteal block and femoral nerve block
D. sciatic nerve block (classic posterior)

Answer: C

4. Which of the following nerves would **LEAST** likely not be affected in a popliteal block of the sciatic nerve?

A. deep peroneal
B. posterior tibial
C. saphenous
D. sural

Answer: C

5. Five minutes after a popliteal block has been performed under general anesthesia, the 9-year-old patient becomes increasingly hypotensive. On the EKG monitor, the patient has developed a ventricular arrhythmia. You suspect local anesthetic toxicity. Which of the following is the **BEST** medication to give during resuscitation?

A. epinephrine 10 mcg/kg
B. intralipid (20%) 1.5 mL/kg
C. propofol 2 mg/kg
D. vasopressin 0.4 units/kg

Answer: B

6. Signs and symptoms **LEAST** consistent with a diagnosis of acute compartment syndrome are

A. burning sensation.
B. compartment pressure of 3 mmHg.
C. pain out of proportion to the injury.
D. paresthesias/pulselessness/pallor.

Answer: B

7. Which of the following is the **MOST** commonly used adjunct in a single -shot peripheral nerve block?

A. dexmedetomidine 20 mcg
B. epinephrine 1:200,000
C. magnesium sulfate 10%
D. neostigmine 0.5 mg

Answer: B

QUESTIONS AND ANSWERS

This chapter has accompanying questions and answers which are available to subscribers as part of the Oxford eLearning platform. To access the questions, go to ✅ http:// oxfordmedicine. com/pediatricanesthesiaPBL

REFERENCES

1. Gan TJ, Habib AS, Miller TE, White W, Apfelbaum JL. Incidence, patient satisfaction, and perceptions of post-surgical pain: results from a US national survey. *Curr Med Res Opin.* 2014 Jan;30(1):149–160.
2. Yeung JH, Gates S, Naidu BV, Wilson MJ, Gao Smith F. Paravertebral block versus thoracic epidural for patients undergoing thoracotomy. *Cochrane Database Syst Rev.* 2016 Feb 21;2:CD009121.
3. Fowler SJ, Symons J, Sabato S, Myles PS. Epidural analgesia compared with peripheral nerve blockade after major knee surgery: a systematic review and meta-analysis of randomized trials. *Br J Anaesth.* 2008 Feb;100(2):154–164.
4. Patel N, Solovyova O, Matthews G, Arumugam S, Sinha SK, Lewis CG. Safety and efficacy of continuous femoral nerve catheter with single shot sciatic nerve block vs epidural catheter anesthesia for same-day bilateral total knee arthroplasty. *J Arthroplasty.* 2015 Feb;30(2):330–334.
5. Sakai N, Inoue T, Kunugiza Y, Tomita T, Mashimo T. Continuous femoral versus epidural block for attainment of 120° knee flexion after total knee arthroplasty: a randomized controlled trial. *J Arthroplasty.* 2013 May;28(5):807–814.
6. Williams BA. For outpatients, does regional anesthesia truly shorten the hospital stay, and how should we define postanesthesia care unit bypass eligibility? *Anesthesiology.* 2004;101:3–6.
7. Young MJ, Gorlin AW, Modest VE, Quraishi SA. Clinical implications of the transversus abdominis plane block in adults. *Anesthesiol Res Pract.* 2012;2012:1–11.
8. Horlocker TT, Wedel DJ, Rowlingson JC, et al. Regional anesthesia in the patient receiving antithrombotic or thrombolytic therapy: American Society of Regional Anesthesia and Pain Medicine

evidence-based guidelines (3rd ed). *Reg Anesth Pain Med.* 2010 Jan-Feb;35(1):64–101.
9. Harrop-Griffiths W, Cook T, Gill H, et al. Regional anaesthesia and patients with abnormalities of coagulation. *Anaesthesia.* 2013;68:966–972.
10. Ivani G, Suresh S, Ecoffey C, et al. The European Society of Regional Anaesthesia and Pain Therapy and the American Society of Regional Anesthesia and Pain Medicine Joint Committee Practice Advisory on Controversial Topics in Pediatric Regional Anesthesia. *Reg Anesth Pain Med.* 2015 Sep-Oct;40(5):526–532.
11. Giaufre E, Dalens B, Gombert A. Epidemiology and morbidity of regional anestheisa in children: a one-year prospective survey of the French-Language Society of Pediatric Anesthesiologists. *Anesth Analg.* 1996 Nov;83(5):904–912
12. Llewellyn N, Moriarty A. The National Pediatric Epidural Audit. *Paediatr Anaesth.* 2007 Jun;17(6):520–533.
13. Ecoffey C, Lacroix F, Giaufre E, Orliaguet G, Courreges P. Epidemiology and morbidity of regional anesthesia in children: a follow-up one-year prospective survey of the French-Language Society of Paediatric Anaesthesiologists (ADARPEF). *Paediatr Anaesth.* 2010 Dec;20(12):1061–1069.
14. Taenzer AH, Walker BJ, Bosenberg AT, et al. Asleep versus awake: does it matter? Pediatric regional block complications by patient state: a report from the Pediatric Regional Anesthesia Network. *Reg Anesth Pain Med.* 2014 Jul-Aug;39(4):279–283.
15. Ting PL, Sivagnanaratnam V. Ultrasonographic study of the spread of local anaesthetic during axillary brachial plexus block. *Br J Anaesth.* 1989 Sep;63(3):326–329.
16. Kapral S, Krafft P, Eibenberger K, Fitzgerald R, Gosch M, Weinstabl C. Ultrasound-guided supraclavicular approach for regional anesthesia of the brachial plexus. *Anesth Analg.* 1994 Mar;78(3):507–513.
17. Neal JM, Brull R, Horn JL, et al. The Second American Society of Regional Anesthesia and Pain Medicine Evidence-Based Medicine Assessment of Ultrasound-Guided Regional Anesthesia: executive summary. *Reg Anesth Pain Med.* 2016 Mar-Apr;41(2):181–194.
18. Robards C, Hadzic A, Somasundaram L, et al. Intraneural injection with low-current stimulation during popliteal sciatic nerve block. *Anesth Analg.* 2009 Aug;109(2):673–677.
19. Suresh S, Simion C, Wyers M, Swanson M, Jennings M, Iyer A. Anatomical location of the bifurcation of the sciatic nerve in the posterior thigh in infants and children: a formula derived from MRI imaging for nerve localization. *Reg Anesth Pain Med.* 2007 Jul-Aug;32(4):351–353.
20. Horlocker TT, Wedel DJ. Regional anesthesia in the immunocompromised patient. *Reg Anesth Pain Med.* 2006 Jul-Aug;31(4):334–345.
21. Suresh S, Sawardekar A, Shah R. Ultrasound for regional anesthesia in children. *Anesthesiol Clin.* 2014 Mar;32(1):263–279.
22. Neal JM, Bernards CM, Butterworth JF 4th, et al. ASRA practice advisory on local anesthetic systemic toxicity. *Reg Anesth Pain Med.* 2010 Mar-Apr;35(2):152–161.
23. Mulroy MF, Hejtmanek MR. Prevention of local anesthetic systemic toxicity. *Reg Anesth Pain Med.* 2010 Mar-Apr;35(2):177–180.
24. Berde CB. Convulsions associated with pediatric regional anesthesia. *Anesth Analg.* 1992 Aug;75(2):164–166.
25. McCartney CJ, Patel S. Local anesthetic volume for peripheral nerve blocks: how low can (or should) we go? *Reg Anesth Pain Med.* 2012 May-Jun;37(3):239–241.
26. Choi S, Rodseth R, McCartney CJ. Effects of dexamethasone as a local anaesthetic adjuvant for brachial plexus block: a systematic review and meta-analysis of randomized trials. *Br J Anaesth.* 2014 Mar;112(3):427–439.
27. Desmet M, Braems H, Reynvoet M, et al. IV and perineural dexamethasone are equivalent in increasing the analgesic duration of a single-shot interscalene block with ropivacaine for shoulder surgery: a prospective, randomized, placebo-controlled study. *Br J Anaesth.* 2013 Sep;111(3):445–452.
28. Hong JY, Han SW, Kim WO, Kim EJ, Kil HK. Effect of dexamethasone in combination with caudal analgesia on postoperative

pain control in day-case paediatric orchiopexy. *Br J Anaesth*. 2010 Oct;105(4):506–510.

29. Kirksey MA, Haskins SC, Cheng J, Liu SS. Local anesthetic peripheral nerve block adjuvants for prolongation of analgesia: a systematic qualitative review. *PLoS One*. 2015 Sep 10;10(9):e0137312.

30. Williams BA, Hough KA, Tsui BY, Ibinson JW, Gold MS, Gebhart GF. Neurotoxicity of adjuvants used in perineural anesthesia and analgesia in comparison with ropivacaine. *Reg Anesth Pain Med*. 2011 May-Jun;36(3):225–230.

31. Neal JM, Bernards CM, Butterworth JF 4th, et al. ASRA practice advisory on local anesthetic systemic toxicity. *Reg Anesth Pain Med*. 2010 Mar-Apr;35(2):152–161.

32. Suresh S, Sarwark J, Bhalla T, Janicki J. Performing US-guided nerve blocks in the postanesthesia care unit (PACU) for upper extremity fractures: is this feasible in children? *Pediatr Anesth*. 2009 Dec;19(12):1238–1240.

33. McQueen MM, Gaston P, Court-Brown CM. Acute compartment syndrome. Who is at risk? *J Bone Joint Surg*. 2000 Mar;82(2):200–203.

34. Joseph J, Giannoudis PV, Hinsche A, Cohen A, Matthews SJ, Smith RM. Compartment syndrome following isolated ankle fracture. *Int Orthop*. 2000 Jul;24(3):173–175.

35. McQueen MM, Court-Brown CM. Compartment monitoring in tibial fractures: the pressure threshold for decompression. *J Bone Joint Surg*. 1996;78-B:99–104.

36. Staudt JM, Smeulders MJ, van der Horst CM. Normal compartment pressures of the lower leg in children. *J Bone Joint Surg*. 2008;90:215–219.

37. Broom A, Schur MD, Arkader A, Flynn J, Gornitzky A, Choi PD. Compartment syndrome in infants and toddlers. *J Child Orthop*. 2016;10(5):453–460.

38. Walker BJ, Noonan KJ, Bosenberg AT. Evolving compartment syndrome not masked by a continuous peripheral nerve block: evidence-based case management. *Reg Anesth Pain Med*. 2012 Jul-Aug;37(4):393–397.

39. Mar GJ, Barrington MJ, McGuirk BR. Acute compartment syndrome of the lower limb and the effect of postoperative analgesia on diagnosis. *Br J Anaesth*. 2009;102:3–11.

40. Walker BJ, Long JB, De Oliveira GS, et al. Peripheral nerve catheters in children: an analysis of safety and practice patterns from the Pediatric Regional Anesthesia Network (PRAN). *Br J Anaesth*. 2015 Sep;115(3):457–462.

SECTION 11

MISCELLANEOUS

57.

PSYCHOLOGICAL PREPARATION OF THE PEDIATRIC PATIENT FOR SURGERY

Haleh Saadat and Zeev N. Kain

STEM CASE AND KEY QUESTIONS

An otherwise healthy 4-year-old boy is booked for outpatient tonsillectomy. The child has no other medical problems but had right inguinal hernia repair at age 3. The child is hiding behind his mother and does not make any eye contact. Both parents are extremely anxious.

WHAT IS THE BEST WAY TO IDENTIFY PREOPERATIVE ANXIETY?

Studies based on Piaget's model show that 2- to 6-year-olds are at the highest risk for the development of extreme anxiety. Factors such as situational anxiety of the mother, child's age and temperament, and the quality of previous medical experiences predict a child's preoperative anxiety. Children who are timid and lack adoptive abilities with behavioral inhibition are significantly more likely to develop anxiety disorders than children with other temperaments. During the preoperative visit one must pay attention to both the verbal and nonverbal communication of the child (eye contact, playfulness, timidity, etc.), assess parents' anxiety, and inquire about past experiences. Items associated with preoperative anxiety can be divided into two categories.

1. Issues that are beyond the anesthesiologist's control:

   Whether the mother practices a religion
   How many times the child has been to the hospital
   Whether the previous admission was pleasant/unpleasant
   Whether any of child's family members/friends have been hospitalized
   Whether the child visited them in the hospital
   Whether the child attended the preadmission tour/clinic
   How long child has known about this procedure
   The mother's prediction of the child's anxiety
2. Controllable issues:

   Waiting period prior to surgery
   Number of people in induction room (large numbers of people with masks overwhelm the child)
   Efforts to build a rapport with the child

HOW DOES A PAST MEDICAL EXPERIENCE AFFECT ANXIETY?

Children with a history of previous stressful medical encounters are likely to be more anxious and require more intense preparation. In contrast, a child with a history of "good experiences" during medical encounters is likely to be less anxious.[7-9] A child who has previously undergone surgery or has been hospitalized may develop an exaggerated emotional response to an information-based preparation program.

This child had a previous surgery during which he had a traumatic experience at the induction of anesthesia. He also has a 5-year-old sister who had a similar distressing experience during her tonsillectomy (rough induction and untreated postoperative pain). According to the mother, the sister suffered from night terrors and bedwetting for almost a month postoperative. The parents are extremely anxious about repeating the experience.

DOES THE PARENTS' ANXIETY AFFECT THE OUTCOME?

Yes, parental anxiety needs to be addressed since it can affect the child's attitude toward the process and the development of postoperative maladaptive behaviors.

Following admission to the hospital, the child and his parents wait in the holding area for about an hour, during which the mother becomes more agitated and the child feels steadily more uncomfortable as he recalls the experience of his previous surgery. He remembers the separation from his parents and mask induction, and he anticipates pain and overall loss of control.

DISCUSSION

THE IMPORTANCE OF IDENTIFYING PREOPERATIVE ANXIETY

Recognizing vulnerable children who are at higher risk for development of preoperative anxiety is the key to directing appropriate resources toward them. Factors such as child's age and temperament, mother's anxiety, and the quality of previous medical experiences predict the extent of a child's preoperative

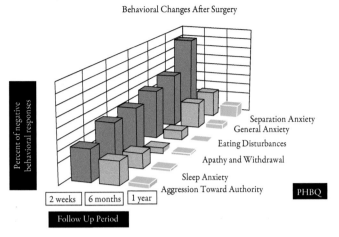

Behavioral Changes After Surgery

Fig. 57.1 Behavioral Changes after surgery. Source: Kain ZN, Wang SM, Mayes LC, Caramico LA, Hofstadter MB. Distress during the induction of anesthesia and postoperative behavioral outcomes. *Anesth Analg.* 1999;88(5):1042–1047.

anxiety. Moreover, it has been shown that preoperative distress in highly anxious children significantly increases the incidence of emergence delirium, sleep disturbances, nightmares, separation anxiety, eating problems, and postoperative pain and delays hospital discharge. Kain et al. (Figure 57.1) showed new negative behaviors in 67% of children on the first day after surgery, while close to 23% continued negative behaviors up to 2 weeks after surgery. These changes persisted for up to 1 year in 7.3% of children.[11] Preoperative fear has also been shown to be associated with a sympathetic discharge and increased serum cortisol, epinephrine, growth hormone, interleukin-6, and natural killer cell activity.

THE PSYCHOBIOLOGY OF SEPARATION ANXIETY

Studies demonstrate that preoperative preparation programs reduce parental anxiety and decrease preoperative anxiety in children.[12] However, the overwhelming majority of families in the United States receive no preparation for preoperative anxiety.

Experiencing separation in a novel situation such as a perioperative event can lead to confusion and create psychobiological stress. The intensity of separation anxiety decreases as a child's cognitive skills and memory expand. However, the increase in abilities does not immunize toddlers and preschoolers against the distress of separation. Children, who are sensitive to transitions, are more vulnerable to stress.[13] Parents have a crucial role in mediating a separation experience and parental anxiety. Therefore reducing parental anxiety decreases preoperative anxiety in children.[14–15] Most parents who participate in preoperative preparation programs display reduced anxiety on the day of surgery. Nevertheless, surveys show that the overwhelming majority of families in the United States receive no preoperative preparation. In summary factors such as parenting, genetics, personality types, and previous medical experiences evoke different adaptive responses in children.

CHILD'S AGE

Starting at 3 months of age, infants start to respond differently to familiar versus unfamiliar faces. And, as they grow up, they tend to smile and engage more with faces they recognize versus strangers.[16] Separation anxiety typically starts in 7- to 8-month-olds and intensifies around 12 months of age. Learning to cope with separation from a parent is essential for a child's development.[12] Piaget's model of childhood psychological development divides it into three periods:

1. Sensorimotor period (birth to 2 years)

2. Preoperational thought period (3–6 years)

3. Concrete operational period (7–12 years)

Piaget's model provides an accurate conceptual framework for the way children process new information and perceive pain, which is closely correlated with preoperative fears and anxiety.[17–19] Studies based on Piaget's model show that 2- to 6-year-olds are at the highest risk for the development of extreme anxiety. It has been shown that older children (>6 years old) who participate in the preparation program 5 to 7 days prior to the procedure are least anxious about separation from their parents, while they show more anxiety if they receive the preparation only 1 day prior to their procedure.[20]

CHILD'S TEMPERAMENT

Data from developmental research show significant individual differences in behavioral reactions to novel social events in infants and toddlers.[21,22] Some children are calm and do not display distress in unfamiliar situations. In contrast, children who are identified as vigilant and behaviorally inhibited stay close to their mothers, refuse to engage, and usually are inclined to show high anxiety in novel social situations.[23] Behavioral inhibition is associated with social wariness in the preschool years and reserved behaviors in adolescence.[24,25] Therefore, behavioral inhibition plays a critical role in social and emotional development. Children's temperament and coping styles are important factors in their response to a preparation program Scientific studies measure children's temperament on four factors of

1. Approach (approach vs. withdrawal from new people/situations).

2. Persistence (tendency to persevere with activities or tasks).

3. Rhythmicity (regularity of biological and behavioral functions).

4. Inflexibility (vs. adaptability).[26]

Children with behavioral inhibition are significantly more likely to develop anxiety disorders than children with other temperaments.[27,28] Obtaining information on a child's temperament helps the process of tailoring the program to the needs of the child. Children who are timid and lack adaptive abilities are at increased risk for perioperative anxiety.

ANXIETY AT PREVIOUS MEDICAL ENCOUNTERS

Children with a history of previous stressful medical encounters are likely to be more anxious and require more intense preparation. In contrast, a child with a history of "good experiences" during medical encounters is likely to be less anxious.[29] A child who has previously undergone surgery or has been hospitalized with pain may develop an exaggerated emotional response to an information-based preparation program.

COPING STYLE

Early studies of communication assumed that all individuals seek information. This assumption is rooted back to 330 BC based on Aristotle's statement that "all men, by nature, desire to know."[30] Yet some individuals *avoid* information to prevent psychological discomfort. Maslow states that "we can seek knowledge in order to reduce anxiety and we can also avoid knowing in order to reduce anxiety."[31] Individuals' sense of locus of control (the degree to which one's fate is governed externally vs. controlled by one's self) affects their perception of self-efficacy. Individuals with an external locus of control believe that searching for information is relatively pointless, since the outcomes in life are out of their control and determined only by external factors; therefore they tend to avoid seeking information in response to a threat.[32] Similarly, providing preoperative information to children and parents with different coping styles will have different effects on their anxiety. *Information-seekers* will require more detailed information as compare to *information-blunters*, as the latter group may exhibit increased anxiety if given too much information.[33]

TYPE OF SURGERY

Different types of surgery will result in different perioperative experiences, particularly in regards to the quality and intensity of postoperative pain. Studies show that negative past experiences such as the history of multiple surgical procedures, pain, hospitalization, and lack of pain relief from large doses of analgesics are likely to sensitize the child, while positive or neutral past experiences do not have a significant impact on subsequent reactions. This effect occurs independently of the coping style of the child (sensitizing vs. repression).[34]

PARENTS' CHARACTERISTICS

Parental perioperative anxiety is strongly related to a child's perioperative anxiety and thus we need to treat both children and parents. High parental anxiety is related to the development of postoperative maladaptive behavior changes in children.[6] Data suggest that parents with higher anxiety

do not respond to the traditional pamphlets and preparation programs, as they do not address how to deal with their anxiety.[10]

STRATEGIES TO ADDRESS CHILDREN'S PREOPERATIVE ANXIETY

BEHAVIORAL MODALITIES

Preoperative preparation programs have evolved significantly over recent decades. A variety of modalities (such as the orientation tours, information pamphlets, rehearsals with dolls, video presentations, child life, music therapy, acupuncture, hypnosis, etc.) have been used throughout past decades. Each modality has its merits, but a program is more effective if it is tailored specifically to the child's age, developmental stage, temperament, and past history of previous experiences. The development of coping skills followed by modeling, play therapy, operating room tour, and printed materials are considered the most effective preoperative preparation interventions.[35] Recently Kain et al. designed a fully animated web-based program that contained educational material, skill training, and interactive games for both children and parents. The program contained coping strategies to manage perioperative anxiety and pain in children and provided a variety of information for parents on modeling techniques, skills training, and anxiety management. The program (Figure 57.2) was tailored to demographic, personality, and surgical characteristics of the parent and child.[36]

Parental presence during induction of anesthesia (PPIA)

It is well established that most parents favor staying with their children as long as possible during visits, invasive/ noninvasive procedures such as vaccinations, diagnostic imaging, dental treatments, and anesthesia. Studies found that an overly anxious parent can increase anxiety in a calm child, while calm parents reduce it. Induction of anesthesia is the most stress-inducing experience during the preoperative period. Some children verbalize their fear, while others become agitated, cry, urinate, or attempt to escape.[6,8,10,11] In 1995 only 26% of US hospitals allowed parental presence during induction of anesthesia, while it was against hospital policy in 32%. However, another study in 2002 showed a significant increase in the use of PPIA compare to the decade earlier.[37]

Initial observational studies suggested decreased anxiety with PPIA, but more recent trials did not find the simple act of parental presence beneficial. An anxious parent can disrupt the induction process, create more anxiety for the child and medical staff, and negatively influence the child's experience.[38,39] Therefore, rather than asking parents to be simply present, they must be prepared with (i) a description of the different stages of induction of anesthesia and (ii) instructions on how to be actively engaged (reassuring touch, eye contact, using distractions such as singing songs, calm conversations, reading, etc. to their child).[40] Since assessment

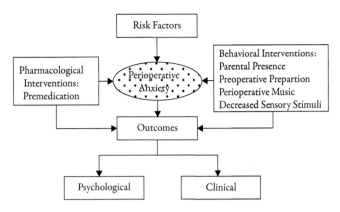

Fig. 57.2 Conceptual framework of preoperative anxiety. Source: McCann ME, Kain ZN. The management of preoperative anxiety in children: an update. *Anesth Analg.* 2001;93(1):98–105.

of anxiety with scientific instruments is not practical in busy perioperative settings, anesthesiologists need to use their clinical judgment with regard to the suitability of PPIA. The practitioner can indicate to very anxious parents that their presence may result in an increase in their child's anxiety and offer instead to administer a premedication.[41] It is important to note that the combination of midazolam and PPIA has no additive anxiolytic effects for children. Nonetheless, parents who accompany their sedated children into the operating room seem to be significantly less anxious and more satisfied.

Hypnosis

Hypnosis is a "therapeutic procedure in which a health care professional makes suggestions that will help a patient experience alterations in perception, sensation, emotion, thought, and/or behavior."[42] The term "hypnosis" is different from the term "hypnotherapy," as hypnosis itself is not a treatment but rather a tool. Hypnotherapy, in contrast, describes the clinical use of specific *suggestions* in order to achieve a specific therapeutic goal (e.g., alleviate pain).[43] Over the past few decades, hypnosis has been utilized in children undergoing painful medical treatments in the emergency room, during invasive diagnostic procedures such as bone marrow aspiration and lumbar puncture, and for the management of preoperative anxiety and postoperative pain. Natural, spontaneous hypnotic states are common in children, and they can be recognized by some physiological indicators such as fixed gaze with eyes open, staring without blinking, or closed eyes with fluttering eyelids followed by eye movement under closed eyelids, slowing of the respiratory rate, and stillness. Children in this state have focused attention and are absorbed in fantasy and imagination. During these states, whether spontaneous or induced by hypnosis, children are intensely focused on the clinician's communication and have a tendency to interpret each word in a literal manner. A clinician's ultimate goal in the use of hypnosis is to alter the child from the relatively passive state to a state of empowerment, self-mastery, and control. Practitioners must tailor the hypnotic strategies to meet the child's particular developmental level and avoid

the temptation to impose their own imagery on the child. They should use child's interests, strengths, and internal resources to solve problems. Brief examples of hypnotic induction techniques are using imagery, favorite place, favorite activity, ideomotor techniques (hand movements), progressive muscle relaxation, and so on. A comprehensive description of different hypnotic inductions and suggestions for a variety of medical disorders can be found in the book *Hypnosis and Hypnotherapy with Children.*[44]

Web-based tailored intervention program (WebTIPS)

Growing access to the Internet generates an opportunity to create a tailored, web-based behavioral preparation program to provide easily accessible information on coping skills and modeling based on child and parent characteristics.

In 2015, Fortier and Kain[36] designed a tailored web-based behavioral intervention that was based on

1. Child's variables, such as developmental abilities, temperament, and coping style.

2. Family variables, such as parental trait anxiety, coping style, and attitude toward pain.

3. The surgical procedure.

This multimedia intervention was comprised of audio, visual, and animation features that addressed both the parents and the child in five different timelines:

1. Home; prior to surgery

2. Holding area

3. Anesthesia induction and surgery

4. Recovery room

5. Home; following the surgery

The child component provided age-appropriate animated information, modeling, and coping skills training. The parent component included the two concepts of (i) information and (ii) coping skills education and practice.[45]

The program also delivered important information about the child and parent to the anesthesiologists and nurses before the day of surgery that served to build rapport. The efficacy of this intervention was evaluated in 2 different phases. Phase I enrolled 13 children aged 2 to 7 years and their parents to inquire about their perceptions and attitudes regarding the product. Phase II evaluated the efficacy of the intervention on preoperative anxiety as compared to standard of care in 2 different medical centers.

Parents found the intervention to be both helpful and easy to use during the first phase of the study. Phase II showed that children in the WebTIPS group were less anxious compare to those in the standard of care group at two stages: (i) entrance to the operating room and (ii) introduction of the anesthesia mask. Furthermore, parents in the WebTIPS group experienced less anxiety compared to the control group.[36]

PHARMACOLOGICAL MODALITIES

Midazolam

Midazolam is the most commonly used sedative in the holding area (85%), followed by ketamine (4%) and transmucosal fentanyl (3%). Oral is the most preferred route in the United States (80%), followed by intranasal (8%), intramuscular(IM; 6%), and rectal (3%).[37]

Midazolam is a short-acting benzodiazepine derivative with an imidazole ring and rapid onset of action. Intranasal administration of 0.2 to 03 mg/kg midazolam is effective in reducing children's anxiety within 10 to 12 minutes; however, it can irritate the nasal passage and thus upset children.[46] The same dose can be administrated sublingually, but it is difficult to prevent small children from swallowing or spitting it out. The rectal dose of 0.5 to 1.0 mg/kg decreases the anxiety of children before induction of anesthesia, but it may cause hiccups in 20% of children, which can be treated by ethyl chloride nasal spray.[47,48] Oral midazolam 0.5 mg/kg is effective in reducing both separation and induction anxiety in children, with minimal effect on recovery time. Disadvantages include restlessness, paradoxical reaction, and amnesia.[49–52] The oral dosage can range between 0.25 and 1.0 mg/kg up to a total dose of 20 mg based on child's anxiety level and the duration of surgery. The timing of administration is important. Suresh et al. showed that 0.25 mg/kg ensues reasonable sedation in 20 minutes.[53,54] There still is a heated debate on the subject of delay in discharge after the oral-dose midazolam. While several studies did not find any association between oral midazolam and delay in discharge,[55,57] some reported delayed emergence and recovery in children undergoing adenoidectomy.[58,59] There has been a significant decrease in incidences of negative behavioral changes in children who used midazolam as a premedication.[6] Amnesia is thought to be the responsible mechanism in decreasing the incidence.[11]

Midazolam can be reversed with flumazenil, which antagonizes benzodiazepines competitively. The initial recommended dose in children is 0.05 mg/kg intravenous (IV) in a titrated fashion of up to 1.0 mg total. Due to re-sedation children need to be monitored for at least 1 to 2 hours after reversal.[60]

Fentanyl

Oral transmucosal fentanyl citrate (OTFC) is a water-soluble salt that when mixed with saliva becomes 80% nonionized, making it the only opioid suitable for transmucosal absorption. OTFC has a rapid onset of action (3–5 minutes) with a peak effect at 20 to 40 minutes and total duration of activity of 2 to 3 hours. OTFC in the form of a lozenge was approved by the Food and Drug Administration in 1993 for use as a sedative in children. OTFC has a sedative effect; however, it does not decrease anxiety or improve cooperation.[61,62] OTFC is mixed in a raspberry-flavored candy matrix in 200-, 300-, and 400-mg dosage units. The dose in children is 10 to 15 mg/kg for transmucosal absorption. OTFC has been shown to significantly decrease the postoperative narcotic requirement in children undergoing tonsillectomy.[63] Side effects include

facial pruritus that usually occurs 30 to 40 minutes after consumption, as well as an increase in postoperative nausea and vomiting. In addition, a small percentage of patients develop respiratory depression, therefore it has to be used in an area with airway management readily available. .

Ketamine

Ketamine is an arylcycloalkylamine that produces profound analgesia, amnesia, sedation, and immobility without cardiorespiratory depression. Its disadvantage as compared with other sedatives is its association with increased salivary and bronchial secretions that can lead to laryngospasm.[64] In addition, children may develop muscle rigidity, emesis, agitation, hallucinations, and nystagmus, which can make uninformed parents apprehensive. These side effects are mostly dose dependent and can be diminished with the use of a small dose of orally administered ketamine (3-4 mg/kg).[65]

The onset of the action of oral ketamine is also dose dependent with large doses (6–8 mg/kg) being effective within 10 minutes, versus 20 minutes in smaller doses (3–4 mg/kg).[66] Higher doses of ketamine (8–10mg/kg) provide rapid-onset sedation, less anxiety during parental separation and insertion of IV lines, as well as less anxiety about the application of the facemask.[67,68]

The IV preparation of ketamine can be mixed with cola or fruit syrup to create an acceptable taste for children. Ketamine can be also given intranasally (3–5 mg/kg), transmucosally (5–6 mg/kg), rectally (5 mg/kg), and IM (2–5 mg/kg).[69,70] The discharge of children who received oral ketamine has not been shown to be prolonged compared to midazolam for procedures that last longer than 30 minutes. However, the IM administration of ketamine significantly delayed discharge and increased costs compared with intranasal or rectal midazolam.[71] An oral ketamine midazolam mixture was also found to provide superior sedation and amnesia as well as less need for propofol rescue as compared to either drug alone.

Clonidine

Clonidine is a centrally active, α^2 selective agonist with a α^1: α^2 selectivity ratio of approximately 200:1. It was found to have analgesic, anxiolytic, and sedative properties in addition to its antihypertensive actions.[72] Its analgesic effect is mediated via brainstem and spinal α^2 adrenergic receptors, which are associated with descending pain inhibitory pathways originating in areas such as the locus ceruleus.[73] These pathways control the release of neurotransmitters from primary afferent neurons in the dorsal horn of the spinal cord. Orally administered clonidine in a dose of 4 mcg/kg reduces neuroendocrine responses to stressful stimuli, causes sedation, reduces anesthetic requirements, and decreases the requirement for postoperative analgesics.[74–77] A study on 105 children ages 4 to 12 years old showed that 4 mcg/kg of clonidine produced significant sedation, provided for easier separation from parents, and allowed easier acceptance of the mask. It also attenuated the increases in blood pressure and heart rate after tracheal intubation without significant perioperative hypotension or bradycardia.[78] Another study comparing midazolam to clonidine showed an increased need for oxygen supplementation in the postanesthesia care unit (PACU) in the midazolam group, consistent with a shorter time to discharge from PACU in the clonidine group.[79] Oral clonidine has also been shown to reduce the incidence of sevoflurane-induced emergence agitation.[80]

Dexmedetomidine

Dexmedetomidine is a more selective α^2 drug with more favorable pharmacokinetic properties than clonidine and a shorter half-life. A study on healthy adult volunteers demonstrated that intranasal 1 to 1.5 mcg/kg dexmedetomidine produces sedation in 45 to 60 minutes and peaks in 90 to 105 minutes. In addition, it caused a modest reduction of heart rate and arterial blood pressure.[81] Another study showed 1 mcg/kg intranasal dexmedetomidine was comparable to midazolam in children 2 and 12 years of age. It produced significant sedation at parental separation as well as induction of anesthesia. The hemodynamic effects on blood pressure and heart rate were modest.[82]

REVIEW QUESTIONS

1. Which age group is at the **HIGHEST** risk for preoperative anxiety?

    A. 6 to 12 months old
    B. 12 to 24 months old
    C. 2 to 6 years old
    D. 7 to 15 years old

Answer: C
Studies based on Piaget's model show that 2- to 6-year-olds are at the highest risk for the development of extreme anxiety. It has been shown that older children (>6 years old) who participate in the preparation program 5 to 7 days prior to the procedure are least anxious on separation from their parents, while they show more anxiety if they receive the preparation only 1 day prior to their procedure.[20]

2. Which is the **MOST** common premedication/route delivered preoperatively in children?

    A. fentanyl, IV
    B. ketamine, intranasal
    C. midazolam, oral
    D. midazolam, rectal

Answer: C
Midazolam is the most commonly used sedative in the holding area (85%), followed by ketamine (4%) and transmucosal fentanyl (3%). Oral is the most preferred route in the United States (80%), followed by intranasal (8%), IM (6%), and rectal (3%).[37]

3. Which of the following statements is the **MOST** accurate?

    A. Hypnosis has no place or use in treating pediatric anxiety.
    B. Preoperative anxiety can cause behavioral changes for a year.

C. Preoperative anxiety is normal and is no cause for concern.
D. Ketamine IM is the best way to handle preoperative anxiety.

Answer: B
Preoperative distress in highly anxious children significantly increases the incidence of emergence delirium, sleep disturbances, nightmares, eating problems, and postoperative pain and delays hospital discharge. More than half of children show new negative behaviors on the first day after surgery, while in 20% it can persist for up to 6 months and even up to a year in 7% of children. Preoperative fear also affects sympathetic discharge, increased serum cortisol, epinephrine, growth hormone, interleukin-6, and natural killer cell activity.

4. Which child, seen preoperatively in the holding area, is **MOST** likely to have preoperative anxiety?

    A. baby cooing, drooling, and smiling
    B. child hiding behind the mom, refusing to make eye contact
    C. child who is friendly, smiling, and asks you your name
    D. toddler waving bye-bye in the middle of your interview

Answer: B
Children, who are sensitive to transitions, are more vulnerable to stress. Children who are timid and lack adoptive abilities with behavioral inhibition are significantly more likely to develop anxiety disorders than children with other temperaments. During the preoperative visit one must pay attention to both verbal and nonverbal communications of the child (eye contact, playfulness, timidity, etc.), assess parents' anxiety, and inquire about past experiences.

5. Of the following statements regarding dexmedetomidine, which is the **LEAST** accurate?

    A. It is equivalent to midazolam.
    B. Hemodynamic effects are possible.
    C. Pharmacokinetics are better than clonidine.
    D. It has a rapid onset.

Answer: A
Dexmedetomidine is a more selective α^2 drug with more favorable pharmacokinetic properties than clonidine and a shorter half-life. A study on healthy adult volunteers demonstrated that intranasal 1 to 1.5 mcg/kg dexmedetomidine produced sedation in 45 to 60 minutes and peaked in 90 to 105 minutes. In addition, it caused a modest reduction of heart rate and arterial blood pressure.[81] Another study showed 1 mcg/kg intranasal dexmedetomidine was comparable to midazolam in children 2 and 12 years old. It produced significant sedation at parental separation as well as induction of anesthesia. The hemodynamic effects on blood pressure and heart rate were modest.[82]

QUESTIONS AND ANSWERS

This chapter has accompanying questions and answers which are available to subscribers as part of the Oxford eLearning platform. To access the questions, go to ✔ http:// oxfordmedicine. com/pediatricanesthesiaPBL

REFERENCES

1. Munafo MR, Stevenson J. Anxiety and surgical recovery: reinterpreting the literature. *J Psychosom Res.* 2001;51(4):589–596.
2. Vaughn F, Wichowski H, Bosworth G. Does preoperative anxiety level predict postoperative pain? *AORN J.* 2007;85(3):589–604.
3. Gouin JP, Kiecolt-Glaser JK. The impact of psychological stress on wound healing: methods and mechanisms. *Immunol Allergol Clin North America.* 2011;31(1):81–93.
4. Broadbent E, Koschwanez HE. The psychology of wound healing. *Curr Opin Psychiatry.* 2012;25(2):135–140.
5. Chen E, Zeltzer LK, Craske MG, Katz ER. Children's memories for painful cancer treatment procedures: implications for distress. *Child Dev.* 2000;71:933–947
6. Kain ZN, Mayes LC, Caramico LA. Preoperative preparation in children: a cross-sectional study. *J Clin Anesth.* 1996; 8:508–514.
7. Melamed BG, Dearborn M, Hermecz DA. Necessary considerations for surgery preparation: age and previous experience. *Psychosom Med.* 1983;45:517–525.
8. Kain Z, Mayes L, Borestein M, Genevro J. Anxiety in children during the perioperative period. In: Anonymous. *Child Development and Behavioral Pediatrics.* Mahwah, NJ: Lawrence Erlbaum; 1996:85–103.
9. Wolfer JA, Visintainer MA. Pediatric surgical patients' and parents' stress responses and adjustment as a function of psychologic preparation and stress-point nursing care. *Nurs Res.* 1975;24:244–255.
10. Kain Z, Wang S, Caldwell-Andrews A, et al. Pre-surgical preparation programs for children undergoing outpatient surgery: current status. Paper presented at American Society of Anesthesiology, Chicago; 2006.
11. Kain ZN, Wang SM, Mayes LC, Caramico LA, Hofstadter MB. Distress during the induction of anesthesia and postoperative behavioral outcomes. *Anesth Analg.* 1999;88(5):1042–1047.
12. Provence S, Mayes L. Separation and deprivation. In: Lewis M, ed. *Child and Adolescent Psychiatry: A Comprehensive Textbook.* Philadelphia, PA: Williams and Wilkins; 1996:382–394.
13. Pinto RP, Hollandsworth JG Jr. Using videotape modeling to prepare children psychologically for surgery: influence of parents and costs versus benefits of providing preparation services. *Health Psychol.* 1989;8:79–95.
14. Karl HW, Pauza KJ, Heyneman N, et al. Preanesthetic preparation of pediatric outpatients: the role of a videotape for parents. *J Clin Anesth.* 1990;2:172–177.
15. Kain Z, Caramico L, Mayes L, et al. Preoperative preparation programs in children: a comparative study. *Anesth Analg.* 1998;87:1249–1255.
16. Lamb M, Hwang C, Frodi A, Frodi M. Security of mother and father infant attachment and its relation to sociability with strangers in traditional and nontraditional Swedish families. *Infant Behav Dev.* 1982;5:355–367.
17. Ross DM, Ross SA. *Childhood Pain.* Baltimore: Urban & Schwarzenberg; 1988.
18. Lavigne JV, Schulein MJ, Hahn YS. Psychological aspects of painful medical conditions in children. I. Developmental aspects and assessment. *Pain.* 1986;27:133–146.
19. Lavigne JV, Hannan JA, Schulein MI, Hahn YS. Pain and the pediatric patient: psychological aspects. In: Ecternach JL, ed. *Pain.* New York: Churchill Livingstone; 1987:267–296.
20. Vetter, TR. The epidemiology and selective identification of children at risk for preoperative anxiety reactions. *Anesth Analg.* 1993;77(1):96–99.
21. Kagan J, Reznick JS, Clarke C, Snidman N, Garcia Coll C. Behavioral inhibition to the unfamiliar. *Child Dev.* 1984;55:2212–2225.
22. Kagan J, Reznick JS, Snidman N, Gibbons J, Johnson MO. Childhood derivatives of inhibition and lack of inhibition to the unfamiliar. *Child Dev.* 1988;59:1580–1589.
23. Fox N, Calkins S. Relations between temperament, attachment, and behavioral inhibition: two possible pathways to extroversion and social withdrawal. In: Rubin KH, Asendorpf J, eds. *Social Withdrawal, Inhibition, and Shyness in Childhood.* Chicago: University of Chicago Press; 1993:81–100.
24. Kagan J. Temperamental contributions to social behavior. *Am Psychol.* 1989;44:668–674.
25. Asendorpf J. Development of inhibited children's coping with unfamiliarity. *Child Dev.* 1991;62:1460–1474.
26. Prior M, Sanson A, Oberklaid F. The Australian temperament projects. In: Kohnstamm GA, Bates JE, Rothbart MK, eds. *Temperament in Childhood.* Chichester, UK: Wiley; 1989:537–554.
27. Perez-Edgar K, Fox NA. Temperament and anxiety disorders. *Child Adolesc Psychiatr Clin.* 2005;14:681–706.
28. Pine DS. Research review: a neuroscience framework for pediatric anxiety disorders. *J Child Psychol Psychiatry.* 2007;48:631–638.
29. Melamed BG, Dearborn M, Hermecz DA. Necessary considerations for surgery preparation: age and previous experience. *Psychosom Med.* 1983;45:517–525.
30. Aristotle. *Metaphysics.* Apostle HG, trans. Grinnell, IA: Peripatetic Press; 1979.
31. Maslow AH. The need to know and the fear of knowing. *J Gen Psychol.* 1963;68:111–125.
32. Suls J, Wan CK. Effects of sensory and procedural information on coping with stressful medical procedures and pain: A meta-analysis. *J Consult Clin Psychol.* 1989;57(3):372–379.
33. Case DO, Andrews JE, Johnson JD, Allard SL. Avoiding versus seeking: the relationship of information seeking to avoidance, blunting, coping, dissonance, and related concepts. *J Med Lib Assoc.* 2005;93(3):353–362.
34. Bijttebier P, Vertommen H. The impact of previous experience on children's reactions to venepunctures. *J Health Psychol.* 1998;3(1):39–46.
35. O'Byrne K, Peterson L, Saldana L. Survey of pediatric hospitals' preparation programs: evidence of the impact of health psychology research. *Health Psychol.* 1997;16:147–154.
36. Fortier MA, Bunzli E, Walthall J, et al. Web-based tailored intervention for preparation of parents and children for outpatient surgery (WebTIPS): formative evaluation and randomized controlled trial. *Anesth Analg.* 2015;120(4):915.
37. Kain ZN, Caldwell-Andrews AA, Krivutza DM, et al. Trends in the practice of parental presence during induction of anesthesia and the use of preoperative sedative premedication in the United States, 1995–2002: results of a follow-up national survey. *Anesth Analg.* 2004;98(5):1252–1259.
38. Hickmott KC, Shaw EA, Goodyer I, Baker RD. Anaesthetic induction in children: the effect of maternal presence on mood and subsequent behavior. *Eur J Anaesth.* 1989;6:145–155.
39. Bevan JC, Johnston C, Haig MJ, et al. Preoperative parental anxiety predicts behavioral and emotional responses to induction of anesthesia in children. *Can J Anaesth.* 1990;37:177–182.
40. Blount R, Bachanas P, Powers S: Training children to cope and parents to coach them during routine immunizations: effects on child, parent, and staff behaviors. *Behav Ther.* 1992;23:689–705.
41. Bevan JC, Johnston C, Haig MJ, et al. Preoperative parental anxiety predicts behavioral and emotional responses to induction of anesthesia in children. *Can J Anaesth.* 1990;37:177–182.
42. Rhue JW, Lynn SJ, Kirsch I. Introduction to clinical hypnosis. In: Rhue JW, Lynn SJ, Kirsch I, eds. *Handbook of Clinical Hypnosis.* Washington, DC: American Psychological Association; 1993:3–22.
43. Raz A, Shapiro T. Hypnosis and neuroscience: a crosstalk between clinical and cognitive research. *Arch Gen Psychiatry.* 2003;59:85–90.
44. Kohen DP, Olness K. *Hypnosis and Hypnotherapy with Children.* New York: Routledge; 2012.
45. McCann, ME, Kain ZN. The management of preoperative anxiety in children: an update. *Anesth Analg.* 2001;93(1):98–105.
46. Griffith N, Howell S, Mason DG. Intranasal midazolam for premedication of children undergoing day-case anaesthesia: comparison of

two delivery systems with assessment of intra-observer variability. *Br J Anaesth*. 1998;81(6):865–869.

47. Karl HW, Rosenberger JL, Larach MG, Ruffle JM. Transmucosal administration of midazolam for premedication of pediatric patients—comparison of the nasal and sublingual routes. *Anesthesiology*. 1993;78:885–891.

48. Marhofer P, Glaser C, Krenn CG, et al. Incidence of therapy of midazolam induced hiccups in paediatric anaesthesia. *Paediatr Anaesth*. 1999;9:295–298.

49. Cox RG, Nemish U, Ewen A, Crowe M-J. Evidence-based clinical update: does premedication with oral midazolam lead to improved behavioural outcomes in children? *Can J Anaesth*. 2006;53:1213–1219.

50. Lonnqvist PA, Habre W. Midazolam as premedication: is the emperor naked or just half-dressed? *Paediatr Anaesth*. 2005;15:263–5 13

51. Kanegaye JT, Favela JL, Acosta M, Bank DE. High-dose rectal midazolam for pediatric procedures: a randomized trial of sedative efficacy and agitation. *Pediatr Emerg Care*. 2003;19:329–336.

52. Watson AT, Visram A. Children's preoperative anxiety and postoperative behaviour. *Paediatr Anaesth*. 2003;13:188–204.

53. Suresh S, Cohen IJ, Matuszczak M, et al. Dose ranging, safety, and efficacy of a new oral midazolam syrup in children [abstract]. *Anesthesiology*. 1998;89:A1313.

54. Levine M, Spahr-Schopfer I, Hartley E, MacPherson B. Oral midazolam premedication in children: the minimum time interval for separation from parents. *Can J Anaesth*. 1993;40:726–729.

55. McGraw T, Kendrick A. Oral midazolam premedication and postoperative behavior in children. *Paediatr Anaesth*. 1998;8:117–121.

56. Lewyn MJ. Should parents be present while their children receive anesthesia? *Anesth Malpract Protect*. 1993;56–57.

57. Lynn, Steven, Kirsch, Irving, Rhue, Judith W. Rhue, Judith W. (Ed); Lynn, Steven Jay (Ed) & Kirsch, Irving (Ed). (1993). Handbook of clinical hypnosis. (pp. 3–22). Washington, DC, US: American Psychological Association, xxv, 765 pp.

58. Viitanen H, Annila P, Viitanen M, Tarkkila P. Premedication with midazolam delays recovery after ambulatory sevoflurane anesthesia in children. Anesth Analg 1999;89:75–9.

59. Viitanen H, Annila P, Viitanen M, Yli-Hankala A. Midazolam premedication delays recovery from propofol-induced sevofluraneanaesthesia in children 1–3 yr. *Can J Anaesth*. 1999;46:766–771.

60. Shannon M, Albers G, Burkhart K, et al. Safety and efficacy of lumazenil in the reversal of benzodiazepine-induced conscious sedation. *J Pediatr*. 1997;131:582–586.

61. Tamura M, Nakamura K, Kitamura R, Kitagawa S, Mori N, Ueda Y. Oral premedication with fentanyl may be a safe and effective alternative to oral midazolam. *Eur J Anaesthesiol*. 2003;20(6):482–486.

62. Epstein RH, Mendel HG, Witkowski TA, et al. The safety and efficacy of oral transmucosal fentanyl citrate for preoperative sedation in young children. *Anesth Analg*. 1996;83:1200–1205.

63. Dsida RM, Wheeler M, Birmingham PK, et al. Premedication of pediatric tonsillectomy patients with oral transmucosal fentanyl citrate. *Anesth Analg*. 1998;86:66–70.

64. Filatov SM, Baer GA, Rorarius G, Oikkonen M. Efficacy and safety of premedication with oral premedication for day-case adenoidectomy compared with rectal diazepam/diclofenac and EMLA. *Acta Anaesthesiol Scand*. 2000;44:118–124.

65. Sekerci CM, Donmez A, Ates Y, Okten F. Oral ketamine premedication in children (placebo controlled double blind study). *Eur J Anaesthesiol*. 1996;13:606–611.

66. Funk W, Jakob W, Reidl T, Taeger K. Oral preanaesthetic medication for children: double-blind randomized study of a combination of midazolam and ketamine vs midazolam or ketamine alone. *Br J Anaesth*. 2000;84:335–340.

67. Tobias JD, Phipps S, Smith B, Mulhern RK. Oral ketamine premedication to alleviate the distress of invasive procedures in paediatric oncology patients. *Pediatrics*. 1992;90:537–541.

68. Turhanoilu S, Ozyilmaz Kararmaz MA, Tok Kaya D. Effects of different doses of oral ketamine for premedication of children. *Eur J Anaesthesiol*. 2003;20:56–60.

69. Diaz JH. Intranasal ketamine preinduction of paediatric outpatients. *Paediatr Anaesth*. 1997;7:273–278.

70. Cioaca R, Canavea I. Oral transmucosal ketamine: an effective premedication in children. *Paediatr Anaesth*. 1996;6:361–365.

71. Lawrence LM, Wright SW. Sedation of pediatric patients for minor laceration repair: effects on length of emergency department stay and patient charges. *Pediatr Emerg Care*. 1998;14:393–395.

72. Nishina K, Mikawa K, Shiga M, Obara H. Clonidine in paediatric anaesthesia. *Paediatr Anaesth*. 1999;9:187–202.

73. Gentili F, Pigini M, Piergentili A, Giannella M. Agonists and antagonists targeting the different alpha2-adrenoceptor subtypes. *Curr Top Med Chem*. 2007;7(2):163–186

74. Segal IS, Jarvis DJ, Duncan SR, et al. Clinical efficacy of oral transdermal clonidine combinations during the perioperative period. *Anesthesiology*. 1991;74:220–225.

75. Ghignone M, Calvilla O, Quintin L. Anesthesia and hypertension: the effect of perioperative hemodynamics on isoflurane requirements. *Anesthesiology*. 1987;67:3–10.

76. Ghinghone M, Quintin L, Duke PC, et al. Effects of clonidine on narcotic requirements and hemodynamic response during induction of anesthesia and endotracheal intubation. *Anesthesiology*. 1986;64(1):36–42.

77. Ghinghone M, Noe C, Calvillo O, Quintin L. Anesthesia for ophthalmic surgery in the elderly: the effects of clonidine on intraocular pressure, perioperative hemodynamics and anesthetic requirement. *Anesthesiology*. 1988;68:707–716.

78. Mikawa K, Maekawa N, Nishina K, Takao Y, Yaku H, Obara H. Efficacy of oral clonidine premedication in children. *Anesthesiology* 1993;79(5):926–931.

79. Fazi L, Jantzen EC, Rose JB, Kurth CD, Watcha MF. A comparison of oral clonidine and oral midazolam as preanesthetic medications in the pediatric tonsillectomy patient. *Anesth Analg*. 2001;92(1):56–61.

80. Tazeroualti N, De Groote F, De Hert S, De Ville A, Dierick A, Van der Linden P. Oral clonidine vs midazolam in the prevention of sevoflurane-induced agitation in children. A prospective, randomized, controlled trial. *Br J Anaesth*. 2007;98:667–671.

81. Yuen VM, Hui TW, Yuen MK, Irwin MG. A double blind crossover assessment of the sedative and analgesic effects of intranasal dexmedetomidine. *Anesth Analg*. 2007;105:374–380.

82. Yuen VM, Hui TW, Irwin MG, Yuen MK. A comparison of intranasal dexmedetomidine and oral midazolam for premedication in pediatric anesthesia: a double-blinded randomized controlled trial. *Anesth Analg*. 2008;106(6):1715–1721.

58.

GOLDENHAR SYNDROME

Amy Soleta and Joelle Karlik

STEM CASE AND KEY QUESTIONS

A 3-year-old female with Goldenhar (GH) syndrome presents to your preoperative clinic prior to a vertical expandable prosthetic titanium rib (VEPTR) expansion. Due to severe scoliosis, she has pulmonary insufficiency syndrome and had VEPTR placement 1 year ago. She has been growing well and is in need of an expansion.

WHAT PREOPERATIVE EVALUATION WOULD YOU LIKE FOR THIS CHILD? WHAT ARE COMMON MEDICAL PROBLEMS ASSOCIATED WITH GH SYNDROME?

Her past medical history includes GH syndrome with facial asymmetry, epibulbar dermoids, pulmonary insufficiency syndrome, sleep apnea, severe thoracic scoliosis, and hearing loss. In the past, she has had multiple respiratory infections. Currently, she is well. Albuterol and chest percussion are part of her pulmonary regimen. She was known to have severe obstructive sleep apnea (documented polysmography). However, the parents report this has resolved after adenotonsillectomy. Per her parents, her infant cardiac echocardiogram was unremarkable. Other than scoliosis, patient has no known renal or vertebral anomalies.

WHAT EFFORT SHOULD BE MADE TO GET OLD RECORDS? WOULD YOU CANCEL THIS CASE IF RECORDS CANNOT BE OBTAINED? DOES IT MAKE A DIFFERENCE IF THIS CHILD SHOWED UP AT A PREOPERATIVE CLINIC VERSUS A HOLDING AREA?

Her previous surgeries include cleft palate, adenotonsillectomy, and VEPTR placement. She always wakes up with "something in her nose." She is usually admitted to the hospital for monitoring after anesthesia.

This is a shy 3-year-old female sitting on her mother's lap. There is notable facial asymmetry, right-sided mandibular hypoplasia, and an abnormal right pinna. Lung sounds are rhonchorous bilaterally. Cardiac auscultation is unremarkable. She does not tolerate an abdominal exam and soon refuses to participate in any further exam.

HOW CAN YOU EVALUATE THIS YOUNG CHILD'S AIRWAY PREOPERATIVELY? OTHER THAN HISTORY AND PHYSICAL EXAM, DO YOU NEED ANY FURTHER IMAGING OR TESTS? DOES A PREVIOUSLY REASSURING AIRWAY GIVE YOU CONFIDENCE IN THIS SCENARIO? WOULD IT MAKE A DIFFERENCE IF YOU RECEIVED HISTORY OF A DIFFICULT AIRWAY?

The child proceeds to the operating room. Standard American Society of Anesthesiologists monitors are placed. The patient undergoes a smooth inhalational induction via mask with an oral airway. After the intravenous (IV) line is placed you proceed with a fiberoptic intubation.

WOULD YOU CONSIDER STANDARD LARYNGOSCOPY IN THIS PATIENT GIVEN THIS HISTORY AND PHYSICAL EXAM? IS THIS AN ELECTIVE FIBEROPTIC? WOULD YOU PREPARE FOR A DIFFICULT AIRWAY?

The endotracheal cuff is confirmed visually for correct placement. There seems to be an upstroke in end-tidal CO_2 waveform indicating obstruction. Four puffs of albuterol are given and the surgeon begins. Suddenly, the patient desaturates despite increasing the fraction of inspired oxygen (FiO_2). Pulse oximetry is consistently 85% despite 100% FiO_2. The $ETCO_2$ waveform has not changed.

HOW WOULD YOU EVALUATE DESATURATION IN THIS PATIENT? SHOULD THE SURGEON STOP?

You ensure that there are no leaks in the anesthesia circuit and that you are delivering 100% oxygen. When listening, you find unilateral breath sounds despite an endotracheal tube (ETT) at its previously taped depth. You suction the ETT and repeat inhaled albuterol. You perform a gentle recruitment maneuver. The pulse oximetry continues to decrease to 80% and peak pressures start to rise. In addition, the patient is becoming hypotensive despite giving a 20 mL/kg IV fluid bolus.

WHAT ARE THE TOP 3 THINGS ON YOUR DIFFERENTIAL? HOW WOULD YOU PROCEED IN THIS SCENARIO?

With the fiberoptic bronchoscope, you quickly confirm the ETT position above the carina with no appreciable mucus plugs. At this point, you inform the surgeon that you are concerned about an evolving tension pneumothorax. You perform needle decompression and hear a rush of air. The pulse oximetry, peak pressures, and hypotension quickly resolve. You ask the surgeon for a chest tube. He agrees and suggests that the patient's underlying lung disease likely predisposed this patient to a pneumothorax.

WHAT ARE THE INDICATIONS FOR A VEPTR PLACEMENT? AT WHAT AGE SHOULD IT BE PLACED, AND HOW IS IT MANAGED AFTER PLACEMENT?

After 2 hours of surgery, you fully reverse neuromuscular blockade and extubate the patient with oral-pharyngeal (OP) and naso-pharyngeal (NP) airways in place. She is oxygenating and ventilating well on 6L O2 via facemask in the postanesthesia care unit (PACU) and is sleeping comfortably. You discuss the plan to remove the OP airway once the patient awakes with the PACU nurse, but you request to continue the NP to relieve possible postoperative airway obstruction. The PACU nurse, due to a concern that the patient was uncomfortable, removes both OA and NP airways. The patient immediately begins to look distressed and is soon desaturating. You attempt to replace the NP and OA airways but ventilation is still inadequate. The patient becomes unresponsive and you attempt direct laryngoscopy with a grade IV view.

You call for a GlideScope and place a laryngeal mask airway but the seal is inadequate and you cannot ventilate. The GlideScope arrives but you cannot view the vocal cords due to supraglottic edema from prolonged intubation and prone positioning. The patient starts to become severely bradycardic.

HOW WOULD YOU PROCEED?

Luckily, an otolaryngology surgeon has just finished his cases and runs to bedside. He performs a surgical tracheostomy at bedside with immediate placement of an ETT through the incision.

WHAT ARE YOUR ALTERNATIVES IF YOU DO NOT HAVE AN OTOLARYNGOLOGY SURGEON AVAILABLE FOR SURGICAL AIRWAY?

Oxygenation quickly improves, and slowly heart rate increases. You start sedation and discuss intensive care unit (ICU) admission with the surgeons.

DISCUSSION

GH syndrome (also known as oculo-auriculo-vertebral [OAV] spectrum, facio-auriculo-vertebral syndrome, Goldenhar-Gorlin syndrome) likely was first described in 1845 by Dr. von Arnt.[1,2] However, this syndrome did not gain attention, nor a name, until 1952 when Dr. Maurice Goldenhar reported an additional 3 cases to review along with the 16 previously described cases. Dr. Goldenhar's review of these 19 patients with congenital mandibulo-facial malformations, auricular malformations, and epibulbar dermoids resulted in the eponymous syndrome described today.[3]

Currently, GH syndrome is classified under the OAV spectrum.[4] The OAV spectrum includes three rare congenital disorders: GH syndrome, hemifacial microsomia (HFM), and oculo-auriculo-vertebral disorder (OAVD). The OAV spectrum presents as a wide and varying range of physical features. GH syndrome, a more severe subset of the OVA spectrum, encompasses multiple facial and associated cardiac, spinal, or renal malformations (see Fig. 58.1).[5]

Classically, a diagnosis of GH syndrome is made with the Feingold criteria which requires an eye abnormality (lipoma, lipodermoid, epibulbar dermoid, or upper eyelid coloboma) associated with at least two other ear, mandibular, or vertebral anomalies.[6] Other grading criteria, such as the OMENS system for HFM (see Table 58.1), have been proposed and do not include GH syndrome as a separate entity.[7,8]

GENETICS

OAV syndrome is due to fetal growth disturbances of the first and second brachial arches, leading to head and neck malformations. Most cases occur sporadically with unidentified causes; only 1% to 2% of patients have family members with the syndrome. It is likely multifactorial with both environmental and genetic components. In the case of inherited GH syndrome, it appears to be autosomal dominant. However, autosomal recessive inheritance has also been reported.[4] OAV syndrome is recognized as a syndrome as it includes multiple anomalies that may occur independently and without a known cause. In contrast, a sequence is a collection of malformations with a known inciting event.[9] A good example is Pierre Robin sequence, where mandibular hypoplasia leads to glossoptosis, airway obstruction, and often cleft palate.

PRESENTATION

The presentation of GH syndrome varies from patient to patient but there are multiple common features (see Table 58.2). The syndrome is usually unilateral, but approximately 10% to 33% cases have bilateral involvement.[10] Facial asymmetry, including an underdeveloped mandible, cheekbone, and temple with associated muscular weakness, is very common. Cleft lip and/or palate and dental abnormalities may be present. Ear abnormalities including microtia (partial or absent ear) and hearing loss can be seen on the affected side. Eye disorders can be severe including anopthalmia, microphthalmia, and vision loss. Retinal abnormalities and epibulbar tumors are also seen.[10]

GH syndrome patients can have pulmonary, cardiac, renal, and vertebral abnormalities as well. Vertebral defects include block vertebrae, vertebral hypoplasia, vertebral fusion, scoliosis, and atlanto-axial instability.[4,11] Five to 58% of patients with GH syndrome have cardiovascular malformations

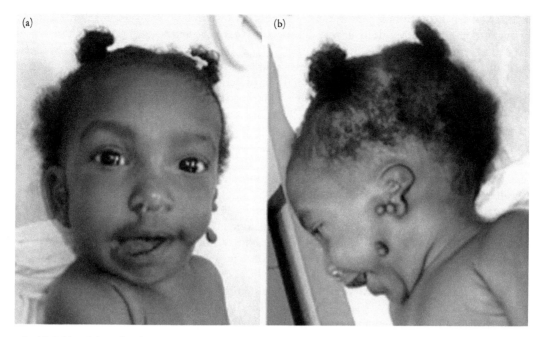

Fig. 58.1 An 8-month-old child with hemifacial microsomia showing facial asymmetry, unilateral microtia, and preauricular tags. Reprinted with permission: Goldenhar Syndrome. In: Chen H, ed. *Atlas of Genetic Diagnosis and Counseling.* New York, NY: Springer US; 2012:971–978.

including tetralogy of Fallot, septal defects, and situs inversus.[11] Other publications report interrupted arch and coarctation of the aorta.[12,13] Renal defects including ectopic kidneys, renal agenesis, vesicoureteral reflux, and ureteropelvic junction obstruction can also occur in GH syndrome.[4,14] Genetic defects in plasma cholinesterase enzymes have been reported in patients with GH syndrome, but this finding is not universal.[15]

ANESTHETIC MANAGEMENT

Preoperative assessment

Due to the multiple craniofacial abnormalities in GH syndrome, airway management can be incredibly challenging.

Table 58.1 OMENS CRITERIA FOR HEMIFACIAL MICROSOMIA

Orbital distortion	
Mandibular hypoplasia	
Ear anomalies	Microtia
	Low-set ears
	Preauricular skin tags/pits
	External auditory canal agenesis/stenosis
	Middle ear malformations with conductive hearing loss
Nerve involvement	Facial nerve palsy
	Auditory nerve dysfunction with sensorineural hearing loss
Soft tissue deficiency	

Adapted from Vento AR, LaBrie RA, Mulliken JB. The O.M.E.N.S. classification of hemifacial microsomia. *Cleft Palate-Craniofacial J.* 1991;28(1):68–76; discussion 77. doi:10.1597/1545-1569(1991)028<0068:tomens>2.3.co;2.

These patients may present for airway management semi-emergently after birth, which limits preoperative assessment. If there is adequate time, a full preoperative airway assessment, including imaging, is recommended.

Preoperative airway evaluation should start with a thorough history and physical. A clear history of snoring, noisy

Table 58.2 COMMON FINDINGS IN GOLDENHAR SYNDROME PATIENTS

APPROXIMATE NUMBER OF PATIENTS	SIGNS AND SYMPTOMS
Very frequent (present in 80%–99% of cases)	Facial asymmetry
	Hearing impairment
	Hypoplasia of the maxilla
	Malar flattening
	Preauricular skin tag
Frequent (present in 30%–79% of cases)	Abnormality of the inner and/or middle ear
	Atresia of the external auditory canal
	Block vertebrae
	Cleft palate
	Epibulbar dermoid
	Feeding difficulties in infancy
	Low-set, posteriorly rotated ears
	Micrognathia
	Microtia
	Neurological speech impairment
	Non-midline cleft lip
	Unilateral external ear deformity
	Vertebral hypoplasia

Adapted from Goldenhar disease Gathersburg, MD: Genetic and Rare Diseases Information Center; 2017. https://rarediseases.info.nih.gov/diseases/6540/goldenhar-disease-ref_11387; and Köhler S, Vasilevsky, N., Engelstad, M., Foster, E. et al. The human phenotype ontology in 2017. *Nucl Acids Res.* 2017.45(1):D865–D876. doi: 10.1093/nar/gkw1039.

breathing, or stridor will help determine the presence of anatomical obstruction or obstructive sleep apnea. Sleep apnea may be related to intrinsic airway abnormalities rather than classic tonsil and adenoid involvement. A proper age-appropriate external airway assessment focusing on the oral cavity, anterior mandibular space, maxilla, temporomandibular joint, and vertebral column should be performed. The Schwartz hyoid maneuver, which measures the anteroposterior distance from the middle of the inside of the mentum of the mandible to the hyoid bone, may be particularly important in GH syndrome patients. Any decrease in this measurement from normative values (about 3 cm in adults and 1.4–1.5 cm in infants) suggests a difficult intubation.[11,17] Airway difficulty can increase with age, so a previously easy airway history is not entirely reassuring.[8,10] Previous surgical mandibular correction may not ease intubation due to scarring and restriction of the temporomandibular joint and soft tissues.[18]

The difficulty of intubation also increases with bilateral mandibular involvement, degree of mandibular hypoplasia, cleft lip/palate, and other craniovertebral anomalies.[8] Early research suggested that severity of mandibular hypoplasia was associated with the degree of difficult intubation.[18] Further case reports suggest that three-dimensional computed tomography (CT) imaging has a role in planning for difficult airways in patients with mandibular hypoplasia.[19] Therefore, airway imaging may be indicated if outside anatomy is suggestive of a severe difficult airway.

Pulmonary hypoplasia can increase the risk for respiratory infections, pulmonary hypertension, and pneumothorax. Plain chest x-rays can evaluate pulmonary branching abnormalities or the preoperative presence of a pneumothorax.[20] In addition, restrictive lung disease may result from severe scoliosis. Restrictive lung disease, when severe, can lead to thoracic insufficiency syndrome and/or resultant atelectasis, bronchiectasis, fibrosis, supplemental oxygen requirement, and an increased risk of pulmonary complications including pneumothorax.

Given the risk of vertebral defects and atlanto-axial instability, a preoperative history and physical to evaluate the cervical spine evaluation is prudent. CT of the spine or cervical flexion-extension x-rays (appropriate after 2 years old) can detect vertebral abnormalities. However, normal imaging does not rule out potential for spinal injury during airway management or surgical positioning.[11]

Echocardiography and abdominal CT may be necessary to rule out any cardiac or renal abnormalities. Also, since the thyroid gland is derived from the 1st through 4th brachial arches, thyroid abnormalities or agensis can occur; therefore, evaluation of thyroid function should be considered with any documented hypotension.[21]

Airway management

Ventilation may range from easy to extremely difficult. Multiple case studies report the use of laryngeal mask airways for successful ventilation.[22–24] Difficulties of ventilation are not limited to craniofacial abnormalities. Pulmonary abnormalities including blind bronchus leading to difficult ventilation have also been reported.[20]

There are multiple case reports detailing various approaches to airway management including laryngeal mask airway, direct laryngoscopy, videolaryngoscope, and fiberoptic intubation.[15,20,22–32] Due to vertebral anomalies, manual in-line stabilization and limited neck extension should be used during all airway management regardless of spinal imaging.[11] These cervical spine precautions may limit direct visualization of the vocal cords so practitioners should be prepared with multiple intubation options.

Surgical airway equipment and an experienced surgical provider should be available for induction and airway manipulation in case of need for surgical airway in a cannot intubate/cannot ventilate situation. A 1998 chart review of 251 patients with major craniofacial abnormalities included 41 patients with OAV syndrome, of which 14 had GH syndrome.[33] Nine patients, or 22% of OAV patients, required a surgical airway. This incidence is clearly markedly increased from the general pediatrics population.

Maintenance

There is no preferred technique for anesthesia maintenance in GH syndrome. Patients with cardiac disease may need limited propofol dosing due to its cardiac depressant properties.[11] Avoidance of long-acting opioids and complete reversal of paralysis is recommended due to the risk of postoperative sleep apnea.[8] Short-acting opioid infusions may be prudent in cases with high stimulation.

Emergence

Airway obstruction is a serious risk in GH syndrome patients during emergence. Opioids, muscle relaxants, and volatile anesthetics add to the risk of obstruction and hypoxia.[8] Placement of a nasopharyngeal and/or oropharyngeal airway prior to extubation, especially in patients with a history suggestive of obstructive sleep apnea, should be considered. Prolonged pulse oximetry may be required with opioid administration. Decision to admit to an ICU depends on patient characteristics such as airway difficulty, cardiac or renal disease, and intraoperative course.

THORACIC INSUFFICIENCY SYNDROME AND VEPTR DEVICE

Thoracic insufficiency syndrome

Thoracic insufficiency syndrome (TIS) is defined as the inability of the thorax to support normal respiration or lung growth.[34] TIS results from restricted biomechanical capabilities of the thorax from fused ribs, scoliosis, or a variety of other orthopedic malformations.[35] These spinal and thoracic abnormalities prevent normal breathing, lung growth, and lung development and predispose patients to recurrent pulmonary infections due to ineffective cough and limited respiratory function. Severe disease can result in atelectasis, bronchiectasis, or fibrosis.[35] TIS is a clinical diagnosis, and complete evaluation may require imaging, blood gases, and pulmonary function testing.

TIS can have a wide spectrum of severity. Mild TIS can present as playtime fatigue and an increased resting respiratory rate.[35] Compensatory mechanisms can avoid hypoxemia but recurrent infections may result in parenchymal lung changes. As TIS progresses, children may develop a supplemental oxygen requirement leading up to a need for positive pressure support and ventilation.

VEPTR

The VEPTR device is an implantable, expandable rod that aims to expand three-dimensional thoracic space and stabilize the diaphragm for improved breathing mechanics.[36] VEPTR is available for use under a US Food and Drug Administration humanitarian device exemption for the treatment of TIS in certain patients (see Table 58.3). The titanium rods are longitudinally attached to the thoracic ribs, lumbar ribs, or ilium.[36] The VEPTR can be expanded as the child grows and reaches adulthood, further promoting proper thoracic and diaphragmatic movement.

The initial VEPTR implantation is a significant surgery often requiring ICU admission and a prolonged hospital stay. Subsequent procedures for VEPTR expansion may be completed with outpatient surgery.[38] Similar models such as the MAGEC™ (MAGnetic Expansion Control) Spinal Growing Rod use magnet-powered expansion that avoids subsequent expansion surgeries.[39]

Anesthetic care generally includes intubation and bilateral pulse oximetry.[40] The patient is placed in the lateral decubitus position and/or prone position with careful attention to avoid brachial plexus injury. Vascular access includes large gauge peripheral IV catheters, arterial cannulation, and central venous cannulation. Somatosensory evoked potentials in all 4 extremities are used to monitor for spinal cord damage and can limit volatile anesthetic use.[40,41] Blood loss is occasionally significant, and surgeons may request autologous

Table 58.3 ANATOMIC INDICATIONS FOR VEPTR US FDA HUMANITARIAN DEVICE USE

DIAGNOSIS	EXAMPLES
Flail Chest	
Constrictive Chest-Wall Syndrome	Fused ribs, scoliosis
Hypoplastic Thoracic Syndrome	Jeune syndrome, achondroplasia, Jarcho-Levin syndrome, Ellis van Creveld syndrome

Note. VEPTR – vertical expandable prosthetic titanium rib; FDA = Food and Drug Administration.

Adapted from Listing of CDRH Humanitarian Device Exemptions. Silver Spring, MD: US Food and Drug Administration; 2017. https://www.fda.gov/MedicalDevices/ProductsandMedicalProcedures/DeviceApprovalsandClearances/HDEApprovals/ucm161827.htm.

hemodilution, tranexamic acid, and/or other anti-fibrinolytic medication. Most patients remain intubated for 2 to 3 days after the initial placement.

TIS patients often have serious comorbidities that predispose them to anesthetic and surgical complications.[34] Complications associated with VEPTR procedures include skin breakdown or infection, dislodgement or migration of devices, device fracture, and spinal cord or brachial plexus injury.[34] In a review of one institution, 33% of patients (22 of 65 patients) had complications ranging from surgical site infection requiring reoperation, device fracture, postoperative pneumonia, and postoperative radiculopathy.[42] The majority of complications were device-related and not related to anesthetic care.

SURGICAL AIRWAY MANAGEMENT

The pediatric cannot intubate/cannot oxygenate (CICO) emergency airway scenario is overall incredibly rare. Fortunately, the development of airway devices such as video and fiberoptic laryngoscopy has made the CICO scenario even more unlikely. A recent multisite review of 1,018 difficult pediatric tracheal intubations showed only 2% (19/1,018) of patients had a surgical or failed airway.[43] Even with this low incidence, airway complications are a large source of morbidity and mortality for pediatric patients. Overall, providing evidence-based research in the pediatric surgical airway is difficult due to the low incidence of pediatric surgical airways and a predominance of animal studies.

In 2015, the Association of Paediatric Anesthetists (APA) and the Difficult Airway Society (DAS) proposed joint guidelines for the situation of "cannot intubate/cannot ventilate" (CICV) in a paralyzed anaesthetized child aged 1 to 8 years (see Fig 58.2).[44] The pediatric guidelines differ from the adult recommendations largely on one topic, the technique for cricothyroidotomy. The DAS recommends cannula technique for pediatric cricothyroidotomy, a deviation from the adult guidelines, which recommend scalpel techniques. The APA recommends using a 14- or 16-gauge cannula with air aspiration to confirm placement (see Fig. 58.2).[44]

Both techniques have a high rate of complications. A rabbit study looking at scalpel airways found a success rate of 100% but with serious complications including tracheal wall damage.[45] Needle cricothyroidtomy is not without similar risks; animal studies have found success rates ranging from 60% to 70% but still with significant complications.[46,47] The small size and varying anatomy of pediatric airways likely add to this high rate of complications.

The (arguably) most critical step in the CICV scenario is calling for help, more specifically, an otolaryngology surgeon. The 4th National Audit Project (NAP4) recorded surgical airway management across the United Kingdom during a 1-year period.[48] Within the NAP4, emergency surgical airways were attempted on 4 children. The 3 successful airways were managed by an otolaryngology surgeon performing an emergency tracheostomy. In contrast, the 1 unsuccessful airway was attempted by an anesthesiologist with a cannula technique.[48] Similar patterns of surgeon versus anesthesiologist success were

APA

Cannot intubate and cannot ventilate (CICV) in a paralysed anaesthetised child aged 1 to 8 years

Failed intubation inadequate ventilation

Give 100% oxygen

Call for help

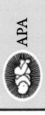

Step A Continue to attempt oxygenation and ventilation

- FiO$_2$ 1.0
- Optimise head position and chin lift/jaw thrust
- Insert oropharyngeal airway or SAD (e.g. LMA™)
- Ventilate using two person bag mask technique
- Manage gastric distension with an OG/NG tube

Step B Attempt wake up if maintaining SpO$_2$ >80%

If rocuronium or vecuronium used, consider sugammadex (16mg/kg) for full reversal

Prepare for rescue techniques in case child deteriorates

Step C Airway rescue techniques for CICV (SpO$_2$ <80% and falling/ and/ or heart rate decreasing

Call for help again if not arrived

Call for specialist ENT assistance

ENT available

ENT not available

Percutaneous cannula cricothyroidotomy/ transtracheal jet ventilation (pressure limited)

Succeed

Fail

Consider:
- Surgical tracheostomy
- Rigid bronchoscopy + ventilate/jet ventilation (pressure limited)

Continue jet ventilation set to lowest delivery pressure until wake up or definitive airway established

- Perform surgical cricothyroidotomy/ transtracheal and insertion of ETT/ tracheostomy tube*
- Consider passive O$_2$ insufflation while preparing

Cannula cricothyroidotomy
- Extend the neck (shoulder roll)
- Stabilise larynx with non-dominant hand
- Access the cricoithyroidotomy membrane with a dedicated 14/16 gauge cannula
- Aim in a caudad direction
- Confirm position by air aspiration using a syringe with saline
- Connect to either:
  - Adjustable pressure limiting device, set to lowest delivery pressure

  or

  - 4Bar O$_2$ source with a flowmeter (match flow l/min to child's age) and Y connector
- Cautiously increase inflation pressure/flow rate to achieve adequate chest expansion Wait for full expiration before next inflation
- Maintain uper airway patency to aid expiration

SAD = supraglottic airway device

---

*Note: Cricothyroidotomy techniques can have serious complications and training is required – only use in life-threatening situations and convert to a definitive airway as soon as possible

Fig. 58.2 Guidelines for the cannot intubate and cannot ventilate (CICV) in a paralyzed anesthetized child 1 to 8 years. Reprinted with permission: Black AE, Flynn PE, Smith HL, Thomas ML, Wilkinson KA. Development of a guideline for the management of the unanticipated difficult airway in pediatric practice. *Paediatr Anaesth.* 2015;25(4):346–362.

also found when looking at adult surgical airways. The 2015 APA/DAS Guidelines reflect these findings by providing an alternate pathway of tracheostomy and/or cricothyroidotomy placed by otolaryngologists (see Fig. 58.2).[44]

CONCLUSION

- GH syndrome is caused by growth abnormalities of the first two brachial clefts often resulting in hemiface hypoplasia. Diagnostic criteria include eye abnormalities (lipoma, lipodermoid, epibulbar dermoid, or upper eyelid coloboma) along with ear, mandibular, or vertebral anomalies.

- Difficult ventilation and/or intubation should be expected in GH syndrome and anesthesia practitioners should be adequately prepared for a difficult airway. Practitioners should also anticipate airway obstruction after extubation.

- GH patients may have vertebral abnormalities and in-line stabilization with neutral cervical spine should be maintained throughout airway manipulation.

- TIS is defined as the inability of the thorax to support normal respiration or lung growth as a result of fused ribs, scoliosis, or other musculoskeletal disease. The VEPTR device is an implantable, expandable rod used to treat TIS.

- Difficult airways requiring surgical intervention are incredibly rare in pediatric anesthesiology practice. Current guidelines recommend cannula approaches and early involvement of otolaryngology surgeons for emergency tracheotomy.

REVIEW QUESTIONS

1. Which common feature of GH syndrome is **LEAST** evident at birth?

 A. cleft palate
 B. micrognathia
 C. microtia
 D. scoliosis

Answer: D

GH syndrome is caused by growth disturbances of first and second brachial arches, leading to head and neck malformations. Spinal abnormalities such as scoliosis and kyphosis tend develop later in life and are not commonly associated with this syndrome.[4]

2. A 5-year-old child with a history of GH syndrome presents for closed reduction and percutaneous pinning of an elbow fracture. Per the parents, the patient has a history of successful intubation as an infant for mandibular surgery. Which of the following statements regarding airway management is **MOST** accurate?

 A. Mandibular hypoplasia presence warrants a three-dimensional computerized tomography scan.
 B. Normal c-spine x-rays rule out major risk of cord injury during laryngoscopy.
 C. Physical exam, after mandibular surgical repairs, will be noncontributory.
 D. Previous successful intubations assure minimal risk of present difficulties.

Answer: A

Patients with GH syndrome can have multiple craniofacial abnormalities resulting in difficult intubation. A focused history and physical is essential to preparing adequately for airway management in these patients. The airway exam should be age appropriate and evaluate the external craniofacial anatomy, with focus on the oral cavity, anterior mandibular space, maxilla, temporomandibular joint, and vertebral column. Difficulty with airway management can increase with age, and previous surgical mandibular correction does not guarantee a straightforward intubation. A previously easy intubation may be more difficult at subsequent presentation due to scar tissue and limited range of motion. Difficult airway predictors include mandibular hypoplasia, bilateral mandibular involvement, cleft lip/palate, or other craniovertebral anomalies.[4,8,18] Case reports suggest that three-dimensional CT imaging can be helpful in planning for airway management in patients with mandibular hypoplasia and may be indicated if exam suggests a difficult intubation.[19] GH syndrome is associated with vertebral anomalies and atlanto-axial instability; therefore, a history of neck pain and physical exam of neck mobility is prudent. Although normal cervical spine flexion-extension imaging may be reassuring, it does not completely rule out risk of spinal cord imaging during positioning for airway management or surgery.[11]

3. Which of the following mechanism is **MOST** accurate about the causes of GH syndrome?

 A. autosomal dominant inheritance
 B. autosomal recessive inheritance
 C. X-linked inheritance
 D. environmental and genetic factors

Answer: D

GH syndrome is due to growth disturbances of the first and second brachial arches which leads to head and neck abnormalities. GH syndrome is associated with both environmental and genetic factors, but most cases occur sporadically. In those cases that are inherited, it is more likely to be autosomal dominant, but cases of autosomal recessive inheritance have been reported. Only 1% to 2% of patients with GH syndrome also have family members who are affected.[4]

4. Which of the following statements regarding airway management in patients with GH syndrome is the **MOST** accurate?

 A. Cervical spine precautions are occasionally necessary during laryngoscopy.
 B. Bag mask ventilation is a reliably achievable element of airway management.

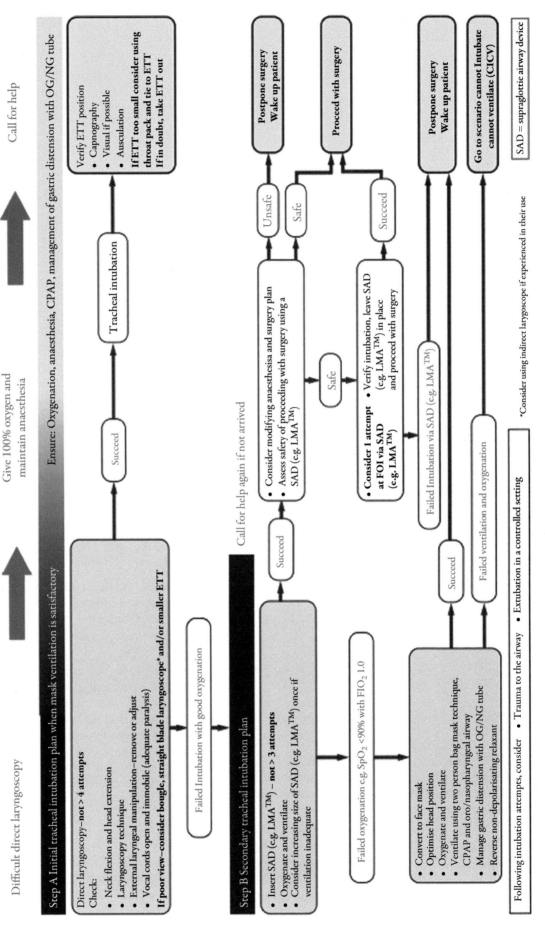

Fig. 58.3 Guidelines for unanticipated difficult tracheal intubation during routine induction of anesthesia in a child aged 1 to 8 years. Reprinted with permission from: Black AE, Flynn PE, Smith HL, Thomas ML, Wilkinson KA. Development of a guideline for the management of the unanticipated difficult airway in pediatric practice. *Paediatr Anaesth*. 2015;25(4):346–362.

C. Multiple options and approaches for intubation should be readily available.

D. Surgical airway occurrences are similar to that of the general pediatric population.

Answer: C

Due to associated vertebral anomalies, patients with GH syndrome may have atlanto-axial instability and cervical spine precautions should be considered when manipulating the head and neck to secure the airway.[11] The craniofacial abnormalities present in GH syndrome increase the likelihood of airway obstruction and difficult bag-mask ventilation and/or intubation. Experienced providers should be prepared for difficult airway management, and many techniques have been described as successful in securing the airway.[15,20,22–29,31,32] In a 1998 chart review of 251 patients with major craniofacial abnormalities (41 with OAV and 14 of those with GH syndrome) 9 patients, or 22% of OAV patients, required a surgical airway.[33]

5. Which of the following statements regarding TIS is the **LEAST** accurate?

A. Expandable titanium rib is a treatment option.

B. Lung development and function are impaired.

C. Mechanical ventilation is rarely indicated.

D. Rib fusion and scoliosis are underlying causes.

Answer: C

Thoracic insufficiency syndrome is caused by musculoskeletal abnormalities such as fused ribs or scoliosis and leads to the inability of the thorax to allow normal lung growth and pulmonary mechanics. TIS presents with varying severity, and symptoms range from playtime fatigue and recurrent pulmonary infections to respiratory failure requiring ventilator support as it progresses.[35] The VEPTR device is an implantable, expandable rod that aims to expand three-dimensional thoracic space and stabilize the diaphragm for improved breathing mechanics.[36]

6. A 2-year-old child with GH syndrome is undergoing an adenotonsillectomy for severe obstructive sleep apnea. You have done an inhalational induction and the patient begins to obstruct while breathing spontaneously. You adjust the chin lift/jaw thrust and insert an oral airway which relieves the obstruction and you are able to bag-mask ventilate. You attempt direct laryngoscopy and can only obtain a view of the epiglottis after multiple attempts before the patient's SpO2 begins to decrease. What would be the next **BEST** step in this situation?

A. Attempt placing a supraglottic airway device.

B. Call for another anesthesiologist or airway expert.

C. Prepare to wake up the patient and end the case.

D. Repeat the laryngoscopy, after repositioning.

Answer: B

In a real scenario, you likely would be doing a few things at once, but after failed intubation the appropriate next step is to call for help while you manage the patient's airway with bag-mask ventilation or a supraglottic airway. According to the unanticipated difficult tracheal intubation guidelines proposed by the DAS, direct laryngoscopy should be limited to 4 attempts while assuring optimal positioning, technique, and external laryngeal manipulation. If intubation is unsuccessful after 4 direct laryngoscoy attempts, the provider should call for help and begin a secondary intubation plan, while inserting a supraglottic airway device to assist with ventilation (see Fig. 58.3). The supraglottic airway can then be used for the case, if appropriate, or as a conduit for fiberoptic intubation. For each case, the risks and benefits of proceeding with the scheduled procedure versus waking up the patient and canceling the case need to be weighed and discussed by the providers involved.[44,49]

7. Of the following signs, which is **LEAST** likely to be found with an intraoperative pneumothorax?

A. hypotension

B. hypoxia

C. pulsus alternans

D. tracheal deviation

Answer: C

A pneumothorax occurs when air becomes trapped in the pleural space due to a defect in the chest wall or lung parenchyma and visceral pleura. This becomes a tension pneumothorax when the defect acts as a one-way valve, allowing air to enter the pleural space with inability to escape. With each breath, more air and subsequent pressure accumulates in the pleural space. This increased intrathoracic pressure leads to increased ventilation pressure, tracheal deviation to the contralateral side, and impaired venous return to the heart resulting in hypotension and increased central venous pressure. Impaired ventilation and absent air exchange on the affected side cause unilateral breath sounds and desaturation. A patient with a tension pneumothorax can deteriorate rapidly, so quick diagnosis and management is essential. However, pneumothorax is a diagnosis of exclusion, so common causes of desaturation and hypotension should be considered as well. An intraoperative chest x-ray can confirm the diagnosis if pneumothorax is suspected but should not delay treatment if the patient is decompensating. Decompression with a needle or angiocatheter should be performed with insertion at the midclavicular line in the second intercostal space.[50,51]

8. Of the following disorders on the OAV spectrum, which is the **MOST** severe?

A. GH syndrome

B. HFM

C. OAVD

D. Pierre Robin sequence

Answer: A

The OAV spectrum consists of three syndromes, GH, HFM, and OAVD. GH syndrome is the most severe and is associated with abnormalities of the eye, ear, mandible, and vertebrae. The OAV spectrum consists of syndromes, which are multiple anomalies occurring together but can also occur independently and without a known cause. Answer D is incorrect because although Pierre Robin sequence is associated with mandibular hypoplasia, it is not part of the OAV spectrum. Also, a sequence is defined as group of malformations that occur due to an inciting event. In Pierre Robin sequence, the mandibular hypoplasia leads to glossoptosis, airway obstruction, and often cleft palate.[4,9]

QUESTIONS AND ANSWERS

This chapter has accompanying questions and answers which are available to subscribers as part of the Oxford eLearning platform. To access the questions, go to ✅ http:// oxfordmedicine. com/pediatricanesthesiaPBL

REFERENCES

1. Mellor DH RJ, Douglas DM. Goldenhar's syndrome: oculoauriculovertebral dysplasia. *Arch Dis Child*. 1973;48(7):537–541.
2. Arnt CFv. *Klinische Darstellung der Krankheiten des Auges*. Vienna: Braumiiler; 1845.
3. Goldenhar M. Associations malformatives de l'oeil et de l'oreille, en particulier le syndrome dermoïde epibulbaire-appendices auriculaires-fistula auris congenita et ses relations avec la dysostose mandibulo-faciale. *J Généti Hum*. 1952;1:243–282.
4. Goldenhar disease. Gathersburg, MD: Genetic and Rare Diseases Information Center; 2017. https://rarediseases.info.nih.gov/diseases/6540/goldenhar-disease#ref_11387
5. Goldenhar syndrome. In: Chen H, ed. *Atlas of Genetic Diagnosis and Counseling*. New York: Springer; 2012:971–978.
6. Feingold M, Baum J. Goldenhar's syndrome. *Am J Dis Child*. 1978;132(2):136–138. doi:10.1001/archpedi.1978.02120270034006
7. Vento AR, LaBrie RA, Mulliken JB. The O.M.E.N.S. classification of hemifacial microsomia. *Cleft Palate-Craniofacial J*. 1991;28(1):68–76; discussion 77.
8. Cakmakkaya OSaK, Kerstin. Anaesthesia recommendations for patients suffering from Goldenhar syndrome. *Orphan Anesthesia* [Internet]; 2014. http://www.orphananesthesia.eu/en/component/docman/doc_download/181-goldenhar-syndrome.html
9. Sifuentes SM, Meeks MN, Tsai A, Elias ER. Genetics & dysmorphology. In: *CURRENT Diagnosis & Treatment Pediatrics* [Internet]. New York: McGraw-Hill; 2016. http://accessmedicine.mhmedical.com.liboff.ohsu.edu/content.aspx?bookid=1795&sectionid=125747809
10. Oculo-auriculo-vertebral spectrum. Danbury, CT: National Organization for Rare Disorders; 2007. https://rarediseases.org/rare-diseases/oculo-auriculo-vertebral-spectrum/
11. Choudhury M, Kapoor PM. Goldenhar syndrome: cardiac anesthesiologist's perspective. *Ann Card Anaesth*. 2017;20(Suppl):S61–S66.
12. Nakajima H, Goto G, Tanaka N, Ashiya H, Ibukiyama C. Goldenhar syndrome associated with various cardiovascular malformations. *Jpn Circ J*. 1998;62(8):617–620.
13. Munoz-Pedroza LA, Arenas-Sordo ML. Clinical features of 149 patients with facio-auriculo-vertebral spectrum. *Acta Otorrinolaringol Espanola*. 2013;64(5):359–362.
14. Ritchey ML, Norbeck J, Huang C, Keating MA, Bloom DA. Urologic manifestations of Goldenhar syndrome. *Urology*. 1994;43(1):88–91.
15. Milne AD, Dower AM, Hackmann T. Airway management using the pediatric GlideScope in a child with Goldenhar syndrome and atypical plasma cholinesterase. *Paediatr Anaesth*. 2007;17(5):484–487.
16. Köhler S, Vasilevsky N, Engelstad M, et al. The human phenotype ontology in 2017. *Nucl Acids Res*. 2017;45(1):D865–D876. doi:10.1093/nar/gkw1039
17. Madan R, Trikha A, Venkataraman RK, Batra R, Kalia P. Goldenhar's syndrome: an analysis of anaesthetic management. A retrospective study of seventeen cases. *Anaesthesia*. 1990;45(1):49–52.
18. Nargozian C. The airway in patients with craniofacial abnormalities. *Paediatr Anaesth*. 2004;14(1):53–59.
19. Suzuki E, Hirate H, Fujita Y, Sobue K. Successful airway management in a patient with Goldenhar syndrome using preoperative three-dimensional computed tomography. *Anaesth Intensive Care*. 2011;39(4):767–768.
20. Hasham F, van Helmond N, Sidlow R. Anaesthesia and orphan disease: difficult ventilation following intubation in Goldenhar syndrome. *Eur J Anaesthesiol*. 2017;34(3):181–183.
21. Khadilkar VV, Khadilkar AV. Goldenhar syndrome with congenital athyrosis. *Indian Pediatrics*. 2001;38(12):1419–1421.
22. Sukhupragarn W, Rosenblatt WH. Airway management in a patient with Goldenhar syndrome: a case report. *J Clin Anesth*. 2008;20(3):214–217.
23. Khan WA, Salim B, Khan AA, Chughtai S. Anaesthetic management in a child with Goldenhar syndrome. *J Coll Physicians Surg Pak*. 2017;27(3):S6–S7.
24. Aydogan MS, Begec Z, Erdogan MA, Yucel A, Ersoy MO. Airway management using the ProSeal laryngeal mask airway in a child with Goldenhar syndrome. *Eur Rev Med Pharmacol Sci*. 2012;16(4):559–561.
25. Vitkovic B, Milic M. Airway management with direct laryngoscopy in a child with Goldenhar syndrome. *Acta Clin Croatica*. 2016;55(Suppl 1):90–93.
26. Sahni N, Bhatia N. Successful management of difficult airway in an adult patient of Goldenhar syndrome. *Saudi J Anaesth*. 2014;8(Suppl 1):S98–S100.
27. Sasanuma H, Niwa Y, Shimada N, et al. [Tracheal intubation using Airtraq optical laryngoscope in an adult patient with Goldenhar syndrome]. *Masui*. 2013;62(7):867–869.
28. Al-Abri AS, Khan RM, Haris A, Kaul N. Successful airway management in patient with Goldenhar's syndrome using Truview PCD (R) laryngoscope. *Paediatr Anaesth*. 2012;22(12):1229–1231.
29. Kaji J, Higashi M, Sakaguchi Y, et al. [Fiberoptic intubation using two tracheal tubes for a child with Goldenhar syndrome]. *Masui*. 2010;59(12):1526–1528.
30. Char DS, Gipp M, Boltz MG, Williams GD. Case report: airway and concurrent hemodynamic management in a neonate with oculo-auriculo-vertebral (Goldenhar) syndrome, severe cervical scoliosis, interrupted aortic arch, multiple ventricular septal defects, and an unstable cervical spine. *Paediatr Anaesth*. 2012;22(9):932–934.
31. Ozlu O, Simsek S, Alacakir H, Yigitkanli K. Goldenhar syndrome and intubation with the fiberoptic broncoscope. *Paediatr Anaesth*. 2008;18(8):793–794.
32. Ahmed Z, Alalami A, Haupert M, Rajan S, Durgham N, Zestos MM. Airway management for rigid bronchoscopy via a freshly performed tracheostomy in a child with Goldenhar syndrome. *J Clin Anesth*. 2012;24(3):234–237.
33. Sculerati N, Gottlieb MD, Zimbler MS, Chibbaro PD, McCarthy JG. Airway management in children with major craniofacial anomalies. *Laryngoscope*. 1998;108(12):1806–1812.
34. Campbell RM Jr., Smith MD, Mayes TC, et al. The characteristics of thoracic insufficiency syndrome associated with fused ribs and congenital scoliosis. *J Bone Joint Surg American*. 2003;85a(3):399–408.
35. Campbell RM Jr., Smith MD. Thoracic insufficiency syndrome and exotic scoliosis. *J Bone Joint Surg American*. 2007;89(Suppl 1):108–122.
36. VEPTR II: Vertical Expandable Prosthetic Titanium Rib. Surgical Technique: DePuy Synthes Spine; 2015. http://sites.synthes.com/mediabin/US%20DATA/Product%20Support%20Materials/Technique%20Guides/DSUSSPN11140557_VEPTR_II_TG.pdf
37. Listing of CDRH Humanitarian Device Exemptions. Silver Spring, MD: U.S. Food and Drug Administration; 2017. https://www.fda.gov/MedicalDevices/ProductsandMedicalProcedures/DeviceApprovalsandClearances/HDEApprovals/ucm161827.htm

38. Research and Clinical Studies: Vertical Expandable Prosthetic Titanium Rib (VEPTR): Seattle Children's Hospital; 1995–2017. http://www.seattlechildrens.org/clinics-programs/orthopedics/research-and-advances/veptr. Accessed June 8, 2017.

39. Patient and Family Guide: MAGEC Noninvasive Growth Modulation: NuVasive; 2016. https://www.nuvasive.com/wp-content/uploads/2017/03/MAGEC-Patient-Education-Brochure-US.pdf. Accessed June 9, 2017.

40. Campbell Jr RM. Operative strategies for thoracic insufficiency syndrome by vertical expandable prosthetic titanium rib expansion thoracoplasty. *Oper Tech Orthop*. 2005;15(4):315–325. https://doi.org/10.1053/j.oto.2005.08.008

41. Schwartz DM, Sestokas AK, Bhalodia VM, et al. The role of neuromonitoring in growing rod and VEPTR surgery: Paper 31. *Spine: Affiliated Society Meeting Abstracts*; September 23–26; San Antonio, TX; 2009:76.

42. Waldhausen JH, Redding G, White K, Song K. Complications in using the vertical expandable prosthetic titanium rib (VEPTR) in children. *J Pediatr Surg*. 2016;51(11):1747–1750. doi:10.1016/j.jpedsurg.2016.06.014.

43. Fiadjoe JE, Nishisaki A, Jagannathan N, et al. Airway management complications in children with difficult tracheal intubation from the Pediatric Difficult Intubation (PeDI) registry: a prospective cohort analysis. *Lancet Resp Med*. 2016;4(1):37–48. doi:10.1016/s2213-2600(15)00508-1

44. Black AE, Flynn PE, Smith HL, Thomas ML, Wilkinson KA. Development of a guideline for the management of the unanticipated difficult airway in pediatric practice. *Paediatr Anaesth*. 2015;25(4):346–362. doi:10.1111/pan.12615

45. Prunty SL, Aranda-Palacios A, Heard AM, et al. The "can't intubate can't oxygenate" scenario in pediatric anesthesia: a comparison of the Melker cricothyroidotomy kit with a scalpel bougie technique. *Paediatr Anaesth*. 2015;25(4):400–404. doi:10.1111/pan.12565

46. Stacey J, Heard AM, Chapman G, et al. The "can't intubate can't oxygenate" scenario in pediatric anesthesia: a comparison of different devices for needle cricothyroidotomy. *Paediatr Anaesth*. 2012;22(12):1155–1158. doi:10.1111/pan.12048

47. Holm-Knudsen RJ, Rasmussen LS, Charabi B, Bottger M, Kristensen MS. Emergency airway access in children—transtracheal cannulas and tracheotomy assessed in a porcine model. *Paediatr Anaesth*. 2012;22(12):1159–1165. doi:10.1111/pan.12045

48. Cook TM, Woodall N, Harper J, Benger J. Major complications of airway management in the UK: results of the Fourth National Audit Project of the Royal College of Anaesthetists and the Difficult Airway Society. Part 2: intensive care and emergency departments. *Br J Anaesth*. 2011;106(5):632–642. doi:10.1093/bja/aer059

49. Weiss M, Engelhardt T. Proposal for the management of the unexpected difficult pediatric airway. *Paediatr Anaesth*. 2010;20(5):454–464. doi: 10.1111/j.1460-9592.2010.03284.x.

50. Bacon AK, Paix AD, Williamson JA, Webb RK, Chapman MJ. Crisis management during anaesthesia: pneumothorax. *Qual Saf Health Care*. 2005;14(3):e18. doi: 10.1136/qshc.2002.004424.

51. Reynolds P, Scattoloni, JA, Ehrlich P, Cladis FP, Davis PJ. Anesthesia for the Pediatric Trauma Patient. In Davis PJ, CF, Motoyama EK., eds. Philadelphia, PA: Elsevier Mosby; 2011

59.

VON WILLEBRAND DISEASE

Laura A. Downey and Nina A. Guzzetta

STEM CASE AND KEY QUESTIONS

A 4-year-old boy with a history of chronic tonsillitis comes to clinic for preoperative evaluation before a tonsillectomy. During the evaluation, his mother tells you that over the past year he has had nosebleeds about every 2 to 3 months. The last episode required a visit to the emergency room (ER). No clear etiology was diagnosed, but the bleeding stopped with pressure and time.

DOES HIS HISTORY OF EPISTAXIS AND ITS FREQUENCY CONCERN YOU REGARDING HIS UPCOMING TONSILLECTOMY? HOW WOULD YOU FURTHER EVALUATE THIS PATIENT PRIOR TO SURGERY?

On further history, you discover that he has a history of easy bruising and his gums often bleed when he brushes his teeth and after he sees the dentist. Mom says that he has not had surgery before. On physical exam, you note small bruises on his shins and arms. You decide to send baseline labs. The results are as follows:

PT 16.1; INR 1.3; aPTT 30.7; fibrinogen 379; Hb 11.7; Hct 33.9; platelets 269

ARE THERE ANY OTHER STUDIES THAT YOU WANT TO SEND? WHAT ARE THE MOST LIKELY DIAGNOSES? HOW DO YOU DIFFERENTIATE BETWEEN THESE?

The clinician should worry about bleeding disorders that may not show up in standard laboratory testing but under the surgical conditions. Bruising and history of bleeding is important to elicit. Specifically designed questionaires can help determine if a bleeding history is reflective of a true bleeding disorder. More specialized testing or a hematology consult may be required.

The diagnosis of von Willebrand disease (vWD) is often not straightforward. It is based on a personal history of bleeding, a family history of bleeding, or both in combination with laboratory tests showing abnormalities in von Willebrand factor (vWF), factor VIII (FVIII), or both. Screening tests include an activated partial thromboplastin time (aPTT), bleeding

time, or platelet function assay (PFA), but these tests lack the sensitivity and specificity for definitive diagnosis. Therefore, assays that measure vWF quantity, function, and structure are used for definitive diagnosis and management.

You consult a hematologist, who decides to send a full hematology panel. Platelet function analyzer (PFA-100') levels were abnormal. Factor activity level of FVIII and factor IX (FIX) were within normal limits. However, vWF levels were 38 IU/dL (normal >60 IU/dL). The vWF-ristocetin cofactor activity to vWF antigen ratio (vWF-ristocetin cofactor [RCo]/vWF antigen [vWF:Ag]) was >0.6, suggesting that the patient has vWD type 1.

WHAT IS VWF? WHAT IS VWD? WHAT ARE COMMON CLINICAL SYMPTOMS OF VWD? WHAT ARE THE DIFFERENT TYPES OF VWD? WHICH ONE IS THE MOST COMMON TYPE?

After diagnosing the patient with type 1 vWD, the hematologist recommends that the patient be treated with epsilon-aminocaproic acid (Amicar') 48 hours prior to the procedure and 48 hours postoperatively. Perioperatively, the patient should receive DDAVP intraoperatively and 24 hours postoperatively.

WHAT IS DDAVP? HOW DOES IT WORK? WHAT ARE THE SIDE EFFECTS OF DDAVP? WHICH TYPE OF VWD IS IT USEFUL FOR AND WHY? WHEN IS IT NOT USEFUL? HOW DO ANTIFIBRINOLYTICS WORK? WHAT OTHER MEASURES SHOULD THE SURGEON TAKE FOR HEMOSTASIS?

DDAVP, a synthetic vasopressin analog, releases vWF from endothelial cells and platelets, and increases plasma levels of vWF and FVIII. There are many routes of delivery. It is contraindicated in type 2B and ineffective in types 2N and 3 vWD. Alternative therapies include plasma and factor replacement. Antifibrinolytics also should be considered. As the name implies, antifibrinolytics prevent the clot from breaking down and fibrinolysis. The surgeon should also consider topical agents such as bovine thrombin, fibrin sealant, and local pressure.

The patient undergoes tonsillectomy without difficulty. At the end of the procedure, the otolaryngology surgeon confirms that he has good hemostasis. You wake the patient up from anesthesia and take him to the postoperative care unit (PACU).

WHAT IS AN APPROPRIATE POSTOPERATIVE PLAN FOR THIS PATIENT? CAN HE GO HOME AFTER DISCHARGE FROM PACU? SHOULD HE BE ADMITTED OVERNIGHT FOR OBSERVATION? WHAT POSTOPERATIVE INSTRUCTIONS SHOULD YOU GIVE THE PATIENT AND HIS FAMILY? WHAT MEDICATIONS WOULD YOU RECOMMEND FOR POSTOPERATIVE PAIN?

In addition to underlying bleeding disorders, patients coming in for adenotonsillectomy may need observation for their underlying obstructive sleep apnea (OSA). The gold standard to diagnose OSA still remains the sleep study. However, patient effort, cost, and availability may limit the patient's access to testing. There is agreement among otolaryngology and anesthesia societies in the United States that any child <3 years old after adenotonsillectomy needs overnight observation. However, there are no established guidelines regarding postoperative admission universally. There should be a low threshold in keeping these children for overnight observation. Discharge instructions should include adequate hydration, signs of bleeding—and if these arise they should come immediately to the ER—and pain management teaching. Children should be given only scheduled narcotics and not given any if sleepy or asleep. Also caution should be used with acetaminophen as many narcotic formulations contain acetaminophen.

The patient was admitted for observation overnight and is discharged on postoperative day (POD) 1 with Amicar˚ and no complications. On POD 6, the patient presents to the ER with recurrent bleeding. His mom reports that he was eating Goldfish crackers, choked, and coughed up a half a cup of blood. The surgeon plans to take him back to the operating room to explore.

DO YOU GET REPEAT LABS PRIOR TO SURGERY? IF SO, WHICH ONES? WHAT IS THE APPROPRIATE HEMOSTATIC MANAGEMENT? DO YOU GIVE MORE DDAVP PRIOR TO SURGERY? DO YOU USE HUMATE-P˚, CRYOPRECIPITATE, OR FRESH FROZEN PLASMA (FFP)?

A complete blood count and coagulation labs, including a vWF profile, should be obtained. If the child needs to go to the operating room emergently, infusion of vWF concentrate (Humate-P˚ or Vonvendi˚) or cryoprecipitate is indicated. Consider consultation with a hematologist to assist.

You discuss the urgency of the procedure with the surgeon, who feels that you can wait a few hours for a hematology consult and laboratory tests. You send a vWF level which is 32 IU/dL. Therefore, you continue Amicar˚, IV DDAVP and consult the hematologist for the appropriate dose of Humate-P˚. The surgery goes smoothly and hemostasis is achieved. The patient emerges uneventfully from anesthesia and is taken to the PACU.

WHAT ABOUT POSTOPERATIVE PAIN MANAGEMENT? WOULD YOU ADMIT THE CHILD FOR OBSERVATION? HOW LONG? WHAT FOLLOW UP SHOULD BE SCHEDULED?

In a procedure with a moderate to severe risk of postoperative bleeding, the child should stay in a monitored setting. In this particular scenario the clinician has to worry about postoperative bleeding as well as any effects from sleep disturbed breathing or OSA.

The patient has an uneventful perioperative course. However, he is admitted for 48 hours to ensure hemostasis, check factor levels, and continue Amicar˚. On discharge he is scheduled to see a hematologist in clinic for follow-up and a DDAVP challenge. He is discharged on POD 2.

DISCUSSION

PATHOPHYSIOLOGY

vWD is an inherited bleeding disorder first described in 1926 by a Finnish physician named Erik von Willebrand. It is the most common inherited bleeding disorder and, thus, a disease that you will likely encounter in your practice. vWD is caused by either a quantitative or a qualitative defect of vWF and displays an autosomal inheritance pattern. vWF is a large multimeric plasma glycoprotein that is synthesized in endothelial cells and released into the circulation in response to activation of the coagulation system or stressful stimuli such as infections, pregnancy, or physical exertion. vWF is also synthesized and stored in platelet α-granules and released into circulation upon platelet activation. vWF plays two essential roles in hemostasis. First, it promotes platelet adhesion to injured blood vessels. Under the turbulent flow conditions seen with vascular injury, vWF undergoes a shear-mediated conformational change thus allowing it to form a strong bond between the glycoprotein Ib platelet receptor and exposed collagen in the subendothelial matrix. In addition, vWF aids in platelet aggregation by mediating interactions between the platelet GpIIbIIIa surface receptor and fibrinogen to promote primary hemostasis.[2] Second, vWF serves as a carrier protein for factor FVIII thus protecting FVIII from degradation by activated protein C.

CLASSIFICATION

vWD is subdivided into three types that vary in clinical severity, quantity of plasma vWF, and defects in vWF structure and function: type I (partially quantitative deficiency), type 2 (qualitative deficiency), and type 3 (total deficiency). Type 1 vWD, the most common of the three subtypes, comprises 65% to 80% of vWD cases and results from mild to moderate quantitative deficiencies of otherwise normal vWF. It is inherited in an autosomal dominant pattern with incomplete penetrance and variable expression. Plasma vWF levels range from 10% to 50% of normal but can be influenced by factors such as age (plasma vWF levels increase 1%–2% per year of age) and the presence of blood group O (where vWF levels are 25% lower than in other blood groups because of deficient carbohydrate content and thus enhanced clearance of vWF).[3,4] The severity of bleeding correlates with the degree of vWF level reduction.

Type 2 vWD, about 20% of vWD cases, results from qualitative abnormalities of vWF and is further classified into four subtypes: types 2A, 2B, 2M, and 2N. Type 2A is caused by a lack of high molecular weight (HMW) vWF multimers, which are the most hemostatically effective forms of vWF. Type 2A results from failure to synthesize vWF multimers or from synthesis of a vWF molecule that is more susceptible to cleavage by ADAMTS13. Type 2B is a "gain of function" mutation that results in an increased affinity of the mutant vWF for platelet glycoprotein Ib (GpIb) receptors. Consequently, the mutant vWF is consumed in spontaneous platelet aggregation. The aggregates are removed from the circulation resulting in decreased vWF levels, thrombocytopenia, and blocked GpIb receptors on remaining platelets thus causing a subsequent bleeding diathesis. Type 2M is due to defects in the collagen-binding and platelet-binding of vWF with preservation of multimer distribution. Types 2A, 2B, and 2M are all inherited in an autosomal dominant pattern with complete penetrance and minimally variable expressivity. Lastly, type 2N (for Normandy) is an autosomal recessive trait that produces a vWF mutant with a reduced ability to bind FVIII. Thus plasma FVIII is cleared quickly resulting in low FVIII levels and a clinical picture resembling hemophilia A with bleeding into joints and muscles.

Type 3 vWD is an autosomal recessive trait characterized by a severe quantitative deficiency of vWF with virtually no vWF found in plasma or platelets. In addition, plasma FVIII levels are also severely depressed so that the clinical picture is one of both mucocutaneous bleeding and bleeding into joints and muscles.[5]

von Willebrand syndrome refers to an acquired form of vWD and is characterized by low plasma vWF levels secondary to autoantibodies against vWF, adsorption of vWF by malignant cell clones, or loss of HMW vWF multimers under conditions of high shear stress. It is rarely associated with anti-vWF inhibitors and is almost always identified by a bleeding diathesis. The etiology of von Willebrand syndrome is usually the result of autoimmune disorders (such as systemic lupus erythematosus), lymphoproliferative disorders, myeloproliferative disorders, Wilms' tumor, and conditions such as congenital heart defects, aortic stenosis, bacterial endocarditis, and atherosclerotic lesions.[6]

CLINICAL PRESENTATION

Clinical manifestations of vWD can be highly variable depending on the individual patient and the degree of quantitative or qualitative deficiencies in vWF.

Patients with type I disease and most variants of type 2 vWD have relatively mild symptoms that usually consist of mucocutaneous bleeding, easy bruising, gingival bleeding,

petechiae, epistaxis, menorrhagia, and gastrointestinal tract bleeding. These patients may have excessive bleeding after dental or surgical procedures resulting from impaired vWF-platelet interactions. For patients with types 2N and 3 vWD, the disordered hemostasis is more severe and includes delayed, deep bleeding into joints and muscles or intracranial bleeding similar to hemophilia patients since these types also have low FVIII levels. The severity of disease may be judged by the age at onset, spontaneous or traumatic triggers for bleeding, frequency of bleeding episodes, number of bleeding sites, and whether blood transfusions have been required.[7]

Diagnosis of vWD is based on personal and family history as well as coagulation tests consistent with the disease. Online assessment tools exist to determine calculated bleeding scores but are strongly dependent on age and previous bleeding episodes and are too time consuming for clinical practice. For patients presenting for preoperative evaluation, one should complete a comprehensive personal and family history and physical exam and consider a hematology consult for further guidance in obtaining an accurate diagnosis.

DIAGNOSIS

The diagnosis of vWD is often not straightforward. It is based on a personal history of bleeding, a family history of bleeding, or both in combination with laboratory tests showing abnormalities in vWF, FVIII, or both. Screening tests include an aPTT, bleeding time, or PFA, but these tests lack the sensitivity and specificity for definitive diagnosis.[8] Therefore, assays that measure vWF quantity, function, and structure are used for a definitive diagnosis and management—see Table 59.1.

Once vWD is suspected, the first level of testing comprises three measurements: (i) vWF:Ag level; (ii) the platelet-binding activity of vWF as measured by a vWF:RCo assay; and (iii) circulating FVIII activity (FVIII:C). If the results of these first level tests are all normal, then vWD is ruled out. However, if the results are in the low end of the normal range and a diagnosis of vWD is suspected, then they should be repeated because of biological variability. If the first level tests are clearly abnormal, then the diagnosis of vWD can be made. However, if the first-level tests are inconclusive, then more sophisticated second-level tests may be required to make the diagnosis.[1] Type 1 vWD will manifest a decrease in vWF:Ag with a proportionate decrease in vWF:RCo (vWF:RCo/vWF:Ag = 1). When interpreting results, one should take into account two caveats: (i) vWF may rise in response to stressful stimuli (i.e., blood draws) and should be rechecked if the tests are normal but the suspicion for vWD remains high, and (ii) patients with type O blood have 25% lower levels of vWF at baseline.[4] Types 2A, 2B, and 2M vWD will show a decrease in vWF:Ag but a disproportionately larger decrease in the functional vWF:RCo assay (vWF:RCo/vWF:Ag < 0.6–0.7). Thrombocytopenia, due to spontaneous binding and consumption of the vWF-platelet complex, may be seen in varying degrees in patients with type 2B vWD. To distinguish between the different type 2A, 2B, and 2M subtypes, second-level tests to assess the distribution pattern of vWF multimers are required.[1] Type 2N vWD is distinguished by a very reduced

Table 59.1 LABORATORY TESTS FOR VON WILLEBRAND DISEASE

LABORATORY TEST	PURPOSE
vWF:Ag	Measures total vWF protein
vWF:RCo	Measures vWF activity in terms of ristocetin-mediated platelet binding
FVIII:C	Measures circulating FVIII levels
vWF multimer distribution	Assesses amount of high molecular weight multimers

Note. vWF = von Willebrand factor; Ag = antigen; RCo = ristocentin cofactor assay; FVIII:C = factor VIII coagulant activity.

FVIII:C assay in the presence of relatively normal values of other first-level tests. Type 3 vWD shows absent vWF:Ag and vWF:RCo with extremely low FVIII:C. A summary of the expected laboratory values seen in the various types of vWD is provided in Table 59.2. Genotyping of the vWF gene is not routinely performed in the diagnosis of vWD. However, genetic analysis is useful to distinguish between subtypes 2B and 2N and for counseling in families with type 3 disease. New innovations in gene sequencing techniques have made genotyping more assessable and easier to perform.[1]

TREATMENT

Treatment of vWD aims to improve hemostatic efficiency by normalizing levels of both vWF and FVIII. This can be achieved by increasing endogenous levels of vWF with the use of desmopressin (1-deamino-8-D-arginine vasopressin [DDAVP]) or by administering exogenous coagulation factors in the form of a low purity FVIII vWF concentrate or a high purity vWF concentrate. Patients with type 1 disease may only require treatment if met with a hemostatic challenge, such as surgery or trauma. However, patients with more severe disease may require routine treatment with vWF and FVIII

Table 59.2 EXPECTED LABORATORY VALUES AND TREATMENT OPTIONS IN THE VARIOUS VON WILLEBRAND DISEASE TYPES

TYPE	CLINICAL MANIFESTATIONS	DEFICIENCY	TESTS	SURGICAL PROPHYLAXIS MINOR	MAJOR
Type 1	Mucocutaneous bleeding; severity determined by vWF levels	Quantitative ß Normal vWF	ßvWF:Ag <40 IU/dL *40-60 IU/dL mild ßvWF:RCo vWF:RCo/vWF:Ag = 1	DDAVP	vWF/FVIII cryo
Type 2A	Mucocutaneous bleeding, severity dependent on vWF function and quantity	Qualitative ß HMW vWF multimers	ßvWF:Ag ßßvWF:RCo vWF:RCo/vWF:Ag = 0.6-0.7	DDAVP	vWF/FVIII cryo
Type 2B	Mucocutaneous bleeding, severity dependent on vWF function and quantity	Function Ý binding of vWF to platelets; Ý vWF-platelet complex clearance	ßvWF:Ag ßßvWF:RCo vWF:RCo/vWF:Ag = 0.6-0.7 Thrombocyotpenia	vWF/FVIII cryo	vWF/FVIII cryo
Type 2N	Mucocutaneous bleeding; delayed deep bleeding in muscles, joints, head	Function ß vWF binding to FVIII, ß FVIII levels	Normal vWF:Ag Normal vWF:RCo ßß FVIII:C	vWF/FVIII cryo	vWF/FVIII cryo
Type 2M	Mucocutaneous bleeding, severity dependent on vWF function and quantity	Function Defective platelet and collagen binding	ßvWF:Ag ßßvWF:RCo vWF:RCo/vWF:Ag = 0.6-0.7	DDAVP	vWF/FVIII cryo
Type 3	Mucocutaneous bleeding; delayed deep bleeding in muscles, joints, head	Quantitative ßßß normal vWF ßßß FVIII	ßßßvWF:Ag <5 IU/dL ßßßvWF:RCo ßßßFVIII:C	vWF/FVIII cryo	vWF/FVIII cryo

Note. vWD = von Willebrand disease; vWF = von Willebrand factor; Ag = antigen; RCo = ristocentin cofactor assay; FVIII:C = factor VIII coagulant activity; HMW = high molecular weight; DDAVP = desmopressin; cryo = cryoprecipitate.

or as prophylaxis prior to surgery. Patients with a known personal or family history of vWD should undergo perioperative consultation with a hematologist at least 1 month prior to a scheduled surgery to allow time for thorough evaluation and planning. The type of vWD will determine the appropriate perioperative management.

The goals of treatment of vWD are to restore the normal platelet adhesion of primary hemostasis and to increase abnormally low levels of FVIII—see Table 59.2. For minor surgery or tooth extraction, levels of 40% to 50% of vWF:RCo and FVIII:C are considered sufficient. For patients requiring major surgery or with life-threatening hemorrhage, levels of 80% to 100% are desired. Postoperatively, levels should be greater than 50% for at least 3 days for vWF:RCo and for 5 to 7 days for FVIII:C.[8]

DDAVP

DDAVP, a synthetic vasopressin analog, releases vWF from endothelial cells and platelets and increases plasma levels of vWF and FVIII. It is effective in treating mucocutaneous bleeding and prophylaxis for minimally invasive procedures in up to 80% of patients with type 1 vWD. It will also restore plasma levels of FVIII and vWF in patients with type 2A and 2M vWD, but the vWF will still be qualitatively deficient so primary hemostasis may continue to be abnormal. DDAVP is contraindicated in type 2B since the release of defective vWF will exacerbate the thrombocytopenia associated with this form of the disease. DDAVP is ineffective in patients with type 2N and type 3 vWD. These patients will require factor replacement of vWF and FVIII.

DDAVP can be administered intranasally, subcutaneously, or intravenously, but its effect on raising vWF and FVIII levels should be measured before it is needed to treat or prevent active bleeding. The National Heart, Lung, and Blood Institute Expert Panel recommends that vWF:RCo and FVIII levels should be measured at baseline, 1 hour after administration, and 2 to 4 hours after administration to determine the effectiveness of DDAVP on elevating vWF levels.[9] It may be re-dosed every 12 to 24 hours depending on the individual response, but repeated use may lead to tachyphylaxis if used for more than 3 to 5 days. DDAVP causes mild side effects such as flushing and hypotension. More serious but rare side effects include volume overload and hyponatremia. Therefore, fluids and serum electrolytes should be monitored and adjusted as necessary to avoid volume overload, hyponatremia, and seizures.

Factor replacement

When DDAVP is contraindicated or ineffective or when prolonged hemostatic coverage is required for major surgeries, virally inactivated plasma-derived vWF concentrates (with or without FVIII) or recombinant vWF may be required. Options for these patients include treatment with a commercially available factor concentrate or cryoprecipitate, which contains both vWF and FVIII as well as fibrinogen and FXIII. Food and Drug Administration (FDA)–approved

concentrates include Humate-P˙ (human derived vWF; CSL Behring, Marburg, Germany), Wilate˙ (human derived vWF/FVIII complex; Octapharma USA, New Jersey, USA) and Vonvendi˙ (recombinant vWF; Shire Pharmaceutical Holdings Ireland Limited, Baxalta Incorporated; Dublin, Ireland). Unfortunately, individuals with type 3 vWD can develop anti-vWF antibodies after repeated infusion of vWF concentrates.

In 2015, Vonvendi˙, a recombinant vWF concentrate, was approved by the FDA for the treatment of bleeding episodes in adults with vWD. It has a low risk of viral transmission and allergic reactions and increases vWF activity in comparison with plasma-derived vWF.[1] An infusion of recombinant vWF in conjunction with a single dose of recombinant FVIII was shown to be highly effective in stopping bleeding without significant side effects in patients with severe vWD.[10]

For patients with deficient vWF, FVIII replacement is also necessary to achieve hemostasis. vWF chaperones FVIII to regulate its half-life, distribution, and activity. vWF also prevents FVIII degradation by activated protein C. In normal plasma, about 95% of FVIII is bound to vWF. However, for patients with type 3 and 2N (a mutation in vWF and FVIII binding site), the half-life of FVIII is reduced from 10 to 14 hours to approximately 3 hours, leaving these patients with 2% to 8% of normal FVIII. Therefore, patients will require replacement of FVIII in addition to vWF. However, supratherapeutic FVIII levels (greater than 150 IU/dL), may increase the risk of thrombosis.[8] As a result, US treatment guidelines recommend that FVIII:C concentrations should remain below 250% for FVIII and 200% for vWF:RCo. European guidelines recommend maintaining FVIII levels between 50 IU/dL and 150 IU/dL perioperatively.[11]

Adjuvant therapies

In patients with oral or mucosal bleeding, antifibrinolytic treatment (e.g., tranexamic acid and epsilon aminocaproic acid) is an important adjuvant therapy to prevent fibrinolysis after hemostasis has been achieved. Antifibrinolytics are typically given for 3 to 7 days following the surgical procedure. Antifibrinolytic use is contraindicated in urinary tract bleeding because of the risk of developing ureteral clots and hydronephrosis. Long-term prophylaxis is recommended for individuals with life-threatening bleeding episodes, severe menorrhagia not responsive to hormonal regulation, or repeated bleeding in joints, muscles, or the gastrointestinal tract.[12–14] If a patient continues to bleed despite adequate vWF and FVIII replacement therapy, platelet transfusions may be required. Consideration should always be given to careful surgical hemostasis which may require topical agents, such as bovine thrombin or fibrin sealant, or local pressure.

PERIOPERATIVE MANAGEMENT

In patients presenting for surgery, the goal is to normalize vWF:RCo and FVIII activity by the administration of either DDAVP or a vWF concentrate. Both values should be greater than 100 IU/dL to ensure normal hemostasis during surgery. For several days after surgery, trough levels should be monitored and maintained at a minimum of 50 IU/dL. Consider further consultation with a hematologist prior to surgery.

Perioperative recommendations for minor surgery:[14]

1. Loading dose: 30–60 IU/kg of vWF

2. Maintenance dose: 20–40 IU/kg of vWF every 12–48 hours

3. Monitoring: vWF:RCo and FVIII troughs at least once

4. Therapeutic goal: Trough vWF:RCo and FVIII >50 U/dL for 3–5 days

Perioperative recommendations for major surgery:[14]

1. Loading dose: 40–60 IU/kg of vWF

2. Maintenance dose: 20–40 IU/kg of vWF every 8–24 hours

3. Monitoring: vWF:RCo and FVIII troughs at least daily

4. Therapeutic goal: Trough vWF:RCo and FVIII >50 U/dL for 7–14 days

POSTOPERATIVE MANAGEMENT

As patients with vWD are at increased risk for bleeding after surgical procedures, the severity of disease and hemostatic challenge should be considered when planning for postoperative monitoring and discharge. These patients may require admission or close follow-up postoperatively for possible re-bleeding, electrolyte abnormalities and volume overload after DDAVP treatment, antifibrinolytic treatment, or continued factor replacement and monitoring.

REVIEW QUESTIONS

1. A 6-year-old 30-kg boy comes to day surgery for bilateral inguinal hernia repairs. During his preoperative evaluation, his mom reports that he bruises easily and his gums bleed when he brushes his teeth. The mother reports that she too bruises easily and has heavy menorrhagia. What is the **BEST** next step in the management of this patient?

    A. cryoprecipitate intravenously 10 mL/kg
    B. desmopressin intranasally 150 ug/kg
    C. desmopressin intravenously 3 ug/kg
    D. reschedule the surgery

Answer: B
Treat the patient with 150ug/kg of intranasal desmopressin preoperatively. Based on the patient and family history, this patient most likely has type 1 vWD. He is scheduled for minor surgery with minimal risk of bleeding. DDAVP, a synthetic analog of antidiuretic hormone, stimulates the release of vWF from storage sites (platelets and endothelial cells), thus raising vWF levels for adequate hemostasis. In patients with type 1 vWD, DDAVP is the first line of treatment for managing hemostasis in minor surgeries and dental extractions. The intranasal dose of DDAVP is 150µg/kg (or 1 puff) for children weighing less than 50 kg and 300ug/kg (2 puffs) for children weighing greater than 50 kg. The intranasal route has a peak onset of 90 to 120 minutes. (C) Intravenous administration is also effective but the appropriate dose is 0.3 ug/kg (not 3µg/kg) over 15 to 30 minutes, with a peak level at 30 to 60 minutes after injection. (D) The case does not need to be rescheduled for type 1 vWD with minimal symptoms and minor surgery. (A) Human derived products, such as cryoprecipitate and FFP, should be avoided if possible.

2. A 4-year-old patient with a history of type 1 vWD undergoes tonsillectomy. She is treated with DDAVP and amino-caproic acid intraoperatively. Postoperatively, she is admitted for monitoring. On POD 1, her platelets are 157K, hematocrit 35%, vWF:RCo 30 IU/dL. What would be the **MOST** appropriate treatment for this patient to prevent bleeding?

    A. Amicar ®
    B. DDAVP
    C. Humate P
    D. platelets

Answer: C
Use Humate P to increase vWF:RCo to >50 IU/dL. For patients requiring major surgery, current guidelines recommend preoperative vWF:RCo and FVIII:C levels to be 100 IU/dL. Postoperatively, vWF:RCo and FVII:C levels should be maintained >50 IU/dL for at least the first few postoperative days. The best way to increase levels of vWF are with factor replacements, such as Humate P. vWF:RCo assays notoriously have a high intra- and interlaboratory variability. FVIII:C assays are less complex and more standardized so it is recommended to monitor both. (B) After the initial dose of DDAVP, it may take 24 to 48 hours to replenish the stores of vWF and therefore a second dose may not achieve adequate levels for hemostasis. (A). Amino-caproic acid (Amicar®) should be continued at 100 mg by mouth every 4–6 hours for 5–7 days postoperatively, but this will not increase the vWF activity adequately. (D) The platelet count is adequate and a transfusion will not increase vWF. While cryoprecipitate will increase vWF and FVIII levels, factor replacements are first line if available.

3. Which of the following is **MOST** likely the result of administration of DDAVP?

    A. dehydration
    B. hypernatremia
    C. seizures
    D. thrombosis

Answer: C
Seizures secondary to hyponatremia are the mostly likely side effect of those listed. (A) DDAVP is an analog to antidiuretic hormone, which results in fluid retention, potential volume overload, and (B) hyponatremia, not hypernatremia. (D) Thrombosis is a very unlikely side effect of DDAVP.

4. A 14-year-old female with a history of vWD presents for spine surgery. She has a history of easy bruising, epistaxis, and heavy menorrhagia. Her laboratory tests demonstrate the following: platelets 110K, vWF:Ag 30 IU/dL; vWF:RCo/vWF:Ag = 0.6. What is the **MOST** appropriate perioperative treatment for a patient with these laboratory findings undergoing major spine surgery?

    A. DDAVP, amino-caproic acid, platelets
    B. DDAVP and amino-caproic acid
    C. FFP, cryoprecipitate, platelets
    D. Humate P, platelets, amino-caproic acid

Answer: D

The answer is Humate P, platelets, Amino-caproic acid. Based on the symptoms and laboratory testing, this patient has type 2B vWD. These patients have a "gain of function" mutation that results in an increased affinity of the mutant vWF for platelet GpIb receptors. Consequently, the mutant vWF is consumed in spontaneous platelet aggregation. The aggregates are removed from the circulation resulting in decreased vWF levels, thrombocytopenia, and blocked GpIb receptors on remaining platelets thus causing a subsequent bleeding diathesis. (A), (B) DDAVP is contraindicated in type 2B vWD since the release of vWF will exacerbate the thrombocytopenia common to these conditions. (C) Although this patient is having major surgery and may require blood products, the low levels of vWF and FVIII should be replaced perioperatively with factor replacement therapy under the guidance of a hematologist.

5. A patient presents to the ER with a diagnosis of vWD and bleeding into his knee. On laboratory tests, the vWF:Ag and vWF:RCo are normal. What is the **MOST** likely pathophysiology of this patient with normal levels of vWF and a bleeding diathesis?

    A. FVIII low due to ineffective FVIII binding causing increased clearance
    B. multimers hemostatically ineffective in spite of normal v-WF levels
    C. platelet aggregates consumption increased due to platelets v-WF binding
    D. platelet aggregation decreased by collagen and platelet binding deficiencies

Answer: A

The correct answer is normal vWF levels but defective FVIII binding site that results in increased FVIII clearance and therefore defective thrombin generation. This patient is presenting with symptoms similar to hemophilia, suggestive of a FVIII deficiency, as seen in type 2N and type 3 vWD. However, his vWF level is normal, confirming the diagnosis of type 2N. Therefore, his vWF level may be normal, but he has a defective FVIII binding site, leading to very low levels of FVIII. Like hemophilia, decreased FVIII levels prevent the formation of the FVIIIa/FIXa complex that activates FX and subsequent thrombin generation. (B) Type 2A has decreased levels of vWF and inability to form hemostatically effective multimers. (C) Type 2 B vWD patients have low levels of vWF

and increased binding of vWF to platelets causing increased clearance of vWF-platelet complex. (D) Type 2M patients also have decreased vWF levels and defective platelet and collagen binding.

6. Of the following laboratory testing for suspected vWD, which would **MOST** likely be performed first?

    A. FVIII (circulating) activity
    B. platelet function assay
    C. vWF antigen level
    D. vWF multimer distribution

Answer: B

Platelet function assays, such as the platelet analyzer 100 (PFA-100), have a high sensitivity for detecting vWD and are often used as a screening test. Once vWD is suspected, the first level of testing comprises laboratory testing to measure the following: (i) vWF:Ag level; (ii) the platelet-binding activity of vWF as measured by a vWF:RCo assay; (iii) FVIII:C activity. If the results of these first level tests are all normal, then vWD is ruled out. Once the diagnosis is made, second-level tests to assess the distribution pattern of vWF multimers are necessary to distinguish between the different type 2A, 2B, and 2M subtypes.

QUESTIONS AND ANSWERS

This chapter has accompanying questions and answers which are available to subscribers as part of the Oxford eLearning platform. To access the questions, go to ✔ http://oxfordmedicine. com/pediatricanesthesiaPBL

REFERENCES

1. Longo DL, Leebeek FWG, Eikenboom JCJ. Von Willebrand's disease. *N Engl J Med*. 2016;375:2067–2080.
2. Jackson SP. The growing complexity of platelet aggregation. *Blood*. 2007;109:5087–5095.
3. Kumar R, Carcao M. Inherited abnormalities of coagulation: hemophilia, von Willebrand disease, and beyond. *Pediatr Clin North Am*. 2013;60:1419–1441.
4. Gill JC, Endres-Brooks J, Bauer PJ, et al. The effect of ABO blood group on the diagnosis of von Willebrand disease. *Blood*. 1987;69:1691–1695.
5. Flood V.H. Perils, problems, and progress in laboratory diagnosis of von Willebrand disease. *Semin Thromb Hemost*. 2014;40:41–48.
6. Federici AB, Budde U, Castaman G. Current diagnostic and therapeutic approaches to patients with acquired von Willebrand syndrome: a 2013 update. *Semin Thromb Hemost*. 2013;39:191–201.
7. James AH, Eikenboom J, Federici AB. State of the art: von Willebrand disease. *Haemophilia*. 2016;22:54–59.
8. Miesbach W, Berntorp W. Von Willebrand disease—the "dos" and "don'ts" in surgery. *Eur J Haematol*. 2016;98:121–127.
9. Nichols WL, Rick ME, Ortel TL, et al. Clinical and laboratory diagnosis of von Willebrand disease: a synopsis of the 2008 NHLBI/NIH guidelines. *Am J Hematol*. 2009;84:366–370.
10. Gill JC, Castaman G, Windyga J, et al. Hemostatic efficacy, safety, and pharmacokinetics of a recombinant von Willebrand factor in severe von Willebrand disease. *Blood*. 2015;126:2038–2046.

11. Miesbach W, Berntorp E. Interaction between vWf and FVIII in treating vWd. *Eur J Haematol*. 2015;95:449–454.
12. Lillicrap D. von Willebrand disease: advances in pathogenetic understanding, diagnosis, and therapy. *Blood*. 2013;122:3735–3740.
13. James PD, Lillicrap D. von Willebrand disease: clinical and laboratory lessons learned from the large von Willebrand disease studies. *Am J Hematol*. 2012;87:S4–S11.
14. Castaman G, Goodeve A, Eikenboom J. Principles of care for the diagnosis and treatment of von Willebrand disease. *Haematologica*. 2013;98:667–674.

60.

TRAUMA

David A. Young

STEM CASE AND KEY QUESTIONS

Your patient is a 10-year-old male who is the victim of gun violence. The patient and his father were apparently involved in a road rage incident earlier today. It appears that they were followed home by the suspects; multiple gunshots were then heard by several of the neighbors. A neighbor found your patient and his father located just outside their house with multiple gunshot wounds. The father was taken to the local community hospital in stable condition with an isolated gunshot wound (GSW) to the arm.

Your patient was taken to your institution which is the nearest Level 1 trauma center. According to the prehospital report from the paramedics, your patient is reported to have a Glasgow Coma Scale (GCS) score of 12. Your patient has the following known injuries: 2 GSWs to the left abdomen and a GSW to the left femur. Supplemental oxygen via a non-rebreather face mask, cervical spine immobilization, and intravenous access have all been obtained.

Vital signs en route to your facility include: temperature (axillary) 35.1°C, respiratory rate 36, heart rate 134, blood pressure 80/48, oxygen saturation 99%. The paramedics have no additional information about this patient. Estimated time for arrival is 7 minutes.

You have been called to the emergency department (ED) for possible airway management. This is standard practice in your institution for all pediatric trauma patients. Upon arrival to the ED, you are the only physician available to care for this patient; the two ED physicians are currently caring for two other patients who are both in critical condition. You have been asked to initiate the evaluation and resuscitation of this trauma patient using Advanced Trauma Life Support (ATLS) principles.

WHY DO YOU THINK THAT THE PRINCIPLES OF ATLS ARE RELEVANT AND BENEFICIAL TO ALL ANESTHESIA PROVIDERS WHO CARE FOR PEDIATRIC TRAUMA PATIENTS?

The patient has arrived at your facility. Vital signs are currently: temperature (axillary) 35.0°C, respiratory rate 34, heart rate 138, blood pressure 84/46, oxygen saturation 99%; GCS Score 12.

WHAT WOULD BE YOUR STRATEGY FOR THE INITIAL EVALUATION AND MANAGEMENT OF THIS TRAUMA PATIENT? WHAT IS THE GCS AND HOW IS THIS SCORE USEFUL IN THE CARE OF PEDIATRIC TRAUMA PATIENTS?

Upon arrival, the patient was receiving an intravenous fluid bolus. This fluid bolus has just completed. The patient has the following vital signs:

Temperature (axillary) 35.1°C, respiratory rate 30, heart rate 136, blood pressure 70/38, oxygen saturation 98% (non-rebreather face mask)

Patient's estimated weight: 30 kg

GCS score: 11

Last oral intake: solid food 3 hours ago

IF YOU THINK THAT THE ADMINISTRATION OF ADDITIONAL VOLUME PRODUCTS IS INDICATED, HOW WILL YOU DECIDE BETWEEN ADMINISTERING CRYSTALLOID, COLLOID, OR BLOOD PRODUCTS? WHAT TYPE(S) AND AMOUNTS OF VOLUME PRODUCTS WILL YOU ADMINISTER? ARE THERE ANY ADVANTAGES TO ONE PRODUCT? WHAT IS YOUR NEXT STEP IN MANAGEMENT IF THE ADDITIONAL FLUID BOLUS IS INEFFECTIVE?

The patient's mother was contacted by the charge nurse. Additional medical history was obtained from mother including:

No known drug allergies

Medications: Albuterol only as needed, last administration 2 months ago

Past medical history: well-controlled asthma

Past surgical history: none

DESCRIBE YOUR STRATEGY TO EVALUATE THE CERVICAL SPINE IN THIS PATIENT. SUPPOSE THE COMPUTED TOMOGRAPHY (CT) SCAN OF THE CERVICAL SPINE IS NEGATIVE; IS THIS INFORMATION SUFFICIENT TO CLEAR THE CERVICAL SPINE? IF NOT, WHAT ADDITIONAL INFORMATION WOULD BE REQUIRED TO CLEAR THE CERVICAL SPINE? IF THE CERVICAL SPINE IS NOT CLEARED PREOPERATIVELY, HOW WOULD A MAGNETIC RESONANCE IMAGING (MRI) STUDY BE USEFUL IN THE *POSTOPERATIVE* EVALUATION OF THIS PATIENT'S CERVICAL SPINE?

You perform a physical examination of the patient and order laboratory as well as imaging studies.

Physical Examination was performed and is significant for the following:

Airway: externally appears adequate; cervical collar in place

Chest/Heart: bilaterally equal breath sounds; heart sounds normal; no wheezing

Two GSWs to the left anterior abdomen; no GSW wounds present on posterior back

Abdomen is tender and mildly distended

Left femur with GSW and deformity present

Remainder of the physical exam is grossly negative

Imaging studies are significant for the following:

Chest x-ray: grossly clear; no pneumothorax or rib fractures

Left leg x-ray: left femur shaft fracture

Focused Assessment with Sonography for Trauma (FAST) exam: free fluid identified in the abdomen

CT scan of the head-brain and cervical spine without contrast: brain grossly normal without fracture, bleed, or midline shift; cervical spine grossly normal

Laboratory studies are all pending.

WHAT IS THE DIFFERENCE BETWEEN BLUNT AND PENETRATING TRAUMA? IN GENERAL, HOW DOES THE ANESTHETIC AND SURGICAL MANAGEMENT DIFFER FOR PENETRATING VERSUS BLUNT TRAUMATIC INJURIES?

The patient is now scheduled for an emergent exploratory laparotomy and a left femur intramedullary (IM) rod placement. You have no additional preoperative information on this patient. No previous medical records are found on this patient within your hospital's electronic medical record. Induction of general anesthesia was uneventful using cervical spine immobilization and a rapid sequence induction technique. The patient has 2 peripheral intravenous lines and a radial arterial line. Significant blood loss occurs during the commencement of the exploratory laparotomy. Estimated blood loss is suddenly 800 cc; you promptly resume fluid resuscitation.

WHAT IS A MASSIVE TRANSFUSION? HOW DOES THE USE OF A MASSIVE TRANSFUSION PROTOCOL (MTP) DIFFER FROM A TRADITIONAL TRANSFUSION? WHAT ARE SOME OF THE CONSEQUENCES FROM ADMINISTERING LARGE VOLUMES OF BLOOD PRODUCTS?

Intraabdominal bleeding continues despite the administration of blood products. The surgeons have decided to pack the abdomen and strongly feel that the bleeding is not due to surgical causes.

WHAT IS DAMAGE CONTROL SURGERY (DCS)? WHAT ADDITIONAL DIAGNOSTIC AND TREATMENT STRATEGIES TO CONTROL THE BLEEDING SHOULD BE CONSIDERED? DO YOU THINK THAT THE ADMINISTRATION OF RECOMBINANT FACTOR VIIA AND/OR FACTOR EIGHT INHIBITOR BYPASSING ACTIVITY (FEIBA) WOULD BE BENEFICIAL FOR THIS CLINICAL SETTING?

The abdominal bleeding has been controlled after the administration of multiple types of blood products. The vital signs are stable and age appropriate; however, the temperature has decreased to 34.5°C. The most recent arterial blood gas with metabolic panel is within normal limits including a normal pH, P_aO_2, P_aCO_2, hemoglobin, electrolytes, and lactate level. The laparotomy portion has been completed; the IM rod placement is now ready to begin.

WHAT CARDIOPULMONARY CONDITION(S) IS THIS PATIENT AT ADDITIONAL RISK FOR DURING IM ROD PLACEMENT? HOW WOULD THESE ADDITIONAL CARDIOPULMONARY CONDITION(S) BE RECOGNIZED IF THEY OCCURRED? WHAT WOULD THE MANAGEMENT BE FOR THESE CARDIOPULMONARY CONDITION(S)? WHAT ARE THE POTENTIAL CONSEQUENCES FROM THE PATIENT'S DECREASED TEMPERATURE VALUE?

The case is complete and the patient is in stable condition. The patient was extubated in the operating room uneventfully and transferred to the pediatric intensive care unit (PICU) with stable vital signs. Report to the PICU team as well as transfer of care was completed.

DISCUSSION

Pediatric patients with traumatic injuries can vary in complexity ranging from an adolescent with a simple, isolated forearm fracture to an infant with a life-threatening abdominal hemorrhage requiring emergent surgery. Several studies have shown that unintentional firearm injuries in children predominantly involve the home, family-owned weapons, and younger aged children and consist of male shooters; most importantly, they can be prevented through adult responsibility for minimizing child access and having secure storage of firearms.[1] Trauma patients may present hemodynamically unstable and with unpredictable circumstances. Patient information may be limited or unknown including important details such as past medical history, past surgical history, and drug allergies. Although the general principles of resuscitation for pediatric trauma patients are like those for adults, effective management of the pediatric trauma patient also requires understanding of the anatomical, physiological, developmental, and emotional differences that differentiate children from adults.

The management of pediatric trauma patients typically includes the contribution from a multidisciplinary team.[2] Anesthesiologists comprise a critical role within this team in many capacities. Anesthesiologists may be summoned unexpectedly to the ED to assist with airway management as well as the unplanned emergent operative case. Anesthesiologists, surgeons, and other personnel should work together as a coordinated team when managing children with traumatic injuries. This collaborative approach can optimize the prompt and consistent identification of traumatic injuries so that the anesthesiologist can more effectively anticipate future bleeding, possible physiologic consequences, and nature of the planned surgical procedures. Once the decision that the pediatric trauma patient requires operative intervention, the anesthesiologist should perform a preoperative evaluation that focuses on the items listed in Table 60.1.

The principles of ATLS[3] closely resemble established teaching philosophies within anesthesiology training regarding the resuscitation of a critically ill patient. ATLS principles are widely accepted within the medical community as well as required certification for many surgeons and emergency medicine physicians. Anesthesiologists should be familiar with the initial evaluation and management of pediatric traumatic injuries to continue this care effectively into the perioperative setting; this can be accomplished by being cognizant of the ATLS guidelines.[4] The initial prioritizing of a trauma patient follows the order of "ABCs," which is typically utilized by many anesthesiologists for the initial evaluation of any critically ill patient. In addition, recognition of the ATLS guidelines currently being performed by other providers may influence perioperative system utilization more effectively.[5]

Based on the most recent ATLS guidelines,[6,7] which were last updated by the American College of Surgeons in 2012, the initial evaluation of the pediatric trauma patient is termed the primary survey. The sequence of the primary survey can be remembered as "ABCDE" and includes: A (airway), B (breathing), C (circulation), D (disability), and E (exposure/environment). The A (airway) should be examined for patency and opened using a jaw-thrust technique as opposed to using maneuvers which utilize head extension. Immobilization of the cervical spine should be maintained at all times including during airway management. Suctioning of secretions from the oral and/or nasal cavities may also be required. The patient's B (breathing) and ventilation should be evaluated and prompt intervention should take place such as providing bag-mask ventilation. C (circulation) is evaluated by blood pressure, palpation of pulses, sensorium, and skin turgor. Control of hemorrhage should also take place; this can typically be achieved by the placement of direct pressure to the area that is bleeding. If the patient is found to be pulseless, chest compressions should be started immediately. The key components of Pediatric Basic Life Support are listed in Table 60.2. D (disability) is evaluated by looking for potential neurological injuries. The GCS is one of the most common scales used to estimate the severity of neurological injury; a modified pediatric version is also available. E (exposure) of the entire patient should occur. The environment (E) should consist of providing a heated treatment area to reduce hypothermia as well as evaluating for environment threats such as chemical contamination of the patient. Table 60.3 depicts the ATLS management categories and corresponding anesthetic implications during the primary survey.

Table 60.1 ITEMS THAT SHOULD BE OBTAINED DURING THE PREOPERATIVE EVALUATION OF THE PEDIATRIC TRAUMA PATIENT

PREINJURY ITEMS	CURRENT ITEMS
Medical history	Vital signs
Surgical history	Airway/c-spine evaluation
Drug allergies	Planned surgical procedure(s)
Current medications	List of known injuries
Fasting time	Treatment(s) since arrival
Anesthetic history	Relevant laboratory/imaging results

Table 60.2 KEY COMPONENTS OF PEDIATRIC BASIC LIFE SUPPORT

1. Determine responsiveness and if palpable pulse

2. Call for help and emergency equipment

3. If pulseless, promptly begin chest compressions
   (15:2 ratio compressions to breaths, if multiple rescuers)
   Compression rate goal of 100–120/minute
   Breathing rate goal of 12–20/minute

4. Re-evaluate patient every 2 minutes

5. Analyze heart rhythm when equipment arrives

6. Transition care to Advanced Life Support when available

Table 60.3 ADVANCED TRAUMA LIFE SUPPORT MANAGEMENT CATEGORIES AND CORRESPONDING ANESTHETIC IMPLICATIONS DURING THE PRIMARY SURVEY

CATEGORY	ANESTHETIC IMPLICATIONS
Airway	In-line stabilization of cervical spine
	Evaluate for airway patency and use jaw-thrust if indicated
	Consider placement of advanced airway
Breathing	Consider bag-mask ventilation
Circulation	Hemorrhage control/obtain hemostasis using direct pressure
	Administration of blood products if refractory to crystalloids
	Evaluate peripheral pulses, blood pressure, heart rate, sensorium
Disability	Calculate Glasgow Coma Scale score
	Assess neurologic status and deficits
Environment	Heated treatment area to reduce hypothermia
	Assess for environment threats to patient and care team

The secondary survey is a comprehensive head-to-toe patient examination. It is not begun until the primary survey is complete and the patient is in an overall stable condition. If clinical deterioration should occur at any time, practitioners must return to the primary survey and reinstituting resuscitation should ensue. A complete neurological exam and imaging studies such as CT scans and FAST exams are completed during the secondary survey. Laboratory studies are also completed during the secondary survey and characteristically include hemoglobin/hematocrit, serum chemistries, coagulation profiles, and blood product cross-matching.

The GCS is the most common scale utilized to estimate the severity of neurological injury among trauma patients. A GCS score of 8 or less implies severe neurological injury and, if present, immediate placement of a secured airway (i.e., tracheal intubation) is strongly recommended. The GCS has modifications for use in younger children (Table 60.4) and is often combined with other scales such as the Pediatric Trauma Score for overall pediatric trauma patient stratification.

In pediatric trauma patients, shock is initially assumed and most commonly the result of hypovolemia. Cardiogenic shock, although rare in children, if present may be associated with chest trauma or preexisting cardiovascular disease. Attempts should be made to place at least 2 large-gauge intravenous lines that are appropriate for age. One strategy for a pediatric trauma patient with hypotension is to administer an initial bolus of 20 mL/kg of an isotonic crystalloid solution such as lactated Ringer's or normal saline. Fluid administration should be repeated with additional boluses of isotonic crystalloid solutions as required to stabilize the blood pressure into an acceptable age-appropriate range. Glucose-containing solutions typically are not administered for volume resuscitation because they may produce hyperglycemia and potentially worsen neurologic outcome.

Hypotension in pediatric trauma patients should be promptly and aggressively managed.[8] If the blood pressure is refractory after 2 fluid boluses of isotonic crystalloid, strong consideration should be given to the administration of blood products. The typical dose for administration of packed red blood cells is 10 mL/kg. Colloid has not been demonstrated to be superior to the administration of crystalloid solutions for volume resuscitation of the pediatric trauma patient. Hypertonic saline has also not been established to have any beneficial effect when compared to standard crystalloid resuscitation. The strategy for administering blood products earlier in the resuscitation process has now been emphasized in the updated ATLS guidelines. However, no specific pediatric guidelines or blood product ratios have been recommended. If the patient's blood pressure is not increasing after multiple fluid boluses including blood products, strong consideration should be given to emergent transfer to the operating room or the angiography suite for the control of hemorrhage. The differential diagnosis for a patient with refractory hypotension despite aggressive therapy includes ongoing hemorrhage, tension pneumothorax, pericardial tamponade, cardiac contusion, neurogenic shock, and preexisting medical conditions such as congenital heart disease and adrenal insufficiency. Specific diagnostic testing that may be helpful to determine the source of hemodynamic instability may include CT, echocardiography, and angiography. However, the risks versus the benefits of transfer for diagnostic testing needs to be carefully considered, especially if the patient remains hemodynamically unstable.

Cervical spine injuries in children commonly occur in different locations than adults.[9] These injuries occur less often in children but tend to be located at a higher level, which is usually at or above cervical spine level C-3. Figure 60.1 illustrates a fracture at cervical spine level 3 on a CT of the cervical spine. In addition, pseudosubluxation of the cervical spine is a common and benign finding in children which can add considerable confusion to the diagnosis of a genuine injury. Pseudosubluxation is usually seen as the anterior displacement of cervical spine level C-2 onto C-3.

History and physical examination are the initial steps in the evaluation of the cervical spine for the pediatric trauma patient.[10] Particular attention should be given to the mechanism of injury, level of consciousness, gross neurological deficits, and the presence of midline cervical tenderness. If neck tenderness, decreased sensorium, or neurological deficits are present, one must assume a cervical spine injury exists. A CT scan of the cervical spine may be helpful in the identification of lesions not visible on plain cervical radiographs. However, spinal cord injury without radiographic abnormality (SCIWORA) is a functional ligamentous injury that is estimated to occur in approximately 25% to 50% of pediatric patients with spinal cord injuries. SCIWORA can only be diagnosed with an MRI.

The cervical spine cannot be cleared exclusively using diagnostic imaging; cervical spine imaging must be used in conjunction with physical examination.[11] Appropriate spine

Table 60.4 COMPARISON OF THE ADULT AND PEDIATRIC GLASGOW COMA SCALES

	RESPONSE TYPE					
	EYE OPENING		VERBAL RESPONSE		MOTOR RESPONSE	
SCORE	ADULT	PEDIATRIC	ADULT	PEDIATRIC	ADULT	PEDIATRIC
6					Follows Commands	Normal spontaneous movement
5			Oriented	Coos, babbles	Localizes pain	Withdraws to touch
4	Spontaneous	Spontaneous	Confused	Irritable, cries	Withdraws to pain	Withdraws to pain
3	To verbal stimuli	To speech	Inappropriate words	Cries to pain	Flexion to pain	Abnormal flexion
2	To pain	To pain	Incomprehensible sounds	Moans to pain	Extension to pain	Abnormal extension
1	None	None	None	None	None	None

immobilization must continue during the intraoperative and postoperative periods if the cervical spine of the patient cannot be cleared in the preoperative period.[12] MRI of the cervical spine may be indicated in the postoperative period if the cervical spine cannot be cleared by physical examination (i.e., patient remains unconscious, patient uncooperative with exam, distracting injuries) in a reasonable time frame.

Traumatic injuries can be classified as either blunt or penetrating. Examples of blunt traumatic injuries can range from simple contusions from a fall to severe liver lacerations from a motor vehicle incident associated with internal bleeding and hemodynamic instability. Severe injuries from blunt force trauma can also occur in children due to nonaccidental causes. Blunt abdominal trauma in pediatric patients can occasionally be treated with close observation and lack of mandatory operative intervention. Penetrating traumatic injuries can range from a superficial puncture wound to multiple GSWs or knife wounds resulting in hypovolemic shock. In contrast to blunt traumatic injuries, penetrating traumatic injuries typically require surgical exploration. For example, exploration is commonly performed for penetrating abdominal trauma that is suspected to have entered the peritoneum. However, if the patient is hemodynamically stable, surgical exploration may initially consist of diagnostic laparoscopy as opposed to a traditional exploratory laparotomy.[13]

Massive transfusions are typically defined as situations in which 100% of the estimated blood volume (EBV) is expected to be administered in less than 24 hours or 50% of the EBV within 3 hours. The EBV for pediatric patients can range from 75 mL/kg for an adolescent to 100 mL/kg for a premature neonate. MTPs have been widely adopted by many hospitals to facilitate the acquisition and administration of several types and large quantities of blood products for massive transfusions.[14] Activation of the MTP commonly results in the ongoing and prompt availability of several types of blood components including packed red blood cells, fresh frozen plasma, cryoprecipitate, and platelets. In addition, many institutions will also notify the blood bank pathologist that a massive transfusion is in progress. The pathologist can be utilized as a consultant regarding interpretation of laboratory values (i.e.,

thromboelastographs [TEGs]) as well as the most appropriate therapies to administer.

The administration of blood products can result in several detrimental conditions including transfusion reactions and electrolyte disorders. Increased vigilance should always occur during the administration of all blood products for hemodynamic instability (i.e., hypotension) and signs of a suspected transfusion reaction (i.e., hemolysis, bronchospasm, urticaria). The administration of large quantities of blood products can be associated with several conditions including[3] hypothermia, dilutional coagulopathy, hypocalcemia, hyperkalemia, as well as the development of transfusion-related acute lung injury (TRALI) and transfusion-associated circulatory overload (TACO).

Children with substantial anatomic lesions associated with uncontrollable hemorrhage and cardiopulmonary instability usually require emergent operative intervention. In many trauma centers, these hemodynamically unstable children are initially managed using DCS.[15] DCS is based on the principle that rapid control of abdominal bleeding by placement of abdominal packing and coverage of the open abdomen enables more effective resuscitation prior to exposing the child to a more prolonged definitive repair. DCS refers to packing of the abdomen either temporarily, which perhaps allows volume resuscitation to occur prior to resuming surgical procedures, or as a short-term definitive measure. Patients receiving DCS may then be subsequently transferred to the intensive care unit for further nonsurgical critical care and possible return to the operating room at a future point for additional exploration and/or definitive surgical care. Acute abdominal packing and coverage avoids the development of abdominal compartment syndrome, allows reevaluation of the injured tissue, and provides access for repeated lavage of contaminated spaces. DCS has demonstrated to be a life-saving technique in limited circumstances by allowing an unstable child to receive comprehensive resuscitation under more controlled circumstances.

If uncontrolled bleeding is still present after surgical causes have been minimized, several options should be considered. The patient should be evaluated for etiologies including hypothermia, acidosis, dilutional coagulopathy, and traumatic

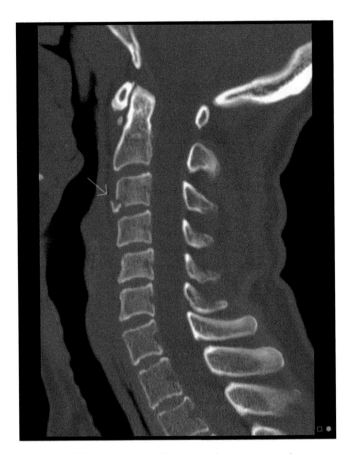

Fig. 60.1 CT of the cervical spine illustrating a fracture at cervical spine level 3. (Creative Commons License; Case courtesy of Dr. Chris O'Donnell, Radiopaedia.org, rID: 20304. https://radiopaedia.org/cases/extension-teardrop-fracture-cervical-spine; accessed June 2017).

coagulopathy. These conditions may be identified by review of the vital signs and laboratory testing results. Traditional laboratory tests in this situation should include an arterial blood gas, hemoglobin/hematocrit, platelets, prothrombin, and partial thromboplastin. Additionally, TEG can be utilized to identify specific coagulopathic abnormalities which can result in providing the most appropriate management.[16] TEG utilizes whole blood to evaluate several parameters of the coagulation process which is depicted as a real-time tracing of coagulation function.[3] The characteristics of the TEG tracing is used to determine the type of coagulation disorder and the most appropriate form of therapy. Figure 60.2 illustrates a characteristic thromboelastography tracing. Four items that represent clot formation are identified with a TEG: the reaction time (R value), the K value, the alpha angle and the maximum amplitude (MA); the LY30 represents the percentage of clot which has lysed after 30 minutes. The R value reflects coagulation factor activity and plasma would be the targeted therapy for a prolonged R value. The K value is the time from the end of R until the clot attains 20 mm; this represents the speed of clot formation. The alpha angle represents the transformation of fibrinogen to fibrin; a reduced alpha angle would be best treated with cryoprecipitate. The MA is derived predominantly from platelet function; a reduced MA is best managed by a platelet transfusion or medications that improve platelet function such as desmopressin. Elevation to the LY30 suggests fibrinolysis and should be treated with an antifibrinolytic such as tranexamic acid.

During treatment of refractory traumatic coagulopathy, the administration of hemostatic agents may also be considered. FEIBA is one type of prothrombin complex concentrate which can be considered in the management of bleeding patients with hemophilia, for the acute reversal of warfarin,[17] and for treatment of traumatic coagulopathy. The available data regarding the effectiveness of FEIBA for the management of bleeding in the pediatric trauma patient is extremely limited. Recombinant factor VIIa has also been used in the treatment of traumatic coagulopathy[18] with limited success. It is proposed that the key mechanism of action for recombinant factor VIIa involves the activation of factor X and thrombin generation on the surface of activated platelets. The use of recombinant factor VIIa for uncontrolled bleeding is typically reserved for refractory cases after several alternative therapies have been ineffective; this is due to limited success in reducing bleeding as well as the risk for the development of thrombotic events. The antifibrinolytic agents (i.e., tranexamic acid) and desmopressin have also been studied in trauma patients, and their use is limited to patients with elevated fibrinogen levels and inherited platelet diatheses, respectively.

Patients undergoing orthopedic surgical procedures, such as IM rod placement, are at increased risk for several conditions including hemorrhage, neurovascular compromise, and the development of fat embolism. Hemorrhage can be typically recognized by awareness of the surgical field, and neurovascular compromise would be identified in the postoperative period. Treatment of hemorrhage would include volume administration which may include blood products. Treatment of neurovascular compromise is typically supportive particularly for pudendal nerve injuries which characteristically resolve spontaneously over a period of several weeks. Subclinical fat embolism is commonly present in patients with long bone fractures. Figure 60.3 illustrates a section from a blood vessel within the lung containing lipid material (arrow) due to a fat embolism.

Fat embolism syndrome (FES) is also a relatively rare but potentially life-threatening condition. FES may occur as a result of orthopedic traumatic injuries especially in patients with long bone fractures of the femur.[19] The diagnosis of FES is nonspecific and may be suspected by the presence of hypoxemia, tachypnea, hypotension, or dyspnea. However, the previously mentioned signs and symptoms are all nonspecific and may occur in several other conditions. Intraoperatively, FES may be suspected by the development of an acute decrease in the end-tidal CO_2, hypoxemia, tachycardia, petechial rash, and the development of cardiovascular collapse. Management of FES is supportive which may range from only providing supplemental oxygen to performing cardiopulmonary resuscitation. Figure 60.4 illustrates the presence of diffuse patchy ground-glass opacities on a CT chest examination which is strongly suspicious for a fat embolism based on the clinical facts of the case.

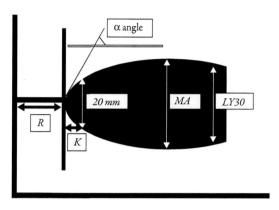

Fig. 60.2 Illustration of a characteristic thromboelastography tracing. Four items that represent clot formation are identified by this test: the reaction time (R value), the K value, the alpha angle, and the maximum amplitude (MA); the LY30 represents the percentage of clot that has lysed after 30 minutes. (Creative Commons Attribution 2.0 Generic license. Luis Teodoro da Luz, Bartolomeu Nascimento, and Sandro Rizoli; https://commons.wikimedia.org/wiki/File:Thromboelastography_Waveform.jpg; accessed June 2017).

An important principle of trauma anesthesia management is the maintenance of body temperature. Hypothermia occurs commonly in patients with major traumatic injuries. Hypothermia may potentiate neuromuscular blockade, exacerbate coagulopathy, and contribute to delayed emergence as well as surgical site infections. Measures to warm the child should be instituted as early as possible. These measures include[20] warming of blood products and intravenous fluids, using forced-air warming devices (which is one of the most effective strategies to treat hypothermia), wrapping the head and extremities in plastic bags, and increasing the ambient temperature of the operating room. Ideally, the operating room should be warmed in advance of the child's arrival to minimize radiant heat loss.

CONCLUSIONS

- Traumatic injuries in children are the most common cause of death in the United States for children above 1 year of age.

- Prevention needs to be emphasized as one of the most important strategies available to reduce the occurrence of injuries to children.

- ATLS guidelines are relevant to anesthesia providers and can be very effective in the perioperative management of the pediatric trauma patient.

- MTPs are systematic processes that are designed to facilitate the prompt administration of large quantities of blood products.

- DCS should be strongly considered as an effective technique in appropriate situations to allow adequate resuscitation of the pediatric trauma patient.

- Hemostatic agents should also be considered during the management of uncontrolled bleeding in the pediatric trauma patient.

- Fat embolism is a rare but potentially life-threatening condition that occurs more commonly during repair of long bone fractures.

- The GCS is composed of three parameters: Best Eye Response, Best Verbal Response, and Best Motor Response. The GCS has a range between 3 and 15. The GCS is calculated by adding the scores from the 3 parameters to produce a total GCS score. A GCS Score of 13 or higher correlates with a mild brain injury, 9 to 12 with a moderate brain injury, and <8 with a severe brain injury.

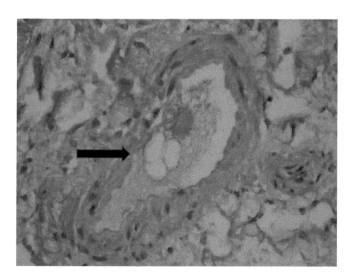

Fig. 60.3 Illustration of a section from a blood vessel within the lung containing lipid material (arrow) due to a fat embolism. (Creative Commons Attribution 2.0 Generic license. Boris L Kanen, Ruud JLF Loffeld. https://commons.wikimedia.org/wiki/File:Fat_embolism.JPEG; accessed June 2017).

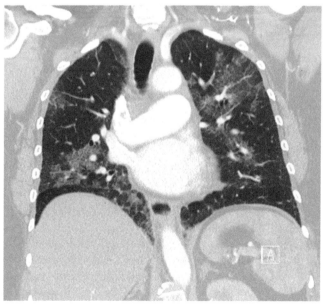

Fig. 60.4 Illustration of diffuse patchy ground-glass opacities on a CT chest examination which is strongly suspicious for a fat embolism based on the clinical facts of the case. (Creative Commons License; Case courtesy of Dr Charlie Chia-Tsong Hsu, Radiopaedia.org, rID: 19157. https://radiopaedia.org/cases/suspected-fat-embolism; accessed June 2017).

1. Which of the following conditions is the **MOST** common cause of mortality for patients >1 year of life?

    A. congenital heart disease
    B. drownings
    C. motor vehicle incidents
    D. sudden infant death syndrome (SIDS)

Answer: C

For pediatric patients that are >1 year of life, motor vehicle incidents are the leading cause of mortality.[2] For pediatric patients that are <1 year of life, SIDS is typically the most common cause of mortality. Drownings and congenital heart disease contribute significantly to mortality of pediatric patients but neither is the most frequent cause.

2. Which of the following interventions is **MOST** appropriate to perform during the primary survey?

    A. CT
    B. Foley catheter placement
    C. laboratory studies
    D. tracheal intubation

Answer: D

The purpose of the primary survey is a focused evaluation to identify life-threatening conditions and to initiate resuscitation if necessary. The main components of the primary survey[3] include: A (airway), B (breathing), C (circulation), D (disability), and E (exposure/environment). The secondary survey is a comprehensive head-to-toe patient examination. It is not begun until the primary survey is complete and the patient is in overall stable condition. Imaging studies such as CT scans, laboratory testing, and placement of Foley catheters would all be expected to be performed during the secondary survey.

3. The administration of 20 cc/kg for which of the following solutions would be **MOST** appropriate to administer to a pediatric trauma patient who remains hypotensive after receiving 20 cc/kg of lactated ringer's solution?

    A. 5% albumin
    B. 5% dextrose in lactated ringer's
    C. lactated ringer's
    D. packed red blood cells

Answer: C

Pediatric patients who remain hypotensive require aggressive and prompt treatment.[8] In pediatric trauma patients, shock is initially assumed and most commonly the result of hypovolemia. One strategy for a pediatric trauma patient with hypotension is to administer an initial bolus of 20 mL/kg of an isotonic crystalloid solution such as lactated ringer's or normal saline. Fluid administration should be repeated with additional boluses of isotonic crystalloid solutions as required to stabilize the blood pressure into an acceptable age-appropriate range. Glucose-containing solutions typically are not administered for volume resuscitation because they may produce hyperglycemia and potentially worsen neurologic outcome. If the blood pressure is refractory after 2 fluid boluses of isotonic crystalloid, strong consideration should be given to the administration of blood products. The typical dose for administration of packed red blood cells is 10 mL/kg. Colloid has not been demonstrated to be superior to the administration of crystalloid solutions for volume resuscitation of the pediatric trauma patient, and the typical initial dose is 10 mL/kg.

4. Which of the following is the **MOST** appropriate to utilize for the <u>initial evaluation</u> of a cervical spine injury in a pediatric trauma patient?

    A. CT
    B. MRI
    C. physical examination
    D. plain film radiography

Answer: C

History and physical examination are the initial steps in the evaluation of the cervical spine for the pediatric trauma patient.[10] If neck tenderness, decreased sensorium, or neurological deficits are present, one must assume a cervical spine injury exists. A CT scan of the cervical spine may be helpful in the identification of lesions not visible on plain cervical radiographs. However, SCIWORA is a functional ligamentous injury that has been estimated to occur in approximately 25% to 50% of pediatric patients with spinal cord injuries. SCIWORA can only be diagnosed with MRI. The cervical spine cannot be cleared exclusively using diagnostic imaging; cervical spine imaging must be used in conjunction with physical examination.[11]

5. The utilization of which of the following devices is expected to **MOST** effectively manage a patient with hypothermia?

    A. forced air warming device
    B. humidifier moisture exchanger
    C. triple lumen fluid warmer
    D. overhead heat lamps

Answer: A

An important principle of trauma anesthesia management is the maintenance of body temperature. Hypothermia occurs commonly in pediatric patients with major traumatic injuries. Hypothermia may potentiate neuromuscular blockade, exacerbate coagulopathy, and contribute to delayed emergence as well as surgical site infections. Measures to prevent hypothermia should be instituted as early as possible. These measures include[20] warming of blood products and intravenous fluids, using forced-air warming devices (which is one of the most effective strategies to treat hypothermia), wrapping the head and extremities in plastic bags, and increasing the ambient temperature of the operating room. Ideally, the operating room should be warmed in advance of the child's arrival to minimize radiant heat loss. Other strategies such as heat lamps, fluid warmers, and humidifier moisture exchangers are helpful to prevent hypothermia but not as effective as forced air warmers and control of the ambient room temperature.

6. Which of the following conditions is **MOST** likely to be present after the development of a fat embolism in the perioperative period?

    A. hypercarbia
    B. hypotension

C. normothermia
D. tachycardia

Answer: C

Subclinical fat embolism is commonly present in patients with long bone fractures. Most patients with fat embolism, in contrast to FES, will exhibit no significant changes in the perioperative period. FES is also a relatively rare but potentially life-threatening condition. FES may occur as a result of orthopedic traumatic injuries especially in patients with long bone fractures of the femur.[19] The diagnosis of FES is nonspecific and may be suspected by the presence of hypoxemia, tachypnea, hypotension, or dyspnea. However, the previously mentioned signs and symptoms are all nonspecific and may occur in several other conditions. Intraoperatively, FES may be diagnosed by the development of an acute decrease in the end-tidal CO_2, hypoxemia, tachycardia, petechial rash, and the development of cardiovascular collapse. Management of FES is supportive which may range from only providing supplemental oxygen to performing cardiopulmonary resuscitation.

7. Which of the following medications is **MOST** appropriate to administer for the acute reversal of warfarin in a pediatric trauma patient?

A. factor VIIa
B. FEIBA
C. desmopressin
D. tranexamic acid

Answer: B

FEIBA is one type of prothrombin complex concentrate which is indicated in the management of bleeding patients with hemophilia, for the acute reversal of warfarin,[17] and perhaps in the treatment of traumatic coagulopathy. The available data regarding the effectiveness of FEIBA for the management of bleeding in the pediatric trauma patient is extremely limited. The antifibrinolytic agents (i.e., tranexamic acid) and desmopressin have also been studied in trauma patients and their use is limited to patients with elevated fibrinogen levels and inherited platelet diatheses, respectively. Factor VIIa would not be the most appropriate medication to administer for the reversal of warfarin.

8. Placement of which of the following devices is the **MOST** appropriate initial management for a pediatric trauma patient with a GCS score of 6?

A. central venous catheter
B. Foley catheter
C. oral gastric tube
D. tracheal tube

Answer: D

The GCS is the most common scale utilized to estimate the severity of neurological injury among trauma patients. A GCS score of 8 or less implies severe neurological injury and, if present, immediate placement of a secured airway (i.e., tracheal intubation) is strongly recommended.[3] The placement of a central venous catheter, oral gastric tube, or Foley catheter would not take priority over placement of a tracheal tube in a patient with a GCS score of 6.

9. Which of the following signs is **MOST** likely to develop from a suspected transfusion reaction?

A. hemoglobinuria
B. hyperkalemia
C. hypertension
D. hypocalcemia

Answer: A

The administration of blood products can result in several detrimental conditions including transfusion reactions and electrolyte disorders. Increased vigilance should always occur during the administration of all blood products for hemodynamic instability (i.e., hypotension) and signs of a suspected transfusion reaction (i.e., hemolysis, hemoglobinuria, bronchospasm, urticaria). The administration of large quantities of blood products can be associated with several conditions including[3] hypothermia, dilutional coagulopathy, hypocalcemia, hyperkalemia, as well as the development of TRALI and TACO. Hypocalcemia and hypertension would not be expected from the administration of blood products. Hyperkalemia would be expected to develop from the administration of large quantities of blood products, particularly if given rapidly; this would not be due to a transfusion reaction.

10. Which of the following components would be **MOST** appropriate to administer in a pediatric trauma patient who has a reduced maximum amplitude (MA) on thromboelastography?

A. factor VIIa
B. fresh frozen plasma
C. packed red blood cells
D. platelets

Answer: D

TEG can be utilized to identify specific coagulopathic abnormalities which can then be used to provide the most appropriate and targeted management.[16] TEG utilizes whole blood to evaluate several parameters of the coagulation process which is depicted as a real-time tracing of coagulation function.[3] The characteristics of the TEG tracing is used to determine the type of coagulation disorder and the most appropriate form of therapy. Four items that represent clot formation are identified with a TEG: the reaction time (R value), the K value, the alpha angle and the maximum amplitude (MA); the LY30 represents the percentage of clot which has lysed after 30 minutes. The R value reflects coagulation factor activity and plasma would be the targeted therapy for a prolonged R value. The K value is the time from the end of R until the clot attains 20 mm; this represents the speed of clot formation. The alpha angle represents the transformation of fibrinogen to fibrin; a reduced alpha angle would be best treated with cryoprecipitate. The MA is derived predominantly from platelet function; a reduced MA is best managed by a platelet transfusion or medications that improve platelet function such as desmopressin. Elevation to the LY30 suggests fibrinolysis and should be treated with an antifibrinolytic such as tranexamic acid. The use of recombinant factor VIIa for uncontrolled bleeding is typically reserved for refractory cases after several alternative therapies have been ineffective; this is due to limited success in reducing bleeding as well as the risk for the development of thrombotic events. Packed red blood cells and fresh frozen plasma would not be the most appropriate components to administer for a patient with a reduced maximum amplitude on thromboelastography.

QUESTIONS AND ANSWERS

This chapter has accompanying questions and answers which are available to subscribers as part of the Oxford eLearning platform. To access the questions, go to ✔ http:// oxfordmedicine. com/pediatricanesthesiaPBL

REFERENCES

1. Faulkenberry JG, Schaechter J. Reporting on pediatric unintentional firearm injury—who's responsible. *J Trauma Acute Care Surg*. 2015 Sep;79(3 Suppl 1):S2–S8.
2. Young DA, Wesson DE. Trauma. In: Cote CJ, Lerman J, Anderson BJ, eds. *A Practice of Anesthesia for Infants and Children*. 5th ed. Philadelphia, PA: Churchill Livingstone Elsevier; 2013:789–802.
3. American College of Surgeons, Committee on Trauma. *ATLS: Advanced Trauma Life Support for Doctors*. 9th ed. Chicago: American College of Surgeons; 2012.
4. Mohammad A, Branicki F, Abu-Zidan FM. Educational and clinical impact of Advanced Trauma Life Support (ATLS) courses: a systematic review. *World J Surg*. 2014 Feb;38(2):322–329.
5. Ivashkov Y, Bhananker SM. Perioperative management of pediatric trauma patients. *Int J Crit Illn Inj Sci*. 2012 Sep;2(3):143–148.
6. Ross AK. Pediatric trauma: anesthesia management. *Anesthesiol Clin North America*. 2001 Jun;19(2):309–337.
7. Kortbeek JB, Al Turki SA, Ali J, et al. Advanced Trauma Life Support, 8th Edition: the evidence for change. *J Trauma*. 2008 Jun;64(6):1638–1650.
8. Carcillo JA. Intravenous fluid choices in critically ill children. *Curr Opin Crit Care*. 2014 Aug;20(4):396–401.
9. Rozzelle CJ, Aarabi B, Dhall SS, et al. Management of pediatric cervical spine and spinal cord injuries. *Neurosurgery*. 2013 Mar;72(Suppl 2):205–226.
10. Booth TN. Cervical spine evaluation in pediatric trauma. *AJR Am J Roentgenol*. 2012 May;198(5):W417–W425.
11. Tat ST, Mejia MJ, Freishtat RJ. Imaging, clearance, and controversies in pediatric cervical spine trauma. *Pediatr Emerg Care*. 2014 Dec;30(12):911–915.
12. Liu YX, Young DA. Anesthesia for pediatric trauma. In: Wesson DE, Naik-Mathuria B, eds. *Pediatric Trauma: Pathophysiology, Diagnosis and Treatment*. 2nd ed. New York: CRC Press Taylor and Francis Group; 2017:167–184.
13. Pearson EG, Clifton MS. The role of minimally invasive surgery in pediatric trauma. *Surg Clin North Am*. 2017 Feb;97(1):75–84.
14. Hwu RS, Spinella PC, Keller MS, et al. The effect of massive transfusion protocol implementation on pediatric trauma care. *Transfusion*. 2016 Nov;56(11):2712–2719.
15. Villalobos MA, Hazelton JP, Choron RL, et al. Caring for critically injured children: an analysis of 56 pediatric damage control laparotomies. *J Trauma Acute Care Surg*. 2017 May;82(5):901–909.
16. Leeper CM, Gaines BA. Viscoelastic hemostatic assays in the management of the pediatric trauma patient. *Semin Pediatr Surg*. 2017 Feb;26(1):8–13.
17. Smith AT, Wrenn KD, Barrett TW, et al. Delayed intracranial hemorrhage after head trauma in patients on direct-acting oral anticoagulants. *Am J Emerg Med*. 2017 Feb;35(2):377.e1–377.e2.
18. Grounds M. Recombinant factor VIIa (rFVIIa) and its use in severe bleeding in surgery and trauma: a review. *Blood Rev*. 2003 Sep;17(Suppl 1):S11–S21.
19. Blokhuis TJ, Pape HC, Frölke JP. Timing of definitive fixation of major long bone fractures: can fat embolism syndrome be prevented? *Injury*. 2017 Jun;48(Suppl 1):S3–S6.
20. Madrid E1, Urrútia G, Roqué i Figuls M, et al. Active body surface warming systems for preventing complications caused by inadvertent perioperative hypothermia in adults. *Cochrane Database Syst Rev*. 2016 Apr 21;4:CD009016.

61.

NONACCIDENTAL TRAUMA

Alyssa Padover and Jennifer K. Lee

STEM CASE AND KEY QUESTIONS

A 2-year-old girl is brought to the emergency department by her grandmother. The grandmother states that the girl seemed "sleepy" all day at home and then started vomiting but that she has not had a fever. Primary survey by the emergency room physicians reveals bruising on the child's forehead and left eye and bilateral burns on her extremities and buttocks. She is lethargic but withdraws to painful stimuli. Head computed tomography (CT) shows a subdural hematoma with midline shift. The neurosurgeons want to emergently take the patient to the operating room for cranial decompression.

WHAT IS ABUSIVE HEAD TRAUMA (AHT)?

AHT, the most common cause of death from child abuse,[1] refers to brain injury from nonaccidental, intentional, or inflicted trauma. Because of the multifactorial mechanisms behind AHT—including blunt force trauma, diffuse axonal injury, shaking, hypoxia-ischemia, and multiorgan injury—AHT has replaced the term "shaken baby syndrome." For unclear reasons, outcomes after AHT are worse than those after accidental traumatic brain injury (TBI), even when the injuries are of similar severity as scored by the Glasgow Coma Scale and injury classification.[2]

WHAT ELSE SHOULD BE CONSIDERED IN THE DIFFERENTIAL DIAGNOSIS?

Diagnosing abuse is difficult because the signs and symptoms may mimic those of accidental trauma. The differential diagnosis also includes infection, coagulopathy, congenital vascular malformation, birth trauma, spontaneous subdural hemorrhage, seizure disorder, cardiac arrest and other causes of hypoxia, cerebral venous thrombosis, retinal hemorrhage from accidental trauma, and metabolic deficiencies such as glutaric aciduria type 1.

WHAT IS THE INCIDENCE OF AHT?

The incidence of child abuse is difficult to measure given the high risk of underreporting and challenges in diagnosing abuse. AHT is estimated to occur in 27.5 to 32.2 cases per 100,000 infants per year,[3] but this is likely a conservative estimate.

WHAT ARE THE PRESENTING SIGNS OF CHILD ABUSE AND AHT?

Abuse victims may suffer multiple episodes of trauma across time in addition to the acute event that brings them to the hospital. This acute-on-chronic injury makes diagnosing and determining the severity of abuse difficult. Acute and healing bone fractures may be evident on radiographic examination, but identifying subtle fractures and periosteal healing around growth plates may require expertise from a pediatric radiologist. Injury to any organ system or body part can occur, including trauma to the oropharynx, chest, abdomen, and extremities. AHT may manifest as altered consciousness, seizures, vomiting, poor feeding, lethargy, irritability, or apnea. Chronic subdural hematomas may cause macrocephaly. Some children will have developmental delay.

WHAT CONSIDERATIONS SHOULD BE GIVEN FOR AIRWAY MANAGEMENT?

Because the oropharynx and face may be injured, a thorough airway exam should be conducted. For example, the oropharynx may be injured if the perpetrator forcefully pushes an object into the child's mouth, such as a utensil during forceful feeding. Injuries to the lips, oral mucosa, teeth, tongue, and frenulum should be clearly documented prior to intubation.

If the airway anatomy seems normal, a rapid sequence induction should be performed, given the risk of full stomach, decreased gastrointestinal motility, and potential for abdominal injury. Videoscopic laryngoscopy may be helpful to reduce neck and head movement during intubation with in-line cervical stabilization. Young children are at high risk of cervical spine injury, and normal plain radiographs of the neck cannot be used alone to rule out cervical injury. A properly sized, microcuffed endotracheal tube should be used to regulate CO_2 and to avoid the need for an endotracheal tube change if a glottic leak develops. The endotracheal tube cuff should be inflated only as needed, and intracuff pressures should be checked regularly. Proper preparations should be made, including plans for a surgical airway, if a difficult mask ventilation or intubation is anticipated. Nasal instrumentation should be avoided in cases of cranial or upper face injury.

WHAT INDUCTION AGENTS SHOULD BE USED FOR INTUBATION?

Etomidate, propofol, barbiturates, and ketamine are all commonly used for induction and intubation in pediatric TBI cases. The anesthesiologist must keep in mind the importance of maintaining cerebral perfusion pressure (CPP) during induction. CPP is the difference between the mean arterial blood pressure (MAP) and intracranial pressure (ICP). Etomidate and ketamine have the advantage of maintaining some hemodynamic stability during intubation, although the risk of future adrenal suppression must be considered with etomidate. Boluses of propofol or barbiturate will rapidly provide intubating conditions but increase hypotension risk. The ideal vasopressor for the treatment of hypotension in pediatric TBI is unclear. Neuromuscular blockade is appropriate for rapid sequence induction if the airway anatomy appears normal. Succinylcholine may be used safely. The slight increase in ICP from succinylcholine-induced fasciculations must be weighed against the potential for catastrophic increase in ICP from aspiration.

WHAT PHYSIOLOGIC PARAMETERS SHOULD BE MAINTAINED DURING ANESTHESIA AND SURGERY?

Factors that could exacerbate secondary brain injury must be avoided, including hypoxia and hypotension. The pediatric TBI treatment guidelines from 2012[4,5] recommend maintaining ICP <20 mmHg and CPP >40 to 50 mmHg. Higher CPP may be needed in older patients to support cerebral blood flow–blood pressure autoregulation. The anesthesiologist should maintain a deep plane of anesthesia for painful stimuli while avoiding hypotension. Normocarbia with $PaCO_2$ >30 mmHg must be maintained, and hyperventilation should be reserved for treatment of intracranial hypertension. Intracranial hypertension can be treated by administering hypertonic saline 3%, deepening the anesthetic, administering barbiturates, using hyperventilation, elevating the head of the bed, draining cerebrospinal fluid (CSF), and/or performing a decompressive craniectomy. Hyperthermia should be strictly avoided.

DISCUSSION

SUSPICION OF ABUSE

Anesthesiologists play critical roles in identifying and treating children suffering from abuse. Intentional trauma must be considered in all trauma cases. The diagnosis can be challenging because children may have nonspecific clinical histories and vague symptoms. For instance, the details of a fall may be unclear or the provided history may be inconsistent with the child's injury. Children may not articulate details or they may avoid discussing events surrounding the abuse, particularly if a caretaker was the perpetrator. Recurrent injuries, delays in seeking medical care, and explanations for the injury that are inconsistent with the child's developmental age (i.e., an infant climbing into a bathtub of hot water or bruising in a child who is not yet mobile) should raise concern for abuse.

The mechanisms of child abuse are complex and synergistic. They include blunt force trauma, shaking, diffuse axonal injury, hypoxia-ischemia, brainstem and spinal cord injuries, and multiorgan trauma. Child abuse may mimic accidental trauma or involve multiple episodes of inflicted trauma over a long period, with an acute-on-chronic injury profile. In a study of 188 children with abusive trauma at a single institution, 48% had multiple injuries. AHT, lower extremity fracture, skull fracture, and retinal hemorrhage were the most common.[6] More than half of the children presented with a single injury, thereby emphasizing the importance of evaluating for abuse even in the absence of multiple injuries.

Stereotypical injuries associated with abuse, such as long-bone fractures, may or may not be present. Fractures can occur anywhere in the body, including the ribs if the child is forcefully grabbed or squeezed. Identifying evidence of healing fractures on radiographic examination may require the expertise of a pediatric radiologist. Subtle growth plate irregularities, subperiosteal new bone formation, and faint fracture fragments on radiologic examination may be difficult to diagnose. Although abdominal injuries can be life threatening, more than half of children with abdominal trauma will not have bruising, distension, tenderness, or abnormal bowel sounds.[7,8] The duodenum is the most commonly injured section of bowel, and a bowel obstruction from posttraumatic stricture or hematoma may be the primary indication for surgery. Cardiovascular, pulmonary, pharyngeal, and esophageal injuries can also occur from abuse.

ALL CHILDREN ARE AT RISK OF ABUSE

Though intentional trauma is most frequently reported in infants and young children, older and larger children are also at risk and may suffer more severe injury. In a case series of children 2.5 to 7 years old (12–22 kg) who died from AHT, none of the victims had bone fractures on radiologic examination or autopsy but all showed evidence of retinal hemorrhages and acute subdural hematoma.[9]

The anesthesiologist must remain vigilant to signs of abuse, engage the institutional trauma service, and alert the proper authorities. All clinicians have the legal and ethical responsibility to report suspected child abuse. As long as the report is made in good faith, physicians are protected by law from potential ramifications of the report.[10] The fear of misdiagnosing a medical condition as abuse should never dissuade clinicians from documenting and reporting their concerns. The consequences of misdiagnosing or failing to report child abuse are severe and sometimes fatal.

SKIN LESIONS

Clinicians in the operating rooms have the opportunity to conduct a full skin examination. This is a critical time to identify and document skin injuries because the lesions will evolve over time and fade. Injuries should be photographed for the medical record before surgical incision and before bandages,

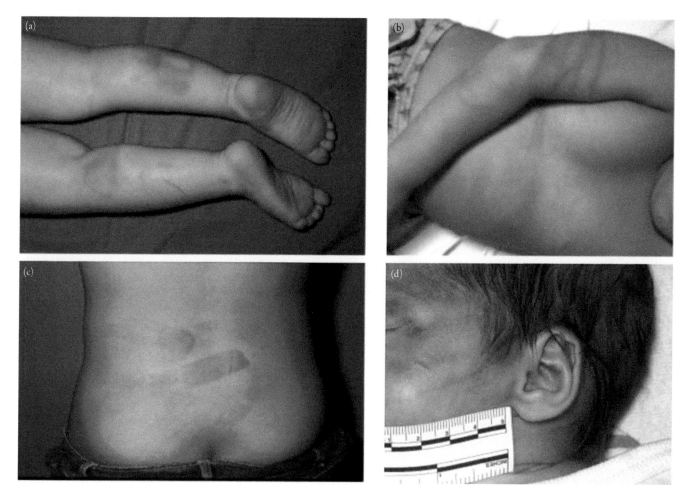

Fig. 61.1 Examples of skin injury patterns consistent with abuse. A. Bruises of different ages. B. Linear, wrap around marks suggest injury from a belt. C. The back is a common location for injury. D. Hand slap injury. Panels A–C are reprinted from *Actas Dermo-Sifiliográficas*, volume 103, edition number 2, Pau-Charles I, Darwich-Soliva D, Grimalt R. Skin signs in child abuse, pp. 94–99, ©2012, with permission from Elsevier. Panel D is reprinted from *Pediatric Clinics of North America*, volume 61, Petska HW, Sheets LK, Sentinal injuries: subtle findings of physical abuse, pp. 923–935, ©2014, with permission from Elsevier.

splints, or casts are applied. The anesthesiologist should also document the skin lesions, including size, character, and location, using terminology that a person without a medical background can understand. For instance, using descriptive and common terminology, such as "a quarter-sized bruise on the right lower back" and "bleeding" rather than "ecchymosis" and "hemorrhage" may assist the investigation. In urgent situations, the anesthesiologist can simply draw an outline of a body, mark the skin lesions' locations, and scan the drawing into the medical record for future use during the investigation. Patterned skin lesions and burns, bruised or boxed ears, bruises of different ages, oral injuries from objects being forcing into the child's mouth, adult bite marks, and injuries to the buttocks or genital region raise the suspicion for abuse (Figure 61.1). Injuries to the genital and anal areas should be documented before Foley insertion.

ANESTHESIA FOR THE DIAGNOSTIC WORKUP

A child with suspected abuse is a trauma victim, and one should assume that he or she has a full stomach and potential cervical spine injury. If the airway anatomy appears normal, the airway should be secured with cervical in-line stabilization and rapid sequence induction used for intubation. Infants and young children are at higher risk of cervical spinal cord injuries than adults owing to their cervical ligamentous laxity, poor muscle development and control, and orientation of the spine to the large head.[11] Plain radiographs may be normal in children with cervical spine injuries.[12] A thorough evaluation of the oropharynx, face, and mandible should be conducted and documented before intubation. Appropriate precautions, including preparation for a surgical airway, should be taken if there is concern for difficult mask ventilation or intubation.

Because thoracolumbar spinal injuries are relatively common in children with AHT,[13] anesthesiologists should take precautions during positioning to protect against further spinal injury. A blood sample for type and crossmatch should be obtained early. The anesthesiologist should also be aware if the child received mydriatic eye drops for pupillary dilation for ophthalmic examination.

The anesthesiologist should coordinate with surgeons, intensivists, and other members of the institutional trauma service to obtain all diagnostic imaging for abuse evaluation during one anesthetic if the patient is hemodynamically stable. Delaying imaging could delay the diagnosis of abuse, impede the patient's treatment, and prevent authorities from ensuring the safety of other children in the home. For instance, a skeletal survey and neurologic, thoracic, and abdominal imaging can be conducted immediately after emergency surgery, provided that the child is hemodynamically stable.

Once the period of acute trauma has passed, the anesthesiologist can consider using sedation, rather than general anesthesia, in older and hemodynamically stable children for diagnostic evaluation, including sexual assault examinations. He or she must carefully weigh the risks and benefits of sedating the child without a protected airway and take into account the duration since the injury, slowed gastrointestinal motility, and potential airway obstruction.

AHT

AHT is the most common cause of death from child abuse.[1] The complex and synergistic injury mechanisms alongside recurrent trauma over time make AHT difficult to treat. Shaking and blunt force trauma cause rapid movement of the brain within the cranial vault, tearing of bridging vessels, and subdural hemorrhages. The acute-on-chronic nature of abuse may cause acute and chronic subdural hematomas. Shear forces can cause retinal hemorrhages in some cases but not all. The absence of retinal hemorrhages should not exclude a diagnosis of AHT, and retinal hemorrhages are not diagnostic of abuse. Hypoxic-ischemic brain injury from respiratory insufficiency or cardiac arrest, disruptions in cerebral blood flow during rapid head rotation,[14] and delays in seeking medical care compound the TBI. The developing brain is particularly susceptible to injury from AHT, including a rapidly progressing form of brain atrophy reported in young survivors of AHT.[15]

ANESTHESIA FOR AHT

Anesthetic management of AHT as a separate entity from accidental TBI has not been well studied. Therefore, the pediatric TBI treatment guidelines[4,5] should be followed for AHT (Table 61.1).

Factors that could worsen secondary brain injury must be avoided, including hypoxia, hypotension, and inadequate depth of anesthesia. Normothermia should be maintained and hyperthermia avoided. Normocarbia should be maintained with $PaCO_2$ >30 mmHg. Hyperventilation should be reserved for intracranial hypertension given the risk of cerebral vasoconstriction and ischemia with prolonged or severe hyperventilation. A properly sized endotracheal tube is critical for CO_2 regulation.

ICP AND CPP

Because children with AHT often experience both trauma and hypoxia-ischemia, it remains controversial whether they should receive ICP monitoring. Specific recommendations for ICP monitoring after brain hypoxia do not exist. Nonetheless,

ICP monitoring is indicated in all infants and children with TBI and a Glasgow Coma Score <9, including those with open cranial sutures or fontanelles. The open fontanelle does not protect the infant brain from intracranial hypertension during cerebral swelling. Younger children are at greater risk of intracranial hypertension than older children after severe TBI.[16]

An extraventricular drain for ICP monitoring can drain CSF during intracranial hypertension. During transport, positioning, and surgery, the extraventricular drain must be leveled appropriately with the patient to prevent over- or underdrainage of CSF. Preoperative communication with the neurosurgeons on managing the extraventricular drain is crucial. If the patient must be intubated, it is reasonable to leave the extraventricular drain open during induction to allow for CSF drainage if hypercapnia and increased ICP occur before or during intubation.

The CPP can be calculated from invasive MAP and ICP monitoring. Hemorrhage, hypovolemia, brain stem injury, and pulmonary injury from neurogenic pulmonary edema or aspiration may cause profound hemodynamic instability. The pediatric TBI guidelines from 2012[4] provide level III recommendations to maintain ICP <20 mmHg and CPP >40 to 50 mmHg. The target CPP may need to be increased in older children and adolescents to support cerebral blood flow–blood pressure autoregulation. Although ICP and CPP are interrelated, both ICP-directed and CPP-directed goals must be met concurrently. For example, increasing MAP alone is not sufficient to support the CPP; ICP must also be decreased. Because intracranial compliance decreases as ICP rises, any further increase in intracranial volume—such as from hypercapnia, seizures, or pain—would substantially increase the ICP and risk brain herniation. The optimal vasopressor to support MAP remains unclear in pediatric TBI.

INTRACRANIAL HYPERTENSION

Intracranial hypertension should be treated with a multipronged approach. Although hypertonic saline 3% is the recommended hyperosmolar treatment in pediatric TBI cases,[5] the risks and benefits for patients with AHT require additional investigation. One single-institution pediatric TBI study, in which 29% of cases were AHT, reported associations between greater cumulative volume of hypertonic saline 3%, higher peak sodium level, and deep vein thrombosis.[17] Barbiturates decrease the ICP but should be used with caution given the risk of hemodynamic depression that could lower CPP. The evidence for or against decompressive craniectomy is primarily limited to case series and single-institution studies.

SEIZURES

Seizures are common after AHT and must be treated early. In a study of >400 children with AHT, including 95% younger than 1 year, more than 70% had clinical seizures. Abnormal electroencephalography and seizures were associated with poor neurologic outcomes. Some children died with refractory status epilepticus or associated intracranial hypertension.[18]

Table 61.1 SUMMARY OF RECOMMENDATIONS FROM THE 2012 GUIDELINES FOR THE ACUTE MEDICAL MANAGEMENT OF SEVERE TRAUMATIC BRAIN INJURY (TBI) IN INFANTS, CHILDREN, AND ADOLESCENTS

PHYSIOLOGIC PARAMETERS	RECOMMENDATIONS	LEVEL OF EVIDENCE
Intracranial pressure	Consider ICP monitoring in infants and children with severe TBI	III
	Treatment of ICP may be considered at a threshold of 20 mmHg	III
Cerebral perfusion pressure	A minimum CPP of 40 mmHg may be considered in children with TBI	III
	A CPP threshold of 40–50 mmHg may be considered; age-specific thresholds may exist, with infants at the lower end of the range and adolescents at the upper end	III
Hyperosmolar therapy	Hypertonic saline should be considered to treat intracranial hypertension. Acute dosing range is 6.5 to 10 mL/kg.	II
	3% hypertonic saline (0.1–1 mL/kg/h infusion) should be considered for the treatment of intracranial hypertension.	III
	Note: no studies of mannitol met the inclusion criteria as evidence for this topic	
Hyperventilation	Consider avoiding prophylactic severe hyperventilation to a $PaCO_2 < 30$ mmHg in the initial 48 hours after injury	III
	If hyperventilation is used in the management of refractory intracranial hypertension, advanced neuromonitoring for evaluation of cerebral ischemia may be considered	III
Temperature control	Moderate hypothermia (32–33°C) beginning early after severe TBI for only 24-hour duration should be avoided	II
	Moderate hypothermia (32–33°C) beginning within 8 hours after severe TBI for up to 48 hours duration should be considered to reduce intracranial hypertension	II
	If hypothermia is induced for any reason, rewarming at a rate >0.5°C/h should be avoided	II
CSF drainage	CSF drainage through an external ventricular drain may be considered for management of elevated ICP	III
	The addition of a lumbar drain may be considered in patients with refractory intracranial hypertension, a functioning external ventricular drain, open basal cisterns, and no evidence of a mass lesion or shift on imaging studies	III
Barbiturates	High-dose barbiturate therapy may be considered in hemodynamically stable patients with refractory intracranial hypertension despite maximal medical and surgical management	III
	When high-dose barbiturate therapy is used to treat refractory intracranial hypertension, continuous arterial blood pressure monitoring and cardiovascular support are required to maintain adequate CPP	III
Corticosteroids	The use of corticosteroids is not recommended to improve outcome or reduce ICP for children with severe TBI	II
Antiseizure prophylaxis	Prophylactic use of antiseizure therapy is not recommended for preventing late posttraumatic seizures in children with severe TBI	III
	Prophylactic antiseizure therapy may be considered as a treatment option to prevent early posttraumatic seizures in young pediatric patients and infants at high risk of seizures after head injury	III
Decompressive craniectomy	Decompressive craniectomy with duraplasty may be considered for patients who are showing early signs of neurologic deterioration or herniation or are developing intracranial hypertension refractory to medical management during the early stages of their treatment	

Note. ICP = intracranial pressure; TBI = traumatic brain injury; CPP = cerebral perfusion pressure; CSF = cerebrospinal fluid.

Source. Adapted from Hardcastle N, Benzon HA, Vavilala MS. Update on the 2012 guidelines for the management of pediatric traumatic brain injury-information for the anesthesiologist. *Pediatr Anesth.* 2014;24:703–710.

SPECIFIC ANESTHETIC AGENTS

During AHT treatment, the anesthetic regimen is at the discretion of the anesthesiologist. Some preclinical data suggest that an intravenous technique with benzodiazepines and opiates may preserve cerebral blood flow autoregulation better than volatile agents.[19] However, recommendations cannot be made regarding the superiority of intravenous or inhaled anesthesia due to insufficient research on this topic. Etomidate, propofol, and barbiturates lower ICP by decreasing the cerebral metabolic rate and oxygen demand and inducing cerebral vasoconstriction. Etomidate may maintain MAP and CPP better than boluses of propofol and barbiturates, which can cause hypotension that requires immediate treatment. However, the risk of adrenal suppression after etomidate must be considered. Ketamine does not raise the ICP and may lower it in some cases while supporting CPP in patients with TBI.[20] For rapid sequence induction, concern for small increases in ICP from succinylcholine-induced fasciculations[21] must be weighed against the potential for catastrophic elevations in ICP with aspiration.

DEBRIEFING AFTER A BAD OUTCOME

The stress on clinicians from witnessing the consequences of child abuse is compounded by emergent surgical situations that carry a high risk of patient injury or death, whether from the abusive injuries or the medical procedures themselves. The term "second victim" was coined to describe clinicians who suffer distress after a medical error or unanticipated poor patient outcome.[22] Clinicians who treat abuse victims may suffer psychological and physical symptoms similar to those described in the second-victim phenomenon. Symptoms include depression, insomnia, anxiety, insecurity about one's clinical capabilities, and concern that similar child abuse situations could affect the clinician's loved ones. Additional research is needed on how to support clinicians after emotionally charged and high-stress cases. Organized support and counseling services and group discussions among health care providers are helpful but may not be readily available at all institutions. The stigma of needing support may also prevent clinicians from seeking help.

Clinicians have a duty to support each other, particularly when faced with the high emotional toll of child abuse. Forums for supportive, nonjudgmental, and open discussions should be readily available with the goal of supporting the clinical team who cared for the abused child. Medical debriefings are as important as ensuring that clinicians receive support. Informal emotional support and peer support are among the most useful strategies for helping clinicians cope with adverse events.[23] Methods should be available to refer clinicians for confidential professional support, without negative consequences, immediately after provision of clinical coverage.

CONCLUSIONS

- The anesthesiologist plays a critical role in the diagnosis, treatment, and reporting of suspected child abuse and AHT.

- Young children are at high risk of cervical spine injury, and in-line neck stabilization should be provided during intubation. Facial and oropharyngeal airway injuries should be documented before intubation. Proper preparation is warranted if difficult mask ventilation or intubation is anticipated.

- Until clinical studies focused on management of AHT are conducted, anesthesiologists should follow the pediatric TBI guidelines.

- Hypoxia, hypocarbia, hypotension, and hyperthermia must be avoided in patients with AHT. CPP must be maintained by simultaneously supporting MAP and decreasing ICP to support cerebral blood flow–blood pressure autoregulation.

REVIEW QUESTIONS

1. A 6-month-old boy is brought to the emergency department with a Glasgow Coma Scale of 7 and vomiting. He is intubated. Brain CT imaging shows a subdural hemorrhage, and an ophthalmic examination reveals bilateral retinal hemorrhages. The infant is taken to the operating room for evacuation of the subdural hematoma. Postoperatively, which additional diagnostic studies are **LEAST** appropriate?

    A. brain magnetic resonance imaging (MRI)
    B. bone densitometry scan
    C. electroencephalogram (EEG)
    D. radiographic skeletal series

Answer: B

B is correct because this diagnostic test is not required in the early evaluation for abuse. A bone densitometry scan as well as skin biopsy and genetic analysis might be indicated later in the patient's treatment course to evaluate for other causes of subdural hemorrhage, such as connective tissue disorder or coagulopathy. However, in the acute treatment period, diagnostic tests should focus on identifying other injuries that may have occurred from trauma and documenting early physical findings that could be related to abuse.

If the patient is hemodynamically stable, all diagnostic imaging should be performed under the same anesthetic as soon as possible. Delays in diagnosing abuse can impede the patient's care and prevent authorities from ensuring the safety of other children in the home environment. Typical diagnostic imaging modalities in the evaluation for abuse include a full-body, radiographic skeletal series to identify new and healing bone fractures and a brain MRI. Seizures are common in patients with AHT and are associated with worse neurologic outcomes. Therefore, seizures must be diagnosed and treated early. Intracranial hypertension may also require barbiturate coma to reduce the ICP. Both of these medical conditions would involve EEG monitoring.

2. Which of the following anatomical differences place infants and children, compared to adults, at **GREATER** risk for severe neurologic injury from AHT?

A. Heads are proportionally larger
B. Necks are shorter and less flexible
C. Brains have lower water content
D. Blood supply is less vulnerable

Answer: A

The large head, relatively underdeveloped cervical muscula-ture, cervical ligamentous laxity, and physiology of the de-veloping brain make young children particularly susceptible to severe and persistent neurologic injury after AHT. The infant's blood vessels and axonal processes are highly suscep-tible to rotational shearing forces and tearing. The developing brain has higher water content and less myelination than the adult brain. AHT consists of a constellation of brain injuries from intentional trauma. It is the leading cause of death from TBI in children under 2 years.

3. Which of the following reported scenarios would be **MOST** suspicious for possible child abuse?

A. femur fracture in a 1-month-old after rolling off a bed
B. humerus fracture in a 2-year old after falling down steps
C. scald burn in a 1-year old after grabbing a hot tea pot
D. tibial spiral fracture in a 3-year-old after a tricycle accident

Answer: A

Anesthesiologists need to maintain high suspicion for child abuse given the severe consequences of misdiagnosing abused children. Rolling is not a typical developmental milestone in most 1-month-old infants. Moreover, fractures are uncommon in nonmobile infants. This report should prompt clinicians to consider nonaccidental trauma.

Answers B, C, and D are incorrect because these are plausible scenarios and within age-appropriate developmental activities.

4. A 6-week-old infant is admitted to the emergency depart-ment with altered level of consciousness after "rolling off the changing table." His mother states that he has not been well for the past 5 days. Gradually, he has become progressively irri-table and then started to vomit. In the emergency department, a brain CT scan shows the image in Figure 61.2.

Which of the following is the **MOST** appropriate next step in caring for this infant?

A. consultation with a pediatric neurology department
B. intubation for intracranial hypertension management
C. observation for significant neurologic status changes
D. reassurance; open fontanelles mitigate herniation risk

Answer: B

The CT shows evidence of subdural hematoma with cere-bral edema and midline shift. The infant's irritability and vomiting are clinical indications of intracranial hypertension. The apparent high ICP must be emergently managed, in-cluding through intubation to protect the airway and control PaCO$_2$. In addition, hypoxia must be avoided because it will cause acute cerebral vasodilation with an increase in cerebral blood volume that could raise the ICP further. Strategies to manage the intracranial hypertension include hypertonic sa-line 3%, hyperventilation, deep sedation, barbiturate coma, CSF drainage, and decompressive craniectomy.

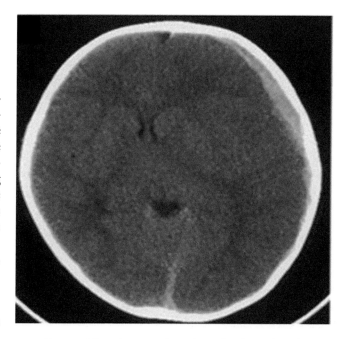

Fig. 61.2 Reprinted from *Progress in Brain Research*, volume 161, Duhaime AC, Durham S. Traumatic brain injury in infants: the phenomenon of subdural hemorrhage with hemispheric hypodensity ("big black brain"), pp. 293–302, ©2007, with permission from Elsevier.

Emergency treatment is warranted, so answers C and D are incorrect. In addition, answer D is incorrect because an open fontanelle or open cranial sutures do not protect the infant brain from intracranial hypertension. A consultation from pediatric neurology should be obtained after the patient is stabilized.

5. You are inducing a 6-month-old boy before exploratory lap-arotomy for a small bowel obstruction. He had been vomiting for a few days and has been "lethargic." You also notice that the patient has bruises of varying ages on his back and abdomen. Airway examination was normal. After inducing anesthesia, the anesthesia resident complains that the cervical collar is too large and is blocking his access to the patient's mouth with the laryngoscope. The **MOST** appropriate course of action in re-gard to the cervical collar is

A. change to a soft collar, if the boy reported no neck pain
B. maintain and perform a nasal fiberoptic intubation
C. open, if the plain radiograph showed no injuries
D. remove, if in-line cervical stabilization is maintained

Answer: D

Infants and young children are at high risk of cervical in-jury because of their immature cervical musculature devel-opment, cervical ligamentous laxity, and large heads. This anatomy makes them prone to neck injury during trauma from acceleration-deceleration, shaking, blunt force injury, and so on. Therefore, in-line cervical stabilization must be maintained. Video laryngoscopy may be used to decrease head and neck movement, and a more experienced practitioner may be needed to do the intubation. An airway exam should have been conducted before induction to evaluate for oral injuries that might also make intubation difficult. A bowel obstruction from posttraumatic stricture or hematoma may be the presenting indication for surgery after abdominal trauma in abuse.

Because the risk of cervical injury is high, answers A and C are incorrect. Lack of pain is an unreliable finding to rule out serious neck injuries, especially in trauma patients in which other injuries could be distractors. Answer C is incorrect because children may have cervical injury even though the plain radiograph does not identify a bony injury. Answer B is incorrect because the child may have cranial injuries. He was vomiting and had lethargy. Nasal instrumentation is contraindicated in suspected cranial injuries.

6. You are transporting a 7-year-old patient to the operating room for emergent cranial decompression. The patient has been undergoing evaluation for child abuse in the intensive care unit. He has been hemodynamically unstable with low blood pressure despite dopamine. During the transport, the patient's heart rate decreases from 110 to 80 beats per minute. The **MOST** appropriate response is

    A. phenobarbital push
    B. hypertonic saline bolus
    C. mannitol injection
    D. pupillary response check

Answer: B

The acute decrease in heart rate may be related to intracranial hypertension. Hypertonic saline is the recommended hyperosmolar therapy for intracranial hypertension in pediatric TBI.

Answer A is incorrect because a bolus of barbiturate might cause hemodynamic suppression with a decrease in blood pressure. Reducing MAP during elevated ICP would cause a significant fall in CPP with risk of cerebral hypoperfusion and ischemia.

Answer C is incorrect because mannitol is not the recommended therapy for intracranial hypertension in pediatric TBI. Limited evidence supports the use of mannitol for pediatric TBI.[5] Risks from mannitol include natriuresis and dehydration with a subsequent decrease in blood pressure and therefore, potentially, CPP.

Answer D is incorrect because the patient may have received mydriatic drops to dilate the pupils for ophthalmic examination. Whether the child's pupils were pharmacologically dilated should be clarified before transport to the operating room.

7. You induce anesthesia in an 8-year-old child for reduction of a tibial fracture. You heard that the child fell while playing soccer. After intubation, the clinical team removes the child's clothing. You note linear marks along the abdomen with a square pattern that looks similar to a belt. The **MOST** appropriate action is

    A. assume the admitting team knows
    B. direct the surgeon to call pediatrics
    C. document the lesions
    D. phone child protective services

Answer: C

Many child abuse victims will suffer life-threatening abdominal injuries but lack clear signs of abdominal injury on physical exam, such as bruising, distension, or decreased bowel sounds. In this situation, however, there is clear evidence of possible abdominal injury that warrants evaluation. The duodenum is the most commonly injured section of bowel in abusive trauma. In addition, the skin lesion must be documented photographically for the medical record with details about the size, shape, and location. The skin markings may fade, and the opportunity to document the findings will be lost if the operating room team fails to record them. This is a critical time window to document potential evidence of abuse.

Answer A is incorrect. Assuming is rarely a good idea.

Answer B is incorrect because the anesthesiologist, as well as all treating clinicians, is ethically and legally obligated to report suspicion of abuse. This includes personally ensuring that a proper report is made and that the appropriate authorities are notified.

Answer D is incorrect because you should proceed with the patient's care, including evaluation for possible gastrointestinal and abdominal organ injury. The anesthesiologist and treating team should notify the institutional trauma service and go through the institution's protocols to activate a child abuse investigation. "Child protective services" is typically the name of a government agency responsible for responding to reports of child abuse; the names of the entities that respond within an institution vary from hospital to hospital.

QUESTIONS AND ANSWERS

This chapter has accompanying questions and answers which are available to subscribers as part of the Oxford eLearning platform. To access the questions, go to ✔ http://oxfordmedicine.com/pediatricanesthesiaPBL

REFERENCES

1. Nuno M, Pelissier L, Varshneya K, Adamo MA, Drazin D. Outcomes and factors associated with infant abusive head trauma in the US. *J Neurosurg Pediatr*. 2015;16:515–522.
2. Beers SR, Berger RP, Adelson PD. Neurocognitive outcome and serum biomarkers in inflicted versus non-inflicted traumatic brain injury in young children. *J Neurotrauma*. 2007;24(1):97–105.
3. Ellingson KD, Leventhal JM, Weiss HB. Using hospital discharge data to track inflicted traumatic brain injury. *Am J Prev Med*. 2008;34(4 Suppl):S157–S162.
4. Kochanek PM, Carney N, Adelson PD, et al. Guidelines for the acute medical management of severe traumatic brain injury in infants, children, and adolescents—second edition. *Pediatr Crit Care Med*. 2012;13(Suppl 1):S1–S82.

5. Hardcastle N, Benzon HA, Vavilala MS. Update on the 2012 guidelines for the management of pediatric traumatic brain injury—information for the anesthesiologist. *Paediatr Anaesth.* 2014;24(7):703–710.

6. Ward A, Iocono JA, Brown S, Ashley P, Draus JM Jr. Non-accidental trauma injury patterns and outcomes: a single institutional experience. *Am Surg.* 2015;81(9):835–838.

7. Lindberg DM, Shapiro RA, Blood EA, Steiner RD, Berger RP, ExSTRA Investigators. Utility of hepatic transaminases in children with concern for abuse. *Pediatrics.* 2013;131(2):268–275.

8. Maguire SA, Upadhyaya M, Evans A, et al. A systematic review of abusive visceral injuries in childhood—their range and recognition. *Child Abuse Negl.* 2013;37(7):430–445.

9. Salehi-Had H, Brandt JD, Rosas AJ, Rogers KK. Findings in older children with abusive head injury: does shaken-child syndrome exist? *Pediatrics.* 2006;117(5):e1039–e1044.

10. Berger RP, Simon D, Wolford JE, Bell MJ. Abusive head trauma. In: Nichols DG, Shaffner DH, eds. *Rogers' Textbook of Pediatric Intensive Care.* 5th ed. Amsterdam, The Netherlands: Wolters Kluwer; 2016:982–989.

11. Vanderhave KL, Chiravuri S, Caird MS, et al. Cervical spine trauma in children and adults: perioperative considerations. *J Am Acad Orthop Surg.* 2011;19(6):319–327.

12. Nigrovic LE, Rogers AJ, Adelgais KM, et al. Utility of plain radiographs in detecting traumatic injuries of the cervical spine in children. *Pediatr Emerg Care.* 2012;28(5):426–432.

13. Choudhary AK, Bradford RK, Dias MS, Moore GJ, Boal DK. Spinal subdural hemorrhage in abusive head trauma: a retrospective study. *Radiology.* 2012;262(1):216–223.

14. Clevenger AC, Kilbaugh T, Margulies SS. Carotid artery blood flow decreases after rapid head rotation in piglets. *J Neurotrauma.* 2015;32(2):120–126.

15. Duhaime AC, Durham S. Traumatic brain injury in infants: the phenomenon of subdural hemorrhage with hemispheric hypodensity ("big black brain"). *Prog Brain Res.* 2007;161:293–302.

16. Guerra SD, Carvalho LF, Affonseca CA, Ferreira AR, Freire HB. Factors associated with intracranial hypertension in children and teenagers who suffered severe head injuries. *J Pediatr (Rio J).* 2010;86(1):73–79.

17. Webster DL, Fei L, Falcone RA, Kaplan JM. Higher-volume hypertonic saline and increased thrombotic risk in pediatric traumatic brain injury. *J Crit Care.* 2015;30(6):1267–1271.

18. Bourgeois M, Di Rocco F, Garnett M, et al. Epilepsy associated with shaken baby syndrome. *Childs Nerv Syst.* 2008;24(2):169–172; discussion 173.

19. Bruins B, Kilbaugh TJ, Margulies SS, Friess SH. The anesthetic effects on vasopressor modulation of cerebral blood flow in an immature swine model. *Anesth Analg.* 2013;116(4):838–844.

20. Zeiler FA, Teitelbaum J, West M, Gillman LM. The ketamine effect on ICP in traumatic brain injury. *Neurocrit Care.* 2014;21(1):163–173.

21. Minton MD, Grosslight K, Stirt JA, Bedford RF. Increases in intracranial pressure from succinylcholine: prevention by prior nondepolarizing blockade. *Anesthesiology.* 1986;65(2):165–169.

22. Burlison JD, Scott SD, Browne EK, Thompson SG, Hoffman JM. The Second Victim Experience and Support Tool: validation of an organizational resource for assessing second victim effects and the quality of support resources. *J Patient Saf.* 2017;13(2):93–102.

23. Edrees HH, Paine LA, Feroli ER, Wu AW. Health care workers as second victims of medical errors. *Pol Arch Med Wewn.* 2011;121(4):101–108.

62.

BURNS

Sanjay Bhananker and Paul Bhalla

STEM CASE AND KEY QUESTIONS

A 3-year-old, 18-kg toddler is brought into the emergency department after an accidental house fire. Initial assessment estimates partial and full thickness burns to approximately 45% of his body surface area, including face, anterior and posterior chest wall, and both upper extremities. There is soot seen in his mouth and he has a hoarse voice with stridor. He is responsive only to painful stimulus.

WHAT SHOULD THE PRIORITIES BE FOR INITIAL MANAGEMENT OF THIS CHILD IN THE EMERGENCY DEPARTMENT? ARE THERE ANY DRUGS THAT ARE CONTRAINDICATED?

Intravenous access is attempted in both lower extremities but after several failed attempts, an intraosseous cannula is placed in the left proximal tibia. With progressive airway compromise and decreased level of consciousness, he is intubated and mechanically ventilated with 100% oxygen. Pulse oximetry shows an oxygen saturation of 93%. Fluid resuscitation is commenced with Ringer's lactate. Blood samples are drawn and co-oximetry shows hypoxemia (PaO_2 68 mmHg), a metabolic acidemia (pH 7.21) with high lactate (6 mmol/L), and a carboxyhemoglobin level of 22%. One of the paramedics accompanying the child reports that he had been trapped for a short period in a smoke-filled bedroom before being rescued.

WHAT IS THE DIFFERENTIAL DIAGNOSIS? WHAT, IF ANY, FURTHER INFORMATION IS REQUIRED BEFORE ASSUMING CYANIDE POISONING? WHAT TREATMENT SHOULD BE CONSIDERED?

A secondary survey is undertaken and some minor non-burn injuries are noted and documented. A more detailed assessment of the burn is undertaken using a Lund-Browder chart for estimation of percent of total body surface area (TBSA) burned. A Foley catheter is placed in the bladder and a nasogastric tube inserted. It is now 5 hours since the injury and the child has had 1000 mL of Ringer's lactate. The Foley catheter drains 20 mL of urine on insertion.

WHAT CALCULATIONS CAN BE MADE TO MANAGE FLUID ADMINISTRATION? WHAT ENDPOINTS SHOULD BE USED TO GUIDE THIS? WHEN SHOULD ENTERAL FEEDING COMMENCE?

The patient is moved to the pediatric burns intensive care unit where a double lumen central venous line is placed in his right femoral vein. High calorie enteral feeding is commenced via a naso-jejunal tube. Pain is controlled by a morphine infusion with nurse-administered boluses, plus scheduled acetaminophen. Fluid balance is carefully monitored with urine output maintained at greater than 1 mL/kg/hour by adjusting the rate of infusion of Ringer's lactate. Bladder pressure is measured every 2 hours as a surrogate for intra-abdominal pressure. Base deficit, lactate, and central venous oxygen saturations ($ScvO_2$) are also monitored regularly. Fiberoptic bronchoscopy is performed through the endotracheal (ET) tube and reveals evidence of inhalation injury.

WHAT ARE THE PATHOPHYSIOLOGIC ALTERATIONS INDUCED BY BURNS? HOW IS TEMPERATURE REGULATION AFFECTED? HOW DOES BURN AFFECT THE METABOLIC AND CALORIC REQUIREMENTS?

His airway edema improves and his trachea is extubated after 72 hours. Postextubation hematocrit is 23%; the carboxyhemoglobin level is 1% and lactate is normal. Other laboratory results are normal. He is scheduled to have excision and grafting to all the burn areas early the next morning. You see the patient in the preoperative waiting area with his mother. The patient is crying and difficult to calm down, and his femoral central line has fallen out so he has no intravenous (IV) access. He had a dose of oral morphine at 5 AM. The child was previously healthy and has no known allergies. He has never needed any medicines in the past. When he cries, he opens his mouth to about more than 3 cm. He does not allow you to auscultate his chest, but the cry is loud enough to suggest good air entry. Oxygen saturation on 1L per minute of oxygen by nasal cannulae is 94% and his heart rate is 148 bpm. His tympanic temperature is 38°C.

HOW DO YOU HANDLE THE ISSUE
OF CONTINUOUS ENTERAL FEEDS
IN THE PERIOPERATIVE PERIOD?
WHAT ADDITIONAL PREOPERATIVE
INFORMATION WOULD YOU LIKE TO
HAVE BEFORE PROCEEDING WITH THE
ANESTHETIC? HOW WOULD YOU LIKE TO
PREMEDICATE THIS CHILD?

After discussion with the surgical team, the decision is made to continue enteral feeds throughout the perioperative period in order to avoid interruptions in nutritional intake. The child is premedicated with oral midazolam and oral ketamine. His mother is grateful to you for calming him down. He has a dry cough, and auscultation of his lungs reveals a few crackles bilaterally. SpO_2 now reads 91% and his heart rate is 136 bpm.

You proceed with an inhalational induction with sevoflurane in oxygen. Intravenous access is obtained with a 16-gauge cannula in the left femoral vein. The trachea is then intubated with a cuffed 4.0 mm ET tube. Bilateral breath sounds are present and end-tidal CO_2 is confirmed. A 22-gauge arterial line is sited in the left posterior tibial artery. A sample is sent for arterial blood gas (ABG) estimation, electrolytes, hematocrit, and a type-and-screen. The surgical team inspects the wounds and decides to harvest split thickness skin graft from the back and the scalp. They use bupivacaine and epinephrine added to the tumescent infiltration solution. The initial ABG shows pH 7.35, $PaCO_2$ 48 mmHg, PaO_2 345 mmHg, Na^+ 137 mEq/L, K^+ 4.5 mEq/L, hematocrit 21%, lactate 1.1 mmol/L.

WHAT IS YOUR TRANSFUSION
TRIGGER FOR THIS CHILD? HOW
WOULD YOU MONITOR THE BLOOD LOSS
IN THIS PATIENT? WHAT INTRAOPERATIVE
ANALGESIA WOULD BE APPROPRIATE? HOW
WOULD YOU MANAGE THE FLUID BALANCE?
WHAT IS THE ALLOWABLE CONCENTRATION
AND DOSE OF LOCAL ANESTHETICS AND
EPINEPHRINE?

Excision and grafting is completed over the next 3 hours. He received 2 adult units of packed red blood cells, and the hematocrit is 20% at the end of surgery. His heart rate is 155 bpm, blood pressure 70/34 mmHg, SpO_2 98%, temperature 35.2°C. Total urine output is 60 mL over the 5-hour procedure.

The patient is scheduled for removal of staples and change of dressings two days later in the procedure room on the burn floor. Since you are familiar with the patient, you are scheduled to provide sedation for the procedure.

Four days later, it is noted that the patient's abdomen is distended and he is no longer tolerating enteral feeding, indicated by high returns on gastric aspiration. He is increasingly tachycardic (170 bpm) and his blood sugar levels have been uncontrollably high (220 mg/dL).

Sepsis is high on the list of differential diagnoses at this stage, but diagnosis is difficult in the setting of a hypermetabolic state. Evidence of infection is sought by sending wound and blood cultures. A complete blood count is also sent. Management of the patient is supportive, with antibiotics started once clear evidence of infection emerges.

DISCUSSION

Roughly 15,000 children require hospitalization for burn injuries each year in the United States. About 1,100 children per year die from fires and burn injuries. Burns are second only to motor vehicle crashes as the leading cause of death in children older than 1 year. Younger children tend to suffer more scalds, while flame burns are more common in older children. Flame burns are often more severe and frequently involve concomitant inhalation injury.

Generally, the principles of burn treatment for children are similar to that for adults. However, the smaller TBSA of a child means a given burn area inflicts a greater percentage injury. On the other hand, older children demonstrate a greater physiological reserve and adaptability to injury, making them more likely to survive extensive burns than adults.

PATHOPHYSIOLOGY OF BURNS

The skin is the largest organ of the body, and large burns (greater than 20% TBSA) alter the physiological function of virtually all organs. Increasing burn size correlates directly with an increased risk of infection and death. Injury severity is therefore determined mainly by the size and depth of the burned area. However, patient age, body part burned, presence of inhalation injury, pre-existing disease, and associated non-burn injuries have an important impact on morbidity and mortality. Children younger than 2 years of age have a high surface area to body mass ratio, thin skin, and reduced physiologic reserves, resulting in worse outcomes than older children.

Severe dermal injury initiates a stress response with release of inflammatory mediators, pyrexia, catabolism, hyperglycaemia, increased capillary permeability, and a progressively hyperdynamic circulation. Fluid shifts are complicated further by evaporative losses from damaged areas of skin, and this combination may result in hypovolemic shock.

Catabolism can be marked, even with small burns, and close attention to nutritional intake is a management priority.

The services of a specialist burn center should be sought for full-thickness burns exceeding 5% TBSA, partial thickness exceeding 10% inhalation burns, or burns to the airway, face, hands, feet, and perineum.

FLUID RESUSCITATION IN MAJOR PEDIATRIC BURNS

Fluid resuscitation and control of edema are vital aspects of early burn management. Volume calculations are guided by the size of the burn as a percentage of TBSA, so it is important to estimate this as accurately as possible. The Rule of Nines is used to rapidly estimate burn size in adults, but the disproportionate ratio of head to body size in small children often results in overestimation. The Lund and Browder burn chart (Fig. 62.1) divides TBSA into smaller units and makes age-appropriate corrections. The Rule of Hands may also be used for smaller burn areas, with the area of the hand representing 1% of TBSA.

Once the burn area has been estimated, the next step is to initiate fluid resuscitation using a formula. The Baxter (Parkland) formula for fluid resuscitation of burn victims is 4 mL Ringer's lactate per kilogram body weight per percent TBSA burned, one half to be given during the first 8 hours after injury and the rest in the next 16 hours. Hypertonic saline may be useful in early shock, and colloids are most effective when used in the 12- to 24-hour period of resuscitation. It is widely believed that the Parkland formula underestimates resuscitation volumes, particularly when concomitant smoke inhalation is present. Allowances should be made for daily maintenance fluids in infants and toddlers. Adequate resuscitation is reflected by normal mentation, stable vital signs, and a urine output of 0.5 to 1.0 mL/kg/hr in children and 1 to 2 mL/kg/hr in infants.

In infants, blood sugar should be monitored and glucose-containing solutions added as necessary.

Overaggressive fluid resuscitation can result in *resuscitation morbidity*, a term used to describe the adverse effects of the large volumes of fluid given during resuscitation.[1] These sequelae include extremity ischemia, pulmonary edema, acute respiratory distress syndrome, and abdominal compartment syndrome. Increased intra-abdominal pressure can lead to decreased splanchnic blood flow, decreased renal perfusion, difficulty in ventilation, and cardiac preload. Bladder pressure measurement can be used to diagnose increasing intra-abdominal pressures. Bladder pressure in the 12 to 20 mmHg range may be considered indicative of intra-abdominal hypertension. Sustained pressures over 20 mmHg with evidence of organ dysfunction or failure (such as falling urine output) suggest abdominal compartment syndrome, which needs immediate treatment with abdominal decompression and is associated with a high mortality.

METABOLIC CHANGES

In burns greater than 40% TBSA, thermal injury leads to hypermetabolism and a hypercatabolic state, mediated by catecholamines and corticosteroids.[2] This hypermetabolic state can last up to 9 months following the injury.[3] Sequelae include increased resting energy expenditure, increased myocardial oxygen consumption, lipolysis, liver dysfunction, muscle catabolism, protein degradation, insulin resistance, and growth retardation.[4]

Blunting of the immune response, with consequent sepsis, can exaggerate these metabolic demands by up to 40% when compared to similar burn TBSA without the development of

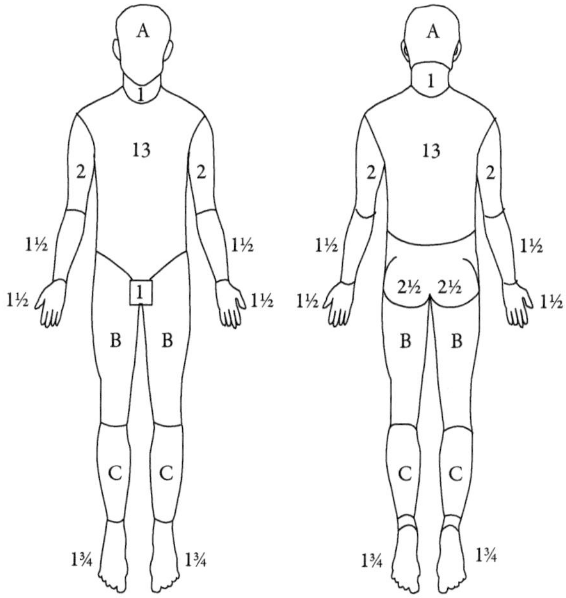

Region	Partial thickness (%) [NB1]	Full thickness (%)
Head		
Neck		
Anterior trunk		
Posterior trunk		
Right arm		
Left arm		
Buttocks		
Genitalia		
Right leg		
Left leg		
Total burn		
NB1: Do not include erythema		

Area	Age 0	1	5	10	15	Adult
A = Half of head	9½	8½	6½	5½	4½	3½
B = Half of one thigh	2¼	3¼	4	4½	4½	4¼
C = Half of one lower leg	2½	2½	2¾	3	3¼	3½

Fig. 62.1 Lund and Brower chart, used for estimating burn size in children.

sepsis.[5] Translocation of bacteria across gastrointestinal mucosa, disruption of the protective skin barrier, and the use of vascular catheters may also be contributory to the development of sepsis.

Management of the hypermetabolic response to a burn focuses on a number of factors, including early excision and grafting, thermoregulation, nutritional support and adequate pain relief.

Early excision and grafting

For burns that encompass over 50% TBSA, there is a 40% decrease in metabolic rate for patients totally excised and covered within 3 days of injury compared to those patients with like-size burns excised and covered 1 week after injury.[6] Excision and grafting of partial thickness burns involves tangential excision of the burn wound, in which the eschar is shaved off from the burn until a plane of viable tissue is reached. The excised wound is then covered with semisynthetic artificial skin, processed pig skin (xenograft), human cadaveric skin (allograft), or a split thickness skin graft (autograft). Excision of full-thickness burns requires fascial excision, where the overlying burned skin and subcutaneous fat are excised down to muscle fascia.

Thermoregulation

Thermal maintenance is critical in young children, especially those with burns of more than 10% TBSA. Immediate cooling of a burn is required to reduce tissue damage but may contribute significantly to hypothermia. Severely burned patients lose the ability to autoregulate core body temperature and often maintain core and skin temperatures at 2°C above baseline. This coupled with the loss of skin from the burn itself results in huge evaporative losses, estimated at up to 4L/m²/day. Maintaining a thermoneutral environment allows the energy from evaporative loss to come from the environment rather than the patient. Increasing the ambient temperature to 28° to 33°C therefore reduces metabolic rate and subsequent catabolism. Forced-air warmers may not be used directly over burned areas due to the risk of tissue desiccation.

Nutritionnal support

Aggressive, early enteral feeding improves outcomes in severely burned patients, partly by reducing the impact of hypermetabolism. Children require 1800 kilocalories (kcal) per meter squared TBSA plus 2200 kcal per meter squared of burn area per day.[7] Early enteral feeding also decreases the risk of sepsis, improves wound healing and nitrogen balance, and reduces stress ulceration and duration of hospitalization.[8] For this reason, traditional perioperative fasting guidelines may be relaxed for pediatric patients with major burns so that enteral feeding time can be maximized.

Hyperglycemia can occur as a result of feeding in the context of insulin resistance after injury. Glucose levels should be controlled with insulin before, during, and after surgery to improve wound healing and decrease wound infection risk. Electrolytes should be checked and replaced as necessary. Hyponatremia and hypophosphatemia are particularly common during the early post-burn period.[9]

Adequate pain control and alleviation of anxiety

Analgesia and anxiolysis, using a combination of pharmacological and non-pharmacological techniques, are important in order to limit the sympathetic emotional response to injury. Balanced multimodal systemic analgesia depends on a number of patient factors and comorbidities, and includes acetaminophen, non-steroidal anti-inflammatory drugs, opioids, low-dose ketamine infusions and gabapentinoids. Regional analgesia using peripheral nerve catheters or neuraxial blockade may also be indicated depending on the location of the burn. Non-pharmacological approaches include play therapy, visualization and meditation, music therapy and hypnosis. In complex patients, the involvement of a specialist acute pain service is paramount to coordinate pain therapy through the hospital stay.

INHALATIONAL INJURY

While children are less likely than adults to experience significant smoke inhalation, it remains a serious and life-threatening problem in the pediatric population. About a third of patients with a burn injury have concomitant inhalation injury,[10,11] and, in children, most fire-related deaths are attributable to smoke inhalation rather than burns.[12] The severity of inhalation injury depends on the precise fuels

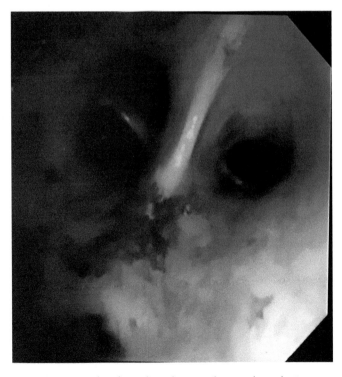

Fig. 62.2 An image taken during bronchoscopy showing thermal injury to the lower airway. (Image courtesy of Dr. Saman Arbabi, Professor of Surgery, Trauma, Burn and Critical Care Division, Harborview Medical Center, Seattle, WA).

burned, intensity of combustion, duration of exposure, and confinement. Inhalation of superheated air, particulate matter in smoke, and toxic gases cause direct injury to the airway and lung parenchyma (Fig. 62.2), as well as systemic toxicity from absorption of hydrogen cyanide and carbon monoxide.

Direct pulmonary injury

Direct pulmonary injury results from both thermal injury and chemical irritation. Unless steam is involved, heat injury to the airway is generally supraglottic, causing swelling of the posterior pharynx and supraglottic regions, leading to potential upper airway obstruction. The natural history of upper airway inhalation injury is edema formation that narrows the airway over the initial 12 to 24 hours. Intubation with a cuffed ET tube is recommended in patients who present with stridor, wheeze, or voice changes. Burns to the face and neck can result in tight eschar formation that, combined with pharyngeal edema, can cause difficult airway management. Lower airway or pulmonary parenchymal damage results from inhalation of the chemical constituents of smoke, usually becoming apparent 24 to 48 hours after the injury.

Pulmonary complications from inhalation injury markedly increase the morbidity and mortality from burn injury from 3% to 10% to 20% to 30%, so early recognition is vital.[10,13]

Signs suggestive of inhalation injury include singed hair, soot in the airway, stridor, hoarseness, dyspnea, wheezing, and facial burns. The clinical picture is identical to that of acute respiratory distress syndrome and is caused by chemical irritation of the terminal bronchiolar tree. Bronchoscopy reveals carbonaceous endobronchial debris and/or mucosal ulceration. Meticulous pulmonary toilet is the cornerstone of early care. Tracheal secretions are often very viscous, and the small internal diameter of pediatric ET tubes increases the risk of obstruction by these secretions.

Carbon monoxide poisoning

Carbon monoxide and cyanide poisoning should be suspected in any child with inhalational injury or with burns from open fires.

Carbon monoxide has an affinity for heme-containing proteins, such as hemoglobin, that is 250 times higher than oxygen.[14] It displaces oxygen from hemoglobin and cytochromes and shifts the oxygen dissociation curve to the left, decreasing oxygen delivery to the tissues. Pulse oximetry is a poor indicator of tissue hypoxia in carbon monoxide poisoning as the standard oximeter interprets carboxyhemoglobin as oxyhemoglobin and thus yields a falsely high value. Carbon monoxide poisoning is diagnosed by co-oximetry to measure carboxyhemoglobin levels. Normal carboxyhemoglobin levels are in the range of 1% to 3%. Children with a level less than 20% usually present with mild symptoms such as lightheadedness, nausea, and headache. At 20% to 40% carboxyhemoglobin the child may be confused and disoriented and at higher levels (>60%–70%) develop ataxia, collapse, and coma with resultant seizures, cardiopulmonary arrest, and death.[14] The half-life of carboxyhemoglobin is 240 minutes when breathing air. Administration of 100% oxygen reduces this to 40 to 60 minutes and facilitates the elimination of carbon monoxide. Hyperbaric oxygen therapy may be considered, as the half-life of carboxyhemoglobin reduces to 20 minutes at 2.5 to 3 atmospheres, but this therapy has limited indications due to the logistical challenges presented by transport of a patient with concomitant burns to a suitable facility.

Cyanide poisoning

Confirmed cyanide poisoning in children is quite uncommon, but as cyanide is a potent and deadly poison it should be considered in the context of inhalation of fire smoke in enclosed spaces, with family homes representing particularly high-risk situations.[15]

Cyanide binds to cytochrome oxidase and causes tissue hypoxia by uncoupling oxidative phosphorylation in mitochondria, thereby converting intracellular aerobic metabolism to anaerobic metabolism.[16]

Cyanide poisoning manifests in respiratory distress, neurological impairment, and metabolic acidosis. Signs and symptoms include cherry-red skin, headache, agitation, disorientation, confusion, weakness, malaise, dizziness, lethargy, and coma.[17] Due to the diminished level of aerobic metabolism there is characteristic venous hyperoxemia and red venous blood due to decreased oxygen consumption. Other possible manifestations are nausea and vomiting, abdominal pain, and, in a few patients, bitter almond breath odor.[18]

Three kinds of antidote are available to treat cyanide poisoning: methemoglobin-forming agents, sulfur donors (thiosulfate), and cobalt compounds (dicobalt edetate hydroxocobalamin).[17] Hydroxocobalamin is the antidote of choice as it is considered the safest and the most effective of those available. Treatment should be considered for victims of fires where cyanide gas exposure is more probable, particularly in pediatric patients. While unexplained elevated lactate may prompt hydroxocobalamin treatment, it should be administered on suspicion of cyanide poisoning, without waiting for laboratory test confirmation.

INITIAL MANAGEMENT OF A BURN VICTIM

The initial management of a burn victim is the same as for any presentation of a critically ill patient. The ABCDE approach prioritizes identification and management of life-threatening issues first. Exposure allows assessment of the site, depth, and extent of the burn to guide further early resuscitation. Background history should include events leading up to the injury, other injuries, conscious state, smoke inhalation or thermal injury of the upper airway, medical problems, vaccination status, and allergies.

Airway

Thermal and chemical airway injury rapidly causes airway edema, which is then potentially worsened by fluid resuscitation. The already narrow pediatric airway is vulnerable to critical obstruction, and so airway control with intubation of the trachea is often warranted at an early stage.

Breathing

All burn patients should be given 100% oxygen due to the risk of smoke inhalation and carbon monoxide poisoning. Ventilation may be impaired by thoracic and abdominal burns, requiring early escharotomy. Inflammation of the lung parenchyma may impair lung compliance and alveolar gas exchange.

Circulation

Loss of circulating volume occurs rapidly following a burn greater than 10%. Prompt fluid replacement by formula is necessary, as discussed previously in this chapter. Early wide-bore IV access may be hindered by the burn itself. Securing an IV cannula around burned tissue may also be problematic. Intraosseus fluid resuscitation is an alternative.

Disability

The AVPU (alert, voice, pain, unresponsive) scale is a common method for measuring and communicating responsiveness during a pediatric resuscitation. A decreased level of consciousness should always prompt suspicion of hypoxia, head injury, or inhalation of toxic gas.

Exposure and environmental control

Children with extensive burns lose the ability to thermoregulate and are at high risk of hypothermia. Cooling of the burn to limit tissue damage also promotes hypothermia. The entire body should be examined as soon as the patient is stable enough to do so. Clothing should be removed and careful attention paid to the possibility of peripheral edema formation in the peripheries, which can precipitate compartment syndrome.

Assessment of the burn

This phase should take into account any available background history such as the circumstances of the burn, presence of other injuries, evidence of smoke inhalation, or thermal airway injury. The burn itself should be examined for site, depth, and extent using standardized assessment tools. Many burn centers use high-resolution photography to record the extent of injury.

CLINICAL COURSE OF CUTANEOUS BURNS AND SUBSEQUENT ANESTHETIC MANAGEMENT

Fasting requirements

Gastric emptying may not be delayed in burn patients, and gastric acid production may actually be reduced in the early

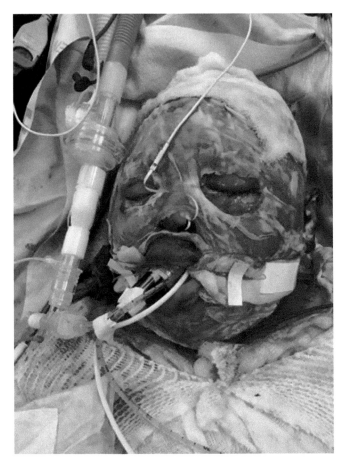

Fig. 62.3 A pediatric patient with facial burns causing difficulty with endotracheal tube fixation.

post-burn period. The safety and advantages of perioperative enteral feeds have been reported.[8] Enteral feeds may be continued throughout the perioperative period in patients who come to the operating room intubated. In non-intubated patients, shorter fasting times, typically 2 to 4 hours, may be acceptable.

Airway management

Airway management in pediatric burn patients can be challenging. Mask ventilation may be a problem with facial burns. Depending on the age of the burns, edema, scarring, or contractures may narrow the mouth opening and limit the neck movements. Location of burns and donor skin sites indicate the need for special positioning, for repositioning the patient during operation, or both. Securing an ET tube by taping or tying may be challenging in the presence of facial burns (Fig. 62.3).

Fixing the ET tube for prone positioning in the presence of facial burns is best achieved by wiring it to the teeth or stitching it to the nares.

In critically ill children requiring high inspiratory pressures during mechanical ventilation, a cuffed ET tube is indicated. Frequent suctioning helps clear mucus and debris from the tracheal tree, and a high index of suspicion should be maintained for plugging of the tracheal tube. A combination of prolonged prone positioning and relatively high fluid volume administration may cause significant airway swelling. It is best to wait until an air leak is present around the ET tube before tracheal extubation, because this indicates resolution of edema. If there is still no air leak and the patient is deemed ready for tracheal extubation, direct laryngoscopy may be necessary to determine the extent of residual edema. Once extubated, the patient should be closely monitored for progressive airway obstruction during the subsequent 24 to 48 hours.

Blood loss

Burn excision can result in massive and sudden blood loss. Quantifying blood loss is typically difficult in pediatric patients, and transfusion is best guided by serial hematocrit estimations. Adequate venous access is a prerequisite to burn excision and grafting procedures. At least 2 IV access routes should be established (peripheral or central), and blood products should be available in the room before excision begins. One study estimated a mean blood loss of 2.8% of blood volume for each percent TBSA excised.[19]

Intraoperative tourniquet use on burned extremities reduces overall blood loss. A tumescent technique with subcutaneous crystalloid injected in generous amounts can facilitate donor skin harvesting and reduce blood loss. Post-excision compression dressings and topical epinephrine have been used to reduce blood loss during excision and grafting procedures. Application of bandages soaked in 1:10,000 epinephrine after excision of burned skin is effective in producing a bloodless surface for placement of skin grafts. Although extremely high levels of catecholamines in the blood have been measured with this technique, complications such as dysrhythmias are uncommon. The hematocrit should be maintained between 20% and 25% to help with high metabolic demands for oxygen. If blood loss is excessive, it is prudent to rule out coagulation abnormalities. Platelets or coagulation factors may need to be replaced.

Anesthetic technique

General anesthesia with the combination of an opioid, a muscle relaxant, and a volatile agent is the most widely used technique for burn excision and grafting. Succinylcholine administration to patients more than 24 hours after burn injury is unsafe, due to the risk of hyperkalemic ventricular dysrhythmias. Patients with thermal injury are resistant to the action of nondepolarizing muscle relaxants. This is because the burn injury causes acetylcholine receptors in muscle to proliferate under the burn and at sites distant from the burn injury.

Tumescent local anesthesia with a maximum dose of 7 mg/kg lidocaine has been shown to be a safe and effective topical anesthetic technique for the surgical treatment of pediatric burns.

Regional anesthesia

Regional anesthesia, alone or in combination with general anesthesia, can be used in patients with small burns or for reconstructive procedures. For procedures on lower extremities, lumbar epidural or caudal catheters can be used to provide intra- and postoperative analgesia. The greatest limitation to the use of regional techniques is the extent of surgical field; most patients with major burns have a wide distribution of injuries and/or need skin harvesting from areas too large to be blocked by a regional technique. Presence of a coagulopathy or systemic or local infection may also contraindicate regional anesthetic techniques in these patients.

Analgesia

Severe pain is an inevitable consequence of a major burn injury, and perioperative analgesic requirements are frequently underestimated. Anxiety and depression are common components in a major burn and can further decrease the pain threshold. Pain management should be based on an understanding of the types of burn pain (acute or procedure-related pain versus background or baseline pain versus postoperative pain), frequent patient assessment by an acute pain service team, and the development of protocols. Acetaminophen is routinely used, but opioids are often needed to manage pain associated with burn procedures, and morphine is currently the most widely used drug. There is an interindividual variation in response to morphine, so titration to effect and frequent reassessment are important. Furthermore, most burned patients rapidly develop tolerance to opioids. Nonsteroidal anti-inflammatory drugs may be extremely useful for burn pain, but this class of drug has antiplatelet effects and may not be appropriate for patients who require extensive excision and grafting procedures. In addition, burn patients can also manifest the nephrotoxic effects of nonsteroidal anti-inflammatory drugs, so careful attention must be paid to fluid balance and renal function monitoring.

Procedural sedation

Procedures such as dressing changes and wound care frequently require sedation and analgesia in pediatric burn patients. These procedures are often performed on a daily basis on the burn ward, making the involvement of a dedicated anesthesia team impractical. Nurse-administered opioid medication (IV, oral, or transmucosal) is typical for analgesia and sedation. However, when wound care procedures are extensive, more potent anesthetic agents may be of benefit. An IV propofol infusion may be administered by an anesthesia provider with American Society of Anesthesiologists minimum standard monitoring. Ketamine offers the advantage of stable hemodynamics and analgesia and has been used extensively as the primary agent for both general anesthesia and analgesia for burn dressing changes. Nitrous oxide with oxygen has been used effectively for analgesia during burn wound dressing changes as well. However, scavenging of the gas when administered outside of an operating room is problematic.

The use of alpha-2 agonist dexmedetomidine, administered as an infusion, is gaining popularity.[20]

BURNS-ASSOCIATED SEPSIS

Sepsis is a leading cause of death in patients who survive the acute burn injury. Burn wound infection, IV catheter associated septicemia, and ventilator-associated pneumonia are particularly common in burned children. Loss of the barrier function of skin and blunting of the immune response result in increased susceptibility to infection and bacterial overgrowth within the eschar. Bowel permeability is increased in burn patients, leading to translocation of bacteria and absorption of endotoxins into the bloodstream. Pyrexia, tachycardia, and leukocytosis are part of the hypermetabolic response in burn patients and cannot be considered signs of sepsis. There is no satisfactory biomarker for the confirmatory diagnosis of sepsis, so diagnosis is inconsistent.[21] The American Burn Association defines sepsis in burns based on clinical and laboratory criteria.[5] In children, the presence of at least 3 of the following criteria are suggestive of sepsis: tachycardia, tachypnea, thrombocytopenia, hyperglycemia, inability to continue enteral feeding.[5] The latest international consensus (sepsis-3) uses a more standardized approach to defining organ failure, the Sequential Organ Failure Assessment (SOFA) score, but this is not yet validated in burn patients.[22] Once sepsis is suspected, evidence of infection must be sought, with wound and blood cultures helping to identify offending pathogens and appropriately treat infection. Systemic antibiotics should be reserved for treatment of proven infection and in the perioperative period. Ideally local guidelines should exist in order to promote diagnostic standards, antibiotic prescribing practices, and consistent swabbing techniques.[23]

CONCLUSIONS

- Burn injuries are a leading cause of death and morbidity in children.

- Initial management must focus on assessment and resuscitation, with emphasis on securing an airway, estimation of burn size, providing adequate fluid resuscitation using an established formula, and maintaining normothermia.

- Subsequent management involves treatment of the burned area with excision and skin grafting, which can require multiple procedures.

- Complications include the development of a hypermetabolic state with subsequent catabolism and increased risk of sepsis.

REVIEW QUESTIONS

1. A 9-year-old girl is brought in to the emergency department following a house fire. Carboxyhemoglobin level is 20%. She has carbonaceous deposits in her oropharynx, oxygen saturation is 97% on room air, and she is breathing spontaneously at a rate of 40 breaths per minute with no sign of airway obstruction. The next **BEST** immediate step in management is

   A. endotracheal intubation.
   B. fiberoptic bronchoscopy.
   C. hyperbaric oxygen therapy.
   D. oxygen by non-rebreather mask.

Answer. D
Carbon monoxide poisoning reduces tissue oxygenation by binding hemoglobin with a much stronger affinity than oxygen, reducing overall oxygen content and shifting the oxygen dissociation curve to the left. Increasing levels of carboxyhemoglobin will cause worsening neurological sequelae and eventual cardiac dysfunction and death.

Initial treatment is with 100% oxygen administration, which reduces the half-life of carboxyhemoglobin from approximately 4 hours to under 1 hour. The half-life of carboxyhemoglobin reduces to 20 minutes in the presence of 100% oxygen at 2 atmospheres of pressure. However, the use of hyperbaric oxygen therapy is limited to specialist centers and is not normally a practical option.[24] The patient will likely need tracheal intubation as the next step in management of inhalation injury.

2. A 4-year-old boy weighing 16 kg presents as a transfer from an outside hospital. They have estimated his burn size as 25% TBSA using the Rule of Nines. Using the Parkland formula, fluid resuscitation is commenced at 800 mL Ringer's lactate over the first 8 hours (starting rate of 100 mL/hr). Later, when the burns team assesses him using a Lund and Brower chart, his burn size is estimated at 15%. Which of the following burn estimating techniques is **MOST** appropriate to calculate ongoing fluid management?

   A. Rule of Nines
   B. Lund and Bower
   C. Rule of Hands
   D. 4-2-1 formula

Answer: B
The Rule of Nines is a quicker way of estimating burn size, but in children it is inaccurate and may overestimate by as much as 100%. This could result in overadministration of fluid and subsequent edema. The Rule of Hands is an adequate tool for estimating the size of smaller burns, but for a burn TBSA over 10% in children the Lund and Brower chart is recommended.

There are 2 commonly used formulae to estimate fluid administration. The modified Brooke formula estimates the first 24-hour fluid requirement at 2 mL/kg/%TBSA, and the Parkland formula uses 4 mL/kg/%TBSA. Both formulae divide the requirement in 2, with half given in the first 8 hours and half given over the next 16 hours. There are no direct comparisons of the 2 methods, and the American Burn Association consensus is to start at 2 to 4 mL/kg/%TBSA.[1] Regardless of the formula used, vigilance for signs and symptoms of hypo- and hypervolemia are key, with a target urine output of 1 mL/kg/hr.

3. A 13-year-old girl presents with 60% flame burns to her torso, face, and upper extremities. After 5 days in the burn unit, she is started on a broad-spectrum antibiotic for presumed sepsis. Which of the following finding is the **LEAST** appropriate in diagnosing sepsis?

- A. enteral feed intolerance >24 hours
- B. hyperglycemia >140 mg/dL (non-fasting)
- C. hypotension <5th percentile for age and gender
- D. tachycardia >85% of age-corrected maximum bpm

Answer: C

The diagnosis of sepsis in the presence of a significant burn injury is difficult, as clinical indicators such as pyrexia and leucocytosis are common to both. The American Burn Association consensus (2007) suggested the following as triggers for suspicion of sepsis: progressive tachycardia, progressive tachypnea, thrombocytopenia, hyperglycemia, inability to continue enteral feeding. A definitive diagnosis of sepsis requires identification of a causative pathogen (e.g., a positive blood culture) or a clinically significant improvement with antimicrobial treatment.[21]

4. A 7-year-old boy is being taken to the operating room 4 days after a 50% scald burn to his abdomen and back for debridement and skin grafting. Preoperatively he is breathing spontaneously with adequate oxygenation and ventilation. He is being fed via a nasogastric tube, which was stopped 2 hours ago per local guidelines. Which is the **MOST** appropriate plan for initiation of anesthesia?

- A. epidural block, catheter placement with propofol sedation
- B. inhalation induction with sevoflurane and cricoid pressure
- C. modified rapid sequence induction with propofol and rocuronium
- D. rapid sequence induction with propofol and succinylcholine

Answer: C

Approximately 24 hours after a significant burn injury, upregulation of extrajunctional nicotinic acetylcholine receptors occurs in muscle, which may cause life-threatening hyperkalemia if succinylcholine is administered. Furthermore, there is resistance to nondepolarizing muscle relaxants, so neuromuscular monitoring is vital if any muscle relaxants are used.

Victims of burn injuries can become hypermetabolic, and adequate nutritional support is vital; therefore fasting guidelines are frequently relaxed in this population in order to maximize enteral feeding time. This patient is at risk of aspiration in the presence of nasogastric feeding, making a laryngeal mask airway potentially risky. Feeding via the nasojejunal route would be preferred if frequent visits to the operating room are anticipated.

Regional anesthesia may be a reasonable option in burn injury surgery but would be limited in this patient by the presence of burned skin on his back.[9]

QUESTIONS AND ANSWERS

This chapter has accompanying questions and answers which are available to subscribers as part of the Oxford eLearning platform. To access the questions, go to ✅ http://oxfordmedicine. com/pediatricanesthesiaPBL

REFERENCES

1. Cancio LC. Initial assessment and fluid resuscitation of burn patients. *Surg Clin North America*. 2014;94(4):741–754. doi:10.1016/j.suc.2014.05.003
2. Wilmore DW, Long JM, Mason AD, Skreen RW, Pruitt BA. Catecholamines: mediator of the hypermetabolic response to thermal injury. *Ann Surg*. 1974;180(4):653–669.
3. Jeschke MG, Chinkes DL, Finnerty CC, et al. The pathophysiologic response to severe burn injury. *Ann Surg*. 2008;248(3):387–401. doi:10.1097/SLA.0b013e3181856241
4. Williams FN, Herndon DN, Jeschke MG. The hypermetabolic response to burn injury and interventions to modify this response. *Clin Plast Surg*. 2009;36(4):583–596. doi:10.1016/j.cps.2009.05.001
5. Greenhalgh DG, Saffle JR, Holmes JH, et al. American Burn Association consensus conference to define sepsis and infection in burns. *J Burn Care Res*. 2007;28:776–790. doi:10.1097/BCR.0b013e3181599bc9
6. Hart DW, Wolf SE, Chinkes DL, et al. Determinants of skeletal muscle catabolism after severe burn. *Ann Surg*. 2000;232(4):455–465. doi:10.1097/00000658-200010000-00001
7. Hildreth MA, Herndon DN, Desai MH, Duke MA. Reassessing caloric requirements in pediatric burn patients. *J Burn Care Rehab*. 1988;9(6):616–618. doi:10.1097/00004630-198811000-00009
8. Jenkins ME, Gottschlich MM, Warden GD. Enteral feeding during operative procedures in thermal injuries. *J Burn Care Rehab*. 1994;15(2):199–205. doi:10.1097/00004630-199403000-00019
9. Fuzaylov G, Fidkowski CW. Anesthetic considerations for major burn injury in pediatric patients. *Paediatr Anaesth*. 2009;19(3):202–211. doi:10.1111/j.1460-9592.2009.02924.x
10. Clark WR Jr. Smoke inhalation: diagnosis and treatment. *World J Surg*. 1992;16(1):24–29. doi:10.1007/BF02067110
11. Barrow RE, Spies M, Barrow LN, Herndon DN. Influence of demographics and inhalation injury on burn mortality in children. *Burns*. 2004;30(1):72–77. doi:10.1016/j.burns.2003.07.003
12. Committee on Injury and Poison Prevention. Reducing the number of deaths and injuries from residential fires. *Pediatrics*. 2000;105(6):1355–1357. doi:10.1542/peds.105.6.1355
13. Edelman DA, White MT, Tyburski JG, Wilson RF. Factors affecting prognosis of inhalation injury. *J Burn Care Res*. 2006;27(6):848–853. doi:10.1097/01.BCR.0000245493.26814.CE
14. Kao LW, Nañagas KA. Carbon monoxide poisoning. *Med Clin North America*. 2005;89(6):1161–1194. doi:10.1016/j.mcna.2005.06.007
15. Grabowska T, Skowronek R, Nowicka J, Sybirska H. Prevalence of hydrogen cyanide and carboxyhaemoglobin in victims of smoke inhalation during enclosed-space fires: a combined toxicological risk. *Clin Toxicol*. 2012;50(8):759–763. doi:10.3109/15563650.2012.714470

16. Geller RJ, Barthold C, Saiers JA, Hall AH. Pediatric cyanide poisoning: causes, manifestations, management, and unmet needs. *Pediatrics*. 2006;118(5):2146–2158. doi:10.1542/peds.2006-1251

17. Mintegi S, Clerigue N, Tipo V, et al. Pediatric cyanide poisoning by fire smoke inhalation: a European expert consensus. Toxicology Surveillance System of the Intoxications Working Group of the Spanish Society of Paediatric Emergencies. *Pediatr Emerg Care*. 2013;29:1234–1240. doi:10.1097/PEC.0b013e3182aa4ee1

18. Nelson L. Acute cyanide toxicity: mechanisms and manifestations. *J Emerg Nurs*. 2006;32(4):S8–S11. doi:10.1016/j.jen.2006.05.012

19. Housinger TA, Lang D, Warden GD. A prospective study of blood loss with excisional therapy in pediatric burn patients. *J Trauma*. 1993;34(2):262–263. doi:10.1097/00005373-199302000-00015

20. Anderson TA, Fuzaylov G. Perioperative anesthesia management of the burn patient. *Surg Clin North America*. 2014;94(4):851–861. doi:10.1016/j.suc.2014.05.008

21. Nunez Lopez O, Cambiaso-Daniel J, Branski LK, Norbury WB, Herndon DN. Predicting and managing sepsis in burn patients: current perspectives. *Ther Clin Risk Manag*. 2017;13:1107–1117. doi:10.2147/TCRM.S119938

22. Singer M, Deutschman CS, Seymour CW, et al. The Third International Consensus Definitions for Sepsis and Septic Shock (Sepsis-3). *JAMA*. 2016;315(8):801. doi:10.1001/jama.2016.0287

23. Davies A, Spickett-Jones F, Brock P, Coy K, Young A. Variations in guideline use and practice relating to diagnosis and management of infection in paediatric burns services in England and Wales: a national survey. *Burns*. 2017;43(1):215–222. doi:10.1016/j.burns.2016.07.032

24. Fidkowski CW, Fuzaylov G, Sheridan RL, Coté CJ. Inhalation burn injury in children. *Paediatr Anaesth*. 2009;19(s1):147–154. doi:10.1111/j.1460-9592.2008.02884.x

63.

ANESTHESIA FOR THE CHILD WITH AUTISM SPECTRUM DISORDER

Bistra G. Vlassakova

STEM CASE AND KEY QUESTIONS

A 15-year-old, 93-kg boy diagnosed with autism at age 5 is scheduled for dental rehabilitation under general anesthesia.

WHAT IS AUTISM SPECTRUM DISORDER (ASD)? HOW DO THE FOURTH AND FIFTH EDITION OF THE *DIAGNOSTIC AND STATISTICAL MANUAL OF MENTAL DISORDERS* (DSM-IV, DSM-V) DIFFER IN THE DIAGNOSIS OF AUTISM?

The patient was diagnosed with autism based on observations made mostly at school by his teachers. He has relatively poor language skills for his age. He is able to communicate simple needs. He lives at home with his parents and 2 siblings.

WHAT IS THE CLINICAL PRESENTATION OF CHILDREN WITH ASD? WHAT ARE THE CHALLENGES THEY FACE DURING HOSPITAL VISITS AND WHY?

Upon review of the patient's medical record, you note that he has emotional outbursts when he becomes angry or anxious and will hit other people and/or throw objects. He dislikes loud noises and too many unfamiliar people around him; when severely anxious, he will bite himself or try to hit his head against the wall. He does not tolerate restrictions on his meals.

WHAT ARE SOME OF THE COMMON BEHAVIORAL CHARACTERISTICS OF CHILDREN WITH ASD? WHAT INFORMATION WOULD YOU LIKE TO HAVE IN ADVANCE TO HELP WITH PLANNING FOR THE CASE?

The patient has a monozygotic twin, also with a diagnosis of autism. He was born at 33 weeks gestational age and was small for his age. He had a prolonged neonatal intensive care unit stay secondary to respiratory problems.

WHAT ARE KNOWN RISK FACTORS FOR AUTISM? WHAT IS THE PATHOGENESIS OF AUTISM?

Following the diagnosis of autism, the patient was placed in a special education program and currently receives scheduled teaching sessions of applied behavioral analysis (ABA) therapy. He is also undergoing occupational therapy and speech sessions.

At age 8, he was also diagnosed with attention deficit hyperactivity disorder (ADHD). He was started on risperidone with some improvement of his symptoms. He also takes melatonin and clonidine for sleep. At age 13, he presented with seizures and has been on levetiracetam since then. His seizures are well controlled. The patient has frequent gastrointestinal (GI) complaints of bloating, constipation, and diarrhea. He has many food aversions and a very specific and limited diet. He also has a prescription for lorazepam as needed for anxiety.

WHAT ARE COMMON COMORBIDITIES IN CHILDREN WITH ASD? WHAT MEDICATIONS ARE COMMON IN THIS PATIENT POPULATION? WHAT ARE THE ANESTHETIC IMPLICATIONS OF THESE DRUGS?

During the preoperative conversation, the mother expresses severe anxiety about the upcoming procedure. The child had anesthesia at age 4 years for tonsillectomy and adenoidectomy with a very difficult perioperative period. According to the mother, he woke up with severe, prolonged agitation, necessitating physical restraints and additional medications. At home, he experienced night terrors and behavioral regression for approximately 2 weeks postoperatively. He has also undergone several upper endoscopies under general anesthesia, and the experience has always been somewhat traumatic to him.

GIVEN THIS INFORMATION, HOW WOULD YOU PREPARE FOR THE CASE? WHAT RESOURCES WILL YOU UTILIZE?

As per instructions the patient arrives at the hospital 1 hour before the surgical procedure. He is immediately brought into a private room. When you arrive at the patient's bedside, he is sitting on the stretcher, rocking, and his mother is holding him, trying to comfort him. They are looking at the book of social stories the child life specialist has offered them. He has a tablet computer and headphones next to him.

HOW WOULD YOU APPROACH THE PATIENT AND THE FAMILY ON THE DAY OF SURGERY? WHAT SPECIAL PRECAUTIONS WOULD YOU TAKE? WHAT ADVANTAGES ARE OFFERED BY A MULTIDISCIPLINARY APPROACH IN THIS SITUATION?

Your discussion with the mother outside the room reveals that the patient has been getting more anxious over time. His emotional outbursts can be unpredictable. He would not take any oral premedication and would not allow a peripheral intravenous (IV) line to be placed. In the past, when he was younger, mask induction was performed in the operating room (OR), and he was held down while crying and kicking. Mom believes that these experiences contribute to his severe anxiety associated with medical facilities and procedures. You discuss the options and your concerns with the mother. A final decision is made to administer intramuscular injection of ketamine and midazolam. You explain to the mother in detail how the premedication will be administered, what the expectations are, and how she can assist you in the process. His mother's suggestion is to try to engage her son and explain in very simple language what will happen. He does well with directions like "first . . ., then . . .". Receiving a toy for positive reinforcement is also discussed.

WHAT PREMEDICATION OPTIONS EXIST, AND HOW WOULD YOU MAKE YOUR CHOICE OF MEDICATION/ADMINISTRATION ROUTE? WHAT ARE THE POTENTIAL ADVERSE EFFECTS?

To help with administration of premedication, you bring another anesthesia provider into the room. The mother is instructed to talk to the boy and to continue to comfort him. His favorite show is playing on the tablet, and he is listening with his headphones on. You introduce yourself to him; he shakes your hand, does not make eye contact, and turns his attention back to the tablet. You explain to him that he will get a small injection in his arm and then he will get a squishy toy—one of his favorite types of toys.

The boy holds his mother's hand tightly and keeps watching the tablet screen but screams and tries to pull away from you when you do the injection. You give him the new toy, and he takes it, but starts rocking even more on the bed while crying. As per initial discussion with the mother, you leave the room.

WHAT IS YOUR PLAN NOW FOR THE ANESTHESIA INDUCTION? HOW WILL YOU PROCEED?

After 5 minutes, the boy appears well sedated, and you are able to roll the bed to the OR without a parent. As per initial discussion with the OR team, the light in the room is low, and only essential personnel for the induction of the anesthetic are in the room. The patient is positioned on the operative table, and smooth induction with O_2 / N_2O is initiated. A peripheral IV line is started, and fentanyl, propofol, and rocuronium are administered. Atraumatic nasal intubation is performed to accommodate the surgical procedure.

WHAT ARE YOUR INTRAOPERATIVE GOALS FOR THIS PATIENT? ARE THERE MEDICATIONS YOU WILL AVOID AND WHY?

The surgical procedure lasts 3.5 hours. It involves multiple fillings and extractions of all four wisdom teeth. One of the extractions is complicated by breaking a root, necessitating additional surgical work. A significant amount of bleeding is encountered. You decide to wake up the patient at the end of the procedure. On emergence, the patient becomes very combative, and it is difficult to control him. Help is called to the room. You administer a large bolus of propofol to calm him down and to be able to transport the patient to the recovery room.

WHAT COMMUNICATION WILL YOU HAVE WITH THE RECOVERY ROOM TEAM? WHAT GOALS WILL YOU SET FOR THIS PATIENT?

As per initial discussion with the mother, she is in the recovery room already awaiting the arrival of her son. Mom states that he would be very aggravated by the monitors and by the peripheral IV line. A decision is made to take a set of vital signs while the patient is still asleep and then to remove them before he wakes up. Since the patient has been well hydrated intraoperatively, the peripheral IV is capped, wrapped well, and covered.

WHAT WOULD BE YOUR INSTRUCTIONS TO THE NURSING TEAM AND THE MOTHER REGARDING DISCHARGE FROM THE RECOVERY ROOM?

The patient wakes up after 15 minutes. His mother is sitting next to him, and he is given his new toy and his tablet. He is somewhat irritable, but the mother is able to comfort him. After 30 minutes and discussion with the mother and the surgical and recovery room team, the decision is made to discharge him home. He remains calm and content on the way to the car. A postoperative call the next day reveals a difficult first night with a tantrum over dessert but no other issues. On postoperative day 2, the patient is able to go to school and to follow his daily routine. The mother is satisfied with her son's clinical care.

DISCUSSION

DEFINITIONS, CLASSIFICATION, AND CLINICAL FEATURES

ASD is a neurodevelopmental disorder associated with deficits in social communication and interaction and the presence of repetitive behaviors and interests. DSM-V, adopted in 2013, significantly changed the diagnosis of autism. Previous categories of autism, such as Asperger syndrome and pervasive developmental disorders not otherwise classified (PDDNOC) from DSM-IV, are now incorporated in the single diagnosis of ASD. The condition manifests early in childhood and impacts quality of life.

To be diagnosed with ASD, the child should have developmental disturbances in 2 main categories: (i) social interactions and communication and (ii) repetitive and restrictive interests and behaviors. (Table 63.1)

In addition to these signs and symptoms, a significant percentage of patients with ASD have some degree of abnormal sensory perception. This can present as under- or overresponsiveness and/or an abnormal response to sensory stimuli.

INCIDENCE AND PREVALENCE

According to the Center for Disease Control and Prevention report from 2014, 1:59 children is diagnosed with ASD in the United States. A significant increase in the number of cases was noted between 2000 and 2010, but no change was observed in newly diagnosed cases between 2010 and 2012 (Table 63.3).

ASD occurs in all races and socioeconomic groups. It affects boys more often than girls at a 4:1 ratio. Worldwide, 1% of the population is affected by the condition.

Table 63.1 **DSM-V AUTISM SPECTRUM DISORDER DIAGNOSTIC CRITERIA**

I. Persistent deficit in social communication and social interactions, not accounted by general developmental delays (3 out of 3 symptoms)	
1. Deficits in normal social-emotional reciprocity	– Abnormal social approach – Failure of normal back and forth conversation – Reduced sharing of interest – Reduced sharing of emotions/affect – Lack of initiation of social interaction – Poor social imitation
2. Deficits in nonverbal communicative behaviors used for social interaction	– Impairment with use of eye contact as social cue – Impairment in use and understanding of body language—postures and gestures – Abnormal volume, pitch, rate, rhythm of voice – Lack of coordinated verbal and nonverbal communication
3. Deficits in developing and maintaining relationships	– Deficits developing friendships – Difficulties adjusting behaviors to suit social context – Difficulties sharing imaginative play – Difficulties in making friends – Absence of interest in others
II. Restricted, repetitive pattern of interest, activities or behavior (2 out of 4 symptoms)	
1. Stereotyped or repetitive speech, movements or use of objects	– Stereotyped/repetitive speech—echolalia, pedantic or formal language; idiosyncratic or metaphoric language – Stereotyped/repetitive motor movements—grimacing, intense body language, rocking, flapping – Stereotyped use of objects—repetitively turns light on/off, repetitively opens and closes doors, aligns toys the same way
2. Excessively adheres to routines, ritualized patterns of verbal and nonverbal communication, or excessive resistance to change	– Adherence to routines—change in route, specific patterns of behavior – Ritualized patterns of verbal and nonverbal behavior – Rigid thinking – Extreme resistance to change
3. Highly restricted, fixed interests that are abnormal in intensity and focus	– Narrow range of interest – Preoccupations, obsessions – Having to carry around a specific object – Unusual fear
4. Hyper- or hyporeactivity to sensory input	– High tolerance to pain – Preoccupation with textures to touch – Unusual visual exploration/activity
III. Symptoms must be present in early childhood (may not be clinically present before the social expectations exceed the limited capabilities)	

Note. DSM-V = *Diagnostic and Statistical Manual of Mental Disorders* (5th ed.).

DSM-V also offers 3 levels of severity based on the degree of support and individual needs. (see Table 63.2).

Table 63.2 **SEVERITY OF ASD ACCORDING TO DSM-V**

SEVERITY	SOCIAL INTERACTIONS AND COMMUNICATIONS	RESTRICTED INTERESTS AND REPETITIVE BEHAVIORS
Level 1 " Requiring support"	Difficulties initiating social interactions May appear to have decreased interest in social interactions	RRB cause interference with functioning Resists attempts from others to break RRB or to be redirected
Level 2 " Requiring substantial support"	Marked deficit in verbal and nonverbal communication skills Abnormal reaction to social overtures by others	RRB appear frequent and interfere with daily functioning Distress or frustration with interruptions of RRB
Level 3 " Requiring very substantial support"	Severe impairment in social and language skills Minimal or no response to social interactions by others	RRB markedly interferes with functioning on all levels Very difficult to redirect from and/or comes back to RRB quickly

Note. ASD = autism spectrum disorder; DSM-V = *Diagnostic and Statistical Manual of Mental Disorders* (5th ed.); RRB = ritualistic and repetitive behaviors.

SCREENING AND DIAGNOSIS

Many of the clinical symptoms of autism are obvious around 2 years of age. They may present earlier but might not be apparent until the social environment exhausts the limited social abilities of the individual. Capabilities of these children may vary from those who never achieve any developmental milestones to others who will plateau after reaching some language skills and then show regression in their language and social skills between 15 and 24 months of age.

Screening is indicated for children with delayed neurodevelopment, per recommendations of teachers or due to parental concerns. The American Academy of Pediatrics (AAP) recommends ASD-directed screening to be conducted between 18 and 24 months of age because this is a critical time for social and language development, and early interventions with ABA therapy and other behavioral techniques have shown promising results.[1,2] Screening is usually done using a tiered approach: tier 1 helps identify children at risk for ASD and tier 2 is geared toward differentiating between children with ASD and other developmental disorders. Multiple scales have been used to screen for ASD. Some of the commonly used screening tools for children under 3 years are the Modified Checklist for Autism in Toddlers (CHAT) and Parent's Observation of Social Interactions. Tools for preschool and school age children include the Social Communication Questionnaire, Autism Spectrum Screening Questionnaire, and others.

Evaluation for ASD should be a comprehensive assessment conducted by a multidisciplinary team. The evaluation has several objectives:

– Definitive diagnosis of ASD.

– Exclusion of other conditions that might present with symptoms similar to ASD.

– Genetic evaluation to rule out other conditions that might present with ASD.

Table 63.3 **IDENTIFIED PREVALENCE OF ASD: ADDM NETWORK 2000–2012**

SURVEILLANCE YEAR	PREVALENCE PER 1,000 CHILDREN (RANGE)	INCIDENCE 1/ PER
2000	6.7 (4.5–9.9)	1:150
2002	6.6 (3.3–10.6)	1:150
2004	8.0 (4.6–9.8)	1:125
2006	9.0 (4.2–12.1)	1:110
2008	11.3 (4.8–21.2)	1:88
2010	14.7 (5.7–21.9)	1:68
2012	14.6 (8.2–24.6)	1:68
2014	16.8 (13.1–29.3)	1:59

Note. ASD = autism spectrum disorder; ADDM = Autism and Developmental Disabilities Monitoring.

Adapted from Autism Spectrum Report: Data and Statistics. Athens, GA: Centers for Disease Control and Prevention. https://www.cdc.gov/ncbddd/autism/data.html

– Determination of the child's level of functionality.

The diagnosis is based on the physical exam, history, and observation of behavior.

PATHOGENESIS

1. **Genetic factors**: There is increasing evidence for a genetic component for ASD. It is also clear that ASD is not a single gene defect disorder. At the moment, 800 ASD predisposing genes have been identified. Many studies are focused on finding a connection between clinical phenotypes with specific genetic profiles. Duplication of the long arm of chromosome 15 has been associated with 1% to 2% of the children with ASD, usually presenting with moderate to severe intellectual disability. Children with ASD and macrocephaly have a higher frequency of PTEN mutations. Other potential loci are located on chromosomes 16p and 17.

   Further proof for a genetic basis for ASD is familial inheritance. Monozygotic twin studies have shown that, if one child is affected, the other twin has a 36% to 95% chance of also being diagnosed with autism. In nonidentical twins, if one child is affected, the other will be affected 0% to 31% of the time.[3] The risk for a couple that already has a child with autism to have another one with ASD is 2% to 18%.

2. **Neurobiological factors**: Neuroimaging and autopsies have found brain anomalies in patients with ASD. These include, but are not limited to, decreased volume of gray and white matter and abnormalities in neuronal networks and cortical structure and function.

3. **Environmental and parental factors**: A meta-analysis by Gardener et al. did not identify one single factor contributing to the development of ASD. Among the ones that were found to contribute were umbilical cord complications, early birth, low birth weight, and low 5-minute Apgar scores. Anesthesia assisted vaginal delivery, postterm delivery, head circumference, and large birth weight were not found to be associated with ASD. Advanced maternal and paternal age has been associated with a risk of having offspring with ASD.[4]

ASD AND COEXISTING CONDITIONS

Many children with ASD have other coexisting medical diseases. Optimization of general health is likely to have a positive effect on habilitative progress, functional outcome, and quality of life. Therefore, important issues, such as management of associated medical problems, pharmacologic and nonpharmacologic intervention for challenging behaviors, and coexisting mental health conditions, are of paramount importance.

1. **Chromosomal abnormalities**: Investigators have found that a significant number of ASD patients, 8% to more than 40%, had some additional genetic or chromosomal abnormalities. Specific disorders include Down syndrome, Fragile X chromosome, 22q deletion syndrome, tuberous sclerosis, Angelman syndrome, and maternally derived duplication of chromosome 15q11-q13.

2. **GI problems**: Many children with ASD have GI problems. A meta-analysis from 2014 found significant prevalence of GI problems in children with ASD in comparison with the control group.[5] A wide range of symptoms from food intolerance, food allergies, malabsorption, celiac disease, and inflammatory bowel disease necessitated frequent GI procedures. The exact cause of these symptoms is not identified. Environmental factors, gut micro flora abnormalities, and mitochondrial dysfunction have all been hypothesized to cause GI dysfunction.[6]

3. **Psychiatric disorders**: ADHD is often comorbid with ASD, and recent studies have found an association of ADHD as a predictor for ASD.

4. **Sleep disturbances**: Sleep problems in children with ASD include increased bedtime resistance, insomnia, sleep-disordered breathing, and daytime somnolence. Polysomnography studies have shown abnormal sleep architecture, including shorter total sleep time and longer sleep latency, when compared to children with normal development..[7]

5. **Mitochondrial disorders**: Rossigniol and Frye conducted a meta-analysis to evaluate the incidence of mitochondrial disorders (MD) in children with ASD. They found a significantly higher percentage of patients with ASD (5%) also had MD in compared with the general population (0.01%). In addition, they also found abnormal biomarkers in these patients. They concluded that ASD/MD represents a distinct subgroup of children with MD.[8]

Another review by Rossigniol et al. looked at the association of ASD with oxidative stress, immune dysregulation, mitochondrial dysfunction, and environmental exposures. They found significant prevalence of all of these, with immune dysfunction and inflammation and oxidative stress showing the strongest evidence.[9]

MANAGEMENT OF PATIENTS WITH ASD

ASD is a chronic condition with a very diverse presentation and thus requires a comprehensive treatment plan. An individualized approach is required for best results.

Behavioral interventions

The main objectives of the different educational programs for children with ASD are to maximize functionality, to increase the child's independence, and to improve quality of life for the child and the family. Management includes behavioral therapy and educational interventions oriented toward improving the core symptoms (i.e., deficiency in social skills and interactions and repetitive, restrictive behaviors and interests). It is well documented that early initiation of behavioral interventions improves outcomes for individuals with ASD. ABA therapy has been considered the "gold standard" for children with ASD, but many other techniques have been utilized with promising results. No matter the educational program used, what is most important is early initiation of interventions.

Pharmacologic interventions

Pharmacologic options for children and adults with ASD include psychiatric medications to target certain non-core behavioral symptoms: hyperactivity and impulsivity, aggression, outbursts, self-injury, sleep disturbances, anxiety, and depressive conditions. Since one of the common problems of patients with ASD is poor communication skills, it might be difficult to identify a particular symptom to target. The same is true with identifying some of the side effects of medications (i.e., dry mouth, dizziness). The literature shows that older patients with more severe symptoms of ASD receive psychotropic medications more often.

Among the most commonly used medications are antipsychotics, ADHD medications, and antidepressants. In a systematic review by Jobski et al., the prevalence of psychotropic medication use ranged from 2.7% to 80% with psychotropic polypharmacy ranging 5.4% to 54%.[10]

Antipsychotic medications. Only 2 antipsychotic drugs are approved by the Food and Drug Administration (FDA) for use in children with ASD — risperidone and Aripiprazole, they are atypical antipsychotics. They are dopamine receptor antagonists but also have effects on histamine, serotonin, acetylcholine (muscarinic), and alpha-adrenergic receptors. The indication is autism-related irritability, and they are approved for children aged 5 to 16 years and 6 to 17 years, respectively.

These medications should be continued in the perioperative period, as withdrawal may result in recurrence or exacerbation of negative behaviors. Antipsychotics can potentiate the hypotensive effects of general anesthetic agents, and close attention needs to be paid to blood pressure during induction of anesthesia. Risperidone can be associated with prolonged Q-T interval, and avoidance of other medications with similar effects (ondansetron) may be advisable. Adverse effects, such as weight gain, gynecomastia, and postural hypotension, are very common. Side effects are summarised in Table 63.4.

ADHD medications. ADHD drugs are used to treat the hyperactivity often seen in children with ASD.

In a review of 32 studies, the use of ADHD medications by patients with ASD ranged from 6.6% to 52.4% and was more common among children. Methylphenidate (Ritalin, Concerta) is one of the most commonly used medications, but the results are less promising when compared to children without ASD.[10] Randomized trials and meta-analyses have shown that different stimulants can improve symptoms in 80% of patients with ASD.

Another stimulant that is often used is atomoxetine (Strattera). The studies are small, and results are better for children without ASD (the same as with methylphenidate). In a randomized trial, moderate improvement in ADHD symptoms was seen, but the effect was greater on the hyperactivity-impulsivity than on the inattention subscore.[11]

Antidepressants. Selective serotonin reuptake inhibitors (SSRIs) are commonly used for treatment of obsessive-compulsive symptoms, anxiety, and depression. The few studies that evaluated SSRI treatment for patients with ASD used fluoxetine, fluvoxamine, fenfluramine, and citalopram. In one study, fluoxetine was found to be beneficial in reducing repetitive behaviors in children with ASD, based on the Children's Yale-Brown Obsessive Compulsive Scale. The results are less impressive when compared with adults with ASD. Children treated with SSRIs present with side effects at lower doses.[12] The risk for serotonin syndrome needs to be taken into consideration, and exposure to other potentially offending drugs, such as fentanyl, should be avoided.

Alpha 2-adrenergic agonists. Guanfacine and clonidine have been evaluated. A placebo study of children with ASD (62 patients) showed improvement in behavioral symptoms in treated children. In another study, children who had no response to methylphenidate had an improved behavior profile after treatment with guanfacine.[13]

Complementary and alternative treatment

Complementary and alternative medicine have been used with questionable and, in some cases, even harmful results. Such interventions range from dietary supplements and multivitamins to chelation therapy to remove heavy metals, bleach ingestion, and hyperbaric oxygen therapy. It is important to have information about all therapies a child has been receiving, since some can be associated with adverse events under anesthesia.

Table 63.4 **SIDE EFFECTS OF ASD ANTIPSYCHOTIC MEDICATION**

MEDICATION	SEDATION	ANTICHOLINERGIC	HYPOTENSION	PROLONG Q-T	IMPAIRED GLUCOSE TOLERANCE	WEIGHT GAIN
Risperidone	+	+	++	+	+	++
Aripiprazole	−	+/−	+	−	−	+

Note. ASD = autism spectrum disorder.

Many authors have discussed the need for an individualized management plan for children with ASD.[14–16] One of the first reports is by Van der Walt and Moran. They discuss the need for early communication with the patients' families and flexibility to individualize the admission schedule, anesthetic management, and even some of the existing guidelines.[16] In a recent publication by Swartz et al., the perioperative management of the child was based on the level of functionality, previous experiences, and parental suggestions; 98% of the parents that responded to the follow-up interview were satisfied with the perioperative experience and appreciated the acknowledgment of their child's specific needs.[17] For optimal management of children with ASD, a multidisciplinary team approach is essential. Nurses from the preoperative area, postanesthesia care unit (PACU), and OR; surgeons; child life specialists; and the anesthesia team all need to be informed and attuned to the particular needs of the patient and the management plan at every point.

Preoperative preparation

Children with ASD often need general anesthesia for surgical and nonsurgical procedures. The rigidity and adherence to routines and relatively high levels of baseline anxiety typical in ASD patients make visits to the hospital extremely stressful for the patients and their families. Due to the uniqueness of the patient population, a standard approach is often inapplicable.

Different behavioral, desensitizing and distraction techniques, social stories, daily schedules, and symbol timelines have been used. A study by Isong et al. demonstrates that certain electronic media technologies can decrease anxiety and unwanted behaviors in children with ASD in preparation for dental visits.[18] Using a TEACCH program-based approach has also been shown to improve the compliance of adults and children with ASD significantly during dental examination.[19]

Preoperative evaluation

In many instances, the first encounter the anesthesiologist has with the patient is on the day of the procedure. Lacking in-depth information on the behavior profile of the patient may present significant problems and lead to an unsatisfactory outcome. Box 63.1 lists questions that can help the anesthesiologist collect valuable information from the parent or caregiver as part of the preoperative evaluation.

Early involvement of the child life specialist is of great importance. In many hospitals, the child life specialist spends time with the child and the family while they are awaiting the procedure.[17] These specialists have skills and tools that can be helpful in early communication with patients and their caregivers. In an abstract presented by Riosa et. al. from a Canadian Hospital, the consensus was that the approach to the patient with ASD requires a multidisciplinary team, and child life specialists have the tools, knowledge, and skills to help with ameliorating the anxiety and uncertainties associated with hospital visits and stays.[20]

Muskat et al. emphasized the need for close communication between parents and caregivers. The parents are seen as "key interpreters for their children with ASD."[21]

Premedication options

To accomplish a smooth transition to the OR, many children with ASD need some premedication. It is important to discuss with the caregiver options for medication and routes of administration. Previous experiences in the perioperative setting can also be used to guide decision-making. It is important to keep in mind that children with ASD often have very particular tastes. Sometimes flexibility is needed to allow mixing medication with a favorite drink to ensure successful administration.[16,22]

A mixture of ketamine and midazolam is usually used for more severe cases of ASD. This can be administered orally or by intramuscular injection. Dexmedetomidine has also been used as a premedication. Unfortunately, its oral bioavailability is quite low, leading to delayed onset. Intramusular injection of Dexmedetomidine with or without Ketamine or Midazolam can be another option.

Table 63.5 describes the most commonly used sedative medications, routes of administration and doses.

Table 63.5 **COMMONLY USED SEDATIVE MEDICATIONS TO TREAT ASD**

DRUGS	ROUTE	DOSES (MG/KG)
Benzodiazepines	Oral	0.1–0.5
Diazepam	Oral	0.25–1 (max 20 mg)
Midazolam	Intranasal	0.2
Lorazepam	Intramuscular	0.1–0.2
	Intravenous	0.01–0.1
	Oral	0.05 (max 2 mg)
Phencyclidine	Oral	3–6
Ketamine	Nasal	3
	Intramuscular	3–6
Alpha-2 adrenergic	Oral	0.004
agonist	Oral	0.004
Clonidine	Intranasal	0.001
Dexmedetomidine	Intramusular	0.001–0.002

Note. ASD = autism spectrum disorder.

Intraoperative management

Induction of general anesthesia in the OR can be another stressful moment for patients with ASD. To decrease unnecessary stimulation, providing a quiet environment with low light and minimal personnel is advisable.

Successful intraoperative management of children with ASD relies on keeping the anesthetic simple, providing good analgesia, and effective postoperative nausea and vomiting (PONV) prophylaxis, ultimately allowing for a smooth and fast recovery.

Regional anesthesia techniques, nonsteroidal anti-inflammatory drugs, and acetaminophen should be utilized to provide adequate analgesia and to decrease the need for opioids, which can be associated with excessive sedation, nausea, vomiting, and constipation.

Ondansetron is best avoided in children treated with atypical antipsychotic agents, but other prophylactic agents for PONV are indicated. Adequate intraoperative hydration will allow for early removal of the peripheral intravenous cannula (PIV)—the presence of which is a known trigger for progressively escalating negative behavior in the recovery room.

Emergence agitation can be associated with maladaptive behaviors in children with normal development. Some parents of children with ASD are convinced that, after general anesthesia, their children suffer regression, and the results of months of hard work with behavioral specialists are lost. While there are no studies confirming a link between general anesthesia and behavioral regression, avoiding or at least decreasing the incidence of emergence agitation should be attempted. Administering additional sedation with dexmedetomidine, clonidine, ketamine, or boluses of propofol have all been described.[23]

There are no studies suggesting superiority of one general anesthetic agent over another in children with ASD. A recent animal study by Li et al. suggests that ASD patients with a certain mutation might be more sensitive to isoflurane when compared

---

Box 63.2 GENERAL GOALS OF THE INTRAOPERATIVE MANAGEMENT OF CHILDREN WITH ASD

Provide a quiet environment for induction of general anesthesia.

Maintain communication with parents and child throughout the process, if possible.

Smooth induction of general anesthesia.

Intraoperative PONV prophylaxis.

Adequate analgesia.

Adequate hydration.

Additional sedation for smooth postoperative recovery.

Use medications known to decrease the incidence of emergence delirium.

Secure PIV well and attempt to hide. Consider PIV on lower extremities.

Box 63.3 GENERAL GOALS FOR PACU STAY FOR CHILDREN WITH ASD

Provide a quiet environment—isolated rooms, dimmed lights.

Have the parents in the room as early as possible.

Provide favorite and comforting items upon arrival.

Minimize recovery room stay, if possible.

Minimize vital signs checks.

If possible, remove PIV early. If not possible, ensure PIV is well secured and camouflaged.

If needed, administer additional sedation for emergence agitation.

---

to sevoflurane. Further studies are needed in that direction. For summary of intraoperative goals please refer to Box 63.2.

Considerations for the PACU

For children with ASD, waking up in an unfamiliar environment can be extremely stressful. The PACU is a very stimulating area with various noises, bright lights, a busy work flow, and multiple unfamiliar people. Providing a private room with diminished light and minimal noise might be beneficial. Bringing the parent early to the room upon the child's awakening may help alleviate anxiety and avoid negative behavioral outbursts. The goals of care for children with ASD in the recovery room are summarized in Box 63.3. The parents' involvement is essential for assessment of pain, communicating needs, and providing comfort.[24] In a retrospective review by Arnold et al., no difference in the perioperative experience was found between children with ASD and healthy controls undergoing dental rehabilitation. The only significant difference was found in the type and the route of administering the premedication—children with ASD had a higher rate of "atypical premedication" compared to the control group.[25] Further work is needed to address the effect of general anesthetic agents on long-term recovery and behavioral outcomes in children with ASD.

CONCLUSION

ASD is the fastest growing neurodevelopmental disorder. Children with ASD exhibit specific signs and deficits in social interaction and communication as well as repetitive habits, activities, and interests. Children with ASD present significant challenges for the anesthesiologist, and a well-defined individualized perioperative plan is advisable. Detailed information about the patient's baseline behavior, triggers for emotional deterioration, and past successful coping techniques are of paramount importance.

REVIEW QUESTIONS

1. According to DSM-V, which of the following symptoms is essential in making the diagnosis of ASD?

A. persistent disturbances in the social interaction and communications
B. inflexible adherence to routines
C. highly restricted, fixated interests
D. stereotyped or repetitive movements

Answer: A

ASD replaced 3 conditions in DSM-IV: classic autism, Asperger syndrome, and PDDNOC. According to DSM-V, symptoms need to be present in early childhood. To be diagnosed with ASD, a patient needs to exhibit 3 out of 3 symptoms in the category "Persistent disturbances in the social interaction and communications" which cover deficits in (i) social-emotional reciprocity; (ii) nonverbal communication; and (iii) developing, maintaining, and understand relationships. They also have to exhibit 2 out of 4 symptoms in the category "Repetitive and restrictive behaviors" which includes (i) inflexible adherence to routines; (ii) highly restricted, fixated interests; (iii) stereotyped or repetitive movements; and (iv) hyper- or hyporeactivity to sensory input.

2. You are scheduled to take care of a 4-year old boy who had recent onset of fever and presents with left-sided neck swelling. A computed tomography scan showed a neck abscess. During the preoperative interview, the mother tells you he was recently diagnosed with ASD. She is still apprehensive about the diagnosis and is asking if you are planning anything special for her child. Which of the following would be the **BEST** response?

A. Arrange a consultation with developmental neuropsychology.
B. Ask for more details about her child's behavioral profile.
C. Reassure her that no special precautions are needed.
D. Request the whole perioperative team participate in the discussion.

Answer: B

A diagnosis of ASD can be very stressful for parents. Taking care of children with ASD necessitates a general understanding of the condition and of the particular behavioral profile of the patient. Addressing the parental concerns will provide for good parent-provider relationship and is of great importance when caring for children with ASD. This will help you structure a better perioperative plan. Bright lights, loud noises, and too many unfamiliar people can often be an emotional trigger for these children. Discussion with the parents and the perioperative care team should be done outside the room.

3. The mother of a child recently diagnosed with autism is concerned about having another child with autism. Which of the following percentage is the **CLOSEST** approximate incidence of autism in siblings?

A. 0.5%–2.5%
B. 1.5%–4%
C. 2%–18%
D. 36%–95%

Answer: C

The exact etiology of ASD is not known. Multiple factors, including environmental, neurobiological, and familial, have been studied, but not a single one has been established as a sole cause. Genetic predisposition is highly suspected in the pathogenesis of ASD;[3] however, more than 800 genes have been found to possibly contribute to it. In a family with 1 child with ASD, the risk of having another offspring with the same condition is 2% to 18%. The incidence of ASD in the general population is 0.5% to 2.5%, in boys is 1.5% to 4%, and in identical twins is 36% to 95%.

4. The diagnosis of ASD is **PRIMARILY** based upon which of the following assessments?

A genetic screening
B. observation of behavior
C. parental concerns
D. validated ASD scales

Answer B

Screening for ASD should be attempted as early as 18 months of age, and a diagnosis should be established as early as possible per AAP recommendations. The initial evaluation is usually based on parental concerns or school referral and signs of delayed development. The screening and diagnosis is conducted by a multidisciplinary team and include an exam, a history of the patient's development, and observation of the child.

5. You are consulted on a 15-year old boy who is scheduled for upper endoscopy under general anesthesia. He has ASD, ADHD, anxiety related to medical visits and procedures, and a history of bolting. He is on clonidine, risperidone, and lorazepam as needed for anxiety. Which of the following is the **BEST** preoperative approach for this patient?

A. early arrival for acclimation
B. last case of the day assignment
C. lorazepam before leaving home
D. multiple distraction technique

Answer: C

Obtaining a detailed history of the behavior of a child with ASD is of great importance.[3] The information helps planning and anticipating potential problems. In children with severe anxiety, administration of antianxiety medication before arriving to the hospital might help with ameliorating stress, help with the admission process, and smooth the induction of general anesthesia. These patients should be scheduled early in the day and have a minimal wait period. Discontinuation of certain medications, in this case, both antipsychotics and an alpha-2-agonist, can have deleterious results.

6. Which of the following psychopharmacologic medications is the **MOST** recognized in the treatment of non-core symptoms in ASD?

A. antidepressants
B. antipsychotics
C. cholinesterase inhibitors

D. NMDA antagonists

Answer: B

Psychopharmacologic treatment for patients with ASD is used for non-core symptoms, such as hyperactivity and impulsivity, aggression, outbursts and self-injury, sleep disturbances, anxiety, and depressive conditions, rather than existing behavioral problems. It is instituted after all behavioral and educational strategies have been utilized and maximized. Risperidone is 1 of 2 medications approved by the FDA for treatment of irritability in children with ASD.

7. You are scheduled to take care of an 8-year old child with ASD. He has an additional diagnosis of ADHD and seizures. Which of the following would be the **MOST** appropriate to include in the preoperative preparation for this child?

    A. discontinuation of all patient's medications the morning of surgery

    B. discussion of plan with the child life specialist and perioperative teams

    C. instruction to the parents on hospital rules for preoperative preparation

    D. request for the child to change out of his street clothes to a hospital gown

Answer: B

A multidisciplinary approach for the child with ASD results in better outcomes.[17] The child's previous experiences and parental opinion should be taken into consideration when the plan is made. A detailed medication history needs to be obtained, and ASD medications should be taken in the morning.

8. You are taking care of a 6-year-old boy with ASD and ADHD for tonsillectomy and adenoidectomy. The child has a history of emergence agitation with a previous procedure at age 2. He was anxious before the procedure, and mask induction required physical restraint. Which of the following is the **MOST** appropriate to include as part of your intraoperative plan?

    A. dexmedetomidine, intraoperatively.

    B. IV catheter removal, postemergence.

    C. opioid avoidance, perioperatively

    D. physical restraints, postoperatively

Answer: A

Children with a previous history of emergence agitation are at higher risk for another episode after anesthesia. Different medications have been used in children with ASD, including propofol boluses, dexmedetomidine, and ketamine.[22] Opioids can cause airway obstruction, but tonsillectomy and adenoidectomy is a very stimulating surgery. ASD patients can have severe behavior outbursts in the face of pain, especially if they have difficulties with communication. Ensuring adequate analgesia intraoperatively should be one of the main goals. The IV should be covered well and removed only after complete confidence that adequate hydration, analgesia, and nausea prophylaxis have been achieved. Restraints will most likely increase the risk for agitation and harm.

9. You are the PACU anesthesiologist of the day, and your colleague transfers care to you of an 18-year-old patient with ASD who had esophagogastroduodenoscopy under general anesthesia. The patient is nonverbal, lives in a special-needs home, and can be aggressive. Which of the following would be the **MOST** appropriate to include in your postanesthesia care plan?

    A. PACU bed space directly across from nursing station

    B. hospital clowns to entertain patient while in the PACU

    C. parents/guardian in PACU before patient arrival

    D. fast-track discharge to avoid disturbance to the PACU

Answer: C

The PACU can be a very stimulating environment for children with ASD with various loud noises, bright lights, and a busy workflow. Anticipating the arrival of this patient to the PACU necessitates certain preparations: providing an isolated room, having parents and caregivers in the room before the patient's arrival, and minimizing disturbances if the patient is still asleep or sedated. Discussion with the anesthesiologist of the case and the admitting nurse is of paramount importance.

10. You have a 10-year-old, 56-kg child with ASD scheduled for orchidopexy, who is very anxious, walks in circles in the room, screams, and tries to escape. The mother is trying to calm him unsuccessfully. He has an oral aversion to many fluids and has had a bad experience with mask induction in the past. Which of the following would be the **MOST** appropriate to discuss with his mother, while seeking her participation?

    A. intramuscular injection of sedative(s)

    B. IV start and induction

    C. mask induction with personnel restraining

    D. oral anxiolytic premedication

Answer: A

Visits to the hospital can be very stressful for children with ASD. Many different premedication options are available.[14–16] Swartz et al. in their recent study suggested using different options based on the patient's level of functionality. Many children have an oral aversion to food, and oral premedication is not an option in these cases. For the uncooperative, severely anxious child with ASD, intramuscular premedication is an option, but, in many cases, parents need to accept the plan and physically help during the administration. Repeating previous stressful and traumatizing experiences is not advisable.

QUESTIONS AND ANSWERS

This chapter has accompanying questions and answers which are available to subscribers as part of the Oxford eLearning platform. To access the questions, go to ✅ http:// oxfordmedicine. com/pediatricanesthesiaPBL

REFERENCES

1. Dreyer B. *AAP Statement on U.S. Preventive Services Task Force Final Recommendation Statement on Autism Screening*. American Academy of Pediatrics; 2016.
2. Plauche' Johnson C, Myers SM, Council on Children With Disabilities. Identification and evaluation of children with autism spectrum disorders. *Pediatrics*. 2007;120(5).
3. Hallmayer J, Cleveland S, Torres A, et al. Genetic heritability and shared environmental factors among twin pairs with autism. *Arch Gen Psychiatry*. 2011;68(11):1095–1102.
4. Gardener H, Spiegelman D, Buka SL. Perinatal and neonatal risk factors for autism: a comprehensive meta-analysis. *Pediatrics*. 2011;128(2):344–355.
5. McElhanon BO, McCracken C, Karpen S, Sharp WG. Gastrointestinal symptoms in autism spectrum disorder: a meta-analysis. *Pediatrics*. 2014;133(5):872–883.
6. Frye RE, Rose S, Slattery J, MacFabe DF. Gastrointestinal dysfunction in autism spectrum disorder: the role of the mitochondria and the enteric microbiome.. *Microb Ecol Health Dis*. 2015;26.
7. Klukowski M, Wasilewska J, Lebensztejn D. Sleep and gastrointestinal disturbances in autism spectrum disorder in children. *Dev Period Med*. 2015;19(2):157–161.
8. Rossignol DA, Frye RE. Mitochondrial dysfunction in autism spectrum disorders: a systematic review and meta-analysis. *Mol Psychiatry*. 2012;17(3):290–314.
9. Rossignol DA, Frye RE. A review of research trends in physiological abnormalities in autism spectrum disorders: immune dysregulation, inflammation, oxidative stress, mitochondrial dysfunction and environmental toxicant exposures. *Mol Psychiatry*. 2012;17(4):389–401.
10. Jobski K, Höfer J, Hoffmann F, Bachmann C. Use of psychotropic drugs in patients with autism spectrum disorders: a systematic review. *Acta Psychiatr Scand*. 2017;135(1):8–28.
11. Harfterkamp M, van de Loo-Neus G., Minderaa RB, et al. A randomized double-blind study of atomoxetine versus placebo for attention-deficit/hyperactivity disorder symptoms in children with autism spectrum disorder. *J Am Acad Child Adolesc Psychiatry*. 2012;51(7).
12. McPheeters M, Warren Z, Sathe N, et al. A systematic review of medical treatments for children with autism spectrum disorders. *Pediatrics*. 2011;127(5):e1312–e1321.
13. Scahill L, McCracken JT, King BH, et al. Extended-release guanfacine for hyperactivity in children with autism spectrum disorder. *Am J Psychiatry*. 2015;172(12):1197–1206.
14. Vlassakova BG, Emmanouil DE. Perioperative considerations in children with autism spectrum disorder. *Curr Opin Anaesthesiol*. 2016;29(3):359–366.
15. Taghizadeh N, Davidson A, Williams K, Story D. Autism spectrum disorder (ASD) and its perioperative management. *Paediatr Anaesth*. 2015;25(11):1076–1084.
16. van der Walt JH, Moran C. An audit of perioperative management of autistic children. *Paediatr Anaesth*. 2001;11(4):401–408.
17. Swartz JS, Amos KE, Brindas M, Girling LG, Graham MR. Benefits of an individualized perioperative plan for children with autism spectrum disorder. *Paediatr Anaesth*. 2017;27(8):856–862.
18. Isong IA, Rao SR, Holifield C, et al. Addressing dental fear in children with autism spectrum disorders: a randomized controlled pilot study using electronic screen media. *Clin Pediatr*. 2014;53(3):230–237.
19. Orellana LM, Martinez-Sanchis S, Silvestre FJ. Training adults and children with an autism spectrum disorder to be compliant with a clinical dental assessment using a TEACCH-based approach. *J Autism Dev Disord*. 2014;44(4):776–785.
20. Riosa B, Muskat B, Nicolas DB, Zwaigenboum L. Autism comes to the hospital: the prospective of a child life specialist. International Meeting for Autism Research Conference presentation, 2014.
21. Muskat B, Riosa PB, Nicholas DB. Autism comes to the hospital: the experiences of patients with autism spectrum disorder, their parents and health-care providers at two Canadian paediatric hospitals. *Autism*. 2015;19:482–490.
22. Shah S, Shah S, Apuya J, Gopalakrishnan S, Martin T. Combination of oral ketamine and midazolam as a premedication for a severely autistic and combative patient. *J Anesth*. 2009;23(1):126–128.
23. Short JA, Calder A. Anaesthesia for children with special needs, including autistic spectrum disorder. *Contin Educ Anaesth Crit Care Pain*. 2013;2(6).
24. Ely E, Chen-Lim ML, Carpenter KM, et al., Pain assessment of children with autism spectrum disorders. *J Dev Behav Pediatr*. 2016;37(1):53–61.
25. Arnold B, Elliott A, Laohamroonvorapongse D, Hanna J, Norvell D, Koh J. Autistic children and anesthesia: is their perioperative experience different? *Paediatr Anaesth*. 2015;25(11):1103–1110.

64.

ANESTHESIA FOR ADOLESCENT BARIATRIC SURGERY

Elizabeth Q. Starker, Staci N. Allen, and Debnath Chatterjee

STEM CASE AND KEY QUESTIONS

A 16-year-old female with severe obesity is scheduled for laparoscopic sleeve gastrectomy. Her comorbidities include severe obstructive sleep apnea (OSA), insulin dependent diabetes mellitus, pre-hypertension, hyperlipidemia, non-alcoholic fatty liver disease, and polycystic ovarian disease.

What are the current trends of childhood obesity in the United States?

How is pediatric obesity defined?

What is the definition for severe obesity in children?

What is the relationship between obesity and obstructive sleep apnea?

How does obesity affect the cardiovascular system?

What are the effects of obesity on pulmonary mechanics and what are the anesthetic implications?

What is the relationship between obesity and asthma?

What are the effects of obesity on the endocrine system?

How does obesity affect liver function?

What are the psychosocial effects of childhood obesity?

What bariatric surgical procedures are commonly performed in adolescents?

What are the benefits of performing bariatric surgery in adolescents?

What criteria must be met before bariatric surgeries are performed on adolescents?

You are scheduled to meet this patient in the preoperative clinic a week before surgery. Her vital signs are: weight 130 kg, height 1.4 meters, blood pressure (BP) 134/84 mmHg, heart rate (HR) 78 beats/min, respiratory rate 26 breaths/minute, and SpO_2 94% on room air.

WHAT WOULD YOU FOCUS ON DURING THE PREOPERATIVE EVALUATION? WHAT LABORATORY INVESTIGATIONS WOULD YOU ORDER PREOPERATIVELY? WHAT NIL PER OS (NPO) INSTRUCTIONS WOULD YOU GIVE THIS PATIENT?

You are setting up the operating room on the day of surgery.

WHAT AIRWAY EQUIPMENT WOULD YOU HAVE AVAILABLE? WHAT BODY SCALAR WOULD YOU USE TO CALCULATE DOSING OF MEDICATIONS?

The patient is appropriately NPO, and her vital signs are unchanged from last week. She is very nervous about her upcoming surgery.

WOULD YOU ADMINISTER AN ANXIOLYTIC PREMEDICATION? HOW WOULD YOU INDUCE GENERAL ANESTHESIA IN THIS PATIENT? WHAT WOULD BE YOUR APPROACH TO MANAGING THIS PATIENT'S AIRWAY? WHAT MONITORS DO YOU PLAN TO USE? HOW WOULD YOU MAINTAIN GENERAL ANESTHESIA?

As you are positioning this patient for surgery, her only intravenous access gets dislodged, and you are not able to obtain intravenous access using your standard technique.

WHAT ARE THE OTHER OPTIONS FOR SECURING INTRAVENOUS ACCESS?

After successfully obtaining intravenous access, the patient is positioned supine, and her BP falls to 90/50 mmHg and HR increases to 110 beats/min. Her SpO_2 is 90% on FiO_2 of 1.0.

The surgery proceeds uneventfully, and the surgeons perform a laparoscopic sleeve gastrectomy. Upon completion of the surgical procedure:

How would you determine timing for extubation?

What extubation criteria are you going to use?

Are the extubation criteria different for a severely obese patient?

What complications can you expect in the early postoperative period?

Does this patient need to be monitored in the intensive care unit postoperatively?

What is your plan for postoperative analgesia?

DISCUSSION

The global epidemic of obesity has affected both adults and children. According to 2015–2016 data from the United States, the prevalence of obesity was 39.8% in adults and 18.5% in youths.[1] The prevalence of obesity was higher among youths aged 6 to 11 years (18.4%) and adolescents aged 12 to 19 years (20.6%), compared with children aged 2 to 5 years (13.9%). Higher rates of childhood obesity are seen among Hispanic, non-Hispanic black, and American Indian children, especially in low-income populations.

Body mass index (BMI) relates weight to height and is commonly used as a screening tool for obesity in adults. BMI is calculated by dividing the patient's weight (in kilograms) by the square of the height (in meters). However, in children, the BMI varies by age, sex, and maturity.[2–4] To take these changes into consideration, the child's BMI is plotted on the Centers for Disease Control and Prevention's gender-specific growth chart to determine the corresponding BMI-for-age percentile. Cut-offs of 85th, 95th, and 99th percentiles for age and weight are used to define overweight, obesity, and severe obesity (Table 64.1).[2–4] Severe obesity in children is also defined as BMI ≥120% of the 95th percentile for age and sex or a BMI ≥35 kg per m². There are approximately 4.4 million severely obese children and adolescents in the United States.

COMORBIDITIES OF CHILDHOOD OBESITY

Obesity affects every major organ system in the body, resulting in immediate and long-term consequences. Childhood obesity typically tracks into adulthood, and obese adolescents are likely to become obese adults.[2–4] Obesity markedly decreases life expectancy, especially among young adults. The

Table 64.1 **CLASSIFICATION OF CHILDHOOD OBESITY BASED ON BMI-FOR-AGE PERCENTILE**

BMI-for-age percentile	Definition
85th–95th percentile	Overweight
≥95th percentile	Obese
≥120% of 95th percentile or BMI ≥35 kg per m², whichever is lower. Represents ≥99th percentile	Severely obese

Note. BMI = body mass index.

comorbidities resulting from obesity and their anesthetic implications are listed in Table 64.2.

ADOLESCENT BARIATRIC SURGERY

Currently, bariatric surgery is considered a valid treatment option in severely obese adolescents in whom lifestyle interventions are not successful. A multidisciplinary, team-based approach involving a bariatric surgeon, anesthesiologist, pediatric obesity specialist, registered dietitian, pediatric psychologist/psychiatrist, and exercise specialist is strongly recommended. Surgical practice guidelines based on expert opinion have outlined criteria for selecting severely obese adolescents for bariatric surgery.[5,6]

1. BMI ≥35 kg/m² with major comorbidities (diabetes mellitus type 2 [T2DM], moderate to severe OSA with apnea-hypopnea index [AHI] >15, pseudotumor cerebri, or severe and progressive non-alcoholic steatohepatitis) or BMI ≥40 kg/m² with minor comorbidities (hypertension, insulin resistance, glucose intolerance, impaired quality of life, dyslipidemia, OSA with AHI ≥5).

2. Physical maturity, defined as completing 95% of predicted adult stature based on bone age or reaching Tanner stage IV.

3. Psychological maturity, demonstrated by motivation, understanding of surgery, and compliance with preoperative therapy.

4. Documented failure with an organized and sustained weight management program.

Contraindications for bariatric surgical procedures include[5,6]

1. Medically correctable causes of obesity.

2. Active substance abuse disorder.

3. Psychosocial, medical, or cognitive conditions that prevent adherence to recommendations or impair decision-making ability.

4. Current or planned pregnancy within 18 months of surgery.

Table 64.2 COMORBIDITIES OF CHILDHOOD OBESITY AND ANESTHETIC IMPLICATIONS

SYSTEM	EFFECTS OF OBESITY	ANESTHETIC IMPLICATION
Cardiovascular	Increased risk of hypertension, left ventricular hypertrophy, dyslipidemia, carotid intima-media thickening, and coronary atherosclerosis Pulmonary hypertension with OSA	Preoperative echocardiography Risk of biventricular failure
Respiratory	OSA: 4 times increased risk secondary to airway narrowing, increased critical airway closing pressures, decreased chest wall compliance, and abnormal ventilatory control For each unit increase in BMI, the risk of OSA increases by 12%	Airway concerns Polysomnography/CPAP use Minimizing opioids Postoperative monitoring
	Decreased lung and chest wall compliance Increased work of breathing Decreased FRC and FVC	Decreased time to desaturation with apnea Increased risk of hypoxemia and atelectasis
	Increased prevalence of asthma	Increased symptoms and exacerbations
Endocrine	Increased risk of T2DM Earlier onset of microvascular and macrovascular complications (neuropathy, nephropathy, retinopathy, and atherosclerosis)	Perioperative glucose control Increased risk for infection
	Metabolic syndrome with 3 out of 5 criteria: elevated TG, low HDL, central obesity, elevated fasting glucose, and hypertension	Increased perioperative morbidity
	Early-onset polycystic ovary syndrome and hyperandrogenism	Risk factor for metabolic syndrome and T2DM
Hepatic	Non-alcoholic fatty liver disease, progressing to NASH and cirrhosis	Elevated liver function tests Need for liver transplantation with NASH/cirrhosis
Renal	Enlarged kidneys	Delayed drug clearance
Psychosocial	Depression, lower self-esteem, subject of teasing and bullying, lower health-related quality of life scores	Preoperative counseling
Orthopedic	Slipped capital femoral epiphysis Increased musculoskeletal pain, gait abnormalities	Need for urgent surgery
Neurologic	Pseudotumor cerebri in female adolescents	Unexplained increase in ICP

Note. OSA = obstructive sleep apnea; CPAP = continuous positive airway pressure; BMI = body mass index; FRC = functional residual capacity; FVC = forced vital capacity; T2DM = type 2 diabetes mellitus; TG = triglycerides; HDL = high density cholesterol; NASH = non-alcoholic steatohepatitis; ICP = intracranial pressure.

Adapted from Chidambaran V, Tewari A, Mahmoud M. Anesthetic and pharmacologic considerations in perioperative care of obese children. *J Clin Anesth.* 2017;45:39–50.

The three most commonly performed adolescent bariatric surgical procedures are Roux-en-Y gastric bypass (RYGB), adjustable gastric band (AGB), and vertical sleeve gastrectomy (VSG; Fig. 64.1).[6] All three procedures are typically performed under laparoscopic guidance. RYGB involves creation of a small gastric pouch (approximately 30 mL) and anastomosis to a Roux limb of jejunum that bypasses 75 to 100 cm of small bowel. AGB is a purely restrictive procedure that involves placement of an adjustable silicone band around the gastric inlet that is attached to a small subcutaneous reservoir. The use of an AGB in adolescents has not been approved by the US Food and Drug Administration. VSG involves resection of most of the greater curvature of the stomach, leaving behind a tubular stomach that is 10% to 15% of its original size. VSG is gaining popularity as the bariatric surgical procedure of choice in obese adolescents.

There is limited data regarding long-term weight loss following bariatric surgery in adolescents. The Teen-Longitudinal Assessment of Bariatric Surgery, a prospective, multicenter study of bariatric surgery in 242 obese adolescents, found significant improvements in weight, cardiometabolic health, and weight-related quality of life at 3 years after the procedure.[7] The average weight loss was 28% among all the participants. The study also found remission of T2DM in 95% of participants, remission of abnormal kidney function in 86%, normalization of elevated blood pressure in 74%, and remission of dyslipidemia in 66%, leading the authors to hypothesize that adolescents may have a greater potential than adults for reversal of cardiometabolic consequences of obesity.[7] Weight-related quality of life also improved significantly.

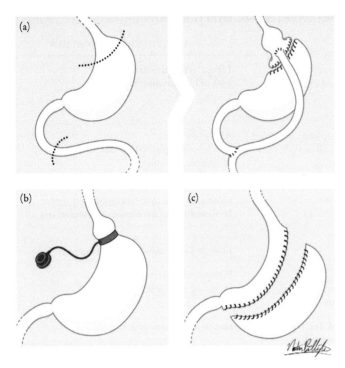

Fig. 64.1 Bariatric surgical procedures: A. Roux-en-Y gastric bypass, B. Adjustable gastric band, C. Vertical sleeve gastrectomy. Reproduced with permission from Chatterjee D. Anesthesia and childhood obesity. In: Holzman RS, Mancuso TJ, Polaner DM, eds. *A Practical Approach to pediatric Anesthesia.* 2nd ed. Philadelphia, PA: Wolters Kluwer; 2016: 806–820.

PREOPERATIVE EVALUATION

Most bariatric surgery programs include a referral to the anesthesiology preoperative clinic for a comprehensive preoperative evaluation. A thorough history and physical examination targeting obesity-related diseases should be performed. Symptoms of sleep-disordered breathing, prior diagnosis of OSA, baseline oxygen requirement, continuous positive airway pressure (CPAP), and bilevel positive airway pressure (BiPAP) requirements should be elucidated. The current status of other associated comorbidities should also be thoroughly evaluated. Baseline vital signs (including room air oxygen saturation), height, and weight should also be obtained. A targeted physical examination should be performed, focusing on the airway and cardiopulmonary systems. For patients with known comorbidities, medical optimization prior to surgery will help minimize perioperative complications.[3,4]

Baseline investigations should include a complete blood count, comprehensive metabolic panel, lipid profile, coagulation profile, glycosylated hemoglobin, type and screen, electrocardiogram, transthoracic echocardiogram, and polysomnography study. Additional studies, such as glucose tolerance tests, pulmonary function tests, and thyroid function tests, may be ordered, if necessary. The patient's ideal body weight (IBW) should be calculated during the preoperative assessment to determine proper dosing of medications during and after surgery.

Preoperative fasting instructions should be provided to the patient during the preoperative evaluation. Obese and overweight children are not at an increased risk for pulmonary aspiration and should be counseled with standard NPO guidelines. Patients should be instructed to continue their current medications up to the time of surgery and bring their CPAP machine from home.

INTRAOPERATIVE MANAGEMENT

On the day of surgery, in addition to the standard operating room set-up, extra laryngoscope blades, oral airways, and a video laryngoscope should be readily available. It is important to ensure that the operating table can accommodate the severely obese patient, and a ramp should be created for appropriate positioning during intubation. An ultrasound machine to assist with vascular access and longer intravenous catheters should also be available. Arterial and central venous catheters are rarely necessary during bariatric surgery procedures. Surgeons will also request availability of various sizes of bougie dilators and air insufflation through an orogastric tube to check for anastomotic leaks.

Medication dosing in obese patients is difficult, as standard dosing recommendations may over- or underdose patients. Scalars such as total body weight (TBW), lean body weight (LBW), and IBW are used to adjust medication dosing and provide an appropriate dose based on pharmacokinetics of the drug. LBW is the difference between TBW and fat mass. Obesity increases both lean body mass (by 20%–40%) and fat mass.[2,3] IBW does not take into account the increase in lean body mass in obesity. Although LBW may be the most reliable scalar for dosing in obese patients, it is difficult to calculate, and IBW is often used in its place. IBW in children can be calculated using the BMI method, which involves multiplying the BMI at the 50th percentile for the child's age by the square of the height in meters.[3] Nomograms have also been published to simplify determination of weight scalars in obese pediatric patients. Recommended body scalars for common anesthetic drugs are listed in Table 64.3. Two pharmacokinetic parameters, volume of distribution (V_d) and clearance, are important to consider in dosing of obese patients. V_d of a drug is increased with lipophilic drugs and remains unchanged with water-soluble drugs. Lipophilic drug loading should be based on TBW, and water-soluble drug dosing should be based on IBW.[2,3] Drug clearance determines a drug's maintenance dose. It is dependent on hepatic and renal function, which is altered in obese children.[2,3]

Administration of preoperative anxiolytics in obese patients must be approached with caution. Benzodiazepines, such as midazolam, increase the risk of respiratory depression in obese patients, especially those with OSA. If it is necessary to administer premedication, a smaller dose should be used, and oxygen saturation monitoring should be utilized until the patient is transferred to the operating room. Intramuscular administration of premedication should be avoided in obese patients due to the unreliability of drug absorption.

Intraoperative monitoring should include standard American Society of Anesthesiologists monitors, consisting

Table 64.3 DRUG DOSING IN OBESE PATIENTS

DRUG	RECOMMENDED SCALAR DOSING
Propofol	
Induction dose	LBW
Maintenance infusion	TBW
Morphine	IBW
Fentanyl	LBW
Succinylcholine	TBW
Non-depolarizing muscle relaxants (vecuronium, rocuronium, cisatracurium)	IBW
Neostigmine	TBW

Note. LBW = lean body weight; TBW = total body weight; IBW = ideal body weight.

of electrocardiogram, pulse oximetry, noninvasive blood pressure monitoring, end-tidal carbon dioxide, and temperature. An appropriate-sized blood pressure cuff should be used, and the conical shape of the upper arm often necessitates the use of alternate sites, such as the forearm or lower leg. The temperature probe should be placed in the axilla instead of the esophagus during bariatric surgery to avoid accidental inclusion within the surgical anastomosis.

Induction of general anesthesia in obese pediatric patients should be approached with caution. The patient should be placed in a ramped position prior to direct laryngoscopy to horizontally align the patient's external auditory meatus to his or her sternal notch using pillows or blankets (Fig. 64.2). The ramped position has been found to improve laryngeal views in obese patients undergoing direct laryngoscopy.[3,4] Prior to intravenous induction, the patient should be preoxygenated using tidal volume breathing with 100% oxygen for 3 minutes in a 25-degree head-up position. Adequate preoxygenation with this technique prolongs time to desaturation during induction in obese children.[3] The addition of CPAP (10 cm H_2O) during spontaneous ventilation and positive end expiratory pressure (PEEP; 10 cm H_2O) during controlled ventilation also decreases time to desaturation.[3]

Obesity is a risk factor for difficult intravenous catheter placement secondary to excess adipose tissue increasing the depth of vessels or obscuring the landmarks. Difficult intravenous access is associated with complications including failed vascular access, increased number of attempts, prolonged time to cannulation, pain, thrombosis, infection, hematoma, infiltration, and low patient satisfaction. In an effort to decrease complications and increase success rate, many practitioners are beginning to utilize technology to aid with vascular access in obese patients. Scoring systems such as the Difficult Intravenous Access Scoring System (which includes criteria of vein palpability, vein visibility, patient age, and history of prematurity) have been devised to indicate when technology should aid a practitioner with intravenous access.[8] Ultrasonography, the most popular and well-studied technology, has been shown to increase success rates and patient satisfaction, while decreasing time to cannulation and the number of punctures required in patients with a history of difficult intravenous access.[9] Infrared, transillumination, and

vein entry indicator devices have also been utilized with success.[10–12] An anesthesiologist should be adept at multiple advanced technologies for vascular access.

Maintenance of general anesthesia in the obese child should include a combination of insoluble volatile agents and intravenous agents that are short acting, hydrophilic, or degrade spontaneously. Desflurane has a lower blood-gas solubility coefficient compared to other volatile anesthetic agents, which may allow for faster wake-ups due to its insolubility in adipose tissue. Remifentanil is an opioid with fast onset and offset, has a half-life of 5 minutes, and is degraded by plasma esterases. Dexmedetomidine has an opioid-sparing effect when used as an adjunct during maintenance of anesthesia. Neuromuscular blocking agents may be chosen based on the patient's comorbidities. Cisatracurium, degraded by Hoffman elimination, has a predictable duration of action. Rocuronium is dependent on hepatic metabolism and should be used with caution in patients with hepatic dysfunction.

Intraoperative ventilation strategies should include low tidal volumes (6–8 mL/kg IBW), modest levels of PEEP (8–10 cm H_2O), maintenance of normocapnia, FiO_2 0.5 to 0.8, and intermittent alveolar recruitment maneuvers to improve oxygenation and prevent atelectasis.[3] The differential diagnosis for an obese patient with hypotension and hypoxemia after induction of general anesthesia includes endobronchial intubation, endotracheal tube obstruction, bronchospasm, anaphylaxis, extensive surgical pneumoperitoneum, and positional hypoventilation. Obese patients have a decreased functional residual capacity and lung compliance due to intra-abdominal adipose tissue displacing the diaphragm upwards toward the chest. These patients may require ventilation at higher airway pressures and modest levels of PEEP to maintain normocapnia. Patients may become hypotensive when ventilated at high airway pressures secondary to decreased venous return and cardiac output. The supine or Trendelenberg position worsens this effect.[3] Positioning the patient in reverse Trendelenberg (head positioned up 25–30 degrees) during surgery will improve ventilation by decreasing the intra-abdominal pressure on the lungs. Hypotension during bariatric surgery can also be treated with a fluid bolus, vasoactive medications or by decreasing the pneumoperitoneum pressure.

Extubation of severely obese children can be done with acceptable risk once strict criteria are met. The criteria are the same for a non-obese patient, just more rigorously adhered to. Prior to evaluating respiratory criteria, all other organ systems should be optimized: hemodynamics, temperature, gastric suctioning as allowed by surgeons, and positioning. Neuromuscular blockade should be completely reversed to promote and assess respiratory mechanics (negative inspiratory force ≤ -25 cm H_2O, respiratory rate 12 to 26 breaths/min, vital capacity >10 mL/kg IBW). Oxygenation and ventilation as gauged by pulse oximeter and end-tidal carbon dioxide should be optimized compared to the patient's baseline ($SpO_2 >95\%$ and $PaCO_2 <50$), considering the sequela of OSA and obesity hypoventilation syndrome. Postoperative pain control should be in effect. A plan for airway management, including emergent reintubation, should be devised

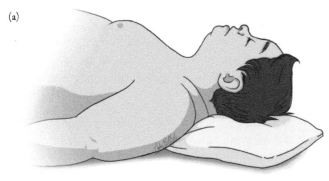

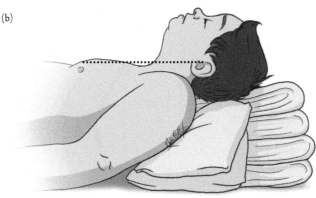

Fig. 64.2 Positioning the obese patient for intubation (A) sniffing position and (B) ramped position. Reproduced with permission from Chatterjee D. Anesthesia and childhood obesity. In: Holzman RS, Mancuso TJ, Polaner DM, eds. *A Practical Approach to Pediatric Anesthesia*. 2nd ed. Philadelphia, PA: Wolters Kluwer; 2016: 806–820.

with patient positioning acknowledged, equipment arranged, and medications readily available. Once the patient is fully awake and all of these criteria are met, extubation may proceed. If the surgical procedure was particularly challenging, intraoperative fluid shifts were large, or the patient is not progressing toward extubation, then arterial blood gas labs should be drawn to aid diagnosis and treatment.

Despite prolonged emergence from anesthesia due to protracted redistribution of anesthetics from the adipose into the central compartment, most pediatric patients meet extubation criteria in the operating room. Extensive multidisciplinary preparation with improved surgical and anesthetic techniques contribute to successful extubation in the operating room. A very difficult surgical procedure in a patient with complex and severe comorbidities may require prolonged intubation at the discretion of the attending anesthesiologist.

POSTOPERATIVE COMPLICATIONS

Obesity, OSA, and bariatric surgery, while intimately related, are each independent risk factors for postoperative respiratory complications. Obese children have a greater incidence of airway obstruction, bronchospasm, major oxygen desaturation, and overall critical respiratory events.[13] The incidence of apnea, hypopnea, oxygen desaturation, or hypercarbia are reported to be as high as 27% in children with OSA.[14]

Furthermore, because the prevalence of OSA among obese children is high, the risk for respiratory complications is compounded.[4] Extensive communication with the patient, parents, nurses, and surgeons regarding adherence to optimal positioning, pulmonary toilet, supplemental oxygen, CPAP/BiPAP, and pain medication regimen is paramount to ameliorate respiratory complications.

Multiple adult studies have demonstrated that preoperative diagnosis of OSA and treatment with CPAP decrease the incidence of postoperative respiratory complications.[15,16] It is reasonable to extrapolate that obese adolescents with OSA would also have a decrease in postoperative respiratory complications if CPAP was utilized preoperatively. The American Society of Anesthesiologists Task Force on Perioperative Management of Patients with Obstructive Sleep Apnea recommends that noninvasive positive pressure ventilation (NIPPV) should be continuously administered postoperatively to patients who were using this modality preoperatively, unless contraindicated by the surgical procedure.[17] Additional studies demonstrate that CPAP blunts the respiratory depressant effects of opioids after bariatric surgery.[15,18] The controversy lies in the timing of initiation of NIPPV after bariatric surgery. Conventional wisdom was that CPAP elevated pressures in the esophagus and stomach, translating to stress on the fresh suture line. Published data does not support this concern;[15,18,19] however, risk of stomach insufflation persuades many physicians to wait several hours before initiating NIPPV.

Other postoperative complications include hemodynamic instability, pressure sores, and thromboembolic events.[13] Surgical complications consist of bowel obstruction from an anastomotic closure, anastomotic leak, bleeding, and wound infection.

POSTOPERATIVE MONITORING

While obese patients are at increased risk for postoperative respiratory events, there are no consensus guidelines regarding method, location, or duration of respiratory monitoring. This requires the anesthesiologist to formulate an individualized monitoring plan adopted from recommendations in the OSA and adult bariatric literature. The American Society of Anesthesiologists Task Force on Perioperative Management of Patients with Obstructive Sleep Apnea recommends that patients at increased risk of respiratory compromise have continuous pulse oximetry monitoring and that it be maintained as long as the patient remains at increased risk.[17] To establish resolution of risk, patients should be observed in an unstimulated environment, preferably while asleep. Thus patients with simple obesity who are otherwise healthy can be monitored with continuous pulse oximetry on a standard hospital ward. For obese patients with OSA, it is important to determine the severity of the disease and the degree of compliance with CPAP therapy and allow these factors to guide postoperative monitoring. Early utilization of NIPPV has decreased the need for direct intensive care unit (ICU) admissions and respiratory related transfers to the ICU,[16] reserving ICU postoperative care for the most complex bariatric patients. Capnometry is the standard of care for monitoring ventilation and should be also be considered in patients with significant comorbidities. As pediatric bariatric surgery becomes more common, development of bariatric care teams and wards can normalize postoperative care for these patients.

POSTOPERATIVE ANALGESIA

An effective perioperative pain plan will provide good analgesia with minimal respiratory depression and increase adherence to respiratory therapies. The discussion of pain management should start in the outpatient setting with a conversation on expectations for pain and a demonstration of nonpharmacologic distraction techniques. The plan should continue with individualized medication choices using a multimodal analgesic approach. While the data in adults is more robust, pediatric studies demonstrating the opioid-sparing effects of acetaminophen, nonsteroidal anti-inflammatory drugs (NSAIDs), clonidine, ketamine, and dexmedetomidine is mounting.[20,21] Preoperative acetaminophen and gabapentin should be considered with both being scheduled to continue after surgery.[22] Scheduled NSAIDs, such as ketorolac, ibuprofen, or naproxen, also decrease the need for postoperative opioids and increase participation in respiratory therapy.[23] Low-dose dexmedetomidine or ketamine infusions can be initiated intraoperatively and continued through the immediate postoperative period to assist in basal pain control. Neuraxial anesthesia (thoracic epidural) provides excellent coverage for open procedures with large incisions, and regional anesthesia (transversus abdominis, quadratus lumborum, erector spinae plane blocks) can be employed for laparoscopic procedures. While there is a higher failure and complication rate for regional anesthesia in obese patients, the benefits of improved analgesia and preserved respiratory mechanics warrant strong consideration. Opioid analgesics should be titrated to effect, with constant reevaluation of their sedative and respiratory effects. Basal infusions should be avoided if patient-controlled analgesia pump is chosen over as-needed bolus dosing of opioids. Lastly, symptoms of nausea, anxiety, and depression can increase the perception of pain; thus it is important to anticipate a need for antiemetics and continue home antidepressants.

REVIEW QUESTIONS

1. Which of the following statements **MOST** accurately describes the calculation of BMI?

   A. weight in kilograms divided by height in centimeters.
   B. weight in kilograms divided by height in centimeters squared
   C. weight in kilograms divided by height in meters
   D. weight in kilograms divided by height in meters squared

Answer: D
BMI relates weight to height and is commonly used as a screening tool for obesity. BMI is calculated by dividing the patient's weight (in kilograms) by the square of the height (in meters). Alternatively, it can also be calculated by dividing the patient's weight (in pounds) by the square of the height (in inches) and then multiplying the answer by 703.

2. The dosing of rocuronium for neuromuscular blockade in a severely obese adolescent is **MOST** appropriately based on which of the following body scalars?

   A. BMI
   B. IBW
   C. LBW
   D. TBW

Answer: B
The V_d of a drug determines its loading dosage. The V_d of lipophilic drugs is increased in obesity, and so TBW should be used to calculate its loading dose. On the other hand, partially lipophilic or water-soluble drugs, like non-depolarizing muscle relaxants, show very little change in V_d, and, therefore, the loading dose of these drugs should be based on IBW. The dosing of these drugs, on the basis of TBW, results in a prolonged duration of action.

3. A 15-year-old obese female with acute perforated appendicitis is scheduled for laparoscopic appendectomy. The dosing of succinylcholine for rapid sequence induction in this patient is **MOST** appropriately based on which of the following body scalars?

   A. BMI
   B. IBW
   C. LBW
   D. TBW

Answer: D
The dosing of succinylcholine for rapid sequence induction in obese patients should be based on TBW secondary to increases in both volume of distribution and pseudocholinesterase levels. Administration of succinylcholine (1 mg/kg) based on TBW results in a more profound block and better intubating conditions compared with dosing by IBW or LBW.

4. A 6-year-old obese boy with obstructive sleep apnea is status post-tonsillectomy and adenoidectomy for sleep-disordered breathing symptoms. Which of the following would be the **MOST** appropriate decision for postoperative discharge?

   A. 4 hours after monitoring in recovery room
   B. 8 hours after monitoring in recovery room
   C. 12 hours after monitoring in recovery room
   D. overnight after monitoring in the ICU

Answer: D
The American Society of Anesthesiologists Task Force on Perioperative Management of Patients with Obstructive Sleep Apnea recommends that patients at increased risk of respiratory compromise should have continuous pulse oximetry monitoring and that it should be maintained as long as the

patient remains at increased risk. Obese children with severe OSA are at an increased risk of respiratory compromise and should be observed overnight in a hospital setting.

5. A 15-year-old, 112-kg female with central obesity and asthma underwent an uneventful laparoscopic sleeve gastrectomy. She is breathing spontaneously and has stable hemodynamics. Which of the following is the **MOST** appropriate plan for extubation?

    A. awake extubation in reverse Trendelenburg position

    B. awake extubation, pooling secretions in Trendelenburg position

    C. deep extubation to prevent bronchospasm

    D. continued ventilation in the ICU

Answer: A

Obese children should be extubated awake after observation of strict criteria. Obese children are at increased risk for critical respiratory events, and awake extubation mitigates some of this risk. Standard extubation criteria include reversal of neuromuscular blockade, neurologic exam appropriate for developmental level, negative inspiratory force ≤25 cm H_2O, age-appropriate respiratory rate, vital capacity >10 mL/kg IBW, and oxygen saturation and expired carbon dioxide approximating the patient's baseline. Extubating an asthmatic deep may reduce the likelihood of bronchospasm. This patient's obesity and likelihood of respiratory decomposition are more concerning than her well-controlled asthma, making an awake extubation preferable. Additionally, if an opioid bolus is to be given, it should be after the patient has demonstrated adequate upper airway tone with a natural airway. An uneventful sleeve gastrectomy is not an indication, in and of itself, for a prolonged intubation. While steep Trendelenburg would allow pooling of oral secretions, this position would be counterproductive when trying to optimize an obese patient's respiratory mechanics. In steep Trendelenburg, the abdominal contents push on the diaphragm and encroach upon the chest cavity, which decreases lung volumes. A head-up or reverse Trendelenburg position will have the opposite affect and improve respiratory mechanics.

QUESTIONS AND ANSWERS

This chapter has accompanying questions and answers which are available to subscribers as part of the Oxford eLearning platform. To access the questions, go to ✓ http:// oxfordmedicine. com/pediatricanesthesiaPBL

REFERENCES

1. Hales CM, Carroll MD, Fryar CD, Ogden CL. Prevalence of obesity among adults and youth: United States, 2015-16. *NCHS Data Brief.* 2017;288:1–8.
2. Chidambaran V, Tewari A, Mahmoud M. Anesthetic and pharmacologic considerations in perioperative care of obese children. *J Clin Anesth.* 2017;45:39–50.
3. Chatterjee D. Anesthesia and childhood obesity. In: Holzman RS, Mancuso TJ, Polaner DM, eds. *A Practical Approach to Pediatric Anesthesia.* 2nd ed. Philadelphia, PA: Wolters Kluwer; 2016: 806–820.
4. Samuels PJ, Sjoblom MD. Anesthetic considerations for pediatric obesity and adolescent bariatric surgery. *Curr Opin Anesthesiol.* 2016;29:327–336.
5. Michalsky M, Reichard K, Inge TH, et al. ASMBS Pediatric Committee best practice guidelines. *Surg Obes Relat Dis.* 2012;8(1) 1–7.
6. Desai NK, Wulkan ML, Inge TH. Update on adolescent bariatric surgery. *Endocrinol Metab Clin N Am.* 2016;45 67–676.
7. Inge TH, Courcoulas AP, Jenkins TM, et al. Weight loss and health status 3 years after bariatric surgery in adolescents. *N Engl J Med.* 2016;374(2):113–123.
8. Yen K, Riegert A, Gorelik MH. Derivation of the DIVA score: a clinical prediction rule for the identification of children with difficult IV access. *Pediatr Emerg Care.* 2008;24(3):143–147.
9. Ueda K, Hussey P. Dynamic ultrasound-guided short axis needle tip navigation technique for facilitating cannulation of peripheral veins in obese patients. *Anesth Analg.* 2017;124:831–833.
10. Sun C-Y, Lee KC, Lin IH, Wu CL, Huang HP, Lin YY. Near-infrared light device can improve intravenous cannulation in critically ill children. *Pediatr Neonatol.* 2013;54(3):194–197.
11. Simhi E, Kachko L, Bruckheimer E, Katz J. A vein entry indicator device for facilitating peripheral intravenous cannulation in children: a prospective, randomized, controlled trial. *Anesth Analg.* 2008;107(5):1531–1535.
12. Belotti G, Bedford R, Arnold A. Fiberoptic transillumination for intravenous cannulation under general anesthesia. *Anesth Analg.* 1981;60(5):348–351.
13. Tait AR, Voepel-Lewis T, Burke C, Kostrezwa A, Lewis I. Incidence and risk factors for perioperative adverse respiratory events in children who are obese. *Anesthesiology.* 2008;108(3):375–380.
14. Patino M, Sadhasivam S, Mahmoud M. Obstructive sleep apnoea in children: perioperative considerations. *Br J Anaesth.* 2013;111(Suppl 1):i83–i95.
15. de Raaff C, de Vries N, van Wagensveld BA. Obstructive sleep apnea and bariatric surgical guidelines: summary and update. *Curr Opin Anesthesiol.* 2018;31(1):104–109.
16. Hallowell P, Stellato TA, Petrozzi MC, et al. Eliminating respiratory intensive care unit stay after gastric bypass surgery. *Surgery.* 2007;142(4):608–612.
17. Practice guidelines for the perioperative management of patients with obstructive sleep apnea: an updated report by the American Society of Anesthesiologists Task Force on Perioperative Management of Patients with Obstructive Sleep Apnea. *Anesthesiology.* 2014;120(2):268–286.
18. Zaremba S, Shin CH, Hutter MM, et al. Continuous positive airway pressure mitigates opioid-induced worsening of sleep-disordered breathing early after bariatric surgery. *Anesthesiology.* 2016;125(1):92–104.
19. de Raaff C, Klaff MC, Coblijn UK, et al. Influence of continuous positive airway pressure on postoperative leakage in bariatric surgery. *Surg Obes Relat Dis.* 2018;14(2):186–190.
20. Zhu A, Benzon H, Anderson T. Evidence for the efficacy of systemic opioid-sparing analgesics in pediatric surgical populations: a systematic review. *Anesth Analg.* 2017;125(5):1569–1587.
21. Bamgbade OA, Oluwole O, Khaw RR. Perioperative analgesia for fast-track laparoscopic bariatric surgery. *Obes Surg.* 2017;27(7):1828–1834.
22. Hassani V, Pazouki A, Nikoubakht N, Chaichian S, Sayarifard A, Shakib Khankandi A. The effect of gabapentin on reducing pain after laparoscopic gastric bypass surgery in patients with morbid obesity: a randomized clinical trial. *Anesth Pain Med.* 2015;5(1):e22372.
23. Govindarajan R, Ghosh B, Sathyamoorthy MK, et al. Efficacy of ketorolac in lieu of narcotics in the operative management of laparoscopic surgery for morbid obesity. *Surg Obes Relat Dis.* 2005;1:530–535.

65.

PERIOPERATIVE CARE OF PATIENTS WITH EPIDERMOLYSIS BULLOSA

Alyssa M. Burgart and Louise K. Furukawa

STEM CASE AND KEY QUESTIONS

A 6-year-old male with recessive dystrophic epidermolysis bulls (RDEB) and severe anxiety is scheduled for circumcision due to phimotic scarring sequela of RDEB. There is no history of esophageal strictures. The patient is noncooperative with exam but, per parent report, can be coaxed to take oral medications. He had dental rehabilitation at age 3 with no reported complications. His physical exam is notable for chronic wounds on both shoulders and has no digits due to pseudosyndactyly. Therapeutic protective dressings cover his extremities and the patient will not allow them to be removed. The patient will not cooperate with a thorough airway exam, but you note trismus and poor dentition. He appears to have no better than 1.5 cm interdental distance mouth opening. The case is scheduled at a mixed pediatric-adult free standing surgicenter.

WHILE EPIDERMOLYSIS BULLOSA (EB) IS GENERALLY THOUGHT OF AS A DERMATOLOGIC DISEASE, WHAT OTHER ORGAN SYSTEMS ARE AFFECTED?

Extracutaneous involvement of EB include the eternal eye, airway (oral mucosa, larynx, and trachea), gastrointestinal (GI) system (esophagus, small and large intestine, anus), and genitourinary system (kidney, genitourinary tract, including the vagina). Some patients will develop renal failure or dilated cardiomyopathy, and one subtype of EB is associated with muscular dystrophy. Patients with EB are at high risk of developing life-threatening cancers, especially aggressive squamous cell carcinoma in chronic wound sites. Sequela of this chronic disease with frequent bleeding and healing wounds include osteopenia, contractures, anemia, hypermetabolism, and failure to thrive. These manifestations may vary significantly based on patient age and the type of EB.

HAS THIS PATIENT HAD A SUFFICIENT PREOPERATIVE WORKUP? WHAT ADDITIONAL INFORMATION SHOULD BE SOUGHT?

The dermatology notes should be reviewed in detail, especially for further information about his chronic wounds. The parents should be asked about chronic wound locations, evidence of infection, and dressing change routine, which products work well, and when dressings were last changed. The history should include information about chronic pain and anxiety and how is it currently treated. The patient's kidney function should be evaluated and his nutritional status assessed. The patient's airway should be meticulously assessed and old anesthetic records reviewed with particular attention to vascular access and airway manipulation. Relevant laboratory evaluation at a minimum includes complete blood count (to evaluate for chronic anemia) and metabolic panel including creatinine.

GIVEN THIS PATIENT'S DIAGNOSIS AND ITS ATTENDANT MANIFESTATIONS, IS THIS CASE BOOKED IN AN APPROPRIATE LOCATION?

No, an outpatient surgical center is unlikely to have the necessary support staff and supplies. The patient has an anticipated difficult airway and his management will require significant additional resources (such as specialized wound dressings) that are unlikely to be found at this location. When patients with EB are treated at centers with adequate expertise in their care, the rate of adverse events is quite low.[1]

YOU ARE CONCERNED THAT OTHER STAFF MEMBERS IN THE ROOM ARE NOT AWARE OF THIS PATIENT'S UNIQUE NEEDS. HOW CAN YOU HELP EDUCATE THE APPROPRIATE PEOPLE? WHAT INFORMATION WILL BE IMPORTANT FOR THE NURSING, SURGICAL, AND ANCILLARY STAFF, LIKE ANESTHESIA TECHS?

It is necessary to avoid trauma throughout the preoperative period and is therefore vital that all staff be prepared and skilled in the care of patients with EB. We recommend a preprocedure huddle and periodic in-service learning opportunities to ensure that all care providers in the room (including the surgeon) understand the patient's unique needs. The discussion should include the patient's relevant physical exam findings, the anesthetic plan, materials in the room for monitors and draping (ensuring no adhesives are accidentally applied), use of electrocautery, and a review of how to touch the patient to reduce shear force injury. The patient's disease influences all aspects of the operating room (OR) environment. Ahead of time, determine who will manage the airway and apply the monitors. Additionally, detailed contingency plans should be discussed, ensuring the circulating nurse knows who to call if a crisis occurs.

YOU PREMEDICATE THE PATIENT WITH ORAL MIDAZOLAM 0.5 MG/KG. THE PATIENT SEPARATES EASILY FROM HIS PARENTS BUT IN THE OR WILL NOT PERMIT YOU TO PLACE YOUR MONITORS. YOU WORRY ABOUT DAMAGE TO HIS SKIN IF YOU FORCE HIM TO COMPLY. WHAT CAN YOU DO?

It is important to place monitors, but this patient's RDEB places him at exceptional risk for injury. If you can only place one monitor before induction, focus on the pulse oximeter, and place other monitors after induction. If the patient will not tolerate a mask for induction, or will fight and risk additional injury, you may consider giving him intranasal midazolam or intramuscular or oral ketamine to deepen his sedation and maximize compliance.

YOUR CIRCULATING NURSE TELLS YOU THAT, AT HER PREVIOUS HOSPITAL, THESE CASES WERE DONE WITH ONLY A PULSE OXIMETER. IS THAT APPROPRIATE?

When providing any type of sedation, the use of American Society of Anesthesiologists standard monitors should be used. Given the risk of cardiomyopathy in this population, the use of electrocardiography (ECG) and noninvasive blood pressure monitors is certainly important. End-tidal carbon dioxide ($ETCO_2$) and oxygen monitoring will confirm ventilation.

WHAT ARE YOUR OPTIONS FOR AIRWAY MANAGEMENT? WHAT AIRWAY EQUIPMENT SHOULD BE IN THE ROOM?

This patient has an anticipated difficult airway secondary to trismus. Further physical exam may demonstrate other conditions, such as oral scarring leading to microstomia, poor dentition, and possible posterior pharyngeal scarring. Intubation will be difficult and may be impossible. As with all difficulty airways, the anesthesiologist should be prepared for a "cannot ventilate, cannot intubate" scenario and have a contingency plan prepared. Fully prepared difficult airway equipment should be in the room, including a small-size fiberoptic scope. Noninvasive management of this difficult airway may be both the least invasive and the safest approach. However, this will require that hypoventilation be avoided at all costs. A noninvasive approach (nasal cannula oxygen and CO_2 monitoring) will require extra vigilance but will also allow you to avoid the difficulties of intubation. If intubation cannot be avoided, oral or nasal intubation is usually possible though typically requiring a smaller tube than predicted by age due to reduced mouth opening or small nasal aperture.

Microlaryngoscopy tubes may be necessary for additional length.

IF THE PATIENT LARYNGOSPASMS, CAN SUCCINYLCHOLINE BE GIVEN?

The use of succinylcholine is not contraindicated. While there are concerns that succinylcholine-induced fasciculations could induce trauma and that the risk of hyperkalemia may be increased in patient with dystrophic musculature or renal insufficiency, 2 large case series have not demonstrated this effect.[2] In patients who require rapid sequence induction due to aspiration risk, it is certainly an option.

MIGHT REGIONAL ANESTHESIA BE HELPFUL IN THIS CASE?

Yes, the provision of a dense regional block of the penis will make it possible to reduce the amount of sedation required to maintain patient comfort, provide a safe surgical environment, and avoid hypoventilation. Regional anesthesia is generally well tolerated in EB patients and tends to be technically easy due to the patients' lean habitus. Contraindications to regional anesthesia are the same as for patients without EB. Once the patient's intravenous (IV) line is in place, the judicious use of ketamine before injection can help the patient remain comfortable and maintain respiratory stability.

DISCUSSION

TYPES OF EB AND COMMON PRESENTATIONS

EB is a disorder of epithelial adhesion due to mutations producing abnormal proteins involved in anchoring the skin layers. There are over 20 subtypes of EB, with varying degrees of severity and impact on quality of life, morbidity, and mortality.[3] The 4 main subtypes include dystrophic, simplex, junctional (JEB), and acquired (see Table 65.1). Recessive dystrophic EB, most commonly associated with extensive skin blistering and scarring, affects most epithelial surfaces resulting in a multitude of systemic disturbances. Ocular manifestations include corneal drying and abrasions resulting in corneal and conjunctival scarring. Oral sequelas of RDEB include mucosal blistering, ankyloglossia, and obliteration of vestibular sulci, all of which can result in a dramatic reduction in mouth opening. Extensive intraoral scarring can result in pharyngeal stenosis although this scarring generally maintains a patent natural airway.

Esophageal strictures and webs are common, with half of RDEB patients symptomatic by age 10. Patients are at high risk for esophageal shortening and gastroesophageal reflux disease (GERD). Cardiomyopathy, typically presenting between the ages of 9 and 12 is uncommon but serious, and the presence of concomitant renal failure portends a worse prognosis. A diagnosis of RDEB greatly increases the risk of clinically aggressive squamous cell carcinoma. Malignant melanoma is rare but

Table 65.1 EPIDERMOLYSIS BULLOSA TYPES AND FEATURES

EB TYPE[3,4]	SUBTYPES/BLISTER FORMATION SITES	LOCATION OF LESIONS	GENETICS	SPECIAL CONCERNS	SURVIVAL
Dystrophic	Recessive Hallopeau, non-Hallopeau, inversa Dominant Lamina densa and upper dermis	Skin and mucosal surfaces Severe scarring—digits may autoamputate or fuse into mitten shape	Collagen VII—encodes anchoring fibril	SCC tends to develop in second or third decade MM rare but onset at earlier age Rare but serious development of cardiomyopathy	Survival past second decade is rare
Simplex Most common form of EB	Basal Suprabasal Epidermis	Most common location for blisters are hands and feet Onset may be at birth or later in life Rare mucosal involvement	Autosomal dominant Genes encoding K5 or K14 Recessive subtype more severe Recessive subtype can have muscular dystrophy or pyloric atresia	Infections are common Outbreaks precipitated by stress, warm climates, infections, puberty Not associated with SCC or MM	
Junctional	JEB-H (severe form) JEB-nH Junctional with pyloric atresia Skin separation at the lamina lucida of BMZ	Non-scarring form Skin tightening and thinning Blistering present at birth; spontaneous blistering and ulceration Involves mucosal and perioral surfaces May affect respiratory tissue	Autosomal recessive JEB-H: Genes encoding collagen XVII, alpha 6, beta 4 integrin, or Laminin 5 JEB-nH: collagen XVII, occasionally Laminin 5	Tracheal involvement. Death due to airway issues	JEB-H in particular rarely survive past childhood Death from sepsis
Acquisita	Mechano-bullous (resembles RDEB) Inflammatory (resembles bullous pemphigoid)	Auto-antibodies that bind to collagen VII	Not inherited	Treated with steroids Associated with other systemic disorders—inflammatory bowel disease (especially Crohns disease) and plasma cell dyscrasias	Normal lifespan; mortality directly from disease is rare

Note. EB = epidermolysis bullosa; SCC = squamous cell carcinoma; MM = malignant melanoma; BMZ = basement membrane zone; JEB-H = junctional epidermolysis bullosa–Herlitz; JEB-nH = junctional epidermolysis bullosa–Non-Herlitz; RDEB = recessive dystrophic epidermolysis bulls.

presents earlier in life.[4] Hematologic risks include a profound multifactorial anemia. Patients are in a hypermetabolic state and require aggressive caloric supplementation while chronic wounds place them at high risk for infection.

To reduce risks to patients with this debilitating disease, anesthesiologists must be familiar with the disease process and prepared to minimize disease-associated morbidity throughout the perioperative period. Anesthesiologists should recognize that patients with inherited EB may express mosaicism, leading to nonuniform cutaneous manifestations, only partial expression in certain organ systems, and siblings with wide variation of disease manifestation.[5] This further contributes to the variety of clinical symptoms patients may experience beyond the individual genetic diagnosis.

COMMON PRESENTATIONS

Common presentations in EB include the following:[6]

Plastics procedures to correct pseudosyndactyly of the hands or feet

Balloon esophageal dilatation (performed under fluoroscopy), GI endoscopy

Gastrostomy (G) tube placement

Dental restorations

Plastics procedures to increase oral opening

Would care or extensive dressing changes

Preoperative assessment

The preoperative evaluation of patient with EB must be thorough and complete, assessing all relevant organ systems including psychosocial needs. Assessments should be completed in-person, preferably with significant time before surgery to

Ocular

The external eye is often involved. Corneal blisters, scaring, and clouding develop over time. Frequently, patients cannot fully close their eyelids.

Airway

Oral examination should assess presence of blistering and scarring (from lips to vocal cords), ankyloglossia, microstomia, the obliteration of vestibular sulci, and dentition. Pre-existing oral lesions should be documented. Of note, pharyngeal scarring tends to create a patent natural airway and patients are not necessarily difficult to ventilate. However, 5% of RDEB patients develop laryngeal stenosis by age 30. The presence of stertor can be a clue to severe laryngeal stenosis. Beware of associating intact external skin with benign airway disease, as milder cutaneous disease does not necessarily correlate well with presence or absence of airway scarring. Trismus and microstomia may significantly reduce mouth opening both horizontally and vertically, and ankyloglossia may limit movement of the tongue. Interincisor distance should be measured. Whenever possible, add a photograph to the medical record demonstrating mouth opening with a ruler for perspective. Such photos assist in monitoring disease progression and providing valuable preoperative information to colleagues. In cooperative patients, it may be possible to conduct a limited fiberoptic exam in the preoperative clinic. Excessive caries are common not because of faulty enamel but rather poor salivary clearance, inability to brush properly, and need for a high-calorie liquid carbohydrate-based diet. Teeth may also be quite crowded. For patients with previous airway manipulations, scarring may worsen with time. Patients with JEB are at higher risk for subglottic and nasal stenosis, as well as peritracheal and intranasal granulation tissue.[7]

GI

Esophageal strictures and webs (typically in the upper third of the esophagus) are common with half of RDEB patients reporting symptoms by age 10.[8] By age 45, the cumulative risk reaches 95%. Scarring may lead to esophageal foreshortening and clinically significant GERD. Patients may have poor intestinal absorption and protein-losing enteropathy. Anal stenosis may be present, so care must be taken if considering any rectal medications. Twenty-five to 35% of patients require supplemental feeding and frequently have G tubes placed.

Skin

A detailed wound history should be obtained, including location of wounds, wound care routine, most recent wound infection, and information regarding which EB products work best for the patient. Patients typically know the best sites on their bodies for IV access.

Cardiac

Patients with RDEB and JEB–non-Herlitz are at risk of developing rare but serious dilated cardiomyopathy with an average of onset between 9 and 12 years of age.[9] As in non-EB patients, cardiomyopathy manifests with dyspnea, tachypnea, tachycardia, and decreased exercise tolerance. Arrhythmias may develop due to electrolyte imbalances. Preoperative ECG and echocardiogram may be indicated and are generally easy to perform in a nontraumatic manner.

Genitourinary

Patients are at risk for urethral strictures and renal failure. Recommended screening for RDEB and JEB patients includes biannual evaluation of electrolytes, urea, urinalysis, and blood pressure.[10] JEB patients should also have an annual renal ultrasound to evaluate scarring. Urethral instrumentation should be avoided when possible, but patients will tolerate short-term urethral catheters. If long-term management of urethral stenosis is needed, a suprapubic catheter may be placed.

Hematologic

Anemia is common in patients with EB, and they should have recent complete blood count and iron studies completed. At times, blood transfusion or iron infusion is indicated. Oral iron supplementation is poorly tolerated, is poorly absorbed, and causes constipation.

Orthopedic

EB patients may develop osteopenia, vertebral compression fractures, and scoliosis. Frequently, due to scarring, patients develop contractures and pseudosyndactyly (fusion of fingers and toes)

PSYCHOLOGICAL ASPECTS AND PAIN

Secondary to repeated hospitalizations in childhood, patients are at risk of developing posttraumatic stress disorder (PTSD) and psychological trauma. In stressful hospital situations, recognize the potential for regression and panic attacks. Additionally, parents/caregivers may find it difficult to relinquish control. Frequently, patients remain dependent on parents/caregivers into adulthood. Chronic pain is common due to painful routine care, such as bathing, wound dressing changes, and management of blistering. Patients may utilize a combination of psychological and pharmacological interventions to treat their pain. Corneal abrasions are common. Patients develop bone pain from compression fractures secondary to osteoporosis.[11]

CANCER EVALUATION

In RDEB-Hallopeau-Siemens squamous cell cancers are especially common and tend to appear in the second decade of life. These malignancies stem from the repeated cycles of cell division. Despite a histopathologically benign appearance, the squamous cell carcinomas are clinically aggressive and metastasize.[12] Malignant melanomas are less common but appear earlier in childhood. Patients should always be evaluated for evidence of metastatic disease, as it will be a contraindication to most elective procedures.

ANESTHETIC PREPARATION

Vigilant protection of the patient's skin is paramount. In the OR, skin integrity protection is challenging and the anesthesiologist may be the person with the most experience in EB skin care. Care of patients with EB requires careful preparation and attention to detail. Adhesives should be avoided at all costs, including tape, ECG electrodes, and pulse oximeter stickers. The facility must have a supply of a variety of specialized materials (see Box 65.1), tools, and staff trained in the needed techniques for management of these patients. The anesthesia provider needs extra time to prepare supplies and equipment. In addition to the work required to conduct a successful anesthetic, the anesthesiologist must also monitor the behavior of other staff in the room, ensuring that they too avoid practices and materials that may injure the patient. If a case requires

---

Box 65.1 EB SUPPLY TOOLBOX

Methylcellulose eye lubricant
Emollients (Albolene®, Aquaphor®)
Webril® cotton undercast padding
Surg-o-Flex® bandages
Coban® wrap
Ace® wrap
Synthetic Sheepskin
Sensi-Care—Sting Free Adhesive Remover Wipes
Mölnlycke® Safetac silicone-based products:
Mepitac®—soft silicone tape
Mepilex Transfer®—foam dressing
Mepilex Border®—foam dressing with silicone adhesive border
Mepitel One®—wound contact layer, prevents adhesive from sticking to open wound
Mepiform®
Vaseline gauze
Covalon® IV Clear—antimicrobial clear silicone adhesive dressing
Suture
3M® Defibrillation Gel Pads
Eye pad gauze rounds
Megadyne® Mega Soft electrocautery return pad

Note there are other products available and international consensus guidelines are available to assist in EB type specific wound care.[13]

---

particularly complex anesthetic management, it can be helpful to have a wound care expert (nurse) in the room to monitor and advise the conduct of others.

GENERAL PRINCIPLES

Friction and shear forces lead to bulla formation, while pressure/compression is typically better tolerated. When touching the patient, wear gloves covered in ointment-based lubricants. It can be convenient to have a small stack of gauze with ointment near the patient for easy reapplication. Touching should be kept to a minimum and when needed gentle touch should be used. Should a blister arise, it should be lanced at the edge (rather than the center) and aspirated. Blisters should not be unroofed. While silicone-based adhesives may be used in EB patients, be aware that removing them should be done with care. When removing bandages, gently apply lubricant to the bandage edge prevent further undermining of the skin.

PREOPERATIVE AREA

A piece of synthetic sheepskin should be used to cover the gurney, unless declined by the patient, as this defuses the shear forces applied to the patient's skin. This sheepskin sheet may be used to cradle the patient when transferring (e.g., onto OR table). Whenever possible, allow the patient to self-position. The patient may need help from a caregiver to successfully change into a gown. No knots should be tied on the gown. Initial vital signs require special modification to obtain, and preoperative nurses may require assistance if they do not yet have significant experience in this arena. The same is true regarding IV placement, as the skin will require special protection and typical adhesives cannot be used.

PULSE OXIMETRY

Pulse oximetry is possible but more difficult in patients who no longer have fingers. Clip oximeters can be very useful as they utilize pressure to stay in place. However, if a clip oximeter is not available or the patient does not have an amenable location on which to place it, a wrap oximeter may be used. The adhesive portion of the oximeter should be covered on both sides with a Tegaderm®, leaving an exposed adhesive tail, which will be applied to the Tegaderm®, rather than the patient's skin (see Fig. 65.1).

ELECTROCARDIOGRAPHY

While cases have been performed without the use of ECG, it is easy to successfully obtain an ECG reading with proper preparation. By placing ECG leads on defibrillation gel pads, an ECG tracing is obtained without exposing the patient to the leads' adhesive backing. Importantly, the edges of the defibrillation pads readily dry, leaving a rough edge that may damage the patient's fragile skin. Pads should be cut significantly larger

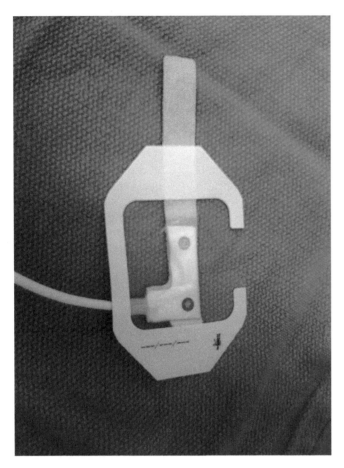

Fig. 65.1 Adhesive pulse oximeters require modification to prevent adhesives from touching the skin of the EB patient.

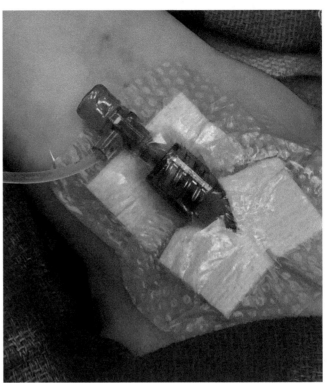

Fig. 65.2 Dressings for IVs can take many forms. Here, a Mepilex Border® has been cut in half, with one half placed under the IV hub to protect the patient's delicate skin. A slit has been placed in the other half and used to hold the IV in position. While difficult to see, a clear adhesive dressing has been placed over the Mepilex Border® material to provide additional stability.

than the lead to account for this issue and in longer cases; the pads may require periodic replacement.

BLOOD PRESSURE

Noninvasive blood pressure monitoring is well tolerated. Blistering is avoided by wrapping the patient's extremity in Webril® prior to cuff placement.

ETCO₂

ETCO$_2$ should be monitored during the anesthetic and does not typically interfere with the patient's skin. It does not require any special modification.

IV ACCESS

Thanks to patient's thin, somewhat translucent skin, IV placement is not necessarily difficult. Appropriate pain reduction should be utilized. EMLA creams and patches are very useful, but pressure-based local anesthetic delivery (i.e., J-tip®, Zingo®) and subcutaneous infiltration should be avoided. Local anesthetic creams may be applied, covered with gauze, and gently wrapped with Coban®. The adhesive portion of any lidocaine patch must be cut away before securing. The anesthesiologist should decide ahead of time who shall place the IV during

induction and notify the preoperative nurse. Though most parents and patients know where the patient's veins are typically found, an ultrasound should be readily available.

Ask the patient about the best ways to prepare his or her skin for procedures (i.e., alcohol pad dab, saline, baby shampoo, Care foam). A tourniquet should be placed over Webril®, rather than directly on the skin. If there is another provider available, that person may apply tourniquet pressure with his or her hand over Webril®. Ask the patient which products work best for him or her to secure the IV. Mepitac® or a Mepitel Border® may be placed under the IV hub. Mepitac® may be used over the IV as well but will not be sufficient on its own to secure the IV. Coban® can be wrapped around the extremity to include the IV. Traditional adhesive tape or Tegaderm® may be used on the dressing (never directly on the patient's skin) (see Fig. 65.2). Unfortunately, the IV will never be as secure as you would normally insist. IVs may be sutured in place.

OR

Never place a traditional adhesive electrocautery pad on a patient with EB. Instead, the patient may lie on a return electrode mat (e.g., Megadyne® Mega Soft), which will allow electrical current to diffuse across any point of contact on its surface. Alternatively, bipolar electrocautery may be used. EB patients suffer from impaired thermoregulation. To reduce thermal losses, fluids should be warmed, the room should be warm, and the patient should be covered with warm blankets. Loss of hair follicles due to scarring leads to the reduced ability to sweat and patients may also overheat. Temperature should be monitored throughout the procedure.

EYE PROTECTION

The patient's eyes should be carefully secured after induction to reduce risk for corneal abrasions and dryness. For eyes that close, they may be secured with silicone tape. Due to scarring, the patient's eyes may not fully close. Methylcellulose eye lubricant should be applied, eyes closed to the degree possible, then wet pads placed over the lids and secured in place with a long piece of Coban® wrapped lightly around the patient's head and eyes. Petroleum-based lubricant is avoided as it can be irritating and if patients rub their eyes to clear their vision, they may cause further blistering and subsequent scarring or abrasions.

DRESSING CHANGES AND ANCILLARY PROCEDURES

If the patient needs wound dressing changes or wound evaluation, a competent practitioner (e.g., wound care nurse) may do so in the OR. Children or teens and young adults with PTSD may require additional procedures in the OR such as blood draws, iron infusions, G tube changes and skin biopsies. If time and safety permits, combining these procedures during one OR visit can spare the patient and family further traumatic medical manipulations.

INDUCTION

IV induction is optimal but not always possible. In patients who will not tolerate being awake for IV placement, mask induction may be safely performed. The mask should be fully inflated and liberally lubricated. Alternatively, the face may be protected with wound care dressings, such as Mepitel® Transfer. One must be cognizant of applying any pressure to the patient's face during mask induction, as bulla may form after only brief application of fingers to the jaw.

AIRWAY MANAGEMENT

Difficult airway equipment should be in the room and prepared for immediate use. Generally, intubation should be avoided when possible given the proclivity for progressive airway disease. In RDEB patients, intubation is not contraindicated but noninvasive management of the airway is possible and preferable when appropriate (see Fig. 65.3). Frequently, however, EB patients present for esophageal stricture dilation, which often necessitates intubation. The strictures in RDEB are typically high in the esophagus behind the larynx and can blister and bleed with dilation. This scenario significantly increases the risk of aspiration of blood and/or contrast. Intubation may be difficult and time-consuming due to small mouth opening, excess saliva, blisters, blood, and/or scarring in the pharynx. The endotracheal

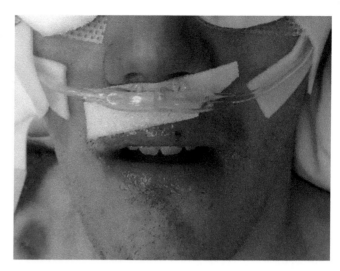

Fig. 65.3 Noninvasive airway management. Silicone foam has been placed to protect the philtrum and cheeks; the nasal cannula prongs have been trimmed to keep them from touching the nostrils.

tube (ETT) should be a reduced size, and, if the cuff must be inflated, it should be done gently. During direct laryngoscopy, the blade and ETT should be well lubricated. Videolaryngoscopy may allow for less force to be used when compared to traditional direct laryngoscopy, but the typical high profile of videolaryngoscopic blades may not fit in a microstomic mouth. If used, the videolaryngoscopy blade should be lubricated. Fiberoptic intubation may also be a good option, allowing for minimal contact with oral mucosa. Nasal mucosa is involved in both RDEB and JEB, but the hairs typically stabilize and protect the mucosal layers. JEB patients form excessive wounds and scarring around the nose, but in other forms of EB, nasal intubation may be considered. Special care must be taken that pressure not be applied to the nasal ala. Blind pharyngeal suctioning must be avoided. Due to the frequently limited mouth opening in this population, laryngeal mask airways may be difficult to place and risk significant oral injury due to prolonged contact.

There are many ways to secure the ETT, yet no method is truly secure. This is especially true during upper endoscopy, where the endoscope may catch on the ETT and extubate the

---

Box 65.2 ENDOSCOPY SPECIFIC ADVICE

Supine self-positioning by patient
Avoid position changes while patient anesthetized
Sheepskin unless declined by patient
If patient has G tube, prepare to vent it
Careful dental exam
Protect the lips against scope friction
Alternative bite blocks available
Small endoscopes available
Never move the scope without the anesthesiologist being aware and prepared
At risk for postoperative nausea

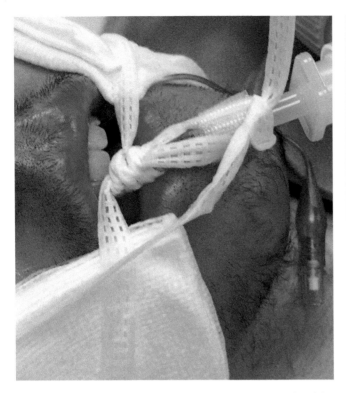

Fig. 65.4 A surgical mask has been placed behind the patient's head and the ties used to wrap around the ETT. Gauzes covered in lubricant have been placed under the ties to prevent friction.

patient (see Box 65.2). Options for securing the ETT include tying a surgical mask with the mask behind the patient's head and using the ties to secure the ETT (see Fig. 65.4). Ensure that wound dressings prevent the ties from contacting the patient's skin. Mepitac® tape may be used to secure the tube, recognizing that it tends to slip (see Fig. 65.5). Suturing the oral or nasal tube may provide a slightly more secure option for longer term intubation such as intensive care unit care. Nasal RAE ETTs can be secured without adhesives by securing with a padded wrap around the head.

MAINTENANCE

For peripheral surgeries, where no muscle relaxation is indicated, remifentanil, propofol, and ketamine infusions are well tolerated with oxygenation via a native airway. For central surgeries, the anesthetic should be tailored to optimize surgical field and allow for rapid emergence. Decreased protein binding due to hypoalbuminemia may lead to increased responsiveness to protein-bound drugs such as muscle relaxants.

REGIONAL ANESTHESIA

Regional anesthesia is well tolerated and usually easy to perform given lean habitus. Ample gel should be used with ultrasound and the probe should be lifted, moved, and reapplied, rather than pulled across the skin. Subcutaneous infiltration should be avoided. Contraindications to regional anesthesia are the same as those for other regional anesthetics.

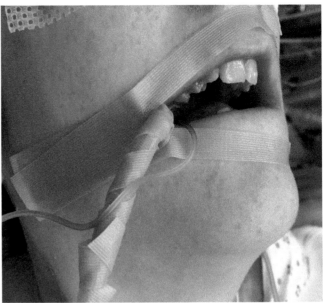

Fig. 65.5 Mepitac® silicon tape has been used to secure the ETT. With an IV induction, such an approach is more feasible. After lubricated mask induction, the patient's face may be too slick for the tape to stick in a secure enough fashion.

EXTUBATION

At the conclusion of surgery, if safe to do so, a deep extubation will reduce potential trauma.

CONCLUSION

EB is a multisystemic disease with diverse presentation. The anesthesiologist must be prepared with highly specialized skills and products to conduct a safe procedure. When proper care is provided, EB patients presenting for surgery have lower rates of morbidity.

REVIEW QUESTIONS

1. Which of the following epithelial tissues is **LEAST** affected in patients with RDEB?

    A. esophagus
    B. small intestine
    C. oral mucosa
    D. trachea

Answer: D
The tracheal mucosa is *not* involved in patients with RDEB, implying that careful intubation is a reasonable option in these patients.

2. Which of the following common characteristics in RDEB patients contributes the **LEAST** to challenges establishing an artificial airway?

    A. markedly poor dentition

B. pharyngeal scar tissue
C. restricted mouth opening
D. thick inflexible neck

Answer: D

The multiple factors relating to the disease process contribute to difficulty in intubating these patients. A thick neck is atypical in EB patients.

3. Which of the following monitoring devices requires the **LEAST** modification for placement in patients with severe generalized forms of EB?

A. arterial catheter
B. bispectral index monitor
C. blood pressure cuff
D. ETCO$_2$ monitor

Answer: D

Most monitors require some modification to application in patients with severe generalized forms of EB, but this does not preclude their use.

4. Which of the following represents the **STRONGEST** contraindication for the use of regional anesthesia in a patient with EB?

A. history of postdural puncture headache
B. neoplasm in the operative limb
C. need to secure catheter with sutures
D. purulent infection at nerve block site

Answer: D

Regional anesthesia is a viable option in most patients with EB. Contraindications are generally the same as in patients without EB.

5. A 17-year-old patient with RDEB is about to undergo esophageal dilatation with contrast study for a high esophageal stricture in the interventional radiology suite. Which of the following concerns **BEST** justifies endotracheal intubation of the patient?

A. difficulty maintaining airway under anesthesia
B. history of "sore throat" with supraglottic airway
C. inability to monitor ETCO$_2$ with nasal cannula
D. significant risk for aspiration of blood or contrast

Answer: D

Most esophageal strictures in patients with RDEB are very proximal in the esophagus. Dilatation of these strictures can induce blisters and bleeding. Blood or contrast may be aspirated in an unprotected airway.

6. A 25-year-old patient with RDEB presents for elective pseudosyndactyly release of the right hand. She has a history of multiple lower extremity squamous cell carcinomas which have been excised. The orthopedic surgeon is enthusiastic about performing the procedure. You see the patient in preoperative evaluation. Which of the following would be the **STRONGEST** contraindication to performing this elective procedure?

A. family history of malignant hyperthermia
B. history of multiple difficult intubations
C. metastatic squamous cell carcinoma
D. patient instance on a inhalation induction

Answer: C

Invasive squamous cell carcinoma is the greatest cause of mortality in RDEB patients surviving into adulthood. Carcinoma arises in chronic wounds due to multiple cycles of cell replication. All RDEB patients should be carefully examined for signs of metastatic disease.

QUESTIONS AND ANSWERS

This chapter has accompanying questions and answers which are available to subscribers as part of the Oxford eLearning platform. To access the questions, go to ✓ http:// oxfordmedicine. com/pediatricanesthesiaPBL

REFERENCES

1. Herod J, Denyer J, Goldman A, Howard R. Epidermolysis bullosa in children: pathophysiology, anaesthesia and pain management. *Paediatr Anaesth.* 2002;12(5):388–397.
2. Griffin RP, Mayou BJ. The anaesthetic management of patients with dystrophic epidermolysis bullosa: a review of 44 patients over a 10 year period. *Anaesthesia.* 1993;48(9):810–815.
3. Fine J-D, Bruckner-Tuderman L, Eady RAJ, et al. Inherited epidermolysis bullosa: updated recommendations on diagnosis and classification. *J Am Acad Dermatol.* 2014;70(6):1103–1126.
4. Fine J-D, Johnson LB, Weiner M, Suchindran C. Cause-specific risks of childhood death in inherited epidermolysis bullosa. *J Pediatr.* 2008;152(2):276–280. http://linkinghub.elsevier.com/retrieve/pii/S0022347607006464
5. Shipman AR, Liu L, Lai-Cheong JE, McGrath JA, Heagerty A. Somatic forward (nonrevertant) mosaicism in recessive dystrophic epidermolysis bullosa. *JAMA Dermatol.* 2014;150(9):1025–1027.
6. Lin Y-C, Golianu B. Anesthesia and pain management for pediatric patients with dystrophic epidermolysis bullosa. *J Clin Anesth.* 2006;18(4):268–271.
7. Liu RM, Papsin BC, de Jong AL. Epidermolysis bullosa of the head and neck: a case report of laryngotracheal involvement and 10-year review of cases at the Hospital for Sick Children. *J Otolaryngol.* 1999;28(2):76–82.
8. Mortell AE, Azizkhan RG. Epidermolysis bullosa: management of esophageal strictures and enteric access by gastrostomy. *Dermatol Clin.* 2010;28(2):311–318.
9. Fine J-D, Hall M, Weiner M, Li K-P, Suchindran C. The risk of cardiomyopathy in inherited epidermolysis bullosa. *Br J Dermatol.* 2008;159(3):677–682.
10. Almaani N, Mellerio JE. Genitourinary tract involvement in epidermolysis bullosa. *Dermatol Clin.* 2010;28(2):343–346.
11. Goldschneider KR, Lucky AW. Pain management in epidermolysis bullosa. *Dermatol Clin.* 2010;28(2):273–282.
12. Venugopal SS, Murrell DF. Treatment of skin cancers in epidermolysis bullosa. *Dermatol Clin.* 2010;28(2):283–287.
13. Denyer J, Pillay E. Best practice guidelines for skin and wound care in epidermolysis bullosa. International Consensus. DEBRA. London: Wounds International; 2012.

66.

ETHICS IN PEDIATRIC ANESTHESIOLOGY

Monica Shah and David Waisel

STEM CASE AND KEY QUESTIONS

A 14-year-old girl presents to the preoperative area after suffering a cervical spine fracture while playing in a soccer game. The surgeon expresses to the anesthesiologist and family the need to proceed urgently to the operating room (OR) to avoid neurological deterioration. After appropriate discussion, the mother gives informed consent. The alert and oriented teenager, however, refuses surgery. She is concerned that the surgery may prevent her from becoming a professional soccer player.

WHAT IS INFORMED CONSENT? CAN THE PATIENT GIVE CONSENT AS AN ADOLESCENT? WHAT IS ASSENT? CAN SHE GIVE INFORMED REFUSAL? IS SHE AN EMANCIPATED MINOR?

When signing the consent forms, the parents mention that they recently became Jehovah's Witnesses and refuse to consent to transfusion of blood products. They insist their daughter shares their beliefs. When the parents step away from the preoperative area to call an elder of the church, the teenager informs the anesthesiologist that she is unsure of her own religious beliefs. She wants to receive blood transfusions if they are needed.

CAN PARENTS REFUSE LIFE-SAVING BLOOD TRANSFUSIONS FOR THEIR CHILDREN BASED ON RELIGIOUS BELIEFS? WHOSE WISHES SHOULD BE FOLLOWED, THOSE OF THE CHILD OR HER PARENTS?

Taking advantage of her parents being out of the room, the teenager confides in the preoperative nurse that she is concerned that she may be pregnant and asks if the pregnancy test was positive.

SHOULD THE PREGNANCY TEST RESULTS BE PROVIDED TO THE PATIENT OR HER PARENTS? DO ADOLESCENTS HAVE A RIGHT TO CONFIDENTIALITY?

As the father is speaking, the anesthesiologist notices that his speech is slurred and his questions are intermittently incoherent. He seems intoxicated.

CAN INTOXICATED PARENTS PROVIDE CONSENT FOR THEIR CHILDREN? SHOULD SURGERY BE DELAYED UNTIL IMPAIRED PARENTS CAN PROVIDE INFORMED CONSENT?

After the mother and patient clearly express their agreement to proceed to the OR, the anesthesiologist prepares to administer intravenous midazolam as an anxiolytic. The teenager then reaches toward the anesthesiologist and states "whatever happens in the OR, please do not let me end up as a vegetable." The teenager's mother overhears and tells the anesthesiologist to "do whatever it takes to keep her alive."

HOW ARE LIMITATIONS ON RESUSCITATION THERAPY REEVALUATED FOR THE PERIOPERATIVE FIELD?

The patient has a successful operation and recovers well. While conducting postoperative rounds, the anesthesiologist notices that the patient qualifies for a postoperative pain management study in neurosurgery patients.

CAN CHILDREN ASSENT TO PARTICIPATE IN RESEARCH?

The teenager asks the research assistant several questions, and she and her parents then agree to participate in the research study.

DISCUSSION

INFORMED CONSENT

To meet the ethical requirements to provide informed consent, (adult) patients must have sufficient decision-making capacity to both understand and appreciate the potential benefits and harms associated with the proposed intervention and to incorporate this knowledge and their values into a decision.[1] Informed consent centers on the concept that patients have a right to self-determination.[2,3] Competency is a legal term, and adult patients are deemed competent unless a court rules otherwise.[4] Adult patients are also considered to have decision-making capacity. Clinicians are obligated to assess decision-making capacity for the specific issue at that specific time.

Most minors do not have the legal authorization to formally provide consent for their health care decisions. But minors do develop varying degrees of decision-making capacity as they get older, and they should be involved in medical decision-making to the best extent of their abilities (Box 66.1). Pediatric informed consent depends on the age of the child (Table 66.1) and consists of the best interest standard, assent, and parental informed consent.[3] For convenience reasons, the term "parent" is used to describe all possible surrogate decision-makers, recognizing that, in practice, the child's legal surrogate decision-maker may not be the parent. The term "decision-maker" refers to those involved in the specific decision and may include parents, children, and their advisors. Anesthesiologists should inform families about the most important aspects of the perioperative experience and then ask whether the decision-makers wish to know more, as 10% to 15% of patients may prefer less information than their peers.[5-7]

BEST INTEREST

The best interest standard guides decision-making for children younger than 6 years of age, as they have insufficient decision-making abilities. The best interest of the child is usually determined by the parent. Parents are given a significant role in decision-making because society places great importance on the role of family and assumes that the parents want the best for their children.[2] Although parents have broad authority, they have less discretion in making medical decisions for their children than for themselves.[8]

Table 66.1 **GRADUATED INVOLVEMENT OF MINORS IN MEDICAL DECISION MAKING[2,3]**

AGE	DECISION-MAKING CAPACITY	TECHNIQUES
Under 6 years	None	Best interest standard
6–13 years	Developing	Informed assent
14–18 years	Mostly developed	Informed assent
Mature minor	Developed, as legally determined by a judge, for a specific decision	Informed consent
Emancipated minor	Developed, as determined by a situation (e.g. being married, in the military, economically independent)	Informed consent

The term "best interest" may be misunderstood because it can be misinterpreted to mean there is one best decision. In reality, there are often a range of acceptable decisions from which families can choose. In situations where parents choose unacceptable overtreatment (persisting with futile or inappropriate care) or undertreatment (redirecting goals of therapy too early), anesthesiologists should seek assistance from other clinicians and the ethics committee to assess the decision.[2] Although clinicians should aim to resolve disagreements without legal intervention, the state, in the end, is obligated to protect vulnerable populations, which includes children. The last step is considering legal intervention. The courts judge whether the parents are suitable decision-makers for this specific situation and the acceptability of the parents' preferred medical care. Considerations may include differing conceptions of benefit and harm. The primary benefit of refusing medical treatment, however, may be religious or spiritual, such as the implications of the treatment on the patient's eternal salvation, such as in children of Jehovah's Witnesses.[8] In those cases, the potential benefit cannot be evaluated using generally accepted criteria. As a general rule, parents may not propose limitations on potentially life-sustaining transfusion therapy. Some suggest that a primary consideration is preserving children's' future ability to decide this issue for themselves.[9] Physicians' personal and professional values can affect their judgment. But when representing the best interest of the child, the physician must ensure that personal values do not restrict or bias options offered to patients and families.[10]

ASSENT

Assent is an agreement to treatment by children and should be obtained from children with sufficient decision-making capacity who desire to participate in discussions about their care.[11] Accurate assessments of children's decision-making capacities help avoid forcing children to participate beyond their preferences or decision-making capacities while ensuring appropriate participation for capable children who want to take part in decision-making.[12] The use of assent improves cooperation with treatment, lessens the child's anxiety, and improves the child's long-term relationship with physicians.[10] What is appropriate to obtain assent for depends in part on the risk of the decision. An otherwise healthy 10-year-old can choose between a mask or intravenous induction of anesthesia, but a 10-year-old does not have sufficient decision-making capacity to reject having an emergent procedure. Age and emotional and intellectual maturity are the factors that explain most of the variance in children's decision-making capacity.[13]

Parents determine what they believe to be in the child's best interests. Children between the ages of 6 and 13 years should give assent and participate in decision-making while the parents provide informed consent.[2] These school-aged children are capable of using logic and reason and are able to relate multiple aspects of a situation.[14] Dissent from these children should be taken seriously, and consideration should

be given to available alternatives and the potential harms of the treatment.[10] Adolescents older than 13 years often have developed adult levels of complex reasoning and abstract thought. Because adolescents do not have the perspective and wisdom that comes with age, they can be emotionally impulsive and may undervalue long-term consequences.[2] In the case presented in this chapter, for example, by expressing a reluctance to have the operation because of her future career as a soccer player, the adolescent is expressing short-term outlook and overvaluing her physical abilities. Her decision-making is limited by her maturity. Although age thresholds are used as measures of a child's ability to assent, they have the potential to ignore the child's cognitive and psychosocial features.[15] Some children and adolescents who are developmentally capable of participating actively in decision-making may choose not to participate.[10]

EMANCIPATED AND MATURE MINORS

Minors can provide their own informed consent for all medical decisions if they are emancipated, either by statute law or as declared by a judge. This status is applied to those who are no longer dependent on their parents and include those who are in the military, who are married, and/or who have children.[2,10] Mature minors are children, often 16 or 17 years old, who wish to have legal informed consent responsibility for a specific or series of medical decisions. The judge factors in the risk of the medical decision as well as the maturity and age of the child in order to determine if the child is legally and ethically capable of giving legal consent.[2]

INFORMED REFUSAL

Children and their parents may refuse medical treatments, but anesthesiologists must first ensure that they are substantially informed about the risks, benefits, and alternatives.[2] This often requires anesthesiologists to more fully inform patients than if the family had followed the original recommendation. If children with sufficient decision-making capacity refuse nonemergent procedures, anesthesiologists should respect the refusal of assent.[2] Children should not be pressured or manipulated into having a procedure as this will damage the child's trust in the medical field. Maintaining trust is especially important in children with chronic medical conditions who will receive ongoing treatment. In order to resolve conflicts, anesthesiologists should focus on maintaining communication, clarifying misunderstandings about the anesthetic and surgical components, and alleviating the anxiety of the child and family members.

But patient education and discussion may not always help resolve the problem. The increasing availability and accessibility of unfiltered and non-evidence-based information obtained from sources on the Internet can negatively affect the ability of physicians to counter preformed and deeply held beliefs with more reliable and trustworthy data.[16-18] The physician must try to ensure that the decision-makers have all the relevant and true information to make an informed decision.

If adolescents still refuse to proceed due to anxiety, pharmacological agents may calm them to enable proceeding, *but only* if the child provides assent to be given the medication. Sedatives and the like should not be used to manipulate the child into proceeding. If anesthesiologists believe parents are refusing necessary medical care for a child with limited decision-making capacity, anesthesiologists should pursue the path of resolving disagreements as described earlier.[2] In cases in which treatment is likely to prevent death, serious disability, or severe pain, the child's health and future ability to make decisions should be protected.[8] Failure to provide children with essential medical care has been increasingly recognized as a form of neglect.[8] The courts consistently order potentially life-saving medical treatment (LSMT) despite parental preferences to decline treatment.[19,20] The US Supreme Court has stated "The right to practice religion freely does not include liberty to expose the community or the child to communicable disease or the latter to ill health or death," and "Parents may be free to become martyrs themselves. But it does not follow they are free, in identical circumstances, to make martyrs of their children before they have reached the age of full and legal discretion when they can make that choice for themselves."[8] Courts, however, should consider the negative psychological effects of court-ordered treatment in their decisions.

JEHOVAH'S WITNESSES

Jehovah's Witnesses may choose to refuse potentially life-sustaining transfusion therapy based on their interpretation of biblical scripture that a blood transfusion "may result in the immediate and very temporary prolongation of life, but at the cost of eternal life for a dedicated Christian."[21] The Watchtower Bible and Tract Society has determined that the choice to receive blood transfusions for Jehovah's Witnesses is a "matter of conscience."[21]

Adults may refuse potentially life-sustaining transfusion therapy because they are presumed to be making informed and voluntary decisions.[2] But since the state is obligated to protect the best interests of incompetent and vulnerable patients, the courts routinely authorize potentially life-sustaining transfusion therapy for children of Jehovah's Witnesses.[2] Anesthesiologists should directly address transfusion therapy when discussing care for these children. As with all patients, attempts should be made to follow the family's wishes within the standard of care. Many clinicians, however, question whether they should change their transfusion triggers for a child of a Jehovah's Witness. Some believe it is appropriate to use their usual transfusion triggers in order to follow the requirement to treat the child of a Jehovah's Witness the same as treating any other child.[14] Others feel that they should make an effort to honor the family's wishes by decreasing their transfusion trigger as much as possible, more than they would do for another child.

Anesthesiologists should have a detailed discussion with the child and family regarding which blood products or fluids are acceptable. Many Jehovah's Witnesses accept synthetic colloid solutions, erythropoietin, and preoperative iron.[2] Some of these followers will accept blood removed and returned in a continuous loop, such as cell saver blood. The anesthesiologist should inform the child and family that, in emergent situations, blood transfusions will be administered while seeking legal authorization. Elective procedures may be postponed until the child matures to decide about transfusion therapy. Older teenagers who are able to express significant decision-making capacity and maturity have been permitted to refuse potentially life-sustaining transfusion therapy.[22]

CONFIDENTIALITY FOR MINORS

In the case presented in this chapter, the adolescent patient confided in the anesthesiologist her wish for life-sustaining transfusion therapy, and she confided in the nurse her concern about being pregnant. Physicians must protect this patient information from unnecessary disclosure. Reassuring the adolescent about appropriate confidentiality enhances trust and supports an open flow of information.[2,14] Anesthesiologists may need to ask sensitive questions without the parents present; otherwise, adolescents are likely to withhold pertinent medical information. Emancipated and mature minors have a right to complete confidentiality.[14]

If a pregnancy test is positive or if other sensitive information is presented, anesthesiologists should encourage adolescents to share that information with their parents. However, anesthesiologists should honor the adolescent's right to confidentiality. Some states limit the clinicians to informing only the adolescent about a positive pregnancy test.[2] Among other reasons, these statutes are in place to address concerns regarding child abuse in pregnant adolescents. However, if a pregnant adolescent does not want to inform her parents, and if the procedure can be postponed, the ethical complexity increases. Anesthesiologists must explain the reason for postponement to the family while maintaining confidentiality. They may need to deceive the parents in order to protect the confidentiality of the adolescent, but they should do so in ways that do not require diagnostic or therapeutic interventions. For example, lying about a newly found murmur could worry parents unnecessarily, but postponing for a questionable upper respiratory infection may minimize concern while allowing for postponement.[2] Although most anesthesiologists would like to encourage adolescents to confide in their parents, they must realize that not all parents or homes are safe.[14] Confidentiality should only be breached when it will prevent serious harm to the patient or another person and when reporting statutes.[2] Anesthesiologists should seek help during these encounters from adolescent and teen pregnancy experts, such as social workers and adolescent medicine clinicians, as they enter this morass.

IMPAIRED DECISION-MAKERS

Chemically impaired parents can be disruptive and may hinder the medical treatment of their children.[23] Although routine treatment ideally is postponed until informed consent can be obtained from an unimpaired parent, anesthesiologists should weigh the benefits of postponement with the risk of not proceeding.[2] But for a child that has missed 3 OR dates and is likely to miss more, it may be in the child's best interest to proceed with a routine procedure even if the impaired parent cannot give informed consent. Anesthesiologists should consult with legal and risk management members as well as the ethics committee in these situations.

PERIOPERATIVE LIMITATIONS ON POTENTIALLY LSMT

Limitations on potentially life-sustaining medical treatment (more commonly known as do-not-resuscitate (DNR) orders, enable patients to forgo LSMT when the burdens of treatment outweigh the potential benefits.[2] Burdens should be viewed from the patient's perspective and include intractable pain, disability, and invasive interventions.[24] The benefits of LSMT include meeting the desires of patients, prolongation of life, and, when applied appropriately, an improved quality of life. Burdens from procedures may be due to resuscitation attempts or to cognitive decrements after resuscitation.

Children with DNR orders may seek benefit from procedures that decrease pain or treat problems unrelated to the primary condition, such as an acute fracture. In these cases, the American Society of Anesthesiologists, the American Academy of Pediatrics, and the American College of Surgeons recommend re-evaluation of the DNR order before proceeding to the OR, because DNR orders are not automatically revoked when patients come to the OR.[24–28] The DNR order re-evaluation should clarify the goals for the procedure and end-of-life care with the patient, parents, and medical team. Discussions should emphasize the differences between the OR and the inpatient units. In the OR, perioperative physicians care for the patient for a specific period of time. Detailed knowledge of the goals for care allows anesthesiologists to resuscitate based on the likelihood of achieving those specific goals.[2] When reevaluating DNR orders, discussions should include likelihood of requiring resuscitation, reversibility of likely causes that require resuscitation, chances of successful resuscitation, response to iatrogenic events, types of postoperative care, and limitations on resuscitation.[2,25] DNR orders that list acceptable interventions, such as tracheal intubation and chest compressions, are not helpful for intraoperative care. Due to unclear distinctions between anesthetic practice and resuscitation, inflexible directives increase the chance that physicians will not honor the patient's desires based on technicalities.[2] For example, a short-term tracheal intubation may be a necessary response for an apneic event due to intraoperative opioid administration. While not intubating would be consistent with an order that prohibits intubation, it is most likely inconsistent with the overall goals of the family. DNR orders should remain modified or suspended until the child recovers fully from anesthesia.[29]

Decision-makers guide their therapy by prioritizing outcomes and developing goal-directed approaches to care.[30] After these goals are defined, anesthesiologists can use their clinical judgment to determine if/how much resuscitation will help achieve these goals.[2] Witnessed arrests in the OR are often from a known cause. Knowing the etiology of the problem and having the ability to provide immediate intervention often leads to better outcome than unwitnessed arrests.[2,31] Therefore, decision-makers may be more likely to modify their previous limits on resuscitation for the perioperative period. Decision-makers who choose goal-directed approaches are more likely to allow temporary therapeutic interventions to manage easily reversible events but will reject interventions that will likely result in permanent sequelae, such as neurological impairment.[2] Documentation is crucial for perioperative DNR orders. For example, the goal-directed preference can be documented as, "The patient desires resuscitative efforts during surgery and in the PACU only if the adverse events are believed to be both temporary and reversible in the clinical judgment of the anesthesiologists and surgeons."[2] In pediatrics, precisely defining postoperative plans is less essential because parents are often available in the postoperative period to make medical decisions.

Honoring perioperative limitations on LSMT is very important, and barriers to doing so often center on insufficient knowledge about law and ethics. Many clinicians worry that honoring limitations on LSMT may result in legal ramifications. However, statutes that address requirements for DNR orders include provisions that protect physicians from liability.[2] The risk of liability for honoring a documented DNR order is likely to be lower than the risk of not honoring it.[2] Another barrier to honoring DNR orders for anesthesiologists is the temporary effects of anesthetic interventions, such as severe hemodynamic instability or cardiac arrest that require interventions including resuscitation.[32] Both inhaled and intravenous anesthetics can lead to hemodynamic instability and cardiac dysrhythmias. The resuscitation administered by the anesthesiologist in response to these events is routine, in contrast to the "heroic" measures taken when a patient needs resuscitation in the inpatient unit.[29] Some anesthesiologists will initiate resuscitation because the etiology was iatrogenic; however, this may be against the wishes of the decision-makers who are only concerned with the physical and mental status following the arrest.[2] The resuscitation may conflict with the ethical principle of patient autonomy.[33] Clinicians also are more likely to honor a refusal of resuscitation for a palliative procedure than for an elective procedure.[25]

RESEARCH IN PEDIATRIC PATIENTS

Research in pediatric patients is an increasingly growing field. Depending on the type of research conducted, children can be exposed to unknown risks of long-term damage as research interventions occur during growth and development of the child, as opposed to research conducted in adults.[2] Due to the risk of harm and possible lack of direct benefit to the child, developmentally appropriate assent should be obtained from the child. US federal law requires assent of minors 7 years of age and older for participation in medical research.[12] Tait and Geisser explained, "If assent is deemed appropriate, children should understand the basic study-specific information, should have a developmentally appropriate awareness of their condition, and be able to appreciate, at a rudimentary level, how the information applies to their own situation. Children should be free to decide whether or not to participate in a study and articulate their choice absent of any undue influence or coercion."[34] Assent may be waived, however, if there is possible direct benefit to the child that is only available by participating in the research.[2] Hein et al. recently used the modified MacArthur Competence Assessment Tool for Clinical Research to determine that children above age of 11.2 years were decision-making competent while children of 9.6 years and younger were not.[4] Hein et al. recommend a dual-consent procedure, for both child and parents, for children from the age of 12 years until they reach adulthood. Federal guidelines for pediatric research emphasize that potential benefits must increase as the potential risks increase.

CONCLUSIONS

- Children and adolescents should be involved in developmentally appropriate decision-making.

- Clinicians should respect families and children and their religious or spiritual beliefs and collaborate with them to develop treatment plans to promote their children's health.

- Clinicians should report suspected cases of medical neglect to state child protective service agencies, regardless of whether the parents' decision is based on religious beliefs.

- End-of-life decisions should be made with the comfort of the dying child as the primary focal point.

- Children older than 7 years old must give assent to participate in clinical research.

- In situations of conflict, anesthesiologists should seek available resources to help resolve that conflict, such as other clinicians, child-life specialists, social work members, legal counsel, and ethics consultants.

REVIEW QUESTIONS

1. A 15-year old girl presents to the hospital to undergo a rhinoplasty under general anesthesia. The preoperative nurse calls you to report the teenager's urine pregnancy test is positive. The teenager is in the preoperative area with both of her parents. Who do you **FIRST** inform of the results?

    A. the parents—have them inform their daughter of her laboratory test results

    B. the patient—encourage her to share with her parents, ensuring confidentiality

    C. the patient and her parents together—so everyone can find out at the same time

    D. risk management—have them disclose the results to the patient and her family

Answer: B

Patients have the right to physician–patient confidentiality. Adolescents need to trust their clinicians before they will fully share information. If maintaining confidentiality may cause harm to the patient, then the physician may be ethically justified in notifying the parents. In this case, the teenager should be informed of the test results in private and be encouraged to inform her parents if she feels safe and supported.[2,12,14]

2. Your pain management team is conducting a research study on postoperative opioid use after posterior spinal fusion surgeries in children 14 to 17 years of age. One of the candidates for participating in the study is 14 years old. She is annoyed when you enter her room, and she is frustrated that she is in the hospital instead of being at home with her friends. She adamantly refuses to participate in the study. What is the next **MOST** appropriate action to take?

    A. Do the study without her consent; it is a minimal risk study.

    B. Get consent from both parents and proceed with the study.

    C. Honor the teenager's decision not to participate in the study.

    D. Obtain consent from 1 parent and proceed with the study.

Answer: C

The requirements for obtaining consent for research is more stringent than for obtaining consent for medical care. Adolescents and teenagers have decision-making capacity and should be involved in their medical care. They should not be coerced into making decisions, and they should be involved in the consent process. Any child who is able to participate in making decisions should provide assent. US federal law requires assent of minors 7 years and older to participate in medical research.[14] A child's refusal to participate in research, regardless of the reason, must be honored.[34]

3. A 16-year old girl with appendicitis presents to the preoperative holding area for a laparoscopic appendectomy. She is with her husband and 2-year-old daughter. While you are obtaining informed consent, she informs you that her mother is incarcerated and her father is not involved in her life. What is the **BEST** course of action to obtain consent for this teenager?

    A. ethics committee to help weigh your options

    B. legal department for local laws and regulations

    C. social work to resolve her family situation

    D. surgeon to obtain a 2-physician consent

Answer: B

Emancipated minors are under the age of 18 years but have the statutory right to make their own health care decisions. Emancipated minors are often adolescents who are financially independent from their parents and who are married, in the military, and/or parents to children of their own. Legal counsel should be able to determine if your state has statutory law regarding emancipated minors.[12,14,22]

4. A 10-year old boy presents with cholelithiasis presents for a laparoscopic cholecystectomy. While obtaining consent from his parents, they inform you that they are Jehovah's Witnesses and will not consent for their child to receive any blood products. You inform them that although cholecystectomies rarely necessitate blood transfusions, you will transfuse in an emergency. The parents eventually give their consent for anesthesia. During the case, the surgeon injures the hepatic vessels, leading to extensive bleeding. Despite treatment with intravenous fluid and vasopressors, the child remains hemodynamically unstable. The hematocrit is 8 g/dL with ongoing bleeding. What is your next **BEST** step?

    A. Acquire verbal consent form the parents.
    B. Respect the parents' religious beliefs.
    C. Initiate transfusion of O-negative blood.
    D. Obtain an emergency court transfusion order.

Answer: C

Jehovah's Witnesses believe that receiving blood products contradicts Biblical teachings. Adults with legal competency are allowed to refuse life-sustaining blood transfusions in regards to their own medical care. The state, however, is obligated to protect the interests of children as they do not have full competence to make their own informed decisions. When parents of Jehovah's Witnesses refuse blood transfusions for their children, physicians can seek the hospital's legal counsel to obtain court orders to allow the necessary transfusion. In emergent life-threatening situations, however, the physician must protect the child and transfuse the blood without the court order. The court order will likely delay care and risk serious harm to the child.[9,14,20]

QUESTIONS AND ANSWERS

This chapter has accompanying questions and answers which are available to subscribers as part of the Oxford eLearning platform. To access the questions, go to ✔ http:// oxfordmedicine. com/pediatricanesthesiaPBL

REFERENCES

1. Rosoff, PM. Do pediatric patients have a right to know? *AMA J Ethics.* 2017;19(5):426–435.
2. Waisel DB. Ethical considerations. In: Gregory GA, Andropoulos DB, eds. *Gregory's Pediatric Anesthesia.* 5th ed. Hoboken, NJ: Blackwell; 2012:1–14.
3. Committee on Bioethics, American Academy of Pediatrics. Informed consent, parental permission, and assent in pediatric practice. *Pediatrics.* 1995;95:314–317.
4. Hein IM, De Vries MC, Troost PW, Meynen G, Van Goudoever JB, Lindauer RJ. Informed consent instead of assent is appropriate in children from the age of twelve: policy implications of new findings on children's competence to consent to clinical research. *BMC Med Ethics.* 2015;16:1–7.
5. Siegal G, Bonnie RJ, Appelbaum PS. Personalized disclosure by attending to patients' needs in the informed consent process. *J Law Med Ethics.* 2012;40(2):359–367. doi:10.1111/j.1748-720X.2012.00669.x
6. Waisel DB. Let the patient drive the informed consent process: ignore legal requirements. *Anesth Analg.* 2011;113(1):13–15. doi:10.1213/ANE.0b013e31821bfc1f
7. Tait AR, Teig MK, Voepel-Lewis T. Informed consent for anesthesia: a review of practice and strategies for optimizing the consent process. *Can J Anaesth.* 2014;61(9):832–842. doi:10.1007/s12630-014-0188-8
8. American Academy of Pediatrics. Conflicts between religious or spiritual beliefs and pediatric care: informed refusal, exemptions, and public funding. *Pediatrics.* 2013;132:962–965.
9. Sheldon M. Ethical issues in the forced transfusion of Jehovah's Witness children. *J Emerg Med.* 1996;14(2):251–257.
10. Canadian Paediatric Society. Treatment decisions regarding infants, children and adolescents, 2004. *Paediatr Child Health.* 2004;(9)2:99–103.
11. Manuel SP, Mai CL. Professional issues. In: Matthes K, Laubach AE, Wang E, Anderson TA, eds. *Pediatric Anesthesiology: A Comprehensive Board Review.* 1st ed. New York: Oxford University Press; 2015:655–663.
12. Joffe S, Fernandez CV, Pentz RD, et al. Involving children with cancer in decision-making about research participation. *J Pediatr.* 2006;149:862–868.
13. Hein IM, Troost PW, Lindeboom R, et al. Key factors in children's competence to consent to clinical research. *BMC Med Ethics.* 2015;16:74.
14. Waisel DB. Ethical issues in pediatric anesthesiology. In: Cote CJ, Lerman J, Anderson BJ, eds. *A Practice of Anesthesia for Infants and Children.* 5th ed. Philadelphia, PA: Saunders/Elsevier; 2013:64–75.
15. Steinberg L. Clinical adolescent psychology: what it is, and what it needs to be. *J Consult Clin Psychol.* 2002;70:124–128.
16. Fisher JH, O'Connor D, Flexman AM, Shapera S, Ryerson CJ. Accuracy and reliability of internet resources for information on idiopathic pulmonary fibrosis. *Am J Respir Crit Care Med.* 2016;194(2):218–225.
17. Ogah I, Wassersug RJ. How reliable are "reputable sources" for medical information on the internet? The case of hormonal therapy to treat prostate cancer. *Urol Oncol.* 2013;31(8):1546–1552.
18. Winship B, Grisell M, Yang CB, Chen RX, Bauer AS. The quality of pediatric orthopaedic information on the internet. *J Pediatr Orthop.* 2014;34(4):474–477.
19. Malecha WF. Faith healing exemptions to child protection laws: keeping the faith versus medical care for children. *J Legis.* 1985;12(2):243–263.
20. Trahan J. Constitutional law: parental denial of a child's medical treatment for religious reasons. *Annu Surv Am Law.* 1989;1989(1):307–341.
21. Watchman Fellowship. New Watchtower Blood Transfusion Policy. 2000. http://www.watchman.org/articles/jehovahs-witnesses/new-watchtower-blood-transfusion-policy/. Accessed June 27, 2017.
22. Coleman DL, Rosoff PM. The legal authority of mature minors to consent to general medical treatment. *Pediatrics.* 2013;131(4):786–793.
23. Fraser JJ, McAbee GN. Dealing with the parent whose judgment is impaired by alcohol or drugs: legal and ethical considerations. *Pediatrics.* 2004;114(3):869–873.
24. Committee on Bioethics, American Academy of Pediatrics. Guidelines on forgoing life-sustaining medical treatment. *Pediatrics.* 1994;93:532–536.
25. Fallat ME, Deshpande JK. Do-not-resuscitate orders for pediatric patients who require anesthesia and surgery. *Pediatrics.* 2004;114:1686–1692.
26. American Society of Anesthesiologists, Committee on Ethics. Ethical guidelines for the anesthesia care of patients with do not resuscitate orders or other directives that limit treatment. www.asahq.org/publicationsAndServices/standards/09.html. Accessed July 1, 2017.
27. American College of Surgeons. Statement of the American College of Surgeons on advance directives by patients. "Do not resuscitate" in the operating room. *Bull Am Coll Surg.* 1994;79(9):29.
28. American Academy of Pediatrics, Committee on Bioethics. Informed consent, parental permission, and assent in pediatric practice. *Pediatrics.* 1995,95:314–317.

29. Sumrall WD, Mahanna E, Sabharwal V, Marshall T. Do not resuscitate, anesthesia, and perioperative care: a not so clear order. *Ochsner J.* 2016;16:176–179.

30. Truog RD, Waisel DB, Burns JP. DNR in the OR: a goal directed approach. *Anesthesiology.* 1999;90:289–295.

31. Brindley PG, Markland DM, Mayers I, Kutsogiannis DJ. Predictors of survival following in-hospital adult cardiopulmonary resuscitation. *CMAJ.* 2002;167(4):343–348.

32. Nurok M, Green DS, Chisholm MF, Fins JJ, Liguori GA. Anesthesiologists' familiarity with the ASA and ACS guidelines on advance directives in the perioperative setting. *J Clin Anesth.* 2014;26(3):174–176.

33. Burkle CM, Swetz KM, Armstrong MH, Keegan MT. Patient and doctor attitudes and beliefs concerning perioperative do not resuscitate orders: anesthesiologists' growing compliance with patient autonomy and self determination guidelines. *BMC Anesthesiol.* 2013;13:2.

34. Tait AR, Geisser ME. Development of a consensus operational definition of child assent for research. *BMC Med Ethics.* 2017;18:1–8.

INDEX

Note: Page numbers followed by *b, t,* and *f* indicate boxes, tables, and figures, respectively.